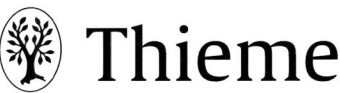

MRI of Bone and Soft Tissue Tumors and Tumorlike Lesions

Differential Diagnosis and Atlas

Steven P. Meyers, MD, PhD

Professor of Radiology,
Imaging Sciences, and Neurosurgery
University of Rochester
School of Medicine and Dentistry
Rochester, NY
USA

2976 illustrations

Thieme
Stuttgart · New York

Library of Congress Cataloging-in-Publication Data is available from the publisher.

Important note: Medicine is an ever-changing science undergoing continual development. Research and clinical experience are continually expanding our knowledge, in particular our knowledge of proper treatment and drug therapy. Insofar as this book mentions any dosage or application, readers may rest assured that the authors, editors, and publishers have made every effort to ensure that such references are in accordance with **the state of knowledge at the time of production of the book.**

Nevertheless, this does not involve, imply, or express any guarantee or responsibility on the part of the publishers in respect to any dosage instructions and forms of applications stated in the book. **Every user is requested to examine carefully** the manufacturers' leaflets accompanying each drug and to check, if necessary in consultation with a physician or specialist, whether the dosage schedules mentioned therein or the contraindications stated by the manufacturers differ from the statements made in the present book. Such examination is particularly important with drugs that are either rarely used or have been newly released on the market. Every dosage schedule or every form of application used is entirely at the user's own risk and responsibility. The authors and publishers request every user to report to the publishers any discrepancies or inaccuracies noticed. If errors in this work are found after publication, errata will be posted at www.thieme.com on the product description page.

© 2008 Georg Thieme Verlag,
Rüdigerstraße 14, 70469 Stuttgart, Germany
http://www.thieme.de
Thieme New York, 333 Seventh Avenue,
New York, NY 10001, USA
http://www.thieme.com

Typesetting by primustype Hurler GmbH, Notzingen
Printed in Germany by Grammlich, Pliezhausen

ISBN 978-3-13-135421-1 (TPS, Rest of World)
ISBN 978-1-58890-251-1 (TPN, The Americas)   1 2 3 4 5 6

Some of the product names, patents, and registered designs referred to in this book are in fact registered trademarks or proprietary names even though specific reference to this fact is not always made in the text. Therefore, the appearance of a name without designation as proprietary is not to be construed as a representation by the publisher that it is in the public domain.

This book, including all parts thereof, is legally protected by copyright. Any use, exploitation, or commercialization outside the narrow limits set by copyright legislation, without the publisher's consent, is illegal and liable to prosecution. This applies in particular to photostat reproduction, copying, mimeographing, preparation of microfilms, and electronic data processing and storage.

To my parents, Morton and Wilma Meyers,
and my uncle, Aaron Fox,
for their unwavering encouragement
along my long journey
through formal education.

And to my wife, Barbara, and son, Noah,
for their continuous love,
support, and patience during this project.

Foreword

MRI has become a widely accepted imaging modality in musculoskeletal radiology. Regarding bone tumors, MRI complements conventional radiography and CT in assessing tissue composition and is unsurpassed in the evaluation of the local tumor extension. For soft tissue lesions, MRI is the imaging modality of choice because of its high soft tissue contrast resolution.

Musculoskeletal tumor evaluation is dependent upon clinical and laboratory data and relevant imaging. Radiologists, clinicians, and pathologists with an interest in bone and soft tissue tumors must work in unison to achieve the best possible outcome for a patient affected with such a disease. This new text facilitates the understanding and interpretation of data provided by the various medical specialists.

I have known Dr. Meyers since he became a staff member of our department 15 years ago. Dr. Meyers is a radiologist with additional fellowship training in MRI and neuroradiology, and has always had a keen interest in musculoskeletal tumors with emphasis on MRI. Over the years he accumulated an outstanding collection of exquisite tumor cases ranging from a complete presentation spectrum of common lesions to the manifestation of the most unusual neoplasm. This collection forms the foundation of this new text.

A few years ago, when I was obliged to seek a new co-author for *Differential Diagnosis in MRI* at short notice, I was extremely fortunate that Dr. Meyers was kind enough to assume the task of writing the "Brain" and "Spine" sections of that text. Dr. Meyers performed this task admirably and at the same time developed a taste for further textbook writing that resulted in the conception and execution of *MRI of Bone and Soft Tissue Tumors and Tumorlike Lesions*.

The book is divided into three main sections. The first section includes an introductory chapter that presents a detailed overview of MRI of musculoskeletal tumors and tumorlike lesions. Multiple tables regarding the WHO classification of bone and soft tissue tumors, their relative frequencies and pertinent immunohistochemical and genetic data round up part one of the book.

The second section of the book contains 20 tables of differential diagnosis of lesions based on anatomic locations and/or specific MRI features. Pertinent radiographic and CT findings and key clinical data are summarized beside the MRI findings.

In the third section of the book, 77 bone and soft tissue lesions are listed in alphabetical order and analyzed in great detail with regard to clinical, pathologic, and imaging findings. A large number of superb state-of-the-art images complement the text throughout the entire book. The photographic quality of the illustrations in the book is outstanding.

Dr. Meyers is to be congratulated for his original approach to this text, the excellent and complete coverage of musculoskeletal tumors and tumorlike lesions, and his succinct presentation of the material. I believe the book will be an invaluable resource for residents, fellows, radiologists, pathologists, orthopedists, and clinicians with an interest in this topic. There is no doubt in my mind that this new text will receive extraordinary acceptance in the medical community.

Francis A. Burgener, MD
Professor of Radiology
University of Rochester Medical Center
Rochester, New York, NY, USA

Preface

Over many decades, conventional radiography has been an important and often critical imaging modality in the evaluation of bone tumors. The radiographic features of various osseous tumors and tumorlike lesions have been well described. Magnetic resonance imaging (MRI), being a relative newcomer to clinical radiology for slightly more than 20 years, has become a widely available imaging modality internationally. It is estimated that there are 20 000 MRI scanners worldwide performing approximately 60 million MRI examinations per year. With its high soft tissue contrast resolution, MRI has been shown to be a very powerful method in the detection of marrow pathology as well as in the evaluation of lesions within soft tissues.

In the daily routine of clinical practice and teaching of physicians-in-training in the medical disciplines of radiology, orthopedics, and neurosurgery, it has become apparent that a need exists for a modern reference book that covers both MRI and radiographic features of neoplasms and tumorlike lesions of bone and adjacent soft tissues as well as providing associated relevant clinical and pathologic data citing recent literature.

The goal of this book is to present the MRI features of bone and soft tissue tumors and tumor mimics in a single easy-to-use resource with extensive utilization of figures for illustration. For consistency purposes, the nomenclature and categorization of the various musculoskeletal tumors and tumorlike lesions in this book are based on the 2002 WHO classification. This book includes soft tissue tumors as well as osseous lesions involving both the appendicular and axial skeleton. For bone tumors and tumorlike lesions, efforts were also made to correlate the conventional radiographic features with the rapidly proliferating data from the published literature using MRI.

The book's unique organization helps the reader obtain desired information efficiently and quickly. It is divided into three main sections. The first portion includes a detailed introductory chapter which presents an overview of MRI in the evaluation of musculoskeletal tumors and tumor mimics. In addition, it contains multiple tables regarding the WHO classification of bone and soft tissue tumors, relative frequencies of malignant and non-malignant lesions, and pertinent immunohistochemical and genetic data.

The second portion of the book contains 20 lists of differential diagnosis of lesions based on anatomic locations and/or specific MRI features in a tabular format. Each of the lesions or musculoskeletal disorders listed in the tables has a column summarizing the MRI features and pertinent radiographic and/or CT findings with associated MR images for illustration, and a comments column summarizing key clinical data. The comments section contains references to the specific Atlas chapters in the subsequent third portion of the book for additional detailed information, or to the literature at the end of each table.

The third portion of the book contains 77 Atlas chapters organized into a routine format that enables the efficient acquisition of specific information regarding each lesion. For the majority of the Atlas chapters, multiple MR images, often with corresponding plain film and/or CT images, are provided to demonstrate the range of imaging findings and locations associated with the lesions. The arrangement of the Atlas chapters in alphabetical order also facilitates easy and quick reference. When using this book, familiarity of the MRI findings for various lesions will allow for a formulation of a reasonable differential diagnosis to guide the clinician.

Acknowledgements

I wish to acknowledge the Thieme staff, in particular Dr. Clifford Bergman, Ms. Rachel Swift, Ms. Stefanie Langner, and Ms. Elisabeth Kurz for their dedication, hard work, and attention to detail. I would also like to thank Ms. Colleen Cottrell for her outstanding secretarial work with this project.

In addition, I wish to acknowledge the following for their contribution of interesting cases: Arun Basu, MD, A. Oscar Beitia, MD, Allan Bernstein, MD, Timothy Bratz, MD, Francis A. Burgerner, MD, Christopher Cerniglia, DO, Gary M. Hollenberg, MD, James J. Lester, MD, Johnny U.V. Monu, MD, David Shrier, MD, Raymond K. Tan, MD, Eric P. Weinberg, MD, Vanessa Zayas, MD, and Andrea Zynda, MD.

I extend my special thanks and appreciation to all of my coworkers and physician colleagues (Drs. Bernstein, Hollenberg, Shrier, Weinberg, Zayas, and Zynda) at University Medical Imaging, the Outpatient Diagnostic Imaging Facility of the University of Rochester Medical Center. I could not ask for a greater group of dedicated people to work with in the clinical practice of Diagnostic Radiology.

Lastly, I would like to give thanks to my former teachers and mentors (Drs. Curtis J. Nelson, Larry E. Schrader, Stephen N. Wiener, and Emanuel Kanal) for their guidance and wisdom; and to the University of Vermont College of Medicine for the opportunity of entering into the great and noble field of Medicine.

Table of Contents

Introduction 1

Differential Diagnosis Tables

1 Tumors and tumorlike lesions involving the skull and facial bones 18
2 Tumors and tumorlike lesions involving the spine 38
3 Paraspinal tumors and tumorlike lesions 64
4 Lesions involving the outer surface of bone 76
5 Lesions associated with thickening of bone cortex 104
6 Intramedullary lesions associated with expansion of intact cortical margins 117
7 Intramedullary lesions associated with cortical destruction and extraosseous extension 128
8 Solitary intramedullary lesions with well-circumscribed margins 140
9 Solitary intramedullary lesions with poorly defined margins of abnormal marrow signal 150
10 Solitary intramedullary lesions located near the ends of tubular bones 163
11 Solitary intramedullary metadiaphyseal lesions 176
12 Solitary intramedullary diaphyseal lesions 189
13 Osseous tumors and tumorlike lesions at the hands and feet 199
14 Diffuse, multiple, poorly defined and/or multi-focal zones of abnormal marrow signal 211
15 Lesions that contain cartilage 236
16 Tumors and tumorlike lesions within joints 247
17 Solitary tumors and tumorlike lesions of the soft tissues located mostly deep to the subcutaneous fat 258
18 Tumors and tumorlike lesions of the superficial soft tissues including subcutaneous fat 280
19 Lesions involving peripheral nervous tissue 305
20 Lesions that contain fat 312

Atlas

A 1 Adamantinoma (Also Referred to as Extragnathic Adamantinoma, Adamantinoma of Long Bones, Juvenile Intracortical Adamantinoma) 325
A 2 Aneurysmal Bone Cyst 328
A 3 Bone Cyst (Also Referred to as Simple Bone Cyst, Unicameral Bone Cyst, Solitary Bone Cyst) 334
A 4 Angiofibroma (Also Referred to as Juvenile Nasopharyngeal Angiofibroma) 340
A 5 Angiomatoid Fibrous Histiocytoma (Also Referred to as Angiomatoid Malignant Fibrous Histiocytoma) .. 342
A 6 Angiosarcoma (Also Referred to as Malignant Hemangioendothelioma, High-Grade Hemangio-endothelioma, Hemangiosarcoma, Angioendo-thelioma, Angiofibrosarcoma, and Hemangio-endotheliosarcoma) 344
A 7 Chondroblastoma 347
A 8 Chondroma, Intramedullary Type: Enchondroma (Also Referred to as Intra-osseous Chondroma or Central Chondroma) 352
A 9 Chondroma, Periosteal or Juxtacortical Type (Also Referred to as Periosteal or Juxtacortical Chondroma, Surface Chondroma, and Juxtacortical/Parosteal Chondroma) 359
A 10 Chondromyxoid Fibroma 364
A 11 Chondrosarcoma 368
A 12 Chordoma 379
A 13 Dermatofibrosarcoma and Dermatofibrosarcoma Protuberans 383
A 14 Dermatomyositis 386
A 15 Dermoid and Epidermoid 390
A 16 Desmoid Tumor (Also Referred to as Fibromatosis, Superficial and Deep Types Involving Soft Tissues; Desmoplastic Fibroma; Desmoid Tumor within Bone) . 396
A 17 Elastofibroma 404
A 18 Eosinophilic Granuloma (Also Referred to as Langerhans Cell Histiocytosis, Formerly Histiocytosis X) 406
A 19 Erdheim–Chester Disease (Also Referred to as Chester–Erdheim Disease, Lipoid Granulomatosis, and Lipogranulomatosis) 413
A 20 Ewing Sarcoma 416
A 21 Nodular Fasciitis (Also Referred to as Pseudo-sarcomatous Fasciitis, Proliferative Fasciitis, Infiltrative Fasciitis, and Pseudosarcomatous Fibromatosis) 423
A 22 Fibrolipomatous Hamartoma (Also Referred to as Nerve Lipoma, Neural Fibrolipoma, Lipofibromatous Hamartoma, Perineural Lipoma, Intraneural Lipoma, Lipofibroma, and Lipomatous Hamartoma) 426
A 23 Fibroma of the Tendon Sheath 428
A 24 Solitary Fibrous Tumor 430
A 25 Fibrosarcoma 433
A 26 Fibrous Cortical Defect and Nonossifying Fibroma (Also Referred to as Metaphyseal Fibrous Defect), Cortical Desmoid (Also Referred to as Periosteal Desmoid or Distal Femoral Cortical Irregularity), and Fibroxanthoma (Also Referred to as Benign Fibrous Histiocytoma) 438
A 27 Fibrous Dysplasia (Also Referred to as Fibro-osseous Dysplasia, Fibrocartilaginous Dysplasia, and Lichtenstein–Jaffe Disease) 449
A 28 Geode (Also Referred to as Subchondral Cyst and Osteoarthritic Cyst); Soft Tissue and Intra-osseous Ganglion (Also Referred to as Intra-osseous Ganglion, Juxta-articular Bone Cyst, and Periosteal Ganglion) 456
A 29 Giant Cell Tumor of Bone 462
A 30 Giant Cell Tumor of the Tendon Sheath and/or Soft Tissue (Also Referred to as Nodular Teno-synovitis, Fibrous Xanthoma, Tenosynovial Giant Cell Tumor, and Benign Synovioma) 469

A 31	Glomus Tumor (Also Referred to as Glomangioma and Angioglomoid Tumor)	476
A 32	Gout	479
A 33	Hemangioendothelioma (Also Referred to as Low-grade Hemangioendothelioma, Low-grade Hemangioendothelial Sarcoma, Low-grade Angiosarcoma, and Myxoid Angioblastoma)	484
A 34	Hemangiomas (Also Referred to as Vascular Hamartomas)	491
A 35	Hemangiopericytoma	502
A 36	Hematoma, Morel–Lavallee Lesion, and Hemophilic Pseudotumor	507
A 37	Bone and Muscle Infarct (Also Referred to as Avascular Necrosis and Osteonecrosis)	512
A 38	Kaposi Sarcoma (Also Referred to as Angiosarcoma Multiplex, Kaposi Disease, Idiopathic Multiple Pigmented Sarcoma of the Skin, and Granuloma Multiplex Hemorrhagicum)	519
A 39	Leiomyoma	521
A 40	Leiomyosarcoma	525
A 41	Leukemia	531
A 42	Lipoblastoma	540
A 43	Lipoma, Atypical Lipoma, and Hibernoma	543
A 44	Liposarcoma	554
A 45	Liposclerosing Myxofibrous Tumor (Also Referred to as Polymorphic Fibro-osseous Lesion of Bone and Polymorphic Fibrocystic Disease of Bone)	563
A 46	Lymphangioma (Also Referred to as Cystic Hygroma)	566
A 47	Lymphoma	570
A 48	Malignant Fibrous Histiocytoma (Also Referred to as Malignant Histiocytoma, Xanthosarcoma, Malignant Fibrous Xanthoma, and Fibroxanthosarcoma)	584
A 49	Meningioma	594
A 50	Metastatic Lesions	601
A 51	Morton Neuroma	609
A 52	Multiple Myeloma (Also Referred to as Myeloma, Kahler Disease, and Plasma Cell Neoplasm; Plasmacytoma Represents a Solitary Neoplastic Variant)	611
A 53	Myositis Ossificans (Also Referred to as Heterotopic Ossification, Reactive Mesenchymal Proliferation, Ossifying Hematoma, and Pseudomalignant Osseous Tumor of Soft Tissues)	618
A 54	Myxoma	624
A 55	Neuroblastoma, Ganglioneuroblastoma, and Ganglioneuroma	627
A 56	Neurofibroma and Malignant Peripheral Nerve Sheath Tumor	633
A 57	Traumatic Neuroma	642
A 58	Osteochondroma (Also Referred to as Osteo-cartilaginous Exostosis)	645
A 59	Osteofibrous Dysplasia (Also Referred to as Ossifying Fibroma of the Tibia and/or Fibula, Cortical Fibrous Dysplasia)	654
A 60	Osteoid Osteoma	660
A 61	Osteoblastoma (Also Referred to as Ossifying Giant Cell Tumor and Giant Osteoid Osteoma)	668
A 62	Osteoma, Enostosis, Osteopoikilosis, and Melorheostosis	674
A 63	Osteomyelitis	679
A 64	Osteosarcoma (Also Referred to as Osteogenic Sarcoma and Osteoblastic Sarcoma)	693
A 65	Paget Disease (Also Referred to as Osteitis Deformans)	713
A 66	Paraganglioma (Also Referred to as Chemodectoma for Carotid Body Tumor and Glomus Jugulare Tumor for Jugulotympanic Paragangliomas)	721
A 67	Pigmented Villonodular Synovitis	726
A 68	Pleomorphic Hyalinizing Angiectatic Tumor	730
A 69	Rhabdomyosarcoma (Also Referred to as Myosarcoma, Malignant Rhabdomyoma, Rhabdosarcoma, and Embryonal Sarcoma)	732
A 70	Rheumatoid Arthritis	738
A 71	Sarcoid	744
A 72	Schwannoma (Also Referred to as Neurilemoma and Neurinoma)	747
A 73	Synovial Chondromatosis (Also Referred to as Primary and Secondary Chondromatosis, and Synovial Chondrometaplasia), and Synovial Osteochondromatosis	753
A 74	Synovial Cyst	758
A 75	Synovial Sarcoma (Also Referred to as Carcinosarcoma and Spindle Cell Carcinoma of Soft Tissue)	762
A 76	Teratoma	769
A 77	Xanthoma	773
Subject Index		775

Abbreviations

ABC	aneurysmal bone cyst	JRA	juvenile rheumatoid arthritis
ABME	acute bone marrow edema	LCH	Langerhans cell histiocytosis
AIDS	acquired immune deficiency syndrome	MDP	methylene diphosphonate
ALL	acute lymphoblastic leukemia	MDS	myelodysplastic syndrome
AML	acute myelogenous leukemia	MFH	malignant fibrous histiocytoma
AP	anteroposterior	MIBG	meta-iodobenzylguanidine
APUD	amine precursor uptake and decarboxylation	MIP	maximum intensity projection
AVN	avascular necrosis	MKI	mitosis karyorrhexis index
Ca	calcium	MPNST	malignant peripheral nerve sheath tumor
CLL	chronic lymphocytic leukemia	MR	magnetic resonance
CML	chronic myelogenous leukemia	MRA	magnetic resonance angiography
CMPD	chronic myeloproliferative disease	MRI	magnetic resonance imaging
CNS	central nervous system	NF1	neurofibromatosis type 1
CPPD	calcium pyrophosphate dihydrate deposition	NF2	neurofibromatosis type 2
CSF	cerebrospinal fluid	NHL	non-Hodgkin lymphoma
CT	computed tomography	NOF	nonossifying fibroma
3DFT	three-dimensional Fourier transform	PCV	polycythemia vera
DFS	dermatofibrosarcoma	PDWI	proton density weighted imaging
DFSP	dermatofibrosarcoma protuberans	PET	positron emission tomography
DTPA	diethylene triamine pentacetic acid	PHAT	pleomorphic hyalinizing angiectatic tumor
DWI	diffusion-weighted imaging	PNET	primitive neuroectodermal tumor
EG	eosinophilic granuloma	PVNS	pigmented villonodular synovitis
EMA	epithelial membrane antigen	RA	rheumatoid arthritis
FCD	fibrous cortical defect	RBC	red blood cell
FISH	fluorescent in situ hybridization	RF	radio frequency
FLAIR	fluid attenuated inversion recovery	RSD	reflex sympathetic dystrophy
FS	frequency selective	SE	spin echo
FS-DFSP	fibrosarcomatous variant of dermato-fibrosarcoma	SFT	solitary fibrous tumor
		SMA	smooth muscle actin
FSE	fast spin echo	STIR	short tau (T1) inversion recovery
FS PDWI	fat-suppressed proton density-weighted imaging	T1	spin-lattice or longitudinal relaxation time
FSPGR	fast spoiled gradient-recalled echo	T2	spin-spin or transverse relaxation time
FS T1WI	fat-suppressed T1-weighted imaging	T2*	effective spin-spin relaxation time using GRE
GCSF	granulocyte colony-stimulating factor	T1WI	T1-weighted imaging
Gd-contrast	gadolinium chelate contrast	T2WI	T2-weighted imaging
GRE	gradient-refocused echo pulse sequence	TB	tuberculosis
HD	Hodgkin disease	TE	echo time
HHV	human herpes virus	TI	inversion time
HPF	high power field	TOF	time-of-flight
HU	Hounsfield unit	TR	repetition time
HVA	homovanillic acid	UBC	unicameral bone cyst
ICA	internal carotid artery	VMA	vanillylmandelic acid
IL	interleukin	WHO	World Health Organization

Introduction

Overview of Magnetic Resonance Imaging and its Role in the Evaluation of Musculoskeletal Abnormalities

Magnetic resonance imaging (MRI) is a powerful medical imaging method that has been used extensively in the evaluation of musculoskeletal tumors and other lesions.[1-3,7-12,20,23-25,29,31,32,36,38-45,47,48] MRI can provide "in vivo" anatomic images of the human body with high, soft tissue contrast resolution. The magnetic resonance (MR) images can be obtained in multiple planes, that is, sagittal, axial, coronal, or various oblique combinations. The "signal" used to generate an MR image comes from hydrogen nuclei (protons) within a human body. In essence, MRI is a hydrogen scan.

The hydrogen nucleus has a net charge of +1 and spins at a frequency that is dependent on the ambient magnetic field and its particular physical characteristic known as the gyromagnetic ratio. The spinning charge of each hydrogen nucleus gives off a tiny magnetic field perpendicular to the axis of spin, thus acting like a tiny bar magnet. Outside the bore of a magnet, the net magnetic properties (magnetic moment) of a person will be zero because the spinning hydrogen nuclei will be oriented randomly, resulting in an overall cancellation of the sum total of tiny magnetic fields. Once placed into a high field-strength magnet, spinning hydrogen nuclei within the human body become aligned or magnetized along its magnetic field. This net magnetization of hydrogen nuclei is oriented in a low-energy alignment (ground state) that is parallel to the magnetic field of the magnet. The hydrogen nuclei spin (precess) at a frequency proportional to their specific gyromagnetic ratio and the magnetic field, in a relationship known as the Larmor equation. The precessional frequency of hydrogen nuclei at 1.5 tesla (T) is 64 megahertz (MHz).

To generate an MR signal, energy is transferred to the hydrogen nuclei within the magnet by using a radio frequency (RF) pulse at the Larmor frequency. The Larmor frequency is dependent on the field strength of the magnetic device and the gyromagnetic ratio, which is specific for the element or molecule of interest. For MRI, that element is the hydrogen nucleus. The hydrogen nuclei absorb this energy and move out of their ground-state alignment. When the RF pulse is turned off, the energy absorbed by the hydrogen nuclei is emitted at the same frequency. This emitted energy, or MR signal, can be detected by the receiver coils (which act like antennae) in the magnet, and used to produce an MR image. Soft tissue contrast results from: (1) the densities of protons (hydrogen nuclei) within different tissues, (2) the different rates which the protons in various tissues realign themselves with the magnetic field of the magnet (also referred to as T1 relaxation, longitudinal or spin lattice relaxation), and (3) rates of signal decay or dephasing (also referred to as T2 relaxation, transverse or spin spin relaxation). Using these biophysical properties of different normal and abnormal tissues allows MRI to have greater soft tissue contrast than computed tomography (CT).

The main components of a typical MRI scanner include: (1) a large-bore magnet with high field strength (0.3–3.0 T); (2) radio frequency (RF) coils within the magnet which can transmit and receive properly-tuned RF pulses, as well as set spatially-dependent magnetic fields (gradients) that allow localization of specific regions of anatomic interest; and (3) a computer which operates the device as well as processes the RF signal data received from the patient to form an anatomic image. To generate an MR image, a person is placed onto a table which can move into specific locations within the bore of the magnet. Once in the magnet, the operator selects programs which include the RF pulse sequences necessary to generate images with the desired contrast parameters based on the proton densities, T1 and T2 values of the various tissues. The data received from the subject or patient are processed by the computer using computer algorithms (2 D or 3 D Fourier transformation). The images are displayed on the monitor console and transferred to film or other computers. Many systems store the image data on digital tape or optical discs for easy retrieval.

Not all patients can have MRI examinations. Intracranial aneurysm clips, cardiac pacemakers, and metallic foreign bodies in the eyes are absolute contraindications for MRI. In addition, the presence of surgical clips, metallic rods, wires, and other orthopedic hardware can produce artifacts obscuring visualization of the anatomic structures in the region of interest.

Major advantages of MRI for musculoskeletal imaging include excellent soft-tissue contrast resolution, multiplanar imaging capabilities, dynamic rapid data acquisition, and various available contrast agents. MRI has proven to be a powerful imaging modality for abnormalities involving fat, muscles, nerves, bone and bone marrow, and has been used in the evaluation of:

- neoplasms of the muscles, fat, nerves, bone, and meninges
- response of neoplasms to neoadjuvant (preoperative chemotherapy) and postoperative chemotherapy and/or radiation treatment
- residual and/or recurrent tumor after surgery
- disorders of histogenesis
- congenital and developmental musculoskeletal anomalies
- traumatic lesions
- hemorrhage
- ischemia and infarction of muscles, fat and bone marrow
- infectious and noninfectious inflammatory diseases
- metabolic disorders.

MR data can also be used to generate images of arteries and veins (MR angiography) in displays similar to conventional angiography. The appearance of blood vessels on MR images depends on various factors such as the type of MRI pulse sequence, pulsatility and range of velocities in the vessels of interest, and size, shape, and orientation of the vessels relative to the image plane. Useful anatomic information of blood vessels can be gained by using spin echo pulse sequences which can display patent vessels as zones of signal void (black-blood images), or gradient recall echo (GRE) pulse sequences which display the moving hydrogen atomic-nuclei (protons) in blood as zones of high signal (bright-blood images). Other options with clinical MRI scanners include: magnetic resonance spectroscopy (acquisition of spectral data to characterize the biochemical properties of selected regions of interest in the soft tissues); diffusion-weighted imaging (evaluation of different rates of proton diffusion between normal and abnormal tissue); and perfusion imaging (evaluation of the differences in rates of contrast enhancement between normal and abnormal tissue).

The appearance of muscle, fascia, tendons, ligaments, and bone cortex and marrow depends on the MRI pulse sequence used as well as the age of the patient imaged. In addition to the standard spin echo or fast spin echo sequences that are commonly used for evaluation of the musculoskeletal system, other MRI pulse sequences or imaging options are sometimes used such as: inversion recovery techniques (STIR—short Tan inversion recovery used for fat signal suppression, FLAIR—fluid attenuated inversion recovery used for fluid signal suppression); GRE imaging with or without MR angiography; magnetic transfer; diffusion/perfusion MR imaging; and frequency selective chemical saturation. Detailed discussions of these sequences and options can be found elsewhere in the literature.

Bone formation occurs by either enchondral or membranous ossification. Longitudinal growth occurs by enchondral bone formation in which a calcified cartilaginous matrix at the growth (physeal) plates is remodeled into bone.[41] The physeal plate contains four parallel zones oriented perpendicular to the long axis of bone. The four zones from peripheral (nearest the epiphysis) to proximal (nearest the metaphysis) are (1) resting zone, (2) proliferating zone, (3) hypertrophic zone, and (4) calcifying zone. Active cartilage cell division and maturation occurs in the proliferating and hypertrophic zones. Osteoid matrix formation and mineralization occurs in the calcifying zone, also referred to as the zone of provisional calcification. At the adjacent metaphyseal region (primary spongiosa), remodeling of bone occurs with osteoclastic activity. The resting, proliferating, and hypertrophic zones are radiolucent, and on MRI have high signal on T2-weighted imaging (WI) and frequency selective (FS) T2WI, whereas the zone of provisional calcification has attenuation similar to mature mineralized bone on radiographs and CT, and has low signal on T2WI and FS T2WI.[41] With membranous bone formation, bone cells form directly from the periosteum (long bones, facial bones, clavicle) for axial growth, or dura (calvarium) without intervening growth plates. The periosteum has low signal on T1WI and T2WI and is attached to the outer surface of the bone cortex in the metadiaphyseal regions by collagen fibers (fibers of Sharpey), but is absent from the articular ends of the bones; it is composed of an outer fibrous layer and an inner cellular layer referred to as the cambrium.[48] Osteoblastic activity occurs in the cambrium, and is responsible for increasing the diameter of bone during growth in childhood. The periosteum is loosely attached to the cortex in children, whereas it is firmly attached in adults. Reactivation of the periosteum in adults can occur as a result of trauma, infection, or neoplasms. Perisoteal membranous bone formation occurs with induction of fibroblasts (in the fibrous layer or adjacent soft tissues) into osteogenic precursor cells that eventually develop into acive osteogenic cells in the cambrium.[48] Hyperemia from fracture, infection or tumor can accelerate new periosteal bone formation which can be seen as a radiodense line superificial to the cortex on radiographs or CT.[48] Perisoteal reaction can have variable configurations related to the disease process.[48] MRI can demonstrate periosteal elevation from diseases as well as subperiosteal abnormalities such as hemorrhage, pus, or tumor.[48]

Within the medullary portion of bone, MRI signal is related to the the presence of hematopoeitic (red) marrow which contains 40% fat, 40% water, and 20% protein, or hematopoeitically-inactive fatty (yellow) marrow containing 80% fat, 15% water, and 5% protein. Fatty marrow usually has a similar signal to subcutaneous fat on T1WI and FS T2WI. Red marrow typically has an intermediate signal on T1WI that is slightly lower than for fat, and an intermediate signal on FS T2WI, which is often similar to muscle. In early childhood, bone marrow is predominantly composed of red (hematopoeitic) marrow.[41,49] Later in childhood, progressive conversion of red to yellow marrow occurs in the hands and feet followed by the distal long bones.[41] In long bones, progressive conversion from red to yellow marrow occurs in the diaphyseal regions during the first decade.[41] The marrow of ossified epiphyses and trochanters is typically fatty.[41] In adults, red marrow is typically found in the spine, flat bones, skull, and proximal portions of the femora and humeri. MRI can demonstrate the process of red to yellow marrow conversion because of the slightly differing signal characteristics on T1WI and FS T2WI.

Most pathologic processes increase the T1 and T2 relaxation coefficients of the involved tissues, resulting in decreased signal on T1WI and increased signal on T2WI relative to adjacent normal tissue. Such processes include ischemia, infarction, inflammation, infection, metabolic or toxic disorders, trauma, neoplasms, and radiation injury. Hemorrhage, however, can have variable appearances depending on the age of the hematoma, oxidation states of the iron in hemoglobin, hematocrit, protein concentration, clot formation and retraction, location, and size.[6] Oxyhemoglobin in a hyperacute blood clot has ferrous iron and is diamagnetic. Oxyhemoglobin does not significantly alter the T1 and T2 values of the tissue environment other than causing possible localized edema. After a few hours during the acute phase of the hematoma, the oxyhemoglobin loses its oxygen to form deoxyhemoglobin which also has ferrous iron, although it has unpaired electrons and becomes paramagnetic. As a result, deoxyhemoglobin shortens the T2 value of the acute clot but does not significantly change the T1 value. On MRI, deoxyhemoglobin in the clot will have intermediate T1 signal and low signal on T2-weighted spin echo or gradient echo images. Later in the early subacute phase of the hematoma, deoyxhemoglobin becomes oxidized to the ferric state in methemoglobin, which is strongly paramagnetic. Methemoglobin shortens the T1 value of hydrogen nuclei resulting in high signal on T1WI. While the red blood cells in the clot are intact, the T2 values of the intracellular methemoglobin will also be decreased resulting in low signal on T2WI. In the late subacute phase, breakdown of the membranes of the red blood cells results in extracellular methemoglobin, which now results in high signal on both T1- and T2WI. In the chronic phase, methemoglobin becomes further oxidized and broken down by macrophages into hemosiderin, which has prominent low signal on T2-weighted images and low-intermediate signal on T1-weighted images.

Other processes which can result in zones of high signal on T1-weighted images are fat, dermoids (intact or ruptured), teratomas, lipomas, cystic structures with high protein concentration or cholesterol, and pantopaque. Lesions or structures with low signal on T1- and T2WI can result from calcifications, very high protein or gadolinium-chelate concentrations, magnetic susceptibility effect especially from metal fragments or surgical clips, and artifacts.

Classification of Bone Tumors and Tumors Involving Musculoskeletal Soft Tissues

The classification of the bone and soft tissue neoplasms has evolved with the combined and coordinated utilization of clinical, imaging, macroscopic, histologic, immunohistochemical cytogenetic, and molecular genetic information.[4,8,12,13,16,17,20,34,35] This book uses the World Health Organization (WHO) classification, which was derived from an Editorial and Consensus Conference of the International Academy of Pathology in Lyon, France, during April 2002. The WHO classification of bone tumors is listed in Table I.1 and that of soft tissue tumors is listed in Table I.2 These classifications incorporate immunohistochemical reactivity profiles to distinguish between lesions that have overlapping morphologic features or have uncertain histogenesis.[14,16,20] Various enzyme-linked antibodies used to

Table I.1 WHO classification of bone tumors

Tumor type	ICD-O Code*
Cartilage tumors	
Osteochondroma	9210/0
Chondroma	9220/0
Enchondroma	9220/0
Periosteal chondroma	9221/0
Multiple chondromatosis	9220/1
Chondroblastoma	9230/0
Chondromyxoid fibroma	9241/0
Chondrosarcoma	9220/3
Central, primary, and secondary	9220/3
Peripheral	9221/3
Dedifferentiated	9243/3
Mesenchymal	9240/3
Clear cell	9242/3
Osteogenic tumors	
Osteoid osteoma	9191/0
Osteoblastoma	9200/0
Osteosarcoma	9180/3
Conventional	9180/3
Chondroblastic	9181/3
Fibroblastic	9182/3
Osteoblastic	9180/3
Telangiectatic	9183/3
Small cell	9185/3
Low grade central	9187/3
Secondary	9180/3
Parosteal	9192/3
Periosteal	9193/3
High-grade surface	9194/3
Fibrogenic tumors	
Desmoplastic fibroma	8823/0
Fibrosarcoma	8810/3
Fibrohistiocytic tumors	
Benign fibrous histiocytoma	8830/0
Malignant fibrous histiocytoma	8830/3
Ewing sarcoma/primitive neuroectodermal tumor	
Ewing sarcoma	9260/3
Hematopoietic tumors	
Plasma cell myeloma	9732/3
Malignant lymphoma, NOS	9590/3
Giant cell tumor	
Giant cell tumor	9250/1
Malignancy in giant cell tumor	9250/3
Notochordal tumors	
Chordoma	9370/3
Vascular tumors	
Haemangioma	9120/0
Angiosarcoma	9120/3
Smooth muscle tumors	
Leiomyoma	8890/0
Leiomyosarcoma	8890/3
Lipogenic tumors	
Lipoma	8850/0
Liposarcoma	8850/3
Neural tumors	
Neurilemmoma	9560/0
Miscellaneous tumors	
Adamantinoma	9261/3
Miscellaneous lesions	
Aneurysmal bone cyst	
Simple cyst	
Fibrous dysplasia	
Osteofibrous dysplasia	
Langerhans cell histiocytosis	9751/1
Erdheim–Chester disease	
Joint lesions	
Synovial chondromatosis	9220/0

* Morphology codes of the International Classification of Diseases for Oncology (ICD-O) and the Systematized Nomenclature of Medicine (http://snomed.org). Behavior is coded /0 for benign tumors, /1 for unspecified, borderline or uncertain behavior, /2 for in-situ carcinomas and grade III intraepithelial neoplasia, and /3 for malignant tumors.
NOS: not otherwise specified.

Table I.2 WHO classification of soft tissue tumors

Tumor type	ICD-O Code
Adipocytic tumors	
Benign	
Lipoma	8850/0
Lipomatosis	8850/0
Lipomatosis of nerve	8850/0
Lipoblastoma/lipoblastomatosis	8881/0
Angiolipoma	8861/0
Myolipoma	8890/0
Chondroid lipoma	8862/0
Extrarenal angiomyolipoma	8860/0
Extra-adrenal myelolipoma	8870/0
Spindle cell/	8857/0
Pleomorphic lipoma	8854/0
Hibernoma	8880/0
Intermediate (locally aggressive)	
Atypical lipomatous tumor/	
Well-differentiated liposarcoma	8851/3
Malignant	
Dedifferentiated liposarcoma	8858/3
Myxoid liposarcoma	8852/3
Round cell liposarcoma	8853/3
Pleomorphic liposarcoma	8854/3
Mixed-type liposarcoma	8855/3
Liposarcoma, not otherwise specified	8850/3

Table I.2 (Continued) WHO classification of soft tissue tumors

Tumor type	ICD-O Code
Fibroblastic/myofibroblastic tumors	
Benign	
Nodular fasciitis	
Proliferative fasciitis	
Proliferative myositis	
Myositis ossificans	
Fibro-osseous pseudotumor of digits	
Ischemic fasciitis	
Elastofibroma	8820/0
Fibrous hamartoma of infancy	
Myofibroma/myofibromatosis	8824/0
Fibromatosis colli	
Juvenile hyaline fibromatosis	
Inclusion body fibromatosis	
Fibroma of tendon sheath	8810/0
Desmoplastic fibroblastoma	8810/0
Mammary-type myofibroblastoma	8825/0
Calcifying aponeurotic fibroma	8810/0
Angiomyofibroblastoma	8826/0
Cellular angiofibroma	9160/0
Nuchal-type fibroma	8810/0
Gardner fibroma	8810/0
Calcifying fibrous tumor	
Giant cell angiofibroma	9160/0
Intermediate (locally aggressive)	
Superficial fibromatoses (palmar/plantar)	
Desmoid-type fibromatoses	8821/1
Lipofibromatosis	
Intermediate (rarely metastasizing)	
Solitary fibrous tumor	8815/1
and hemangiopericytoma	9150/1
(incl. lipomatous hemangiopericytoma)	
Inflammatory myofibroblastic tumor	8825/1
Low-grade myofibroblastic sarcoma	8825/3
Myxoinflammatory	
fibroblastic sarcoma	8811/3
Infantile fibrosarcoma	8814/3
Malignant	
Adult fibrosarcoma	8810/3
Myxofibrosarcoma	8811/3
Low-grade fibromyxoid sarcoma	8811/3
Hyalinizing spindle cell tumor	
Sclerosing epithelioid fibrosarcoma	8810/3
So-called fibrohistiocytic tumors	
Benign	
Giant cell tumor of tendon sheath	9252/0
Diffuse-type giant cell tumor	9251/0
Deep benign fibrous histiocytoma	8830/0
Intermediate (rarely metastasizing)	
Plexiform fibrohistiocytic tumor	8835/1
Giant cell tumor of soft tissues	9251/1
Malignant	
Pleomorphic "MFH"/undifferentiated	
pleomorphic sarcoma	8830/3
Giant cell "MFH"/undifferentiated	
pleomorphic sarcoma with giant cells	8830/3
Inflammatory "MFH"/undifferentiated	
pleomorphic sarcoma with prominent inflammation	8830/3
Smooth muscle tumors	
Angioleiomyoma	8894/0
Deep leiomyoma	8890/0
Genital leiomyoma	8890/0
Leiomyosarcoma (excluding skin)	8890/3

Tumor type	ICD-O Code
Pericytic (perivascular) tumors	
Glomus tumor (and variants)	8711/0
malignant glomus tumor	8711/3
Myopericytoma	8713/1
Skeletal muscle tumors	
Benign	
Rhabdomyoma	8900/0
adult type	8904/0
fetal type	8903/0
genital type	8905/0
Malignant	
Embryonal rhabdomyosarcoma	8910/3
(incl. spindle cell,	8912/3
botryoid, anaplastic)	8910/3
Alveolar rhabdomyosarcoma	
(incl. solid, anaplastic)	8920/3
Pleomorphic rhabdomyosarcoma	8901/3
Vascular tumors	
Benign	
Hemangiomas of:	
subcut/deep soft tissue:	9120/0
capillary	9131/0
cavernous	9121/0
arteriovenous	9123/0
venous	9122/0
intramuscular	9132/0
synovial	9120/0
Epithelioid haemangioma	9125/0
Angiomatosis	
Lymphangioma	9170/0
Intermediate (locally aggressive)	
Kaposiform hemangioendothelioma	9130/1
Intermediate (rarely metastasizing)	
Retiform hemangioendothelioma	9135/1
Papillary intralymphatic angioendothelioma	9135/1
Composite hemangioendothelioma	9130/1
Kaposi sarcoma	9140/3
Malignant	
Epithelioid hemangioendothelioma	9133/3
Angiosarcoma of soft tissue	9120/3
Chondro-osseous tumors	
Soft tissue chondroma	9220/0
Mesenchymal chondrosarcoma	9240/3
Extraskeletal osteosarcoma	9180/3
Tumors of uncertain differentiation	
Benign	
Intramuscular myxoma	8840/0
(Incl. cellular variant)	
Juxta-articular myxoma	8840/0
Deep ("aggressive") angiomyxoma	8841/0
Pleomorphic hyalinizing	
angiectatic tumor	
Ectopic hamartomatous thymoma	8587/0
Intermediate (rarely metastasizing)	
Angiomatoid fibrous histiocytoma	8836/1
Ossifying fibromyxoid tumor	8842/0
(incl. atypical/malignant)	
Mixed tumor	8940/1
Myoepithelioma	8982/1
Parachordoma	9373/1

Table I.2 (Continued) WHO classification of soft tissue tumors

Tumor type	ICD-O Code
Malignant	
Synovial sarcoma	9040/3
Epithelioid sarcoma	8804/3
Alveolar soft part sarcoma	9581/3
Clear cell sarcoma of soft tissue	9044/3
Extraskeletal myxoid chondrosarcoma ("chordoid" type)	9231/3
PNET/extraskeletal Ewing tumor	
pPNET	9364/3
extraskeletal Ewing tumor	9260/3
Desmoplastic small round cell tumor	8806/3
Extrarenal rhabdoid tumor	8963/3
Malignant mesenchymoma	8990/3
Neoplasms with perivascular epithelioid cell differentiation (PEComa)	
clear cell myomelanocytic tumor	
Intimal sarcoma	8800/3

PNET: primitive neuroectodermal tumor.

detect tissue antigens and their clinical applications for diagnosis are listed in Table I.3 In addition, the new WHO classifications of bone and soft tissue tumors also utilize data from cytogenetic and molecular genetic analyses.[4,5,8,12,13,34,35,37] Cytogenetic and gene abnormalities of tumors of bone and soft tissues are listed in Table I.4.

Table I.3 Immunohistochemical markers used in the diagnosis of bone and soft tissue tumors

Marker		Positive immunoreactivity in:
Endothelial markers	**CD 31**-antigen gpIIa, PECAM-1: platelet endothelial cell adhesion	Angiosarcoma, hemangioendothelioma, Kaposi sarcoma, hemangioma
	CD 34; 110 kDa transmembrane glycoprotein that occurs in skin and blood vessels on endothelium cells, stem cells and dendritic cells, marker for endothelial differentiation	Kaposi sarcoma, angiosarcoma, epithelioid hemangioendothelioma, dermatofibrosarcoma protuberans, solitary fibrous tumor, hemangiopericytoma, malignant peripheral nerve sheath tumor, other vascular and fibroblastic tumors
	CD 141	Variable in angiosarcoma, positive in mesothelioma, squamous carcinoma
	FLI-1; type of DNA-binding transcription factor	Angiosarcoma, Ewing sarcoma/PNET [translocation: t(11;22)(q24;q12)], lymphoblastic lymphoma
	Factor VIII antigen (von Willebrand factor); antigen expressed by endothelial cells within Weibel–Palade bodies and mekaryocytes	Endothelial neoplasms
Leukocyte differentiation antigens (CD; clusters of differentiation of monoclonal antibodies to human leukocyte and erythroid antigens)	**CD 1**	CD 1a and S 100 in Langerhans cell histiocytosis
	CD 3	T-ALL/T-LBL (*T cell lymphoblastic lymphoma/leukemia*), NK (*natural killer*) cells
	CD 5	T-ALL/T-LBL, B-CLL (*chronic lymphoid leukemia*), mantle cell lymphoma
	CD 10	B-ALL (*acute lymphoid leukemia*), AML (*acute myeloid leukemia*), follicular lymphoma, Burkitt lymphoma
	CD 11	CD 11c in hairy cell leukemia
	CD 15	Hodgkin disease, granulocytic sarcoma
	CD 20	B cell lymphomas
	CD 23	B cell lymphomas
	CD 25	Adult T-ALL, hairy cell leukemia
	CD 30	Hodgkin disease, anaplastic large cell lymphoma
	CD 38	Plasma cells are characteristically CD 38+/CD 45-
	CD 43	Neoplastic B cell positive, normal B cell negative
	CD 45	T and B lymphomas, plasma cells
	CD 79a	B lymphomas
	CD 99 (MIC-2 gene product): surface glycoprotein 30–32 kDa present in most tissues	Ewing sarcoma/PNET (90%), lymphoblastic lymphoma (90%), synovial sarcoma (75%), mesenchymal chondrosarcoma (50%), neuroepitheliomas, alveolar rhabdomyosarcoma, solitary fibrous tumor, hemangiopericytoma.
	CD 117	Mast cells, gastrointestinal stromal tumors

Table I.3 (Continued) Immunohistochemical markers used in the diagnosis of bone and soft tissue tumors

Marker		Positive immunoreactivity to:
Leukocyte differentiation antigens	CD 138	Plasma cells
Muscle cell markers	**Actin,** consists of contractile filaments in smooth muscle	Smooth muscle and myofibroblastic tumors, primary or metastatic spndle cell and round cell tumors
	Actin, (sarcomeric) consists of contractile filaments in skeletal muscle	Skeletal muscle and rhabdomyosarcoma
	Desmin, intermediate filament protein present in smooth and striated muscle cells and myofibroblasts	Angiomatoid malignant fibrous histiocytoma, Smooth and skeletal muscle tumors, other tumors
	HCD	Smooth muscle and its tumors, myoepithelia, GI stromal tumors
	Calponin: actin-binding protein in smooth muscle associated with regulation of smooth muscle contractility	Smooth muscle, myofibroblasts, myoepithelia, synovial sarcoma (often)
	MyoD 1, myogenin; represent intranuclear MyoD transcription factors that initiate differentiation of striated muscle	Rhabdomyosarcoma (reactive skeletal muscle)
	Myoglobin: an oxygen-binding heme protein in cardiac and skeletal muscle, but not in smooth muscle	Rhabdomyosarcoma (differentiated)
	Myosin	Isoforms for smooth and skeletal muscle tumors
Neural, nerve sheath, and neuroendocrine-specific markers	**Synaptophysin:** glycoprotein in synaptic vesicles, used for cells of neural or neuroendocrine origin	Neuroblastoma, ganglioneuroblastoma, paraganglioma, neuroendocrine carcinoma, rhabdomyosarcoma, peripheral neuroepithelioma
	Chromogranin: family of acidic glycoproteins located in neurosecretory granules	Paraganglioma, neuroendocrine carcinoma (low grade)
	Neuron-specific enolase: enzyme of glycolytic pathway expressed in neural and non-neural tumors	General neuroendocrine marker (poor specificity), Ewing sarcoma
	Neurofilaments (NF proteins): useful in diagnosis of small round-cell tumors	Neuroblastoma, paraganglioma, malignant fibrous histiocytoma, rhabdomyosarcoma, Merkel cell carcinoma
	Glial fibrillary acidic protein (GFAP)	Glial tumors, schwannomas, myoepithelial tumors.
	CD 57 (Leu-7): 110 kDa antigen is present on the surface of natural killer cells and T-lymphocytes	Synovial sarcoma, leiomyosarcoma (relatively nonspecific), round and spindle cells with nerve sheath differentiation
S-100 Protein and other multispecific neural markers	**S-100 protein:** dimeric, acidic calcium-binding protein that is soluble in 100% ammonium sulfate, used for tumors of neural origin, melanoma, and cartilaginous differentiation	Melanoma, schwannoma, neurofibroma, chondroblastoma, chondromyxoid fibroma, ossifying fibromyxoid tumor, chordoma, chondrosarcoma, clear cell sarcomas, Langerhans cell histiocytosis
	Nerve growth factor receptor	Dermatofibrosarcoma protuberans and other nerve sheath tumors
	CD 56: 140 kDa membrane glycoprotein involved in neural cell adhesion molecule	Neuroendocrine carcinoma, rhabdomyosarcoma, synovial sarcoma, chondrosarcoma, osteosarcoma, neuroblastoma, malignant peripheral nerve sheath tumor, schwannoma, rhabdomyosarcoma, leiomyosarcoma, leiomyoma
Melanoma markers other than S-100 protein	**HMB45:** monoclonal antibody for Pmel gene product in immature melanosomes	Melanoma, clear cell sarcoma, angiomyolipoma, perivascular epithelioid cell tumors (PECOmas)
	Tyrosinase; enzyme involved in melanin synthesis	Nevi, melanoma
	Melan-A, marker for melanosomes	Nevi, melanoma, angiomyolipoma
	Microphthalmia-transcription factor; transcription factor involved in melanogenesis and expression of the tyrosinase gene	Melanoma, clear cell sarcoma, osteoclastic giant cells
	CD 63	Melanoma, some carcinomas, alveolar soft parts sarcoma
Histiocytic markers	**Lysozyme**	Histiocytes, myelomonocytic cells
	Factor XIIa	Histiocytes, especially dendritic ones
	CD 68: 110 kDa glycoprotein found in tumors containing lysosomes or phagolysosomes	Histiocytes, melanoma, paraganglioma, schwannoma, granular cell tumor malignant fibrous histiocytoma (50%)
	CD 163	Histiocytes

Table I.3 (Continued) Immunohistochemical markers used in the diagnosis of bone and soft tissue tumors

Marker		Positive immunoreactivity to:
Epithelial markers	**Cytokeratins**: acidic or basic proteins of intermediate sized filaments ranging from 40 to 67 kDa, often allows distinction of epithelial from non-epithelial tumors	Carcinoma, metastatic epithelial carcinoma, synovial and epithelioid sarcoma, chordoma, Merkel cell tumor, adamantinoma
	Epithelial membrane antigen (EMA): transmembrane glycoprotein with high molecular weight that is expressed in epithelial cells and tumor derived from epithelial cells	Epithelial tumors, synovial sarcoma, epithelioid sarcoma, meningioma, perineural tumors, malignant peripheral nerve sheath tumors, leiomyosarcoma
	Carcinoembryonic antigen (CEA)	Many adenocarcinomas, biphasic synovial sarcoma
	Desmoplakin	Epithelial tumors in general, meningioma, Ewing sarcoma
	HBME-1	Mesothelioma, some adenocarcinoma, synovial sarcoma, chondroma
	CD 117: proto-oncogene transmenbrane receptor for stem cell factor on mast cells, melanocytes, hematopoeitic cells, and germ cells	GI stromal tumor, angiosarcoma, Ewing sarcoma, leiomyoma, leiomyosarcoma, nerve sheath tumors
Mesenchymal marker	**Vimentin**: widely distributed intermediate filament (57 kDa) expressed in mesenchymal cells	Sarcomas, melanoma, some carcinomas and lymphomas
Bone tissue markers	**Alkaline phosphatase**: enzyme associated with bone turnover	
	Osteonectin: secreted glycoprotein in the extracellular matrix by bone cells	Osteosarcoma, Malignant fibrous histiocytoma, meningioma, melanoma, breast carcinoma
	Osteocalcin: intraosseous protein associated with osteoblasts and osteoblastic differentiation	Osteosarcoma
	Collagen: many subtypes	Type X collagen is seen only in benign osteochondromas, Type IV seen with glomus tumor
Cell proliferation evaluation	**K_i-67**: 395 kDa specific nuclear antigen only expressed in proliferating cells in late G1, S, G2 and M phases	For sarcomas; aggressive can be related to the K_i-67 index (number of positive cells per 10 high-power fields), >50/10HPFs
	Mutated p53 protein: TP53 gene product consisting of a nuclear phosphorylation protein that suppresses transcription and proliferation of cells with damaged DNA; has a longer half life when mutated and more detectable than wild type	p53 overexpression has been associated with sarcomas with high tumor grade, prognostic utility not proven
	p16 and p27: cyclin-dependent kinase inhibitors	Loss of p16 expression from deletion of CDKN2A/p16 in malignant peripheral nerve sheath tumors but not in neurofibromas; loss of p27 seen with malignant transformation of neurofibromas

Source: Adapted from references 14, 16, and 20.

Table I.4 Genetic abnormalities in bone and soft tissue tumors

Tumor/lesion	Cytogenetic (chromosomal) abnormality	Molecular abnormality	Frequency (%)	Diagnostic utility
Malignant bone tumors				
Osteosarcoma	Loss of heterozygosity (LOH) at 3q, 13q, 17p, and 18q and variable chromosomal changes			Unclear
Parosteal osteosarcoma	Supernumerary ring chromosomes, ring 12q13-15			Unclear
Chondrosarcoma	1, 5, 7, 8, 11, 12, 15, 18, 19, 20			Unclear
Ewing sarcoma and PNET	t(11;22)(q24;q12), t(21;22)(q22;q12), t(7;22)9p22;q22)			Yes
Chordoma	3, 4, 10, 13			No
Adamantinoma	Numerical changes in 2 cases			No

Table I.4 (Continued) Genetic abnormalities in bone and soft tissue tumors

Tumor/lesion	Cytogenetic (chromosomal) abnormality	Molecular abnormality	Frequency (%)	Diagnostic utility
Benign bone lesions				
Chondroma	12q13–15			Unclear
Malignant soft tissue tumors				
Chondrosarcoma, extraskeletal myxoid	t(9;22)(q31;q12) t(9;17)(q22;q11) t(9;15)(q22;q21)	EWS-CHN fusion RBP56-CHN(TEC) TEC-TCF12	>75	Yes
Clear cell sarcoma	t(12;22)(q13;q12)	EWS-ATF1 fusion	>75	Yes
Desmoplastic small round cell tumor	t(11;22)(p13;q12)	EWS-WT1 fusion	>75	Yes
Dermatofibrosarcoma protuberans	Ring form of chromosomes 17q and 22q t(17;22)(q22;q13)	COL 1A1-PDGFB fusion COL 1A1-PDGFB fusion	>75 10	Yes
Ewing sarcoma	t(11;22)(q21;q13) t(21;22)(p22;q12) t(2;22)(q33;q12) t(7;22)(p22;q12) t(17;22)(q12;q12)	EWS-FLI1 fusion EWS-ERG fusion EWS-FEV fusion EWS-ETV1 fusion EWS-E1AF fusion	>80 5–10 <5 <5 <5	Yes Yes Yes Yes Yes
Fibrosarcoma, infantile	t(12;15)(p13;q25) Trisomies 8, 11, 17, and 20	ETV6-NTRK3 fusion	>75 >75	Yes Yes
Gastrointestinal stromal tumor	Monosomies 14 and 22 Deletion of 1p	KIT mutation	>75 >25 >90	Yes No Yes
Malignant Hemangiopericytoma	t(12;19)(q13;q13)			
Inflammatory myofibroblastic tumor	t(2;19)(p23;p13.1) t(1;2)(q22–23;p23)	ALK-TPM4 TPM3-ALK		
Leiomyosarcoma	Deletion of 1p		>50	No
Liposarcoma				
Well differentiated	Ring form of chromosome 12q13–15, 12q21.3–22		>75	
Myxoid/round cell	t(12;16)(q13;p11) t(12;22)(q13;q12)	TLS-CHOP fusion EWS-CHOP fusion	>75 >5	Yes Yes
Pleomorphic	Complex*		90	No
Malignant fibrous histiocytoma				
Myxoid	Ring form of chromosome 12		?	?
High-grade	Complex*		>90	No
Myxofibrosarcoma	See malignant fibrous histiocytoma			
Malignant peripheral nerve sheath tumor				
Low-grade	None		>90	No
High-grade	Complex*			
Mesothelioma	Deletion of 1p Deletion of 9p Deletion of 22q Deletions of 3p and 6q	P15, p16, and p19 inactivation NF2 inactivation	>50 >75 >50 >50	Yes Yes Yes Yes
Neuroblastoma				
Good prognosis	Hyperdiploid, no 1p deletion		90	Yes
Poor prognosis	1p deletion Double minute chromosomes	N-myc amplification	90 >25	Yes Yes
Primitive neuroectodermal tumor	(see Ewing sarcoma)			
Rhabdoid tumor	Deletion of 22q	INI1 inactivation	>90	Yes

Table I.4 (Continued) Genetic abnormalities in bone and soft tissue tumors

Tumor/lesion	Cytogenetic (chromosomal) abnormality	Molecular abnormality	Frequency (%)	Diagnostic utility
Rhabdomyosarcoma				
Alveolar	T(2;13)(q35;q14)	PAX3-FKHR fusion	>75	Yes
	t(1;13)(p36;q14), double minutes	PAX7-FKHR fusion	10–20	Yes
Embryonal	Trisomies 21, 8, and 20	Loss of heterozygosity at 11 p15	>75	Yes
			>75	Yes
Synovial sarcoma				
Monophasic	T(X;18)(p11;q11)	SYT-SSZ1 or SYT-SSX2 fusion	>90	Yes
Biphasic	T(X;18)(p13;q11)	SYT-SSX1 fusion	>90	Yes
Benign soft tissue tumors				
Desmoid tumor	Trisomies 8 and/or 20	APC deletion	25	No
	Deletion of 5 q		10	?
Hibernoma	Translocation at 11 q13		>50	Yes
Leiomyoma, uterine	T(12;14)(q15;q24)	HMGIC and RAD 51 translocation	20	Yes
	Deletion of 7 q		20	?
	Trisomy 12		10	?
Lipoblastoma	Rearrangement of 8 q11–13	PLAG1 fusions	>50	Yes
Lipoma				
Solitary	Rearrangement of 12 q13, t(13–15), t(3;12), 6 p, 13 q	HMGIC fusions	75	Yes
Multiple	None			
Spindle cell lipoma	16 q, 10,13			
Atypical lipoma	Supernumerary ring chromosomes			
Myxoma	Y, telomeric associations			
Neurofibroma	None			
Schwannoma, benign	Deletion of 22 q	NF2 inactivation	>75	Yes

Source: Adapted from references 4, 5, 13, 20, 34, and 37.

Frequency of Occurrence of Bone Tumors

Bone neoplasms can be primary lesions arising from osseous structures or secondary to metastatic disease. Metastatic carcinoma is the most frequent malignant tumor involving bone.[33] In adults, metastatic lesions to bone occur most frequently from carcinomas of the lung, breast, prostate, kidney, thyroid, as well as from sarcomas.[30] The exact incidence of metastatic skeletal disease is unknown.[33] Up to 50% of patients who die from disseminated carcinoma have evidence of skeletal metastases at autopsy.[33] Almost 240 000 patients die in the United States each year from carcinoma of the lung, breast, prostate, kidney, and thyroid.[18] Using these data, up to 120 000 oncology patients who die each year may have metastatic skeletal disease. Metastatic skeletal disease has also been reported to occur in up to 30% of all cancer cases.[15] Thirty per cent of the 1 284 900 annual new cancer cases in the United States[17] is 385 470. In comparison, only 2400 primary malignant bone tumors occur in the United States per year.[19] Metastatic lesions may therefore occur from 50 to 161 times more frequently than primary malignant bone tumors.[15,18,26,31]

Primary bone sarcomas represent only 0.2% of all neoplasms.[8] The incidence of primary bone sarcomas has been reported to be 8 per million.[8] Primary bone sarcomas occur ten times less frequently than sarcomas in the soft tissues.[8] The most frequent type of primary bone sarcoma is osteosarcoma followed by chondrosarcoma and Ewing sarcoma.[8] Bone sarcomas have a bimodal incidence rate with one peak occurring in the second decade (osteosarcoma, chondrosarcoma) and the other in patients over 60 years (chordoma, chondrosarcoma, osteosarcoma).[8] The relative frequencies of primary malignant bone tumors and primary nonmalignant bone tumors are listed in Tables I.5 and I.6, respectively.[27,28,46] The relative frequencies of tumorlike bone lesions are listed in Table I.7.[27,28] Other lesions or abnormalities involving bone are listed in Table I.8. The imaging features of some of these abnormalities may overlap those of bone tumors.

Table I.5 Primary malignant bone tumors

	Mayo Clinic		NCBT		Age range (years): median age
	% malignant (N = 8591)	% total (N = 11 087)	% malignant (N = 3355)	% total (N = 5133)	
Myeloma	44%	34%	2%	1%	16–80:60
Osteosarcoma	19%	15%	34%	22%	2–92:16–39
Chondrosarcoma	12%	9%	21%	14%	7–91:26–59
Lymphoma	8%	6%	3%	2%	18–69
Ewing sarcoma	6%	5%	11%	7%	6–30:14
Chordoma	4%	3%	2%	1%	30–80:58
Fibrosarcoma	3%	2%	5%	4%	10–75:43
Malignant fibrous hist.	1%	<1%	5%	3%	11–80:48
Giant cell tumor	<1%	<1%	2%	1%	10–55:30
Angiosarcoma	<1%	<1%	1%	<1%	10–80:51
Hemangioendothelioma	<1%	<1%	<1%	<1%	15–60:34
Adamantinoma	<1%	<1%	<1%	<1%	10–60:25
Hemangiopericytoma	<1%	<1%	<1%	<1%	1–90:40
Liposarcoma	<1%	<1%	<1%	<1%	Not reported
Synovial sarcoma			2%	1%	5–60:25
Paget sarcoma			1%	<1%	50–80:66

Source: Data for the Mayo Clinic from reference 46. Data for the Netherlands Committee on Bone Tumors (NCBT) from references 27 and 28.

Table I.6 Primary benign bone tumors

	Mayo Clinic		NCBT		Age range (years): median age
	% benign (N = 2496)	% total (N = 11 087)	% benign (N = 1778)	% total (N = 5133)	
Osteochondroma	35%	8%	14%	5%	1–50:20
Giant cell tumor	23%	5%	22%	8%	10–55:30
Enchondroma	12%	3%	17%	6%	3–83:35
Osteoid osteoma	13%	3%	11%	4%	6–30:17
Chondroblastoma	5%	1%	9%	3%	10–30:17
Hemangioma	4%	1%	2%	<1%	1–84:33
Osteoblastoma	3%	<1%	6%	2%	1–30:15
Juxtacortical chondroma	2%	<1%	5%	2%	4–77:26
Chondromyxoid fibroma	2%	<1%	4%	1%	1–40:17
Neurilemoma	<1%	<1%	1%	<1%	2–65:30
Fibrous histiocytoma	<1%	<1%			
Lipoma	<1%	<1%	<1%	<1%	
Hamartoma	<1%	<1%			
Osteoma			<1%	<1%	
Lymphangioma			<1%	<1%	
Desmoplastic fibroma			<1%	<1%	1–71:21

Source: Data for the Mayo Clinic from reference 46. Data for the Netherlands Committee on Bone Tumors (NCBT) from references 27 and 28.

Frequency of Occurrence of Soft Tissue Tumors

Benign tumors of the soft tissues are 100 times more frequent than sarcomas.[13] The annual incidence of benign tumors has been estimated to be 3000 per million, and 30 per million for sarcomas.[12] Sarcomas of the musculoskeletal system account for less than one per cent of all malignant tumors.[12] The relative frequencies of primary malignant tumors and primary non-malignant tumors of the soft tissues are listed in Tables **I.9** and **I.10**, respectively.[21–23]

Grading and Staging of Bone Tumors

Two systems that are currently used for staging of primary malignant bone tumors include the the American Joint Committee on Cancer (AJCC) system that was recently revised in 2002, and the Musculoskeletal Tumor Society (MSTS) system.[8,40]

For the revised AJCC system, four criteria are used for Stages 1A to IVB. T1 refers to tumors measuring less than 8 cm in greatest dimension and T2 for tumors greater than 8 cm. N0 refers to no regional lymph node metastasis and N1 for the occurrence of regional lymph node metastasis. M0 refers to the

Table I.7 Tumorlike bone lesions

	Relative frequency (%) (N = 2287)	Age range (years): median age
Fibrous dysplasia	18%	1–50:20
Osteomyelitis	14%	
Fibrous cortical defect / non-ossifying fibroma	13%	5–20:14
Aneurysmal bone cyst	11%	1–25:14
Traumatic injury (fracture/callus)	10%	
Solitary bone cyst	9%	1–62:11
Eosinophilic granuloma	8%	1–35:10
Heterotopic bone formation/reaction	5%	1–45:22
Pigmented villonodular synovitis	3%	15–60:32
Geode	1%	25–85:52
Brown tumor	1%	40–70:52
Ganglion	<1%	20–70:38
Epidermoid cyst	<1%	19–71:38
Neuropathic arthropathy	<1%	
Melorheostosis	<1%	

Source: Data for the Netherlands Committee on Bone Tumors (NCBT) from references 27 and 28.

Table I.8 Other lesions involving bone

Malignant lesions
Metastatic disease
Leukemia
Desmoid tumors
Benign lesions
Aneurysmal bone cyst
Unicameral bone cyst
Fibrous cortical defect
Non-ossifying fibroma
Fibrous dysplasia
Eosinophilic granuloma
Osteofibrous dysplasia
Paget disease
Plexiform neurofibromas
Ganglion cysts
Geode
Bone island
Melorrheostosis
Metabolic disorders
Thalasemia
Sickle-cell disease
Hemophilia
Osteopetrosis
Gaucher disease
Hyperparathyroidism
Vitamin deficiencies
Radiation injury
Fat conversion
Bone Infarcts
Inflammatory diseases
Pyogenic osteomyelitis
TB osteomyelitis
Fungal osteomyelitis
Langerhans cell histiocytosis / Eosinophilic granuloma
Erdheim–Chester disease
Sarcoid
Traumatic lesions
Fractures
Hematomas
Pseudoarthrosis
Neuropathic joint
Bone infarct
Osteochondritis dissecans

Table I.9 Malignant soft tissue tumors

	% malignant (N = 12 370)	% total (N = 31 047)	Age range (years): median age
Malignant fibrous histiocytoma	24%	10%	32–80; 59
Liposarcoma	14%	6%	18–78; 47
Sarcoma (not further classified)	12%	5%	
Leiomyosarcoma	8%	3%	35–79; 58
Malignant schwannoma	6%	2%	17–70; 42
Dermatofibrosarcoma protuberans	6%	2%	19–60; 38
Synovial sarcoma	5%	2%	14–58; 32
Fibrosarcoma	4%	2%	14–72; 41
Extraskeletal chondrosarcoma	2%	<1%	22–71; 49
Angiosarcoma	2%	<1%	17–77; 49
Rhabdomyosarcoma	2%	<1%	2–40; 18
Epithelioid sarcoma	1%	<1%	15–54; 31
Kaposi sarcoma	1%	<1%	34–84; 64
Malignant hemangiopericytoma	1%	<1%	22–73; 46
Extraskeletal Ewing	1%	<1%	11–42; 25
Clear cell sarcoma	1%	<1%	15–60; 37
Extraskeletal osteosarcoma	<1%	<1%	33–77; 57
Neuroblastoma	<1%	<1%	1–47; 19
Hemangioendothelioma	<1%	<1%	17–60; 40
Malignant granular cell tumor	<1%	<1%	14–70; 39

Source: Data from reference 22.

Table I.10 Benign soft tissue tumors/lesions

	% benign (N = 18 677)	% total (N = 31 047)	Age range (years): median age
Lipoma	16%	10%	26–68; 48
Fibrous histiocytoma	13%	8%	13–57; 33
Nodular fasciitis	11%	7%	11–51; 31
Hemangioma	8%	5%	1–65; 32
Fibromatosis	7%	4%	13–65; 36
Neurofibroma	5%	3%	16–66; 37
Schwannoma	5%	3%	22–72; 46
Giant cell tumor of tendon sheath	4%	2%	18–64; 39
Myxoma	3%	2%	24–74; 52
Granuloma annulare	2%	1%	2–58; 23
Hemangiopericytoma	2%	1%	23–70; 44
Granular cell tumor	2%	1%	15–56; 35
Leiomyoma	2%	1%	14–67; 40
Chondroma	1%	<1%	16–70; 44
Fibroma of tendon sheath	1%	<1%	15–75; 35
Fibroma	1%	<1%	11–67; 40
Myofibromatosis	1%	<1%	<1–52; 14
Glomus tumor	<1%	<1%	19–71; 47
PVNS	<1%	<1%	18–59; 38
Lymphangioma	<1%	<1%	1–50; 19
Ganglion	<1%	<1%	19–65; 40
Proliferative fasciitis	<1%	<1%	33–71; 54
Myositis ossificans	<1%	<1%	13–64; 35
Lipoblastoma	<1%	<1%	1–10; 4
Proliferative myositis	<1%	<1%	
Paraganglioma	<1%	<1%	24–70; 47
Synovial chondromatosis	<1%	<1%	
Ganglioneuroma	<1%	<1%	4–44; 22
Hibernoma	<1%	<1%	21–50; 32

Source: Data from reference 21.
PVNS: Pigmented villonodular synovitis.

Table I.11 American Joint Committee on Cancer Staging system for primary malignant tumors of bone for those tumors diagnosed on or after January 1, 2003[40]

Stage	Tumor	Lymph node	Metastases	Grade
IA	T1	N0	M0	G1 or G2
IB	T2	N0	M0	G1 or G2
IIA	T1	N0	M0	G3 or G4
IIB	T2	N0	M0	G3 or G4
III	T3	N0	M0	Any G
IVA	Any T	N0	M1a	Any G
IVB	Any T	N1	Any M	Any G
IVB	Any T	Any N	M1b	Any G

Classifications: Tx, primary tumor cannot be assessed; T0, no evidence of primary tumor; T1, tumor 8 cm or less in greatest dimension; T2, tumor more than 8 cm in greatest dimension; T3, discontinuous tumors in the primary bone; Nx, regional lymph nodes not assessed; N0, no regional lymph node metastases; N1, regional lymph node metastasis; Mx, distant metastasis cannot be assessed; M0, no distant metastasis; M1, distant metastasis; M1 a, lung; M1 b, other distant sites; and Gx, grade cannot be assessed; G1, well differentiated (low grade); G2, moderately differentiated (low grade); G3, poorly differentiated (high grade); G4, undifferentiated (high grade).

absence of distant metastasis and M1 for the presence of distant metastasis. The last criterion is based on tumor grade: G1 assigned to low grade or well differentiated, G2 for moderately differentiated (also low grade), G3 for poorly differentiated (high grade), and G4 for undifferentiated (high grade) (Table I.11). The AJCC system is used for all primary malignant tumors of bone (osteosarcoma, Ewing sarcoma), except for primary malignant lymphoma or myeloma.[40]

For the MSTS system, three criteria are used for Stages 1A to III. T refers to whether the tumor is localized to a single compartment (T1) or involves more than one compartment (T2); M0 designation for absence of metastases and M1 for the presence of metastases; and G1 for low-grade tumors and G2 for high-grade tumors.[40]

Grading and Staging of Soft Tissue Tumors

The WHO has developed a classification system for soft tissue tumors with lesions assigned to four groups; benign, intermediate (locally aggressive), intermediate (rarely metastasizing), and malignant.[12] Two systems currently used for grading of soft tissue sarcomas include the NCI (United States National Cancer Institute) system and the FNCLCC (French Federation Nationale des Centres de Lutte Contre le Cancer) system (Table I.12). The NCI grading system for tumors takes into account the histologic type, cellularity, pleomorphism, mitotic rate, and presence of necrosis. The FNCLCC system uses tumor differentiation, mitotic rate, and presence/extent of necrosis. Two important histologic features that have been associated with prognosis include high mitotic indices and presence of necrosis. The FNCLCC system has been reported to result in a better correlation with overall and metastasis-free survival than the NCI system.[12] Staging of malignant soft tissue tumors is based on the extent of tumor from imaging, histologic features of the tumors, and clinical data. The main system used for staging for soft tissue sarcomas is the TNM system developed by the American Joint Committee on Cancer (AJCC) and the International Union against Cancer (Table I.13). The TNM system has been shown to be clinically useful for prognostic purposes.[12] The TNM system utilizes data consisting of tumor size and depth, histologic tumor grade, regional lymph node involvement, and presence of distant metastases.

Table I.12 FNCLCC grading system: definition of parameters[12]	
Tumor differentiation	
Score 1:	sarcomas closely resembling normal adult mesenchymal tissue (e. g., low-grade leiomyosarcoma).
Score 2:	sarcomas for which histological typing is certain (e. g., myxoid liposarcoma).
Score 3:	embryonal and undifferentiated sarcomas, sarcomas of doubtful type, synovial sarcomas, osteosarcomas, PNET.
Mitotic count	
Score 1:	0–9 mitoses per 10 HPF*
Score 2:	10–19 mitoses per 10 HPF
Score 3:	≥ 20 mitoses per 10 HPF
Tumor necrosis	
Score 0:	no necrosis
Score 1:	< 50 % tumor necrosis
Score 2:	≥ 50 % tumor necrosis
Histological grade	
Grade 1:	total score 2, 3
Grade 2:	total score 4, 5
Grade 3:	total score 6, 7, 8

* A high power field (HPF) measures 0.1734 mm^2
PNET: primitive neuroectodermal tumor

Imaging Evaluation of Bone and Soft Tissue Tumors Tumorlike Lesions

The diagnosis of bone tumors is often made on conventional radiographs.[4] Osteolytic lesions from tumors, however, may not be visible on conventional radiographs until there is 30–50 % loss of mineralization.[40] Because of superior soft tissue contrast, MRI can detect marrow based tumors before they are evident on radiographs. In addition, MRI can be used to further characterize lesions with regard to extent and extra-osseous extension. With progressive increased utilization of MRI for evaluation of musculoskeletal disorders, tumors and other bone lesions may also be found incidentally.

Features used to characterize bone tumors and other lesions on conventional radiographs include:

- lesion location (metaphyseal/diaphyseal/epiphyseal, cortical, intramedullary, eccentric, central)
- lesion size
- lesion density (radiolucent, sclerotic, presence of matrix mineralization)
- margins (well-defined geographic with or without sclerotic borders, poorly-defined geographic, "moth-eaten" and/or "permeative" radiolucent patterns)
- presence of cortical destruction with or without extra-osseous tumor extension
- presence of periosteal reaction (interrupted vs. noninterrupted pattern, lamellated/onion-skin pattern, perpendicular pattern, sunburst pattern, Codman triangles).[4,8,32,48]

Table I.13 TNM classification of soft tissue sarcomas

Primary tumor (T)	TX:	primary tumor cannot be assessed		
	T0:	no evidence of primary tumor		
	T1:	tumor ≤5 cm in greatest dimension		
		T1 a: superficial tumor*		
		T1 b: deep tumor		
	T2:	tumor >5 cm in greatest dimension		
		T2 a: superficial tumor		
		T2 b: deep tumor		
Regional lymph nodes (N)	NX:	regional lymph nodes cannot be assessed		
	N0:	no regional lymph node metastasis		
	N1:	regional lymph node metastasis		
Distant metastasis (M)	M0:	no distant metastasis		
	M1:	distant metastasis		
G Histopathological Grading				
Translation table for three- and four-grade to two-grade (low vs. high-grade) system				
TNM two-grade system	Three-grade systems		Four-grade systems	
Low-grade	Grade 1		Grade 1	
			Grade 2	
High-grade	Grade 2		Grade 3	
	Grade 3		Grade 4	
Stage IA	T1 a	N0, NX	M0	Low-grade
	T1 b	N0, NX	M0	Low-grade
Stage IB	T2 a	N0, NX	M0	Low-grade
	T2 b	N0, NX	M0	Low-grade
Stage IIA	T1 a	N0, NX	M0	High-grade
	T1 b	N0, NX	M0	High-grade
Stage IIB	T2 a	N0, NX	M0	High-grade
Stage III	T2 b	N0, NX	M0	High-grade
Stage IV	Any T	N1	M0	Any grade
	Any T	Any N	M1	Any grade

Source: Reference 12.
* Superficial tumor is located exclusively above the superficial fascia without invasion of the fascia; deep tumor is located either exclusively beneath the superficial fascia, or superficial to the fascia with invasion of or through the fascia. Retroperitoneal, mediastinal and pelvic sarcomas are classified as deep tumors.
Note: Regional node involvement is rare and cases in which nodal status is not assessed either clinically or pathologically could be considered N0 instead of NX or pNX.

On conventional radiographs, most bone tumors are radiolucent.[8,32] The appearance of the tumor margins on conventional radiographs is often predictive of the aggressiveness of the neoplasms. Radiolucent lesions with margins that appear as abrupt zones of transition relative to normal-appearing bone are referred to as having a geographic destructive pattern (type 1), usually indicating a slow growing lesion.[8,32] A "moth-eaten" radiolucent pattern (type 2) consists of multiple radiolucent foci separated by normal-appearing bone. A "permeative" radiolucent pattern (type 3) consists of poorly defined radiolucent zones with indistinct margins. The "moth-eaten" and "permeative" radiolucent patterns are often associated with aggressive lesions, including malignant neoplasms.[8,32] There can be, however, occasional overlapping patterns of bone destruction with benign and malignant neoplasms.[8,32] The presence of matrix mineralization (calcification, ossification) in tumors may allow a narrowing of the differential diagnosis. The presence of arc or ring shaped calcifications is highly suggestive of a cartilaginous tumor, whereas amorphous, cloud-like, ill-defined densities can be seen with osteosarcomas.[8,32]

Patterns of periosteal reaction can also vary related to tumor growth as well as occur with other disorders.[8] Slow-growing tumors (osteoma, osteoid osteoma, etc.) and inflammatory lesions (osteomyelitis, Langerhans cell histiocytosis) that cross the cortex can elevate the periosteum, resulting in noninterrupted layers of periosteal formation and cortical thickening.[8,32,48] Single layered noninterrupted periosteal reaction can also occur with healing fractures, hypertrophic pulmonary osteoarthropathy, venous stasis, myositis ossificans, thyroid acropachy, and Gaucher disease. Zones of cortical destruction are commonly seen with malignant neoplasms as well as extra-osseous tumor extension.[8,32,48] Aggressive and/or malignant tumors (osteosarcoma, Ewing sarcoma, chondrosarcoma, lymphoma) can elevate the periosteum as well as eventually destroy and interrupt portions of the elevated periosteum.[8,32,48] Tumor-induced bone formation can occur within medullary bone as well as within extra-osseous portions of neoplasms. Tumor-induced bone formation within extra-osseous portions of the neoplasms, also referred to as periosteal reaction, can have various configurations. Tumor-induced bone formation from malignant neoplasms can be oriented perpendicular to the long axis of bone with "velvet," "hair on end," "sunburst," "cumulus cloud" or disorganized/complex configurations.[8,32,48] Multilayered zones of periosteal reaction with an "onion-peel" or lamellated appearance can also be seen with aggressive tumors and inflammatory lesions. Triangular zones of periosteal reaction may be seen at the borders of cortical destruction and extra-osseous tumor extension, and are referred to as Codman triangles.[8,32,48] Codman triangles can be seen with malignant primary bone neoplasms, osteomyelitis, or trauma.[48] Various types of interrupted periosteal may be coexistent in malignant bone tumors.

With MRI, features used to evaluate and characterize bone and soft tissue tumors include:
- lesion location
- lesion size
- margins (well-defined geographic with or without low signal margins versus poorly-defined margins)
- signal of the lesion on T1-weighted images, proton-density weighted images with and/or without fat-suppression, T2-weighted images with and/or without fat-suppression, STIR images
- enhancement after intravenous administration of Gadolinium-based contrast material
- presence of cortical destruction.

For bone tumors, MRI can accurately demonstrate the size, configuration, and margins of extra-osseous neoplastic extension from the medullary canal through sites of cortical destruction.

MRI findings may be useful for diagnosis and narrowing the list of differential possibilities of bone and soft tissue tumors. For example, extra- and intra-osseous lipomas have signal similar to fat, and unicameral bone cysts usually have circumscribed margins and contain fluid signal. Nonossifying fibromas in bone often have circumscribed margins and have internal low signal on T2-weighted images, reflecting their histological features. The locations of lesions combined with MRI features may also be highly suggestive of specific lesions, such as with osteofibrous dysplasia, osteoid osteoma, juxtacortical chondroma, enchondroma, osteochondroma, chondroblastoma, fibrous dysplasia, chordoma, chondromyxoid fibroma, and Paget sarcoma. Features commonly associated with malignant bone tumors include: poorly-defined margins, extension of tumor from marrow through sites of cortical destruction, irregular contrast enhancement with zones of necrosis, and skip lesions. Overlapping MRI features of many malignant tumors require biopsies for diagnosis and treatment planning. MRI is, however, recommended and routinely used for staging of bone and soft tissue tumors because of its superior contrast resolution and multi-planar imaging capabilities in determining tumor size and extent.[8,32] MRI provides a more accurate assessment of tumor volume compared with radiographs and CT, and is also useful in detecting fluid-fluid levels in tumors as well as nonenhancing necrotic zones.[8] MRI also provides detailed information regarding tumor margins, presence of tumor invasion of neurovascular structures and bone;[12] MRI can also confirm the presence of hemorrhage, cystic, fibrotic and/or myxoid changes within tumors.[12]

Contrast-enhanced MRI often provides useful information in the evaluation of musculoskeletal lesions.[9-11,23, 24,43-45] For evaluation of musculoskeletal neoplasms, dynamic MR imaging after bolus intravenous administration of gadolinium-chelate contrast can sometimes be useful in distinguishing between rapidly enhancing tumor and initially nonenhancing perineoplastic edema and/or necrosis.[9-11] Combining information from static and dynamic contrast-enhanced MRI with results from nonenhanced MRI may allow improved differentiation between benign and malignant soft tissue tumors.[44] The presence of liquefaction, large tumor size and early patterns of dynamic contrast enhancement were features that were commonly associated with malignant than benign soft tissue tumors.[44] Responses of malignant tumors such as osteosarcomas and Ewing sarcomas to chemotherapy can also be assessed by detecting nonenhancing zones of necrosis or sites of persistent early enhancement that are typically associated with remaining viable tumor. Newer MRI techniques, such as diffusion weighted imaging and MR spectroscopy, have been used in clinical research studies for the evaluation of musculoskeletal neoplasms, although their clinical relevance requires further study.[38,47]

The information provided by MRI is valuable for the planning of biopsies and surgical resection.[12] Knowledge of the MRI features and associated findings from conventional radiographs and/or CT scans can provide comprehensive and detailed evaluation of musculoskeletal tumors and tumorlike lesions.

This book is focussed on the description and categorization of the MRI features of both benign and malignant bone and soft tissue tumors of the musculoskeletal system. The actual definition of the English word "tumor" is derived from the Latin word "tumere," which is translated as "swelling." The lesions described in this book include both neoplasms and tumorlike masses involving the appendicular skeleton/extremities as well as the axial skeleton (spine, paraspinal soft tissues, and skull).

The portion of this book immediately following this introductory chapter groups musculoskeletal lesions into 20 lists of differential diagnoses based on anatomic locations and/or MRI features illustrated with MR images. This approach is intended to provide the reader with an easy-to-use format to help guide the evaluation of lesions that can be encountered in clinical practice. It is similar to the author's prior collaboration for the book *Differential Diagnosis in Magnetic Resonance Imaging* by Frances Burgener, Steven P. Meyers, Raymond K. Tan, and Wolfgang Zaubauer (Thieme, 2002). One substantial change that has been made for the new book is that the references are supplied for each lesion listed in the Comments Section of the tables. References are either made to the last section of the book, wich includes 77 Atlas chapters with illustrations for various lesions, or to publications in the literature at the end of each table for uncommon lesions with no Atlas chapter dedicated to them. Efforts were made to provide the reader with the most current references in the literature at the time of publication. The last portion of this book is organized into an atlas format with chapters that include detailed demographic, pathologic, and clinical information for musculoskeletal lesions as well as multiple MRI examples, often with corresponding plain film and/or CT images, to demonstrate the range of imaging findings and locations associated with each of the lesions. Each Atlas chapter also has references to the literature for each lesion. Some tumors (lipoma, hemangioma, hemangioendothelioma, malignant fibrous histiocytoma, osteosarcoma, chondrosarcoma, leukemia, etc.) and tumorlike lesions (sarcoidosis, Erdheim–Chester, etc.) can occur as primary abnormalities in bone and/or soft tissue. When relevant, the Atlas chapters contain examples of lesions that are primarily located in bone as well as within soft tissue.

For this book, MRI signal of the various entities will be described as low, intermediate, high, or mixed on T1-weighted imaging (T1WI), proton density weighted imaging (PDWI), and T2-weighted imaging (T2WI); and whether there is gadolinium-contrast (Gd-contrast) enhancement or not. When available, comments and examples will be given regarding MRI features with fat-suppression techniques such as frequency-selective (FS) fat-presaturation applied on T1WI, PDWI, T2WI, or utilization of the short TI inversion recovery (STIR) sequence. Both techniques enable distinction of pathologic processes (neoplasm, infection, inflammation, edema, etc.) from normal anatomic structures with high signal from intrinsic fat, such as marrow and subcutaneous soft tissues.

References

1 Arndt CA, Crist WM. Common musculoskeletal tumors of childhood and adolescence. *N Engl J Med* 1999;341(5):342–352.
2 Berquist TH, Ehman RL, King BF, Hodgman CG, Ilstrup DM. Value of MR imaging in differentiating benign from malignant soft-tissue masses: study of 95 lesions. *AJR Am J Roentgenol* 1990;155:1251–1255.
3 Biondetti PR, Ehman RL. Soft-tissue sarcomas: use of textural patterns in skeletal muscle as a diagnostic feature in postoperative MR imaging. *Radiology* 1992;183(3):845–848.
4 Bridge JA, Orndal C. Cytogenetic analysis of bone and joint neoplasms. In: Helliwell TR, ed. *Pathology of Bone and Joint Neoplasms* Philadelphia, Pa: W.B. Saunders; 1999:59–78.
5 Bridge JA, Sandberg AA. Cytogenetic and molecular genetic techniques as adjunctive approaches in thediagnosis of bone and soft tissue tumors. *Skeletal Radiol* 2000;29:249–258.
6 Bush CH. The MRI of hemorrhage. *Skeletal Radiol* 2000;29:1–9.
7 Choi H, Varma Datla GK, Fornage BD, Kim EE, Johnston DA. Soft-tissue sarcoma: MR imaging vs. sonography for detection of local recurrence after surgery. *AJR Am J Roentgenol* 1991;157:353–358.
8 Dorfman HD, Czerniak B, Kotz R, Vanel D, Park YK, Unni KK. WHO classification of tumours of bone: introduction. In: Fletcher CDM, Unni KK, Mertens F, eds. *World Health Organization Classification of Tumours. Pathology and Genetics of Tumours of Soft Tissue and Bone* Geneva: IARC Press; 2002:227–232.
9 Dyke JP, Panicek DM, Healy JH, et al. Osteogenic and ewing sarcomas: estimation of necrotic fraction during induction chemotherapy with dynamic contrast-enhanced MR imaging. *Radiology* 2003;228:271–278.
10 Erlemann R, Reiser MF, Peters PE, et al. Musculoskeletal neoplasms: static and dynamic Gd-DTPA-enhanced MR imaging. *Radiology* 1989;171(3):767–773.
11 Erlemann R. Letters to the Editor – Dynamic, Gadolinium-enhanced MR imaging to monitor tumor response to chemotherapy. *Radiology* 1993;186(3):904–905.
12 Fletcher CDM, Ryholm A, Singer S, Sundaram M, Coindre IM. Soft tissue tumours: epidemiology, clinical features, histopathological typing and grading. In: Fletcher CDM, Unni KK, Mertens F, eds. *World Health Organization Classification of Tumours. Pathology and Genetics of Tumours of Soft Tissue and Bone*. Geneva: IARC Press; 2002:12–18.
13 Fletcher JA. Cytogenetic analysis of soft-tissue tumors. In: Weiss SW, Goldblum JR, eds. *Enzinger and Weiss's Soft Tissue Tumors* 4th ed. St. Louis, Mo: Mosby; 2001:125–146.
14 Folpe AL, Gown AM. Immunohistochemistry for analysis of soft tissue tumors. In Weiss SW, Goldblum JR, eds. *Enzinger and Weiss's Soft Tissue Tumors* 4th ed. St. Louis: Mosby 2001; 199–245.
15 Forest M. Bone metastases. In: Forest M, Tomeno B, Vanel D, eds. *Orthopedic Surgical Pathology: Diagnosis of Tumors and Pseudotumoral Lesions of Bone and Joints* Edinburgh: Churchill Livingstone;1998:501–516.
16 Gao Z, Kahn LB. The application of immunohistochemistry in the diagnosis of bone tumors and tumorlike lesions. *Skeletal Radiol* 2005;34:755–770.
17 Helliwell TR. Classification and diagnosis of bone neoplasms. In: Helliwell TR,ed. *Pathology of Bone and Joint Neoplasms*. Philadelphia, Pa: W.B. Saunders; 1999:1–14.
18 Jemal A, Thomas A, Murray T, Thun M. Cancer statistics 2002. *CA Cancer J Clin* 2002;52:23–47.
19 Kransdorf MJ, Meis JM. From the Archives of the AFIP – Extraskeletal osseous and cartilaginous tumors of the extremities. *Radiographics* 1993;13(4):853–884.
20 Kransdorf MJ, Murphey MD. Origin and classification of soft tissue tumors. In: *Imaging of Soft Tissue Tumors*. 2nd ed. Philadelphia, Pa: Lippincott, Williams & Wilkins; 2006:1–5.
21 Kransdorf MJ. Benign soft-tissue tumors in a large referral population: distribution of specific diagnoses by age, sex, and location. *AJR Am J Roentgenol* 1995;164:395–402.
22 Kransdorf MJ. Malignant soft-tissue tumors in a large referral population: distribution of diagnoses by age, sex, and location. *AJR Am J Roentgenol* 1995;164:129–134.
23 Kransdorf MJ. Questions and Answers – Is it necessary to routinely use gadolinium in the MR imaging evaluation of soft-tissue tumors of the extremities? *AJR Am J Roentgenol* 1995;165(6):1545.
24 Miller SL, Hoffer FA. Malignant and benign bone tumors. *Radiol Clin North Am* 2001;39(4):673–699.
25 Moore SG, Bisset GS III, Siegel MJ, Donaldson JS. Pediatric musculoskeletal MR imaging. *Radiology* 1991;179(2):345–360.
26 Moser RP, Madewell JE. Metastatic bone disease. In: Tavers JM, Ferrucci JT, eds. *Radiology Diagnosis–Imaging-Intervention* Vol 5. Philadelphia, PA: Lippincott Williams & Wilkins; 2002.
27 Mulder JD, Schutte HE, Kroon HM, Taconis WK. Introduction. In: *Radiologic Atlas of Bone Tumors*. Amsterdam: Elsevier; 1993:3–6.
28 Mulder JD, Schutte HE, Kroon HM, Taconis WK. The diagnosis of bone tumors. In: *Radiologic Atlas of Bone Tumors*. Amsterdam: Elsevier; 1993:9–46.
29 Murphey MD, Smith WS, Smith SE, Kransdorf MJ, Temple HT. From the Archives of the AFIP – Imaging of musculoskeletal neurogenic tumors: radiologic-pathologic correlation. *Radiographics* 1999;19(5):1253–1280.

30 Patel SR, Benjamin RS. Sarcomas of soft tissue and bone. In: Fauci AS, Braunwald E, Isselbacher KJ, et al. *Harrison's Principles of Internal Medicine*. 14th ed. New York: McGraw-Hill; 1998:611–615.
31 Pettersson H, Gillespy T III, Hamlin DJ, et al. Primary musculoskeletal tumors: examination with MR imaging compared with conventional modalities. *Radiology* 1987;164(1):237–241.
32 Ritchie DA, Davies AM. Imaging studies in bone neoplasia. In: Helliwell TR, ed. *Pathology of Bone and Joint Neoplasms* Philadelphia, Pa: W.B. Saunders; 1999:106–27.
33 Salisbury JR. Bone neoplasms containing epithelial and epithelioid cells. In: Helliwell TR, ed. *Pathology of Bone and Joint Neoplasms.* Philadelphia, PA: WB Saunders; 1999:345–368.
34 Sandberg AA. Cytogenetic and molecular genetics of bone and soft-tissue tumors. *Am J Med Genet* 2002;115:189–193.
35 Scholz RB, Christiansen H, Kabisch H, Winkler K. Molecular markers in the evaluation of bone neoplasms. In: Helliwell TR, ed. *Pathology of Bone and Joint Neoplasms* Philadelphia, Pa: W.B. Saunders; 1999:79–105.
36 Shuman WP, Patten RM, Baron RL, Liddell RM, Conrad EU, Richardson ML. Comparison of STIR and spin-echo MR imaging at 1.5 T in 45 suspected extremity tumors: lesion conspicuity and extent. *Radiology* 1991;179(1):247–252.
37 Slominski A, Wortsman J, Carlson A, Mihm M, Nickoloff B, McClatchey K. Molecular pathology of soft tissue and bone tumors, a review. *Arch Pathol Lab Med* 1999;123:1246–1259.
38 Sostman HD, Prescott DM, Dewhirst MW, et al. MR imaging and spectroscopy for prognostic evaluation in soft-tissue sarcomas. *Radiology* 1994;190(1):269–275.
39 Stacy GS, Heck RK, Peabody TD, Dixon LB. Pictorial Essay – Neoplastic and tumorlike lesions detected on MR imaging of the knee in patients with suspected internal derangement: Part 1, intraosseous entities. *AJR Am J Roentgenol* 2002;178:589–594.
40 Stacy GS, Mahal RS, Peabody TD. Staging of bone tumors: a review with illustrative examples. *AJR Am J Roentgenol* 2006;186:967–976.
41 States LJ. Imaging of metabolic bone disease and marrow disorders in children. *Radiol Clin North Am* 2001;39:749–772.
42 Vade A, Eissenstadt R, Schaff HB. MRI of aggressive bone lesions of childhood. *Magn Reson Imaging* 1992;10(1):89–96.
43 van der Woude HJ, Bloem JL, Pope TL. Magnetic resonance imaging of the musculoskeletal system: Part 9. Primary tumors. *Clin Orthop Relat Res* 1998;347:272–286.
44 Van Rijswijk CSP, Geirnaerdt MJA, Hogendoorn PCW, et al. Soft-tissue tumors: value of static and dynamic gadopentetate dimeglumine-enhanced MR imaging in prediction of malignancy. *Radiology* 2004;233:493–502.
45 Vanel D, Shapeero LG, De Baere T, et al. MR imaging in the follow-up of malignant and aggressive soft-tissue tumors: results of 511 examinations. *Radiology* 1994;190(1):263–268.
46 Unni KK. Introduction and scope of study. In: *Dahlin's Bone Tumors. General Aspects and Data on 11 087 Cases*. 5th ed. Philadelphia, PA: Lippincott, Williams & Wilkins; 1996:1–9.
47 Wang CK, Li CW, Hsieh SH, Liu GC, Tsai KB. Characterization of bone and soft-tissue tumors with in vivo 1 H MR spectroscopy: initial results. *Radiology* 2004;232:599–605.
48 Wenaden AET, Szyszko TA, Saifuddin. A Imaging of periosteal reactions associated with focal lesions of bone. *Clin Radiol* 2005;60:439–456.
49 Zawin JK, Jaramillo D. Conversion of bone marrow in the humerus, sternum, and clavicle: changes with age on MR images. *Radiology* 1993;188(1):159–164.

Differential Diagnosis Tables

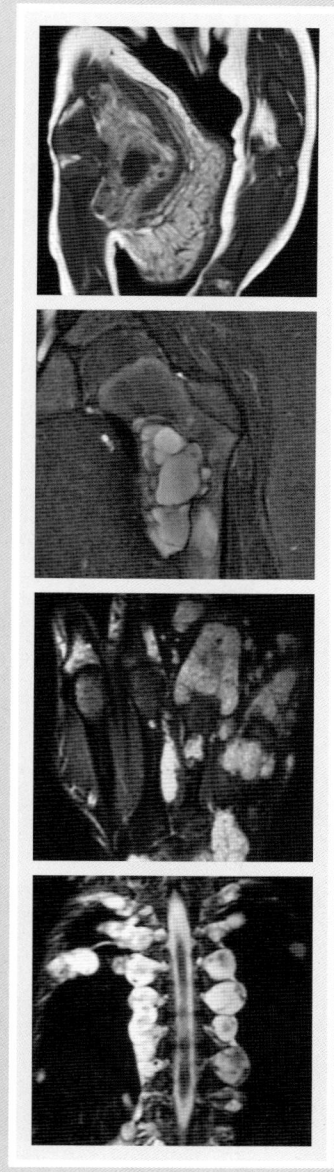

Table 1 Tumors and tumorlike lesions involving the skull and facial bones

Tumor/Tumorlike Lesion	MRI Findings	Comments
Malignant neoplasms		
Metastatic tumor (Figs. 1.1–1.3)	Single or multiple well-circumscribed or poorly defined lesions involving the skull, dura, leptomeninges, and/or choroid plexus; low-intermediate signal on T1WI, intermediate-high signal on T2WI, usually shows Gd-contrast enhancement, +/− bone destruction, +/− compression of neural tissue or vessels. Leptomeningeal tumor often best seen on postcontrast images.	May have variable destructive or infiltrative changes involving single or multiple sites of involvement. Primary tumors are usually from outside of CNS. **(See Atlas Chapter A 50)**
Myeloma/plasmacytoma (Figs. 1.4, 1.5)	Multiple (myeloma) or single (plasmacytoma) well-circumscribed or poorly defined lesions involving the skull, and dura; low-intermediate signal on T1WI, intermediate-high signal on T2WI, usually shows Gd-contrast enhancement + bone destruction.	May have variable destructive or infiltrative changes involving the axial and/or appendicular skeleton. **(See Atlas Chapter A 52)**
Lymphoma (Fig. 1.6)	Single or multiple well-circumscribed or poorly defined lesions involving the skull, dura, and/or leptomeninges; low-intermediate signal on T1WI, intermediate-high signal on T2WI, usually shows Gd-contrast enhancement, +/− bone destruction, leptomeningeal tumor often best seen on postcontrast images.	Extra-axial lymphoma may have variable destructive or infiltrative changes involving single or multiple sites of involvement. **(See Atlas Chapter A 47)**
Leukemia (Fig. 1.7)	Single or multiple well-circumscribed or poorly defined lesions involving the skull, dura, and/or leptomeninges; low-intermediate signal on T1WI, intermediate-high signal on T2WI, may show Gd-contrast enhancement, +/− bone destruction. Leptomeningeal tumor often best seen on postcontrast images.	Extra-axial leukemia may have variable destructive or infiltrative changes involving single or multiple sites of involvement. **(See Atlas Chapter A 41)**

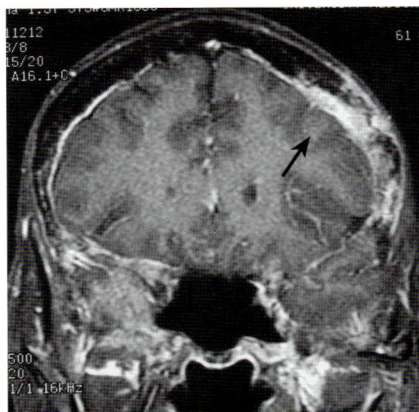

Figure 1.1 A 61-year-old woman with metastatic breast carcinoma involving the skull. The poorly defined metastatic disease shows Gd-contrast enhancement on coronal FS T1WI and extends from the marrow through zones of bone destruction at the inner and outer tables of the skull to involve the intracranial dura and soft tissues of the scalp.

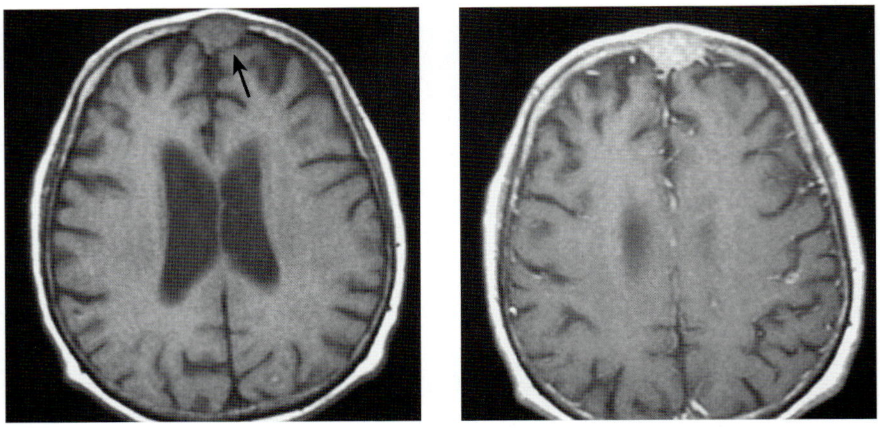

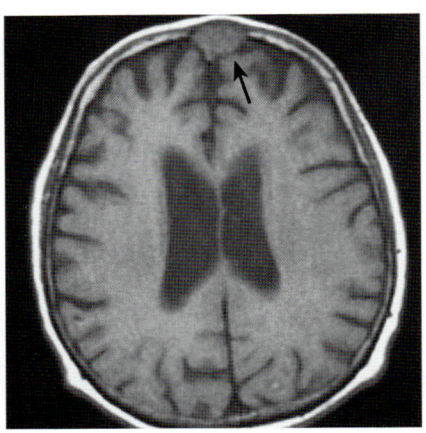

Figure 1.2 a, b Single metastatic lesion in the frontal bone from breast carcinoma has circumscribed margins and extends from the marrow through zones of bone destruction. The tumor has intermediate signal on axial T1WI (**a**) and shows prominent Gd-contrast administration on axial T1WI (**b**).

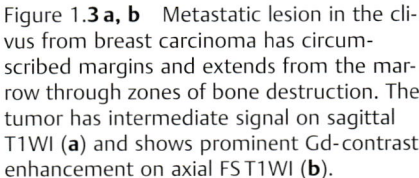

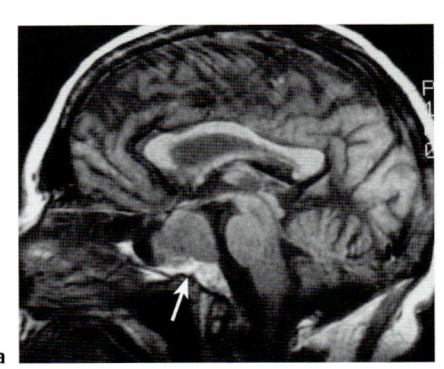

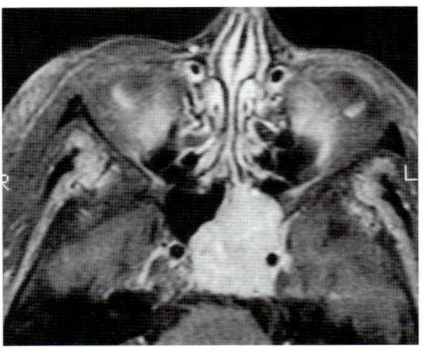

Figure 1.3 a, b Metastatic lesion in the clivus from breast carcinoma has circumscribed margins and extends from the marrow through zones of bone destruction. The tumor has intermediate signal on sagittal T1WI (**a**) and shows prominent Gd-contrast enhancement on axial FS T1WI (**b**).

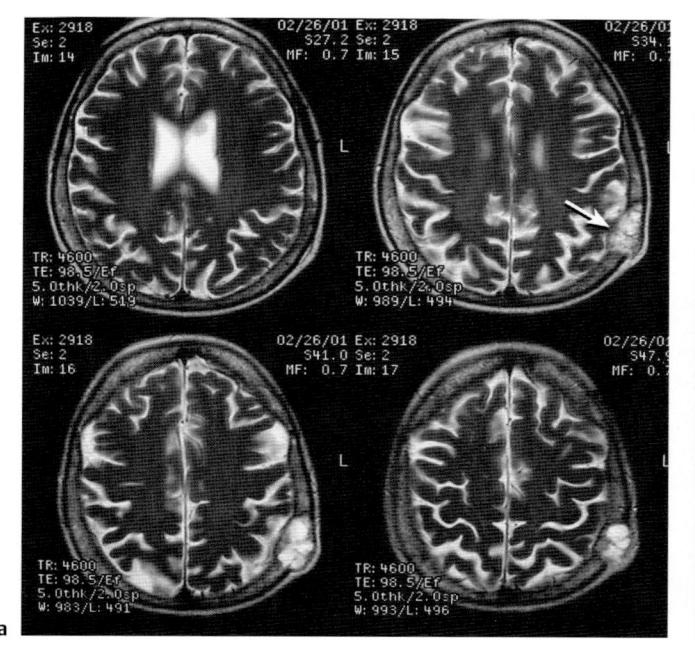

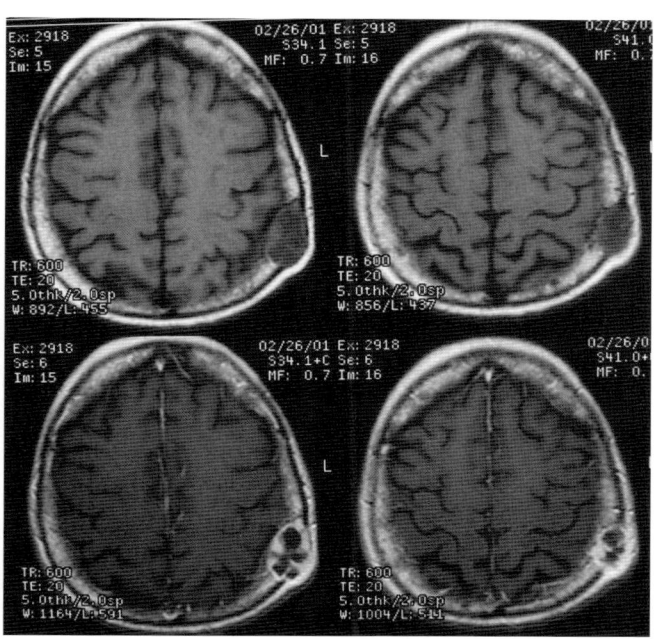

Leukemia 19

Figure 1.**4a, b** A 65-year-old woman with myeloma and a circumscribed lesion involving the skull that has heterogeneous high signal on axial T2WI (**a**). The tumor has low-intermediate signal on axial T1WI (**b**, *top images*) and shows irregular Gd-contrast enhancement on axial T1WI (**b**, *bottom images*).

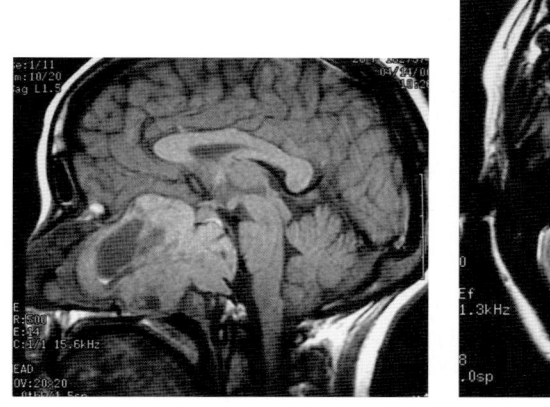

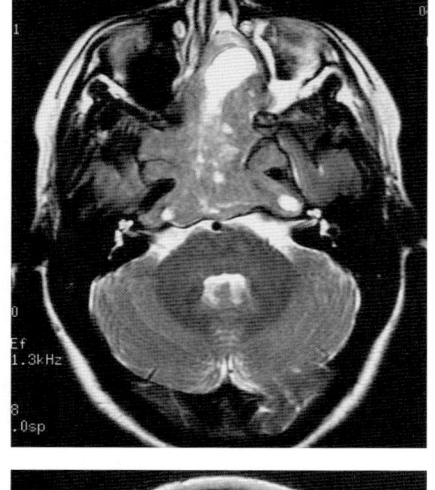

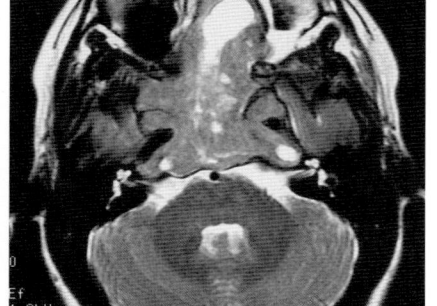

Figure 1.**5a, b** Plasmacytoma involving the nasal cavity, ethmoid and sphenoid sinuses, and skull base in a 28-year-old woman. The tumor has mixed zones of low and intermediate signal on sagittal T1WI (**a**) and zones of intermediate to slightly high signal and high signal on axial T2WI (**b**).

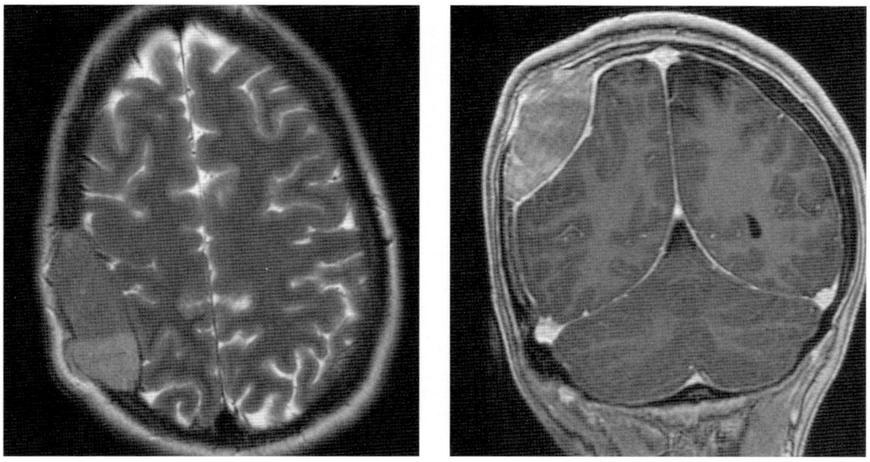

Figure 1.**6a, b** A 46-year-old woman with diffuse large B cell non-Hodgkin lymphoma involving the skull and dura. The lesion has low-intermediate signal on axial T2WI (**a**) and shows heterogeneous Gd-contrast enhancement on coronal T1WI (**b**).

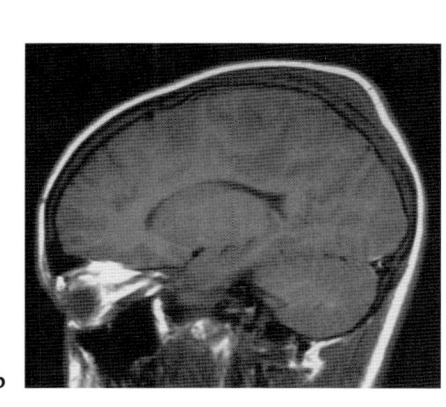

Figure 1.**7** A 12-year-old female with leukemia (ALL) involving the skull, which is seen as zones of low-intermediate signal in the marrow as well as sites of destruction of the inner and outer tables on sagittal T1WI.

Table 1 (Continued) Tumors and tumorlike lesions involving the skull and facial bones

Tumor/Tumorlike Lesion	MRI Findings	Comments
Chordoma (Fig. 1.8)	Well-circumscribed lobulated lesions, low-intermediate signal on T1WI, high signal on T2WI, usually shows Gd-contrast enhancement (usually heterogeneous), locally invasive associated with bone erosion/destruction, encasement of vessels and nerves, skull base–clivus common location, usually in the midline.	Rare, slow-growing tumors at the skull base, detailed anatomic display of extension of chordomas by MRI is important for planning of surgical approaches. **(See Atlas Chapter A 12)**
Chondrosarcoma (Fig. 1.9)	Lobulated lesions, low-intermediate signal on T1WI, high signal on T2WI, +/− matrix mineralization-low signal on T2WI, usually shows Gd-contrast enhancement (often heterogeneous), locally invasive associated with bone erosion/destruction, encasement of vessels and nerves, skull base-petrous-occipital synchondrosis common location, usually off midline.	Rare, slow-growing tumors, detailed anatomic display of extension of chondrosarcomas by MRI is important for planning of surgical approaches. **(See Atlas Chapter A 11)**
Osteogenic sarcoma (Fig. 1.10)	Destructive lesions involving the skull base, low-intermediate signal on T1WI, mixed low, intermediate, high signal on T2WI, usually + matrix mineralization/ossification–low signal on T2W images, typically shows Gd-contrast enhancement (usually heterogeneous).	Rare lesions involving the skull-base and calvaria, more common than chondrosarcomas and Ewing sarcoma, locally invasive, high metastatic potential. Occurs in children as primary tumors and adults (associated with Paget disease, irradiated bone, chronic osteomyelitis, osteoblastoma, giant cell tumor, fibrous dysplasia). **(See Atlas Chapter A 64)**
Ewing sarcoma (Fig. 1.11)	Destructive lesions involving the skull base, low-intermediate signal on T1WI, mixed low, intermediate, high signal on T2WI, typically shows Gd-contrast enhancement (usually heterogeneous).	Usually occurs between the ages of 5 and 30, males > females, rare lesions involving the skull-base, locally invasive, high metastatic potential. **(See Atlas Chapter A 20)**

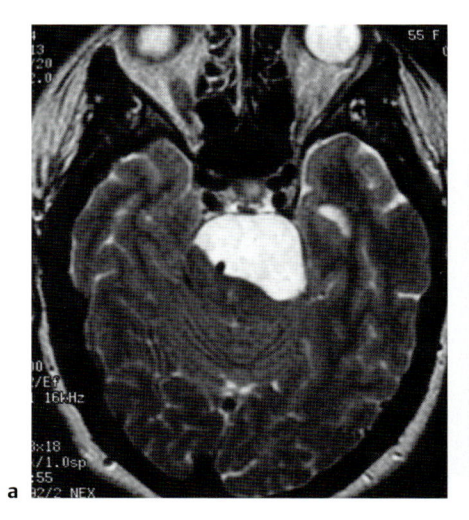

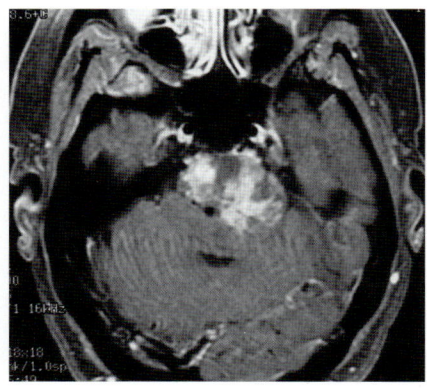

Figure 1.8 a, b A 55-year-old woman with a chordoma involving the endocranial surface of the clivus with intracranial extension causing compression of the brainstem. The tumor has high signal on axial T2WI (**a**) and shows heterogeneous Gd-contrast enhancement on axial FS T1WI (**b**).

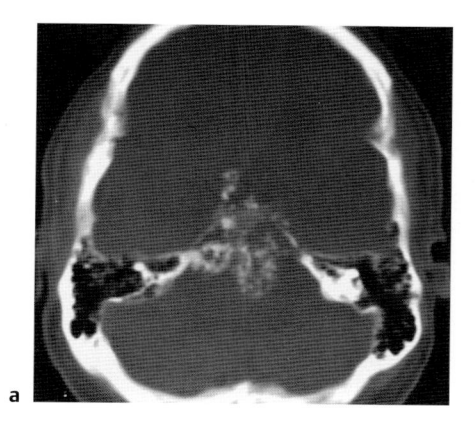

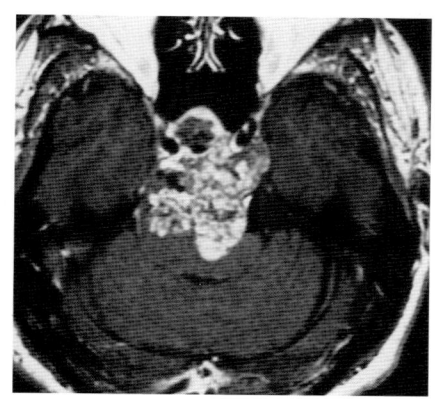

Figure 1.**9 a, b** A 42-year-old woman with a chondrosarcoma involving the clivus. Axial CT image (**a**) shows the lesion to have prominent chondroid matrix mineralization. The tumor shows prominent heterogeneous Gd-contrast enhancement on axial T1WI (**b**).

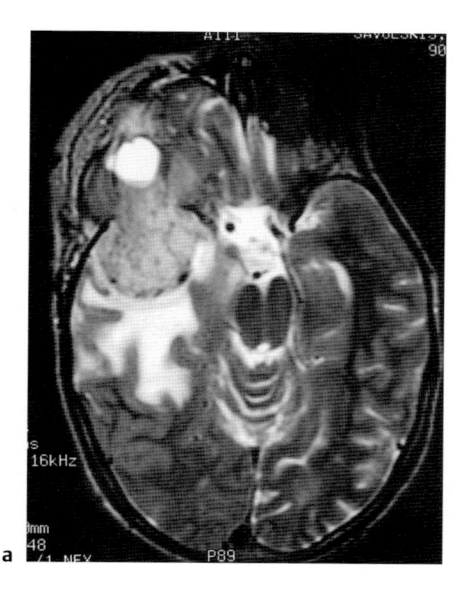

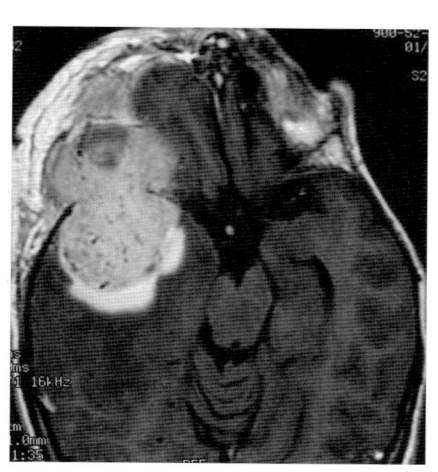

Figure 1.**10 a, b** A 16-year-old female with history of radiation and surgery for retinoblastoma and subsequent development of osteosarcoma involving the right sphenoid and frontal bones. The tumor has mixed intermediate, slightly high, and high signal on axial T2WI (**a**). The tumor is associated with bone destruction as well as intracranial extension resulting in compression and posterior displacement of the right temporal lobe, edema in the brain, and early uncal herniation. The tumor shows prominent heterogeneous Gd-contrast enhancement on axial T1WI (**b**).

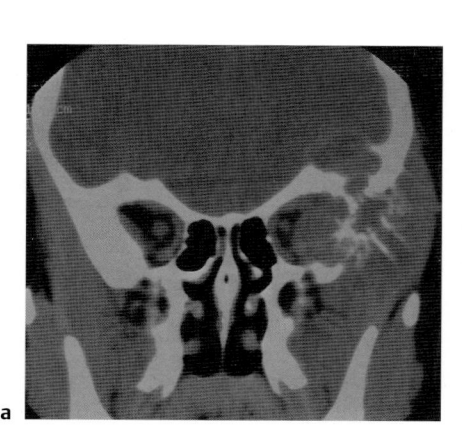

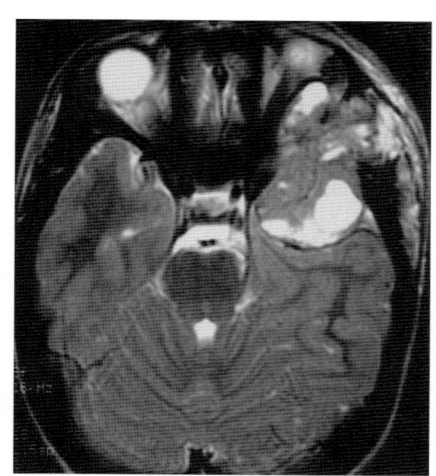

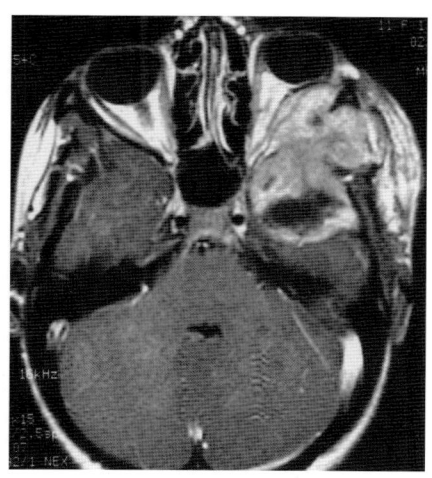

Figure 1.**11 a–c** An 11-year-old girl with Ewing sarcoma involving the left frontal and zygomatic bones with tumor extension intracranially as well as into the left orbit. Coronal CT image (**a**) shows a soft tissue tumor containing perpendicular striated periosteal reaction associated with bone destruction. The tumor has heterogeneous intermediate and high signal on axial T2WI (**b**) with small foci of low signal. The tumor shows prominent irregular Gd-contrast enhancement on axial T1WI (**c**).

Table 1 (Continued) Tumors and tumorlike lesions involving the skull and facial bones

Tumor/Tumorlike Lesion	MRI Findings	Comments
Sinonasal/nasopharyngeal carcinoma (Figs. 1.12, 1.13)	Destructive lesions in the nasal cavity, paranasal sinuses, nasopharynx; +/− intracranial extension via bone destruction or perineural spread; intermediate signal on T1WI, intermediate-slightly high signal on T2WI; often shows Gd-contrast enhancement; large lesions (+/− necrosis and/or hemorrhage).	Occurs in adults usually > 55 years, males > females, associated with occupational or other exposure to: nickel, chromium, mustard gas, radium, manufacture of wood products.
Adenoid cystic carcinoma (Fig. 1.14)	Destructive lesions in the paranasal sinuses, nasal cavity, nasopharynx, +/− intracranial extension via bone destruction or perineural spread, intermediate signal on T1WI, intermediate-high signal on T2WI, variable mild, moderate, or prominent Gd-contrast enhancement.	Account for 10 % of sinonasal tumors, arise any location within sinonasal cavities, usually occurs in adults > 30 years.
Esthesioneuroblastoma (Figs. 1.15)	Locally destructive lesions with low-intermediate signal on T1WI, intermediate-high signal on T2WI, usually show prominent Gd-contrast enhancement, location: superior nasal cavity, ethmoid air cells with occasional extension into the other paranasal sinuses, orbits, anterior cranial fossa, cavernous sinuses.	Tumors also referred to as olfactory neuroblastoma, arise from olfactory epithelium in the superior nasal cavity. Occur in adolescents and adults, males > females.
Rhabdomyosarcoma (Atlas Fig. 459)	Lesions have low-intermediate signal on T1WI and FS-T1WI with circumscribed and/or poorly defined margins. Signal changes from areas of hemorrhage may be present. Lesions usually have heterogeneous signal (various combinations of intermediate, slightly high, and/or high signal) on T2WI and FS T2WI. Zones of edema may occur in the adjacent soft tissues. Tumors can be associated with destructive changes of adjacent bone. Tumors show variable degrees and patterns of contrast enhancement.	Malignant mesenchymal tumors with rhabdomyoblastic differentiation that occur primarily in soft tissue, and only very rarely in bone. Occurs most frequently in children. (See Atlas Chapter A 69)
Hemangiopericytoma (Fig. 1.16)	Extra-axial mass lesions, often well-circumscribed, intermediate signal on T1WI, intermediate-slightly high signal on T2WI, usually show prominent Gd-contrast enhancement (may resemble meningiomas), +/− associated erosive bone changes.	Rare neoplasms in young adults (males > females) sometimes referred to as angioblastic meningioma or meningeal hemangiopericytoma, arise from vascular cells-pericytes, frequency of metastases > meningiomas. (See Atlas Chapter A 35)

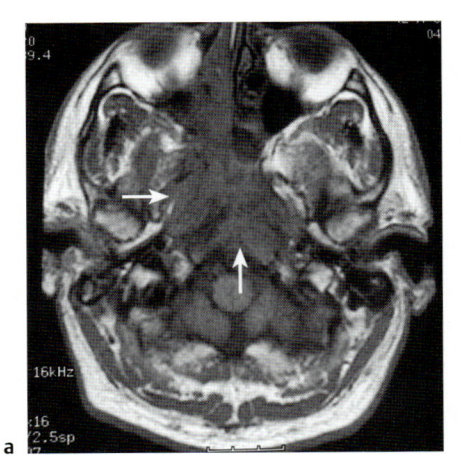

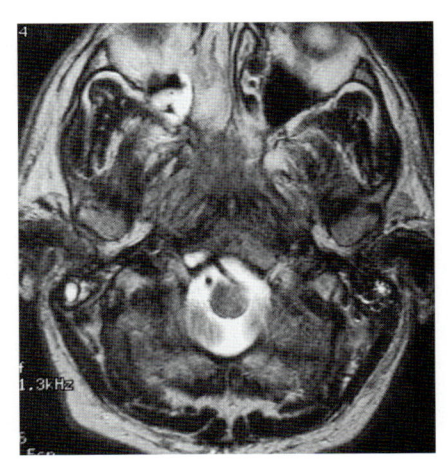

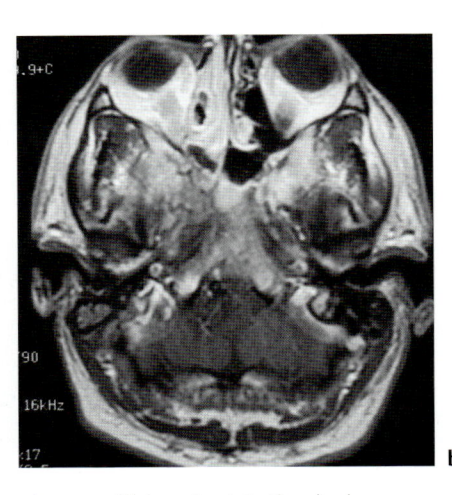

Figure 1.12 a–c Squamous cell carcinoma is seen as a poorly defined tumor in the posterior nasopharynx with invasion into the clival marrow. The tumor has intermediate signal on axial T1WI (**a**) and axial T2WI (**b**), and shows Gd-contrast enhancement on axial T1WI (**c**).

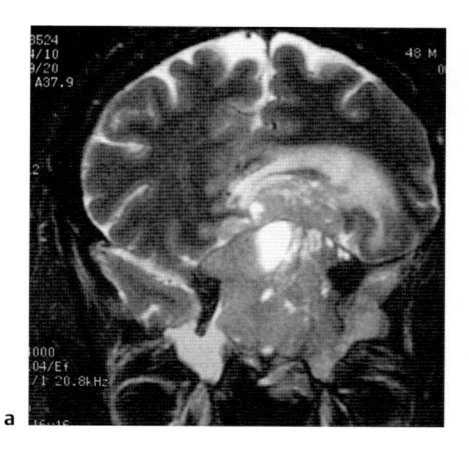

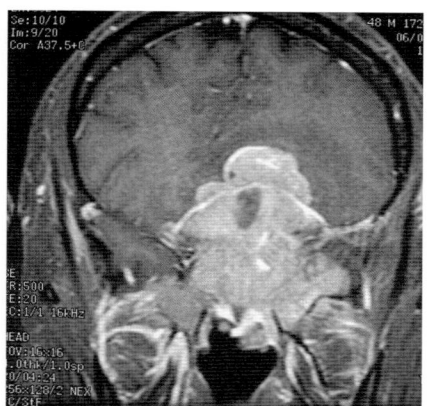

Figure 1.**13 a, b**   A 48-year-old man with a poorly differentiated nasopharyngeal carcinoma in the ethmoid sinus associated with bone destruction and intracranial and left infratemporal extension. The tumor has heterogeneous intermediate and high signal on coronal FS T2WI (**a**) and shows prominent irregular Gd-contrast enhancement on coronal FS T1WI (**b**).

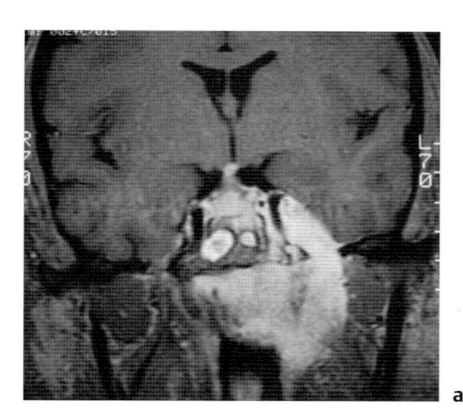

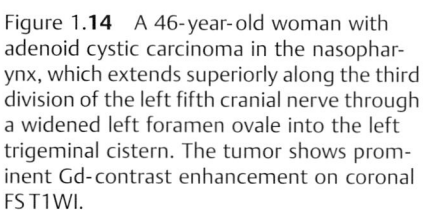

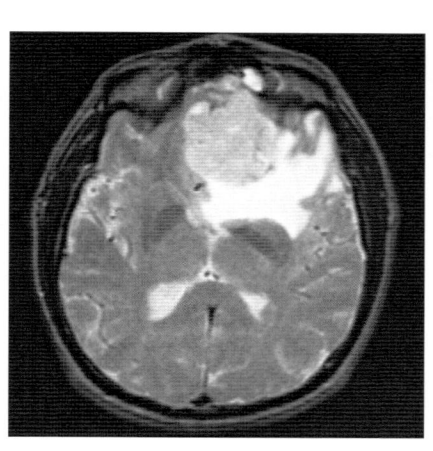

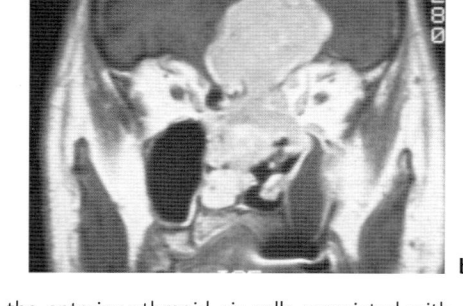

Figure 1.**14**   A 46-year-old woman with adenoid cystic carcinoma in the nasopharynx, which extends superiorly along the third division of the left fifth cranial nerve through a widened left foramen ovale into the left trigeminal cistern. The tumor shows prominent Gd-contrast enhancement on coronal FS T1WI.

Figure 1.**15 a, b**   Esthesioneuroblastoma in the anterior ethmoid air cells associated with bone destruction at the skull base and intracranial tumor extension. The tumor has heterogeneous slightly high to high signal on axial T2WI (**a**). The tumor shows prominent Gd-contrast enhancement on coronal T1WI (**b**).

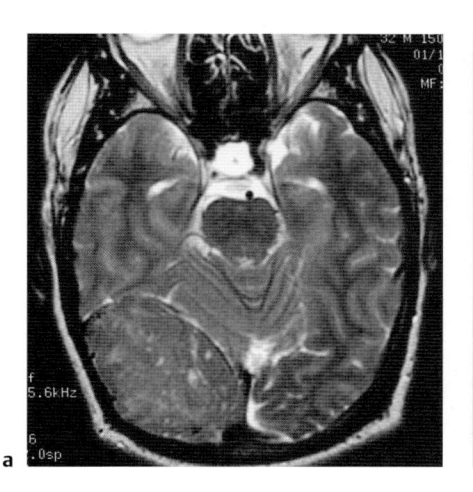

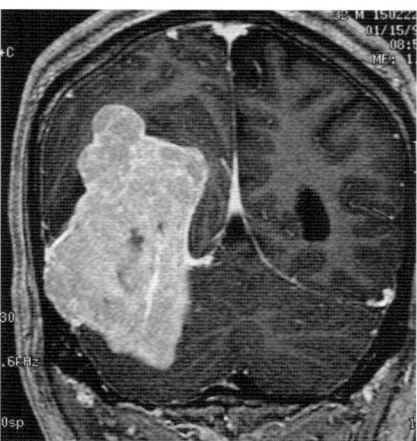

Figure 1.**16 a, b**   A 32-year-old man with a hemangiopericytoma involving the tentorium. The tumor has slightly lobulated margins and mostly intermediate signal on axial T2WI (**a**) as well as small zones with high signal. The tumor shows prominent Gd-contrast enhancement on coronal T1WI (**b**).

Table 1 (Continued) Tumors and tumorlike lesions involving the skull and facial bones		
Tumor/Tumorlike Lesion	MRI Findings	Comments
Benign neoplasms		
Meningioma (Figs. 1.17–1.20)	Extra-axial dural-based lesions, well-circumscribed (supra- > infratentorial, parasagittal > convexity > sphenoid ridge > parasellar > posterior fossa > optic nerve sheath > intraventricular), intermediate signal on T1WI, intermediate-slightly high signal on T2WI, typically shows prominent Gd-contrast enhancement, +/− calcifications, +/− hyperostosis and/or invasion of adjacent skull.	Most common extra-axial tumor, usually benign neoplasms, typically occurs in adults (> 40 years), women > men, multiple meningiomas seen with NF2, can result in compression of adjacent brain parenchyma, encasement of arteries, and compression of dural venous sinuses, rarely invasive/malignant types. **(See Atlas Chapter A 49)**
Hemangioma (Fig. 1.21)	Circumscribed or poorly marginated structures (< 4 cm in diameter) in marrow of skull (often frontal bone) with intermediate-high signal on T1WI (often isointense to marrow fat), high signal on T2WI and FS T2WI, typically show Gd-contrast enhancement, +/− widening of diploic compartment.	Benign skull lesions, adults (> 30 years). **(See Atlas Chapter A 34)**
Ossifying hemangioma (Fig. 1.22)	Zone with low-intermediate signal on T1WI and slightly high to high signal on T2WI and FS T2WI. Lesions usually show prominent Gd-contrast enhancement on T1WI and FS T1WI.	Benign lesions within the temporal bone that involve the facial nerve, and on CT are usually radiolucent containing bone spicules. Lesions can be associated with slowly progressive or recurrent facial paralysis.

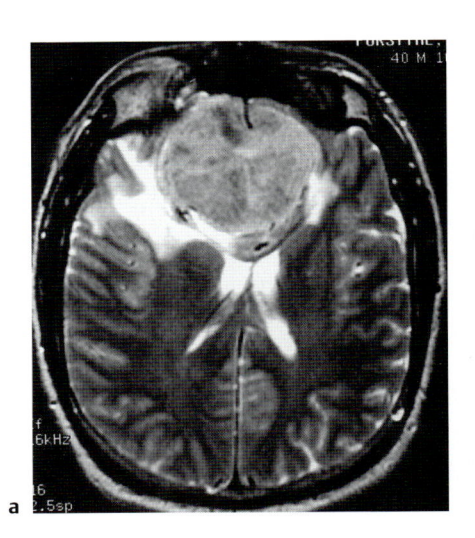

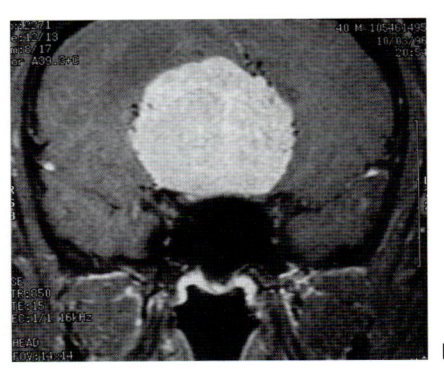

Figure 1.**17 a, b** A 40-year-old man with an olfactory groove meningioma that has heterogeneous slightly high signal on axial T2WI (**a**) as well as several small zones of low signal. Edematous high signal changes on T2WI are seen in the brain compressed by the meningioma. The tumor shows prominent Gd-contrast enhancement on coronal FS T1WI (**b**).

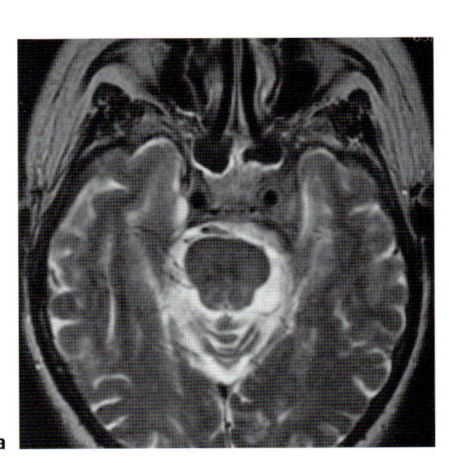

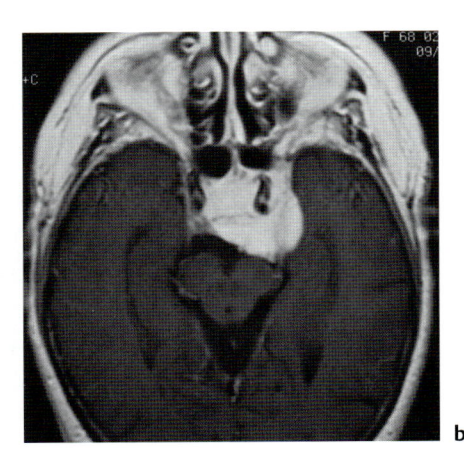

Figure 1.**18 a, b** A 68-year-old woman with a meningioma involving the anteromedial left middle cranial fossa, clivus, left cavernous sinus with encasement of the left internal carotid artery, and left trigeminal cistern. The tumor has heterogeneous intermediate signal on axial T2WI (**a**). The tumor shows prominent Gd-contrast enhancement on axial T1WI (**b**).

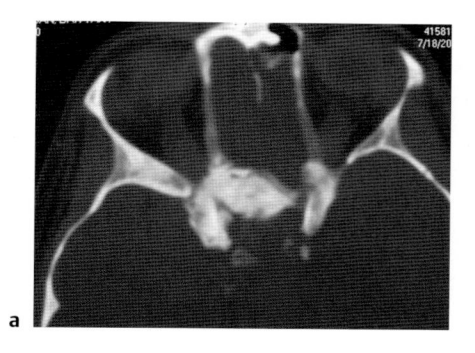

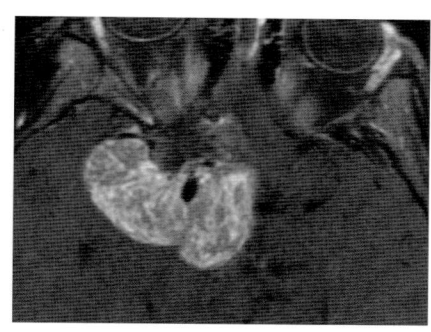

Figure 1.**19 a, b** A 9-year-old girl with neurofibromatosis type II with a large meningioma involving the right sphenoid bone. Axial CT image (**a**) shows reactive hyperostosis at the greater wing and right anterior clinoid process of the sphenoid bone from osseous invasion of the meningioma. The meningioma shows prominent heterogeneous Gd-contrast enhancement on axial FS T1WI (**b**). Minimal irregular Gd-contrast enhancement is seen in the hyperostotic bone.

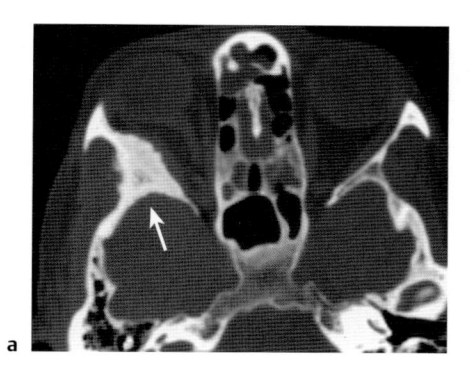

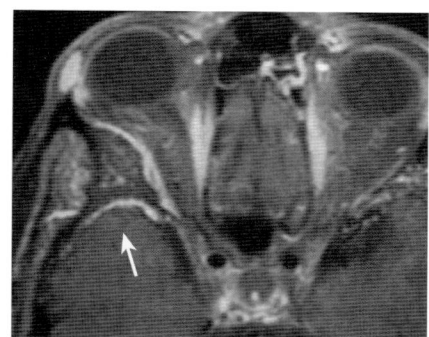

Figure 1.**20 a, b** A 52-year-old woman with an intraosseous meningioma. Axial CT image (**a**) shows thickening and hyperostosis at the posterolateral wall of the right orbit. Small zones of extraosseous tumor at the lateral orbit and anterior middle cranial fossa show Gd-contrast enhancement on axial FS T1WI (**b**).

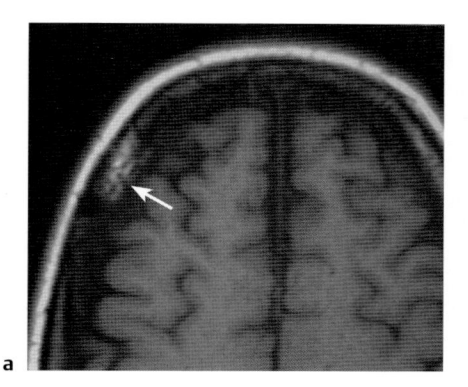

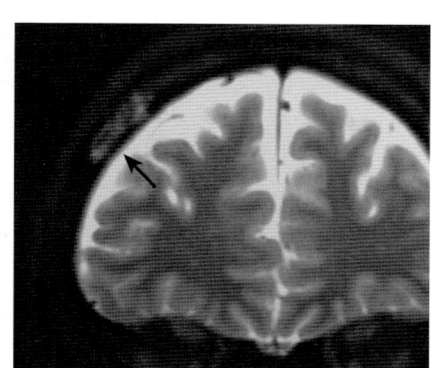

Figure 1.**21 a, b** A hemangioma in the marrow of the right frontal bone has high signal on axial T1WI (**a**) and coronal FS T2WI (**b**).

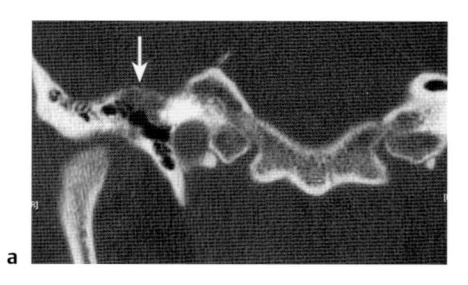

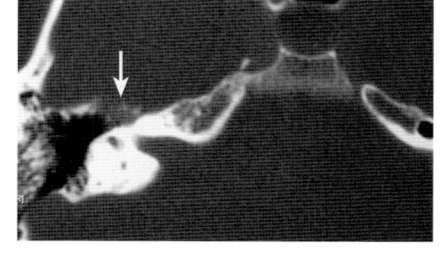

Figure 1.**22 a–d** An ossifying hemangioma in the right temporal bone is seen as a radiolucent lesion containing bone spicules on coronal (**a**) and axial (**b**) CT images. The lesion has slightly high to high signal on axial T2WI (**c**) and shows prominent Gd-contrast enhancement on axial FS T1WI (**d**).

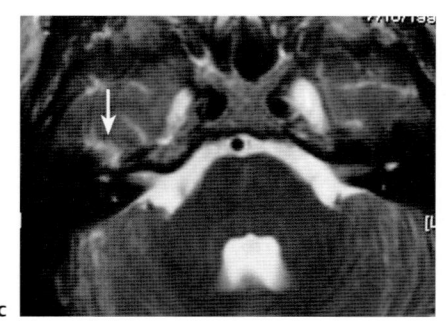

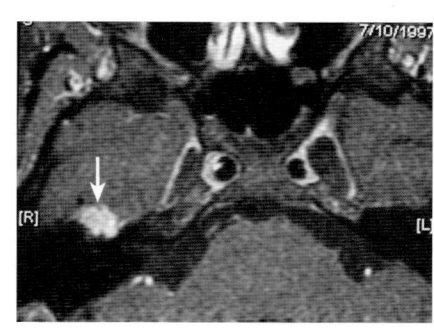

Table 1 (Continued) **Tumors and tumorlike lesions involving the skull and facial bones**

Tumor/Tumorlike Lesion	MRI Findings	Comments
Osteoid osteoma (Fig. 1.23)	Intraosseous circumscribed radiolucent lesion less than 1.5 cm in diameter surrounded by bone sclerosis. Lesions often have low-intermediate signal on T1WI and high signal on T2WI and FS T2WI with prominent Gd-contrast enhancement, surrounded by a peripheral rim of low signal on T1WI and T2WI (bone sclerosis).	Benign osseous lesion containing a nidus of vascularized osteoid trabeculae surrounded by osteoblastic sclerosis, rarely occurs in the skull. Usually occurs between ages of 5 and 25, males > females. Focal pain and tenderness, which is often worse at night, associated with lesion; relieved with aspirin. **(See Atlas Chapter A 60)**
Osteoblastoma	Expansile radiolucent lesion often greater than 1.5 cm surrounded by bone sclerosis. Lesions often have low-intermediate signal on T1WI and intermediate-high signal on T2WI and FS T2WI. Usually show Gd-contrast enhancement, +/− high signal on T2WI and FS T2WI in bone (edema) beyond zone of sclerosis or in adjacent soft tissues.	Rare benign bone neoplasm (2% of bone tumors) usually occurs between ages of 6 and 30. Rarely involves the skull. **(See Atlas Chapter A 61)**
Enchondroma (Fig. 1.24)	Lobulated intramedullary that usually have low-intermediate signal on T1WI and intermediate signal on PDWI. On T2WI and fat-suppressed T2WI, lesions usually have predominantly high signal with foci and/or bands of low signal representing areas of matrix mineralization and fibrous strands. Lesions typically show Gd-contrast enhancement in various patterns (peripheral curvilinear lobular, central nodular/septal, and peripheral lobular, or heterogeneous diffuse).	Benign intramedullary lesions composed of hyaline cartilage, represent ~10% of benign bone tumors. Enchondromas can be solitary (88%) or multiple (12%).
Chondroblastoma	Tumors often have fine lobular margins, and typically have low-intermediate heterogeneous signal on T1WI, and mixed low, intermediate, and/or high signal on T2WI. Areas of low signal on T2WI are secondary to chondroid matrix mineralization, and/or hemosiderin. Lobular, marginal, or septal Gd-contrast enhancement patterns can be seen. Tumors may have thin margins of low signal on T2WI representing sclerotic borders. Cortical destruction is uncommon. Bone expansion can result in spinal cord compression.	Benign cartilaginous tumors with chondroblast-like cells and areas of chondroid matrix formation, rarely occur in the craniofacial bones. The squamous portion of the temporal bone is the most common location of these tumors involving the craniofacial bones. **(See Atlas Chapter A 7)**
Pituitary adenoma (Fig. 1.25)	Macroadenomas (>10 mm): Commonly have intermediate signal on T1WI and T2WI and often similar to gray matter, +/− necrosis, +/− cyst, +/− hemorrhage, usually show prominent Gd-contrast enhancement, extension into suprasellar cistern with waist at diaphragma sella, +/− extension into cavernous sinus, occasionally invades skull base.	Common benign slow-growing tumors representing ~50% of sellar/parasellar neoplasms in adults. Can be associated with endocrine abnormalities related to oversecretion of hormones (prolactin > nonsecretory type > growth hormone > ACTH > others). Prolactinomas: females > males, growth hormone tumors: males > females.
Paraganglioma/glomus jugulare (Fig. 1.26)	Ovoid or fusiform lesions with low-intermediate signal on T1WI and PDWI, and intermediate to high signal on T2WI and FS T2WI. Punctate zones of signal void or low signal on PDWI, T2WI, and FS T2WI can be seen within tumors as a "salt and pepper" pattern. Lesions typically show moderate to prominent Gd-contrast enhancement. Often erode adjacent bone.	Benign encapsulated neuroendocrine tumors that arise from neural crest cells associated with autonomic ganglia (paraganglia) throughout the body. Lesions are also referred to as chemodectomas, and are named according to location (glomus jugulare tympanicum, glomus vagale).
Endolymphatic sac cystadenoma (Fig. 1.27)	Extra-axial retrolabyrinthine lesions involving the posterior petrous bone extending into the cerebellopontine angle cistern. Lesions can have low, intermediate, and or high signal on T1WI and T2WI, and can show Gd-contrast enhancement. May contain blood products.	Rare solid and/or cystic benign or malignant papillary adenomatous tumors arising from the endolymphatic sac in children and adults. Tumors are slow growing and rarely metastasize. May be sporadic or associated with von Hippel–Lindau disease.

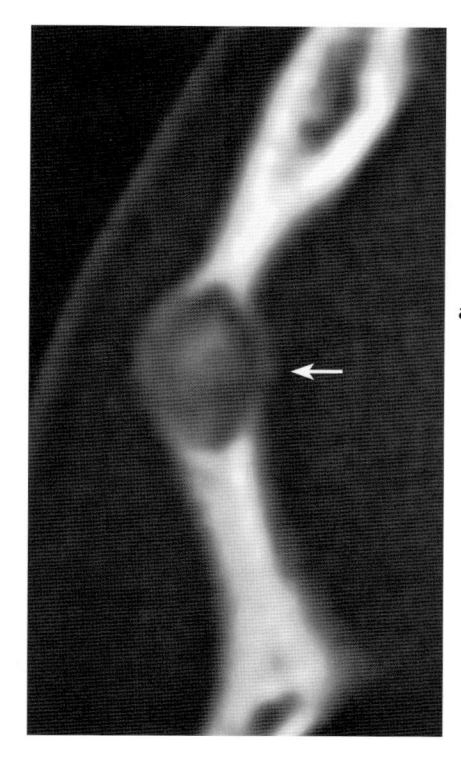

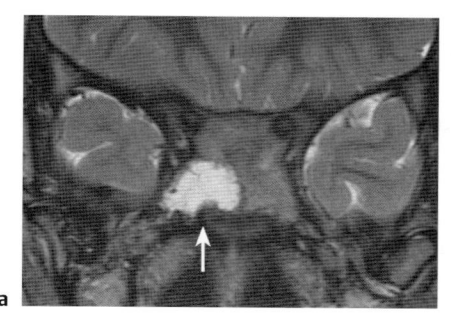

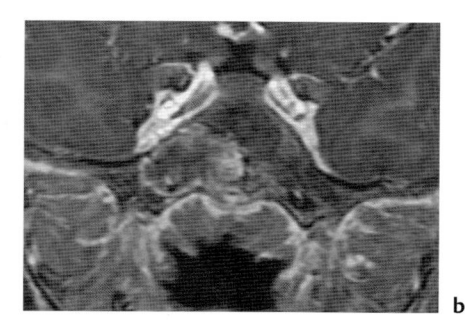

Figure 1.24 a, b   Enchondroma in the sphenoid bone has high signal on coronal T2WI (**a**) and shows mostly peripheral lobular Gd-contrast enhancement on coronal T1WI (**b**).

Figure 1.23   Osteoid osteoma in the right frontal bone in a 16-year-old male. Axial CT shows a small radiolucent lesion containing a central calcification associated with thinning and expansion of the inner and outer tables of the skull.

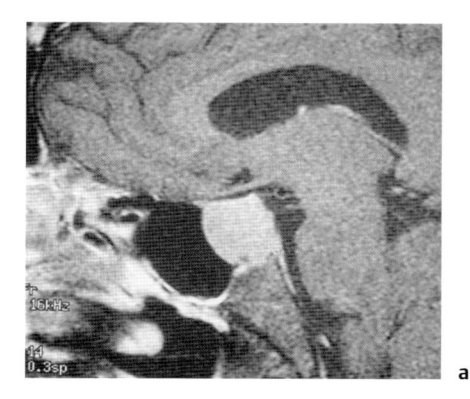

Figure 1.25   A pituitary macroadenoma is seen enlarging the sella with extension into the suprasellar cistern. The lesion shows prominent Gd-contrast enhancement on sagittal FS T1WI.

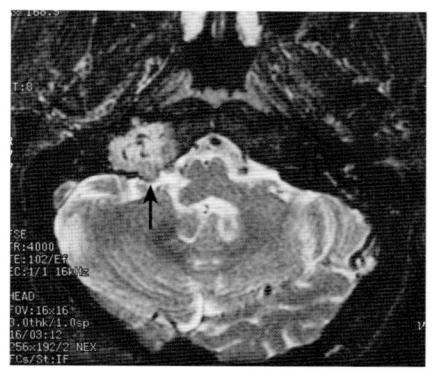

Figure 1.26 a, b   A 55-year-old woman with a glomus jugulare at the right jugular foramen, which has heterogeneous slightly high signal on axial FS T2WI (**a**). Multiple tortuous and punctate zones of signal void are seen representing intratumoral vessels. The tumor shows prominent Gd-contrast enhancement on axial (**b**) FS T1WI.

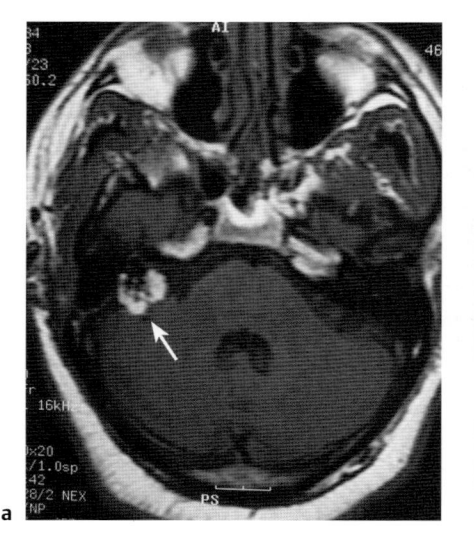

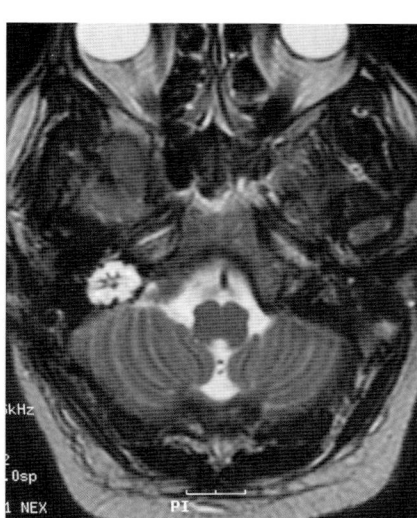

Figure 1.27 a, b   Cystadenoma of the endolymphatic sac involving the right petrous bone has lobulated margins and contains mostly high signal on axial T1WI (**a**) and T2WI (**b**).

Table 1 (Continued) Tumors and tumorlike lesions involving the skull and facial bones

Tumor/Tumorlike Lesion	MRI Findings	Comments
Ameloblastoma (Fig. 1.28)	Lesions occur in the mandible and maxilla, are often radiolucent with associated bone expansion and cortical thinning on CT. Tumors often have circumscribed margins, and can show mixed low, intermediate, and/or high signal on T1WI, T2WI, and FS T2WI. Lesions can show heterogeneous Gd-contrast enhancement.	Slow-growing solid and cystic tumors that contain epithelioid cells (basaloid and/or squamous types) associated with regions of spindle cells and fibrous stroma. These tumors typically lack metastatic potential.
Other lesions		
Osteoma (Fig. 1.29)	Well circumscribed lesions involving the skull with low-intermediate signal on T1WI and T2WI, typically show no significant Gd-contrast enhancement.	Benign proliferation of bone located in the skull or paranasal sinuses (frontal > ethmoid > maxillary > sphenoid). **(See Atlas Chapter A 62)**
Epidermoid (Fig. 1.30)	Well-circumscribed spheroid ectodermal inclusion cystic lesions in the skull associated with chronic bone erosion, low-intermediate signal on T1WI, high signal on T2WI and diffusion weighted imaging, low signal on ADC maps, and no Gd-contrast enhancement.	Non-neoplastic lesions filled with desquamated cells and keratinaceous debris involving the skull. **(See Atlas Chapter A 15)**
Dermoid (Fig. 1.31)	Well-circumscribed spheroid lesions in the skull associated with chronic bone erosion, usually with high signal on T1WI and variable low, intermediate, and/or high signal on T2WI, no Gd-contrast enhancement, +/− fluid–fluid or fluid–debris levels.	Non-neoplastic ectodermal inclusion cystic lesions involving the skull filled with lipid material, cholesterol, desquamated cells, and keratinaceous debris. **(See Atlas Chapter A 15)**

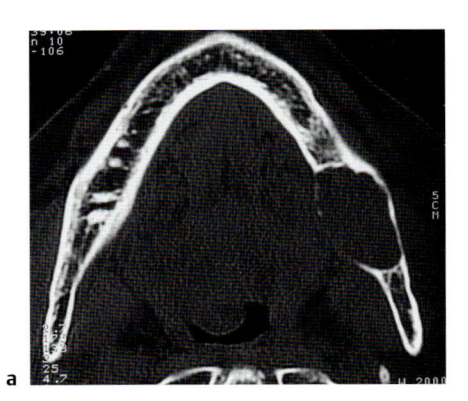

Figure 1.28 a–c Ameloblastoma in the mandible is seen as a radiolucent lesion with associated bone expansion and cortical thinning on axial CT (**a**). The tumor has mixed high and intermediate signal on axial T2WI (**b**). A small fluid–fluid level is also seen. The tumor shows heterogeneous Gd-contrast enhancement on axial FS T1WI (**c**)

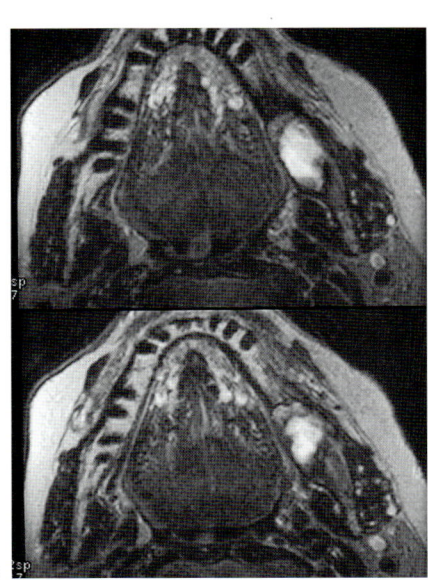

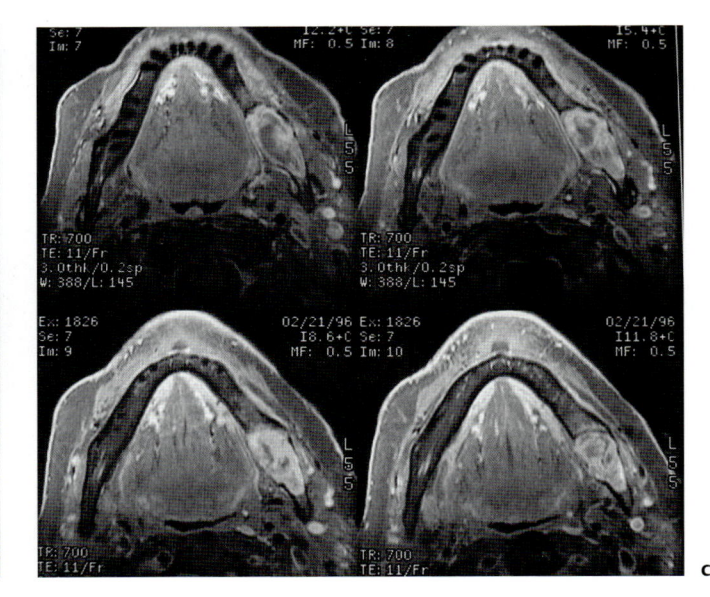

Dermoid 29

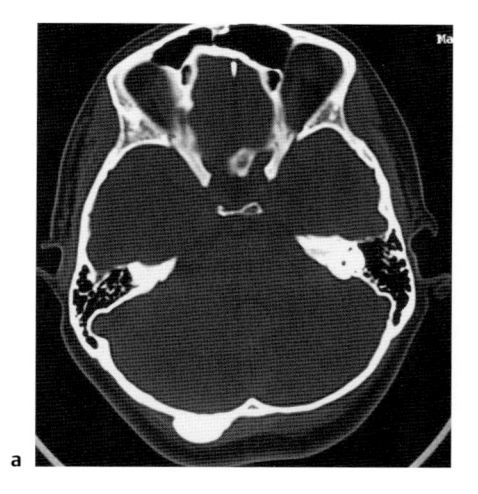

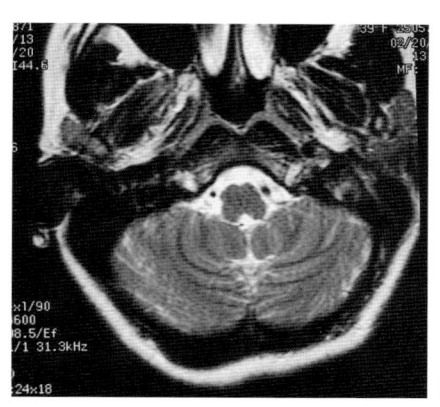

Figure 1.**29 a, b** A 39-year-old woman with an osteoma involving the right occipital bone. Axial CT image (**a**) shows a well-circumscribed ovoid lesion with dense bone attenuation contiguous with the outer table of the right occipital bone via a broad base. The lesion has low signal on axial T2WI (**b**).

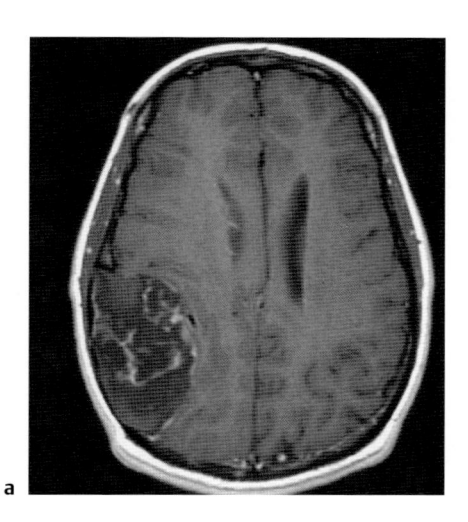

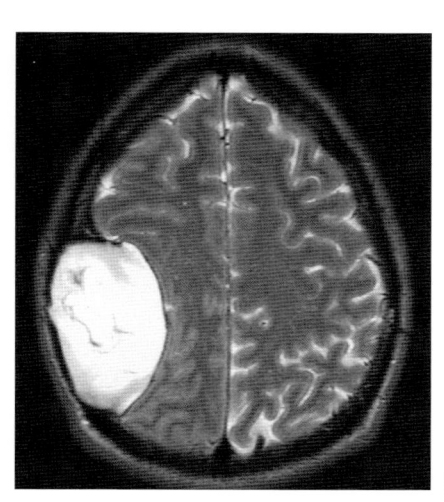

Figure 1.**30 a, b** A 39-year-old man with an epidermoid involving the right parietal bone. The lesion has a mostly intermediate signal as well as zones of high signal on axial T1WI (**a**) associated with marked thinning of the inner and outer tables of the skull. The lesion has high signal centrally surrounded by a thin rim of low signal on axial T2WI (**b**).

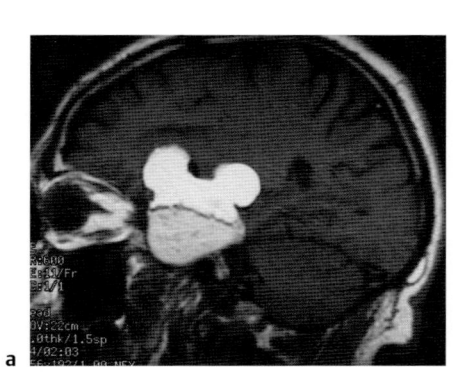

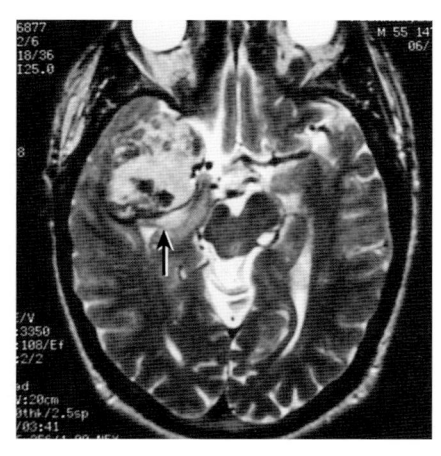

Figure 1.**31 a, b** A 55-year-old man with a dermoid in the right middle cranial fossa. The extra-axial lesion has heterogeneous mostly high signal with a thin low signal septum on sagittal T1WI (**a**). The lesion has mixed low and high signal on axial T2WI (**b**).

Table 1 (Continued) **Tumors and tumorlike lesions involving the skull and facial bones**

Tumor/Tumorlike Lesion	MRI Findings	Comments
Aneurysmal bone cyst (Fig. 1.32)	Circumscribed lesion with variable low, intermediate, high, and/or mixed signal on T1WI and T2WI, +/− surrounding thin zone of low signal on T2WI, +/− lobulations, +/− one or multiple fluid–fluid levels.	Expansile blood/debris-filled lesions that may be primary lesions or occur secondary to other bone lesions such as giant cell tumor, fibrous dysplasia, chondroblastoma. Most occur in patients < 30 years. These lesions rarely involve the skull. **(See Atlas Chapter A 2)**
Giant cell reparative granuloma (Fig. 1.33)	Lesions are radiolucent, and can have heterogeneous low, intermediate, and/or high signal on T1WI, PDWI, and T2WI; as well as peripheral rim-like and central Gd-contrast enhancement on FS T1WI.	Giant cell reparative granulomas are also referred to as solid ABCs. **(See Atlas Chapter A 2)**. Histologic appearance resembles brown tumors.
Arachnoid cyst (Fig. 1.34)	Well-circumscribed extra-axial lesions with low signal on T1WI and FLAIR, and high signal on T2WI and FS T2WI, similar to CSF, no Gd-contrast enhancement. Chronic erosive changes can be seen at the adjacent skull.	Non-neoplastic acquired, developmental, or congenital extra-axial cysts filled with CSF. Cysts can be small or large, asymptomatic or symptomatic.
Inflammatory lesions		
Pyogenic osteomyelitis (Figs. 1.35, 1.36)	Abnormal low signal on T1WI and high signal on T2WI, FS T2WI, diffusion-weighted imaging and low signal on ADC maps in marrow, focal sites of bone destruction, +/− complications including: subgaleal empyema, epidural empyema, subdural empyema, meningitis, cerebritis, intra-axial abscess, venous sinus thrombosis.	Osteomyelitis of the skull can result from surgery, trauma, hematogenous dissemination from another source of infection, or direct extension of infection from an adjacent site such as the paranasal sinuses. **(See Atlas Chapter A 63)**
Eosinophilic granuloma (Fig. 1.37)	Single or multiple circumscribed soft-tissue lesions in the marrow of the skull associated with focal bony destruction/erosion with extension extra-, intracranially or both. Lesions usually have low-intermediate signal on T1WI, mixed intermediate–slightly high signal on T2WI and FS T2WI, usually show Gd-contrast enhancement +/− enhancement of the adjacent dura.	**Single lesion:** Commonly seen in males > females, < 20 years, proliferation of histiocytes in medullary cavity with localized destruction of bone with extension in adjacent soft tissues. **Multiple lesions:** Associated with syndromes such as: Letterer–Siwe disease (lymphadenopathy hepatosplenomegaly), children < 2 years; Hand-Schüller-Christian disease (lymphadenopathy, exophthalmos, diabetes insipidus). children 5–10 years. **(See Atlas Chapter A 18)**

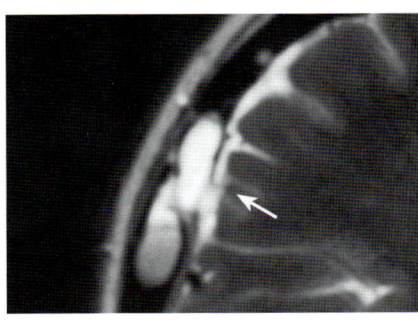

Figure 1.**32** A 47-year-old woman with an aneurysmal bone cyst involving the right frontal bone. The lesion is associated with thinning and slight expansion of the inner and outer tables of the skull, and contains fluid–fluid levels on axial T2WI.

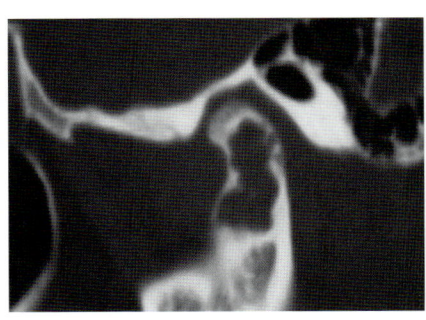

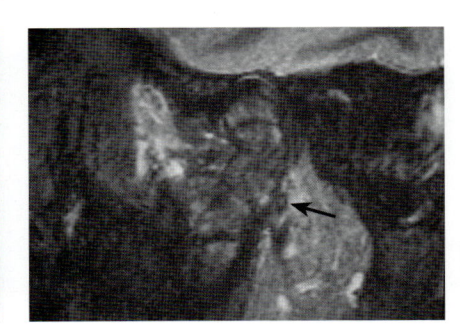

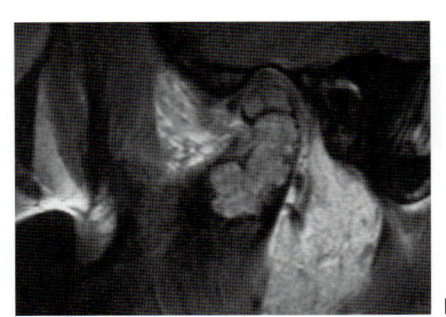

Figure 1.**33 a–c** A 15-year-old female with a giant cell reparative granuloma involving the mandible. The radiolucent lesion has circumscribed margins on sagittal CT (**a**) and heterogeneous intermediate to slightly high signal on sagittal FS T2WI (**b**). The lesion shows Gd-contrast enhancement on sagittal T1WI (**c**).

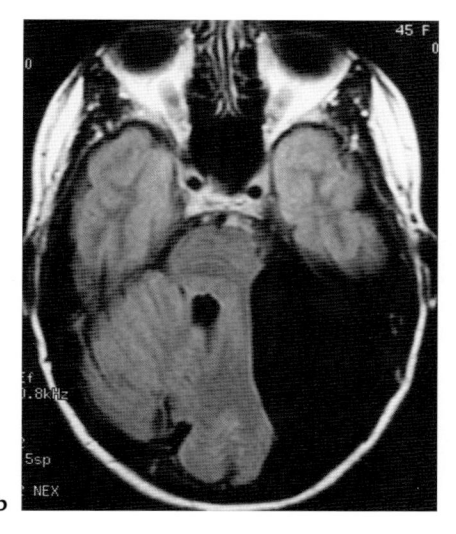

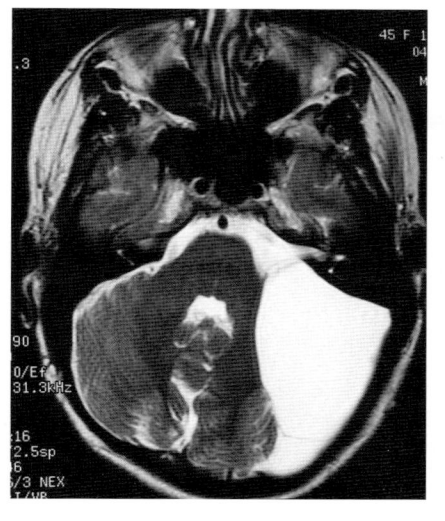

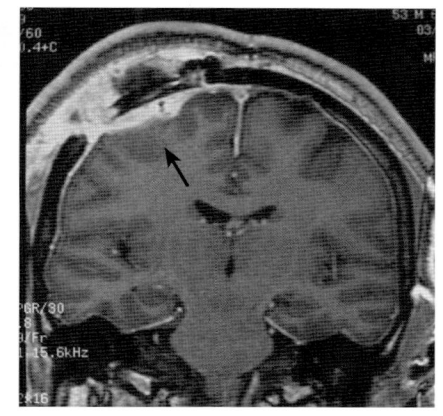

Figure 1.**34 a, b** A large arachnoid cyst is seen in the left side of the posterior cranial fossa resulting in medial displacement and deformation of the left cerebellar hemisphere. The cyst contents have an MRI signal equal to CSF on axial FLAIR (**a**) and axial T2WI (**b**).

Figure 1.**35** A 53-year-old man with pyogenic osteomyelitis involving a craniotomy flap associated with dural inflammation and scalp abscess. Prominent Gd-contrast enhancement is seen in the soft tissues superficial and deep to the infected bone, as well as at the margins and intramedullary portions of the craniotomy flap on coronal T1WI.

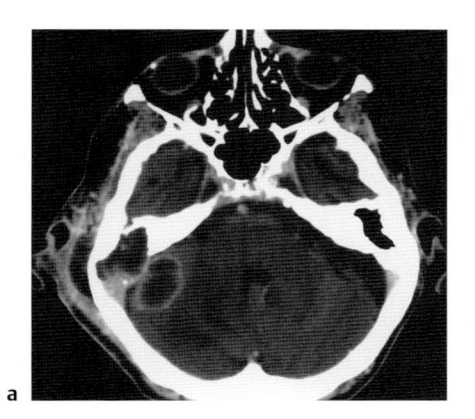

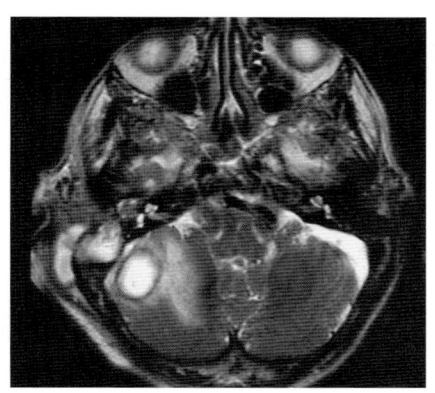

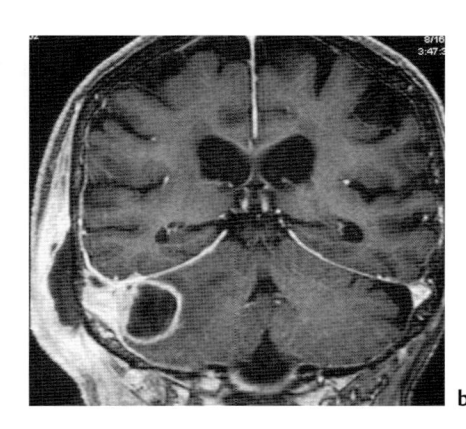

Figure 1.**36 a–c** A 94-year-old woman with pyogenic osteomyelitis involving the mastoid portion of the right temporal bone associated with dural inflammation, and abscesses involving the right cerebellar hemisphere and scalp. Contrast-enhanced axial CT image (**a**) shows an irregular zone of bone destruction with associated dural enhancement, cerebellar and scalp abscesses. The region of osteomyelitis has heterogeneous mostly high signal on axial T2WI (**b**) and the cerebellar and scalp abscesses have high signal centrally surrounded by rims of low signal. The abscesses are surrounded by irregular zones of Gd-contrast enhancement on coronal T1WI (**c**).

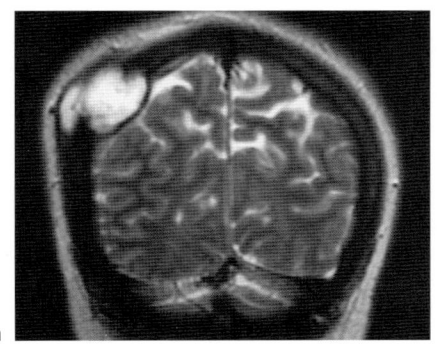

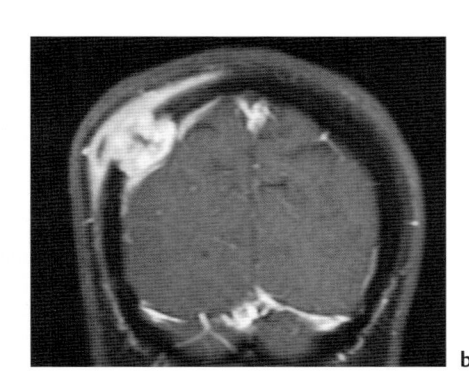

Figure 1.**37 a, b** A 20-year-old woman with an eosinophilic granuloma involving the right parietal bone. The lesion has high signal on coronal T2WI (**a**). Intra- and extracranial extension of the lesion is seen through areas of cortical disruption. The lesion shows prominent Gd-contrast enhancement in the marrow, intra- and extracranial portions of the lesion as well as the dura on coronal FS T1WI (**b**).

Table 1 (Continued) Tumors and tumorlike lesions involving the skull and facial bones

Tumor/Tumorlike Lesion	MRI Findings	Comments
Sarcoidosis (Fig. 1.38)	Sarcoid lesions within marrow may be multiple or solitary, with or without bone expansion and/or erosions or areas of destruction of the inner and/or outer tables with extension intracranially or into the extracranial soft tissues. Lesions can have circumscribed and/or indistinct margins, and usually have low to intermediate signal on T1WI, slightly high to high signal on T2WI and FS T2WI, and show variable degrees of Gd-contrast enhancement.	Chronic systemic granulomatous disease of unknown etiology in which noncaseating granulomas occur in various tissues and organs including bone. **(See Atlas Chapter A 71)**
Paranasal sinus mucocele (Fig. 1.39)	Circumscribed expansile lesion within a paranasal sinus that has variable low, intermediate, and/or high signal on T1WI, T2WI, and FS T2WI depending on contents of mucous, inspissated mucous, and protein concentration.	Lesions occurring from chronic obstruction of a paranasal sinus ostium, results in outward expansion of the osseous margins from remodeling secondary to increased pressure from accumulated secretions from the sinus mucosa. Mucoceles occur most commonly in the frontal sinuses followed by the ethmoid, maxillary, and sphenoid sinuses.
Cholesterol granuloma (Fig. 1.40)	Circumscribed lesion measuring between 2 and 4 cm in the marrow of the petrous bone often associated with mild bone expansion. Lesions usually have high signal on T1WI and FS T1WI. Lesions may have high, intermediate, and/or low signal on T2WI and FS T2WI. A peripheral rim of low signal on T2WI may also be seen from hemosiderin.	Lesions occur in young and middle-age adults and occur when there is obstruction of mucosal-lined air cells in the petrous bone. Multiple cycles of hemorrhage and granulomatous reaction result in accumulation of cyst contents with cholesterol granules, chronic inflammatory cells, red blood cells, hemosiderin, fibrous tissue, and debris.
Aneurysm (Fig. 1.41)	Focal circumscribed lesion with layers of low, intermediate, and/or high signal on T1WI and T2WI secondary to layers of thrombus, as well as a signal void representing a patent lumen if present.	Abnormal dilatation of artery secondary to acquired/degenerative cause, connective tissue disease, atherosclerosis, trauma, infection (mycotic), AVM, drugs, and vasculitis.
Acquired		
Postsurgical pseudomeningocele (Fig. 1.42)	CSF-filled collection contiguous with the subarachnoid space protruding through a surgical bony defect. Gliotic brain tissue may also accompany the dural protrusion.	Usually are not clinically significant unless they become large or infected.

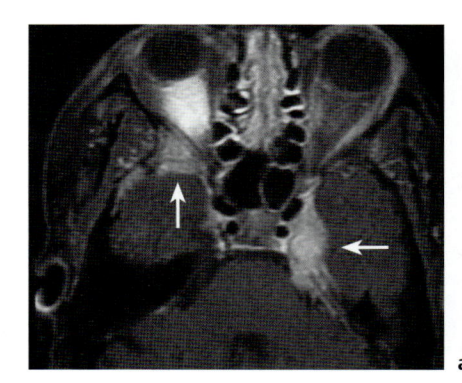

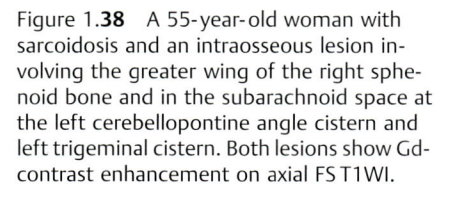

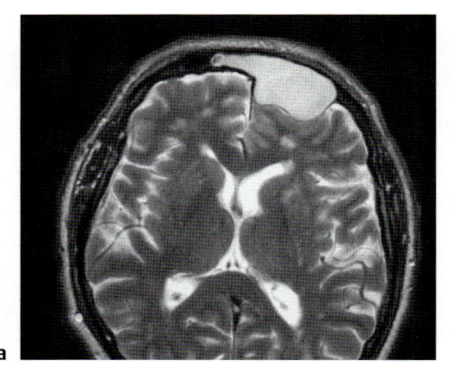

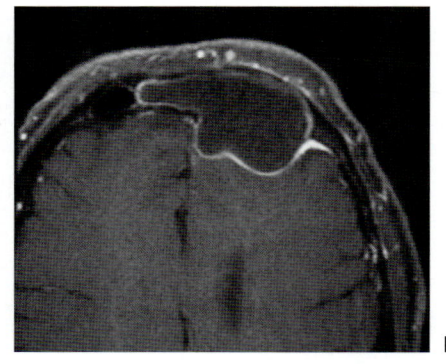

Figure 1.38 A 55-year-old woman with sarcoidosis and an intraosseous lesion involving the greater wing of the right sphenoid bone and in the subarachnoid space at the left cerebellopontine angle cistern and left trigeminal cistern. Both lesions show Gd-contrast enhancement on axial FS T1WI.

Figure 1.39 a, b A mucocele is seen expanding the left frontal sinus associated with remodeling and thinning of the inner table and orbital roof. The mucocele contains high signal on axial T2WI (**a**). Thin peripheral Gd-contrast enhancement is seen surrounding low signal mucous on axial FS T1WI (**b**).

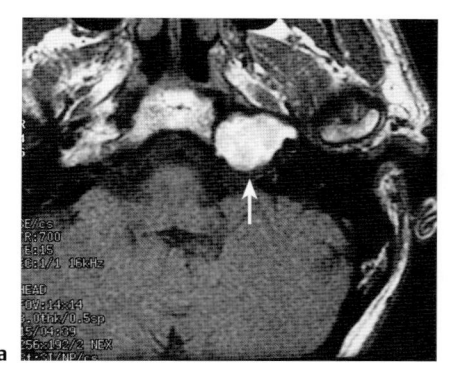

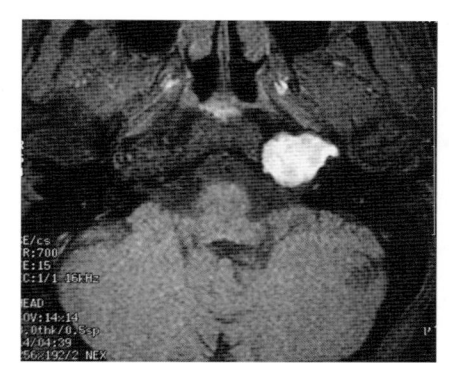

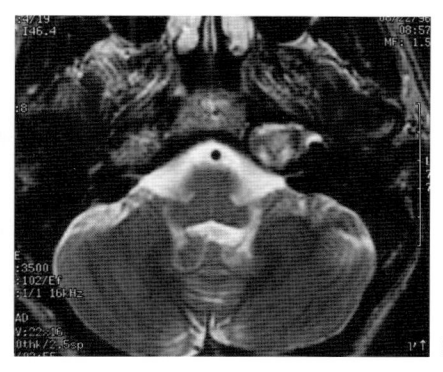

Figure 1.**40 a–c** A cholesterol granuloma is seen in the left petrous apex which has high signal on axial T1WI (**a**) and axial FS T1WI (**b**). The lesion has mixed high, intermediate, and low signal on axial T2WI (**c**). Mild bone expansion and a peripheral rim of low signal on T2WI are also seen.

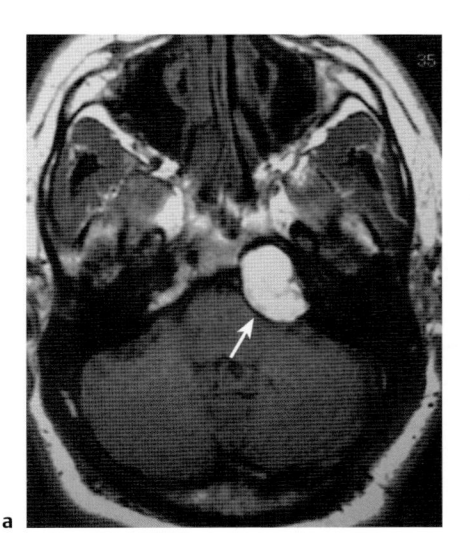

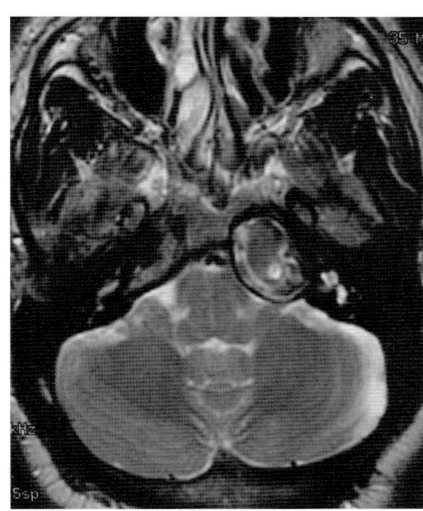

Figure 1.**41 a, b** A 35-year-old man with an intraosseous aneurysm at the left petrous carotid canal, which erodes the petrous bone. The aneurysm has mostly high signal on axial T1WI (**a**) and mixed low, intermediate, and high signal on axial T2WI (**b**).

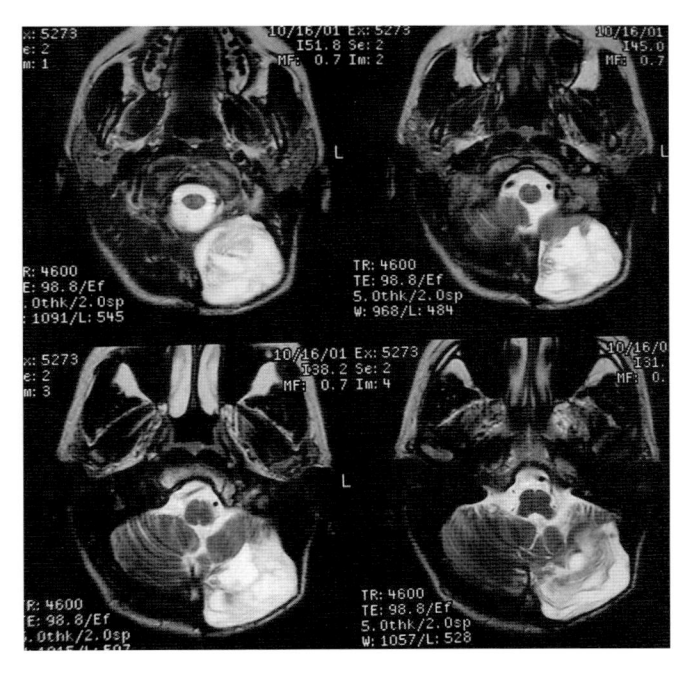

Figure 1.**42** A pseudomeningocele is seen contiguous with the subarachnoid space protruding through a surgical bony defect from a left occipital craniectomy on axial T2WI. Damaged cerebellar tissue (gliosis and localized encephalomalacia) with high signal on T2WI is also seen.

Table 1 (Continued) **Tumors and tumorlike lesions involving the skull and facial bones**

Tumor/Tumorlike Lesion	MRI Findings	Comments
Paget disease (Fig. 1.43)	Expansile sclerotic/lytic process involving the skull with mixed low-intermediate signal on T1WI, variable mixed low, intermediate, high signal on T2WI, variable heterogeneous enhancement. Irregular/indistinct borders between marrow and inner margins of the outer and inner tables of the skull.	Usually seen in older adults, can result in narrowing of neuroforamina with cranial nerve compression, basilar impression +/− compression of brainstem. **(See Atlas Chapter A 65)**
Fibrous dysplasia (Fig. 1.44)	Expansile process involving the skull base with mixed low-intermediate signal on T1WI, variable mixed low, intermediate, high signal on T2WI, usually heterogeneous Gd-contrast enhancement.	Usually seen in adolescents and young adults, can result in narrowing of neuroforamina with cranial nerve compression, facial deformities, mono- and poly-ostotic forms (+/− endocrine abnormalities such as with McCune–Albright syndrome, precocious puberty). **(See Atlas Chapter A 27)**
Hematopoietic disorders (Fig. 1.45)	Enlargement of the diploic space with red marrow hyperplasia (low-intermediate signal on T1WI and intermediate to slightly high signal on T2WI and FS T2WI) with thinning of the inner and outer tables.	Thickening of diploic space secondary to erythroid hyperplasia from anemia related to Sickle cell disease, thalassemia major, hereditary spherocytosis. Similar findings of red marrow expansion can be seen with polycythemia rubra.
Trauma		
Cephalohematoma	Hematoma located beneath periosteum of outer table, does not cross suture lines; +/− skull fracture; +/− subdural hematoma.	Results from birth trauma (complication of forceps delivery), associated with 1 % of births.
Fracture	**Nondisplaced/nondepressed skull fractures:** Abnormal low signal on T1WI and high signal on T2WI in marrow at the site of fracture, +/− subgaleal hematoma, +/− epidural hematoma, +/− subdural hematoma, +/− subarachnoid hemorrhage. **Depressed skull fracture:** Angulation and internal displacement of fractured skull, abnormal low signal on T1WI and high signal on T2WI in marrow at the site of fracture, +/− subgaleal hematoma, +/− epidural hematoma, +/− subdural hematoma, +/− subarachnoid hemorrhage.	Traumatic fractures of the skull can involve the calvaria or skull base, significant complications that can result include: epidural hematoma, subdural hematoma, subarachnoid hemorrhage, CSF leakage/rhinorrhea, otorrhea.
Congenital abnormalities		
Cephaloceles (meningoceles or meningoencephaloceles) (Figs. 1.46, 1.47)	Defect in skull through which there is either herniation of meninges and CSF (meningocele); or meninges, CSF/ventricles, and brain tissue (meningoencephaloceles).	Congenital malformation involving lack of separation of neuroectoderm from surface ectoderm with resultant localized failure of bone formation. Occipital location most common in western hemisphere, frontoethmoidal location most common site in Southeast Asians. Other sites include parietal and sphenoid bones. Cephaloceles can also result from trauma or surgery.

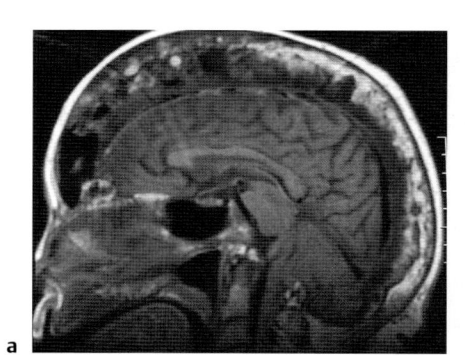

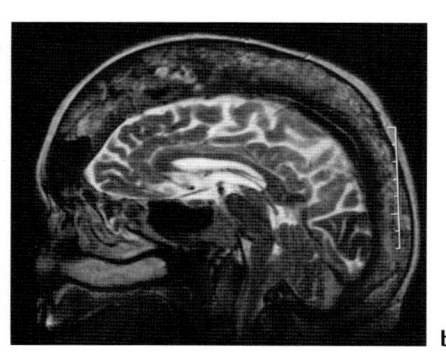

Figure 1.**43 a, b** An 81-year-old woman with Paget disease involving the skull with associated basilar impression. The interface between the diploic space and the inner and outer tables is obscured, and there is marked osseous expansion. The marrow has mixed low, intermediate, and high signal on sagittal T1WI (**a**) and sagittal T2WI (**b**).

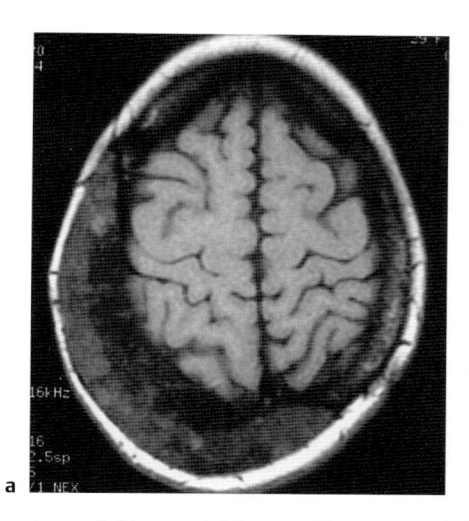

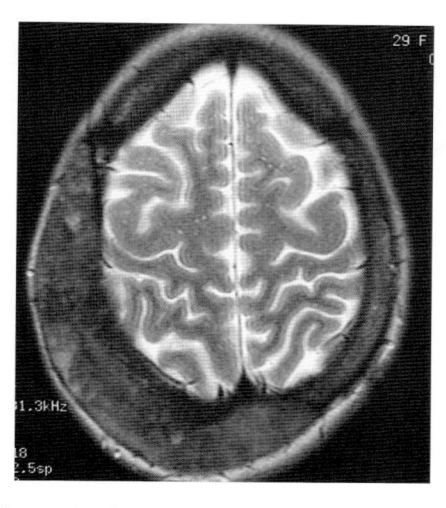

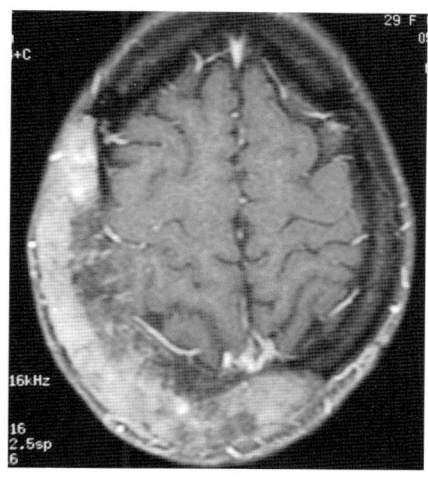

Figure 1.**44 a–c** A 29-year-old woman with fibrous dysplasia expanding the right and posterior portions of the calvarium. The lesion has mixed low and intermediate signal on axial T1WI (**a**) and axial T2WI (**b**), and shows prominent Gd-contrast enhancement on axial FS T1WI (**c**).

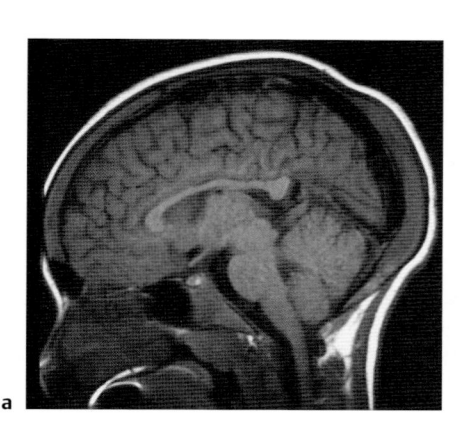

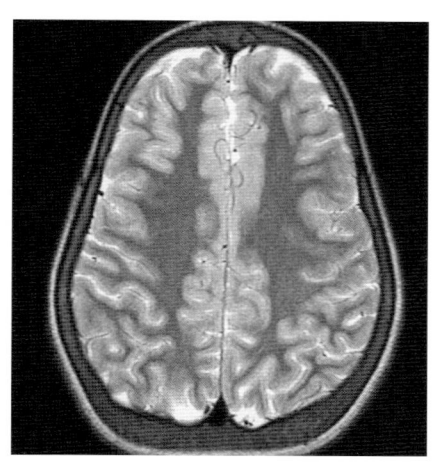

Figure 1.**45 a, b** Patient with sickle cell anemia who has enlargement of the diploic space with red marrow hyperplasia which has low-intermediate signal on sagittal T1WI (**a**) and intermediate signal on axial T2WI (**b**).

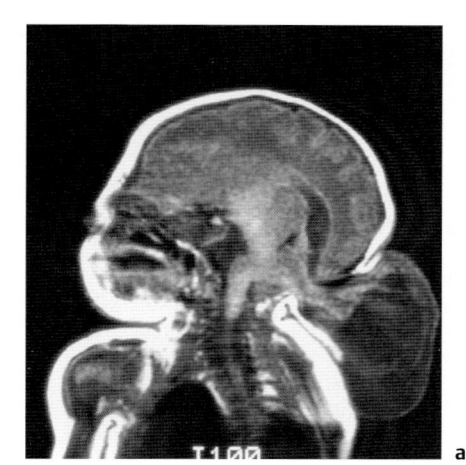

Figure 1.**46** A 1-day-old neonate with an occipital meningoencephalocele containing meninges and damaged brain tissue as seen on sagittal T1WI.

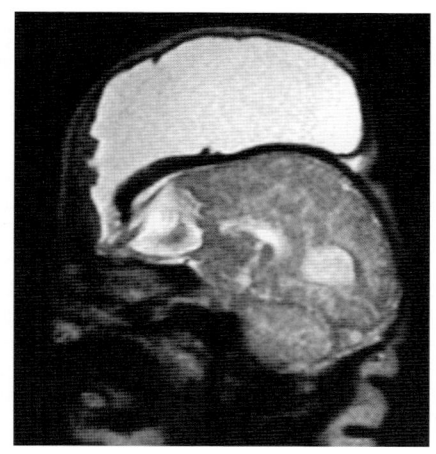

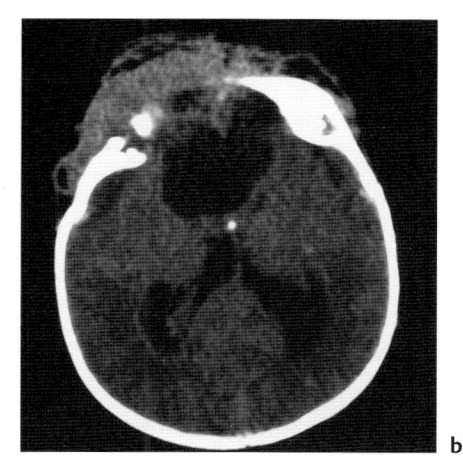

Figure 1.**47 a, b** Neonate with a frontal meningoencephalocele containing meninges and damaged brain tissue as seen on sagittal (**a**) T2WI and axial CT image (**b**).

Table 1 (Continued) **Tumors and tumorlike lesions involving the skull and facial bones**

Tumor/Tumorlike Lesion	MRI Findings	Comments
Neurofibromatosis type 1 (Fig. 1.48)	NF1 associated with: focal ectasia of intracranial dura; widening of internal auditory canals from dural ectasia; dural and temporal lobe protrusion into orbit through bony defect, bony hypoplasia of greater sphenoid wing, bone malformation, or erosion from plexiform neurofibromas.	Autosomal dominant disorder (1/2500 births) representing the most common type of neurocutaneous syndromes, associated with neoplasms of central and peripheral nervous system and skin. Also associated with meningeal and skull dysplasias. **(See Atlas Chapter A 56)**

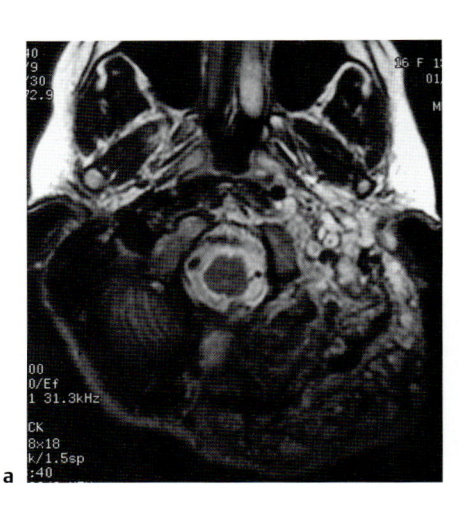

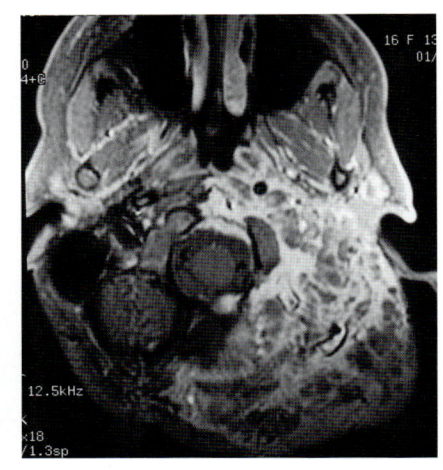

Figure 1.**48 a, b** A 16-year-old female with a plexiform neurofibroma involving the posterior scalp and skull. The lesion appears as curvilinear and multinodular zones with intermediate, slightly high to high signal separated by curvilinear zones of low signal on axial T2WI (**a**). The plexiform neurofibroma shows heterogeneous Gd-contrast enhancement on axial FS T1WI (**b**).

References

Nasopharyngeal Carcinoma
King AD, Vlantis AC, Tsang RKY, et al. Magnetic resonance imaging for the detection of nasopharyngeal carcinoma. *AJNR* Jun–Jul 2006; 27:1288–1291.

Loevner LA, Sonners AI. Imaging of neoplasms of the paranasal sinuses. *Magn Reson Imaging Clin N Am* August 2002;10(3):467–493.

Adenoid Cystic Carcinoma
Sigal R, Monnet O, de Baere T, et al. Adenoid cystic carcinoma of the head and neck: evaluation with MR imaging and clinical-pathologic correlation in 27 patients. *Radiology* 1992;184:95–101.

Triantafillidou K, Dimitrapoulos J, Iordanidis F, Koufogiannis D. Management of adenoid cystic carcinoma of minor salivary glands. *J Oral Maxillofac Surg* 2006;64:1114–1120.

Esthesioneuroblastoma
Bradley PJ, Jones NS, Robertson I. Diagnosis and management of esthesioneuroblastoma. *Otolaryng Head Neck* 2003;11:112–118.

Chirico G, Pergolizzi S, Mazziotti S, Santacaterina A, Ascenti G. Primary sphenoid esthesioneuroblastoma studies with MR. *J Clin Imag* 2003;27:38–40.

Li C, Yousem DM, Hayden RE, Doty RL. Olfactory neuroblastoma: MR evaluation. *AJNR* Sep-Oct 1993;14(5):1167–1171.

Pickuth D, Heywang-Köbrunner SH, Spielmann RP. Computed tomography and magnetic resonance imaging features of olfactory neuroblastoma: an analysis of 22 cases. *Clin Otolaryngol* 1999;24:457–461.

Schuster JJ, Phillips CD, Levine PA. MR of esthesioneuroblastoma (olfactory neuroblastoma) and appearance after craniofacial resection. *AJNR* June 1994;15(6):1169–1177.

Ossifying Hemangioma
Brackman DE, Weisskopf PA, Lo WWM. Ossifying hemangioma of the internal auditory canal. *Otol Neurotol* 2005;26:1239–1240.

Curtin HD, Jensen JE, Barnes L, May M. Ossifying hemangiomas of the temporal bone: evaluation with CT. *Radiology* 1987;164:831–835.

Isaacson B, Telian SA, McKeever PE, Arts HA. Hemangiomas of the geniculate ganglion. *Otol Neurotol* 2005;26:796–802.

Pituitary Adenoma
Elster AD. Modern imaging of the pituitary. *Radiology* 1993;187:1–14.

FitzPatrick M, Tartaglino LM, Hollander MD, Zimmerman RA, Flanders AE. Imaging of sellar and parasellar pathology. *Radiol Clin N Am* January 1999;37(1):101–121.

Pierallini A, Caramia F, Falcone C, et al. Pituitary macroadenomas: preoperative evaluation of consistency with diffusion-weighted MR imaging – initial experience. *Radiology* April 2006;239(1):223–231.

Pisaneschi M, Kapoor G. Imaging the sella and parasellar region. *Neuroimag Clin N Am* February 2005;15(1):203–219.

Endolymphatic Sac Tumor
Baltacioglu F, Ekinci G, Ture U, Sav A, Pamyr N, Erzen C. MR imaging, CT, and angiography features of endolymphatic sac tumors: report of two cases. *Neuroradiology* 2002;44:91–96.

Bonneville F, Sarrazin JL, Marsot-Dupuch K, et al. Unusual lesions of the cerebellopontine angle: a segmental approach. *RadioGraphics* 2002; 21:419–438.

Patel NP, Wiggins RH, Shelton C. The radiologic diagnosis of endolymphatic sac tumors. *Laryngoscope* 2006;116:40–46.

Ameloblastoma
Asaumi J, Hisatomi M, Yanagi Y, et al. Assessment of ameloblastomas using MRI and dynamic contrast-enhanced MRI. *Eur J Radiol* 2005; 56:25–30.

Cihangiroglu M, Akfirat M, Yildirim H. CT and MRI findings of ameloblastoma in two cases. *Neuroradiology* 2002;44:434–437.

Arachnoid Cyst

Bonneville F, Sarrazin JL, Marsot-Dupuch K, et al. Unusual lesions of the cerebellopontine angle: a segmental approach. *RadioGraphics* 2002; 21:419–438.

Cakirer S. Arachnoid cyst of the craniospinal junction: a case report and review of the literature. *Acta Radiol* 2004;45:460–463.

Mukherji SK, Chenevert TL, Castillo M. Diffusion-weighted magnetic resonance imaging. *J Neuro-Ophthalmol* 2002;22(2):118–122.

Rao G, Anderson RCE, Feldstein NA, Brockmeyer DL. Expansion of arachnoid cysts in children. *J Neurosurg (Pediatrics 3)* 2005;102:314–317.

Tang L, Cianfoni A, Imbesi SG. Diffusion weighted imaging distinguishes recurrent epidermoid neoplasm from postoperative arachnoid cyst in the lumbosacral spine. *J Comput Assist Tomogr* 2006;30:507–509.

Paranasal Sinus Mucocele

Bonneville F, Cattin F, Marscot-Dupuch K, Dormont D, Bonneville JF, Chiras J. T1 hyperintensity in the sellar region: spectrum of findings. *RadioGraphics* 2006;26:93–113.

Cholesterol Granuloma

Bonneville F, Sarrazin JL, Marsot-Dupuch K, et al. Unusual lesions of the cerebellopontine angle: a segmental approach. *RadioGraphics* 2002; 21:419–438.

Mosnier I, Cyna-Gorse F, Grayeli AB, et al. Management of cholesterol granulomas of the petrous apex based on clinical and radiologic evaluation. *Otol Neurotol* 2002;23(4):522–528.

Pisaneschi MJ, Langer B. Congenital cholesteatoma and cholesterol granuloma of the temporal bone: role of magnetic resonance imaging. *Top Magn Reson Imag* 2000;11(2):87–97.

Hematologic Disorders

Lorand-Metze I, Santiago GF, Lima CSP, Zanardi VA, Torriani M. Magnetic resonance imaging of femoral marrow cellularity in hypocellular haemopoietic disorders. *Clin Radiol* 2001;56:107–110.

Loevner LA, Tobey JD, Yousem DM, Sonners AI, Hsu WC. MR imaging characteristics of cranial bone marrow in adult patients with underlying systemic disorders compared with healthy control subjects. *AJNR* February 2002;23:248–254.

Tyler PA, Madani G, Chaudhuri R, Wilson LF, Dick EA. The radiological appearances of thalassaemia. *Clin Radiol* 2006;61:40–52.

Table 2 Tumors and tumorlike lesions involving the spine

Tumor/tumorlike lesion	MRI Findings	Comments
Neoplasms		
Metastatic tumor (Figs. 2.1, 2.2)	Single or multiple well-circumscribed or poorly defined infiltrative lesions involving the vertebral marrow, dura, and/or leptomeninges; low-intermediate signal on T1WI, low, intermediate, and/or high signal on T2WI and FS T1WI, usually show Gd-contrast enhancement, +/− bone destruction, +/− pathologic vertebral fracture, +/− compression of neural tissue or vessels. Leptomeningeal tumor often best seen on postcontrast images.	May have variable destructive or infiltrative changes involving single or multiple sites of involvement. **(See Atlas Chapter A 50)**
Myeloma/plasmacytoma (Figs. 2.3, 2.4)	Multiple (myeloma) or single (plasmacytoma) well-circumscribed or poorly defined diffuse infiltrative lesions involving the vertebra(e), and dura; involvement of vertebral body typical, rarely involves posterior elements until late stages, low-intermediate signal on T1WI, intermediate-high signal on T2WI, usually show Gd-contrast-enhancement + bone destruction.	May have variable destructive or infiltrative changes involving the axial and/or appendicular skeleton. **(see Atlas Chapter A 52)**

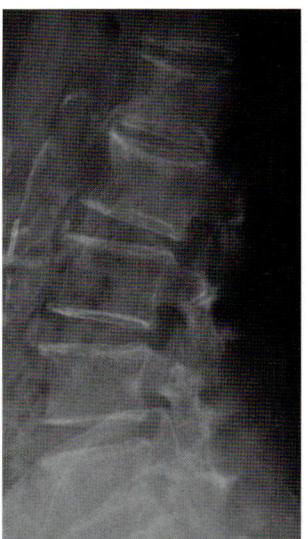

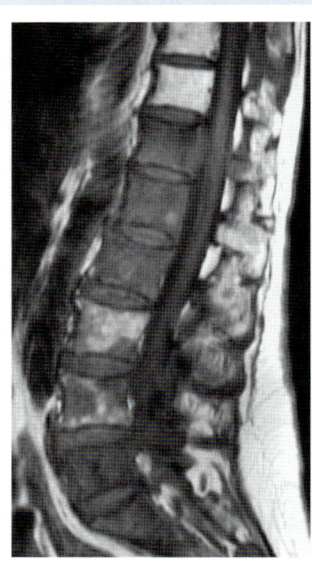

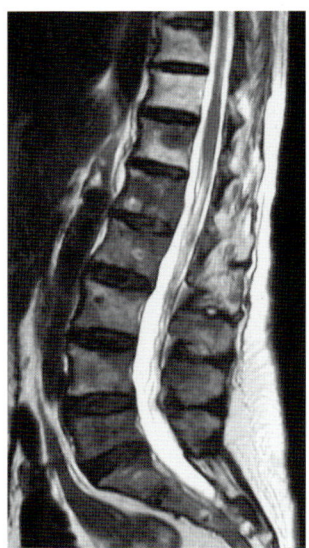

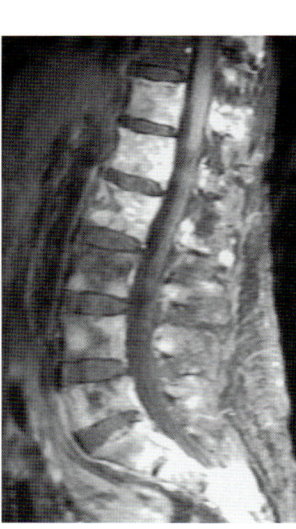

Figure 2.1 a–d An 83-year-old woman with multiple metastases from breast carcinoma involving the lower spine. A lateral radiograph (a) shows multiple radiolucent lesions in the vertebrae. The metastatic lesions have low-intermediate signal on sagittal T1WI (b) and sagittal T2WI (c), and show Gd-contrast enhancement on sagittal FS T1WI (d).

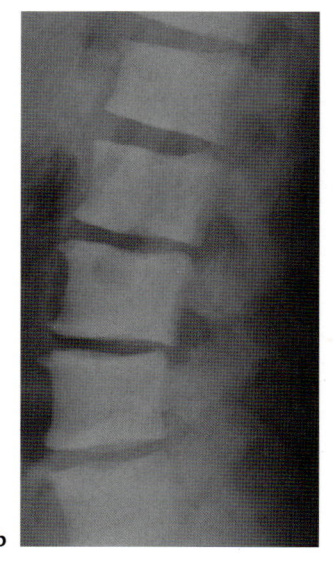

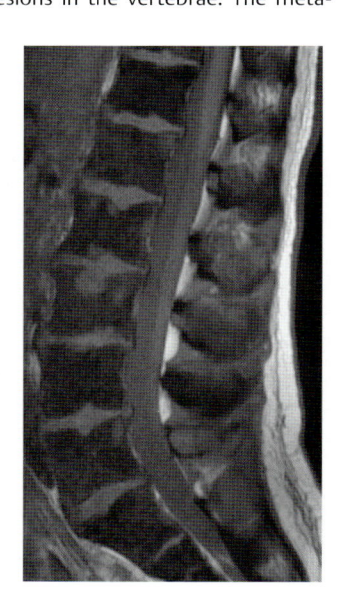

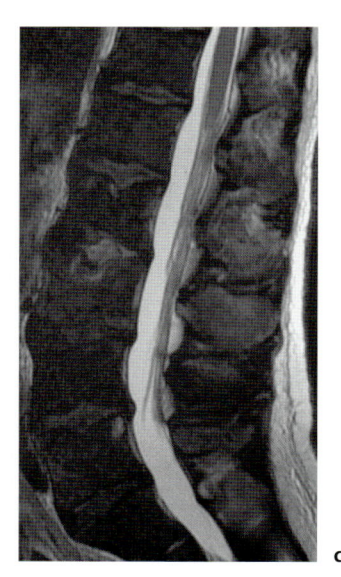

Figure 2.2 a–c A 57-year-old man with diffuse sclerotic metastases from prostate carcinoma involving the thoracic and lumbar spine seen as diffuse increased density on lateral radiograph (a). The neoplastic disease has mostly low signal on sagittal T1WI (b) and sagittal T2WI (c).

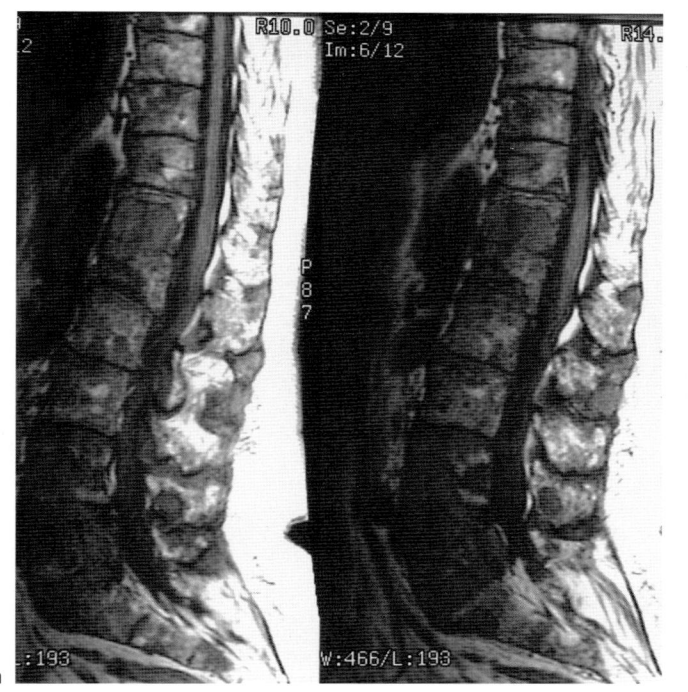

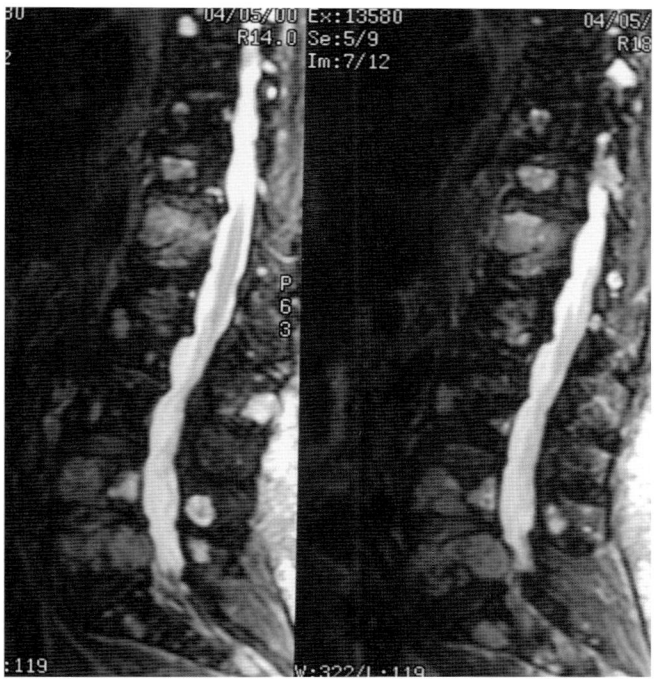

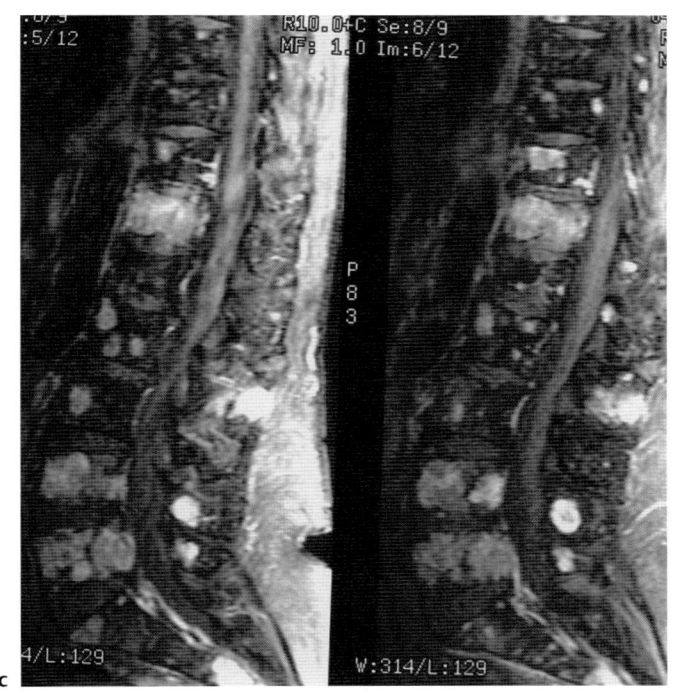

Figure 2.3 a–c Multiple myeloma involving multiple thoracic and lumbar vertebrae. The lesions have low-intermediate signal on sagittal T1WI (**a**) and high signal on sagittal FS T2WI (**b**). The lesions show prominent Gd-contrast enhancement on sagittal FS T1WI (**c**).

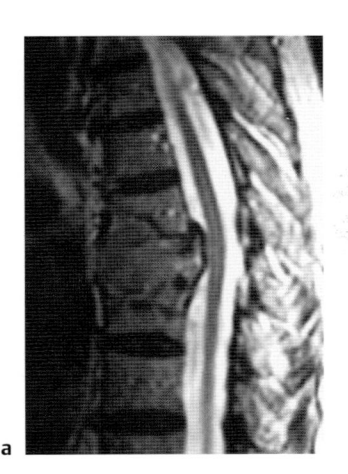

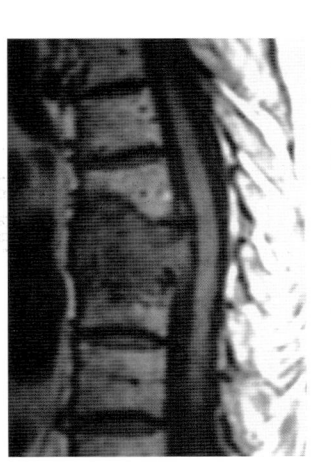

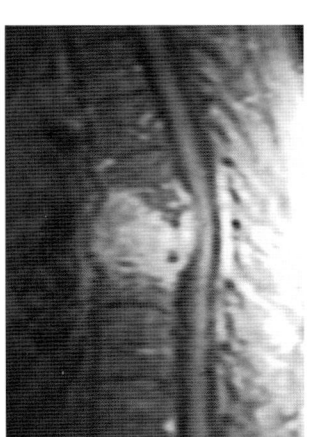

Figure 2.4 a–c Plasmacytoma involving a thoracic vertebral body with associated epidural extension and pathologic fracture. The tumor has diffuse low-intermediate signal on sagittal T1WI (**a**), and intermediate signal on sagittal (**b**) T2WI. The tumor shows prominent Gd-contrast enhancement on sagittal FS T1WI (**c**).

Table 2 (Continued) **Tumors and tumorlike lesions involving the spine**

Tumor/Tumorlike Lesion	MRI Findings	Comments
Lymphoma and leukemia (Figs. 2.5–2.8)	Single or multiple well-circumscribed or poorly defined infiltrative lesions involving the vertebrae, dura, and/or leptomeninges; low-intermediate signal on T1WI, intermediate-high signal on T2WI and FS T2WI, often shows Gd-contrast enhancement, +/− bone destruction. Diffuse involvement of vertebra with Hodgkin lymphoma can produce an "ivory vertebra" that has low signal on T1WI and T2WI. Leptomeningeal tumor often best seen on postcontrast images.	May have variable destructive or infiltrative marrow/bony changes involving single or multiple sites of vertebral involvement. Lymphoma may extend from bone into adjacent soft tissues within or outside of the spinal canal; or initially involve only the epidural soft tissues or only the subarachnoid compartment. Can occur at any age (peak incidence 3rd to 5th decades). **(See Atlas Chapters A 41, A 47)**

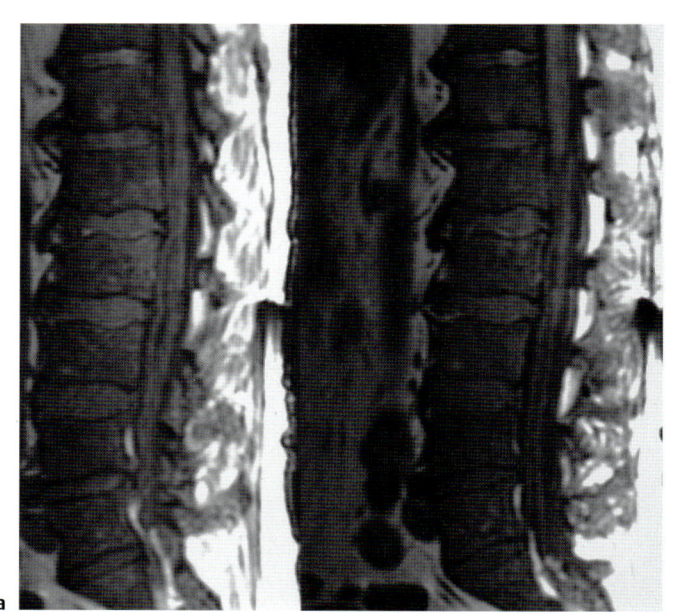

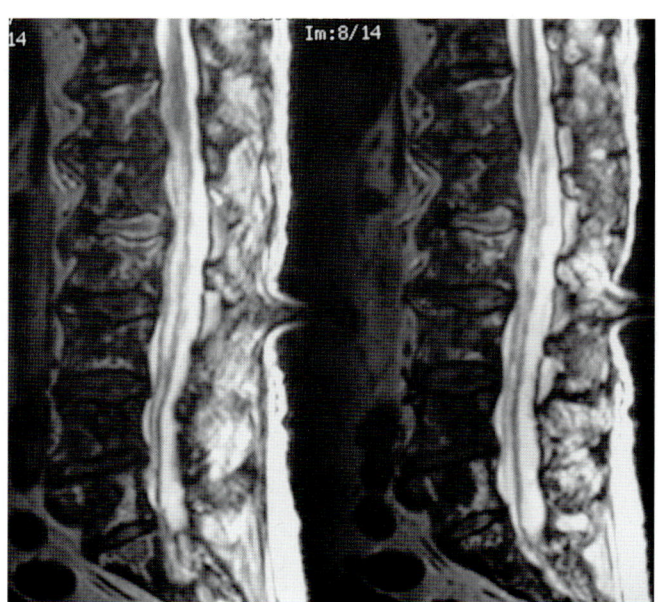

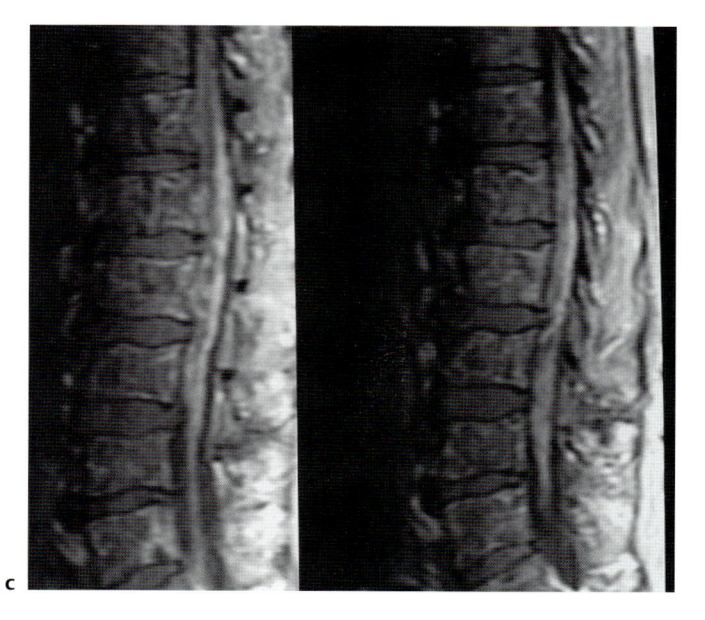

Figure 2.5 a–c   Non-Hodgkin lymphoma involving vertebral marrow as well as within the lumbar subarachnoid space. Diffuse low-intermediate signal on sagittal T1WI (**a**) is seen throughout the marrow. Mostly low signal is seen in the marrow on sagittal T2WI (**b**). Heterogeneous Gd-contrast enhancement is seen throughout the marrow as well as within the thecal sac on sagittal (**c**) FS T1WI.

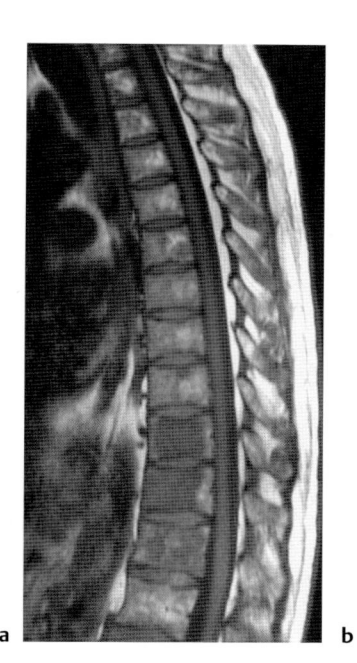

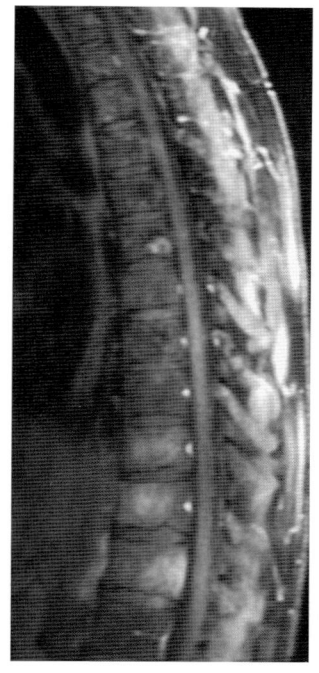

Figure 2.6 a, b A 41-year-old man with Hodgkin lymphoma involving multiple vertebrae. The lymphoma has intermediate signal on sagittal T1WI (a), and shows mild–moderate Gd-contrast enhancement on sagittal FS T1WI (b).

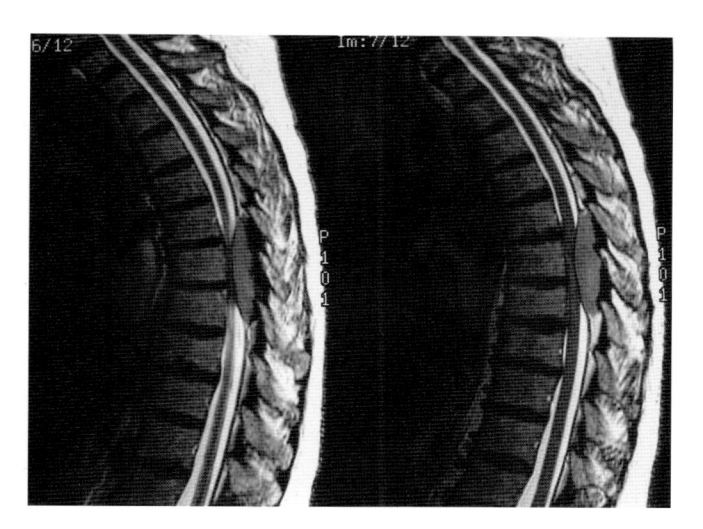

Figure 2.7 Epidural non-Hodgkin lymphoma causing compression of the thoracic spinal cord. The epidural lesion has intermediate signal on sagittal T2WI.

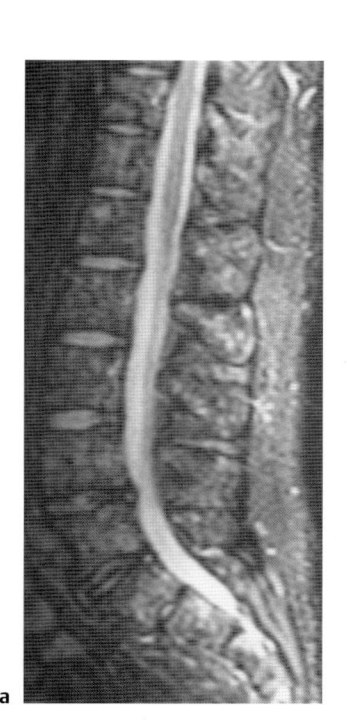

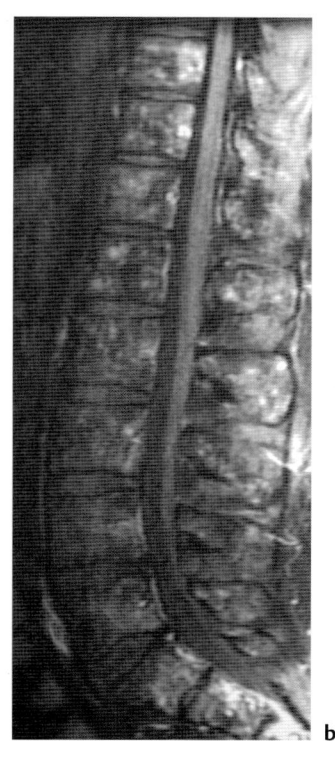

Figure 2.8 a, b A 28-year-old man with AML involving the marrow of the spine. The leukemic tissue has heterogeneous slightly high signal on sagittal FS T2WI (a) and shows mild heterogeneous Gd-contrast enhancement on sagittal FS T1WI (b).

Table 2 (Continued) Tumors and tumorlike lesions involving the spine		
Tumor/Tumorlike Lesion	**MRI Findings**	**Comments**
Chordoma (Fig. 2.9)	Well-circumscribed lobulated lesions, low-intermediate signal on T1WI, high signal on T2WI and FS T2WI, usually show Gd-contrast enhancement (usually heterogeneous), locally invasive associated with bone erosion/destruction, usually involves the dorsal portion of the vertebral body with extension toward the spinal canal. Also occurs in sacrum.	Rare, slow-growing tumors (~3% of bone tumors); usually occur in adults 30 to 70 years; males > females (2/1); sacrum (50%) > skull base (35%) > vertebrae (15%). **(See Atlas Chapter A 12)**
Enchondroma	Lobulated lesions, low-intermediate signal on T1WI, high signal on T2WI and FS T2WI, +/− matrix mineralization, with low signal on T2WI, usually show Gd-contrast enhancement (usually heterogeneous), usually involve posterior elements.	Rare, slow-growing tumors (~12% of bone tumors), usually occur in children and young adults (10–30 years), males = females. **(See Atlas Chapter A 8)**
Chondrosarcoma (Fig. 2.10)	Lobulated lesions, low-intermediate signal on T1WI, high signal on T2WI, +/− matrix mineralization, with low signal on T2WI, usually show Gd-contrast enhancement (usually heterogeneous), locally invasive associated with bone erosion/destruction, encasement of vessels and nerves, can involve any portion of the vertebra.	Rare, slow-growing tumors (~16% of bone tumors), usually occur in adults (peak in 5th to 6th decades), males > females, sporadic (75%), malignant degeneration/transformation of other cartilaginous lesion enchondroma, osteochondroma, etc (25%). **(See Atlas Chapter A 11)**
Chondroblastoma	Tumors often have fine lobular margins and typically have low-intermediate heterogeneous signal on T1WI and mixed low, intermediate, and/or high signal on T2WI. Areas of low signal on T2WI are secondary to chondroid matrix mineralization, and/or hemosiderin. Lobular, marginal, or septal Gd-contrast enhancement patterns can be seen. Tumors may have thin margins of low signal on T2WI representing sclerotic borders. Cortical destruction is uncommon. Bone expansion can result in spinal cord compression.	Benign cartilaginous tumors with chondroblast-like cells and areas of chondroid matrix formation, rarely occur in the spine. Spinal tumors most often involve the thoracic vertebrae and usually involve both the body and pedicles. **(See Atlas Chapter A 7)**
Osteogenic sarcoma (Fig. 2.11)	Destructive malignant lesions, low-intermediate signal on T1WI, mixed low, intermediate, high signal on T2WI, usually + matrix mineralization/ossification, with low signal on T2W images, usually show Gd-contrast enhancement (usually heterogeneous).	Malignant bone lesions rarely occur as primary tumor involving the vertebral column, locally invasive, high metastatic potential. Occur in children as primary tumors and adults (associated with Paget's Paget disease, irradiated bone, chronic osteomyelitis, osteoblastoma, giant cell tumor, and fibrous dysplasia). **(See Atlas Chapter A 64)**

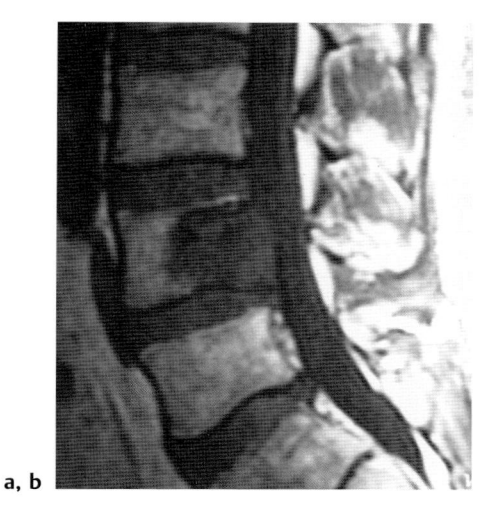

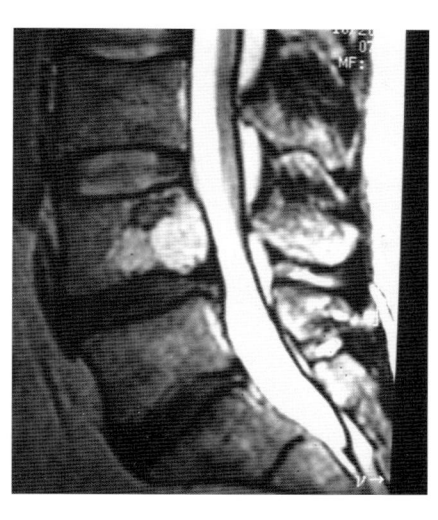

Figure 2.**9 a–c** A 48-year-old man with a chordoma involving the dorsal portion of the L 4 vertebral body. The tumor has low-intermediate signal on sagittal T1WI (**a**) and heterogeneous mostly high signal with small zones of low signal on sagittal T2WI (**b**). The tumor shows Gd-contrast enhancement on sagittal FS T1WI (**c**).

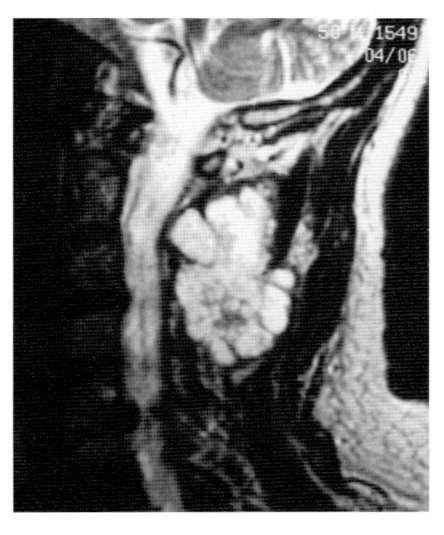

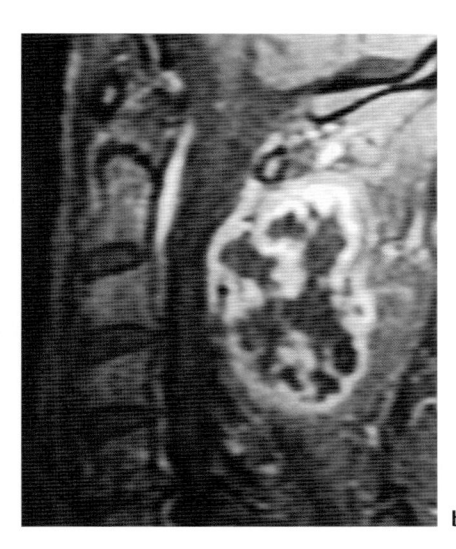

Figure 2.**10 a, b** A 50-year-old man with chondrosarcoma involving the posterior elements of C 3. The tumor has high signal with thin bands of low signal on the sagittal view (**a**) and shows irregular nodular and curvilinear patterns of Gd-contrast enhancement on sagittal FS T1WI (**b**).

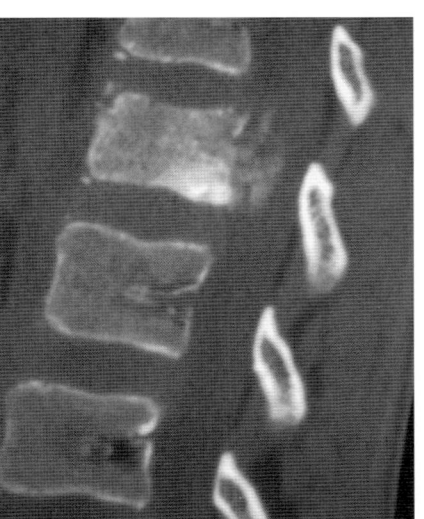

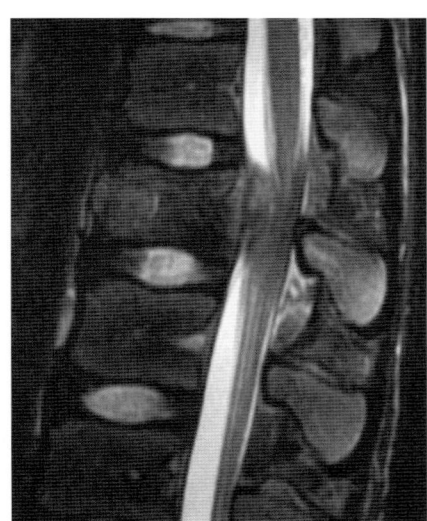

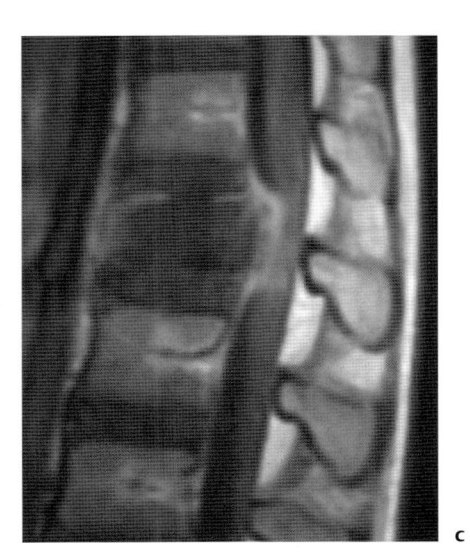

Figure 2.**11 a–c** A 12-year-old boy with osteosarcoma involving the L 1 vertebra. The tumor has heterogeneous mixed sclerotic and lucent zones within the vertebral body with cortical destruction and epidural tumor extension containing cumulus cloud-type matrix ossification on sagittal (**a**) CT. The tumor has mixed low and intermediate signal on sagittal FS T2WI (**b**). The tumor shows heterogeneous Gd-contrast enhancement on sagittal T1WI (**c**). Enhancing tumor extending into the spinal canal compresses the spinal cord.

Table 2 (Continued) Tumors and tumorlike lesions involving the spine		
Tumor/Tumorlike Lesion	**MRI Findings**	**Comments**
Ewing sarcoma (Fig. 2.12)	Destructive malignant lesions involving the vertebral column, low-intermediate signal on T1WI, mixed low, intermediate, and/or high signal on T2WI and FS T2WI, usually show Gd-contrast enhancement (usually heterogeneous).	Usually occurs between the ages of 5 and 30, males > females, rarely occurs as primary tumor involving the spinal column, locally invasive, high metastatic potential. **(See Atlas Chapter A 20)**
Malignant fibrous histiocytoma (MFH) (Fig. 2.13)	Tumors are often associated with zones of cortical destruction and extraosseous soft tissue masses. Tumors have low-intermediate signal on T1WI and heterogeneous intermediate-high signal on T2WI and FS T2WI. Tumors show heterogeneous often prominent enhancement.	Malignant tumors involving soft tissue and rarely bone that are presumed to derive from undifferentiated mesenchymal cells. The World Health Organization (WHO) now uses the term undifferentiated pleomorphic sarcoma for pleomorphic MFH. **(See Atlas Chapter A 48)**
Osteoid osteoma (Fig. 2.14)	Intraosseous circumscribed vertebral lesion often less than 1.5 cm in diameter located in posterior elements, central zone with low-intermediate signal on T1WI and high signal on T2WI and FS T2WI with prominent Gd-contrast enhancement, surrounded by a peripheral rim of low signal on T1WI and T2WI (sclerosis); +/− high signal on T2WI and FS T2WI in bone (edema) beyond zone of sclerosis or in adjacent soft tissues.	Benign osseous lesion containing a nidus of vascularized osteoid trabeculae surrounded by osteoblastic sclerosis, 14 % of osteoid osteomas are located in the spine, usually occurs between ages 5 and 25, males > females. Focal pain and tenderness associated with lesion that is often worse at night, relieved with aspirin. **(See Atlas Chapter A 60)**
Osteoblastoma (Fig. 2.15)	Expansile vertebral lesion often greater than 1.5 cm in diameter located in posterior elements (90 %) +/− extension into vertebral body (30 %), +/− epidural extension (40 %), low-intermediate signal on T1WI and intermediate-high signal on T2WI and FS T2WI, usually show Gd-contrast enhancement. +/− spinal cord/spinal canal compression. +/− high signal on T2WI and FS T2WI in bone (edema) beyond zone of sclerosis or in adjacent soft tissues.	Rare benign bone neoplasm (2 % of bone tumors) usually occurs from 6 to 30 years. One-third of osteoblastomas involve the spine. **(See Atlas Chapter A 61)**

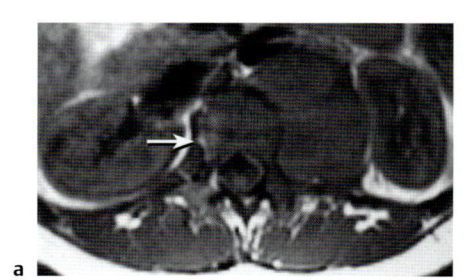

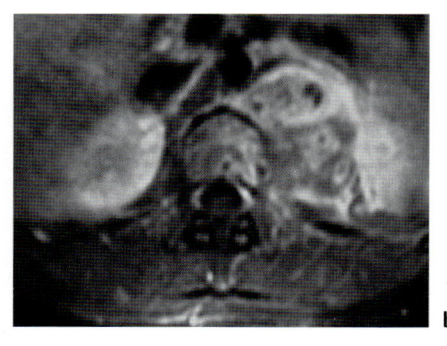

Figure 2.**12 a, b**   A 16-year-old female with Ewing's sarcoma involving a vertebral body with extension laterally into the adjacent soft tissues on the left. Axial (**a**) T1WI shows the tumor to have low-intermediate signal. The tumor shows heterogeneous Gd-contrast enhancement on axial FS T1WI (**b**).

Osteoblastoma 45

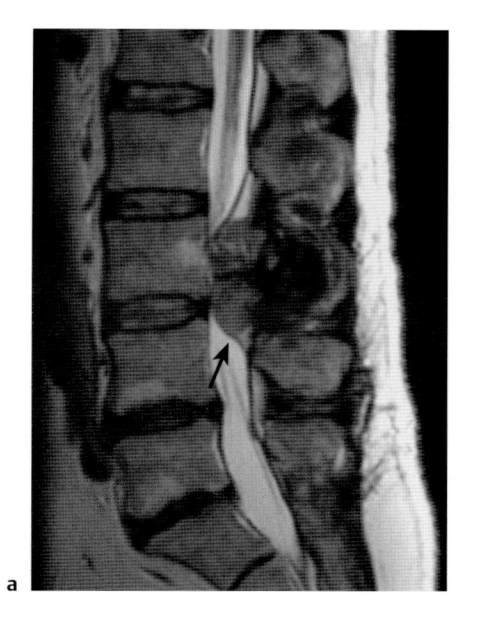

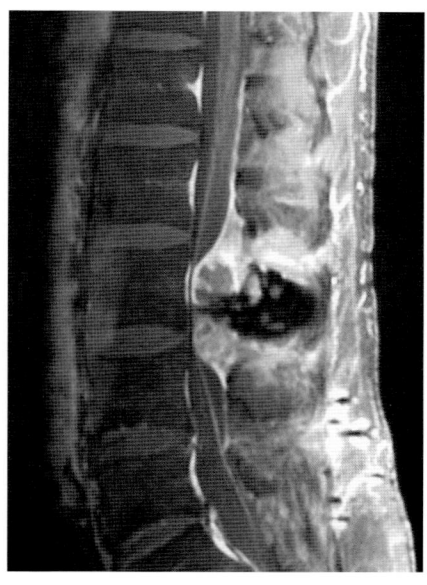

Figure 2.13 a, b A 56-year-old man with malignant fibrous histiocytoma involving the posterior elements at the L3 vertebra with extraosseous extension and spinal canal compression. The tumor has mixed low and intermediate signal on sagittal T2WI (**a**). The tumor shows heterogeneous Gd-contrast enhancement on sagittal FS T1WI (**b**).

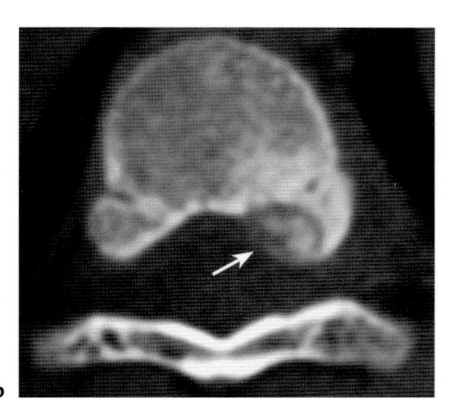

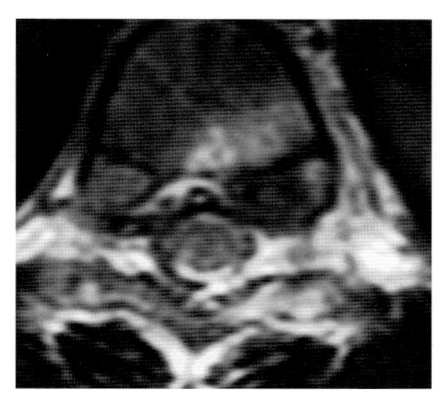

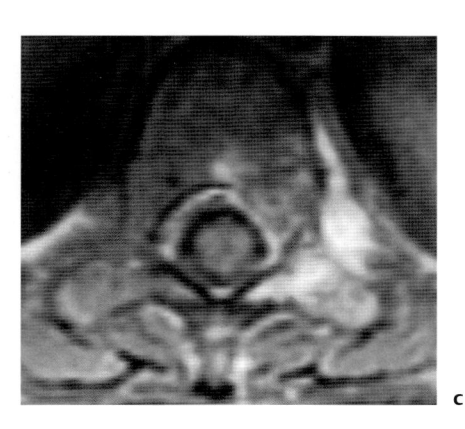

Figure 2.14 a–c A 5-year-old female with an osteoid osteoma involving the left pedicle of the T10 vertebra. Axial CT image (**a**) shows a circumscribed intramedullary lesion with low attenuation surrounding a zone of mineralization/calcification. Sclerotic increased attenuation is seen in the medullary bone adjacent to the lesion. The lesion has low and intermediate signal on axial T2WI (**b**) surrounded by high signal. The lesion shows prominent Gd-contrast enhancement on axial FS T1WI (**c**). In addition, poorly defined zones of Gd-contrast enhancement are seen in the marrow adjacent to the lesion as well as in the extraosseous soft tissues.

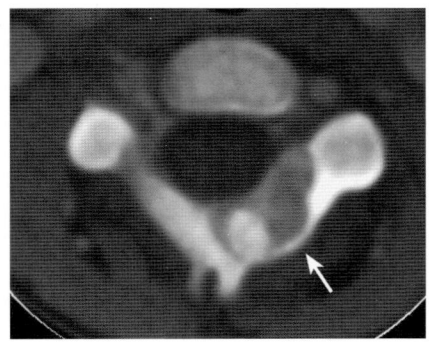

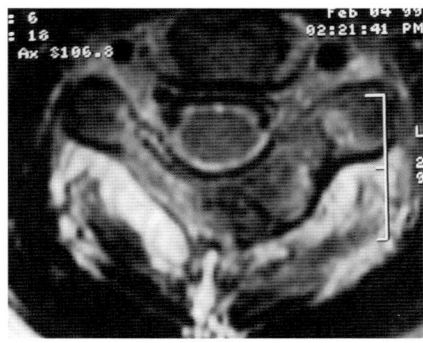

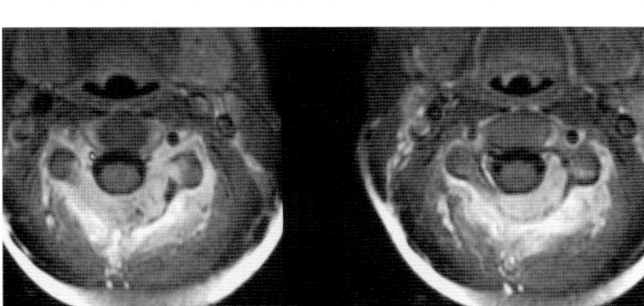

Figure 2.15 a–c A 4-year-old female with an osteoblastoma involving the left lamina of the C3 vertebra. The axial CT image (**a**) shows a circumscribed radiolucent lesion with an internal calcification. Sclerotic reaction is seen in the adjacent bone. Bony expansion with thin peripheral sclerotic rims is seen. The lesion has heterogeneous low-intermediate signal on axial T2WI (**b**). The lesion shows prominent Gd-contrast enhancement on axial FS T1WI (**c**). Poorly defined zones of high signal on T2WI and corresponding Gd-contrast enhancement are seen in the marrow and soft tissues adjacent to the osteoblastoma.

Table 2 (Continued) **Tumors and tumorlike lesions involving the spine**

Tumor/Tumorlike Lesion	MRI Findings	Comments
Giant cell tumor (Fig. 2.16)	Circumscribed extradural vertebral lesion with low-intermediate signal on T1WI, high signal on T2WI +/− surrounding thin zone of low signal on T2WI, usually show Gd-contrast enhancement; Location: vertebral body > vertebral body and vertebral arch > vertebral arch alone. +/− spinal cord / spinal canal compression.	Locally aggressive lesions that rarely metastasize. Account for 5% of primary bone tumors Usually involve lone bones, only 4% involve vertebrae. Occur in adolescents and adults (20–40 years). **(See Atlas Chapter A 29)**
Aneurysmal bone cyst (Fig. 2.17)	Circumscribed extradural vertebral lesion usually involving the posterior elements +/− involvement of the vertebral body; with variable low, intermediate, high, and/or mixed signal on T1WI and T2WI, +/− surrounding thin zone of low signal on T2WI, +/− lobulations, +/− one or multiple fluid–fluid levels.	Expansile blood/debris-filled lesions that may be primary lesions or occur secondary to other bone lesions such as giant cell tumor, fibrous dysplasia, chondroblastoma. Most occur in patients < 30 years. Locations: lumbar > cervical > thoracic. Clinical findings can include neurologic deficits and pain. **(See Atlas Chapter A 2)**
Osteochondroma (Fig. 2.18)	Circumscribed sessile lesion typically arising from posterior elements of vertebrae, central zone with intermediate signal on T1WI and T2WI similar to marrow surrounded by a peripheral zone of low signal on T1WI and T2WI, + cartilaginous cap. Increased malignant potential when cartilaginous cap is > 2 cm thick.	Benign cartilaginous tumors arising from defect at periphery of growth plate during bone formation with resultant bone outgrowth covered by a cartilaginous cap. Usually benign lesions unless associated with pain and increasing size of cartilaginous cap. **(See Atlas Chapter A 58)**
Hemangioma (Fig. 2.19)	Circumscribed or diffuse vertebral lesion usually located in the vertebral body +/− extension into pedicle or isolated within pedicle, typically have intermediate-high signal on T1WI, high signal on T2WI and FS T2W, associated with thickened vertical trabeculae, usually show Gd-contrast enhancement, multiple in 30%, thoracic (60%) > lumbar (30%) > cervical (10%).	Most common benign lesions involving vertebral column, women > men, composed of endothelial-lined capillary and cavernous spaces within marrow associated with thickened vertical trabeculae and decreased secondary trabeculae, seen in 11% of autopsies. Usually asymptomatic, rarely cause bone expansion and epidural extension resulting in neural compression (usually in thoracic region), increased potential for fracture with epidural hematoma. **(See Atlas Chapter A 34)**

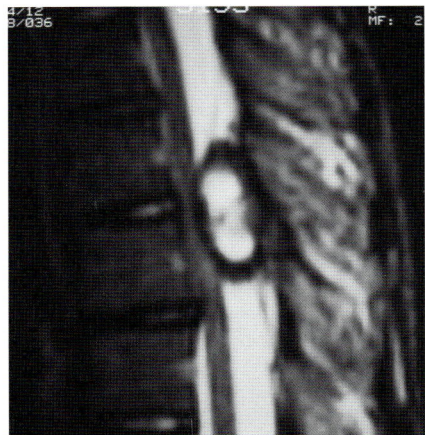

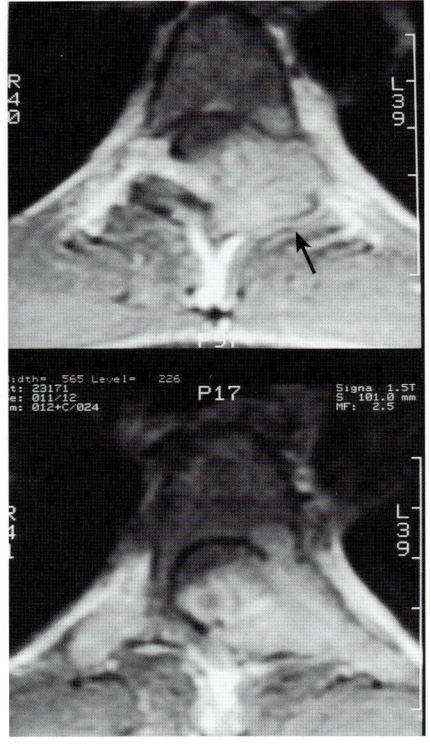

Figure 2.16 a, b Giant cell tumor involving a thoracic vertebra in a 15-year-old male. The lesion involves the vertebral body, left pedicle, left transverse process, and left lamina. Epidural tumor extension causes spinal cord compression. The tumor has well-defined margins, and has a central high signal on sagittal FS T2WI (**a**) surrounded by a rim of low signal. The tumor shows prominent Gd-contrast enhancement on axial T1WI (**b**).

Hemangioma 47

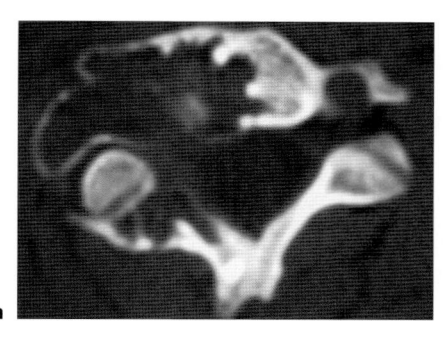

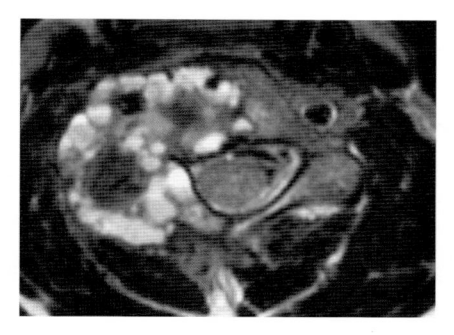

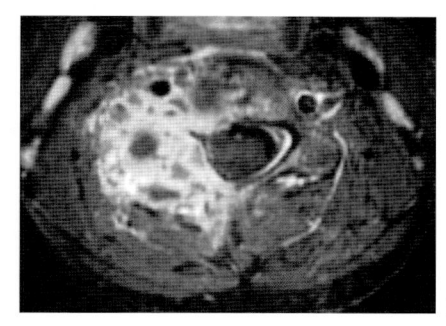

Figure 2.**17 a–c** A 12-year-old girl with an aneurysmal bone cyst seen as a radiolucent expansile lesion involving the right side of the C5 vertebral body, right transverse process, right pedicle, and lamina on axial CT (**a**). The MRI shows the lesion to have mixed low, intermediate, and high signal with multiple fluid–fluid levels on axial T2WI (**b**). The lesion shows multiple lobules with peripheral rim-like Gd-contrast enhancement on axial FS T1WI (**c**).

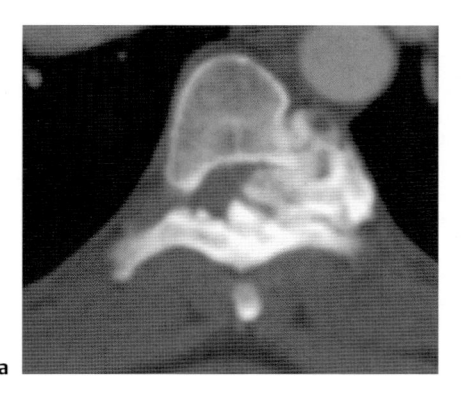

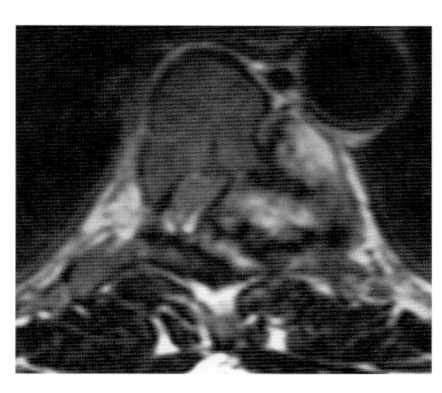

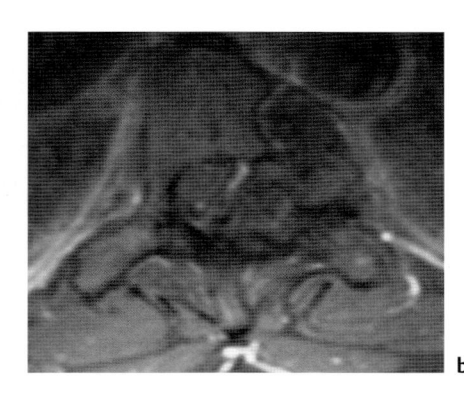

Figure 2.**18 a–c** A 43-year-old woman with an osteochondroma involving the left pedicle of a thoracic vertebra with extension of the lesion into the spinal canal resulting in compression of the spinal cord as seen on axial CT image (**a**) and axial T2WI (**b**). The lesion has a central signal similar and slightly higher to marrow on T2WI surrounded by a thin rim of low signal from subchondral bone. The cartilaginous cap is very thin and shows minimal Gd-contrast enhancement on axial FS T1WI (**c**).

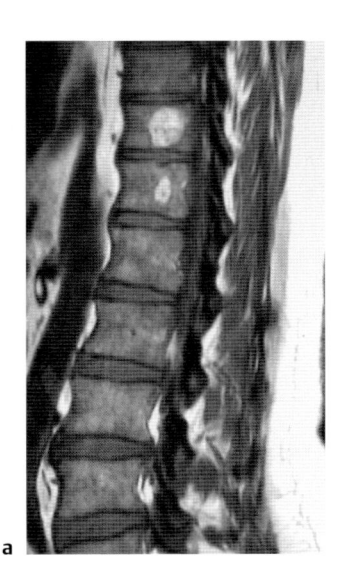

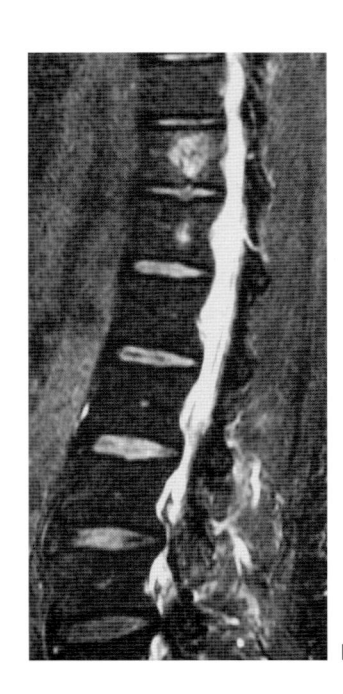

Figure 2.**19 a, b** Hemangiomas in the T12 and L1 vertebral bodies. The hemangiomas have mostly high signal on sagittal (**a**) T1WI, and sagittal FS T2WI (**b**).

Table 2 (Continued) Tumors and tumorlike lesions involving the spine

Tumor/Tumorlike Lesion	MRI Findings	Comments
Hemangioendothelioma (Fig. 2.20)	Lesions usually have sharp margins that may be slightly lobulated and often have low-intermediate signal on T1WI, and heterogeneous intermediate-high signal on T2WI and FS T2WI with zones of low signal. Lesions can be multifocal. Extraosseous extension of tumor through zones of cortical destruction can be seen. Lesions often show prominent heterogeneous Gd-contrast enhancement.	Vasoformative/endothelial low-grade malignant neoplasms that are locally aggressive and rarely metastasize compared with high-grade angiosarcoma. **(See Atlas Chapter A 33)**
Hemangiopericytoma (Fig. 2.21)	Tumors usually have well-defined margins, with or without lobulations, low-intermediate signal on T1WI, intermediate or slightly high to high signal on T2WI, and heterogeneous high signal on FS T2WI. On T2WI, lesions may contain tubular signal voids centrally or peripherally likely representing tumor vessels. Tumors can contain hemorrhagic zones with corresponding MR signal alteration. Tumors often show moderate to prominent Gd-contrast enhancement.	Rare malignant tumors of pericytic origin that occur in soft tissues and less frequently in bone. **(See Atlas Chapter A 35)**
Other tumorlike lesions		
Arachnoid cyst (Fig. 2.22)	Well-circumscribed extra-axial lesions with low signal on T1WI and FLAIR, and high signal on T2WI and FS T2WI, similar to CSF, no Gd-contrast enhancement. Usually cause mass effect on the adjacent spinal cord. Chronic erosive changes can be seen at the vertebrae adjacent to the cyst.	Non-neoplastic acquired, developmental, or congenital extra-axial cysts filled with CSF. Cysts can be small or large, asymptomatic or symptomatic.
Tarlov cyst (perineural cyst) (Fig. 2.23)	Well-circumscribed cysts with MRI signal comparable to CSF involving nerve root sleeves associated with chronic erosive changes involving adjacent bony structures. Sacral (+/− widening of sacral foramina) > lumbar nerve root sleeves. Usually range from 15 to 20 mm in diameter, but can be larger.	Typically represent incidental asymptomatic anatomic variants associated with prior dural injury.

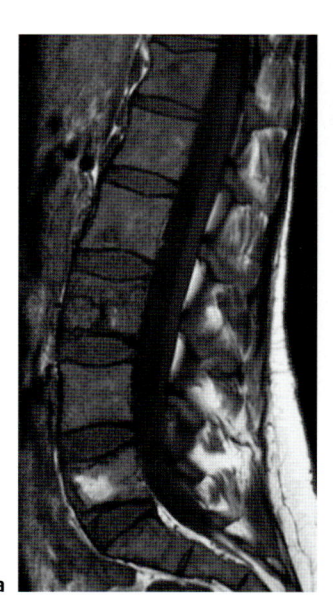

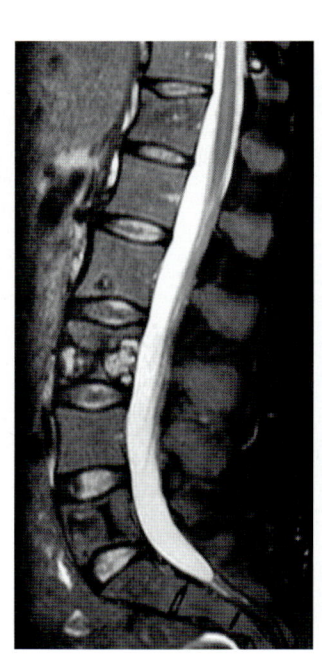

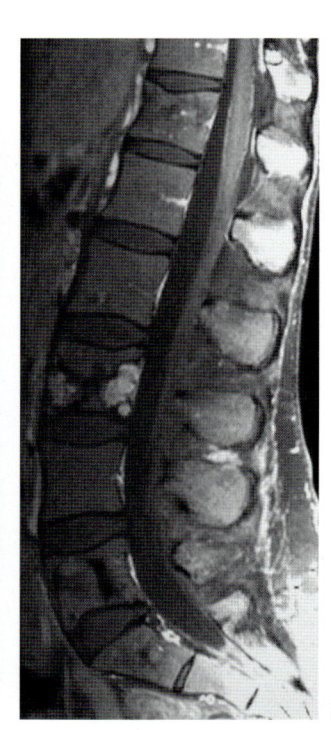

Figure 2.**20 a–d** A 42-year-old woman with multifocal hemangioendotheliomas involving the L2, L3, and L5 vertebral bodies. The lesions have mixed low-intermediate and high signal on sagittal T1WI (**a**), and sagittal FS T2WI (**b**). Lesion in the L3 vertebral body shows Gd-contrast enhancement on sagittal FS T1WI (**c**).

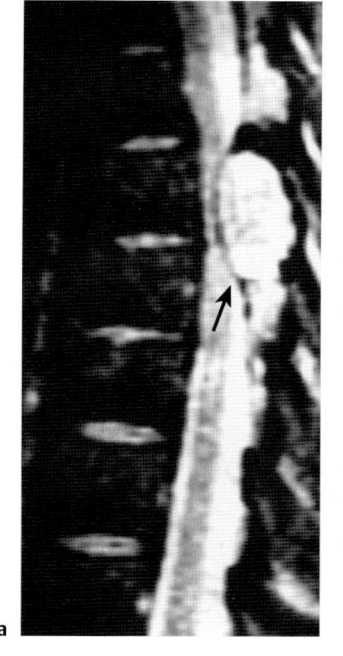

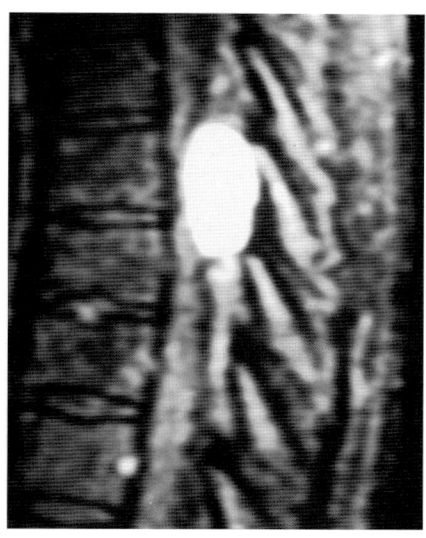

Figure 2.**21 a, b** Posterior epidural hemangiopericytoma involving the thoracic spine with spinal cord compression. The tumor has high signal on sagittal T2WI (**a**) and shows prominent Gd-contrast enhancement on sagittal FS T1WI (**b**).

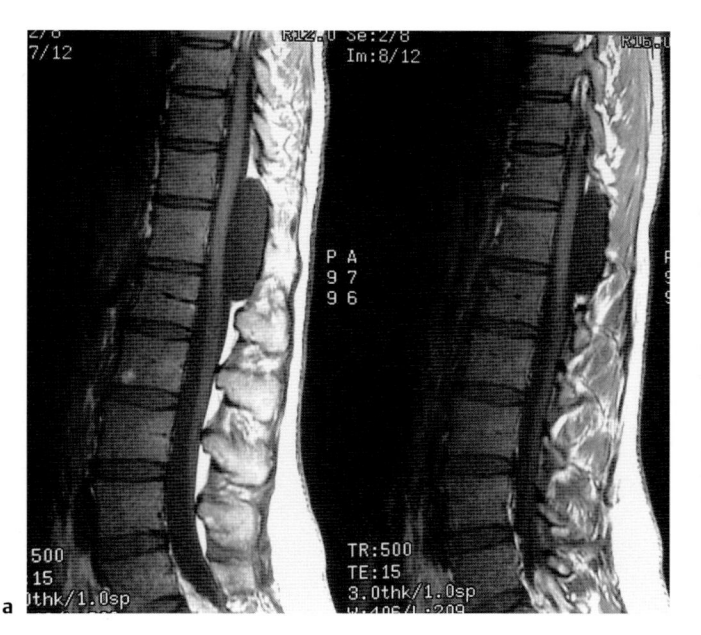

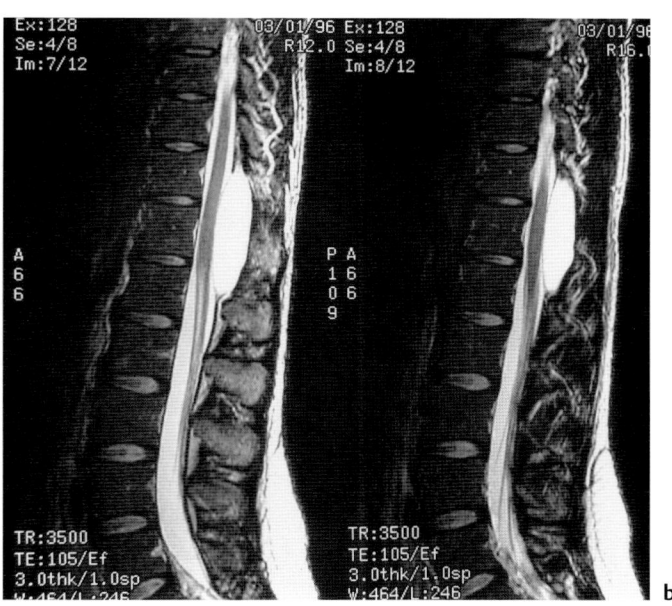

Figure 2.**22 a, b** A 35-year-old woman with an arachnoid cyst at the dorsal portion of the spinal canal at the thoracolumbar junction. The cyst has circumscribed margins and contains fluid with low signal on sagittal T1WI (**a**) and high signal on sagittal (**b**) T2WI.

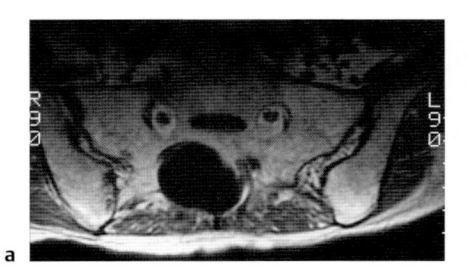

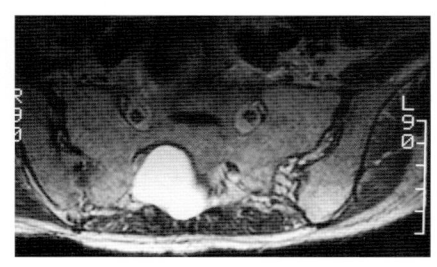

Figure 2.**23 a, b** A well-circumscribed cyst with MRI signal comparable to CSF is seen at the right S 3 nerve root sleeve with associated expansion of the adjacent sacral foramen on axial T1WI (**a**) and axial T2WI (**b**).

Table 2 (Continued)   Tumors and tumorlike lesions involving the spine

Tumor/Tumorlike Lesion	MRI Findings	Comments
Dermoid (Fig. 2.24)	Well-circumscribed spheroid or multilobulated intradural extramedullary or intramedullary lesions, usually with intermediate-high signal on T1WI, and variable low, intermediate, and/or high signal on T2WI. Usually show no Gd-contrast enhancement, +/– fluid–fluid or fluid–debris levels. Lumbar region most common location in spine. Can cause chemical meningitis if dermoid cyst ruptures into the subarachnoid space. Commonly located: at or near midline.	Non-neoplastic congenital or acquired ectodermal inclusion cystic lesions filled with lipid material, cholesterol, desquamated cells, and keratinaceous debris, usually mild mass effect on adjacent spinal cord or nerve roots, adults: males slightly > females, +/– related clinical symptoms. **(See Atlas Chapter A 15)**
Epidermoid	Well-circumscribed spheroid or multilobulated intradural extramedullary lesion with low-intermediate signal on T1WI, and high signal on T2WI and diffusion-weighted images, mixed low, intermediate, or high signal on FLAIR images, typically show no Gd-contrast enhancement.	Non-neoplastic extramedullary epithelial-inclusion lesions filled with desquamated cells and keratinaceous debris, usually mild mass effect on adjacent spinal cord and/or nerve roots. May be congenital (+/– associated with dorsal dermal sinus, spina bifida, hemivertebrae) or acquired (late complication of lumbar puncture). **(See Atlas Chapter A 15)**
Neurenteric (endodermal) cyst (Fig. 2.25)	Well-circumscribed spheroid intradural extramedullary lesions, with low, intermediate, or high signal on T1WI and T2WI, and usually showing no Gd-contrast enhancement. Lesions may extend into the spinal cord in 10 %.	A type of split cord malformation in which there is a persistent communication between ventrally located endoderm and dorsally located ectoderm secondary to developmental failure of separation of notochord and foregut, observed in patients < 40 years. Obliteration of portions of a dorsal enteric sinus can result in cysts lined by endothelium, fibrous cords, or sinuses. Can occur within spinal canal (ventral > dorsal to the spinal cord), commonly in cervical and upper thoracic regions, and are often associated with vertebral anomalies such as hemivertebrae, butterfly vertebrae, clefts in vertebral bodies, and zones of incomplete segmentation. Patients can present with local and distal long tract symptoms and progressive spinal cord compression.

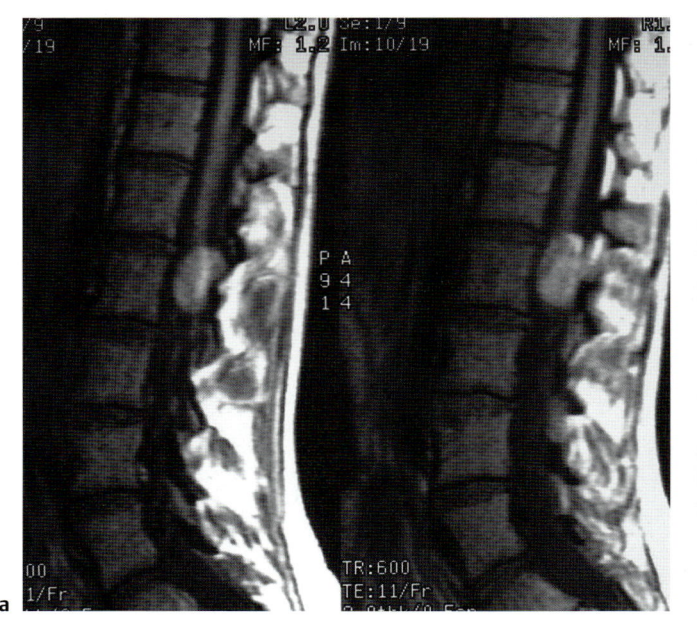

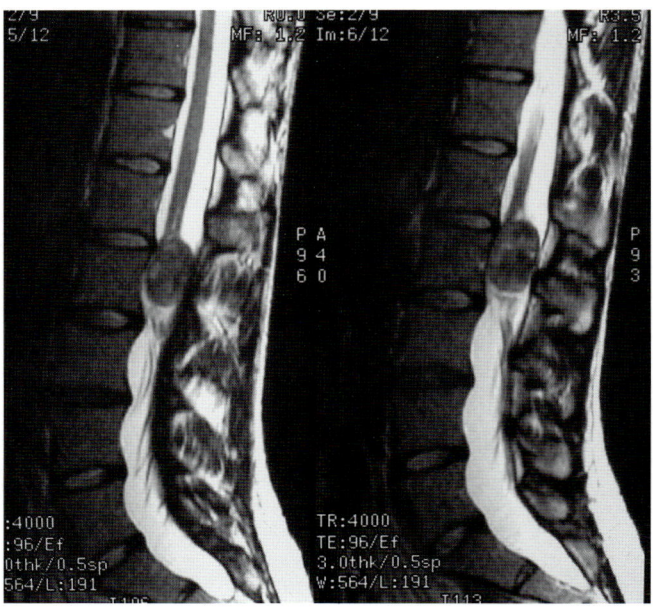

Figure 2.24 a, b   A 27-year-old woman with a dermoid in the posterior lumbar spinal canal. The lesion has high signal on sagittal T1WI (**a**), and low-intermediate signal on sagittal (**b**).

Neurenteric (endodermal) cyst 51

Figure 2.**25 a–e** A 7-year-old girl with a neurenteric cyst in the anterior portion of the cervical spinal canal which compresses the ventral margin of the spinal cord. The lateral radiograph (**a**) and coronal CT image (**b**) show segmentation anomalies and remnants of a midline cleft involving multiple vertebral bodies ventral to the neurenteric cyst. The cyst has high signal on sagittal T1WI (**c**) and FS T1WI (**d**), and low-intermediate signal on FS T2WI (**e**).

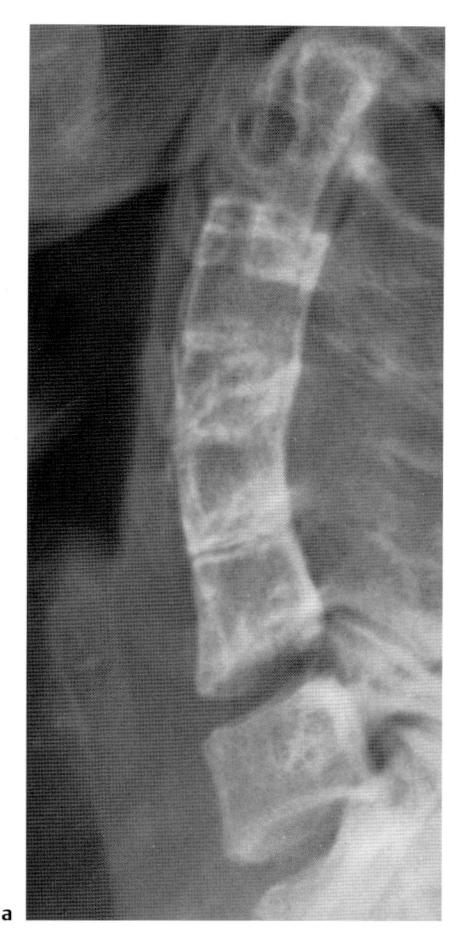

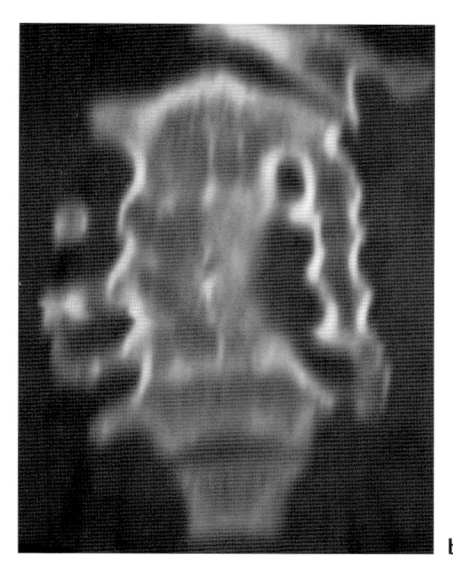

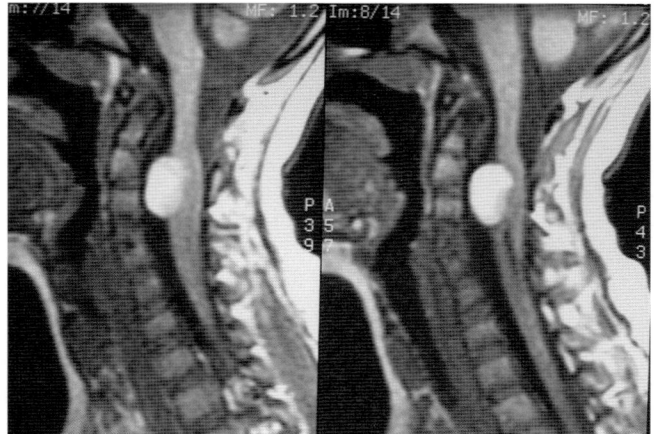

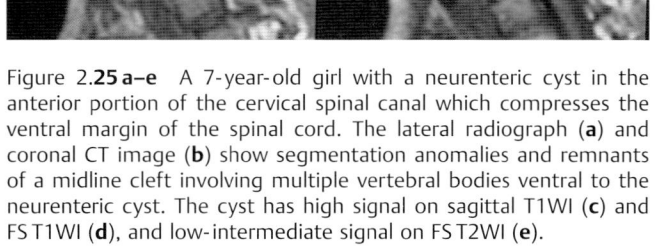

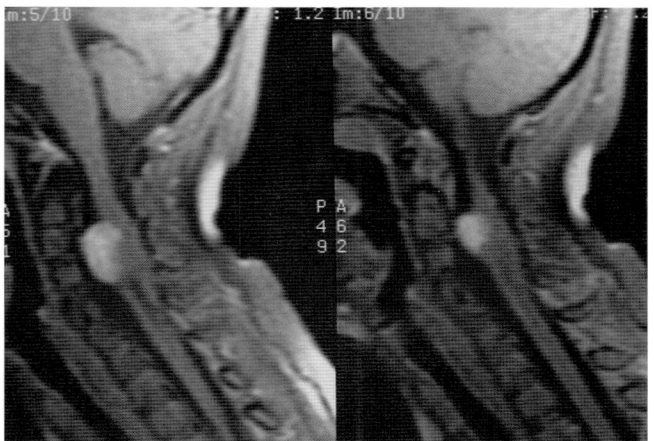

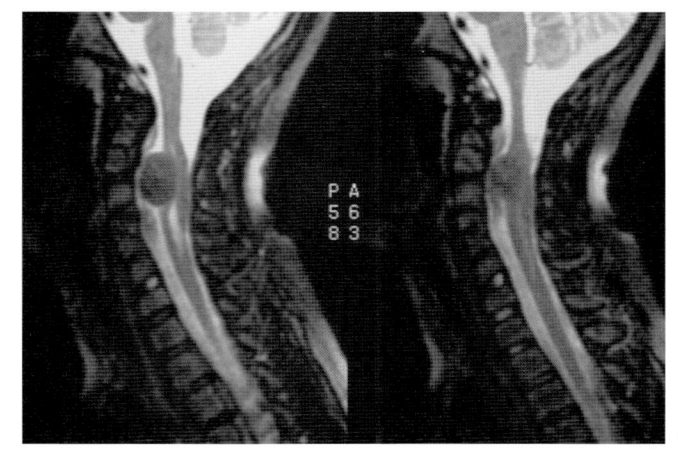

Table 2 (Continued)   **Tumors and tumorlike lesions involving the spine**

Tumor/Tumorlike Lesion	MRI Findings	Comments
Synovial cyst (Fig. 2.26)	Circumscribed lesion located adjacent to the facet joint. A thin rim of low signal on T2WI surrounds a central zone that may have low-intermediate signal on T1WI, and low, intermediate, and or high signal on T2WI. No central Gd-contrast enhancement is usually seen, but a thin rim of peripheral enhancement may be observed.	Represents protrusion of synovium with fluid from degenerated facet joint into the spinal canal medially or dorsally into the posterior paraspinal soft tissues. Variable MRI signal is related to the contents that may include serous or mucinous fluid, blood, hemosiderin, and/or gas. **(See Atlas Chapter A 74)**
Bone island (Fig. 2.27)	Usually appear as a circumscribed radiodense ovoid or spheroid focus in medullary bone that may or may not contact the endosteal surface of cortical bone. Typically have low signal comparable to cortical bone on all pulse sequences.	Bone islands (enostoses) are non-neoplastic intramedullary zones of mature compact bone composed of lamellar bone; considered to be developmental anomalies resulting from localized failure of bone resorption during skeletal maturation. **(See Atlas Chapter A 62)**
Melorheostosis (Fig. 2.28)	MRI signal varies based on the relative proportions of chondroid, mineralized osteoid, and soft tissue components in these lesions. Mineralized zones typically have low signal on T1WI and T2WI, no Gd-contrast enhancement. Nonmineralized portions can have low-intermediate signal on T1WI, intermediate to high signal on T2WI, and show Gd-contrast enhancement.	Rare bone dysplasia with cortical thickening that has a "flowing candle wax" configuration. Associated soft tissue masses occur in ~25%. The soft tissue lesions often contain mixtures of chondroid material, mineralized osteoid, and fibrovascular tissue. Surgery is usually performed only for lesions causing symptoms. **(See Atlas Chapter A 62)**

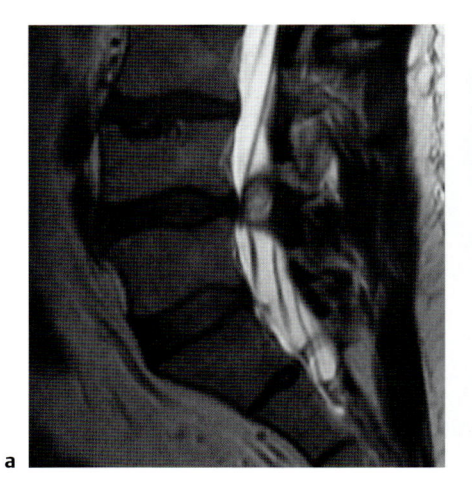

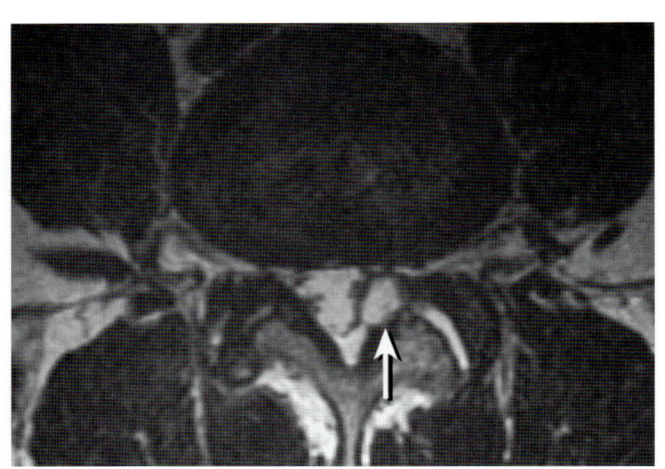

Figure 2.**26 a, b**   A 51-year-old man who has a synovial cyst extending from the medial aspect of the left L 4–L 5 facet joint, which mildly compresses the lateral margin of the thecal sac. The cyst lesion shows slightly high to high signal on sagittal (**a**) and axial (**b**) T2WI. A thin rim of low signal on T2WI is seen at the periphery of the lesion.

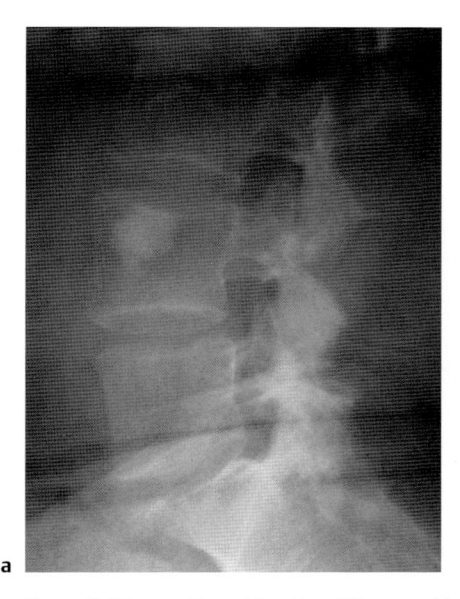

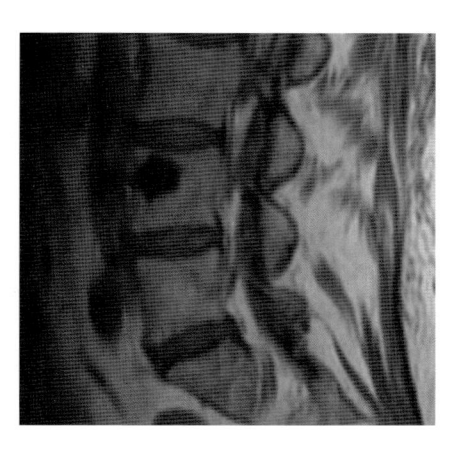

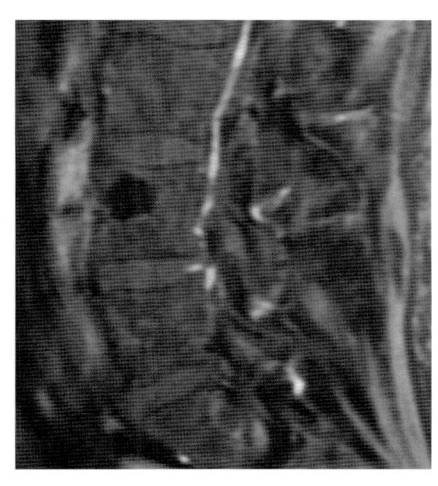

Figure 2.**27 a–c** Bone island in a 70-year-old woman. A circumscribed dense lesion is seen in the L 4 vertebral body on a lateral radiograph (**a**). The lesion has low signal on sagittal T1WI (**b**). The lesion shows no Gd-contrast enhancement on sagittal FS T1WI (**c**).

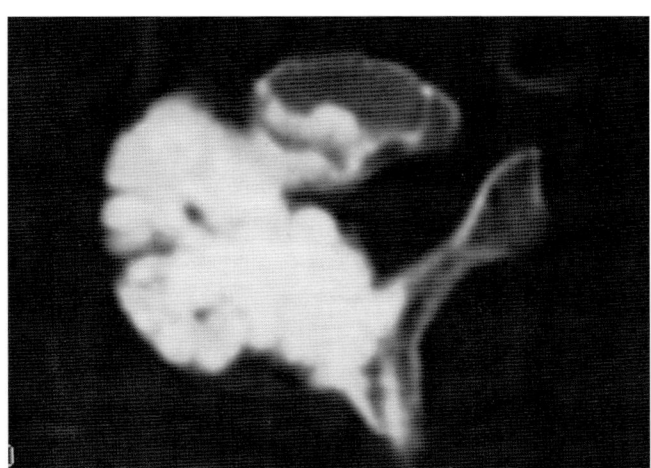

Figure 2.**28 a–c** A 53-year-old man with melorheostosis involving multiple vertebrae at the cervical and upper thoracic spine. The axial (**a**) CT image shows smooth zones of cortical hyperostosis with a "dripping candle wax" appearance at the right sides of the involved vertebrae. The zones of cortical hyperostosis show low signal on the axial (**b**) T2WI. No Gd-contrast enhancement is seen on the axial FS T1WI (**c**).

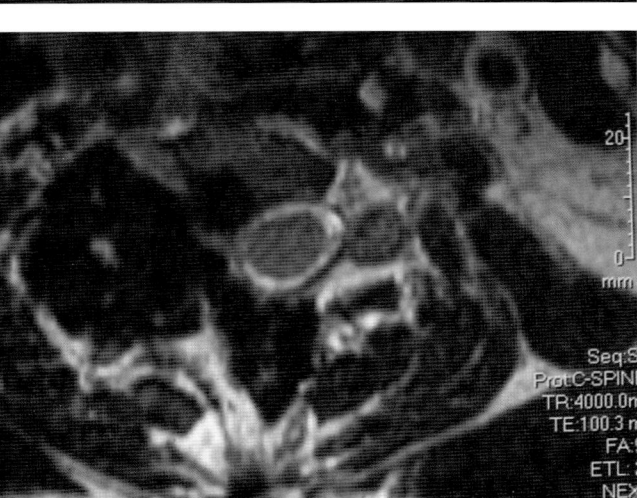

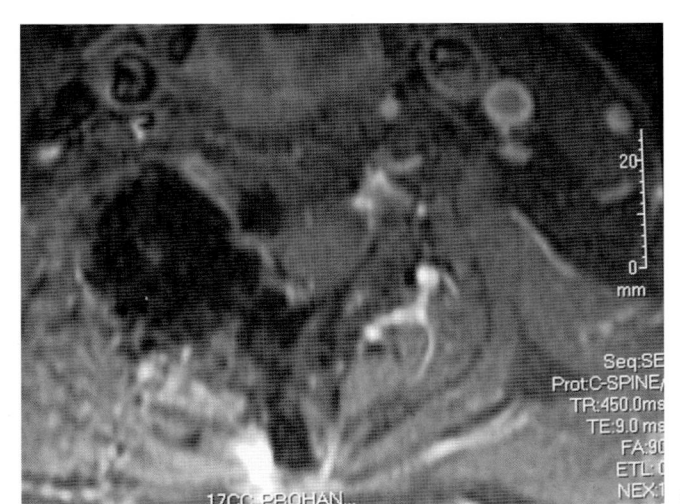

Table 2 (Continued) **Tumors and tumorlike lesions involving the spine**

Tumor/Tumorlike Lesion	MRI Findings	Comments
Trauma		
Fracture	**Traumatic and osteopenic vertebral fracture (Fig. 2.29)** Acute/subacute fractures have sharply angulated cortical margins, near-complete or complete abnormal signal (usually low signal on T1WI, high signal on T2WI, and FS T2WI in marrow of affected vertebral body. Gd-contrast enhancement is seen in the early postfracture period, no destructive changes at cortical margins of fractured endplates. +/− convex outward angulated configuration of compressed vertebral bodies, +/− spinal cord and/or spinal canal compression related to fracture deformity, +/− retropulsed bone fragments into spinal canal, +/− subluxation, +/− kyphosis, +/−epidural hematoma, +/− high signal on T2WI and FS T2WI involving marrow of posterior elements or between the inter-spinous ligaments. Chronic healed fractures usually have normal or near normal signal in compressed vertebral body. Occasionally persistence of signal abnormalities in vertebral marrow results from instability and abnormal axial loading. **Malignancy related vertebral fracture (Fig. 2.30)** Near-complete or complete abnormal marrow signal (usually low signal on T1WI, high signal on T2WI and FS T2WI, occasionally low signal on T2WI for metastases with sclerotic reaction) in involved vertebra(e). Lesions usually show Gd-contrast enhancement, +/− destructive changes at cortical margins of vertebrae, +/−convex outward-bowed configuration of compressed vertebral bodies, +/− paravertebral mass lesions, +/− spheroid or diffuse signal abnormalities/lesions in other noncompressed vertebral bodies.	Vertebral fractures can result from trauma, primary bone tumors/lesions, metastatic disease, bone infarcts (steroids, chemotherapy, and radiation treatment), osteoporosis, osteomalacia, metabolic (calcium/phosphate) disorders, vitamin deficiencies, Paget disease, and genetic disorders (e. g., osteogenesis imperfecta).
Degenerative changes		
Marrow changes related to degenerative disk disease	**Type 1:** Poorly defined zones with low-intermediate signal on T1WI (decreased relative to normal marrow), slightly high signal on T2WI (increased relative to normal marrow), and high signal on FS T2WI in marrow next to intact endplates, often associated with Gd-contrast enhancement, intervening disk usually with degenerative changes. **(Fig. 2.31) Type 2:** Poorly defined zones with intermediate-slightly high signal on T1WI images (increased relative to normal marrow), intermediate-slightly high signal on T2WI (isointense or increased relative to normal marrow), and low or intermediate signal on FS T2WI in marrow next to intact endplates, +/− Gd-contrast enhancement, intervening disk usually with degenerative changes. **(Fig. 2.32) Type 1 and 2 marrow changes** can also be focal in association with degenerative disk disease and Schmorl's nodes.	Reactive changes in marrow from degenerative disk disease can result from fissuring of endplates with edematous changes and/or replacement with fibrovascular tissue in the subjacent marrow. The endplate margins typically appear intact as thin linear zones of low signal on T1WI and T2WI adjacent to a degenerated disk with low signal on T2W images. These latter two findings differ from the MRI features of vertebral osteomyelitis where there is often destruction of the endplates and annulus, as well as high signal on T2WI within the disk.

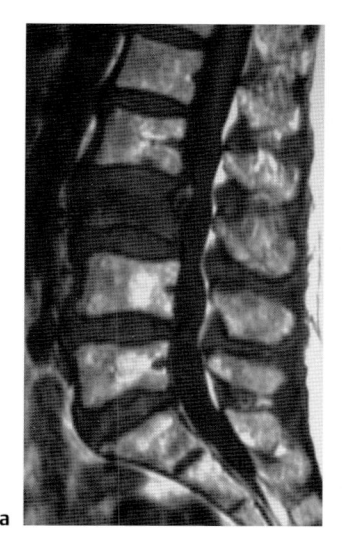

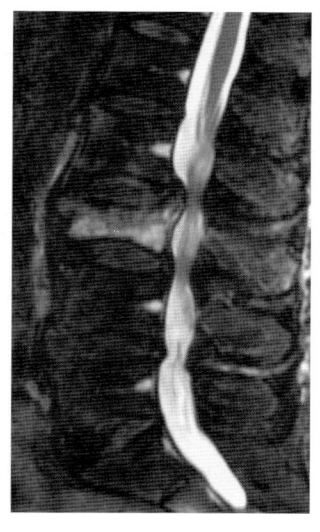

Figure 2.**29 a, b** An 82-year-old woman with a recent osteoporotic compression fracture involving the superior endplate of the L 3 vertebral body. Sharply angulated cortical margins are seen at the fracture site, and the marrow has low signal on sagittal T1WI (**a**) and high signal on sagittal FS T2WI (**b**).

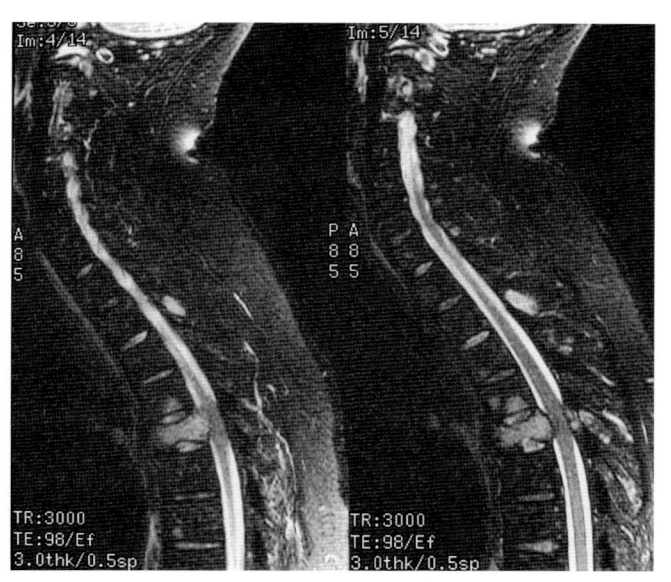

Figure 2.**30** Multiple myeloma involving the spine including one lesion in a thoracic vertebral body that has a pathologic fracture causing spinal cord compression. The lesions including the fractured vertebral body have high signal on sagittal FS T2WI.

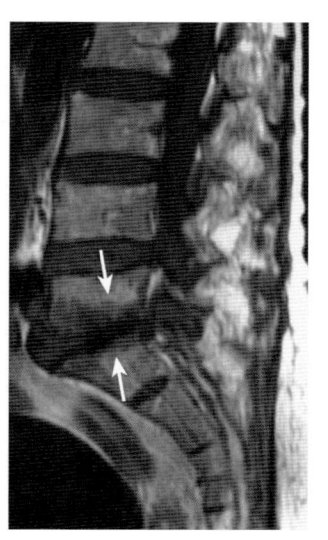

Figure 2.**31 a, b** Poorly defined zones of low-intermediate signal are seen in the marrow adjacent to the endplates at the L 5–S 1 level on the sagittal T1WI (**a**), which have high signal on the sagittal FS T2WI (**b**) representing reactive edematous changes secondary to the degenerative disk disease in this location.

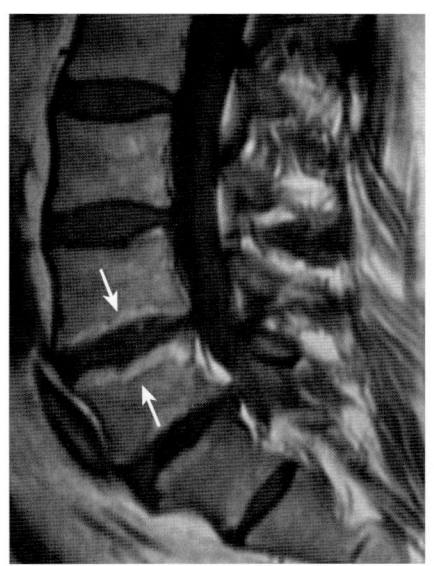

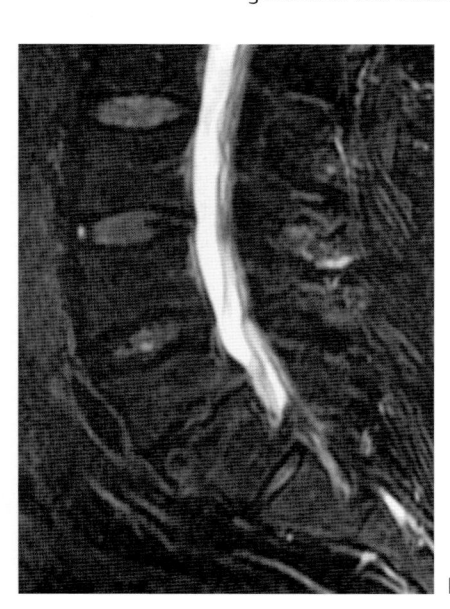

Figure 2.**32 a, b** Poorly defined zones of fatty signal are seen in the marrow adjacent to the endplates at the L 4–L 5 and L 5–S 1 levels secondary to chronic degenerative disk disease in these locations. The fatty marrow has high signal on sagittal T1WI (**a**), which is suppressed on sagittal T2WI (**b**).

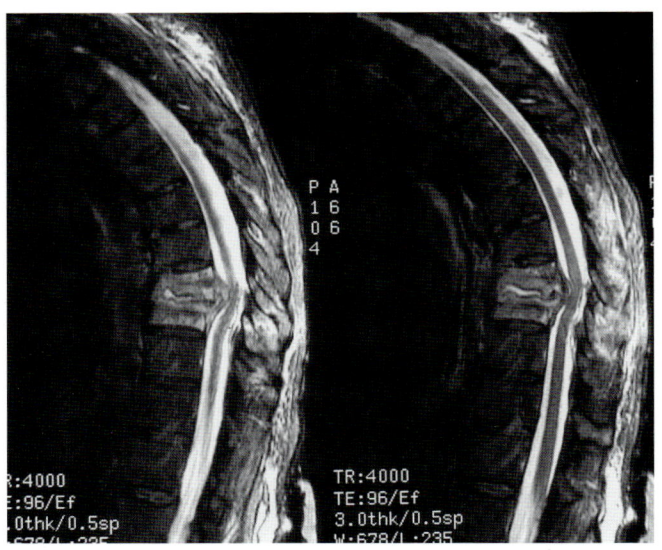

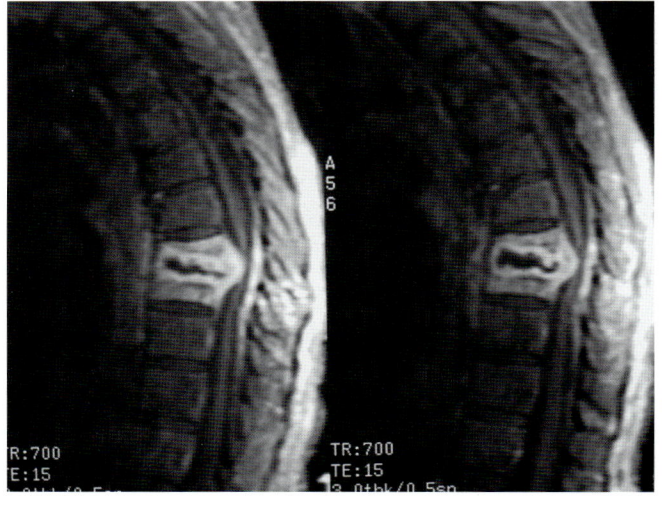

Table 2 (Continued)   Tumors and tumorlike lesions involving the spine

Tumor/Tumorlike Lesion	MRI Findings	Comments
Inflammation/Infection		
Pyogenic vertebral osteomyelitis/diskitis (Fig. 2.33)	Poorly defined zones of low-intermediate signal on T1WI and high signal on T2WI and FS T2WI in marrow of two or more adjacent vertebral bodies and intervening disk(s), and +/− paravertebral soft tissues; +/− irregular deficiencies of endplates (loss of linear low signal on T1WI and T2WI); usually with prominent Gd-contrast enhancement in marrow and paravertebral soft tissues; variable enhancement of disk (patchy zones within disk, and/or thin or thick peripheral enhancement; +/− epidural abscess / paravertebral abscess (high signal collections on T2WI surrounded by a peripheral rim of gadolinium enhancement on T1WI. +/− vertebral compression deformity; +/− spinal cord or spinal canal compression.	Vertebral osteomyelitis represents 3% of osseous infections, results from hematogenous source (most common) from distant infection or intravenous drug abuse; complication of surgery, trauma, diabetes; spread from contiguous soft tissue infection. Initially involves end-arterioles in marrow adjacent to endplates with eventual destruction and spread to the adjacent vertebra through the disk. Children and adults > 50 years. Gram-positive organisms (*Staph. aureus*, *S. epidermidis*, *Streptococcus*, etc) account for 70% of pyogenic osteomyelitis and Gram-negative organisms (*Pseudomonas aeruginosa*, *Escherichia coli*, *Proteus*, etc) represent 30%. Fungal osteomyelitis can appear similar to pyogenic infection of spine. **(See Atlas Chapter A 63)**

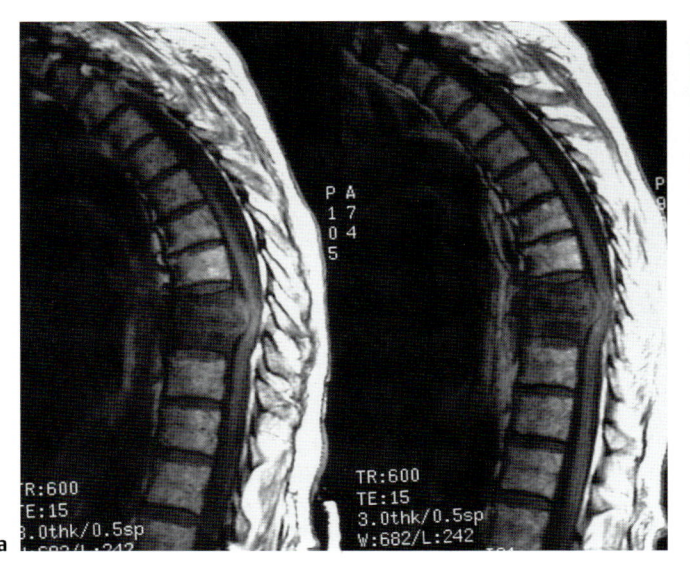

Figure **2.33 a–c**   A 77-year-old woman with pyogenic osteomyelitis involving two adjacent thoracic vertebral bodies and infection of the intervening disk. Poorly defined zones of low signal on sagittal T1WI (**a**) and high signal on sagittal FS T2WI (**b**) are seen throughout the marrow of the vertebral bodies and intervening disk. Loss of definition of the low signal line of the end plates of the vertebral bodies is seen on T1WI and FS T2WI. Prominent diffuse Gd-contrast enhancement is seen in the involved marrow on sagittal FS T1WI (**c**).

Table 2 (Continued) Tumors and tumorlike lesions involving the spine		
Tumor/Tumorlike Lesion	MRI Findings	Comments
Vertebral osteomyelitis-tuberculosis (Fig. 2.34)	Poorly defined zones of low-intermediate signal on T1WI and high signal on T2W and FS T2W images in marrow of two or more adjacent vertebral bodies, Limited disk involvement early in the disease process tends to spare the disk until later in the disease process; +/− paravertebral soft tissues; +/− irregular deficiencies of endplates (loss of linear low signal on T1W and T2W images); usually associated with Gd-contrast enhancement in marrow and paravertebral soft tissues; +/− epidural abscess, often paravertebral abscesses (high signal collections on T2WI surrounded by a peripheral rim(s) of Gd-contrast enhancement on T1WI. +/− vertebral compression deformity; +/− spinal cord or spinal canal compression.	Initially involves marrow in the anterior portion of the vertebral body with spread to the adjacent vertebrae along the anterior longitudinal ligament, often sparing the disk until later in the disease process; usually associated with paravertebral abscesses that may be more prominent than the vertebral abnormalities. (See Atlas Chapter A 63)

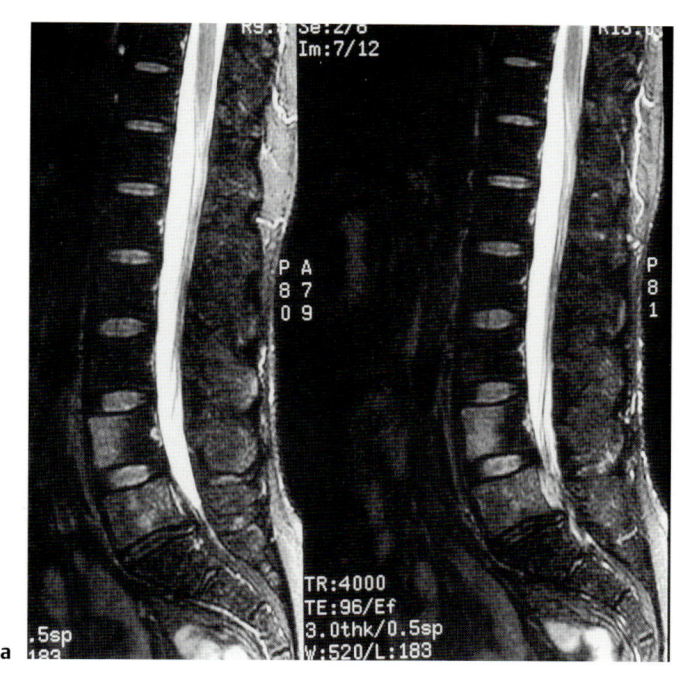

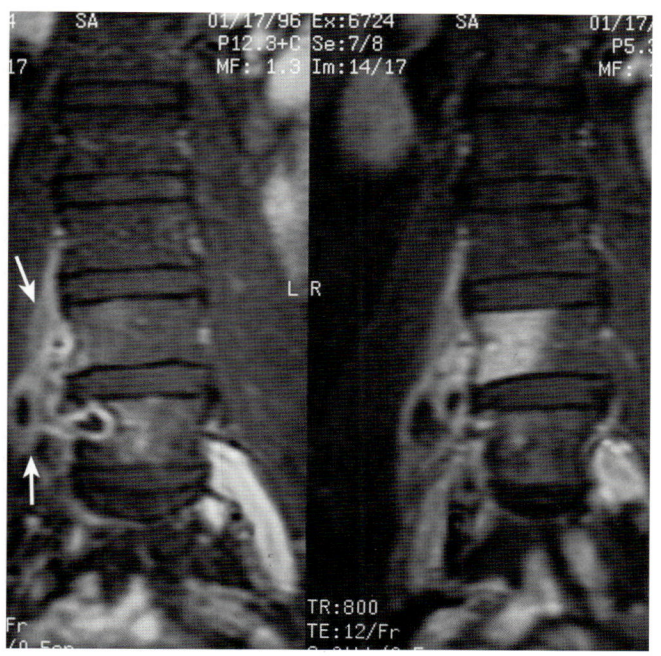

Figure 2.34 a, b A 35-year-old man with tuberculous osteomyelitis involving the L4 and L5 vertebral bodies and paraspinal cold abscesses (arrows). Poorly defined zones of high signal on sagittal FS T2WI (a) are seen in the marrow of adjacent vertebral bodies. No abnormal signal is seen at the intervening disk. The end plates appear intact. Irregular Gd-contrast enhancement is seen in the involved marrow and surrounding paraspinal "cold abscesses" on coronal (b) FS T1WI.

Table 2 (Continued) Tumors and tumorlike lesions involving the spine

Tumor/Tumorlike Lesion	MRI Findings	Comments
Rheumatoid arthritis (Fig. 2.35)	Erosions of vertebral endplates, spinous processes, and uncovertebral and apophyseal joints. Irregular enlarged enhancing synovium (pannus low-intermediate signal on T1WI, intermediate-high signal on T2WI and FS T2WI) at atlanto-dens articulation results in erosions of dens and transverse ligament, +/− destruction of transverse ligament with C1 on C2 subluxation and neural compromise. +/− basilar impression.	Most common type of inflammatory arthropathy that results in synovitis causing destructive/erosive changes of cartilage, ligaments, and bone. Cervical spine involvement in two-thirds of patients, juvenile and adult types. (See Atlas Chapter A70)
Eosinophilic granuloma (Fig. 2.36)	Single or multiple circumscribed lesions in the vertebral marrow associated with focal bony destruction/erosion with extension into the adjacent soft tissues. Lesions usually involve the vertebral body and not the posterior elements, with low-intermediate signal on T1WI, mixed intermediate-slightly high signal on T2WI, usually with prominent Gd-contrast enhancement, +/− enhancement of the adjacent dura. Progression of lesion can lead to vertebra plana (collapsed flattened vertebral body) with minimal or no kyphosis and relatively normal-sized adjacent disks.	**Single lesion:** Commonly seen in males > females, < 20 years, proliferation of histiocytes in medullary cavity with localized destruction of bone with extension into adjacent soft tissues. **Multiple lesions:** Associated with syndromes such as: Letterer-Siwe disease (lymphadenopathy hepatosplenomegaly), children < 2 years; Hand-Schüller-Christian disease (lymphadenopathy, exophthalmos, diabetes insipidus) children 5–10 years. (See Atlas Chapter A18)
Sarcoidosis (Fig. 2.37)	Sarcoid lesions can be multiple with variable sizes or solitary within marrow. Lesions can have circumscribed and/or indistinct margins within marrow and usually have low to intermediate signal on T1WI, and intermediate or slightly high to high signal on T2WI and FS T2WI. Lesions usually show variable degrees of Gd-contrast enhancement.	Chronic systemic granulomatous disease of unknown etiology in which noncaseating granulomas occur in various tissues and organs including bone. (See Atlas Chapter A71)
Hematopoietic		
Hematopoietic disorders (Fig. 2.38)	Red marrow hyperplasia can be seen as diffuse low-intermediate signal on T1WI; slightly high to high signal on FSE T2WI; and low to intermediate signal on FS T2WI with or without thinning of cortical bone.	Red marrow reconversion from erythroid hyperplasia can result from anemia secondary to sickle cell disease, thalassemia major, hereditary spherocytosis. Similar findings of red marrow expansion can be seen with polycythemia rubra. Medications (such as exogenous erythropoietin and granulocyte/macrophage colony-stimulating factor in patients with anemia and neutropenia, respectively) can also cause red marrow reconversion in adults and children.

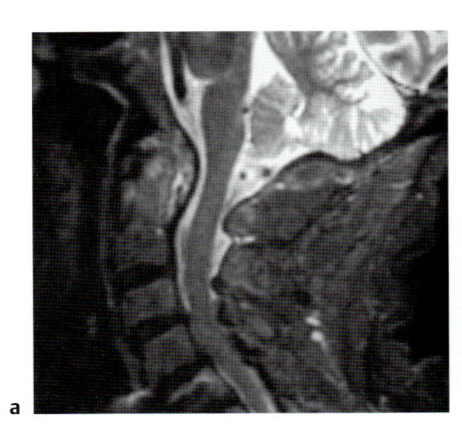

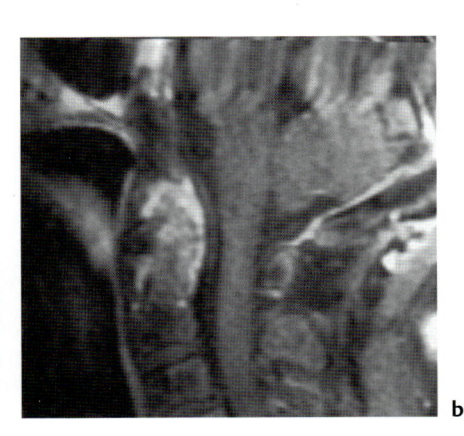

Figure 2.35 a, b A 72-year-old woman with pannus from rheumatoid arthritis causing erosive changes at the upper dens and atlas as seen on sagittal FS T2WI (**a**). The pannus and adjacent marrow have low-intermediate signal on T1WI and heterogeneous intermediate to slightly high signal on FS T2WI. The pannus and adjacent marrow show Gd-contrast enhancement on sagittal FS T1WI (**b**).

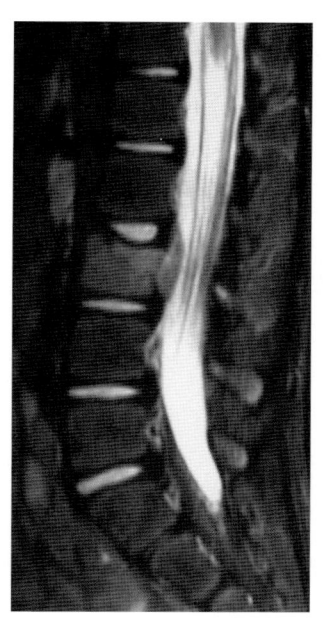

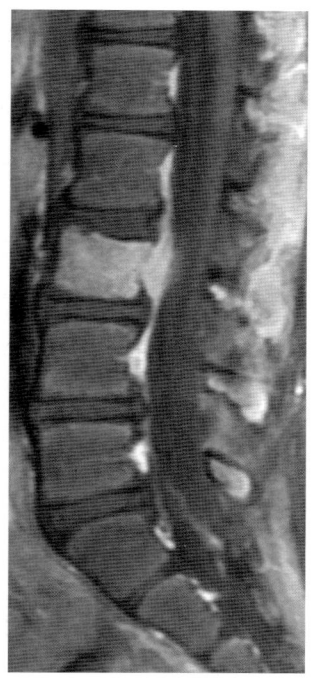

Figure 2.**36 a, b** A 6-year-old boy with an eosinophilic granuloma involving the L3 vertebral body. The lesion has heterogeneous slightly high signal on sagittal FS T2WI (**a**). The lesion shows Gd-contrast enhancement in the marrow as well as an extraosseous portion that extends into the anterior epidural soft tissues on sagittal FS T1WI (**b**).

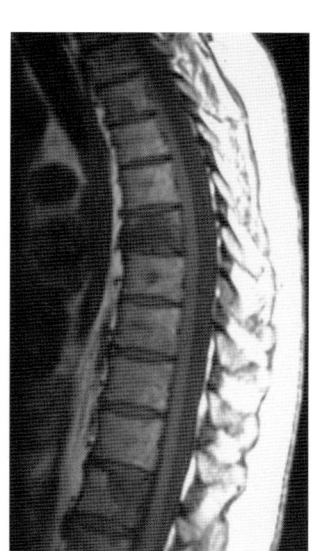

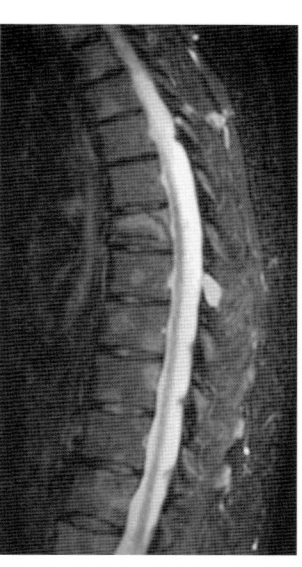

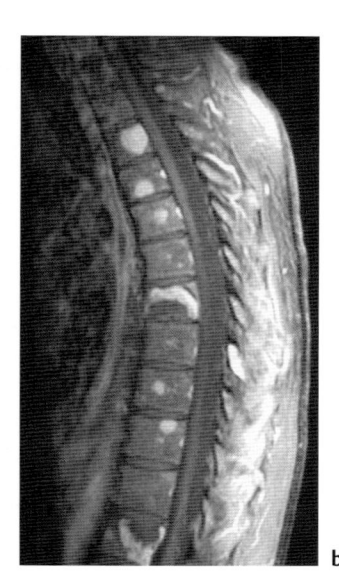

Figure 2.**37 a–c** A 50-year-old man with sarcoidosis and multiple intraosseous spinal lesions. Multiple zones of low-intermediate signal on sagittal T1WI (**a**) and slightly high signal on sagittal FS T2WI (**b**) are seen in multiple vertebrae. The lesions show Gd-contrast enhancement on sagittal FS T1WI (**c**).

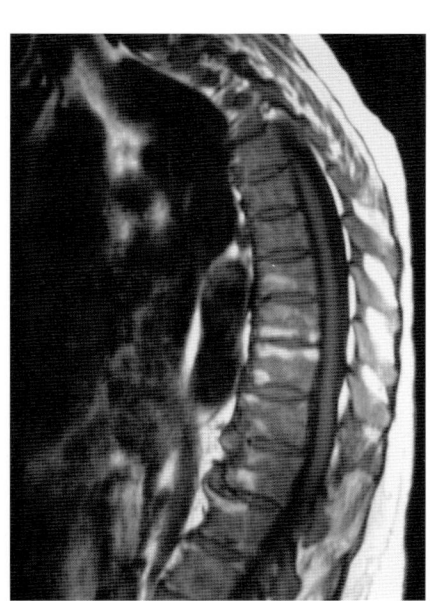

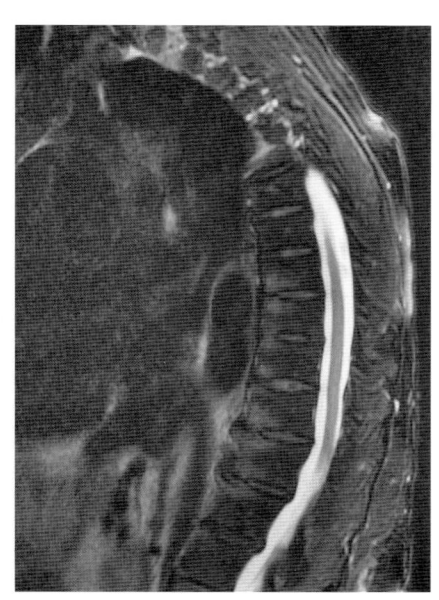

Figure 2.**38 a, b** A 60-year-old woman who has erythroid hyperplasia in the vertebral marrow from exogenous erythropoietin. Red marrow hyperplasia is seen as diffuse low-intermediate signal on sagittal T1WI (**a**) and FS T2WI (**b**).

Table 2 (Continued) Tumors and tumorlike lesions involving the spine

Tumor/Tumorlike Lesion	MRI Findings	Comments
Extramedullary hematopoiesis (Fig. 2.39)	Lesions can have low, intermediate, and/or high signal on T1WI and T2WI depending on the proportions and distribution of fat and red marrow.	Represents proliferation of erythroid precursors outside of medullary bone secondary to physiologic compensation for abnormal medullary hematopoiesis from congenital disorders such as hemoglobinopathies (sickle cell, thalassemia, etc.) as well as acquired disorders such as myelofibrosis, leukemia, lymphoma, myeloma, or metastatic carcinoma.
Amyloidoma (Fig. 2.40)	Amyloid lesions in bone can occur as zones of osteopenia, permeative radiolucent destruction or uni- or multifocal radiolucency. Lesions can have low-intermediate signal on T1WI, and intermediate to slightly high signal on T2WI. Lesions can show Gd-contrast enhancement.	Uncommon disease in which various tissues (including bone, muscle, tendons, tendon sheaths, ligaments and synovium) are infiltrated with extracellular eosinophilic material composed of insoluble proteins with β-pleated sheet configurations (amyloid protein). Amyloidomas are single sites of involvement. Amyloidosis can be a primary disorder associated with an immunologic dyscrasia or secondary to a chronic inflammatory disease.
Bone infarcts (Atlas Figs. 209, 210)	Focal ring-like lesion or poorly defined zone with low-intermediate signal on T1WI, intermediate-high signal on T2WI centrally, variable or no Gd-contrast enhancement involving the marrow depending on age/stage of infarction/healing, +/− associated fracture.	Bone infarcts can occur after radiation treatment, surgery, chemotherapy, or trauma. **(see Atlas Chapter A 37)**
Congenital		
Myelomeningocele/myelocele (Figs. 2.41, 2.42)	MRI is usually performed after surgical repair of myeloceles or myelomeningoceles. Posterior protrusion of spinal contents and unfolded neural tube (neural placode) is seen through defects in the bony dorsal elements of the involved vertebrae or sacral elements. The neural placode is usually located at the lower lumbar–sacral region with resultant tethering of the spinal cord. If the neural placode is flush with the adjacent skin surface, the anomaly is labeled a **myelocele** If the neural placode extends above the adjacent skin surface, the anomaly is labeled a **myelomeningocele** +/− syringohydromyelia.	Failure of developmental closure of the caudal neural tube results in an unfolded neural tube (neural placode) exposed to the dorsal surface in the midline without overlying skin. Other features associated with myelomeningoceles and myeloceles include: dorsal bony dysraphism, deficient dura posteriorly at the site of the neural placode, and Chiari II malformations. By definition the spinal cords are tethered. Usually repaired surgically soon after birth.

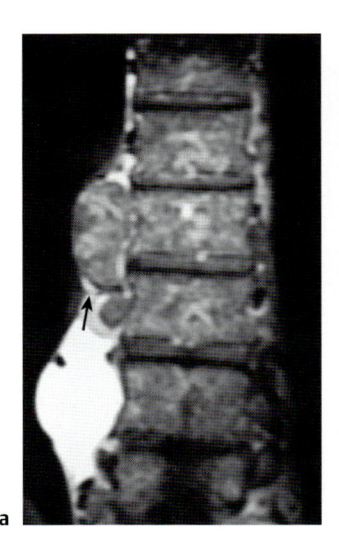

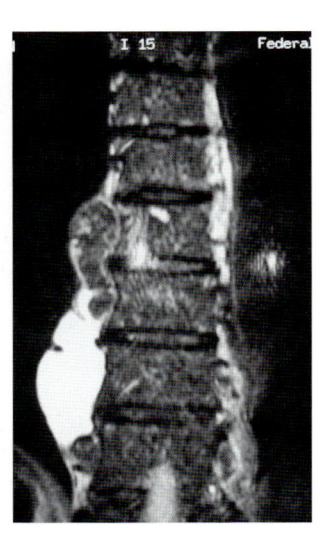

Figure 2.39 a, b A 56-year-old man with sickle cell disease and extramedullary hematopoiesis adjacent to a thoracic vertebra. A right paraspinal lesion is seen that has circumscribed margins and has intermediate signal on coronal T1WI (**a**) and coronal T2WI (**b**) which is similar to the vertebral marrow.

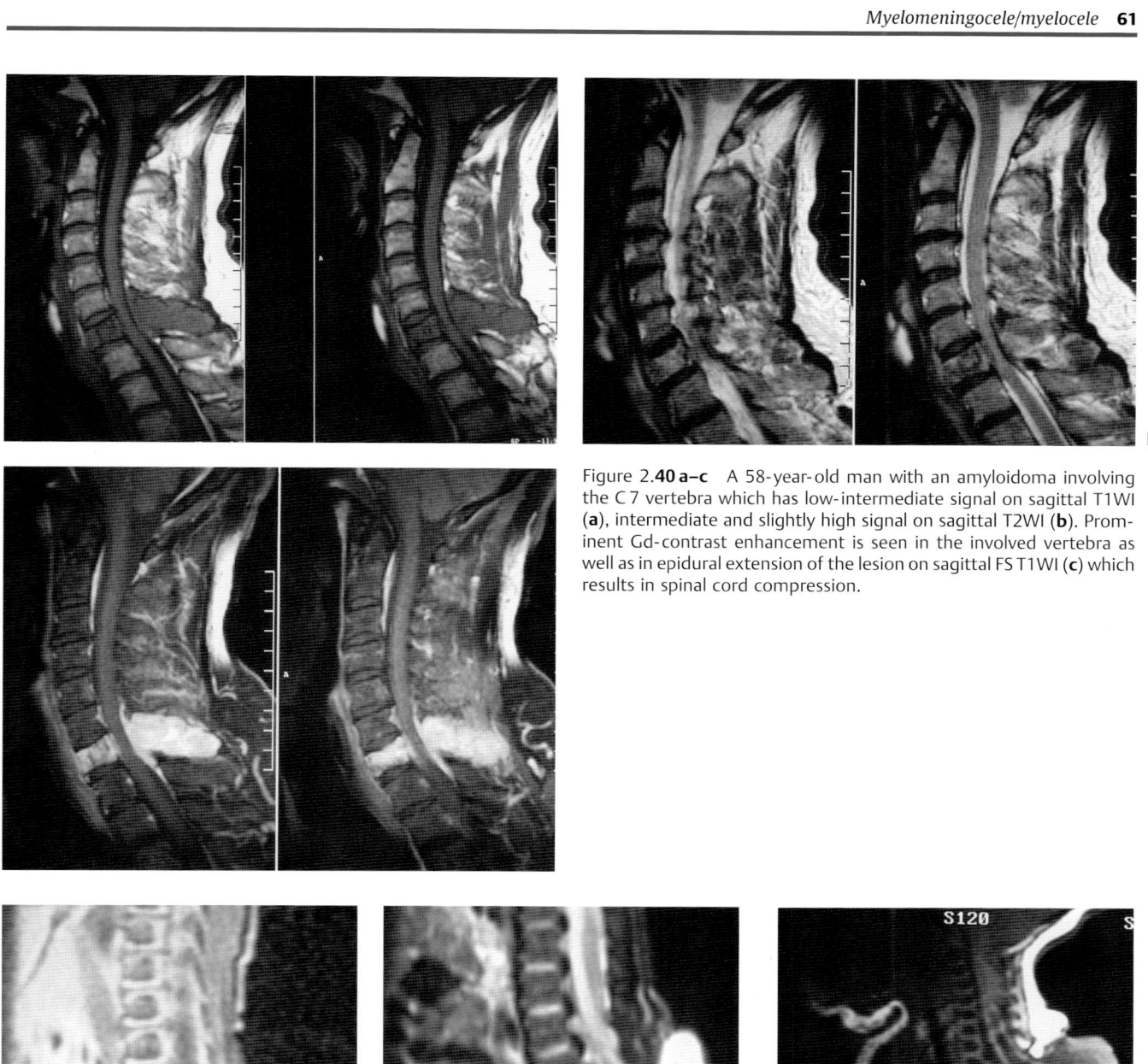

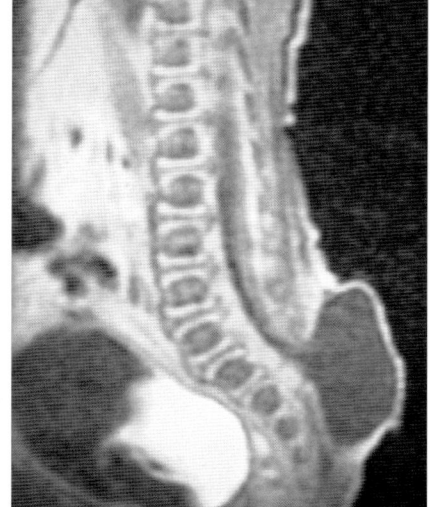

Figure 2.**40 a–c** A 58-year-old man with an amyloidoma involving the C 7 vertebra which has low-intermediate signal on sagittal T1WI (**a**), intermediate and slightly high signal on sagittal T2WI (**b**). Prominent Gd-contrast enhancement is seen in the involved vertebra as well as in epidural extension of the lesion on sagittal FS T1WI (**c**) which results in spinal cord compression.

Figure 2.**41 a–c** Neonate with a sacral myelomeningocele that is seen as a posterior protrusion of spinal contents and unfolded neural tube (neural placode) through defects in the bony dorsal elements of the involved sacral elements on sagittal FS T1WI (**a**) and sagittal FS T2WI (**b**) and axial (**c**) T2WI.

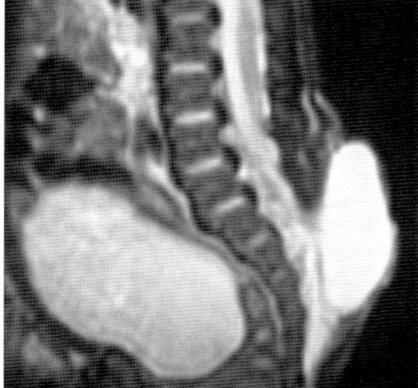

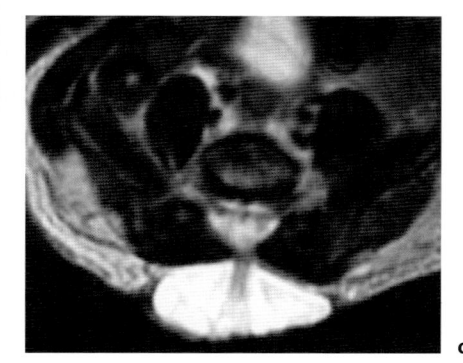

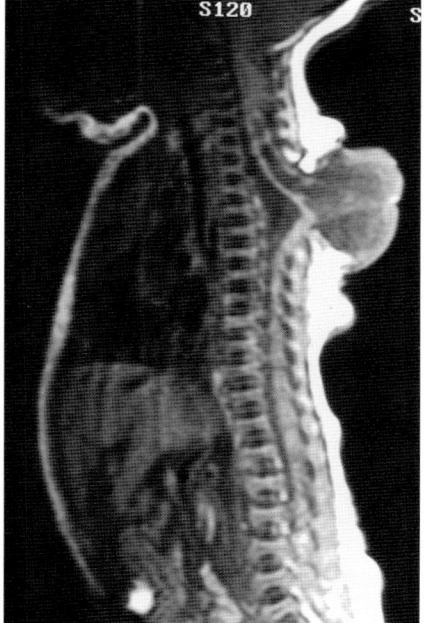

Figure 2.**42** Neonate with a thoracic myelomeningocele that is seen as a posterior protrusion of spinal contents and unfolded neural tube through defects in the bony dorsal elements of the involved thoracic vertebra on sagittal T1WI.

Table 2 (Continued) **Tumors and tumorlike lesions involving the spine**

Tumor/Tumorlike Lesion	MRI Findings	Comments
Meningoceles (Fig. 2.43)	Protrusion of CSF and meninges through a dorsal vertebral defect either from surgical laminectomies or congenital anomaly. Sacral meningoceles can alternatively extend anteriorly through a defect in the sacrum.	Acquired meningoceles are more common than meningoceles resulting from congenital dorsal bony dysraphism. Anterior sacral meningoceles can result from trauma or be associated with mesenchymal dysplasias (NF1, Marfan syndrome, syndrome of caudal regression).
Lipomyelomeningocele (Fig. 2.44)	Unfolded caudal neural tube (neural placode) covered by a lipoma, which is often contiguous with the dorsal subcutaneous fat through defects (spina bifida) involving the bony dorsal vertebral elements. The neural placode is usually located at the lower lumbar–sacral region with resultant tethering of the spinal cord, +/− syringohydromyelia.	Failure of developmental closure of the caudal neural tube results in an unfolded neural tube (neural placode) covered by a lipoma, which is continuous with the subcutaneous fat. The overlying skin is intact, although the lipoma usually protrudes dorsally. The nerve roots arise from the placode. Features associated with lipomyelomeningoceles and lipomyeloceles include: tethered spinal cords, dorsal bony dysraphism, and deficient dura posteriorly at the site of the neural placode. Not associated with Chiari II malformations. Diagnosis often in children, occasionally in adults.
Dural ectasia (Fig. 2.43)	Scalloping of the dorsal aspects of vertebral bodies, dilatation of optic nerve sheaths, dilatation of intervertebral and sacral foraminal nerve sheaths, lateral meningoceles.	Dural dysplasia associated with NF1. Dural ectasia can also result from Marfan syndrome.

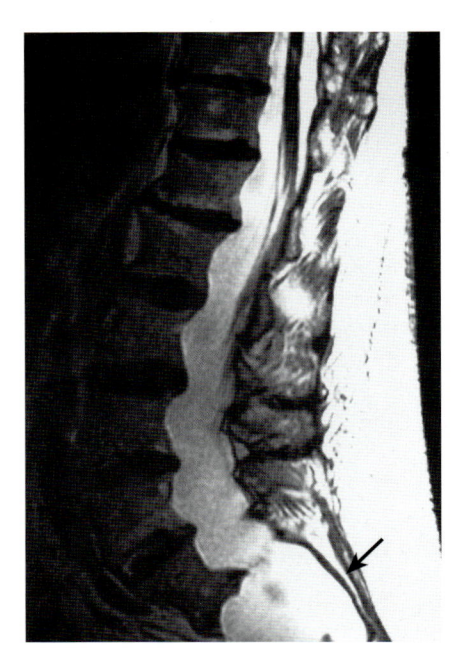

Figure 2.**43** A 67-year-old woman with Marfan syndrome who has dural ectasia and an anterior sacral meningocele as seen on sagittal T2WI.

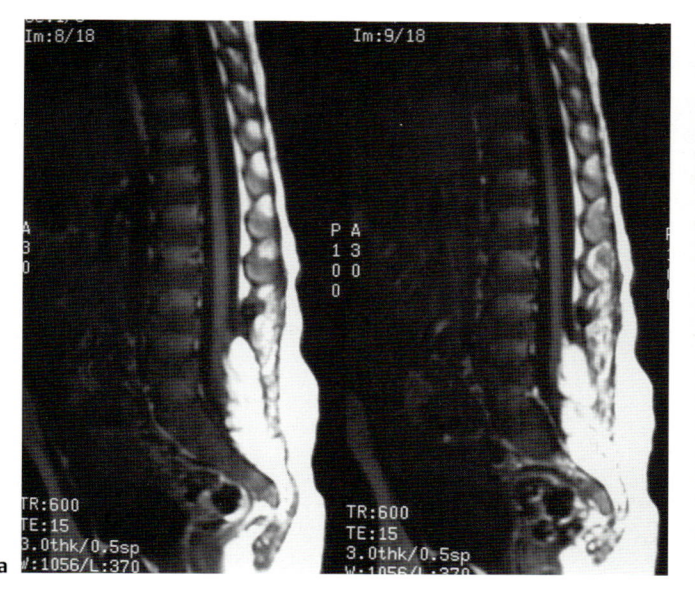

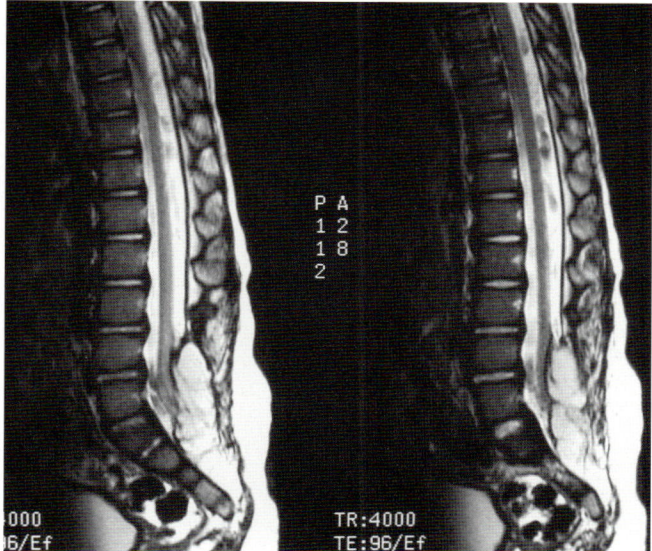

Figure 2.44 a, b   A lipomyelocele, representing an unfolded caudal neural tube covered by a lipoma, is seen located between congenital bony defects at the posterior elements (spina bifida) on sagittal T1WI (a) and sagittal (b) T2WI. Also seen is tethering of the spinal cord.

References

Arachnoid Cyst

Mukherji SK, Chenevert TL, Castillo M. Diffusion-weighted magnetic resonance imaging. *J Neuro-Ophthalmol* 2002;22(2):118–122.

Tali ET, Ercan N, Kaymaz M, Pasaoglu A, Jinkins JR. Intrathecal gadolinium (gadopentetate dimeglumine)-enhanced MR cisternography used to determine potential communication between the cerebrospinal fluid pathways and intracranial arachnoid cysts. *Neuroradiology* 2004;46:744–754.

Tang L, Cianfoni A, Imbesi SG. Diffusion weighted imaging distinguishes recurrent epidermoid neoplasm from postoperative arachnoid cyst in the lumbosacral spine. *J Comput Assist Tomogr* 2006;30:507–509.

Tarlov Cyst

Voyadzis JM, Bhargava P, Henderson FC. Tarlov cysts: a study of 10 cases with review of the literature. *J Neurosurg (Spine1)* 2001;95:25–32.

Neurenteric Cyst

Kumar R, Jain R, Rao KM, Hussain N. Intraspinal neurenteric cysts-report of three pediatric cases. *Child's Nerv Syst* 2001;17:585–588.

Menezes AH, Traynelis VC. Spinal neurenteric cysts in the magnetic resonance imaging era. *Neurosurgery* 2006;58:97–105.

Hematopoietic Disorders

Dibbern DA, Jr., Loevner LA, Lieberman AP, Salhany KE, Freese A, Marcotte PJ. MR of thoracic cord compression caused by epidural extramedullary hematopoiesis in myelodysplastic syndrome. *AJNR* February 1997;18:363–366.

Levin TL, Sheth SS, Hurlet A, et al. MR marrow signs of iron overload in transfusion-dependent patients with sickle cell disease. *Pediatr Radiol* 1995;25(8):614–619.

Niggemann P, Krings T, Hans F, Thron A. Fifteen-year follow-up of a patient with β thalassaemia and extramedullary hematopoietic tissue compressing the spinal cord. *Neuroradiology* 2005;47:263–266.

Salehi SA, Koski T, Ondra SL. Spinal cord compression in β-thalassemia: case report and review of the literature. *Spinal Cord* 2004;42: 117–123.

States LJ. Imaging of metabolic bone disease and marrow disorders in children. *Radiol Clin Am* July 2001;39(4):749–772.

Extramedullary Hematopoiesis

Capelastegui A, Astigarraga E, García-Iturraspe C. MR findings in pulmonary hypertrophic osteoarthropathy. *Clin Radiol* January 2000; 55(1):72–75.

Dibbern DA, Jr., Loevner LA, Lieberman AP, Salhany KE, Freese A, Marcotte PJ. MR of thoracic cord compression caused by epidural extramedullary hematopoiesis in myelodysplastic syndrome. *AJNR* February 1997;18:363–366.

Niggemann P, Krings T, Hans F, Thron A. Fifteen-year follow-up of a patient with β thalassaemia and extramedullary hematopoietic tissue compressing the spinal cord. *Neuroradiology* 2005;47:263–266.

Tan TC, Tsao J, Cheung FC. Extramedullary haemopoiesis in thalassemia intermedia presenting as paraplegia. *J Clin Neurosci* 2002;9(6): 721–725.

Amyloidoma

Haridas A, Basu S, King A, Pollock J. Primary isolated amyloidoma of the lumbar spine. *Neurosurgery* 2005;57(1):E196.

Meyers SP, Mullins J, Kazee AM. Unifocal primary amyloidoma of the spine causing compression of the cervical spinal cord: MR findings. *J Comput Asst Tomogr* 1996;20:592–593.

Unal A, Sutlap PN, Kyyk M. Primary solitary amyloidoma of the thoracic spine: a case report and review of the literature. *Clin Neurol Neurosur* 2003;105:167–169.

Table 3 Paraspinal tumors and tumorlike lesions

Tumors/tumorlike lesions	MRI Findings	Comments
Ependymoma (Fig. 3.1)	Intradural circumscribed lobulated lesions at conus medullaris and/or cauda equina / filum terminale, rarely in sacrococcygeal region; lesions usually have low-intermediate signal on T1WI, intermediate-high signal on T2WI, +/− foci of high signal on T1WI from mucin or hemorrhage, +/− peripheral rim of low signal (hemosiderin) on T2WI, +/− tumoral cysts (high signal on T2WI). Lesions usually show Gd-contrast enhancement.	Ependymomas at conus medullaris or cauda equina / filum terminale usually are myxopapillary type, thought to arise from ependymal glia of filum terminale. Slight male predominance. Usually are slow-growing neoplasms associated with long duration of back pain, sensory deficits, motor weakness, bladder and bowel dysfunction. +/− chronic erosion of bone with scalloping of vertebral bodies and enlargement of intervertebral foramina.
Neurofibroma (Fig. 3.2)	Lobulated extramedullary lesions +/− irregular margins, +/− extradural extension of lesion with dumbbell shape, low-intermediate signal on T1WI, slightly high to high signal on T2WI and FS T2WI, usually show prominent Gd-contrast enhancement. High signal on T2WI and Gd-contrast enhancement can be heterogeneous in large lesions. +/− erosion of foramina, +/− scalloping of dorsal margin of vertebral body (chronic erosion or dural ectasia/NF1).	Unencapsulated neoplasms involving nerve and nerve sheath, common type of intradural extramedullary neoplasms often with extradural extension, usual presentation in adults with pain and radiculopathy, paresthesias and lower extremity weakness. Multiple neurofibromas seen with NF1. **(See Atlas Chapter A 56)**

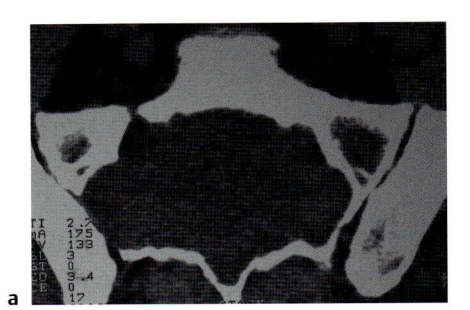

Figure 3.1 a–d A 41-year-old man with a myxopapillary ependymoma eroding the sacrum. The tumor has intermediate attenuation on axial CT (**a**) and intermediate signal on sagittal T1WI (**b**). The tumor has mixed heterogeneous high, intermediate, and low signal on sagittal T2WI (**c**) and shows heterogeneous irregular Gd-contrast enhancement on sagittal FS T1WI (**d**).

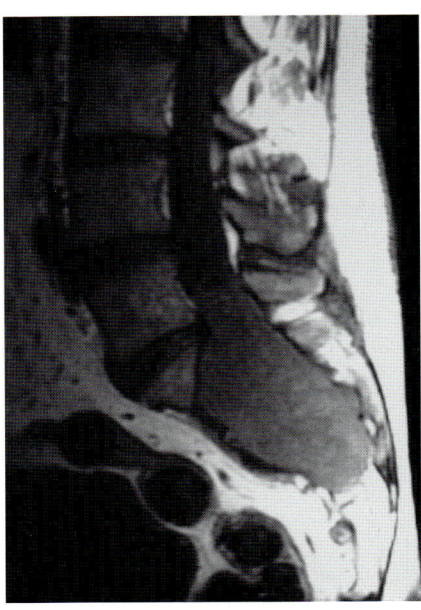

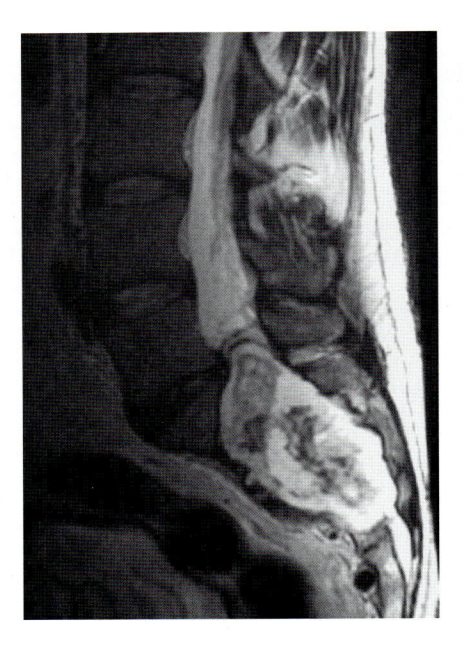

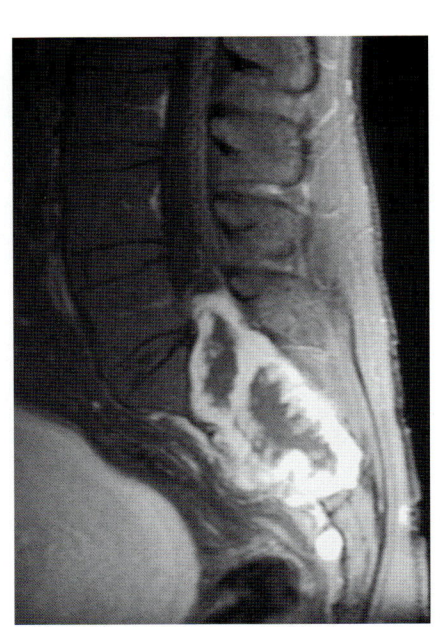

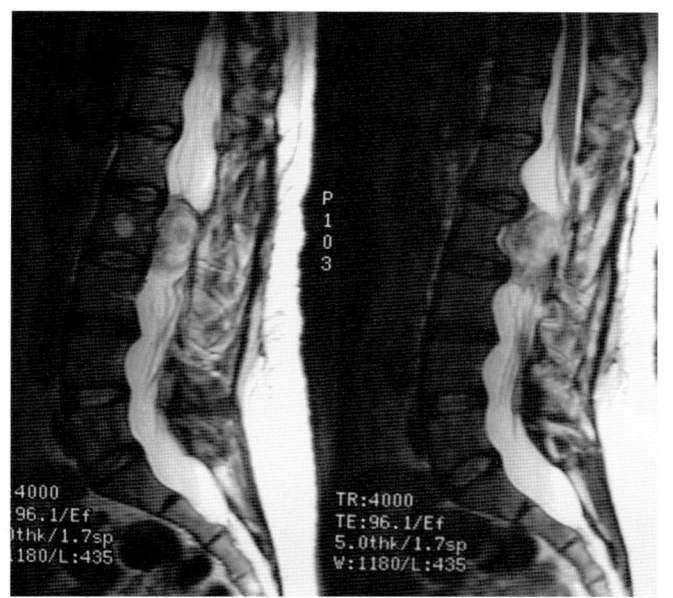

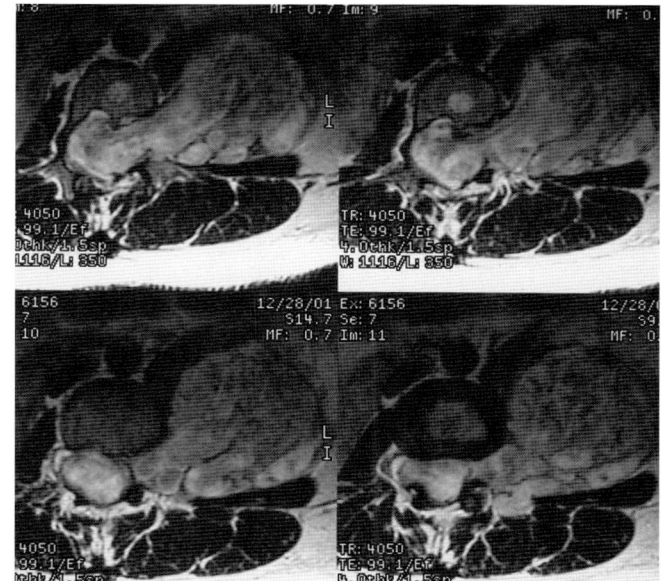

Figure 3.2 a–c A 45-year-old woman with a large left paraspinal neurofibroma extending through a widened intervertebral foramen and severely compressing the thecal sac. The lesion has intermediate, slightly high to high signal with foci of low signal on sagittal (**a**) and axial (**b**) T2WI. The lesion shows heterogeneous Gd-contrast enhancement on axial FS T1WI (**c**). Note also the scalloping of the dorsal margins of the vertebral bodies from dural ectasia.

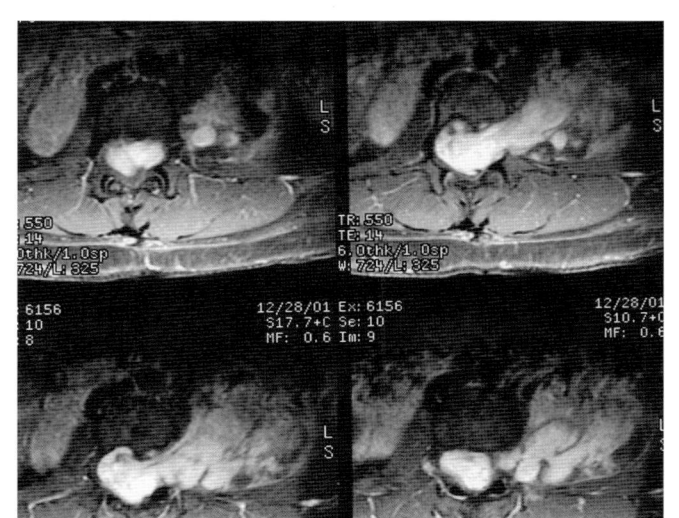

Table 3 (Continued) Paraspinal tumors and tumorlike lesions

Tumors/Tumorlike Lesion	MRI Findings	Comments
Schwannoma (neurinoma) (Fig. 3.3)	Circumscribed or lobulated extramedullary lesions, low-intermediate signal on T1WI, high signal on T2WI and FS T2WI, usually show prominent Gd-contrast-enhancement. High signal on T2WI and Gd-contrast enhancement can be heterogeneous in large lesions due to cystic degeneration and/or hemorrhage.	Encapsulated neoplasms arising asymmetrically from nerve sheath, most common type of intradural extramedullary neoplasms, usual presentation in adults with pain and radiculopathy, paresthesias and lower extremity weakness. Multiple schwannomas seen with NF2. **(See Atlas Chapter A 72)**

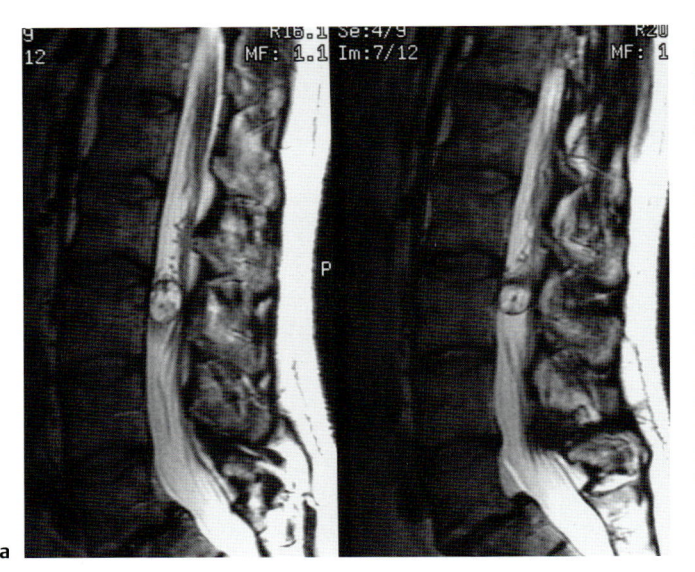

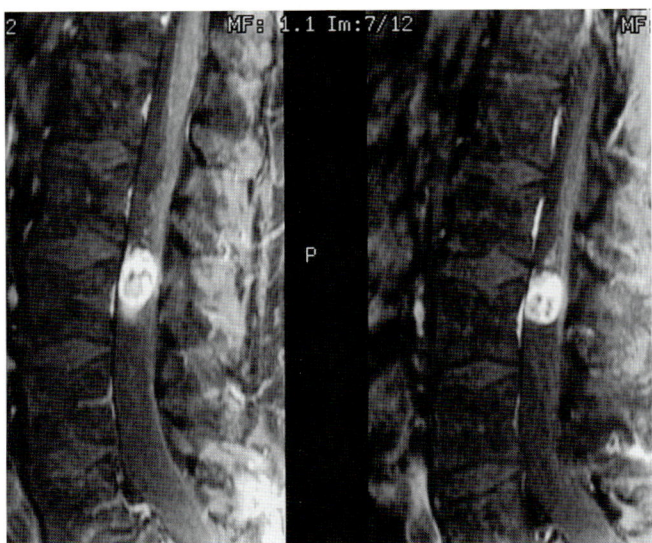

Figure 3.3 a–c Solitary schwannoma in the lumbar spine at the upper L3 level. The lesion has heterogeneous high signal on sagittal (**a**) and axial (**c**, *upper images*) T2WI, and shows heterogeneous Gd-contrast enhancement on sagittal (**b**) and axial (**c**, *lower images*) FS T1WI.

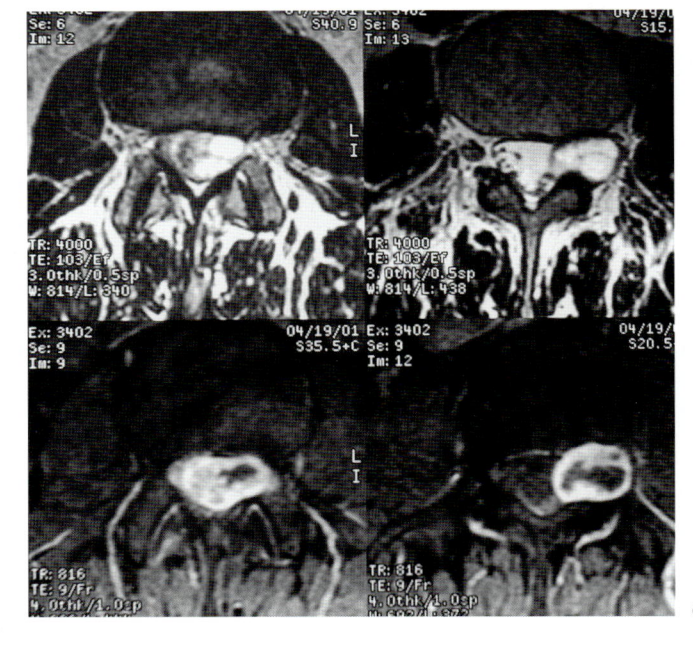

Table 3 (Continued) **Paraspinal tumors and tumorlike lesions**

Tumors/Tumorlike Lesion	MRI Findings	Comments
Malignant peripheral nerve sheath tumor (Fig. 3.4)	These lesions usually have heterogeneous signal on T1WI and T2WI; as well as heterogeneous Gd-contrast enhancement because of necrosis and hemorrhage. Some are similar in appearance to benign nerve sheath tumors.	Malignant tumors of the peripheral nerve sheath that contain mixtures of packed hyperchromatic spindle cells with elongated nuclei and slightly eosinophilic cytoplasm, mitotic figures, and zones of necrosis. Approximately 50% of malignant peripheral nerve sheath tumors occur in patients with NF1, followed by de novo evolution from peripheral nerves. Malignant peripheral nerve sheath tumors infrequently arise from schwannomas, ganglioneuroblastomas/ganglioneuromas, and pheochromocytomas. **(See Atlas Chapter A 56)**
Meningioma (Fig. 3.5)	Extradural or intradural extramedullary lesions, intermediate signal on T1WI, intermediate-slightly high signal on T2WI and FS T2WI, usually show prominent Gd-contrast enhancement, +/− calcifications.	Usually benign neoplasms, typically occurs in adults (>40 years), women > men, multiple meningiomas seen with NF2, can result in compression of adjacent spinal cord and nerve roots, rarely invasive/malignant types. **(See Atlas Chapter A 49)**

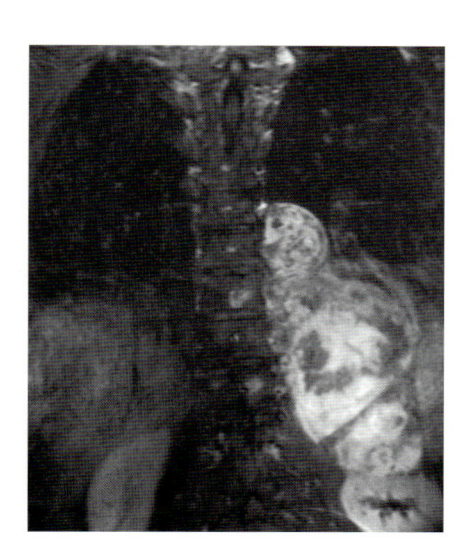

Figure 3.4 A 49-year-old man with a malignant peripheral nerve sheath tumor arising from a benign schwannoma. The large left paraspinal tumor shows irregular Gd-contrast enhancement on coronal FST1WI. Small zones of abnormal contrast enhancement are seen in two vertebral bodies secondary to tumor invasion.

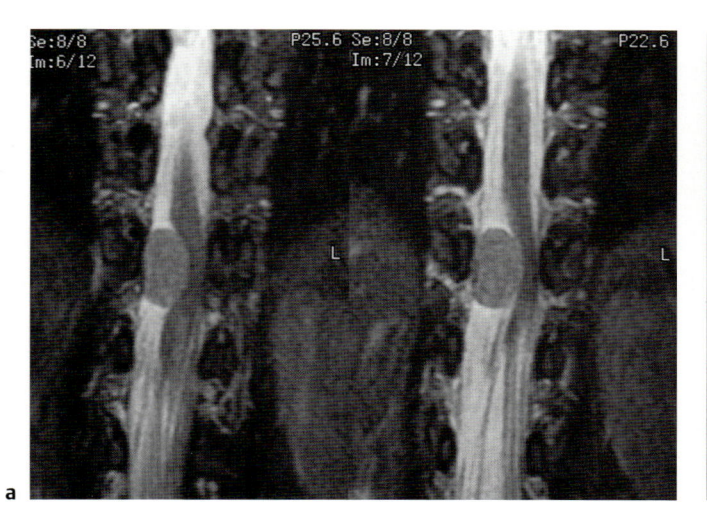

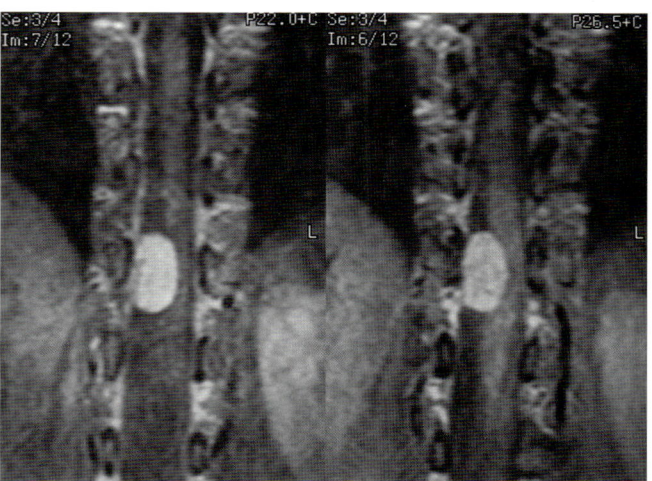

Figure 3.5 a, b A 43-year-old woman with a meningioma causing compression of the lower thoracic spinal cord. The tumor has intermediate signal on coronal FS T2WI (**a**) and shows prominent Gd-contrast enhancement on coronal FS T1WI (**b**).

Table 3 (Continued) Paraspinal tumors and tumorlike lesions

Tumors/Tumorlike Lesion	MRI Findings	Comments
Paraganglioma (Fig. 3.6)	Spheroid or lobulated intradural–extramedullary lesion with intermediate signal on T1WI, intermediate-high signal on T2WI and FS T2WI, +/− tubular zones of flow voids, usually show prominent Gd-contrast enhancement, +/− foci of high signal on T1WI from mucin or hemorrhage, +/− peripheral rim of low signal (hemosiderin) on T2WI, usually located in region of cauda equina and filum terminale.	Neoplasms that arise from paraganglion cells of neural crest origin usually occur at carotid body, jugular foramen, middle ear, and along vagus nerve. Rarely occur in spine. **(See Atlas Chapter A 66)**
Neuroblastoma/ganglioneuroblastoma (Fig. 3.7)	Tumors can have distinct or indistinct margins, and have low-intermediate signal on T1WI, homogeneous or heterogeneous intermediate, slightly high, and/or high signal on T2WI and FS T2WI. Zones of high signal on T2WI may occur from sites of hemorrhage or necrosis. Foci of low signal on T2WI may be seen secondary to calcifications and blood products. Tumors can show mild to marked heterogeneous Gd-contrast enhancement. MRI can show extension of these tumors into the spinal canal as well as into bone marrow.	Neuroblastomas and ganglioneuroblastomas are malignant tumors of the sympathetic nervous system that consist of neuroectodermal cells derived from the neural crest. Neuroblastomas are highly malignant undifferentiated tumors whereas ganglioneuroblastomas are intermediate-grade malignant tumors. **(See Atlas Chapter A 55)**
Ganglioneuroma (Fig. 3.8)	Tumors are well-circumscribed with low-intermediate signal on T1WI, and slightly high to high signal on T2WI and FS T2WI. Small foci or strands of low signal on T2WI may be seen secondary to calcifications and fibrous tissue, respectively. Tumors show mild to marked heterogeneous Gd-contrast enhancement. MRI can show extension of these tumors into the spinal canal.	Rare benign lesions of the sympathetic nervous system composed of ganglion cells and Schwannian stroma and lacking neuroblasts and mitotic figures. **(See Atlas Chapter A 55)**
Lymphoma (Fig. 3.9)	Lymphadenopathy from lymphoma often has low-intermediate signal on T1WI and intermediate to slightly high signal on T2WI. Variability in MRI signal characteristics may be related to differing histologic features (such as the degree of fibrosis). After Gd-contrast administration, extraosseous lymphoma can show Gd-contrast enhancement in varying degrees. Epidural lymphoma can show Gd-contrast enhancement and can cause spinal cord compression.	Lymphoma represents a group of lymphoid tumors whose neoplastic cells typically arise within lymphoid tissue (lymph nodes and reticuloendothelial organs). Unlike leukemia, lymphoma usually arises as discrete masses. **(See Atlas Chapter A 47)**

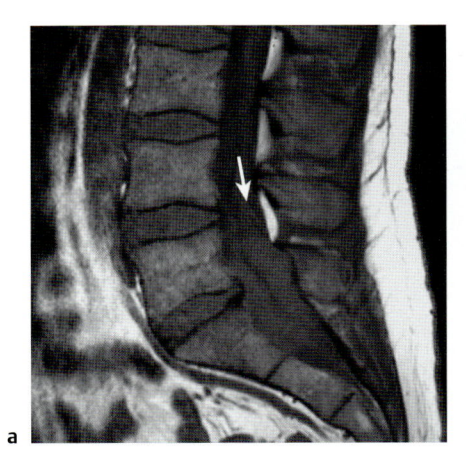

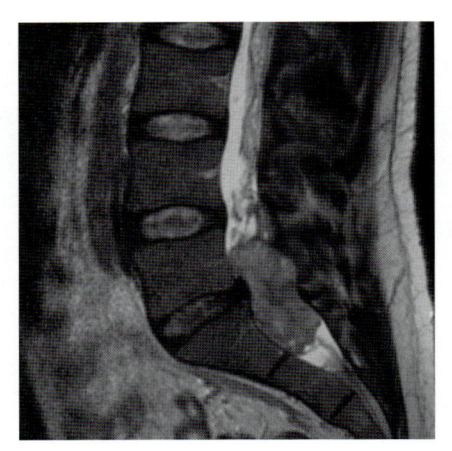

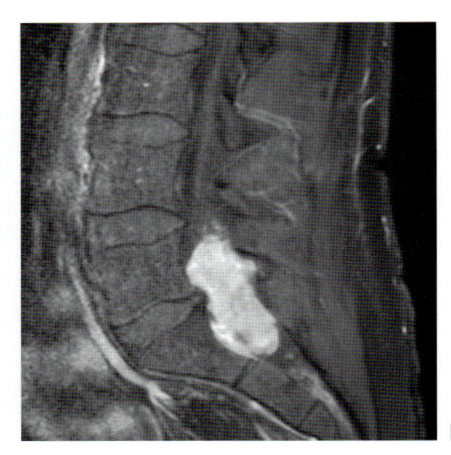

Figure 3.6 A 33-year-old man with an intradural paraganglioma in the distal lumbar thecal sac. The lesion has low-intermediate signal on sagittal T1WI (**a**), and heterogeneous intermediate to slightly high signal on sagittal T2WI (**b**). The tumor shows prominent Gd-contrast enhancement on sagittal FS T1WI (**c**).

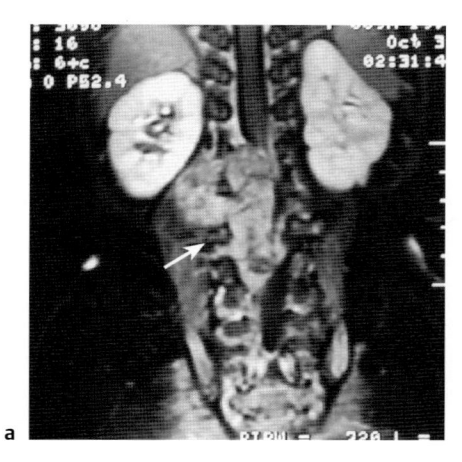

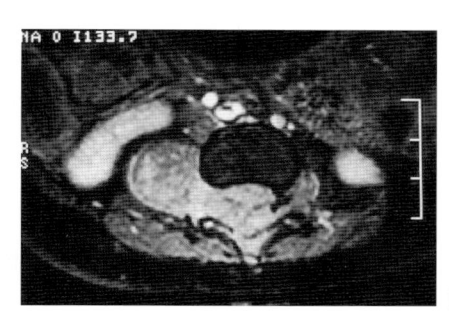

Figure 3.**7 a, b** A 9-month-old female infant with a right infra-renal paraspinal neuroblastoma with extension into the spinal canal resulting in spinal canal compression. The tumor has prominent slightly heterogeneous Gd-contrast enhancement on coronal (**a**) and axial (**b**) FS T1WI.

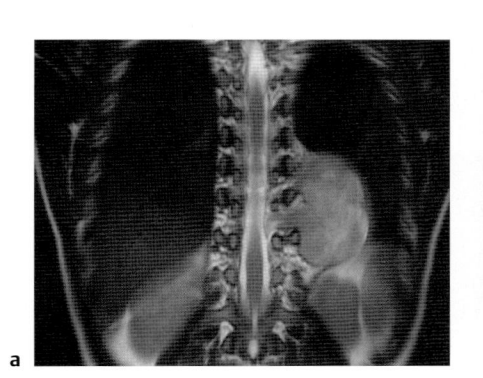

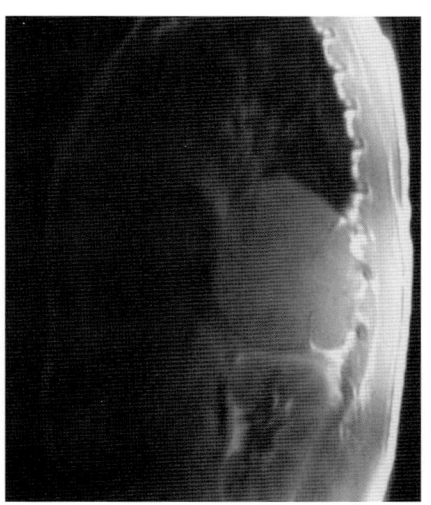

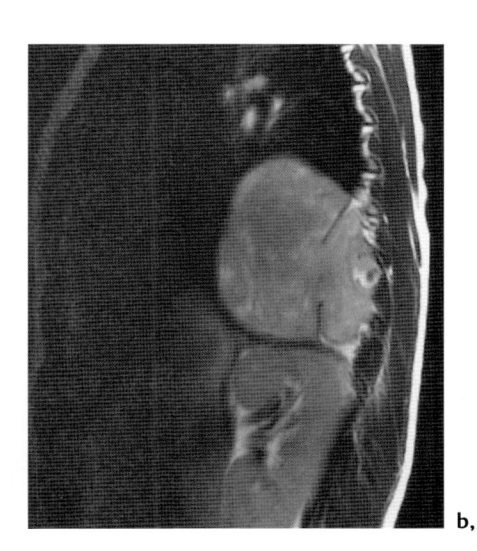

Figure 3.**8 a–c** A 10-year-old boy with a left paraspinal ganglioneuroma. The tumor has heterogeneous intermediate, slightly high to high signal on coronal (**a**) and sagittal (**c**) T2WI and intermediate signal on sagittal T1WI (**b**).

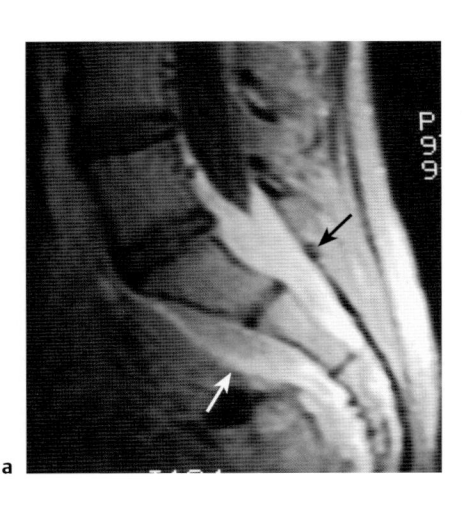

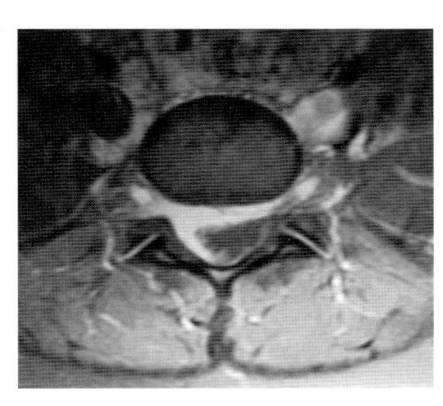

Figure 3.**9 a, b** A 14-year-old female with epidural non-Hodgkin lymphoma that shows prominent Gd-contrast enhancement on sagittal (**a**) and axial (**b**) FS T1WI.

Table 3 (Continued) **Paraspinal tumors and tumorlike lesions**

Tumors/Tumorlike Lesion	MRI Findings	Comments
Metastatic disease	Single or multiple well-circumscribed or poorly defined infiltrative lesions involving the paraspinal soft tissues with eventual involvement of vertebral marrow, dura, and leptomeninges. Lesions often have low-intermediate signal on T1WI, low, intermediate, and/or high signal on T2WI and FS T1WI, and usually show Gd-contrast enhancement. +/− bone destruction, +/− pathologic vertebral fracture, +/− compression of neural tissue or vessels.	Metastatic tumor can involve the paraspinal tissues by direct extension from tumors such as retroperitoneal liposarcoma, lung and renal carcinomas; or from involved adjacent lymph nodes. Metastatic disease may also occur from hematogenous dissemination. **(See Atlas Chapter A 50)**
Hemangiopericytoma (Fig. 1.20)	Extradural or intradural extramedullary lesions, can involve vertebral marrow, often well circumscribed, intermediate signal on T1WI, intermediate-slightly high signal on T2WI and FS T2WI, usually show prominent Gd-contrast enhancement (may resemble meningiomas), +/− associated erosive bone changes.	Rare neoplasms in young adults (males > females) sometimes referred to as angioblastic meningioma or meningeal hemangio-pericytoma, arise from vascular cell-pericytes **(See Atlas Chapter A 35)**
Desmoid tumor (Fig. 3.10)	Lesions can have distinct and/or poorly defined margins, homogeneous or heterogeneous low-intermediate signal on T1WI, and variable intermediate-high signal on T2WI, +/− zones of low signal. Myxoid zones in the lesions can have high signal on T1WI and T2WI. Tumors with high cellularity tend to show higher signal on T2WI than lesions with larger proportions of collagen. Lesions show variable degrees and patterns (heterogeneous versus homogenous) of Gd-contrast enhancement. Pattern or degree of Gd-contrast enhancement by desmoids does not enable prediction of rate of tumor recurrence.	Desmoid tumors or fibromatosis represent a group of soft tissue lesions comprised of benign fibrous tissue with elongated or spindle-shaped cells adjacent to collagen. **(See Atlas Chapter A 16)**

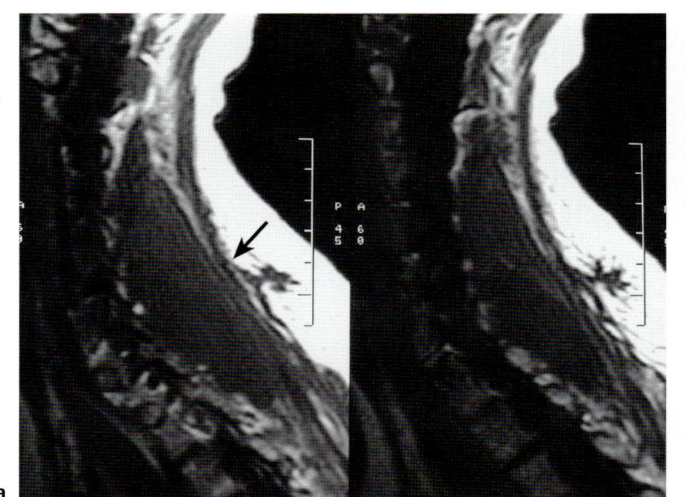

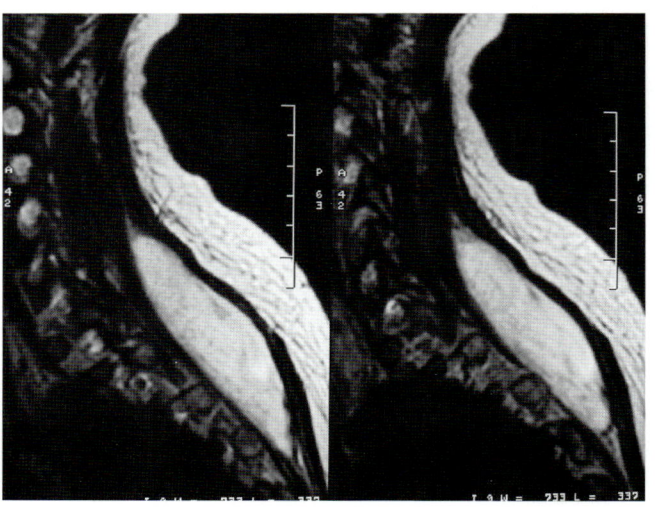

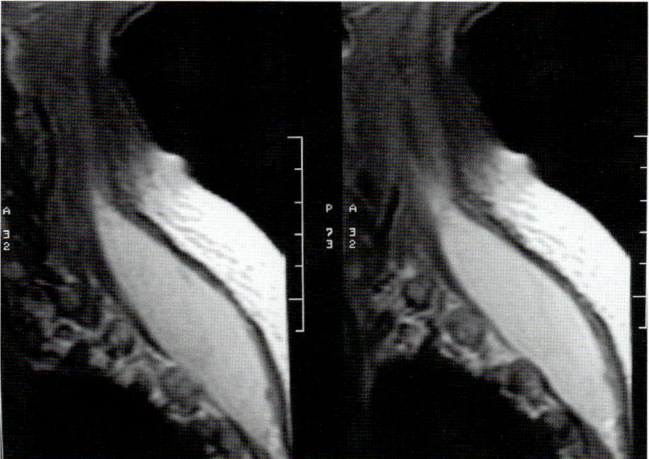

Figure 3.**10 a–c** A 20-year-old woman with a desmoid tumor involving the posterior paraspinal muscles of the cervical and upper thoracic spine. The fusiform lesion has low-intermediate signal on sagittal T1WI (**a**) and high signal on sagittal T2WI (**b**). The lesion shows prominent Gd-contrast enhancement on sagittal FS T1WI (**c**).

Table 3 (Continued) Paraspinal tumors and tumorlike lesions

Tumors/Tumorlike Lesion	MRI Findings	Comments
Primary sarcoma involving the paraspinal soft tissues (Fig. 3.11, 3.12)	Tumors can have regular and/or irregular margins, and often have low-intermediate signal on T1WI, heterogeneous intermediate-high signal on T2WI, and show Gd-contrast enhancement. Signal heterogeneity on T1WI and T2WI is often related to the presence and extent of fibrous components (low signal on T1WI and T2WI), zones of hemorrhage (intermediate or high signal on T1WI; low, intermediate, and/or high signal on T2WI), zones of necrosis and/or myxoid material (low signal on T1WI and high signal on T2WI). Margins of lesions may be indistinct on T2WI for high-grade lesions. Tumors can be associated with erosion, destruction, and invasion of adjacent bone.	Various types of primary sarcomas can occur in the paraspinal soft tissues and subsequently invade the vertebrae, intervertebral foramina, and/or spinal canal.
Lipoblastoma (Fig. 3.13)	Lesions often have mixed low, intermediate, and high signal on T1WI, T2WI, and FS T2WI. Lesions often show heterogeneous Gd-contrast enhancement.	Rare benign mesenchymal tumors that contain embryonal fat. Typically occur in infancy and early childhood. **(See Atlas Chapter A 42)**

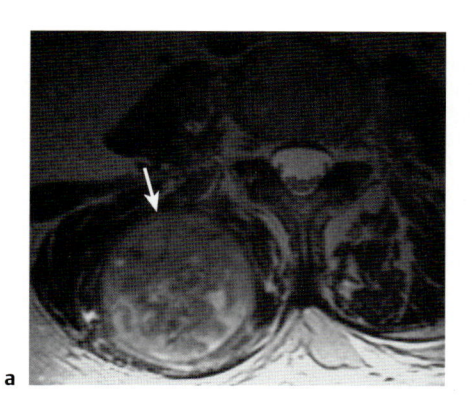

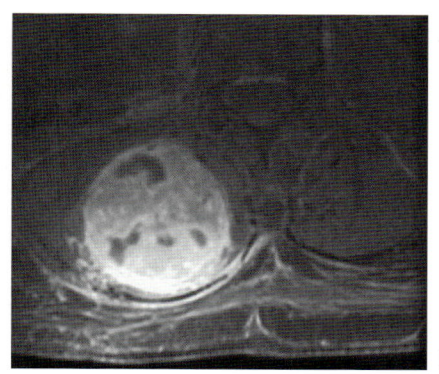

Figure 3.**11 a, b** A 56-year-old woman with a leiomyosarcoma involving the right paraspinal muscles in the lumbar region. The tumor has heterogeneous intermediate and slightly high signal on axial T2WI (**a**), and shows mostly prominent Gd-contrast enhancement on axial FS T1WI (**b**).

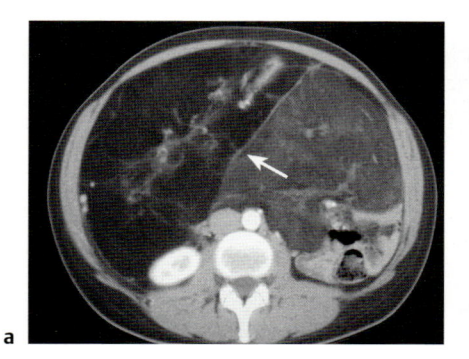

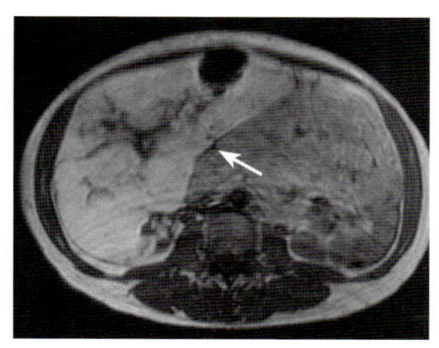

Figure 3.**12 a, b** A 35-year-old woman with a liposarcoma in the right abdomen. The tumor has mostly low attenuation and contains thickened bands of enhancement on CT (**a**). The tumor has mostly a high fatty signal with irregular bands of low signal on axial T1WI (**b**)

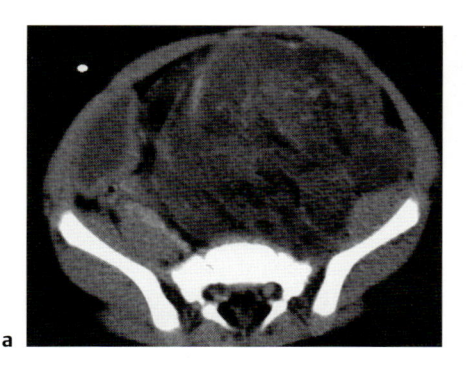

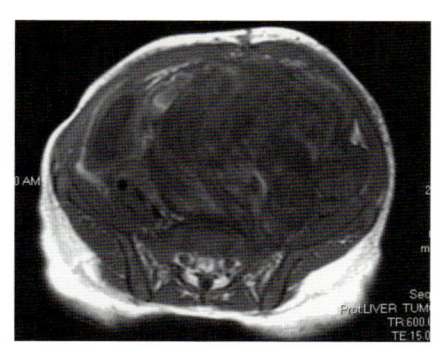

Figure 3.**13 a, b** A 1.5-year-old boy with a large intra-abdominal and pelvic lipoblastoma. The lesion has heterogeneous attenuation with zones of soft tissue, fluid and fat attenuation on axial CT (**a**). The lesion has mixed low-intermediate, intermediate, and high signal on axial T1WI (**b**).

Table 3 (Continued) **Paraspinal tumors and tumorlike lesions**

Tumors/Tumorlike Lesion	MRI Findings	Comments
Epidural abscess (Figs. 3.14, 3.15)	Epidural collection with low signal on T1WI and high signal on T2WI and FS T2WI surrounded by a peripheral rim (thin or thick) of Gd-contrast enhancement, +/− associated vertebral osteomyelitis/diskitis, +/− air collections (signal void on T1 W and T2 W images), often extend over two to four vertebral segments, can result in compression of spinal cord and spinal canal contents.	Epidural abscess can evolve from an inflammatory phlegmonous epidural mass, extension from paravertebral inflammatory process, or vertebral osteomyelitis/diskitis. May be associated with complications from surgery, epidural anesthesia, diabetes, distant source of infection, immuno-compromised status. Organisms commonly involved include *Staph. aureus*, Gram-negative bacteria, Mycobacteria, coccidiomycosis, candidiasis, aspergillosis, blastomycosis. Clinical findings include: back and radicular pain, +/− paresthesias and paralysis of lower extremities.
Epidural hematoma (Fig. 3.16)	**Acute hematoma (< 48 hours):** Epidural collection with low-intermediate signal on T1WI and PDWI, heterogeneous high signal on T2WI. +/− spinal cord compression. +/− minimal central peripheral pattern of Gd-contrast enhancement at hematoma. **Subacute hematoma (> 48 hours):** Epidural collection with intermediate-slightly high signal on T1WI, heterogeneous intermediate to high signal on T2WI. +/− spinal cord compression. +/− mixed central and/or peripheral patterns of Gd-contrast enhancement of hematoma as well as adjacent dura. **Older hematoma:** Epidural collection with variable/heterogeneous signal on T1WI and T2WI. +/− spinal cord compression.	The MR signal of acute epidural hematoma typically is secondary to deoxyhemoglobin, and with subacute hematoma secondary to methemoglobin. Older epidural hematomas have mixed MR signal related to the various states of hemoglobin and breakdown products. Can be spontaneous or result from trauma or complication from: coagulopathy, lumbar puncture, myelography, surgery. **(See Atlas Chapter A 36)**
Teratoma (Fig. 3.17)	Circumscribed lesions variable low, intermediate, and/or high signal on T1WI and T2WI; +/− Gd-contrast enhancement. May contain calcifications, cysts, as well as fatty components that can cause chemical meningitis if ruptured.	Second most common type of germ cell tumors; occur in children, males > females; benign or malignant types, composed of derivatives of ectoderm, mesoderm, and/or endoderm. **(See Atlas Chapter A 76)**

Figure 3.**14** A 34-year-old man with pyogenic osteomyelitis involving the L 4 and L 5 vertebral bodies and intervening disk associated with an epidural abscess. Irregular Gd-contrast enhancement is seen in the involved marrow on sagittal FS T1WI as well as in the anterior epidural soft tissues causing spinal canal compression.

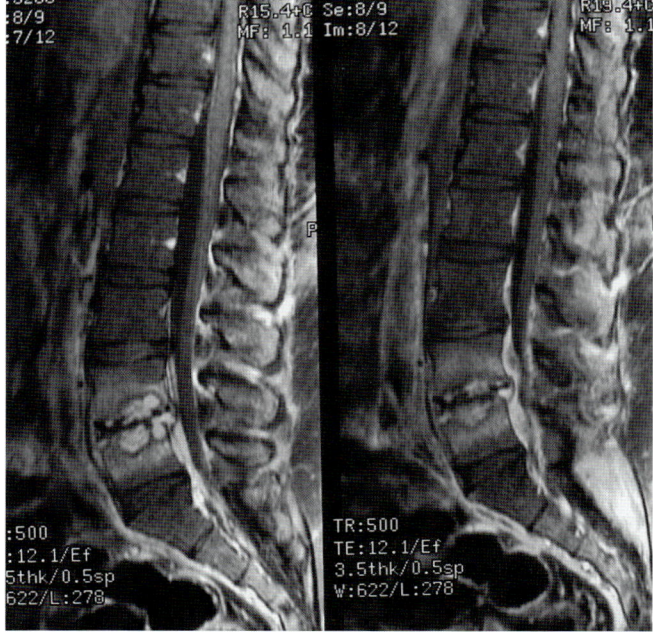

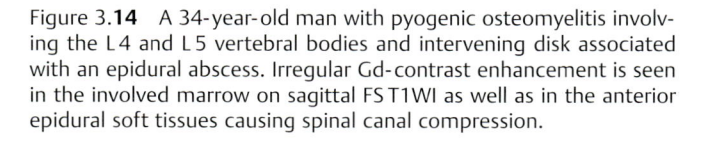

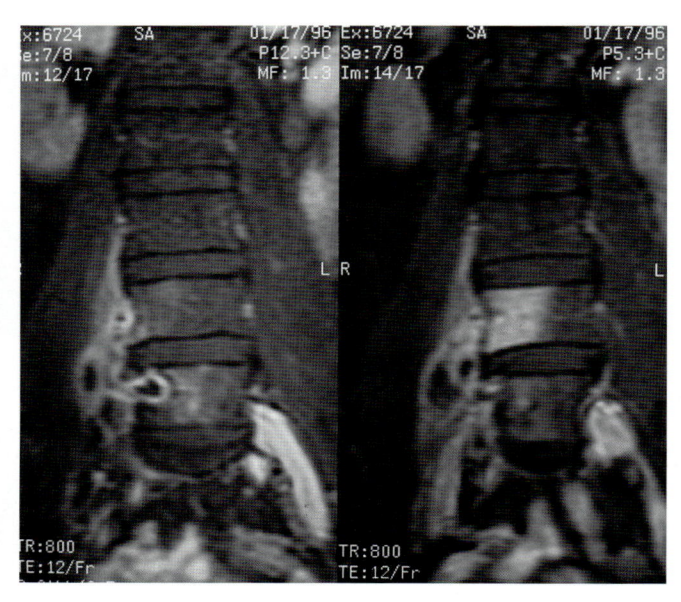

Figure 3.**15** A 35-year-old man with tuberculous osteomyelitis involving the L 4 and L 5 vertebral bodies with right paraspinal cold abscesses. Irregular Gd-contrast enhancement is seen in the involved marrow on coronal FS T1WI. Also seen is subligamentous spread of the paraspinal abscesses that show irregular peripheral zones of Gd-contrast enhancement.

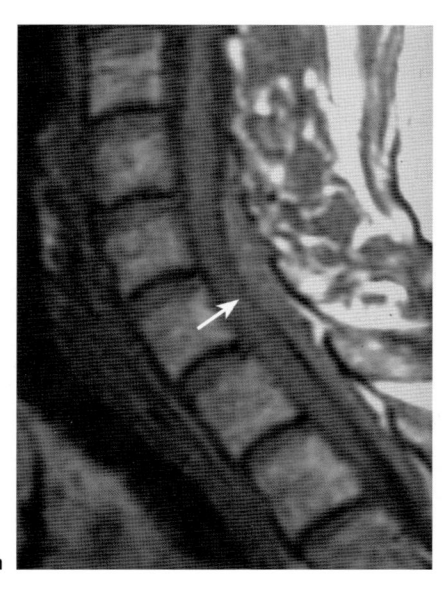

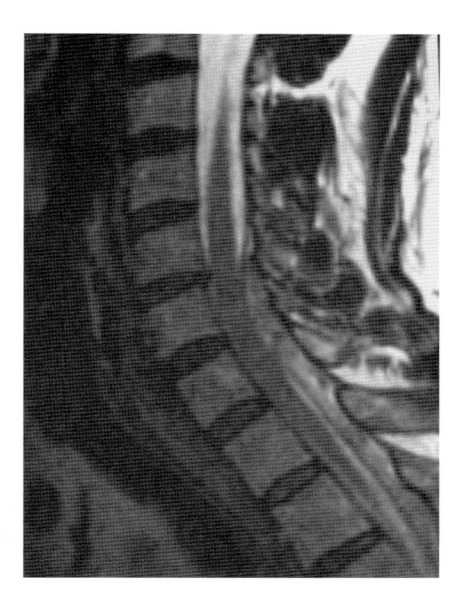

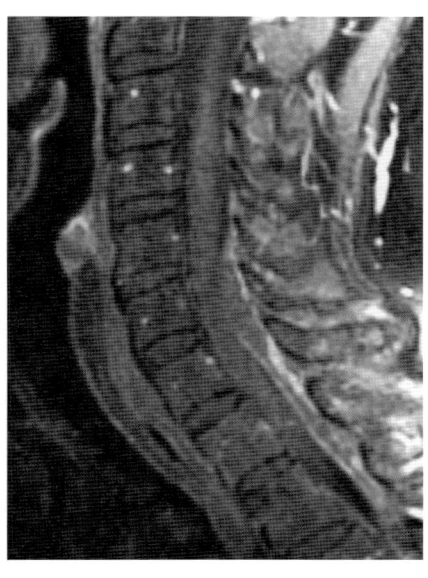

Figure 3.**16 a–c** A 60-year-old man with an epidural hematoma dorsally within the mid and lower cervical spinal canal as well as the upper thoracic spinal canal. The subdural hematoma has mostly intermediate signal and several small zones of slightly high signal on sagittal T1WI (**a**). The hematoma has intermediate, slightly high, and high signal on sagittal T2WI (**b**) and shows peripheral Gd-contrast enhancement on sagittal FS T1WI (**c**).

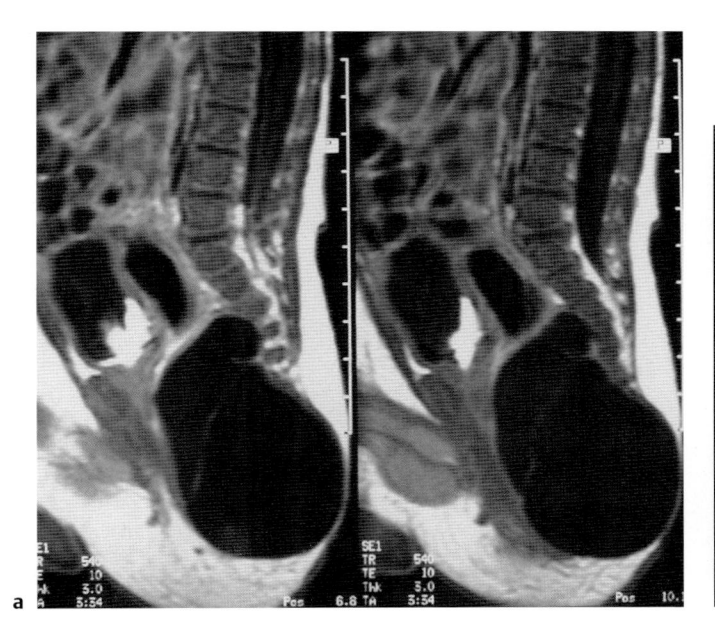

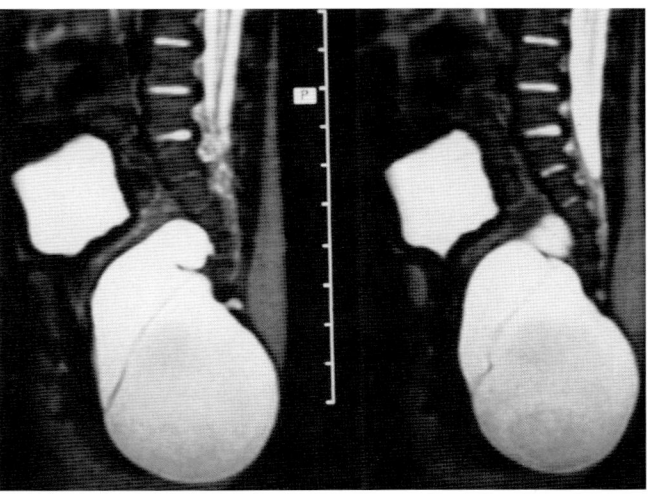

Figure 3.**17 a, b** Sacrococcygeal teratoma in a 2-month-old male infant. The large lesion has low signal on sagittal T1WI (**a**) and high signal on sagittal T2WI (**b**). Two thin septa are seen within the lesion.

Table 3 (Continued) **Paraspinal tumors and tumorlike lesions**

Tumors/Tumorlike Lesion	MRI Findings	Comments
Hiatal hernia (Fig. 3.18)	Circumscribed paraspinal structure contiguous with esophagus and gastric fundus and/or intra-abdominal fat. A low signal rim with rugae may be seen surrounding contents, which can have variable low, intermediate, and/or high signal on T1WI and T2WI. Fluid–fluid or air–fluid levels may be present.	Represent trans-diaphragm communications through which abdominal contents extend into the thoracic cavity. Most occur posterolaterally through the foramen of Bochdalek (left greater than right sides). Anterior hernias occur less commonly through the foramen of Morgagni.
Retroperitoneal fibrosis	Bands or nodular lesions with low-intermediate signal on T1WI, intermediate signal on T2WI, and intermediate to slightly high signal on FS T2WI, can be seen adjacent to or surrounding the aorta, inferior vena cava, and/or ureters. Lesions usually show Gd-contrast enhancement.	Disorder in which there is proliferation of fibrous and inflammatory tissue in the retroperitoneum. Retroperitoneal fibrosis can be a primary disorder or occur secondary to malignancy, aortic aneurysm, or drugs such as methysergide and ergotamine.
Pneumonia (Fig. 3.19)	Infection of lung tissue adjacent to the spine can be seen as poorly defined zones of consolidation with low-intermediate signal on T1WI, intermediate to high signal on T2WI. Lesions can show Gd-contrast enhancement.	Infection of lung tissue adjacent to the spine is infrequently associated with direct extension to the spine.

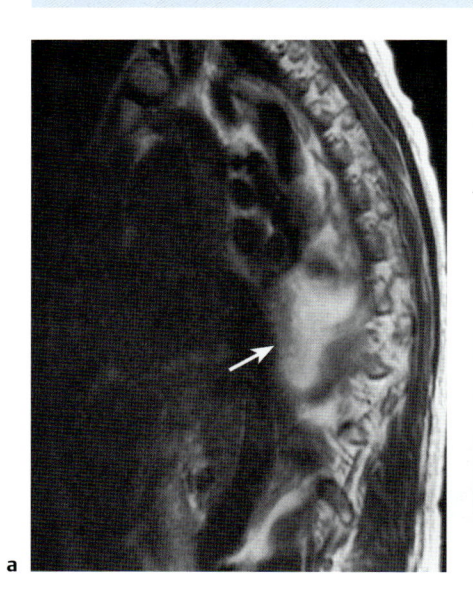

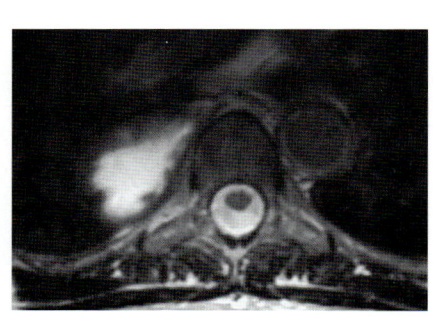

Figure 3.**18 a, b** A hiatal hernia is seen on sagittal (**a**) and axial (**b**) T2WI as a right paraspinal structure that has a low signal wall with rugae, within which are high signal contents.

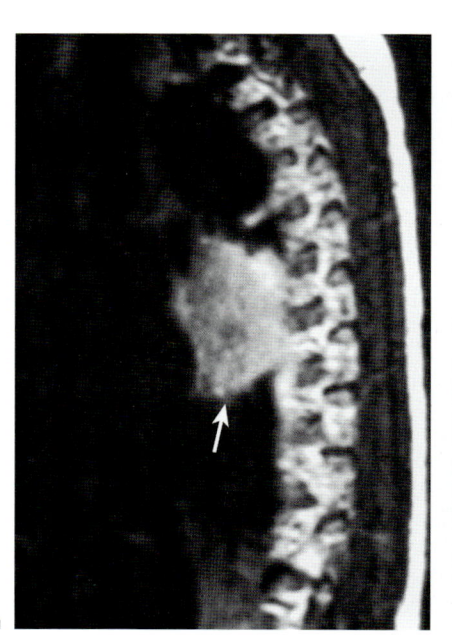

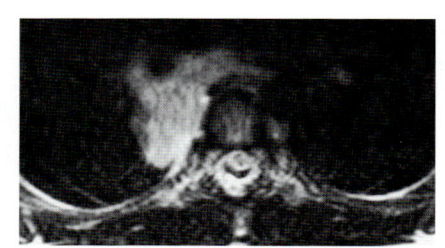

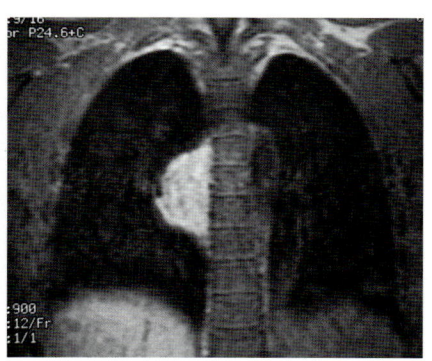

Figure 3.**19 a–c** A 9-year-old boy who is immunocompromised and has a right paravertebral cryptococcal pneumonia. The pulmonary consolidation has high signal on sagittal (**a**) and axial (**b**) T2WI, and shows Gd-contrast enhancement on coronal FS T1WI (**c**).

References

Ependymoma

Biagini R, Demitri S, Orsini U, Bibiloni J, Briccoli A, Bertoni F. Osteolytic extra-axial sacral myxopapillary ependymoma. *Skeletal Radiol* 1999; 28:585–589.

Ginsberg LE, Williams DW, Stanton C. Intrasacral myxopapillary ependymoma. *Neuroradiology* 1994;34:56–58.

Moelleken SM, Seeger LL, Eckardt JJ, Batzdorf U. Myxopapillary ependymoma with extensive sacral destruction: CT and MR findings. *J Comput Assist Tomogr* 1992;16:164–166.

Epidural Abscess

Baleriaux DL, Neugroschl C. Spinal and spinal cord infection. *Eur Radiol* 2004;14:E72–E83.

Ledermann HP, Schweitzer ME, Morrison WB, Carrino JA. MR imaging findings in spinal infections: rules or myths? *Radiology* 2003;228: 506–514.

Soehle M, Wallenfang T. Spinal epidural abscesses: clinical manifestations, prognostic factors, and outcomes. *Neurosurgery* 2002;51: 79–87.

Table 4 Lesions involving the outer surface of bone

Lesion	MRI Findings	Comments
Benign		
Osteophyte (Fig. 4.1)	Bone spurs (osteophytes) occur at the margins of synovial joints and have low peripheral signal on T1WI and T2WI overlying fatty marrow with or without edematous reaction. In the axial skeleton, smooth undulating zones of ossification involving the anterior longitudinal ligament can be seen along the anterior margins of the vertebral bodies and extending across the disks.	Bony outgrowths usually related to degenerative arthropathy at synovial joints, or degenerative disk disease adjacent to the anterior and posterior longitudinal ligaments. At synovial joints, these bony protrusions may be a response to increase the articular surface to reduce load. At the spine, osteophytes occur as a metaplastic bone response related to degenerative disk bulges displacing the longitudinal ligaments. Flowing or bridging osteophytes at four or more adjacent vertebral bodies have been referred to as diffuse idiopathic skeletal hyperostosis (DISH).
Synovial cyst (Fig. 4.2)	Spinal lesions are spheroid or ovoid circumscribed collections that protrude beyond the margins of the facet joints. Spinal synovial cysts typically show a site of communication with the adjacent degenerated facet joint. The contents of the spinal synovial cyst usually have low to intermediate signal on T1WI and PDWI, and high signal on T2WI and FS T2WI. A thin or slightly thick rim of low signal on T2WI and FS T2WI is typically seen at the periphery of the cysts. Some synovial cysts may have intermediate to high signal on T1WI, and/or intermediate or low signal on T2WI secondary to calcifications, cartilage formation, and/or hemorrhage. After Gd-contrast administration, thin marginal enhancement may be seen.	Synovium-lined fluid collections that frequently occur at or near joints of the extremities, occasionally occur at facet joints of the spine, as well as bursae and tendon sheaths. In adults, synovial cysts are often associated with osteoarthritis, rheumatoid arthritis, and trauma. **(See Atlas Chapter A 74)**
Ganglion cyst (Fig. 4.3)	Sharply defined lesions with low signal on T1WI, low-intermediate signal on PDWI, and homogeneous high signal on T2WI. Peripheral rim-like Gd-contrast enhancement can be seen as well as complete lack of enhancement. Lesions can erode and/or invade adjacent bone.	Ganglia are juxta-articular benign myxoid lesions that arise from degeneration of peri-articular connective tissue, prior trauma, or prior inflammation. Ganglia may be derived from tendons, tendon sheaths, joint capsules, bursae, or ligaments. **(See Atlas Chapter A 28)**

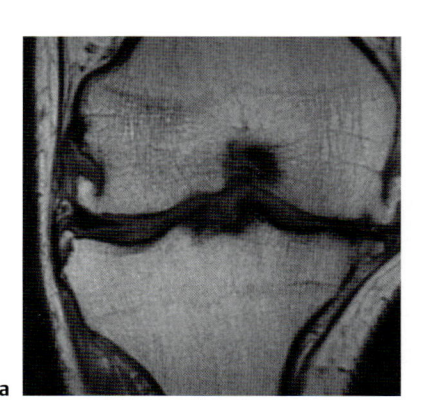

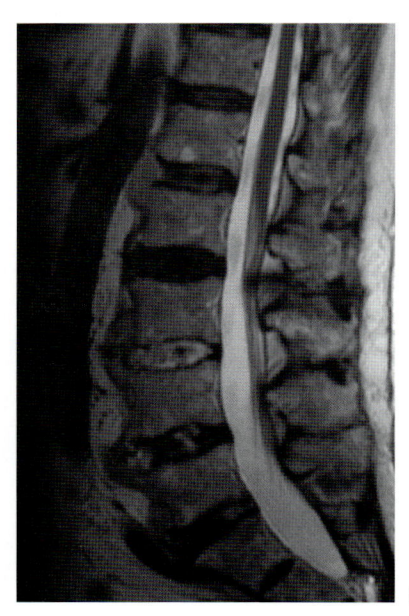

Figure 4.1 a, b A 54-year-old man with degenerative arthropathy at the knee with prominent osteophytes at the distal femur and proximal tibia on coronal PDWI (**a**). Sagittal T2WI showing bridging anterior osteophytes involving adjacent vertebral bodies (DISH) (**b**).

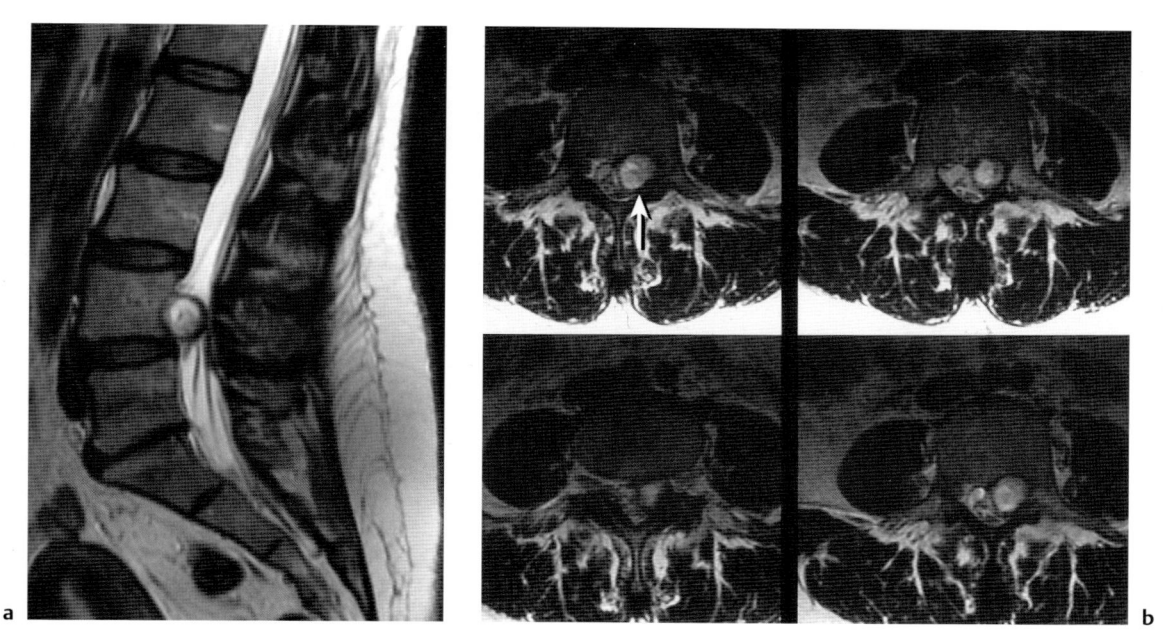

Figure 4.2 a, b Sagittal (a) and axial (b) T2WI shows a synovial cyst at the medial aspect of the left facet joint causing erosive changes at the vertebral body.

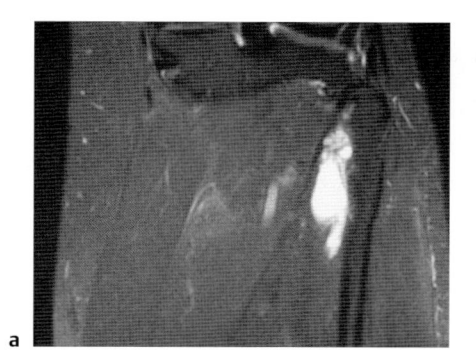

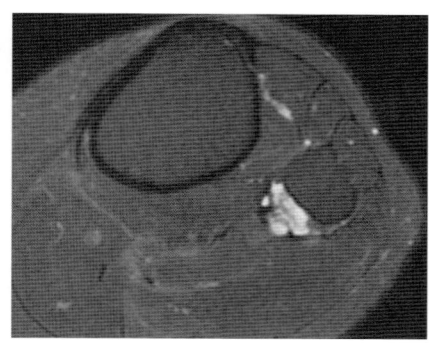

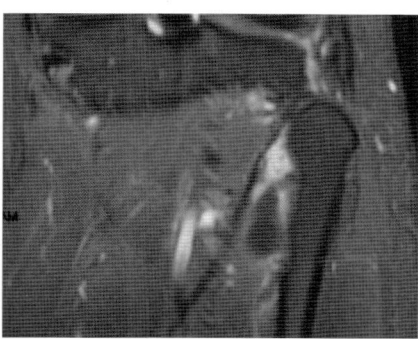

Figure 4.3 a, b Ganglion cyst along the outer surface of the fibula that has high signal on coronal (a) and axial (b) FS T2WI. Thin peripheral Gd-contrast enhancement is seen at the margins on coronal FS T1WI (c).

Table 4 (Continued) Lesions involving the outer surface of bone

Lesion	MRI Findings	Comments
Osteochondroma (Fig. 4.4)	Circumscribed protruding lesion arising from outer cortex with a central zone with intermediate signal on T1WI and T2WI similar to marrow surrounded by a peripheral zone of low signal on T1WI and T2WI, a cartilaginous cap is usually present in children and young adults. Increased malignant potential when cartilaginous cap is >2 cm thick.	Benign cartilaginous tumors arising from defect at periphery of growth plate during bone formation with resultant bone outgrowth covered by a cartilaginous cap. Usually benign lesions unless associated with pain and increasing size of cartilaginous cap. Osteochondromas are common lesions, accounting for 14 to 35% of primary bone tumors. Occur with median age of 20 years, up to 75% of patients are less than 20 years. (See Atlas Chapter A 58)
Juxtacortical chondroma (Fig. 4.5)	Lesions are located at the bone surface and are usually lobulated with low-intermediate signal on T1WI, which is hypo- or isointense relative to muscle. Lesions usually have heterogeneous predominantly high signal on T2WI. Lesions are surrounded by low signal borders on T2WI representing thin sclerotic reaction. Areas of low signal on T2WI are secondary to matrix mineralization. Edema is not typically seen in nearby medullary bone. Lesions often show a peripheral pattern of Gd-contrast enhancement.	Benign protuberant hyaline cartilaginous tumors that arise from the periosteum and superficial to bone cortex. Juxtacortical chondromas account for <1% of bone lesions. Occur with median age of 26 years. (See Atlas Chapter A 9)
Chondromyxoid fibroma (Fig. 4.6)	Lesions are often slightly lobulated with low-intermediate signal on T1WI, intermediate signal on PDWI, and heterogeneous predominantly high signal on T2WI secondary to myxoid and hyaline chondroid components with high water content. MR signal heterogeneity on T2WI is related to the proportions of myxoid, chondroid, and fibrous components within the lesions. Thin low signal septa within lesions on T2WI are secondary to fibrous strands. Lesions are surrounded by low-signal borders representing thin sclerotic reaction. Edema is not typically seen in medullary bone. Lesions show prominent diffuse Gd-contrast enhancement.	Rare, benign, slow-growing bone lesions that contain chondroid, myxoid, and fibrous components. Chondromyxoid fibromas represent 2–4% of primary benign bone lesions, and <1% of primary bone lesions. Most chondromyxoid fibromas occur between the ages of 1 and 40 years, with a median of 17 years, and peak incidence in the 2nd to 3rd decades. (See Atlas Chapter A 10)
Periosteal osteoid osteoma (Fig. 4.7)	Typically shows dense fusiform thickening of the cortex, which has low-intermediate signal on T1W, PDWI, T2WI, and FS T2WI. Within the thickened cortex, a spheroid or ovoid zone (nidus) measuring <1.5 cm is seen in the region of the original external surface of bone cortex. The nidus can have irregular, distinct, or indistinct margins relative to the adjacent region of cortical thickening. The nidus can have low-intermediate signal on T1WI and PDWI, and low-intermediate or high signal on T2WI and FS T2WI. Calcifications in the nidus can be seen as low signal on T2WI. After Gd-contrast administration, variable degrees of enhancement are seen at the nidus and adjacent marrow and cortex.	Benign osteoblastic lesion comprised of a circumscribed nidus <1.5 cm, and usually surrounded by reactive bone formation. These lesions are usually painful and have limited growth potential. Osteoid osteoma accounts for 11 to 13% of primary benign bone tumors. Occurs in patients 6 to 30 years, median=17 years. Approximately 75% occur in patients less than 25 years. (See Atlas Chapter A 60)

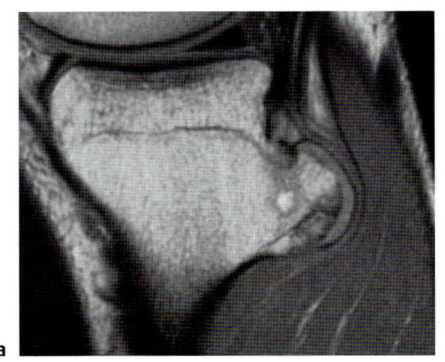

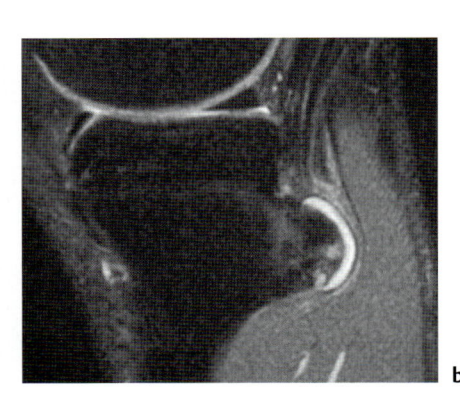

Figure 4.4 a, b A 14-year-old male with an osteochondroma at the proximal dorsal surface of the tibia as seen on sagittal PDWI (**a**) and FS T2WI (**b**).

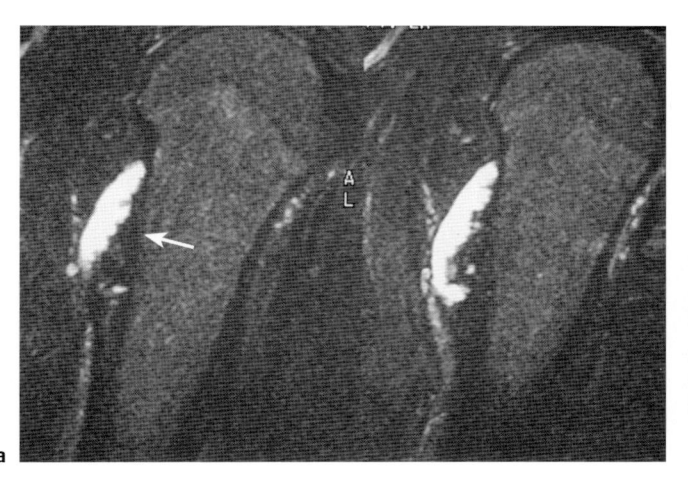

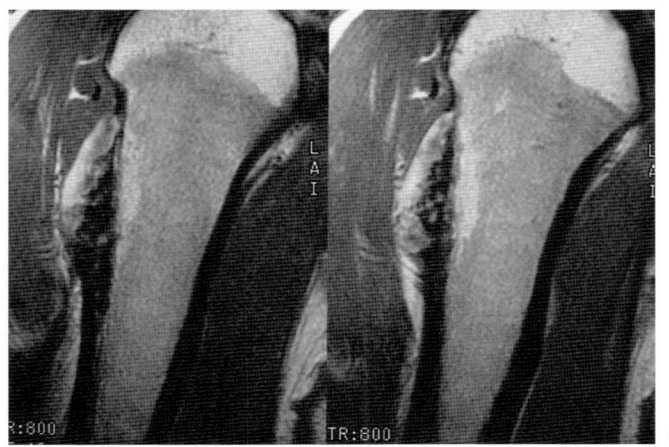

Figure 4.**5 a, b** Juxtacortical chondroma at the outer surface of the proximal humerus as seen on sagittal FS T2WI (**a**). The lesion shows Gd-contrast enhancement on sagittal T1WI (**b**).

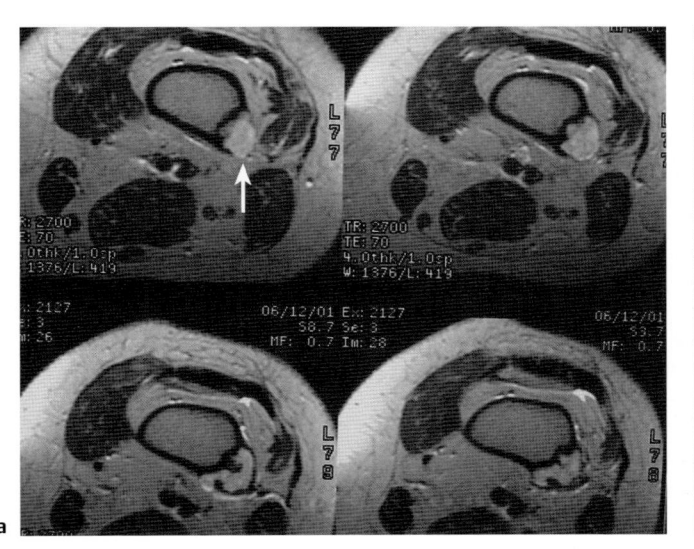

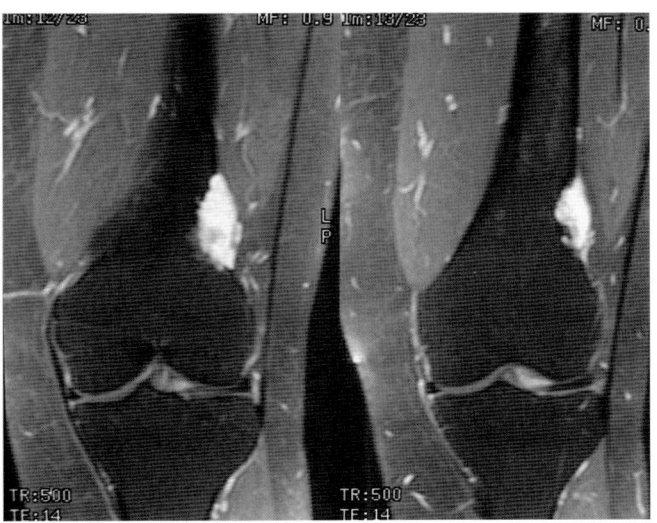

Figure 4.**6 a, b** Chondromyxoid fibroma involving the superficial portion of the distal femur. The expansile lesion has high signal on axial T2WI (**a**) and shows prominent Gd-contrast enhancement on coronal FS T1WI (**b**).

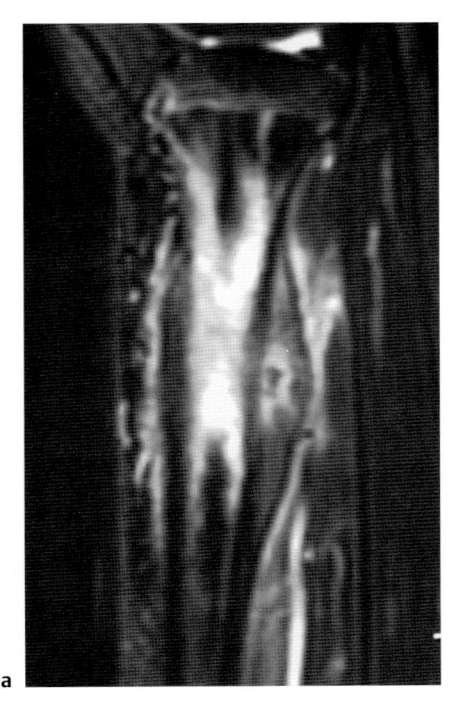

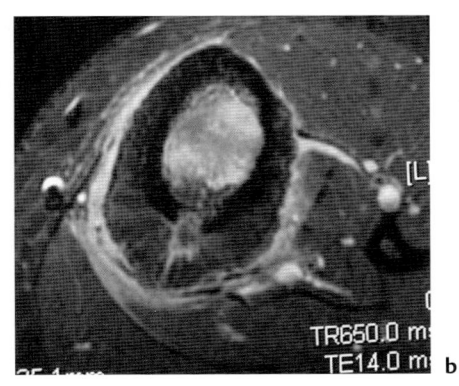

Figure 4.**7 a, b** Periosteal osteoid osteoma involving the tibia has a nidus with high signal on FS T2WI (**a**) that shows prominent Gd-contrast enhancement on axial FS T1WI (**b**). Prominent thickened periosteal bone formation is seen, which has heterogeneous intermediate and low signal on FS T2WI. Zones with high signal on FS T2WI with corresponding Gd-contrast enhancement are seen in the marrow and soft tissues superficial to the periosteal bone formation secondary to inflammatory and edematous changes from prostaglandin production by the lesion.

Table 4 (Continued) **Lesions involving the outer surface of bone**

Lesion	MRI Findings	Comments
Fibrous cortical defect (FCD) and nonossifying fibroma (NOF) (Figs. 4.8, 4.9)	**FCDs:** Circumscribed oval lesions involving bone cortex of long bones, which have low to intermediate signal on T1WI and PDWI, and low, intermediate, and/or high signal on FS T2WI surrounded by varying thickness of low signal from corresponding marginal sclerosis. FCDs with or without fracture can show variable degrees of Gd-contrast enhancement. **NOFs** have MRI features similar to FCDs, although they are larger and eccentrically involve the marrow in the metadiaphyseal regions of long bones. Cortical thinning or thickening, and bone expansion can be seen.	**FCDs** and **NOFs** are benign fibrohistiocytic lesions in the metaphyseal portions of long bones, which are comprised of whorls of fibroblastic cells combined with smaller amounts of multinucleated giant cells and xanthomatous cells. Both lesions have similar pathologic findings although they differ in size. **FCDs** are small lesions in bone cortex, whereas the larger **NOFs** are located eccentrically in the medullary cavity. Both lesions are considered in the spectrum of the same disorder of fibrohistiocytic origins. **FCDs** and **NOFs** are common benign lesions that are usually asymptomatic, and are often detected as incidental findings. Incidence may be up to 30 to 40% of children. Both lesions occur in patients 1 to 45 years, median = 14 years, 95% occur between the ages of 5 and 20. **(See Atlas Chapter A 26)**
Cortical desmoid (Fig. 4.10)	Cortical desmoids are located at the bone cortex at the distal posterior medial portions of the femur, and usually have low to intermediate signal on T1WI and PDWI, and intermediate to slightly high signal on T2WI, and slightly high to high signal on FS T2WI. A thin border of low signal on T1WI and T2WI is often seen at the inner margin of the lesion, which corresponds to a thin zone of sclerosis seen on plain films and/or CT. Bone marrow deep and peripheral to the lesion may have slightly high signal on FS T2WI. After Gd-contrast administration, enhancement can be seen at the lesion and occasionally in the adjacent marrow.	Cortical desmoids (also referred to as periosteal desmoid or distal femoral cortical irregularity) are fibrous defects at the distal posteromedial femur; may occur from an avulsive injury or stress reaction at the insertion site of the medial head of the gastrocnemius muscle or adductor magnus. Similar-appearing irregularities of bone cortex at sites where other tendons attach to bone are referred to as tug lesions. **(See Atlas Chapter A 26)**
Osteoma (Fig. 4.11)	Typically appear as well-circumscribed zones of dense bone with low signal on T1WI, PDWI, T2WI, and FS T2WI. No infiltration into the adjacent soft tissues is seen with osteomas. Zones of bone destruction or associated soft tissue mass-lesions are not associated with osteomas. Periosteal reaction is not associated with osteomas except in cases with coincidental antecedent trauma.	Benign primary bone tumors composed of dense lamellar, woven, and/or compact cortical bone usually located at the surface of bones. Multiple osteomas usually occur in Gardner syndrome, which is an autosomal dominant disorder associated with intestinal polyposis, fibromas, and desmoid tumors. Account for less than 1% of primary benign bone tumors. Occurs in patients 16 to 74 years, most frequent in 6th decade. **(See Atlas Chapter A 62)**

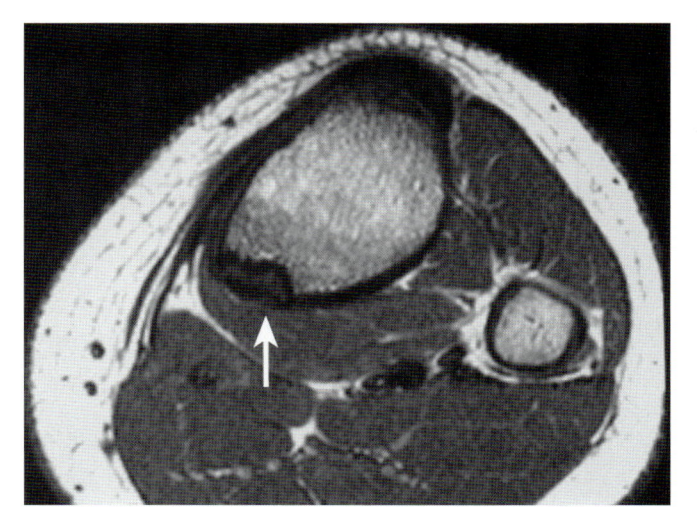

Figure 4.8 Fibrous cortical defect in the tibia on axial T1WI.

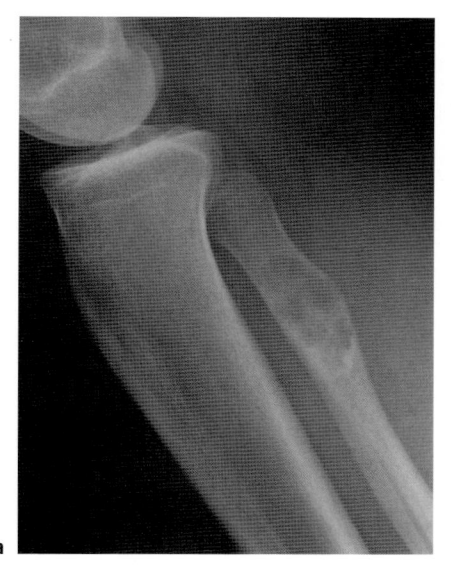

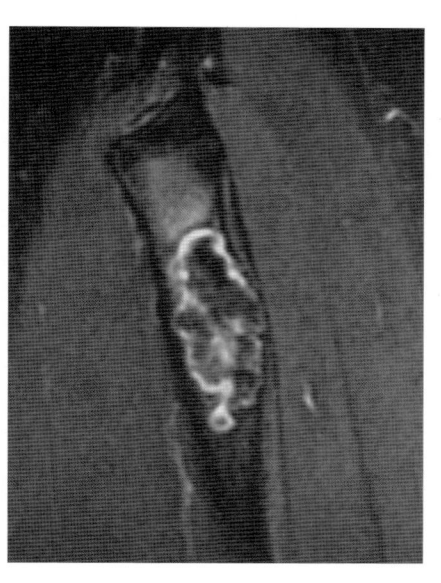

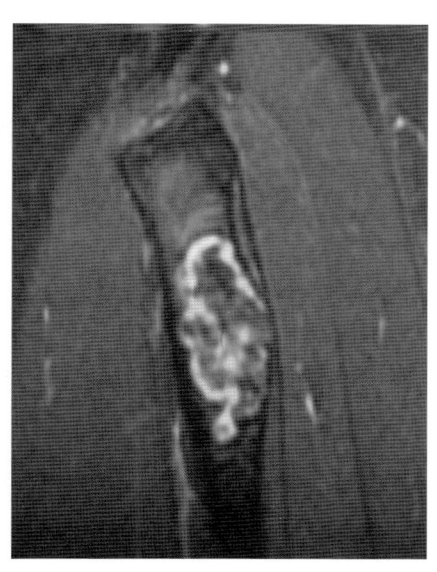

Figure 4.**9 a–c** Nonossifying fibroma in the marrow of the proximal fibula of a 15-year-old female. Oblique radiograph (**a**) shows a circumscribed radiolucent intramedullary lesion associated with thinning and expansion of the outer cortical margin. The lesion has mostly low signal centrally surrounded by thin zones with high signal on sagittal FS T2WI (**b**) and Gd-contrast enhancement on sagittal FS T1WI (**c**). The lesion expands and thins the outer cortical margin.

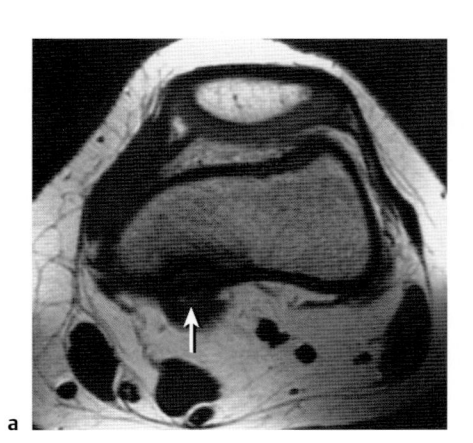

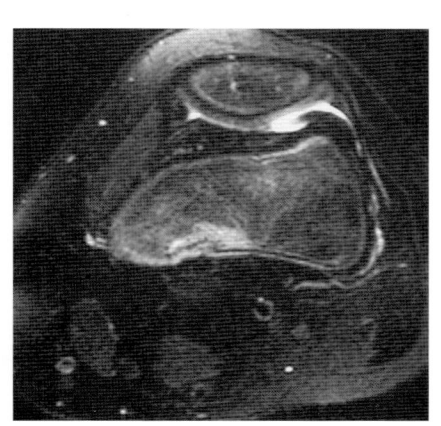

Figure 4.**10** Cortical desmoid at the distal dorsal aspect of the femur medially adjacent to the insertion of the medial gastrocnemius muscle tendon as seen on axial T1WI (**a**) and axial FS T2WI (**b**).

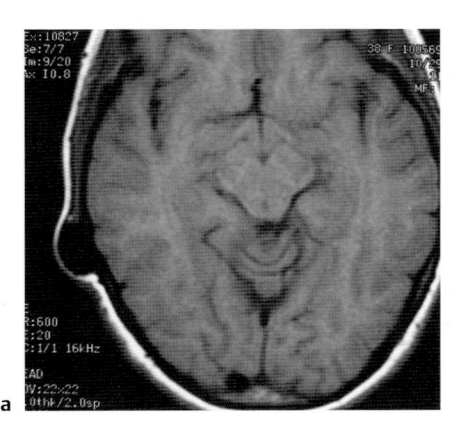

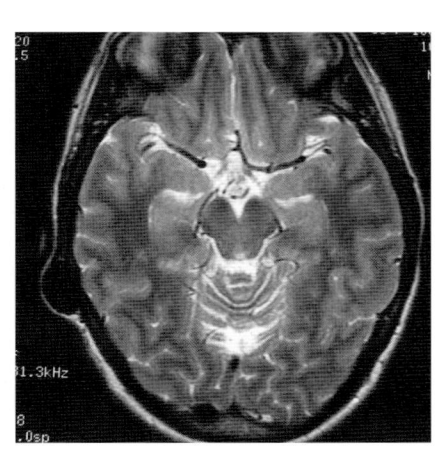

Figure 4.**11 a, b** Osteoma involving the outer table of the calvarium has low signal on axial T1WI (**a**) and T2WI (**b**).

Table 4 (Continued) **Lesions involving the outer surface of bone**

Lesion	MRI Findings	Comments
Parosteal lipoma	Lesions often have lobular margins and are immediately adjacent to the outer intact surface of adjacent bone. Lesions typically have fat signal on MRI, as well as zones of low signal on T1WI and T2WI from ossification changes that can occur within these lesions and at the junction with bone cortex. Zones with intermediate signal on T1WI and high signal on T2WI can occur in these lesions secondary to cartilaginous contents.	Rare, benign, slow-growing painless tumors with mature adipose tissue associated with the periosteum of bone. Account for 0.3% of lipomas, typically occur in patients 40 to 60 years. Common sites include the femur, proximal radius, tibia, and humerus. Other sites have been reported. May be associated with compression of adjacent nerves causing sensory or motor deficits. **(See Atlas Chapter A 43)**
Melorheostosis (Fig. 4.12)	MRI signal varies based on the relative proportions of mineralized osteoid, chondroid, and soft tissue components in these lesions. Mineralized osteoid zones along bone cortex typically have low signal on T1WI and T2WI, no Gd-contrast enhancement. Soft tissue lesions may also occur adjacent to the cortical lesions, which have a mixed signal on T1WI and T2WI.	Melorheostosis is a rare bone dysplasia with cortical thickening that has a "flowing candle wax" configuration. Associated soft tissue masses occur in ~25%. The soft tissue lesions often contain mixtures of chondroid material, mineralized osteoid, and fibrovascular tissue. **(See Atlas Chapter A 62)**
Heterotopic ossification (Fig. 4.13)	Long-standing lesions can have variable low signal on T1WI, PDWI, and T2WI depending on the degree of mineralization/ossification, fibrosis, and hemosiderin deposition. Zones of high signal on T1WI and T2WI may occur from fatty marrow metaplasia. Gd-contrast enhancement in old mature lesions is often minimal or absent. Signal abnormalities within bone marrow are usually absent.	Represents localized non-neoplastic reparative lesions that are comprised of reactive hypercellular fibrous tissue, cartilage, and/or bone. Can arise secondary to trauma (myositis ossificans circumscripta, ossifying hematoma), although may also occur without a history of prior injury (pseudomalignant osseous tumor of the soft tissues). **(See Atlas Chapter A 53)**
Schwannoma (Fig. 4.14)	**Schwannomas** are circumscribed ovoid or fusiform lesions with low-intermediate signal on T1WI, intermediate signal on PDWI, and intermediate to high signal on T2WI and FS T2WI. After Gd-contrast administration, lesions typically show moderate to prominent enhancement. Schwannomas involving spinal nerve roots may be associated with chronic erosive changes of adjacent vertebrae. Lesions may show signal heterogeneity on T2WI and heterogeneous Gd-contrast enhancement secondary to cyst formation, hemorrhage, fibrous/collagenous zones, and/or dense cellularity. Signal heterogeneity on T2WI tends to occur frequently in large schwannomas. Malignant schwannomas (malignant peripheral nerve sheath tumors) can be large lesions that have heterogeneous signal on T1WI, T2WI, and FS T2WI; as well as heterogeneous Gd-contrast enhancement because of necrosis and hemorrhage. These tumors can have irregular margins and associated invasion of adjacent structures.	Benign encapsulated tumors that contain differentiated neoplastic Schwann cells. Multiple schwannomas are often associated with NF2. Account for 5% of benign primary soft tissue tumors and 3% of all primary soft tissue tumors. Occur in patients 22 to 72 years, mean = 46 years. Peak incidence is in the 4th to 6th decades. With NF2, many patients present in the 3rd decade with bilateral vestibular schwannomas. **(See Atlas Chapter A 72)**

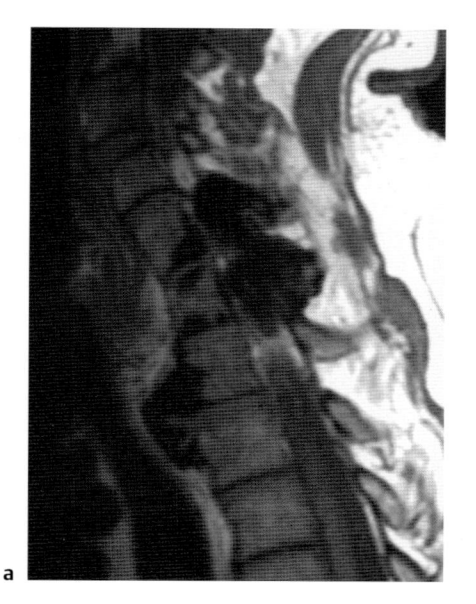

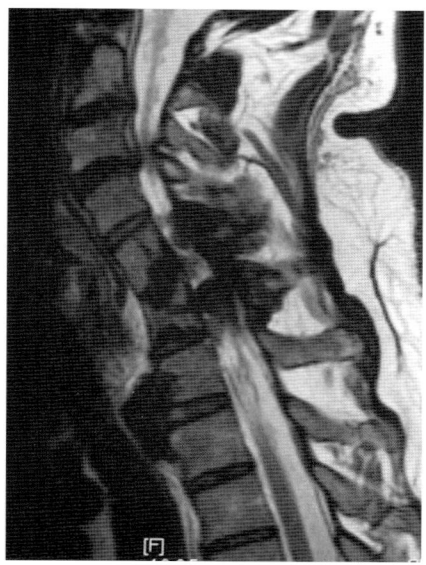

Figure 4.12 Melorheostosis involving multiple vertebrae as seen on sagittal T1WI (**a**) and T2WI (**b**).

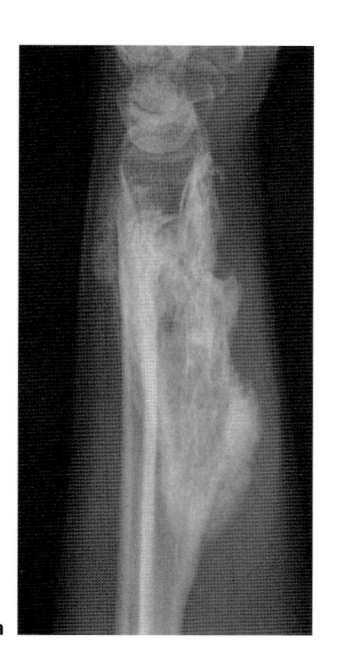

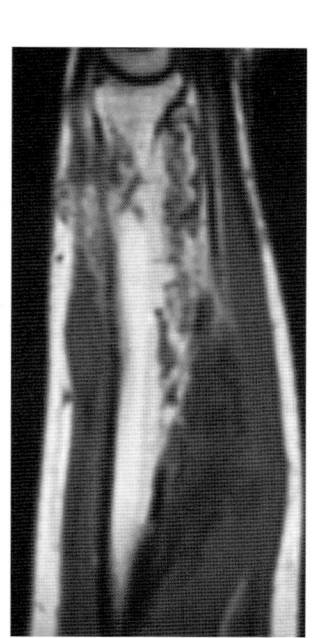

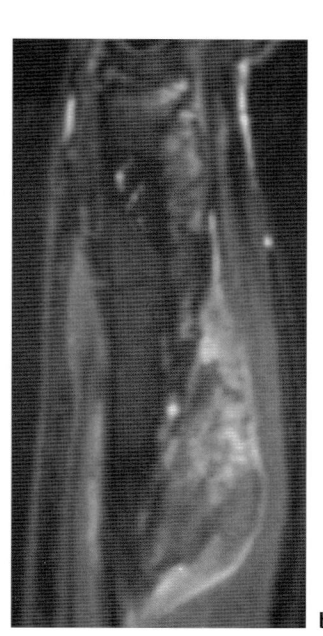

Figure 4.13 Extensive heterotopic ossification with involvement of the cortex of the distal radius as seen on lateral radiograph (**a**), sagittal T1WI (**b**), and FS T2WI (**c**).

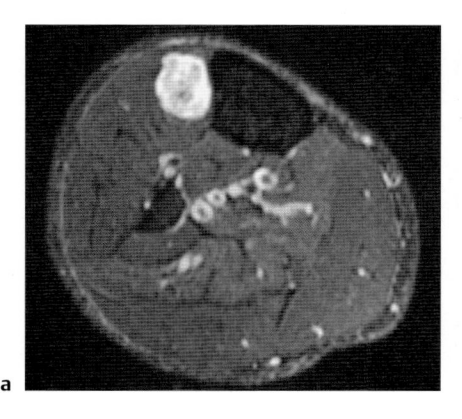

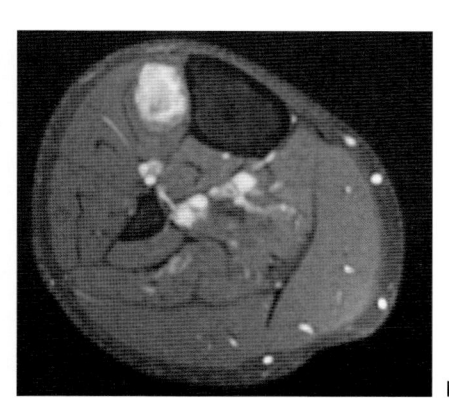

Figure 4.14 Schwannoma adjacent to the outer surface of the tibia as seen on axial FS T2WI (**a**). The lesion shows prominent Gd-contrast enhancement on axial FS T1WI (**b**).

Table 4 (Continued) **Lesions involving the outer surface of bone**

Lesion	MRI Findings	Comments
Neurofibroma (Figs. 4.15, 4.16)	**Localized neurofibromas** are circumscribed ovoid or fusiform lesions with low-intermediate signal on T1WI and intermediate to high signal on T2WI and FS T2WI. After Gd-contrast administration, lesions typically show moderate to prominent enhancement. Large lesions may show signal heterogeneity on T2WI and heterogeneous Gd-contrast enhancement. Neurofibromas involving spinal nerve roots may have a dumb-bell shape with or without associated chronic erosive changes of adjacent vertebrae. **(Fig. 4.15) Plexiform neurofibromas** appear as curvilinear and multinodular lesions involving multiple nerve branches. Lesions usually have low to intermediate signal on T1WI; and intermediate, slightly high to high signal on T2WI and FS T2WI with or without bands or strands of low signal. On T2WI, lesions may show nodules with high signal surrounding a central region of low signal referred to as a "target sign." Lesions typically show Gd-contrast enhancement in a heterogenous pattern. Lesions can be associated with remodeling of adjacent bone **(Fig. 4.16)**	Benign tumors of the peripheral nerve sheath that contain mixtures of Schwann cells, perineural-like cells, and interlacing fascicles of fibroblasts associated with abundant collagen. Unlike schwannomas, neurofibromas lack Antoni A and B regions and cannot be separated pathologically from the underlying nerve. Neurofibromas can be localized lesions (90%), or occur as diffuse or plexiform lesions. The presence of multiple neurofibromas is a typical feature of NF1, which is an autosomal dominant disorder resulting in mesodermal dysplasia affecting multiple organ systems. Plexiform neurofibromas are associated with an increased risk of malignant transformation into malignant peripheral nerve sheath tumors. Solitary neurofibromas account for 5% of primary benign soft tissue tumors and 3% of all primary soft tissue tumors. Lesions occur in patients 16 to 66 years, mean = 37 years. Neurofibromas can also occur in younger children and older adults. NF1 often presents in childhood. **(See Atlas Chapter A 56)**
Meningioma (Fig. 4.17)	Extra-axial dural-based lesions usually with intermediate signal on T1WI, intermediate-slightly high signal on T2WI, typically show prominent Gd-contrast enhancement, +/− calcifications, +/− hyperostosis, and/or invasion of adjacent skull.	Most common extra-axial intracranial tumor, usually benign neoplasms, typically occurs in adults (>40 years), women > men, multiple meningiomas seen with NF2. Can also occur in the spine with osseous erosion or invasion with or without associated hyperostosis. **(See Atlas Chapter A 49)**
Arachnoid cyst (Fig. 4.18)	Well-circumscribed extra-axial lesions with low signal on T1WI and FLAIR, and high signal on T2WI and FS T2WI, similar to CSF, no Gd-contrast enhancement. Chronic erosive changes can be seen at the adjacent skull.	Non-neoplastic acquired, developmental or congenital extra-axial cysts filled with CSF. Cysts can be small or large, asymptomatic or symptomatic.
Perineural, Tarlov cysts (Fig. 4.19)	Well-circumscribed cysts with MRI signal comparable to CSF involving nerve root sleeves associated with chronic erosive changes involving adjacent bony structures.	Typically represent incidental asymptomatic anatomic variants associated with prior dural injury.

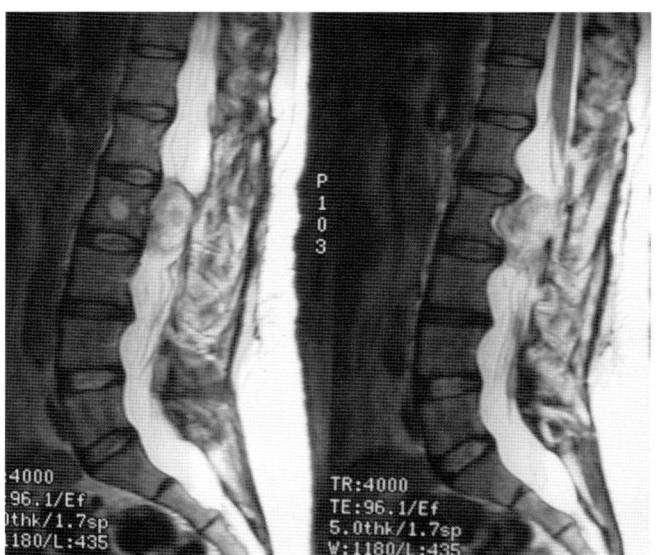

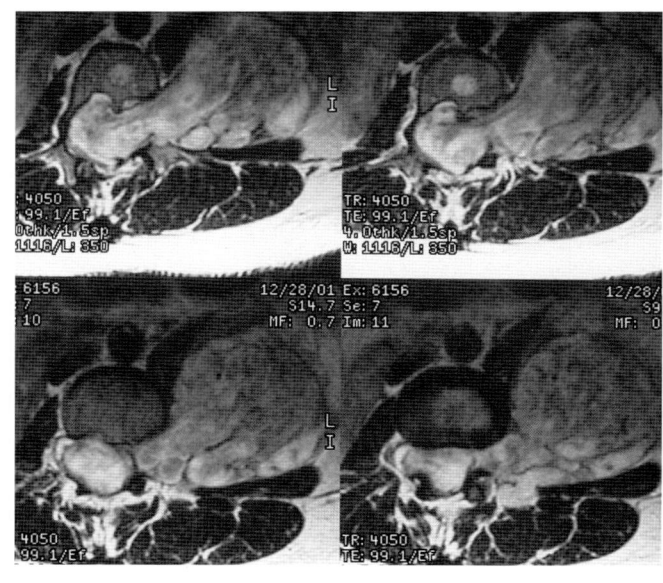

Figure 4.**15 a, b** Neurofibroma within the spinal canal at the L 2 level resulting in remodeling of the adjacent vertebra as seen on sagittal (**a**) and axial (**b**) T2WI.

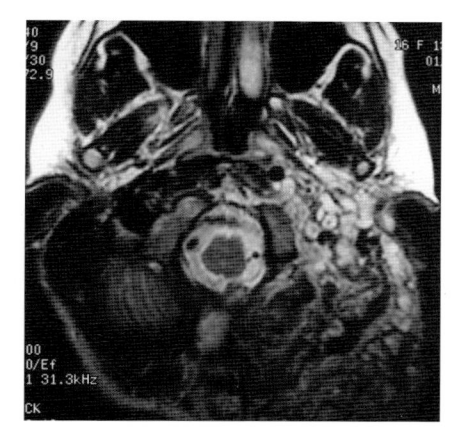

Figure 4.**16** Plexiform neurofibroma in the posterior left scalp and upper neck resulting in remodeling of the occipital bone as seen on axial T2WI.

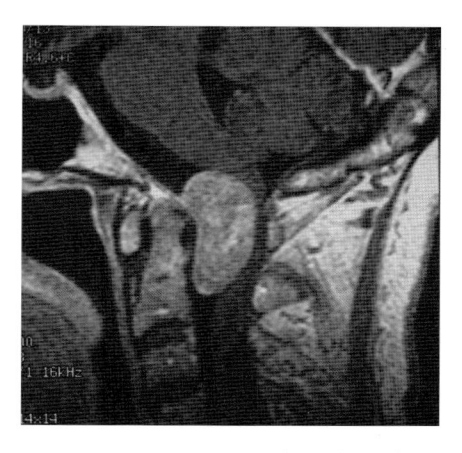

Figure 4.**17** Meningioma along the endocranial surface of the clivus showing prominent Gd-contrast enhancement on sagittal T1WI.

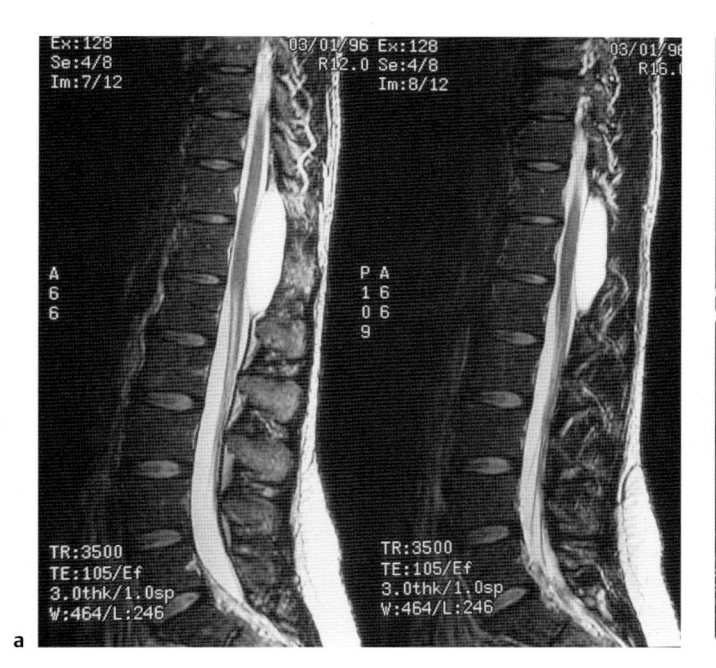

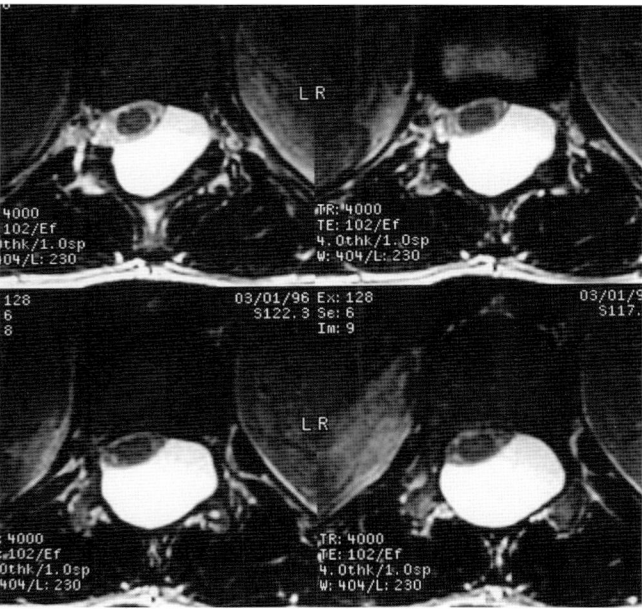

Figure 4.**18 a, b** Arachnoid cyst in the dorsal portion of the spinal canal on sagittal (**a**) and axial (**b**) T2WI that displaces the thecal sac anteriorly and causes thinning and remodeling of the posterior elements.

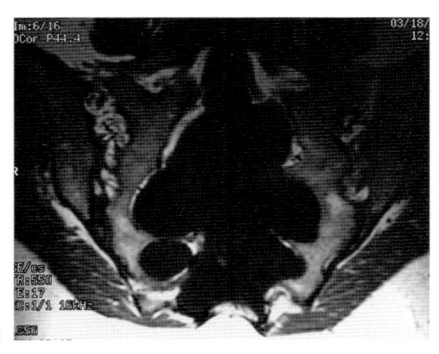

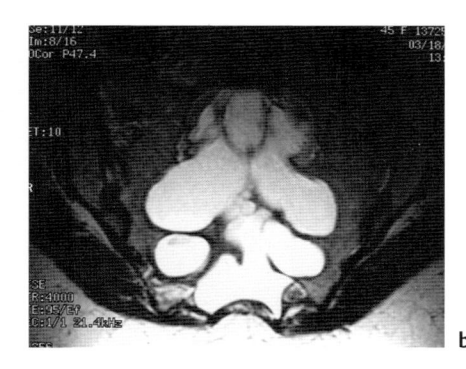

Figure 4.**19 a, b** Tarlov (perineural) cysts involving the sacral nerve root sleeves causing expansile remodeling of the sacral foramina as seen on coronal T1WI (**a**) and T2WI (**b**).

Table 4 (Continued) **Lesions involving the outer surface of bone**

Lesion	MRI Findings	Comments
Giant cell tumor of tendon sheath (Fig. 4.20)	Lesions usually have well-defined margins and are often adjacent to a tendon/tendon sheath. Lesions can be ovoid or multilobulated, and usually have low-intermediate or intermediate signal on T1WI and PDWI that is often similar to or less than muscle. On T2WI and FS T2WI, lesions can have mixed low, intermediate, and/or high signal. Zones of low signal on T2WI often correspond to sites of hemosiderin deposition. Lesions often show Gd-contrast enhancement in either homogeneous or heterogeneous pattern. Erosions of adjacent bone can be seen with some lesions.	Giant cell tumors of the tendon sheath and pigmented villonodular synovitis are benign proliferative lesions of synovium (tendon sheaths, joints, and bursae). Giant cell tumors of the tendon sheaths can occur as localized nodular lesions attached to tendon sheaths outside of joints (hands, feet) or within joints (infrapatellar portion of knee joint); or as a diffuse form near/outside of large joints such as the knee and ankle. Giant cell tumors of the tendon sheath represent 4% of benign soft tissue tumors and 2% of all soft tissue tumors. Occur in patients from 6 to 71 years, mean = 39 to 46 years with peak ages in 3rd to 4th decades. **(See Atlas Chapter A 30)**
Glomus tumor (Fig. 4.21)	Glomus tumors are well-circumscribed ovoid lesions measuring less than 1 cm and are often located under the nail beds at the distal phalanges of fingers and toes. Glomus tumors often have low-intermediate signal on T1WI and PDWI, high signal on T2WI and FS T2WI. A thin rim of low signal on T2WI may be seen secondary to a capsule from reactive tissue surrounding the glomus tumor. Lesions typically show Gd-contrast enhancement. MRI can show erosion of the underlying bone.	Benign mesenchymal hamartomas, composed of round cells derived from the neuromyoarterial apparatus (glomus bodies). that regulate arteriolar blood flow to the skin. **(See Atlas Chapter A 31)**
Nonmalignant giant cell tumor eroding through bone cortex (Fig. 4.22)	Usually well-defined lesions with thin low signal margins on T1WI, PDWI, and T2WI. Solid portions of giant cell tumors often have low to intermediate signal on T1WI and PDWI, intermediate to high signal on T2WI, and high signal on FS PDWI and FS T2WI. Signal heterogeneity on T2WI is not uncommon. Zones of low signal on T2WI and T2* imaging may be seen secondary to hemosiderin. Aneurysmal bone cysts can be seen in 14% of giant cell tumors, resulting in cystic zones with variable signal and fluid–fluid levels. After Gd-contrast administration, mild to prominent enhancement of the solid intraosseous portions of the lesions is seen, as well as peripheral rim-like enhancement around cystic zones/aneurysmal bone cysts. Contrast enhancement is usually seen in the extraosseous portions of the tumors. Poorly defined zones of enhancement and high signal on FS T2WI may also be seen in the marrow peripheral to the portions of the lesions associated with radiographic evidence of bone destruction, indicating reactive inflammatory and edematous changes associated with elevated tumor prostaglandin levels.	Aggressive tumors composed of neoplastic ovoid mononuclear cells and scattered multinucleated osteoclast-like giant cells (derived from fusion of marrow mononuclear cells). Up to 10% of all giant cell tumors are malignant. Benign giant cell tumors account for ~5 to 9.5% of all bone tumors and up to 23% of benign bone tumors. Occurs in patients 4 to 81 years (median = 30 years), 75% occur in patients between 15 and 45 years. **(See Atlas Chapter A 29)**

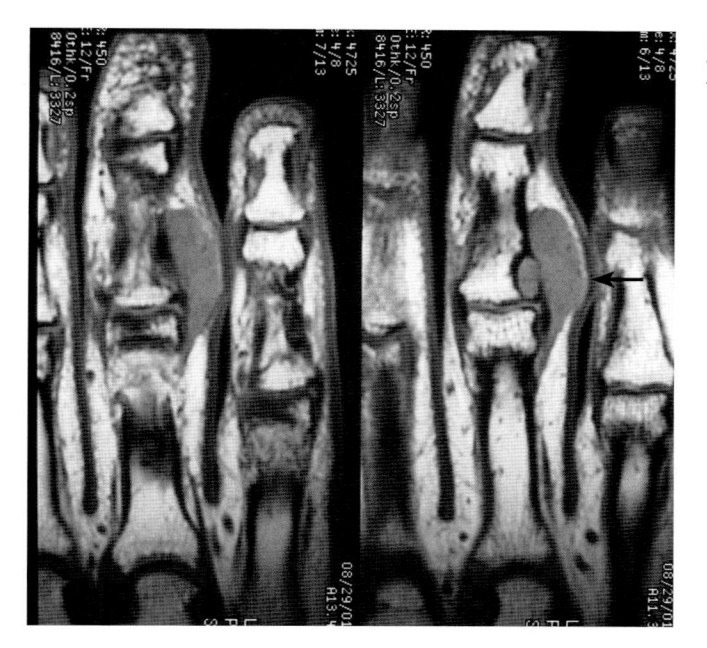

Figure 4.20 Giant cell tumor of the tendon sheath (nodular synovitis) causing focal erosion of the adjacent phalanx as seen on coronal T1WI.

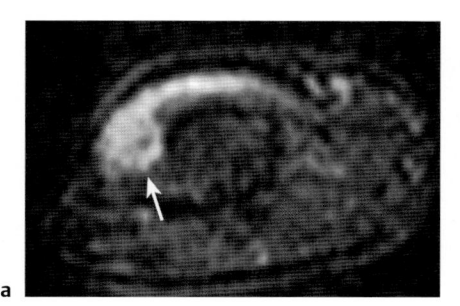

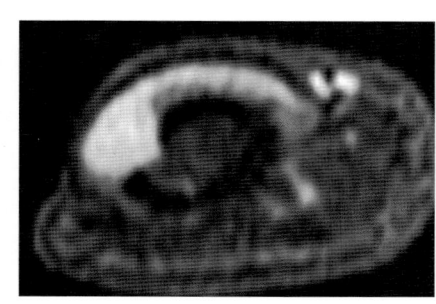

Figure 4.21 a, b Glomus tumor under the fingernail with slightly high signal on axial FS T2WI (**a**) and Gd-contrast enhancement on axial FS T1WI (**b**). The lesion erodes the cortical margin of the adjacent phalanx.

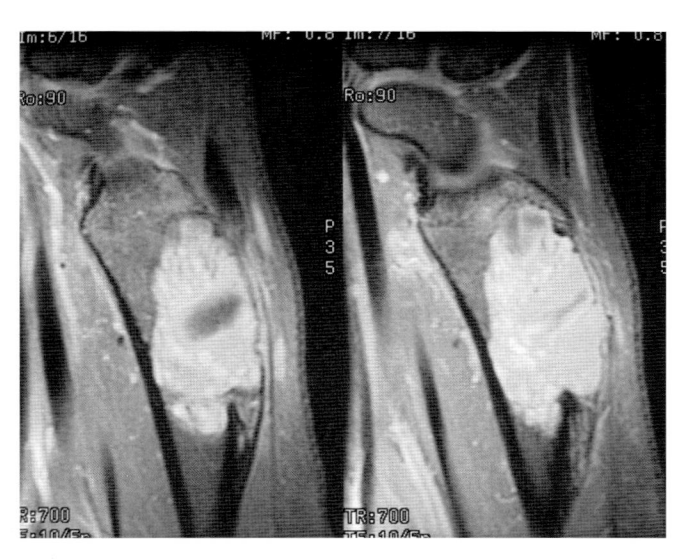

Figure 4.22 Giant cell tumor of bone involving the distal radius. The intramedullary lesion erodes cortical bone and extends into the extraosseous soft tissues. The lesion shows prominent Gd-contrast enhancement on sagittal FS T1WI.

Table 4 (Continued) **Lesions involving the outer surface of bone**

Lesion	MRI Findings	Comments
Eosinophilic granuloma eroding through bone cortex (Fig. 4.23)	Focal intramedullary lesion(s) associated with trabecular and cortical bone destruction that typically have low-intermediate signal on T1WI and PDWI and heterogeneous slightly high to high signal on T2WI. Poorly defined zones of high signal on T2WI are usually seen in the marrow peripheral to the portions of the lesions associated with radiographic evidence of bone destruction, indicating reactive inflammatory and edematous changes. Extension of lesions from the marrow into adjacent soft tissues through areas of cortical disruption are commonly seen as well as linear periosteal zones of high signal on T2WI. Lesions typically show prominent Gd-contrast enhancement in marrow and in extraosseous soft tissue portions of the lesions.	Single or multiple eosinophilic granulomas are benign tumorlike lesions consisting of Langerhans' cells (histiocytes), and variable amounts of lymphocytes, polymorphonuclear cells, and eosinophils. Account for 1 % of primary bone lesions, and 8 % of tumor-like lesions, 5 to 20 per 1 000 000 children per year in the USA. Occurs in patients 1 to 60 years, median = 10 years, average = 13.5 years, peak incidence is between 5 and 10 years, 80 to 85 % occur in patients less than 30 years, and 60 % occur in children less than 10 years. **(See Atlas Chapter A 18)**
Osteomyelitis (Fig. 4.24)	Periosteal reaction associated with osteomyelitis is seen as a peripheral rim of high signal on T2WI and FS T2WI and Gd-contrast enhancement on FS T1WI adjacent to the low signal of cortical bone. A subperiosteal abscess with high signal on T2WI and FS T2WI can be often seen elevating a single low signal thin band of periosteum. Within the underlying marrow, poorly defined zones with high signal on T2WI and FS T2WI and Gd-contrast enhancement are seen with or without associated zones of cortical destruction.	Osteomyelitis refers to infection of bone and can result from hematogenous spread of microorganisms, trauma-direct inoculation, extension from adjacent tissues, and complications from surgery. *Staphylococcus aureus* and *Streptococcus pyogenes* are the most common bacterial infections involving bone. Osteomyelitis can also result from other bacteria as well as from other organisms such as Mycobacteria tuberculosis, fungi, parasites, and viruses. **(See Atlas Chapter A 63)**
Myositis/cellulitis associated with infection of bone (Fig. 4.25)	Irregular poorly defined zones with slightly high to high signal on T2WI and FS T2WI are typically seen with Gd-contrast enhancement. Circumscribed zones with high signal on T2WI and FS T2WI may also be seen with abscess formation.	Infection of soft tissues can result in erosion, destruction, and invasion of adjacent bone.
Rheumatoid pannus adjacent to and eroding bone (Fig. 4.26)	Erosions of cortical bone in large and small joints, vertebral endplates, spinous processes, and uncovertebral and apophyseal joints. Irregular enlarged enhancing synovium (pannus low-intermediate signal on T1WI, intermediate-high signal on T2WI and FS T2WI) in joints results in osseous erosions.	Most common type of inflammatory arthropathy that results in synovitis causing destructive/erosive changes of cartilage, ligaments, and bone. Cervical spine involvement two-thirds of patients, juvenile and adult types. **(See Atlas Chapter A 70)**
Pigmented villonodular synovitis (PVNS) (Fig. 4.27)	Often appears as irregular, multinodular, and/or irregular thickening of synovium with low or low-intermediate signal on T1WI and T2WI. Solitary nodular lesions can also occur. Areas of low signal on T2WI and T2*WI in lesions are secondary to hemosiderin. Joint effusions are usually present, rarely with fluid–fluid levels. PVNS usually shows Gd-contrast enhancement in homogeneous, heterogeneous, and/or septal patterns.	Benign intra-articular lesions of proliferative synovium containing zones of recent or remote hemorrhage. Similar histopathologic features with giant cell tumors of the tendon sheath. Account for < 1 % of benign and all soft tissue tumors. Mean age = 38 years, median age = 32 years. **(See Atlas Chapter A 67)**

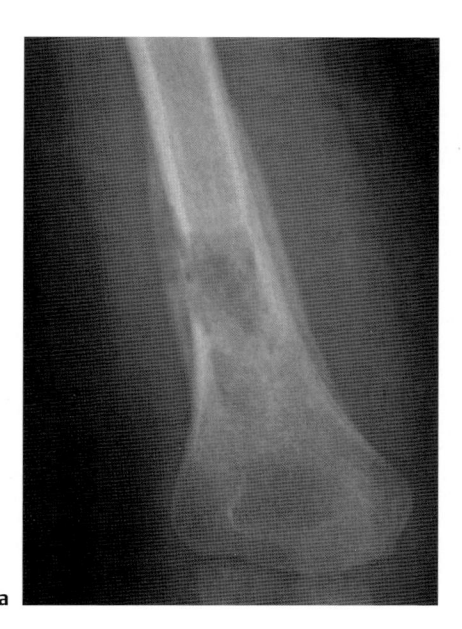

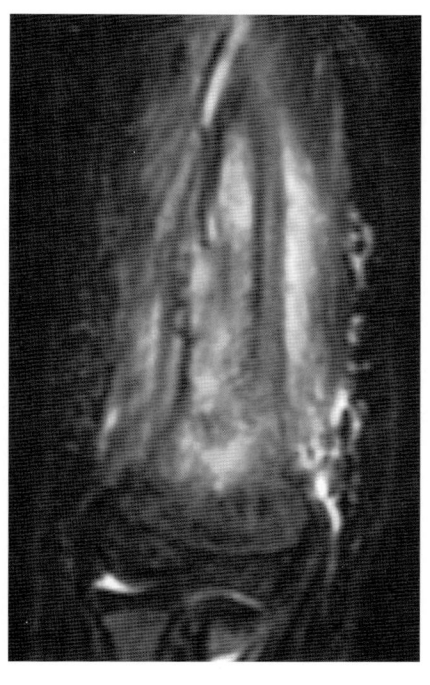

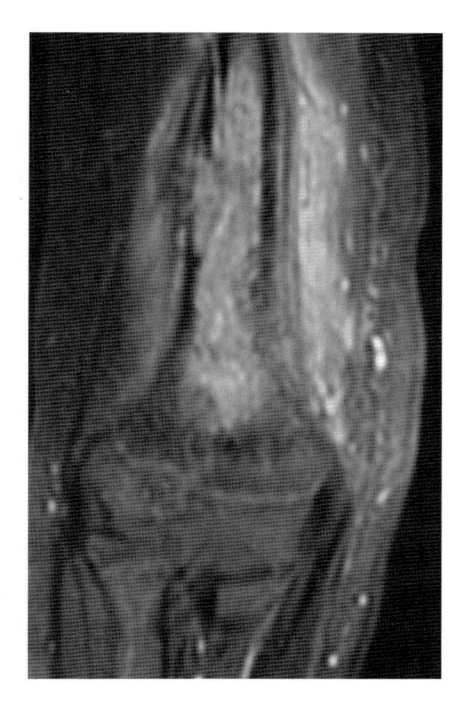

Figure 4.23 a–c Eosinophilic granuloma involving the distal humerus. AP radiograph (**a**) shows a radiolucent intramedullary lesion with irregular margins, cortical disruption medially, and a single layer of smooth periosteal reaction. A zone of disruption of the periosteum is seen medially. MRI shows an intramedullary poorly defined lesion with heterogeneous slightly high to high signal on coronal FS T2WI (**b**) and corresponding Gd-contrast enhancement on coronal FS T1WI (**c**). Extension of the lesion from the marrow into adjacent soft tissues is seen through areas of cortical disruption. Zones of high signal and Gd-contrast enhancement are seen superficial and deep to the elevated periosteum, which is seen as a linear zone of low signal.

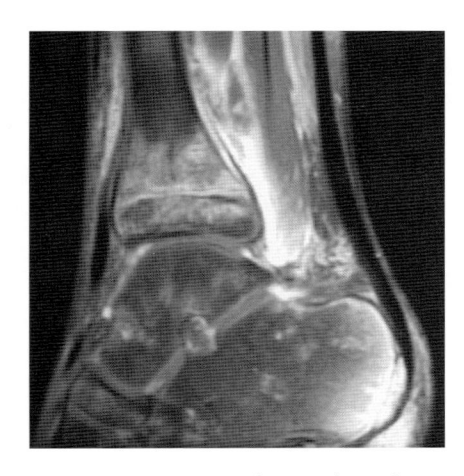

Figure 4.24 Osteomyelitis involving the metaphysis and epiphysis of the distal tibia. The infection is seen as poorly defined zones of Gd-contrast enhancement in the marrow associated with periosteal elevation and poorly defined zones of Gd-contrast enhancement in the adjacent soft tissues on sagittal FS T1WI.

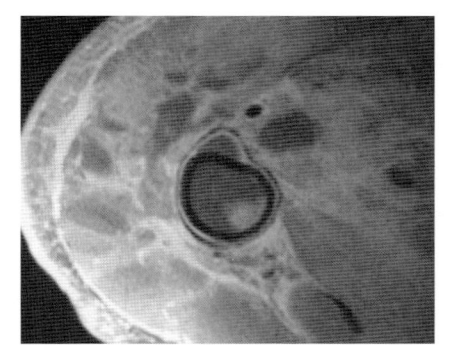

Figure 4.25 Myositis involving the muscles at the shoulder with erosion of cortical bone, intraosseous extension, periosteal reaction, and subperiosteal abscess as seen on post-contrast axial FS T1WI.

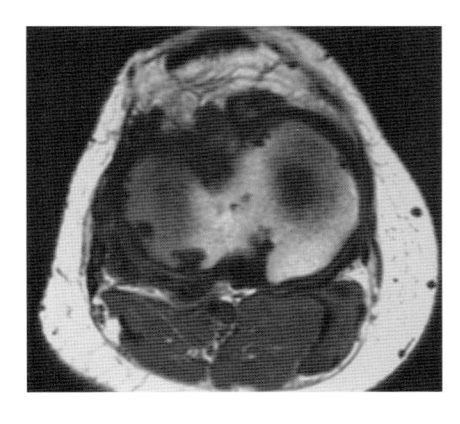

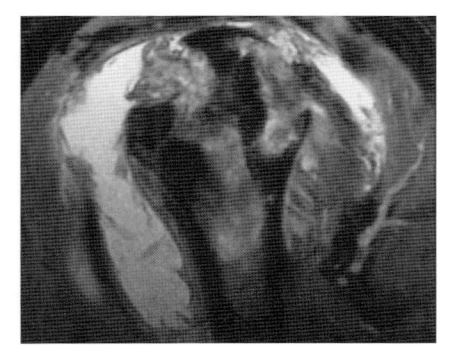

Figure 4.26 Rheumatoid arthritis at the shoulder with pannus eroding the humerus as seen on sagittal FS T2WI. Pannus is seen as poorly defined synovium with mixed intermediate slightly high and low signal. A large joint fluid collection is also present.

Figure 4.27 Pigmented villonodular synovitis in the knee associated with focal erosions of the adjacent tibia as seen on axial T1WI.

Table 4 (Continued) **Lesions involving the outer surface of bone**

Lesion	MRI Findings	Comments
Calcific tendinitis eroding into bone (Fig. 4.28)	Zones with slightly high and low signal on T2WI and FS T2WI are seen in tendons with or without erosion of bone cortex. Intramedullary zones with mixed low, intermediate, and/or high signal on T2WI and FS T2WI may be seen in the adjacent marrow.	Degenerative disorder with amorphous calcifications in tendons or bursa associated with erosion of adjacent bone cortex, with or without marrow invasion. Most common in humerus and femur in patients 16 to 82 years, average = 50 years.
Noninterrupted periosteal reaction from fracture (Fig. 4.29)	Noninterrupted periosteal reaction from stress fractures and healing traumatic fractures typically appear as a linear thin single 1–2-mm band of low signal superficial to bone cortex, which is surrounded by poorly defined zones with high signal on FS T2WI and Gd-contrast enhancement. Poorly defined intramedullary zones with high signal on FS T2WI and Gd-contrast enhancement are usually seen in the underlying bone marrow. A thin linear radiodense line is seen at the elevated periosteum 7 to 10 days later.	48 hours after fracture, extravascular red blood cells lyse causing an intense inflammatory reaction followed by granulation tissue ingrowth. Periosteal reaction occurs when fibroblasts are induced to form osteoblasts in the outer periosteal layer secondary to trauma. Periosteal reaction occurs earlier in children compared with adults.
Subperiosteal hematoma (Fig. 4.30)	Low signal thin bands of periosteum separated from underlying bone cortex can be seen surrounded by irregular zones with intermediate to high signal on T2WI and FS T2WI, and irregular Gd-contrast enhancement.	Subperiosteal hematomas can result from bone fractures or avulsion of periosteum near sites of tendinous insertions.
Hemophilic pseudotumor	Subperiosteal pseudotumors elevate the periosteum from hemorrhage associated with cortical erosion and periosteal reaction. Lesions usually have mixed low, intermediate, and high signal on T1WI and T2WI, as well as fluid–fluid levels.	Lesions can occur within medullary bone or in a subperiosteal location, as well as within soft tissues in 1–2 % of patients with severe factor VIII or IX deficiency. Enlarging lesions may require surgical resection.
Noninterrupted periosteal reaction from primary hypertrophic osteoarthropathy (pachydermoperiostosis)	Linear and/or irregular periosteal and cortical thickening seen in tubular bones of the extremities bilaterally (tibia, fibula, radius ulna are common sites, also seen in other bones and skull). Can involve epiphyseal, metaphyseal, and/or diaphyseal portions of long bones.	Rare clinical syndrome in adolescents or adults with swollen painful joints, enlargement of the extremities from osseous proliferation and periostitis, clubbing of digits, thickening of skin of the face and scalp with excessive sweating and sebaceous secretions. Can be hereditary (autosomal dominant with variable expression) or idiopathic.
Noninterrupted periosteal reaction from secondary hypertrophic osteoarthropathy	Smooth, wavy, and or irregular periosteal and cortical thickening seen in the diaphyseal and metaphyseal portions of long bones of the upper and lower extremities, as well as in other bones.	Clinical syndrome with clubbing of the digits, periostitis, hypertrophic osteoarthropathy, skin thickening, limb swelling, nail bed abnormalities (striations, increased curvature) related to extraskeletal lesions involving the lungs (bronchogenic carcinoma, metastasis, cystic fibrosis, bronchiectasis, infection, lymphoma), pleura (mesothelioma), abdomen (biliary atresia, cirrhosis, tumors, ulcerative colitis, Crohn disease), heart (cyanotic heart disease), or neoplasms at other sites. Regression of hypertrophic osteoarthropathy can occur after thoracotomy in patients with thoracic abnormalities, even in those without complete removal of the intrathoracic lesions.

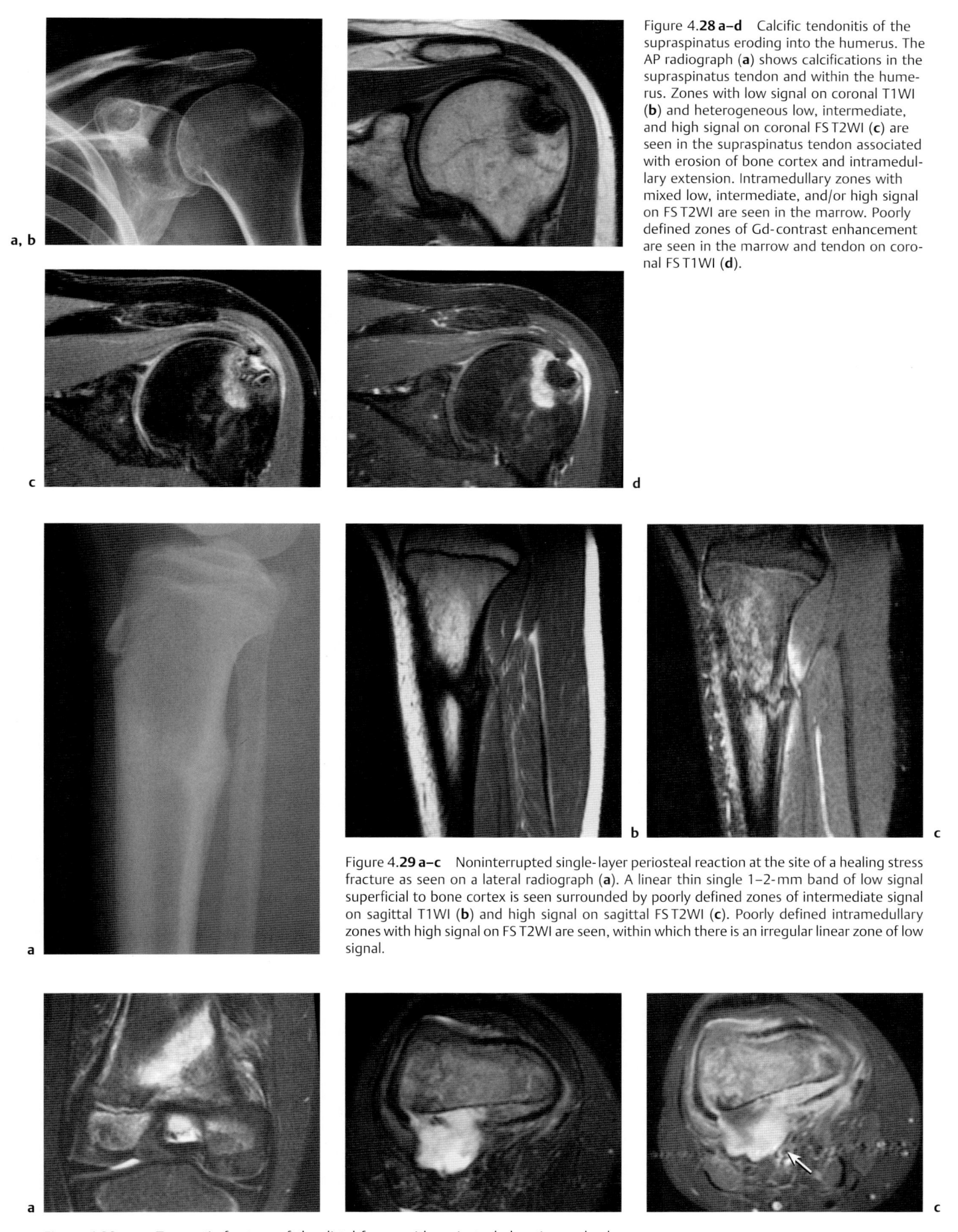

Figure 4.28 a–d Calcific tendonitis of the supraspinatus eroding into the humerus. The AP radiograph (a) shows calcifications in the supraspinatus tendon and within the humerus. Zones with low signal on coronal T1WI (b) and heterogeneous low, intermediate, and high signal on coronal FS T2WI (c) are seen in the supraspinatus tendon associated with erosion of bone cortex and intramedullary extension. Intramedullary zones with mixed low, intermediate, and/or high signal on FS T2WI are seen in the marrow. Poorly defined zones of Gd-contrast enhancement are seen in the marrow and tendon on coronal FS T1WI (d).

Figure 4.29 a–c Noninterrupted single-layer periosteal reaction at the site of a healing stress fracture as seen on a lateral radiograph (a). A linear thin single 1–2-mm band of low signal superficial to bone cortex is seen surrounded by poorly defined zones of intermediate signal on sagittal T1WI (b) and high signal on sagittal FS T2WI (c). Poorly defined intramedullary zones with high signal on FS T2WI are seen, within which there is an irregular linear zone of low signal.

Figure 4.30 a–c Traumatic fracture of the distal femur with periosteal elevation and subperiosteal hematoma as seen on coronal (a) and axial (b) FS T2WI. Focal disruption of the periosteum is also seen dorsally on axial FS T2WI and post-contrast axial FS T1WI (c).

Table 4 (Continued)   **Lesions involving the outer surface of bone**

Lesion	MRI Findings	Comments
Noninterrupted periosteal reaction from venous stasis (Fig. 4.31)	Smooth and wavy periosteal and cortical thickening seen in the diaphyseal and metaphyseal portions of long bones of the lower extremities (tibia, fibula, metatarsal bones, phalanges).	Venous stasis is associated with edematous changes in the soft tissues as well as soft tissue ossification, periostitis, and cortical thickening.
Noninterrupted periosteal reaction from infantile cortical hyperostosis (Caffey disease)	Smooth, wavy, and/or irregular periosteal and cortical thickening seen in the diaphyseal and metaphyseal portions of one or multiple bones.	Clinical disorder that affects infants less than 5 months with findings of soft tissue swelling (commonly over the mandible), fever, hyperirritability, and cortical hyperostosis (ribs, ulna, tibia, fibula, humerus, femur, radius, metacarpal, and metatarsal bones). The clinical course is variable but regression of findings can occur over 3 to 4 years.
Noninterrupted periosteal reaction from thyroid acropachy	Asymmetric, irregular, spiculated periosteal thickening seen in the diaphyseal portions of one or multiple bones (metacarpal and metatarsal bones, phalanges, other bones).	This disorder represents an extreme form of autoimmune thyroid disease with clinical manifestations such as swelling of the digits and toes, digital clubbing, and periosteal reaction. Thyroid dermopathy (pretibial myxedema) occurs in 4% of patients with Graves ophthalmopathy. Pronounced cases of thyroid dermopathy can be associated with thyroid acropachy in 1% of patients with Graves ophthalmopathy.
Noninterrupted periosteal reaction from hypervitaminosis A	Smooth and wavy periosteal and cortical thickening seen in the diaphyseal portions of one or multiple bones (ulna, metatarsal bones, clavicle, tibia, fibula, other bones). Damage to the physeal plates can result in irregularities and premature fusion, as well as splaying and cupping deformities of the metaphyses.	Vitamin A intoxication in children can result in anorexia, dermatologic, and osseous disorders. In children, damage to the physeal plates may be irreversible despite cessation of vitamin A administration. In adults, anorexia, weight loss, and dermatologic disorders are frequently associated with hypervitaminosis A.

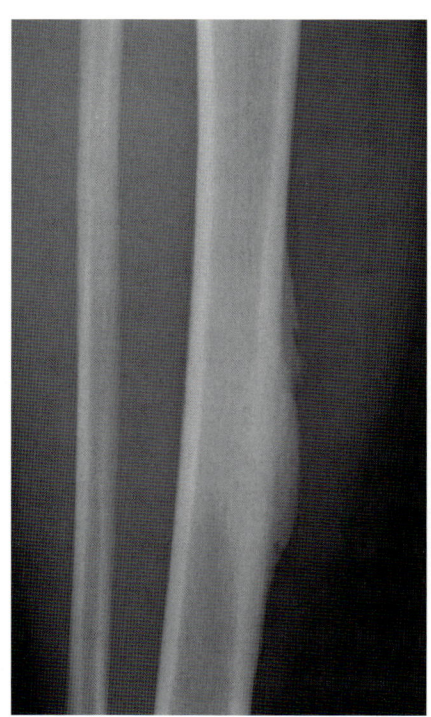

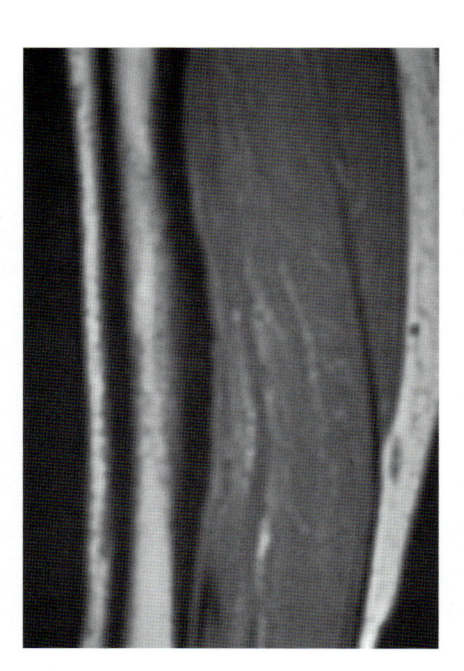

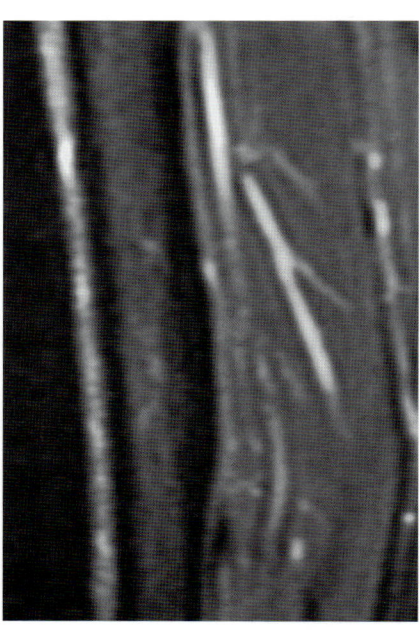

Figure 4.31 a–c   Thickened noninterrupted periosteal reaction from venous stasis as seen on oblique radiograph (**a**). The periosteal bone formation has low signal on sagittal T1WI (**b**) and post-contrast FS T1WI (**c**).

Table 4 (Continued) Lesions involving the outer surface of bone

Lesion	MRI Findings	Comments
Noninterrupted periosteal reaction from hypovitaminosis A	Smooth and wavy periosteal and cortical thickening seen in the diaphyseal portions of one or multiple bones.	Vitamin A deficiency can result in anemia, dermatologic abnormalities (dry and scaly skin), growth retardation, osseous abnormalities, cranial nerve, and visual disorders.
Periosteal reaction from hypovitaminosis C (scurvy)	In children, periosteal elevation with new bone formation can be seen in the diaphyseal and metaphyseal portions of one or multiple bones from subperiosteal hemorrhage. Metaphyseal beak-like bone protrusions can occur from the abnormal zones of provisional calcification at the physeal plate, as well as subepiphyseal fractures. In adults, osteopenia with hemarthrosis can be associated with ischemic necrosis and fractures with mild periosteal reaction.	In young children, vitamin C deficiency after 4 to 10 months can result in infantile scurvy with clinical features including failure to thrive, petechial hemorrhages, ulcerated gingiva, hematemesis, melena, hematuria, and anemia. Clinical features associated with adult scurvy include anorexia, fatigue, weakness, petechial hemorrhages involving gingiva and skin, hemarthrosis, osteoporosis, ischemic necrosis, dermatologic disorders (dry and scaly skin), growth retardation, osseous and nerve disorders.
Syndromes of hyperostosis, osteitis, and skin lesions (SAPHO syndrome)	Periosteal elevation with cortical thickening can be seen as well as syndesmophyte formation at one or multiple levels.	Syndrome that includes abnormalities such as synovitis, acne, pustulosis, hyperostosis with periosteal proliferation (sternum, clavicle, anterior ribs, symphysis pubis, femur, sacrum, iliac bones) and osteitis at the chest wall.
Neurofibromatosis type 1 (Fig. 4.32)	Undulating zones of periosteal bone formation can occur in the lower extremities in patients with NF1.	One of the most common genetic diseases with the involved locus on chromosome 17q12 typically resulting in multiple neurofibromas. This is an autosomal dominant disorder resulting in mesodermal dysplasia affecting multiple organ systems. Can result in periosteal proliferation in the long bones of the lower extremities. **(See Atlas Chapter A 56)**

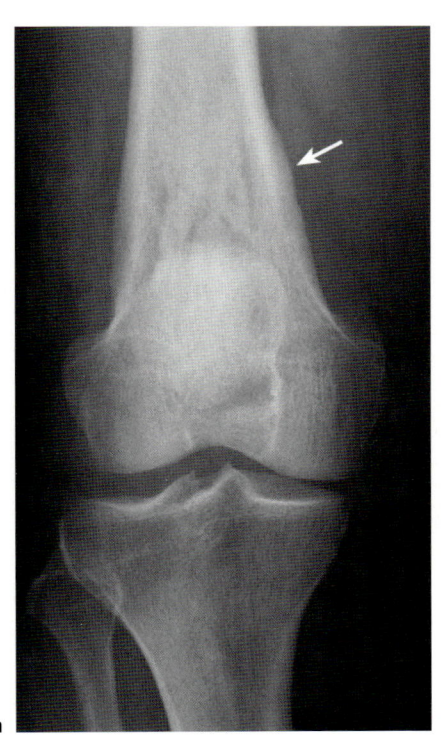

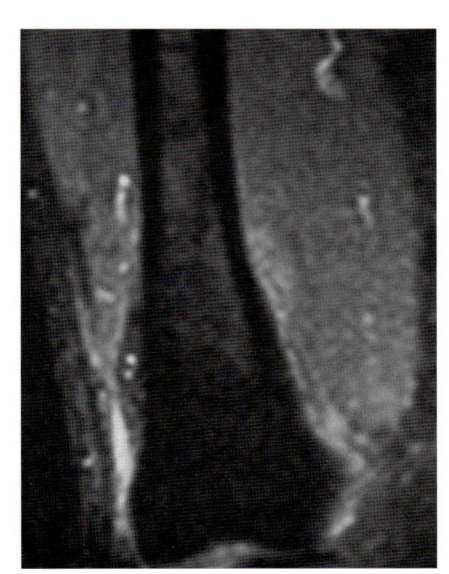

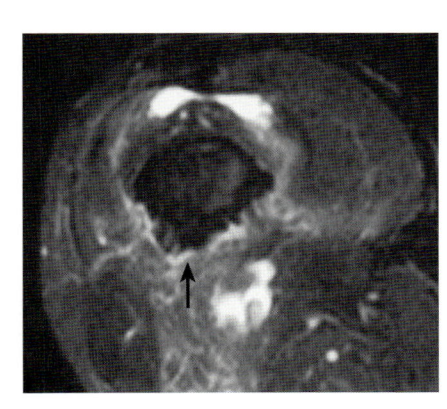

Figure 4.**32 a–c** Thickened irregular noninterrupted periosteal reaction in a patient with NF1 as seen on the AP radiograph (**a**). The periosteal bone formation has low signal on coronal (**b**) and axial (**c**) FS T2WI.

Table 4 (Continued) Lesions involving the outer surface of bone

Lesion	MRI Findings	Comments
Periostitis associated with acute/subacute bone infarction (Fig. 4.33)	Acute and subacute bone infarcts typically show intramedullary zones with low-intermediate signal on T1WI and slightly high to high signal on FS T2WI, often with heterogeneous Gd-contrast enhancement. Elevation of the periosteum surrounded by increased signal on FS T2WI and Gd-contrast enhancement on FS T1WI can also occur from associated periostitis.	Acute and subacute intramedullary bone infarcts can be associated with a periostitis that can be seen on MRI. **(See Atlas Chapter A 37)**

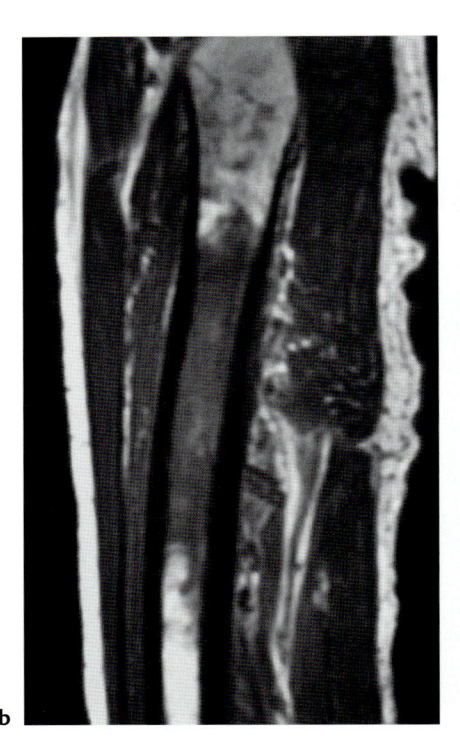

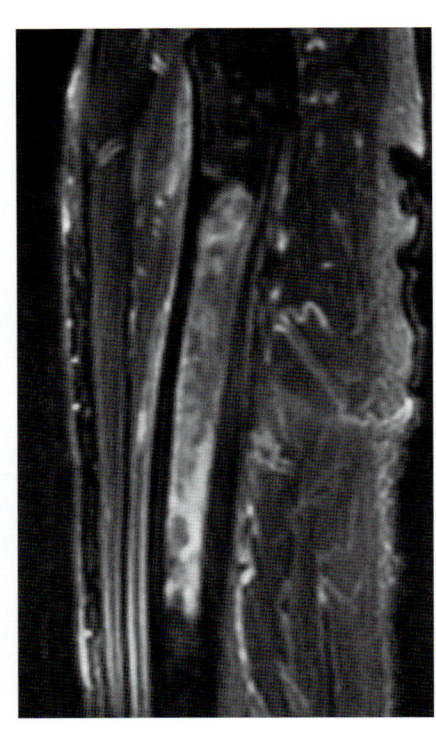

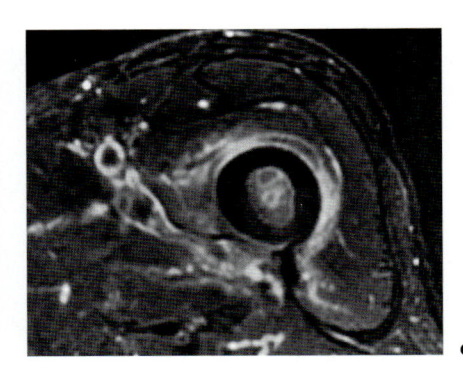

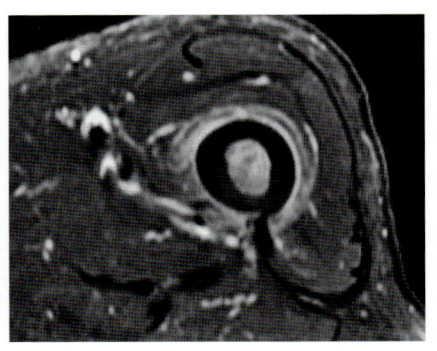

Figure 4.33 a–d Subacute bone infarct involving the diaphyseal marrow of the femur. The involved marrow has heterogeneous intermediate signal on sagittal T1WI (**a**), heterogeneous slightly high and high signal on sagittal (**b**) and axial (**c**) FS T2WI, and shows Gd-contrast enhancement on axial FS T1WI (**d**). A thin linear zone with low signal is seen superficial to the cortex representing elevated periosteum, which is surrounded by zones of Gd-contrast enhancement and high signal on FS T2WI.

Table 4 (Continued) Lesions involving the outer surface of bone

Lesion	MRI Findings	Comments
Malignant		
Parosteal osteosarcoma (Fig. 4.34)	Tumors occur at the surface of bone and extend outward with well-defined and/or indistinct margins. Tumors typically have mixed soft tissue and mineralized components. The mineralized portions of these tumors usually have low signal on T1WI, PDWI, T2WI, and FS PDWI and FS T2WI. The soft tissue portions of these tumors often have low-intermediate signal on T1WI, intermediate to slightly high or high signal on T2WI, and high signal on FS PDWI and FS T2WI. Areas of hemorrhage, cystic change, and/or necrosis with or without associated fluid–fluid levels may be present. Tumor extension into the medullary space can be seen in up to 50% of cases. Nonnecrotic or nonmineralized soft tissue portions of these tumors usually show Gd-contrast enhancement as well as sites of invasion into the medullary space and adjacent soft tissues.	Malignant tumor, comprised of proliferating neoplastic spindle cells, that produce osteoid and/or immature tumoral bone. Parosteal osteosarcomas arise on the external surface of bone and account for 4 to 6% of osteosarcomas, occur in patients 6 to 80 years, median = 27 years. **(See Atlas Chapter A 64)**

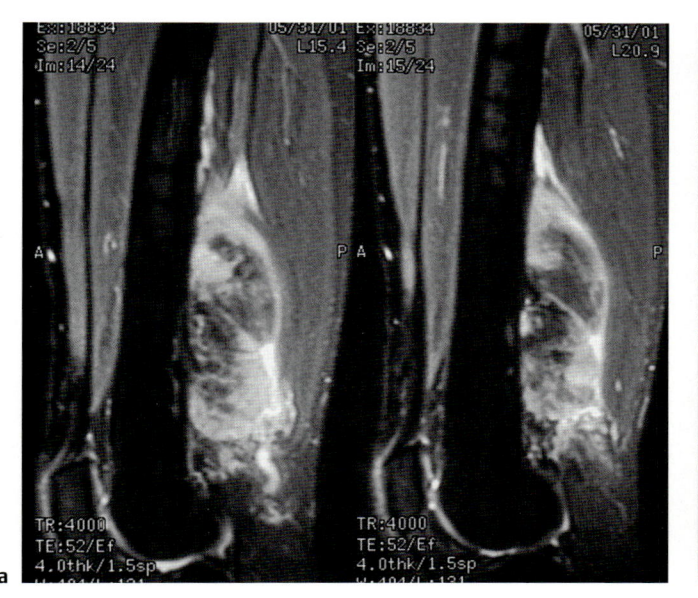

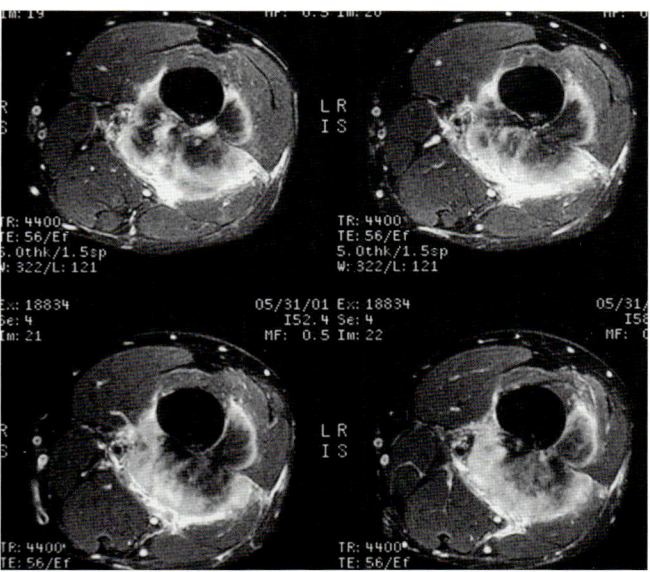

Figure 4.**34 a, b** Parosteal osteosarcoma along the outer dorsal surface of the distal femur that has heterogeneous low, slightly high, and high signal on sagittal (**a**) and axial (**b**) FS T2WI.

Table 4 (Continued)   **Lesions involving the outer surface of bone**

Lesion	MRI Findings	Comments
Periosteal osteosarcoma (Fig. 4.35)	Tumors usually involve the diaphyseal regions (femur > tibia > humerus > other bones) with associated cortical thickening and manifest as low signal on T1WI and T2WI. Tumors often have a broad base along the outer cortex extending outward toward the adjacent soft tissues. Periosteal reaction, seen as linear zones of low signal on T1WI and T2WI, can be associated with these tumors, as well as Codman's triangles. Tumors often have low-intermediate signal on T1WI and heterogenous slightly high to high signal on T2WI and FS T2WI. Tumor extension into the marrow is uncommon, and when present is usually seen associated with a zone of cortical destruction.	Malignant tumor, comprised of proliferating neoplastic spindle cells, that produce osteoid and/or immature tumoral bone. Periosteal sarcoma has been proposed to represent a variant of parosteal osteogenic sarcoma that contains cartilaginous zones. Account for 1 to 2% of osteosarcomas, occur in patients 11 to 57 years, median = 17 to 24 years. **(See Atlas Chapter A 64)**
Chondrosarcoma (Fig. 4.36)	MRI can easily demonstrate the thickness of cartilaginous caps of osteochondromas as well as erosive and/or destructive changes involving osteochondromas. Cartilage cap thickness exceeding 2 cm is commonly associated with malignant degeneration or dedifferentiation of osteochondromas into secondary chondrosarcomas. Secondary chondrosarcomas from osteochondromas and periosteal chondrosarcomas have low-intermediate signal on T1WI, intermediate signal on PDWI, and heterogeneous intermediate-high signal on T2WI. Lesions show heterogeneous contrast enhancement, with or without Gd-contrast enhancement of adjacent soft tissues suggesting tumor invasion.	Malignant tumors containing cartilage formed within sarcomatous stroma. Primary chondrosarcomas represent neoplasms that occur without pre-existent lesions, whereas secondary chondrosarcomas arise from formerly benign cartilaginous lesions. Periosteal chondrosarcomas are rare malignant cartilage tumors that occur on the surface of bone. Account for 12 to 21% of malignant bone lesions, 21 to 26% of primary sarcomas of bone, 5 to 91 years, mean = 40 years, median = 26 to 59 years. **(See Atlas Chapter A 11)**
Chordoma (Fig. 4.37)	Chordomas are often midline in location, and usually have lobulated or slightly lobulated margins. Lesions can occur at the surface of bone, and often erode or destroy bone. Chondroid chordomas are either midline or off-midline in location. Chordomas typically have low-intermediate signal on T1WI and heterogeneous predominantly high signal on T2WI. Chordomas typically enhance with Gd-DTPA, often in a heterogeneous pattern.	Rare, locally aggressive, slow-growing low to intermediate malignant tumors derived from ectopic notochordal remnants along the axial skeleton. Account for 2–4% of primary malignant bone tumors, 1–3% of all primary bone tumors; and <1% of intracranial tumors. Patients range in age from 6 to 84 years, median = 58 years. **(See Atlas Chapter A 12)**
Hemangioendothelioma (Fig. 4.38)	Intramedullary tumors usually have sharp margins that may be slightly lobulated. Lesions often have low-intermediate and/or high signal on T1WI and PDWI, and heterogeneous intermediate-high signal on T2WI and FS T2WI with or without zones of low signal. Lesions can be multifocal. Extraosseous extension of tumor through zones of cortical destruction commonly occur. Lesions often show prominent heterogeneous Gd-contrast enhancement.	Low-grade malignant vasoformative/endothelial neoplasms that are locally aggressive and rarely metastasize compared with the high-grade endothelial tumors such as angiosarcoma. Account for <1% of primary malignant bone tumors. Patients range from 10 to 82 years, median = 36 to 47 years. Patients with multifocal lesions tend to be ~10 years younger on average than those with uni-focal tumors. **(See Atlas Chapter A 33)**

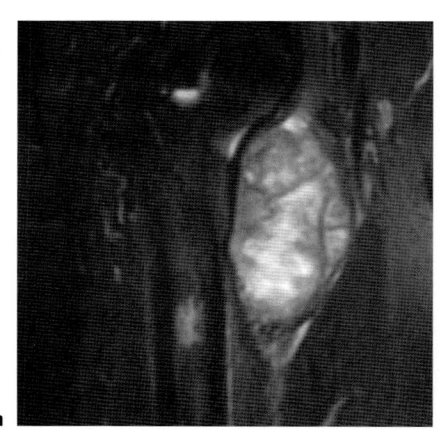

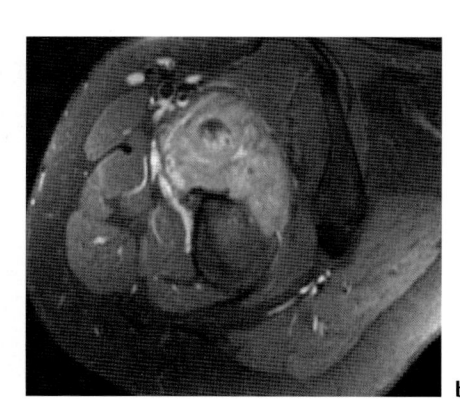

Figure 4.**35 a, b** Periosteal osteosarcoma along the outer anterior and medial margins of the proximal femur that has heterogeneous low, slightly high, and high signal on coronal FS T2WI (**a**), and moderate Gd-contrast enhancement on axial FS T1WI (**b**).

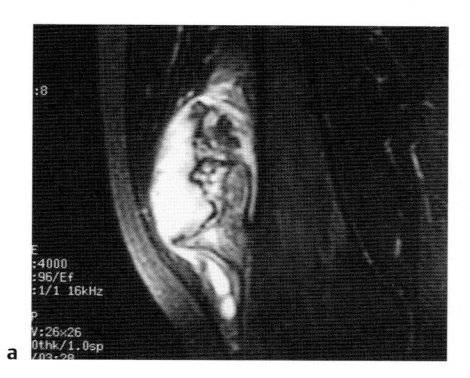

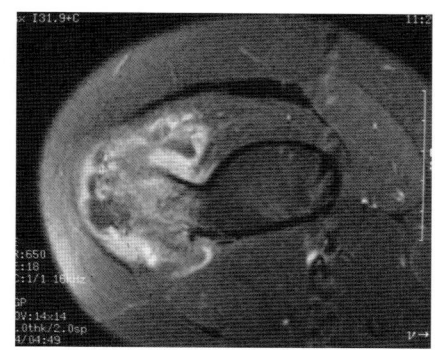

Figure 4.**36 a, b** Chondrosarcoma arising from an osteochondroma at the distal femur. The tumor has heterogeneous slightly high and high signal on coronal FS T2WI (**a**) and shows heterogeneous Gd-contrast enhancement on axial FS T1WI (**b**). Cortical destruction and intramedullary extension of tumor are also seen.

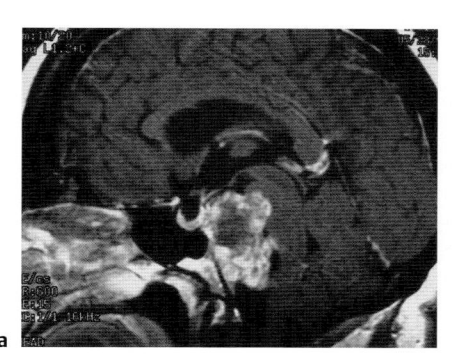

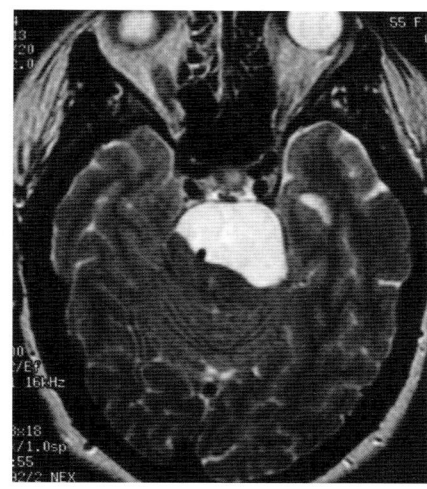

Figure 4.**37 a, b** Chordoma along the endocranial surface of the clivus associated with bone erosion. The tumor shows heterogeneous Gd-contrast enhancement on sagittal T1WI (**a**), and has high signal on axial T2WI (**b**).

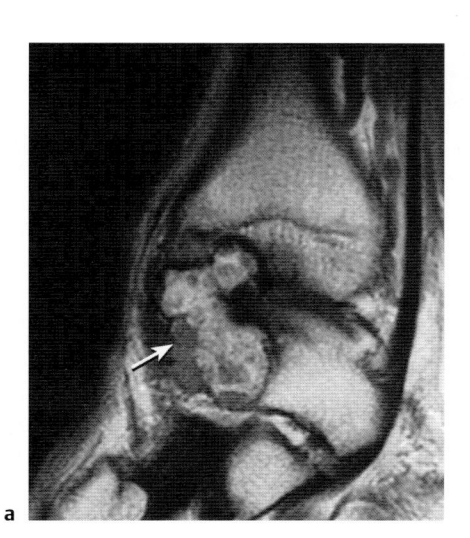

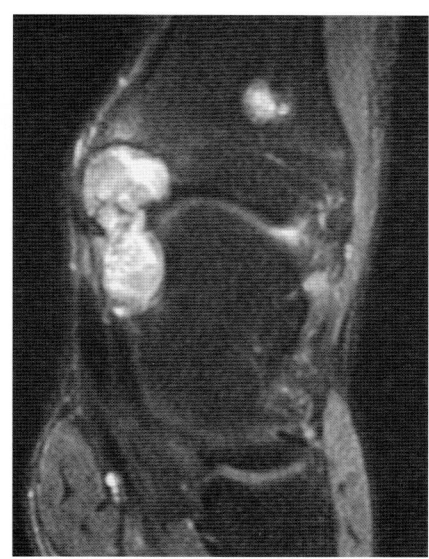

Figure 4.**38 a, b** Hemangioendothelioma involving the marrow of the distal tibia with cortical destruction, extension into the ankle joint and invasion of the talus as seen on sagittal PDWI (**a**) and coronal FS T2WI (**b**). Note that another focus of tumor is seen in the metaphyseal region.

Table 4 (Continued) Lesions involving the outer surface of bone

Lesion	MRI Findings	Comments
Sarcoma of soft tissue eroding into bone (Fig. 4.39)	Lesions with circumscribed or ill-defined margins may be associated with erosions and/or focal destruction of adjacent cortical bone with or without intraosseous extension of tumor.	Malignant tumors in extraosseous soft tissues can erode adjacent cortex and extend into the marrow.
Intramedullary primary sarcoma eroding through bone cortex (Fig. 4.40)	Poorly defined and/or circumscribed lesions in marrow with low-intermediate signal on T1WI; variable low, intermediate, and/or high signal on T2WI and FS T2WI; and variable Gd-contrast enhancement associated with sites of cortical destruction and extraosseous tumor extension.	Malignant primary and metastatic tumors in marrow usually show trabecular bone destruction with frequent eventual cortical destruction and extraosseous tumor extension.
Metastatic lesions (Fig. 4.41)	Metastatic tumor within bone often appears as intramedullary zones with low-intermediate signal on T1WI; low-intermediate to slightly high signal on PDWI; slightly high to high signal on T2WI and FS T2WI. Sclerotic lesions often have low signal on T1WI; and mixed low, intermediate, and/or high signal on T2WI. Cortical destruction and tumor extension into the extraosseous soft tissues frequently occurs. Pathologic fractures can be associated with metastatic lesions involving tubular bones and vertebrae. Lesions show varying degrees of Gd-contrast enhancement. Periosteal reaction can occasionally be seen, but is uncommon.	Metastatic lesions typically occur in the marrow with or without cortical destruction and extraosseous tumor extension. Metastatic lesions occur rarely in the cortex alone. Metastatic lesions infrequently have associated single or multilayered periosteal reaction, (<15 to 21%). (See Atlas Chapter A 50)
Myeloma/plasmacytoma (Fig. 4.42)	Multiple (myeloma) or single (plasmacytoma) are well-circumscribed or poorly defined diffuse infiltrative lesions involving marrow, low-intermediate signal on T1WI, intermediate-high signal on T2WI, usually show Gd-contrast-enhancement, eventual cortical bone destruction and extraosseous extension.	Malignant tumors comprised of proliferating antibody-secreting plasma cells derived from single clones. Most common primary neoplasm of bone in adults. Most patients are older than 40 years, median = 60 years. May have variable destructive or infiltrative changes involving the axial and/or appendicular skeleton. (See Atlas Chapter A 52)
Lymphoma (Fig. 4.43)	Single or multiple well-circumscribed or poorly defined infiltrative lesions involving marrow; low-intermediate signal on T1WI, intermediate-high signal on T2WI and FS T2WI, often shows Gd-contrast enhancement, +/- bone destruction and extraosseous extension. Diffuse involvement of vertebra with Hodgkin's lymphoma can produce an "ivory vertebra," which has low signal on T1WI and T2WI.	Lymphoid tumors with neoplastic cells typically within lymphoid tissue (lymph nodes and reticuloendothelial organs). Unlike leukemia, lymphoma usually arises as discrete masses. Lymphomas are subdivided into Hodgkin disease (HD) and non-Hodgkin lymphoma (NHL). Almost all primary lymphomas of bone are B cell NHL. (See Atlas Chapter A 47)

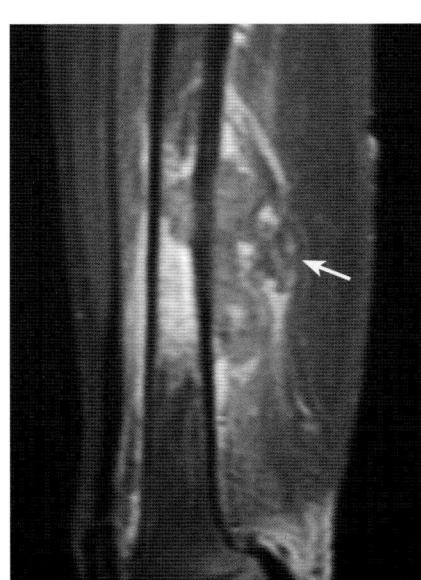

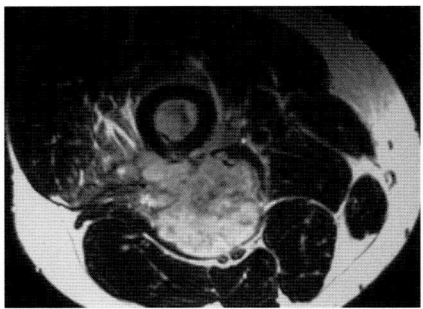

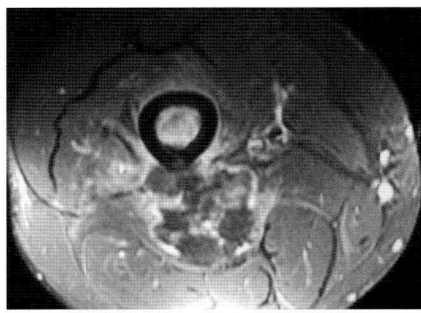

Figure 4.39 a–c Clear cell sarcoma of soft tissue (formerly called malignant melanoma of soft parts) involving the deep soft tissue of the lower thigh. The tumor shows heterogeneous Gd-contrast enhancement on sagittal (a) and axial (c) FS T1WI, and has heterogeneous mostly high signal on axial T2WI (b). The tumor is associated with cortical destruction and intraosseous extension.

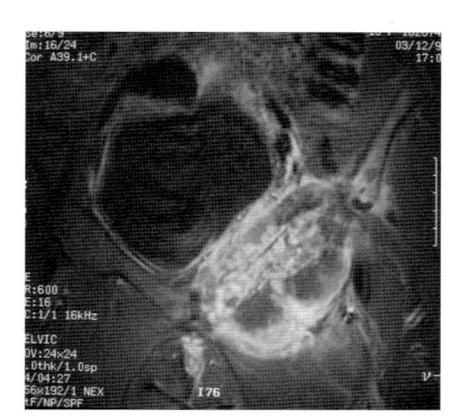

Figure 4.**40** Ewing sarcoma involving the pubic bone, which extends from the marrow through destroyed cortical bone into the adjacent soft tissues. The tumor shows heterogeneous Gd-contrast enhancement on coronal FS T1WI.

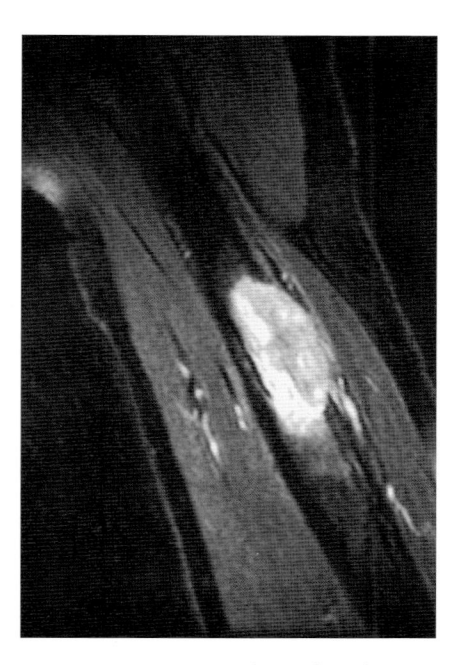

Figure 4.**41** Metastatic lesion from lung carcinoma in the marrow of the humeral diaphysis associated with cortical destruction and extraosseous extension as seen on sagittal FS T2WI.

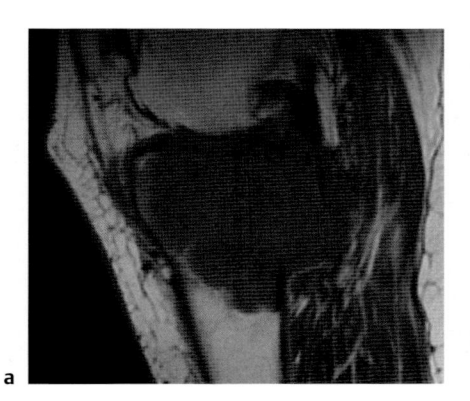

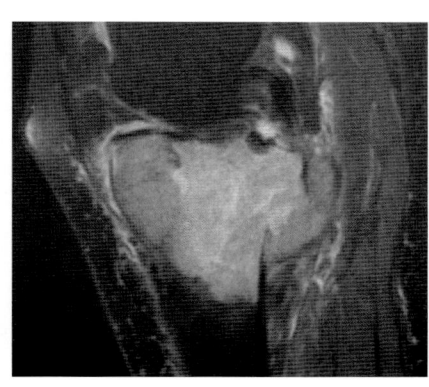

Figure 4.**42** Myeloma involving the marrow of the proximal tibia with intermediate signal on sagittal T1WI (**a**) and heterogeneous high signal on FS T2WI (**b**), associated with cortical destruction and extraosseous extension dorsally.

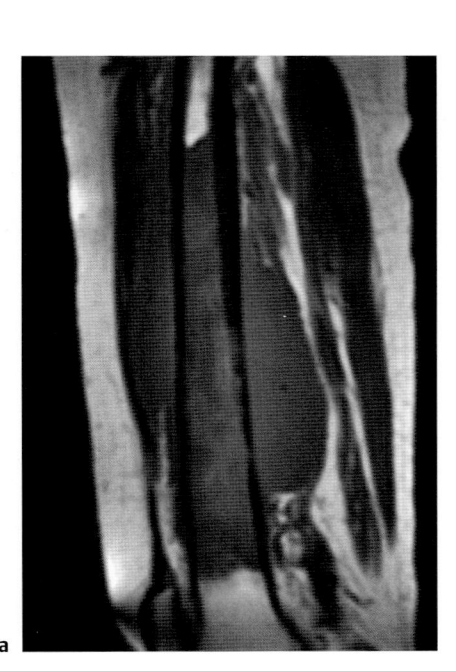

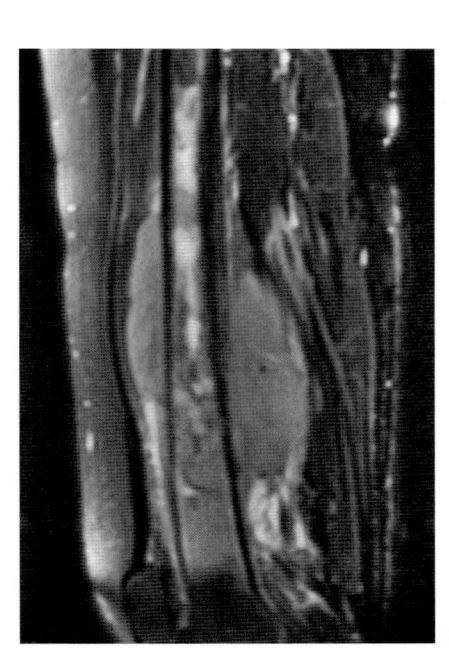

Figure 4.**43** Large cell lymphoma involving the diaphyseal marrow of the femur, which has heterogeneous intermediate signal on sagittal T1WI (**a**) and heterogeneous slightly high and high signal on sagittal FS T2WI (**b**). The tumor is associated with cortical destruction and extensive extraosseous extension.

Table 4 (Continued) **Lesions involving the outer surface of bone**

	MRI Findings	Comments
Leukemia (Fig. 4.44)	Single or multiple well-circumscribed or poorly defined infiltrative lesions involving marrow; low-intermediate signal on T1WI, intermediate-high signal on T2WI and FS T2WI, often shows Gd-contrast enhancement, +/− bone destruction and extraosseous extension.	Lymphoid neoplasms with involvement of bone marrow and with tumor cells in peripheral blood. In children and adolescents, acute lymphoblastic leukemia (ALL) is the most frequent type. In adults, chronic lymphocytic leukemia (small lymphocytic lymphoma) is the most common type of lymphocytic leukemia. Myelogenous leukemias are neoplasms derived from abnormal myeloid progenitor cells. Acute myelogenous leukemia (AML) occurs in adolescents and young adults, and represents ~20% of childhood leukemia. Chronic myelogenous leukemia (CML) usually affects adults older than 25 years. **(See Atlas Chapter A 41)**
Malignant tumor with interrupted periosteal reaction: sunburst or divergent pattern (Fig. 4.45)	Intramedullary neoplasm can be associated with zones of cortical destruction through which the lesion extends into the extraosseous soft tissues. Zones of reactive and/or tumoral bone formation under the elevated periosteum can have a divergent or "sunburst" appearance with low signal within the extraosseous tumor that often has slightly high to high signal on T2WI and FS T2WI with corresponding Gd-contrast enhancement.	Periosteal elevation by tumor results in formation of a "sunburst or divergent pattern" of underlying bone spicules along vascular channels and fibrous bands (Sharpey's fibers) that are stretched out from the outer surface of bone cortex. Typically seen with osteosarcoma, rarely seen with osteoblastoma and osteoblastic metastasis (prostate carcinoma, lung carcinoma, carcinoid, breast carcinoma).
Malignant tumor with interrupted periosteal reaction: Codman's triangle (Fig. 4.46)	Intramedullary neoplasm or infection can be associated with zones of cortical destruction through which the lesions extend into the extraosseous soft tissues. Lamellated and/or spiculated zones of periosteal reaction are often seen secondary to tumor invasion and perforation of bone cortex. Low signal from spicules of reactive and tumoral bone formation may have a "sunburst" appearance. Triangular zones of periosteal elevation (Codman's triangles) can be seen at the borders of zones of cortical destruction and tumor extension.	Codman's triangles are triangular zones of periosteal reaction or reactive bone at the borders of cortical destruction adjacent to extraosseous extension of neoplasms or infections from marrow. Can be seen with malignant primary bone neoplasms and lesions (osteosarcoma, Ewing sarcoma, chondrosarcoma, malignant fibrous histiocytoma, aneurysmal bone cyst, giant cell tumor), metastasis, osteomyelitis, or trauma.
Malignant tumor with interrupted periosteal reaction: disorganized pattern (Fig. 4.47)	Intramedullary neoplasm or infection seen with zones of cortical destruction through which the lesion extends into the extraosseous soft tissues. Irregular disorganized zones of periosteal reaction can be seen below the elevated periosteum.	Extraosseous extension of intramedullary tumor or infection results in disorganized thin and/or thick irregular bone spicules under the elevated periosteum. Disorganized periosteal reaction is often seen with highly aggressive osteosarcomas, but can also be seen with other benign and malignant tumors that have associated complications of pathologic fracture or infection.

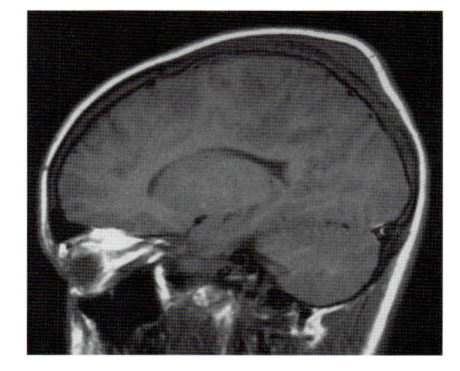

Figure 4.**44** Acute lymphoblastic leukemia involving the marrow of the calvarium associated with cortical destruction and extraosseous extension on sagittal T1WI.

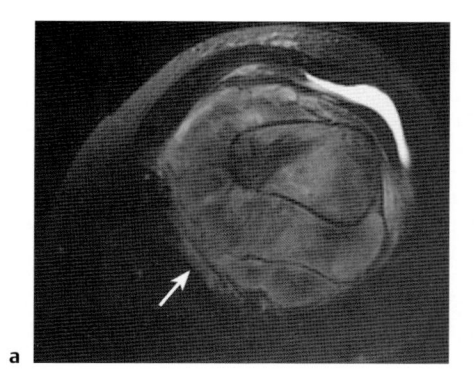

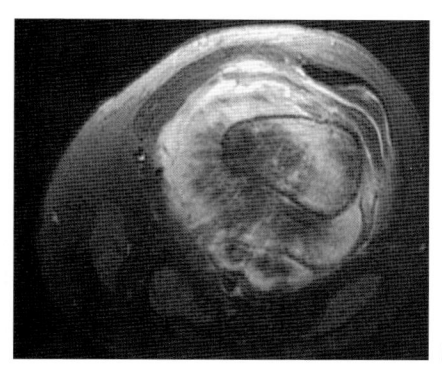

Figure 4.**45 a, b** Intramedullary osteogenic sarcoma with cortical destruction and extraosseous extension under an interrupted elevated periosteum. Beneath the elevated periosteum, divergent striated zones of low signal on FS T2WI (**a**) and post-Gd-contrast FS T1WI (**b**) are seen representing divergent or sunburst tumoral bone formation within the extraosseous neoplasm.

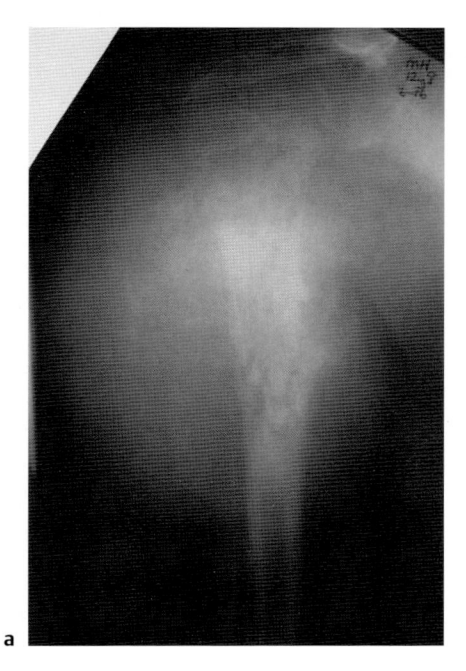

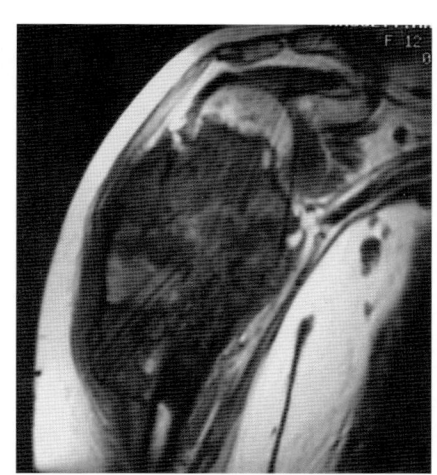

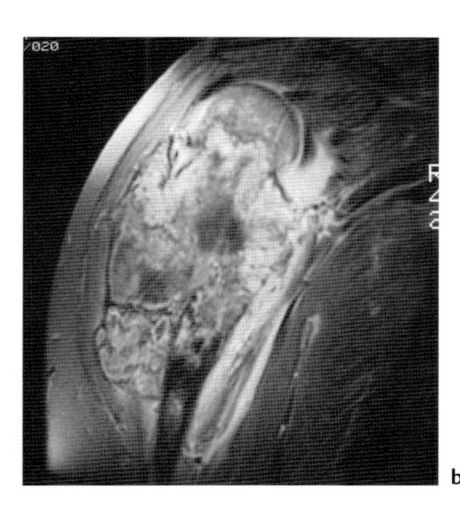

Figure 4.**46 a–c** Intramedullary osteogenic osteosarcoma with cortical destruction, extraosseous extension, and interrupted periosteal elevation. The AP radiograph (**a**) shows a destructive intraosseous lesion with mineralized ossified matrix, cortical destruction, extraosseous tumor extension with disorganized tumoral bone formation, and a Codman's triangle at the inferior borders. The tumor has mixed low, intermediate, and high signal on coronal T1WI (**b**), and shows prominent Gd-contrast enhancement on coronal FS T1WI (**c**).

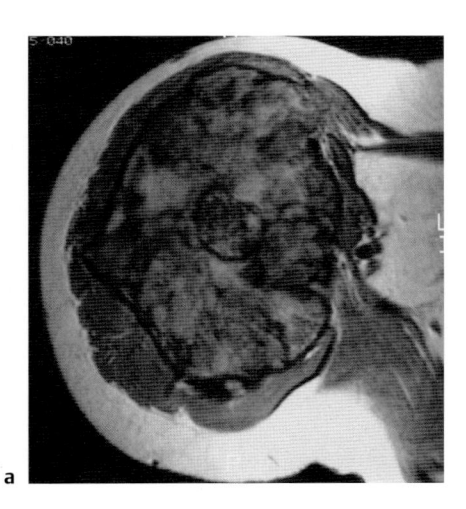

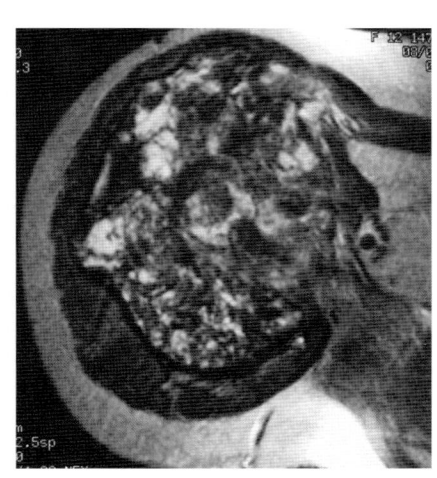

Figure 4.**47 a, b** Intramedullary osteogenic osteosarcoma with cortical destruction, extraosseous extension, and interrupted periosteal elevation. The destructive intraosseous tumor with extensive extraosseous extension contains irregular zones of low signal on axial PDWI (**a**) and axial T2WI (**b**) representing disorganized tumoral/ periosteal bone formation.

Table 4 (Continued) Lesions involving the outer surface of bone

Lesion	MRI Findings	Comments
Malignant tumor with interrupted periosteal reaction: "hair on end" or perpendicular-oriented spicules of periosteal reaction (Fig. 4.48)	Intramedullary neoplasm or infection seen with zones of cortical destruction through which the lesions extend into the extraosseous soft tissues. Parallel spiculated zones ("hair on end" pattern) of periosteal reaction oriented perpendicular to the long axis of bone can be seen within the extraosseous lesion often under an elevated periosteum.	Extraosseous extension of intramedullary tumor or infection results in a perpendicular ("hair on end," or "honeycomb") pattern of thin bone spicules radially oriented under the elevated periosteum. These bone spicules tend to be thin and oriented along radially oriented blood vessels extending from the cortical surface within the lesions. Most frequently seen with Ewing sarcoma, sometimes with osteosarcoma, and rarely with infection.
Malignant tumor with interrupted periosteal reaction: "onion skin" multilayered, or multilamellated periosteal reaction oriented parallel to the long axis of bone (Fig. 4.49)	Intramedullary neoplasm, inflammatory lesion, or infection seen with zones of cortical destruction through which the lesions extend into the extraosseous soft tissues. Multiple layers of periosteal reaction oriented parallel to cortical bone ("onion skin" pattern) can be seen within the extraosseous lesion often under an elevated periosteum.	Extraosseous extension of intramedullary tumor, noninfectious inflammatory lesions, or infection results in a multilayered periosteal reaction. Most frequently seen with Ewing sarcoma, sometimes with osteosarcoma, lymphoma, and rarely with infection.

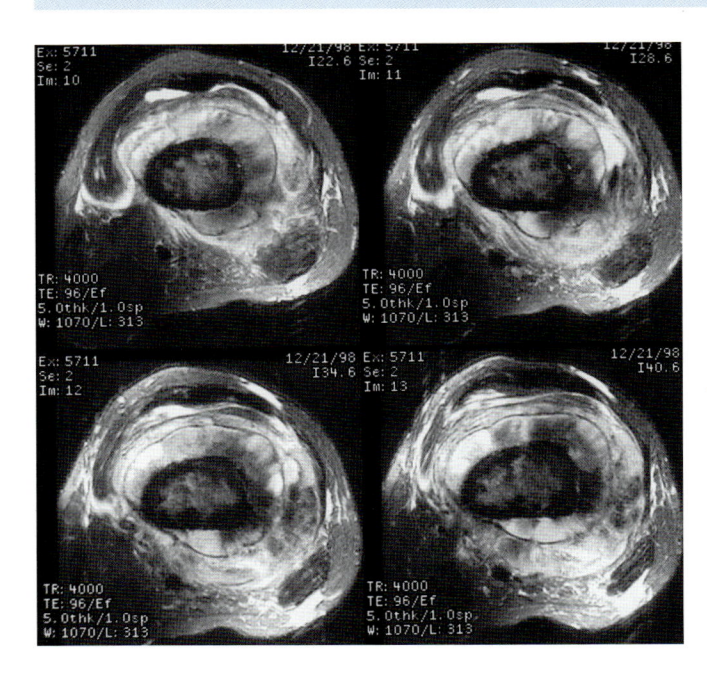

Figure 4.48 Intramedullary osteogenic sarcoma with cortical destruction and extraosseous extension under an interrupted elevated periosteum. Beneath the elevated periosteum, "hair on end" as well as divergent striated/ "sunburst-type" zones of low signal on FS T2WI are seen representing tumoral bone formation within the extraosseous neoplasm.

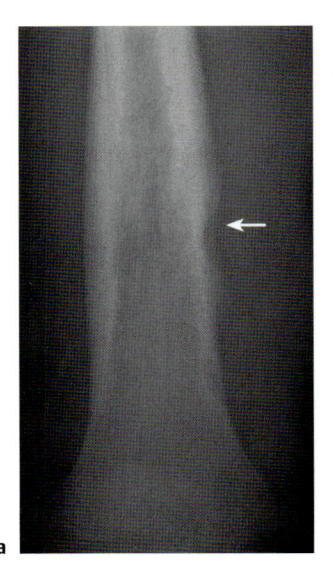

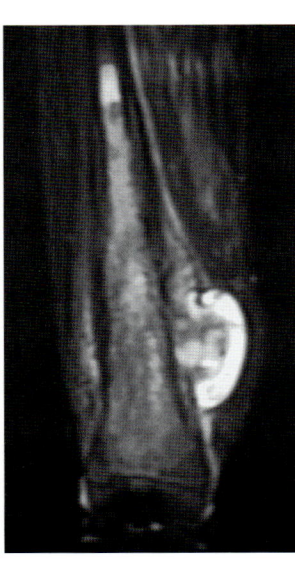

Figure 4.49 a, b Intramedullary telangiectatic osteosarcoma in the distal femur associated with cortical destruction with extraosseous tumor extension. Multiple layers of periosteal reaction oriented parallel to cortical bone (*onion skin* pattern) and a Codman's triangle inferiorly are seen on an AP radiograph (**a**). An intraosseous tumor is seen extending through destroyed cortical bone beneath an interrupted periosteum on coronal (**b**) FS T2WI. Multiple thin layers or periosteal reaction are seen in the extraosseous tumor on axial FS T2WI.

References

Calcific Tendinitis
Flemming DJ, Murphey MD, Shekitka KM, Temple HT, Jelinek JJ, Kransdorf MJ. Osseous involvement in calcific tendonitis: a retrospective review of 50 cases. *AJR* 2003;181:965–972.

Periosteal Reaction
Resnick D. Enostosis, hyperostosis, and periostitis. In: Resnick D, ed. *Diagnosis of Bone and Joint Disorders*, 4th ed. Philadelphia, Pa: W.B. Saunders; 2002:5:4870–4919.

Wenaden AET, Szyszko TA, Saifuddin A. Imaging of periosteal reactions associated with focal lesions of bone. *Clin Radiol* 2005;60:439–456.

Hemophilic Pseudotumor
Geyskens W, Vanhoenacker FM, Van der Zijden T, Peerlinck K. MR imaging of intra-osseous hemophilic pseudotumor: case report and review of the literature. *JBR-BTR* Nov–Dec 2004;87(6):289–293.

Jaovisidha S, Ryu KN, Hodler J, Schweitzer ME, Sartoris DJ, Resnick D. Hemophilic pseudotumor: spectrum of MR findings. *Skeletal Radiol* 1997;26:468–474.

Park JS, Ryu KN. Hemophilic pseudotumor involving the musculoskeletal system: spectrum of radiologic findings. *AJR* 2004;183:55–61.

Primary Hypertrophic Osteoarthropathy
Araki Y, Tsukaguchi I, Nakamura H. Pachydermoperiostosis involving the skull and spine: MR findings. *AJR* March 1993;160(3):664–665.

Capelastegui A, Astigarraga E, García-Iturraspe C. MR findings in pulmonary hypertrophic osteoarthropathy. *Clin Radiol* January 2000;55(1):72–75.

Demirpolat G, Sener RN, Stun EE. MR imaging of pachydermoperiostosis. *J Neuroradiol* March 1999;26(1):61–63.

Loredo R, Pathria MN, Salonen D, Resnick D. Magnetic resonance imaging in pachydermoperiostosis. *Clin Imag* July–September 1996;20(3):212–218.

Resnick D. Enostosis, hyperostosis, and periostitis. In: Resnick D, ed. *Diagnosis of Bone and Joint Disorders*, 4th ed. Philadelphia, Pa: W.B. Saunders; 2002:5:4870–4919.

Secondary Hypertrophic Osteoarthropathy
Capelastegui A, Astigarraga E, García-Iturraspe C. MR findings in pulmonary hypertrophic osteoarthropathy. *Clin Radiol* January 2000;55(1):72–75.

Resnick D. Enostosis, hyperostosis, and periostitis. In: Resnick D, ed. *Diagnosis of Bone and Joint Disorders*, 4th ed. Philadelphia, Pa: W.B. Saunders; 2002:5:4870–4919.

Sainani NI, Lawande MA, Parikh VP, Pungavkar SA, Patkar DP, Sase KS. MRI diagnosis of hypertrophic osteoarthropathy from a remote childhood malignancy. *Skeletal Radiol* 2007 Jun;36 Suppl 1:63–6. Epub Sep 5 2006.

Varan A, Kutluk T, Demirkazik FB, Akyüz C, Büyükpamukçu M. Hypertrophic osteoarthropathy in a child with nasopharyngeal carcinoma. *Pediatr Radiol* 2000;30:570–572.

Periosteal Reaction from Venous Stasis
Resnick D. Enostosis, hyperostosis, and periostitis. In: Resnick D, ed. *Diagnosis of Bone and Joint Disorders*, 4th ed. Philadelphia, Pa: W.B. Saunders; 2002:5:4870–4919.

Wenaden AET, Szyszko TA, Saifuddin A. Imaging of periosteal reactions associated with focal lesions of bone. *Clin Radiol* 2005;60:439–456.

Infantile Cortical Hyperostosis (Caffey Disease)
Katz DS, Eller DJ, Bergman G, Blankenberg FG. Caffey's disease of the scapula: CT and MR findings. *AJR* January 1997;168(1):286–287.

Resnick D. Enostosis, hyperostosis, and periostitis. In: Resnick D, ed. *Diagnosis of Bone and Joint Disorders*, 4th ed. Philadelphia, Pa: W.B. Saunders; 2002:5:4870–4919.

Saatci I, Brown JJ, McAlister WH. MR findings in a patient with Caffey's disease. *Pediatr Radiol* November 1996;26(1):68–70.

Thyroid Acropachy
Fatourechi V, Ahmed DDF, Schwartz KM. Thyroid acropachy: report of 40 patients treated at a single institution in a 26-year period. *J Clin Endocrin Metab* December 2002;87(12):5435–5441.

Vanhoenacker FM, Pelckmans MC, De Beuckeleer LH, Colpaert CG, De Schepper AM. Thyroid acropachy: correlation of imaging and pathology. *Eur Radiol* 2001;11(6):1058–1062.

Hypervitaminosis and Hypovitaminosis
Lips P. Hypervitaminosis A and fractures. *N Engl J Med* 2003;384:347–349.

Romero JB, Schreiber A, Von Hochstetter AR, Wagenhauser FJ, Michel BA, Theiler R. Hyperostotic and destructive osteoarthritis in a patient with vitamin A intoxication syndrome: a case report. *Bull Hosp Jt Dis* 1996;54:169–174.

Jiang YB, Wang YZ, Zhao J, et al. Bone remodeling in hypervitaminosis D3. radiologic-microangiographic-pathologic correlations. *Invest Radiol* 1991;26:213–219.

Resnick D. Hypervitaminosis and hypovitaminosis. In: Resnick D, ed. *Diagnosis of Bone and Joint Disorders*, 4th ed. Philadelphia, Pa: W.B. Saunders; 2002:4:3456–3464.

Syndromes of Hyperostosis, Osteitis, and Skin Lesions (SAPHO Syndrome)
Boutin RD, Resnick D. The SAPHO syndrome: an evolving concept for unifying several idiopathic disorders of bone and skin. *AJR* 1998;170:585–591.

Davies AM, Marino AJ, Evans N, Grimer RJ, Deshmukh N, Mangham DC. SAPHO syndrome: 20 year followup. *Skeletal Radiol* 1999;28:159–162.

Kirchoff T, Merkesdal S, Rosenthal H, et al. Diagnostic management of patients with SAPHO syndrome: use of MR imaging to guide bone biopsy at CT for microbiological and histological work-up. *Eur Radiol* 2003;13:2304–2308.

Resnick D. Enostosis, hyperostosis, and periostitis. In: Resnick D, ed. *Diagnosis of Bone and Joint Disorders*, 4th ed. Philadelphia, Pa: W.B. Saunders; 2002:5:4870–4919.

Interrupted Periosteal Reaction
Resnick D. Enostosis, hyperostosis, and periostitis. In: Resnick D, ed. *Diagnosis of Bone and Joint Disorders*, 4th ed. Philadelphia, Pa: W.B. Saunders; 2002:5:4870–4919.

Wenaden AET, Szyszko TA, Saifuddin A. Imaging of periosteal reactions associated with focal lesions of bone. *Clin Radiol* 2005;60:439–456.

Table 5 Lesions associated with thickening of bone cortex

Lesion	MRI Findings	Comments
Benign		
Osteoid osteoma (Fig. 5.1)	Typically shows dense fusiform thickening of the cortex that has low to intermediate signal on T1W, PDWI, T2WI, and FS T2WI. Within the thickened cortex, a spheroid or ovoid zone (nidus) measuring < 1.5 cm is typically seen. The nidus can have irregular, distinct or indistinct margins relative to the adjacent region of cortical thickening. The nidus can have low-intermediate signal on T1WI and PDWI, and low-intermediate or high signal on T2WI and FS T2WI. Calcifications in the nidus can be seen as low signal on T2WI. After Gd-contrast administration, variable degrees of enhancement are seen at the nidus.	Benign painful osteoblastic lesion comprised of a circumscribed nidus < 1.5 cm usually surrounded by reactive bone formation. Accounts for 11 to 13 % of primary benign bone tumors. Occurs in patients 6 to 30 years, median = 17 years. Approximately 75 % occur in patients less than 25 years. **(See Atlas Chapter A 60)**
Osteoblastoma (Fig. 5.2)	Lesions appear as spheroid or ovoid zone measuring > 1.5 to 2 cm located within medullary and/or cortical bone with low-intermediate signal on T1WI; low-intermediate to slightly high signal on PDWI; and low-intermediate and/or high signal on T2WI and FS T2WI. Calcifications or areas of mineralization can be seen as zones of low signal on T2WI. After Gd-contrast administration, osteoblastomas show variable degrees of enhancement. Zones of thickened cortical bone and medullary sclerosis that are often seen adjacent to osteoblastomas typically show low signal on T1W, T2WI, and FS T2WI. Poorly defined zones of marrow signal alteration consisting of low-intermediate signal on T1WI, high signal on T2WI and FS T2WI, and corresponding Gd-contrast enhancement can be seen in the marrow adjacent to osteoblastomas as well as within the extraosseous soft tissues.	Rare benign bone-forming tumors that are histologically related to osteoid osteomas. Osteoblastomas are larger than osteoid osteomas and show progressive enlargement. Account for 3 to 6 % of primary benign bone tumors and < 1 to 2 % of all primary bone tumors. Occurs in patients 1 to 30 years, median = 15 years, mean age = 20 years. Approximately 90 % of lesions occur in patients less than 30 years. **(See Atlas Chapter A 61)**
Osteoma (Fig. 5.3)	Lesions typically appear as well-circumscribed zones of dense cortical bone with low signal on T1WI, PDWI, T2WI, and FS T2WI. No infiltration into the adjacent soft tissues is seen by osteomas. Zones of bone destruction or associated soft tissue mass lesions are not associated with osteomas. Periosteal reaction is not associated with osteomas except in cases with coincidental antecedent trauma.	Benign primary bone lesions composed of dense lamellar, woven, and/or compact cortical bone usually located at the surface of bones. Account for less than 1 % of primary benign bone tumors. Occur in patients 16 to 74 years, most frequent in 6th decade. **(See Atlas Chapter A 62)**
Juxtacortical chondroma (Fig. 5.4)	Lesions are located at the bone surface and are usually lobulated with low-intermediate signal on T1WI, which is hypo- or isointense relative to muscle. Lesions usually have heterogeneous predominantly high signal on T2WI. Lesions are surrounded by low signal borders on T2WI representing thin sclerotic reaction. Areas of low signal on T2WI are secondary to matrix mineralization. Edema is not typically seen in nearby medullary bone. Lesions often show a peripheral pattern of Gd-contrast enhancement that correlates to fibrovascular bundles surrounding the cartilage lobules.	Benign protuberant hyaline cartilaginous tumors that arise from the periosteum and superficial to bone cortex. Account for < 1 % of bone lesions. Juxtacortical chondromas represent ~5 to 12 % of chondromas. Patients range from 4 to 77 years, median = 26 years. **(See Atlas Chapter A 9)**
Parosteal lipoma	Lesions often have lobular margins and are immediately adjacent to the outer intact surface of adjacent bone. Lesions typically have fat signal on MRI, as well as zones of low signal on T1WI and T2WI from ossification changes that can occur within these lesions and at the junction with bone cortex. Zones with intermediate signal on T1WI and high signal on T2WI can occur in these lesions secondary to cartilaginous contents.	Rare, benign, slow-growing painless tumors with mature adipose tissue associated with the periosteum of bone. Account for 0.3 % of lipomas; typically occur in patients 40 to 60 years. Common sites include the femur, proximal radius, tibia, and humerus. **(See Atlas Chapter A 43)**

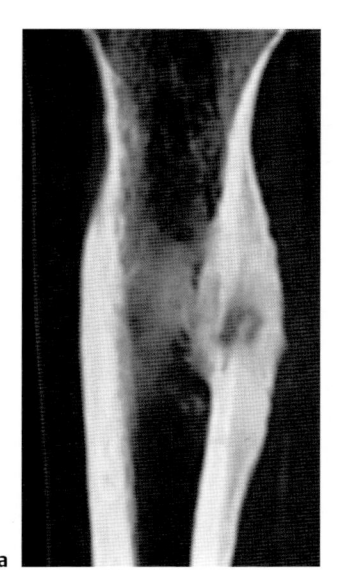

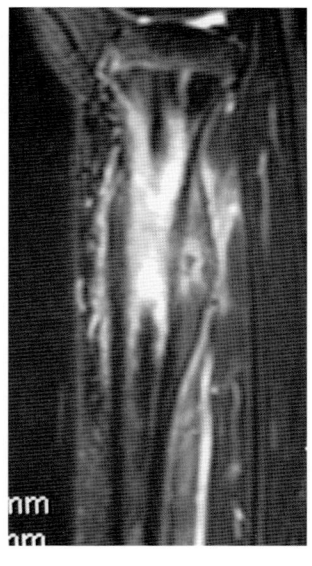

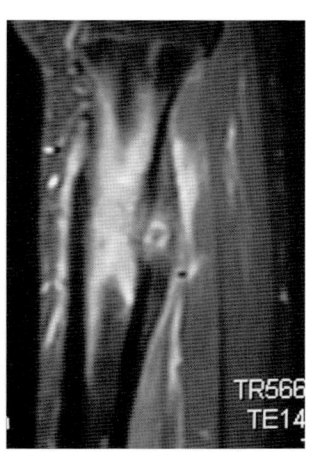

Figure 5.1 a–c   Osteoid osteoma involving the cortex of the proximal tibial shaft in a 15-year-old female. Sagittal CT image (**a**) shows dense fusiform osteosclerosis surrounding a small radiolucent zone (nidus) with a central calcification. The nidus has high signal on sagittal FS T2WI (**b**) and the small central calcification has low signal. The thickened cortex has low-intermediate and slightly high signal on FS T2WI, and is associated with periosteal reaction with high signal. The nidus shows Gd-contrast enhancement on sagittal FS T1WI (**c**). Prominent Gd-contrast enhancement is seen at the periosteal reaction, and mild diffuse enhancement is seen in the cortical thickening adjacent to the nidus. Poorly defined zones of high signal on FS T2WI and corresponding Gd-contrast enhancement on FS T1WI are also seen in the marrow adjacent to the lesion.

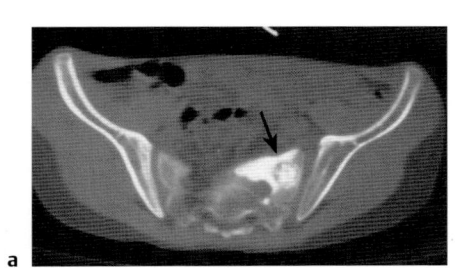

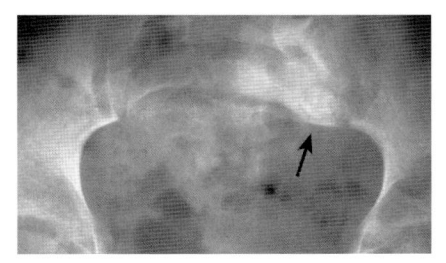

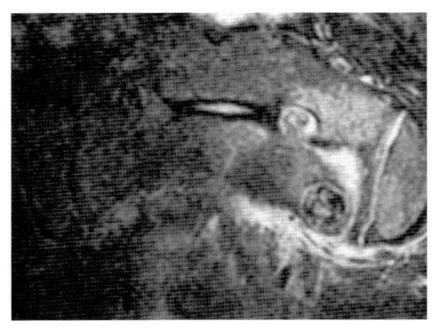

Figure 5.2 a–c   Osteoblastoma in the anterior left sacral alum in a 12-year-old boy. Prominent dense sclerotic reaction is seen in cortical and medullary bone adjacent to the mixed radiolucent and radiodense lesion on the axial CT image (**a**) and AP radiograph (**b**). The lesion has intermediate to slightly high signal peripherally surrounding a central zone with low and slightly high signal on coronal FS T2WI (**c**). Poorly defined zones of high signal on FS T2WI are seen in the marrow and soft tissues adjacent to the lesion.

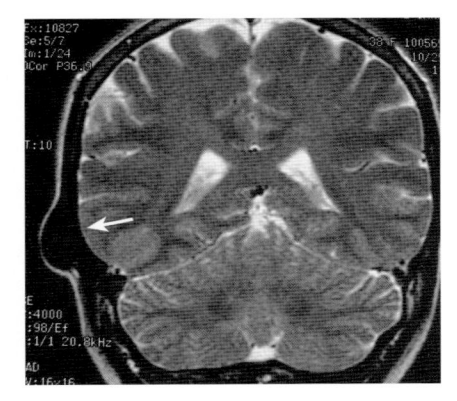

Figure 5.3   Osteoma involving the outer table of the skull. A circumscribed lesion with low signal on coronal T2WI is seen protruding from the right side of the skull.

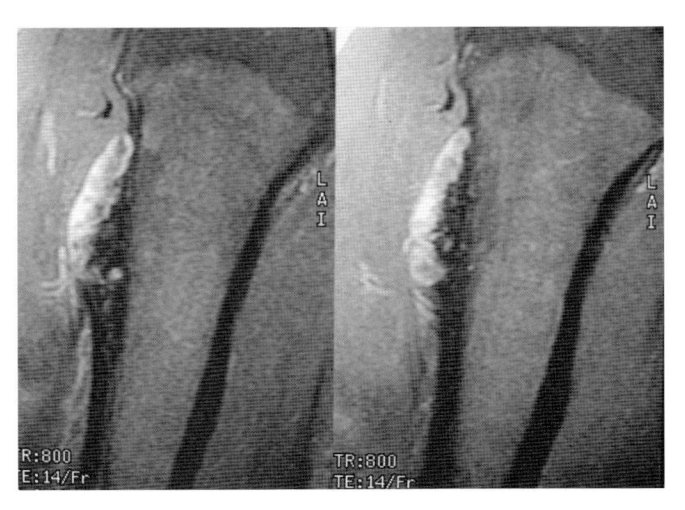

Figure 5.4   Juxtacortical chondroma involving the outer surface of the proximal humerus of a 28-year-old man. Periosteal and cortical bone thickening is seen at the base of the lesion. The lesion shows irregular zones of Gd-contrast enhancement on sagittal FS T1WI.

Table 5 (Continued)   **Lesions associated with thickening of bone cortex**

Lesion	MRI Findings	Comments
Malignant		
Parosteal osteosarcoma (Fig. 5.5)	These tumors occur at the surface of bone and extend outward with well-defined and/or indistinct margins. Portions of these tumors that extend toward the juxtacortical soft tissues typically have mixed soft tissue and mineralized components. The mineralized portions of these tumors tend to be dense centrally and at the sites of contiguity (broad-based or stalk-like) with the outer cortical margins. The mineralized portions of these tumors usually have low signal on T1WI, PDWI, T2WI, FS PDWI and FS T2WI. The soft tissue portions of these tumors often have low-intermediate signal on T1WI, intermediate to slightly high or high signal on T2WI, and high signal on FS PDWI and FS T2WI. Tumor extension into the medullary space seen with MRI can occur in up to 50%. After Gd-contrast administration, non-necrotic or nonmineralized soft tissue portions of these tumors usually show enhancement as well as sites of invasion into the medullary space and adjacent soft tissues.	Malignant tumor comprising proliferating neoplastic spindle cells that produce osteoid and/or immature tumoral bone. Parosteal osteosarcomas arise on the external surface of bone and account for 4 to 6% of osteosarcomas, occur in patients 6 to 80 years, median = 27 years. **(See Atlas Chapter A 64)**
Intraosseous osteosarcoma (Fig. 5.6)	Intramedullary osteosarcomas often have zones of cortical destruction through which tumors extend toward the extraosseous soft tissues under an elevated periosteum. Lamellated and/or spiculated zones of bone formation can occur under the periosteal elevation secondary to tumor invasion and perforation of bone cortex. Low signal from spicules of periosteal, reactive, and tumoral bone formation may have a divergent ("sunburst") pattern, perpendicular ("hair on end") pattern, or disorganized or complex appearance.	Malignant tumor comprised of proliferating neoplastic spindle cells which produce osteoid and/or immature tumoral bone. Intraosseous osteosarcoma accounts for 91 to 95% of osteosarcomas. Osteogenic sarcoma has two age peaks of incidence. The larger peak occurs between the ages of 10 and 20 and accounts for over half of the cases. The second smaller peak occurs in adults over 60 years and accounts for ~10% of the cases. **(See Atlas Chapter A 64)**
Adamantinoma (Fig. 5.7)	Most frequently appear as a solitary lobulated focus versus a multinodular pattern of signal alteration in thickened bone cortex. More than half involve bone cortex and marrow compared with only cortical involvement. Tumor foci in bone typically have low-intermediate signal on T1WI and PDWI, and slightly high to high signal on T2WI and FS T2WI. Lesions usually show prominent Gd-contrast enhancement. Adamantinomas with a multinodular pattern have enhancing nodules which have high signal on T2WI and FS T2WI separated by zones of low signal from intervening cortical bone.	Rare low-grade malignant bone tumors consisting of epithelial cells surrounded by spindle cells and osteo-fibrous tissue that often involve the shaft of the tibia account for <1% of primary bone tumors. Patients range in age from 3 to 86 years, median = 19 to 25 years, average = 35 years, most common in 3rd and 4th decades. **(See Atlas Chapter A 1)**

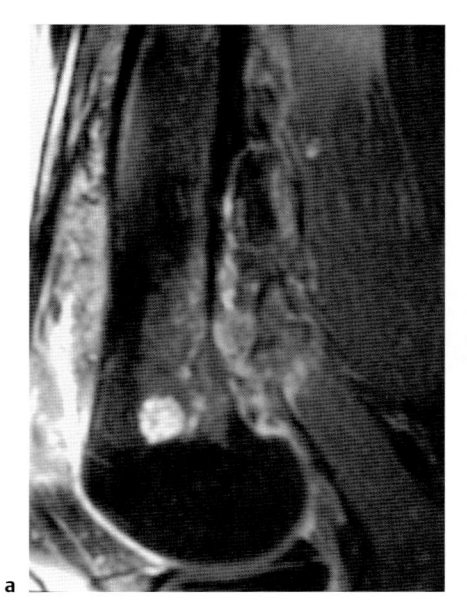

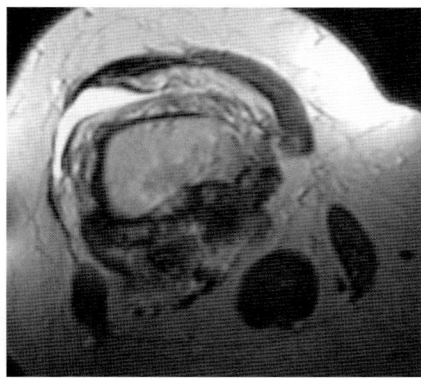

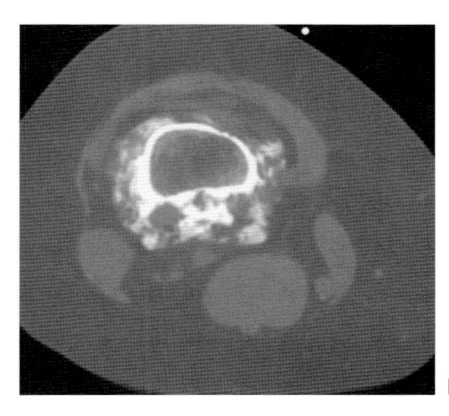

Figure 5.**5 a–c** Parosteal osteosarcoma of the dorsal distal portion of the femur in a 45-year-old woman. The tumor has mixed low, intermediate, slightly high and high signal on sagittal (**a**) FS T2WI and axial T2WI (**b**). The tumor extends into the marrow through a zone of cortical destruction. The mineralized portions of this tumor have low signal on T2WI and FS T2WI. The axial CT image (**c**) shows a soft tissue tumor containing mineralized osteoid along the dorsal, medial, and lateral outer margins of the bone cortex. Small zones of cortical erosion are seen. Slight thickening of the bone cortex is also seen at several sites.

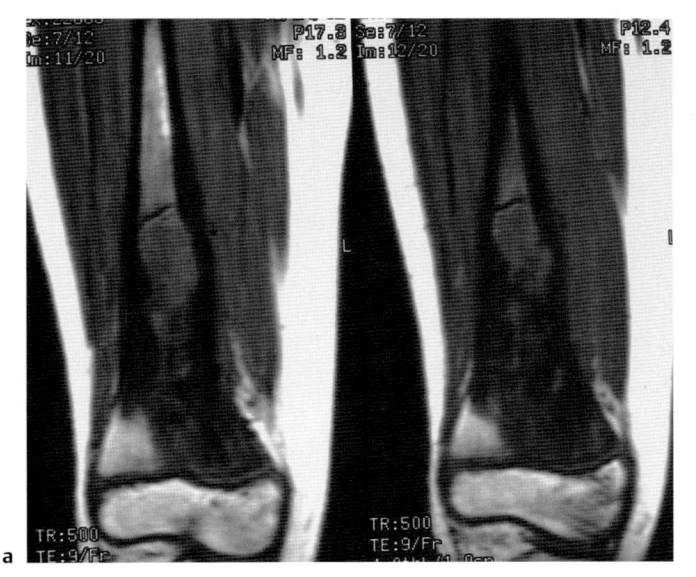

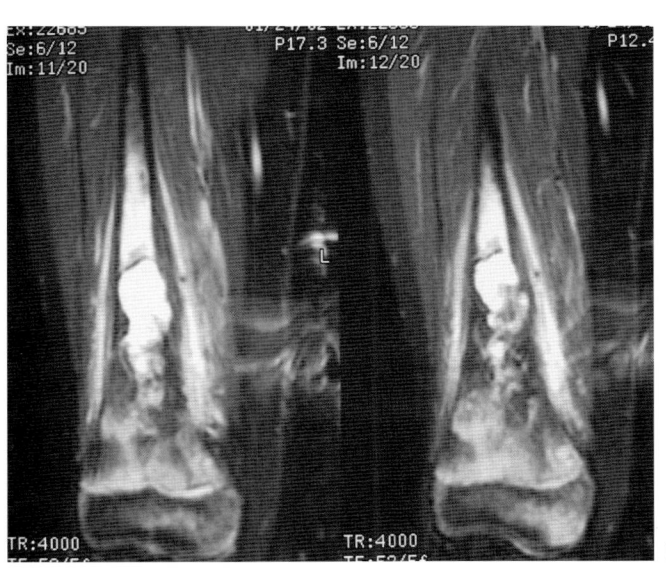

Figure 5.**6 a, b** Conventional intramedullary osteosarcoma in the marrow of the distal metadiaphyseal portion of the femur in a 9-year-old boy. The tumor has heterogeneous intermediate signal on coronal T1WI (**a**) and heterogeneous high signal on coronal FS T2WI (**b**). The intramedullary tumor is associated with zones of cortical destruction, periosteal elevation, and extraosseous extension.

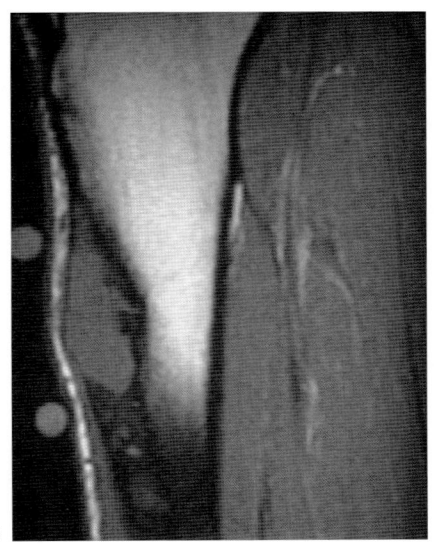

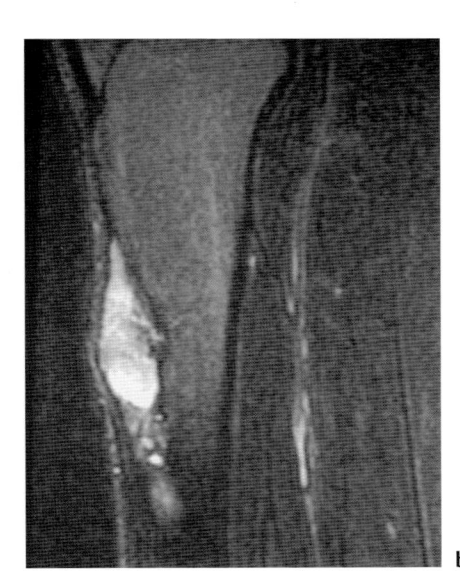

Figure 5.**7 a, b** Adamantinoma involving the anterior cortex of the proximal shaft of the tibia. The lesion expands the cortex and has heterogeneous intermediate signal on sagittal T1WI (**a**) and high signal on sagittal FS T2WI (**b**).

Table 5 (Continued) Lesions associated with thickening of bone cortex		
Lesion	**MRI Findings**	**Comments**
Other lesions		
Heterotopic ossification (Fig. 5.8)	Long-standing lesions can have variable low signal on T1WI, PDWI, and T2WI depending on the degree of mineralization/ossification, fibrosis, and hemosiderin deposition. Zones of high signal on T1WI and T2WI may occur from fatty marrow metaplasia. Gd-contrast enhancement in old mature lesions is often minimal or absent. Signal abnormalities within bone marrow are usually absent.	Represents localized non-neoplastic reparative lesions that are comprised of reactive hypercellular fibrous tissue, cartilage, and/or bone. Can arise secondary to trauma (myositis ossificans circumscripta, ossifying hematoma), although may also occur without a history of prior injury (pseudomalignant osseous tumor of the soft tissues). **(See Atlas Chapter A 53)**
Osteofibrous dysplasia (Fig. 5.9)	Osteofibrous dysplasia often shows multiple irregular intracortical zones of low-intermediate signal on T1W images, intermediate to slightly high signal on PDWI, and high signal on T2WI and FS T2WI separated by irregular zones of low signal on T1WI and T2WI, the latter representing thickened sclerotic cortical bone. The outer cortical margins can be expanded and thinned. Intracortical lesions usually show prominent Gd-contrast enhancement. Thin juxtacortical/periosteal enhancement may be seen in lesions with thinned and expanded cortical margins.	Rare self-limited benign fibro-osseous lesion primarily involving the anterior midshaft of the tibial cortex in children and adolescents. **(See Atlas Chapter A 59)**
Fibrous dysplasia (Figs. 5.10, 5.11)	MRI features depend on the proportions of bony spicules, collagen, fibroblastic spindle cells, hemorrhagic and/or cystic changes, and associated pathologic fracture if present. Lesions are usually well-circumscribed, and have low or low-intermediate signal on T1WI and PDWI. On T2WI, lesions have variable mixtures of low, intermediate, and/or high signal often surrounded by a low signal rim of variable thickness. Internal septations and cystic changes are seen in a minority of lesions. Bone expansion and cortical thickening can be seen. Lesions show Gd-contrast enhancement that varies in degree and pattern. Periosteal and juxtacortical enhancement can be seen in lesions with associated pathologic fractures.	Benign medullary fibro-osseous lesion which can involve a single site (mono-ostotic) or multiple locations (poly-ostotic). Thought to occur from developmental failure in the normal process of remodeling primitive bone to mature lamellar bone with resultant zone or zones of immature trabeculae within dysplastic fibrous tissue. Lesions do not mineralize normally and result in loss of mechanical strength predisposing to deformity and pathologic fracture. Accounts for ~10% of benign bone lesions. Patients range in age from <1 to 76 years. 75% occur before the age of 30 years. **(See Atlas Chapter A 27)**

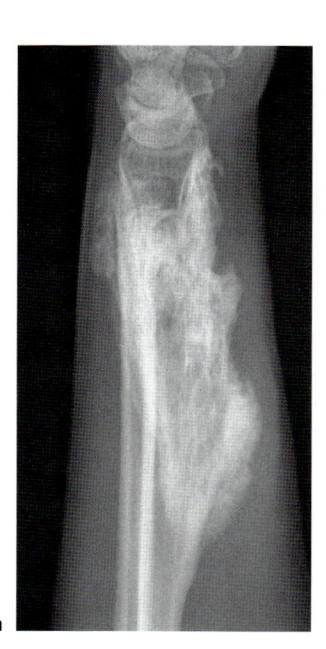

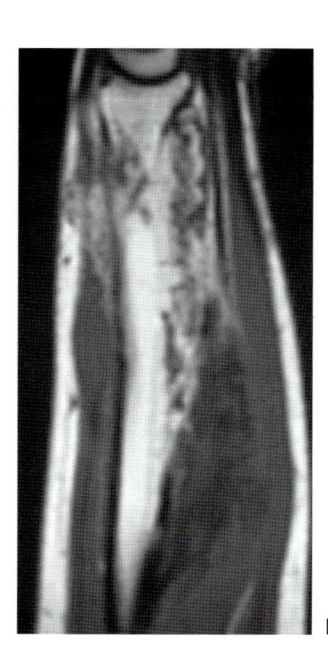

Figure 5.8 a, b Extensive pathologically proven heterotopic ossification that has blended into the outer cortical surface of the distal ulna as seen on the lateral radiograph (**a**) and sagittal T1WI (**b**).

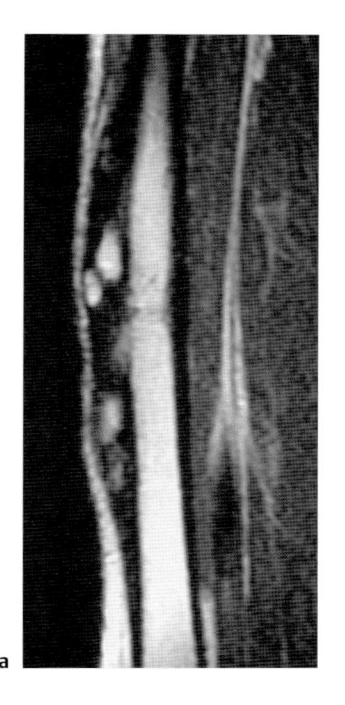

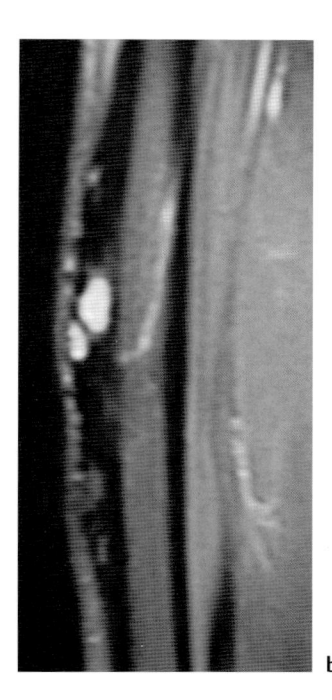

Figure 5.**9 a, b** Osteofibrous dysplasia involving the anterior cortex of the proximal shaft of the tibia. The lesion expands the cortex, within which are multiple zones of heterogeneous high signal on sagittal T2WI (**a**) that shows corresponding Gd-contrast enhancement on sagittal FS T1WI (**b**).

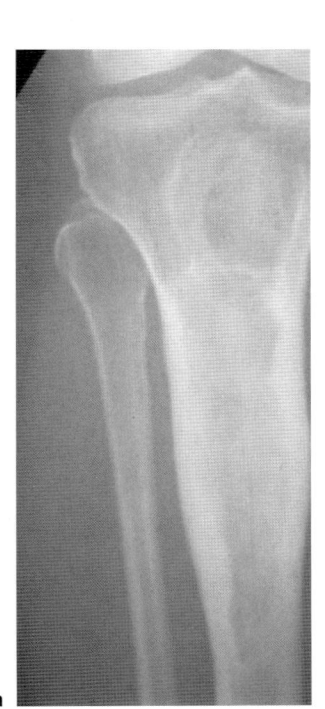

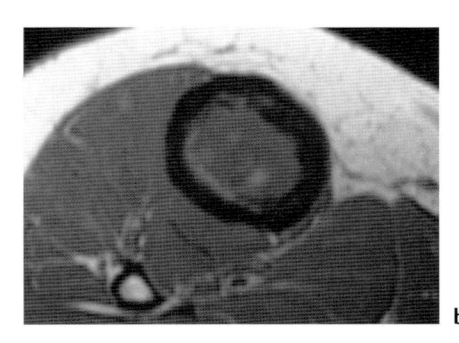

Figure 5.**10 a, b** Fibrous dysplasia involving the proximal shaft of the tibia with cortical thickening as seen on the AP radiograph (**a**) and axial T1WI (**b**). Also seen is the intermediate signal of the lesion within the marrow on axial T1WI.

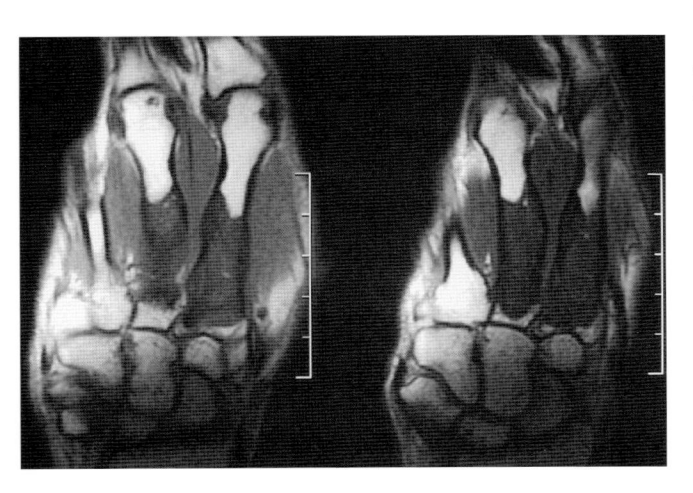

Figure 5.**11** Polyostotic fibrous dysplasia involving adjacent metacarpal bones with cortical thickening and intermediate marrow signal alteration on coronal T1WI.

Table 5 (Continued) **Lesions associated with thickening of bone cortex**

Lesion	MRI Findings	Comments
Focal fibrocartilaginous dysplasia (Fig. 5.12)	Cortical thickening seen along concave side of tibia vara, and asymmetric thickening of the epiphysis medially.	Uncommon benign condition causing deformities of long bones in children. Most frequent at proxial tibia in young children; typically unilateral; results in tibia vara. Also occurs less frequently in femur, humerus, and ulna. Lesions show dense collagenous tissue that may spontaneously regress. Corrective osteomy may be needed for severe and persistent lesions.
Melorheostosis (Fig. 5.13)	MRI signal varies based on the relative proportions of, mineralized osteoid, chondroid, and soft tissue components in these lesions. Mineralized osteoid zones involving bone cortex typically have low signal on T1WI and T2WI, no Gd-contrast enhancement. Soft tissue lesions may also occur adjacent to the cortical lesions, which have mixed signal on T1WI and T2WI.	Rare bone dysplasia with cortical thickening that has a "flowing candle wax" configuration. Associated soft tissue masses occur in ~25%. The soft tissue lesions often contain mixtures of chondroid material, mineralized osteoid, and fibrovascular tissue. **(See Atlas Chapter A 62)**
Healing and healed fractures (Figs. 5.14, 5.15)	Healing stress or traumatic fractures can have periosteal elevation with associated adjacent high signal on T2WI and FS T2WI, as well as poorly defined marrow zones with high signal on T2WI and FS T2WI (**Fig. 5.14**). Poorly defined zones of Gd-contrast enhancement can be seen in the juxtacortical soft tissues and marrow. Maturation of the periosteal reaction can lead to cortical thickening (**Fig. 5.15**).	Fracture results in localized hemorrhage followed by an inflammatory response after 48 hours that leads to granulation tissue ingrowth, and activation of the osteoblasts in the periosteum. Periosteal bone formation results in cortical thickening. In addition endosteal sclerosis with stress fractures can be seen on radiographs, CT, and MRI.

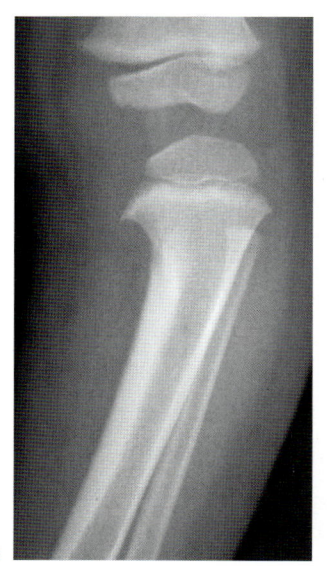

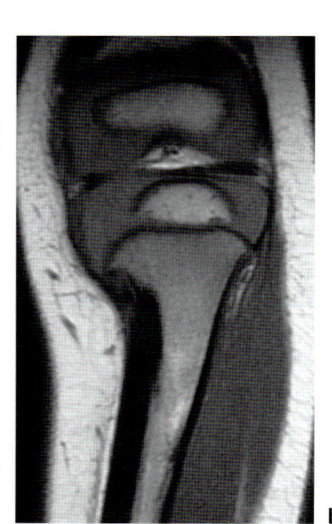

Figure 5.**12 a, b** Focal fibrocartilaginous dysplasia with cortical thickening seen along the concave side of the tibia vara, and asymmetric thickening of the epiphysis medially on the AP radiograph (**a**) and coronal T1WI (**b**).

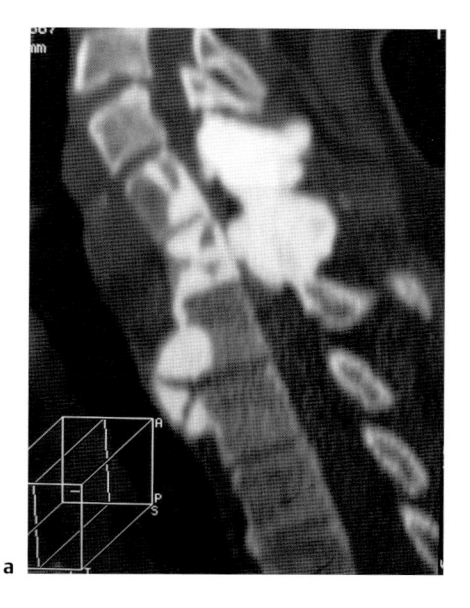

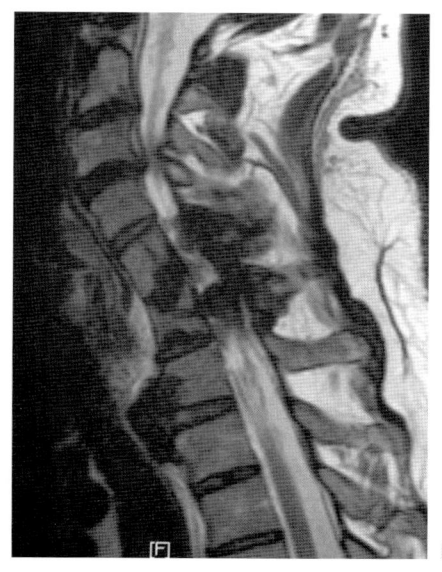

Figure 5.**13 a, b** Melorheostosis involving multiple vertebrae with extensive cortical thickening as seen on the sagittal CT image (**a**). Zones of cortical thickening have low signal on the sagittal T2WI (**b**).

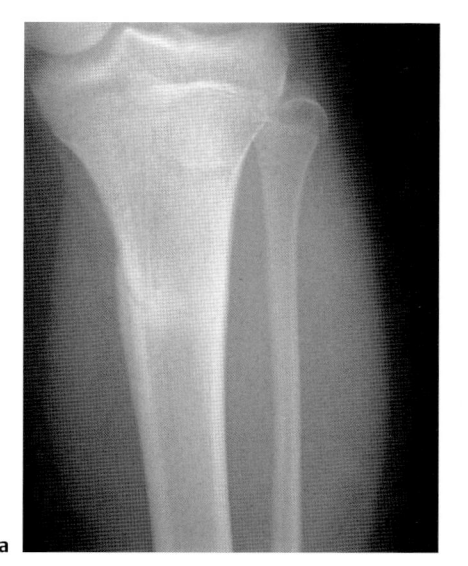

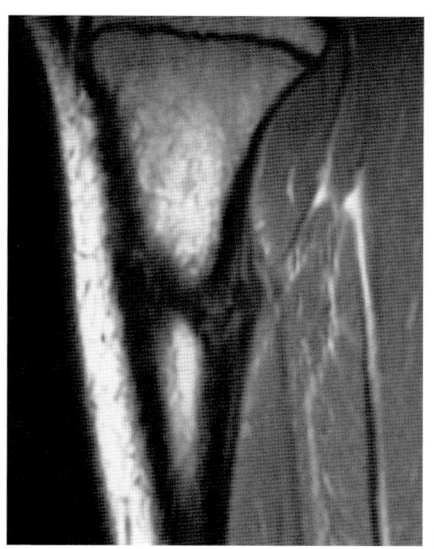

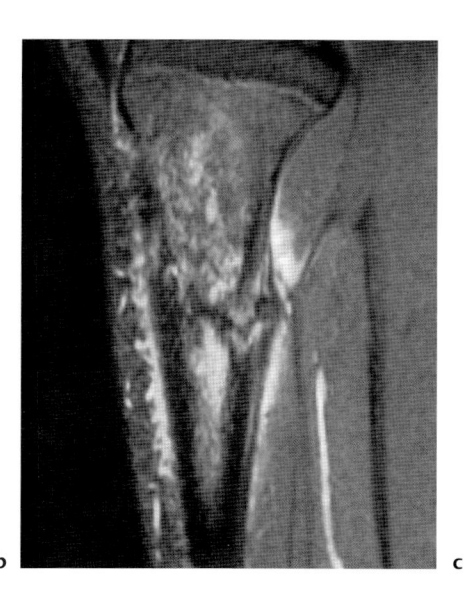

Figure 5.**14 a–d** Healing stress fracture involving the proximal tibial diaphysis with cortical thickening and endosteal sclerosis as seen on an AP radiograph (**a**). The cortical thickening has mixed low and intermediate signal on sagittal T1WI (**b**) and mixed slightly high and low signal on sagittal (**c**) and axial (**d**) FS T2WI. Zones with high signal are seen within the marrow and juxtacortical soft tissues on FS T2WI. A thin zone of low signal is also seen within the marrow.

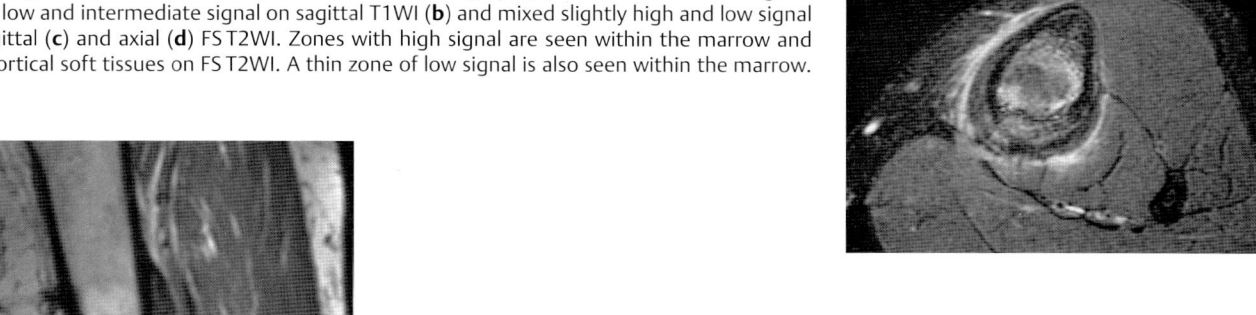

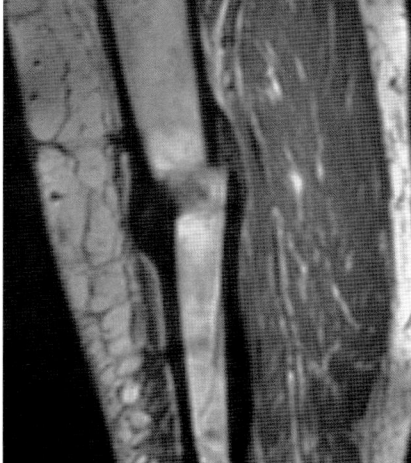

Figure 5.**15** Healed traumatic fracture deformity of the tibial shaft with thickened cortex as seen on sagittal T1WI.

Table 5 (Continued) Lesions associated with thickening of bone cortex		
Lesion	**MRI Findings**	**Comments**
Noninterrupted periosteal reaction and bone formation from secondary hypertrophic osteoarthropathy	Smooth, wavy, and/or irregular periosteal and cortical thickening seen in the diaphyseal and metaphyseal portions of long bones of the upper and lower extremities, as well as in other bones.	Clinical syndrome with clubbing of the digits, periostitis, hypertrophic osteoarthropathy, skin thickening, limb swelling, nail bed abnormalities (striations, increased curvature) related to extraskeletal lesions involving the lungs (bronchogenic carcinoma, metastasis, cystic fibrosis, bronchiectasis, infection, lymphoma), pleura (mesothelioma), abdomen (biliary atresia, cirrhosis, tumors, ulcerative colitis, Crohn disease), heart (cyanotic heart disease), or neoplasms at other sites. Regression of hypertrophic osteoarthropathy can occur after thoracotomy in patients with thoracic abnormalities, even in those without complete removal of the intrathoracic lesions.
Noninterrupted periosteal reaction and bone formation from venous stasis (Fig. 5.19)	Smooth and wavy periosteal and cortical thickening seen in the diaphyseal and metaphyseal portions of long bones of the lower extremities (tibia, fibula, metatarsal bones, phalanges).	Venous stasis is associated with edematous changes in the soft tissues as well as soft tissue ossification, periostitis, and cortical thickening.
Noninterrupted periosteal reaction and bone formation from infantile cortical hyperostosis (Caffey disease)	Smooth, wavy, and/or irregular periosteal and cortical thickening seen in the diaphyseal and metaphyseal portions of one or multiple bones.	Clinical disorder that affects infants less than 5 months with findings of soft tissue swelling (commonly over the mandible), fever, hyperirritability, and cortical hyperostosis (ribs, ulna, tibia, fibula, humerus, femur, radius, metacarpal, and metatarsal bones). The clinical course is variable but regression of findings can occur over 3–4 years.

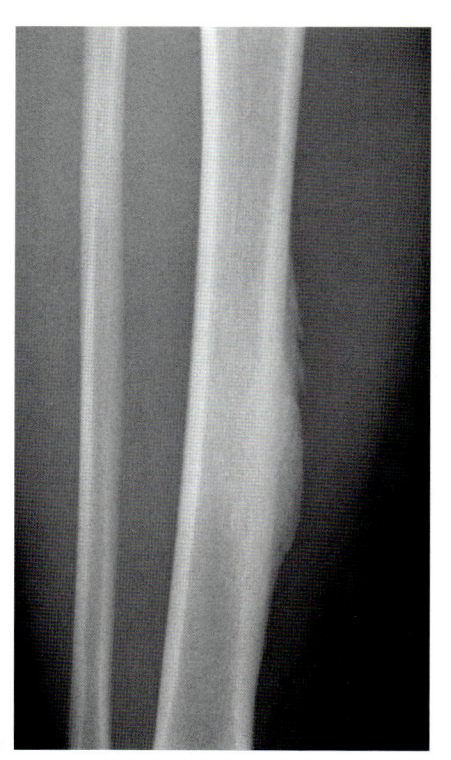

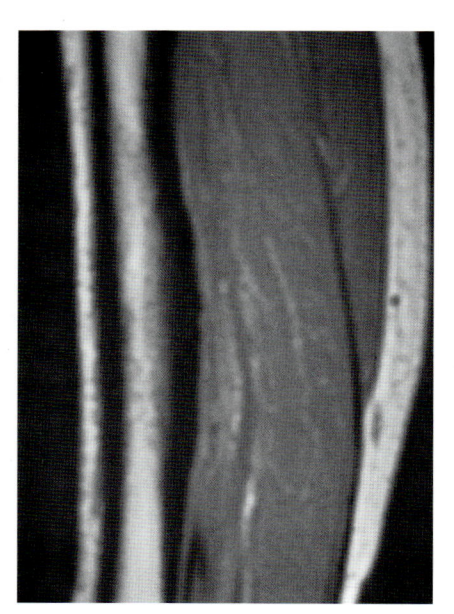

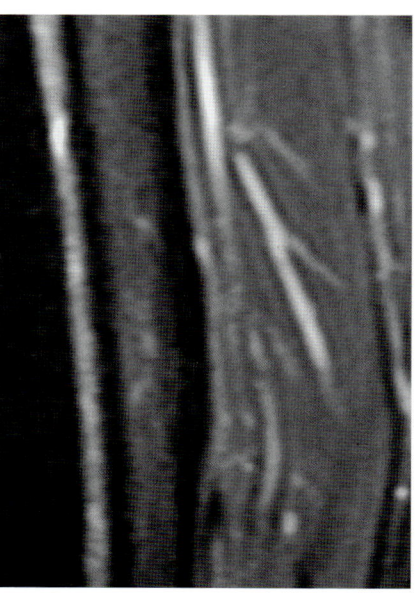

Figure 5.**19 a–c** Undulating solid periosteal bone formation along the tibial shaft as seen on a radiograph (**a**). The periosteal reaction and cortical thickening has low signal on sagittal T1WI (**b**) and post-contrast FS T1WI (**c**).

Table 5 (Continued) Lesions associated with thickening of bone cortex		
Lesion	**MRI Findings**	**Comments**
Noninterrupted periosteal reaction and bone formation from thyroid acropachy	Asymmetric, irregular, spiculated periosteal thickening seen in the diaphyseal portions of one or multiple bones (metacarpal and metatarsal bones, phalanges, other bones).	This disorder represents an extreme form of autoimmune thyroid disease with clinical manifestations such as swelling of the digits and toes, digital clubbing, and periosteal reaction. Thyroid dermopathy (pretibial myxedema) occurs in 4% of patients with Graves ophthalmopathy. Pronounced cases of thyroid dermopathy can be associated with thyroid acropachy in 1% of patients with Graves ophthalmopathy.
Noninterrupted periosteal reaction from hypervitaminosis A	Smooth and wavy periosteal and cortical thickening seen in the diaphyseal portions of one or multiple bones (ulna, metatarsal bones, clavicle, tibia, fibula, other bones). Damage to the physeal plates can result in irregularities and premature fusion, as well as splaying and cupping deformities of the metaphyses.	Vitamin A intoxication in children can result in anorexia, dermatologic and osseous disorders. In children, damage to the physeal plates may be irreversible despite cessation of vitamin A administration. In adults, anorexia, weight loss, and dermatologic disorders are frequently associated with hypervitaminosis A.
Noninterrupted periosteal reaction from hypovitaminosis A	Smooth and wavy periosteal and cortical thickening seen in the diaphyseal portions of one or multiple bones.	Vitamin A deficiency can result in anemia, dermatologic disorders (dry and scaly skin), growth retardation, osseous abnormalities, cranial nerve and visual disorders.
Noninterrupted periosteal reaction from hypovitaminosis C (scurvy)	In children, periosteal elevation with new bone formation can be seen in the diaphyseal and metaphyseal portions of one or multiple bones from subperiosteal hemorrhage. Metaphyseal beak-like bone protrusions can occur from the abnormal zones of provisional calcification at the physeal plate, as well as subepiphyseal fractures. In adults, osteopenia with hemarthrosis can be associated with ischemic necrosis and fractures with mild periosteal reaction.	In young children, vitamin C deficiency after 4 to 10 months can result in infantile scurvy with clinical features including failure to thrive, petechial hemorrhages, ulcerated gingiva, hematemesis, melena, hematuria, and anemia. Clinical features associated with adult scurvy include anorexia, fatigue, weakness, petechial hemorrhages involving gingiva and skin, hemarthrosis, osteoporosis, ischemic necrosis, dermatologic disorders (dry and scaly skin), growth retardation, osseous and nerve disorders.
Syndromes of hyperostosis, osteitis, and skin lesions (SAPHO syndrome)	Periosteal elevation with cortical thickening can be seen as well as syndesmophyte formation at one or multiple levels.	Syndrome including abnormalities such as synovitis, acne, pustulosis, hyperostosis with periosteal proliferation (sternum, clavicle, anterior ribs, symphysis pubis, femur, sacrum, iliac bones) and osteitis at the chest wall.

References

Focal Fibrocartilaginous Dysplasia

Choi IH, Kim CJ, Cho TJ, et al. Focal fibrocartilaginous dysplasia of long bones: report of eight additional cases and literature review. *J Pediatr Orthoped* 2000;20:421–427.

Kim CJ, Choi IH, Chung CY, Chi JG. The histologic spectrum of subperiosteal fibrocartilaginous pseudotumor of long bone (focal fibrocartilaginous dysplasia). *Pathol Int* 1999;49:1000–1006.

Neurofibromatosis

Resnick D. Enostosis, hyperostosis, and periostitis. In: Resnick D, ed. *Diagnosis of Bone and Joint Disorders*, 4th ed. Philadelphia, Pa: W.B. Saunders; 2002:5:4870–4919.

Primary Hypertrophic Osteoarthropathy

Araki Y, Tsukaguchi I, Nakamura H. Pachydermoperiostosis involving the skull and spine: MR findings. *AJR* March 1993;160(3):664–665.

Capelastegui A, Astigarraga E, García-Iturraspe C. MR findings in pulmonary hypertrophic osteoarthropathy. *Clin Radiol* January 2000;55(1):72–75.

Demirpolat G, Sener RN, Stun EE. MR imaging of pachydermoperiostosis. *J Neuroradiol* March 1999;26(1):61–63.

Loredo R, Pathria MN, Salonen D, Resnick D. Magnetic resonance imaging in pachydermoperiostosis. *Clin Imag* July-September 1996;20(3):212–218.

Resnick D. Enostosis, hyperostosis, and periostitis. In: Resnick D, ed. *Diagnosis of Bone and Joint Disorders*, 4th ed. Philadelphia, Pa: W.B. Saunders; 2002:5:4870–4919.

Secondary Hypertrophic Osteoarthropathy

Capelastegui A, Astigarraga E, García-Iturraspe C. MR findings in pulmonary hypertrophic osteoarthropathy. *Clin Radiol* January 2000;55(1): 72–75.

Resnick D. Enostosis, hyperostosis, and periostitis. In: Resnick D, ed. *Diagnosis of Bone and Joint Disorders*, 4th ed. Philadelphia, Pa: W.B. Saunders; 2002:5:4870–4919.

Sainani NI, Lawande MA, Parikh VP, Pungavkar SA, Patkar DP, Sase KS. MRI diagnosis of hypertrophic osteoarthropathy from a remote childhood malignancy. *Skeletal Radiol* 2007 Jun;36 Suppl 1:63–6. Epub Sep 5 2006.

Varan A, Kutluk T, Demirkazik FB, Akyüz C, Büyükpamukçu M. Hypertrophic osteoarthropathy in a child with nasopharyngeal carcinoma. *Pediatr Radiol* 2000;30:570–572.

Periosteal Reaction from Venous Stasis

Resnick D. Enostosis, hyperostosis, and periostitis. In: Resnick D, ed. *Diagnosis of Bone and Joint Disorders*, 4th ed. Philadelphia, Pa: W.B. Saunders; 2002:5:4870–4919.

Wenaden AET, Szyszko TA, Saifuddin A. Imaging of periosteal reactions associated with focal lesions of bone. *Clin Radiol* 2005;60:439–456.

Infantile Cortical Hyperostosis (Caffey Disease)

Katz DS, Eller DJ, Bergman G, Blankenberg FG. Caffey's disease of the scapula: CT and MR findings. *AJR* January 1997;168(1):286–287.

Resnick D. Enostosis, hyperostosis, and periostitis. In: Resnick D, ed. *Diagnosis of Bone and Joint Disorders*, 4th ed. Philadelphia, Pa: W.B. Saunders; 2002:5:4870–4919.

Saatci I, Brown JJ, McAlister WH. MR findings in a patient with Caffey's disease. *Pediatr Radiol* November 1996;26(1):68–70.

Thyroid Acropachy

Fatourechi V, Ahmed DDF, Schwartz KM. Thyroid acropachy: report of 40 patients treated at a single institution in a 26-year period. *J Clin Endocrinol Metab* 2002;87:5435–5441.

Resnick D. Enostosis, hyperostosis, and periostitis. In: Resnick D, ed. *Diagnosis of Bone and Joint Disorders*, 4th ed. Philadelphia, Pa: W.B. Saunders; 2002:5:4870–4919.

Vanhoenacker FM, Pelckmans MC, De Beuckeleer LH, Colpaert CG, De Schepper AM. Thyroid acropachy: correlation of imaging and pathology. *Eur Radiol* 2001;11(6):1058–1062.

Hypervitaminosis and Hypovitaminosis

Jiang YB, Wang YZ, Zhao J, Marchal G, Shen YL, Xing SZ, Li RG, Baert AL. Bone remodeling in hypervitaminosis D3. radiologic-microangiographic-pathologic correlations. *Invest Radiol* 1991;26:213–219.

Lips P. Hypervitaminosis A and fractures. *N Engl J Med* 2003;384: 347–349.

Resnick D. Hypervitaminosis and hypovitaminosis. In: Resnick D, ed. *Diagnosis of Bone and Joint Disorders*, 4th ed. Philadelphia, Pa: W.B. Saunders; 2002:4:3456–3464.

Romero JB, Schreiber A, Von Hochstetter AR, Wagenhauser FJ, Michel BA, Theiler R. Hyperostotic and destructive osteoarthritis in a patient with vitamin A intoxication syndrome: a case report. *Bull Hosp Jt Dis* 1996;54:169–174.

Syndromes of Hyperostosis, Osteitis, and Skin Lesions (SAPHO syndrome)

Boutin RD, Resnick D. The SAPHO syndrome: an evolving concept for unifying several idiopathic disorders of bone and skin. *AJR* 1998; 170:585–591.

Davies AM, Marino AJ, Evans N, Grimer RJ, Deshmukh N, Mangham DC. SAPHO syndrome: 20 year followup. *Skeletal Radiol* 1999;28: 159–162.

Kirchoff T, Merkesdal S, Rosenthal H, et al. Diagnostic management of patients with SAPHO syndrome: use of MR imaging to guide bone biopsy at CT for microbiological and histological work-up. *Eur Radiol* 2003;13:2304–2308.

Resnick D. Enostosis, hyperostosis, and periostitis. In: Resnick D, ed. *Diagnosis of Bone and Joint Disorders*, 4th ed. Philadelphia, Pa: W.B. Saunders; 2002:5:4870–4919.

Table 6 Intramedullary lesions associated with expansion of intact cortical margins

Lesion	MRI Findings	Comments
Benign		
Osteochondroma (Fig. 6.1)	Circumscribed protruding lesion arising from outer cortex with a central zone with intermediate signal on T1WI and T2WI similar to marrow surrounded by a peripheral zone of low signal on T1WI and T2WI, a cartilaginous cap is usually present in children and young adults. Increased malignant potential when cartilaginous cap is >2 cm thick.	Benign cartilaginous tumors arising from defect at periphery of growth plate during bone formation with resultant bone outgrowth covered by a cartilaginous cap. Usually benign lesions unless associated with pain and increasing size of cartilaginous cap. Osteochondromas are common lesions, accounting for 14 to 35 % of primary bone tumors. Occur with median age of 20 years, up to 75 % of patients are less than 20 years old. **(See Atlas Chapter A 58)**
Fibrous dysplasia (Fig. 6.2)	MRI features depend on the proportions of bony spicules, collagen, fibroblastic spindle cells, hemorrhagic and/or cystic changes, and associated pathologic fracture if present. Lesions are usually well-circumscribed, and have low or low-intermediate signal on T1WI and PDWI. On T2WI, lesions have variable mixtures of low, intermediate, and/or high signal often surrounded by a low signal rim of variable thickness. Internal septations and cystic changes are seen in a minority of lesions. Bone expansion with thickened and/or thinned cortex can be seen. Lesions show Gd-contrast enhancement that varies in degree and pattern.	Benign medullary fibro-osseous lesion that can involve a single site **(mono-ostotic)** or multiple locations **(poly-ostotic)**. Thought to occur from developmental failure in the normal process of remodeling primitive bone to mature lamellar bone with resultant zone or zones of immature trabeculae within dysplastic fibrous tissue. Account for ~10 % of benign bone lesions. Patients range in age from <1 to 76 years. 75 % occur before the age of 30 years. **(See Atlas Chapter A 27)**

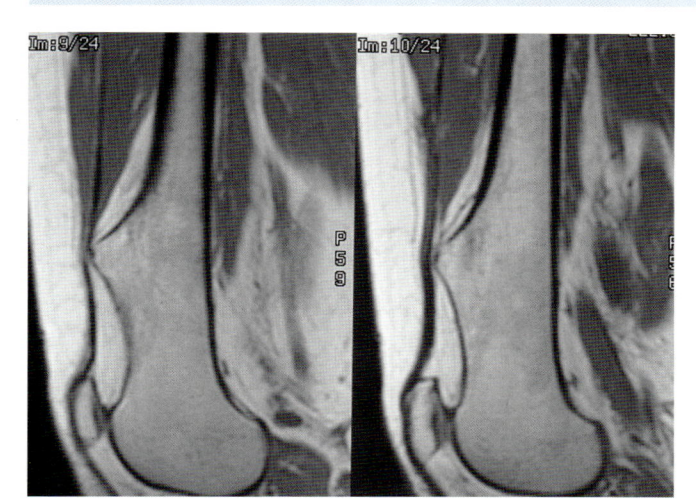

Figure 6.1 A 20-year-old woman with an osteochondroma protruding from the anterior distal femur as seen on sagittal PDWI.

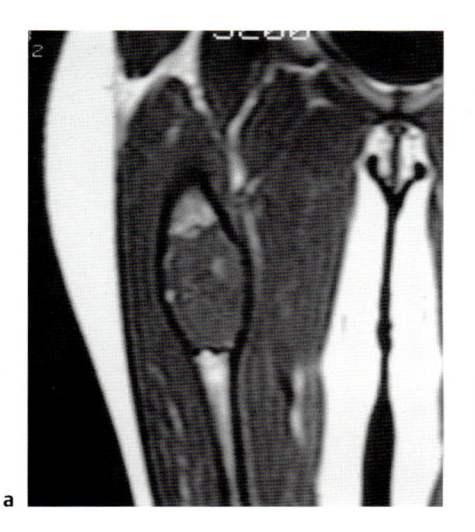

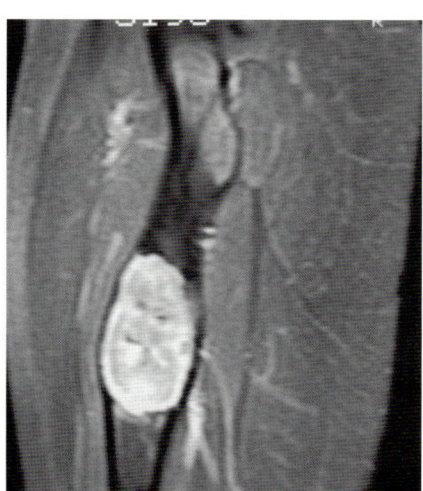

Figure 6.2 a, b A 39-year-old woman with fibrous dysplasia expanding the diaphyseal portion of the femur as seen on coronal T1WI (**a**), and showing Gd-contrast enhancement on sagittal FS T1WI (**b**).

Table 6 (Continued) **Intramedullary lesions associated with expansion of intact cortical margins**

Leson	MRI Findings	Comments
Nonossifying fibroma (fibroxanthoma) (Fig. 6.3)	Well-circumscribed eccentric intramedullary lesions in the metadiaphyseal regions of long bones that have mixed low-intermediate signal on T1WI, and mixed low, intermediate, and/or high signal on T2WI, PDWI, and FS T2WI. Zones of low signal on T1WI, PDWI, and T2WI can be seen in the central portions of the lesions. Zones with varying thickness of low signal on T1WI, PDWI, and T2WI are seen at the margins of the lesions representing bone sclerosis. Internal septations are commonly seen as zones of low signal on T2WI in these lesions. Cortical thinning or thickening and bone expansion can be seen. Lesions can show Gd-contrast enhancement (heterogeneous > homogeneous patterns). Linear periosteal Gd-contrast enhancement can be seen at lesions with associated fracture or marked cortical expansion/thinning.	Fibrous cortical defects (**FCDs**) and **nonossifying fibromas (NOFs)** are well-circumscribed common benign fibrohistiocytic lesions in the metadiaphyseal portions of long bones that are comprised of whorls of fibroblastic cells combined with smaller amounts of multinucleated giant cells and xanthomatous cells. Both **FCDs** and **NOFs** have similar pathologic findings although they differ in size and primary locations in long bones. **FCDs** are small lesions primarily located in bone cortex, whereas the larger **NOFs** are located eccentrically in the medullary cavity. **FCDs** and **NOFs** are usually asymptomatic and are often detected as incidental findings. The true incidence of these lesions is unknown, maybe up to 40% of children. 95% occur between the ages of 5 and 20, median = 14 years. **(See Atlas Chapter A 26)**
Unicameral bone cyst (Fig. 6.4)	Unicameral bone cysts (UBCs) often have a peripheral rim of low signal on T1W, PDWI, and T2W images adjacent to normal medullary bone. UBCs usually contain fluid with low to low-intermediate signal on T1WI; low-intermediate, intermediate or slightly high signal on PDWI; and high signal on T2WI. Fluid–fluid levels may occur. In tubular bones, mild to moderate expansion of bone may occur with variable thinning of the overlying cortex. For UBCs without pathologic fracture, thin peripheral Gd-contrast enhancement can be seen at the margins of lesions. UBCs with pathologic fracture can have heterogeneous or homogeneous low-intermediate or slightly high signal on T1WI, and heterogeneous or homogeneous high signal on T2WI and FS T2WI. UBCs complicated by fracture can have internal septations and fluid–fluid levels, as well as irregular peripheral Gd-contrast enhancement at internal septations.	Intramedullary non-neoplastic cavities filled with serous or serosanguineous fluid. Account for 9% of primary tumor-like lesions of bone. 85% occur in the first two decades, median = 11 years. **(See Atlas Chapter A 3)**
Aneurysmal bone cyst (Fig. 6.5)	Aneurysmal bone cysts (ABCs) often have a low signal rim on T1WI, PDWI, and T2WI adjacent to normal medullary bone, and between extraosseous soft tissues. Various combinations of low, intermediate, and/or high signal on T1WI, PDWI, and T2WI images are usually seen within aneurysmal bone cysts as well as fluid–fluid levels. Variable Gd-contrast enhancement is seen at the margins of lesions as well as involving the internal septae.	Tumor-like expansile bone lesions containing cavernous spaces filled with blood. ABCs can be primary bone lesions (two-thirds) or secondary to other bone lesions/tumors (such as giant cell tumors, chondroblastomas, osteoblastomas, osteosarcomas, chondromyxoid fibromas, nonossifying fibromas, fibrous dysplasia, fibrosarcomas, malignant fibrous histiocytomas, and metastatic disease). Account for ~11% of primary tumor-like lesions of bone. Patients usually range in age from 1 to 25 years, median = 14 years. **(See Atlas Chapter A 2)**

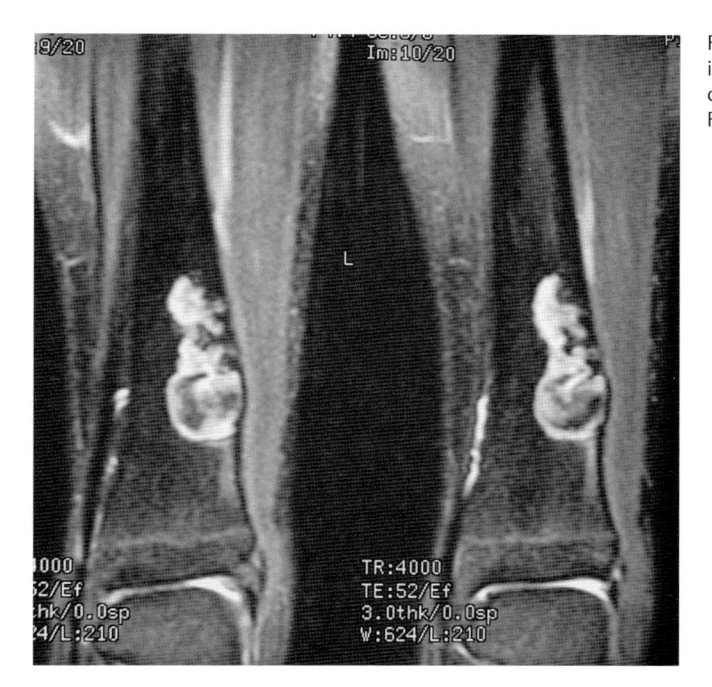

Figure 6.3 A 16-year-old female with a nonossifying fibroma involving the posterior diaphyseal portion of the distal tibia. The lesion has circumscribed margins and has mixed low and high signal on coronal FS T2WI. Cortical thinning and slight expansion are seen.

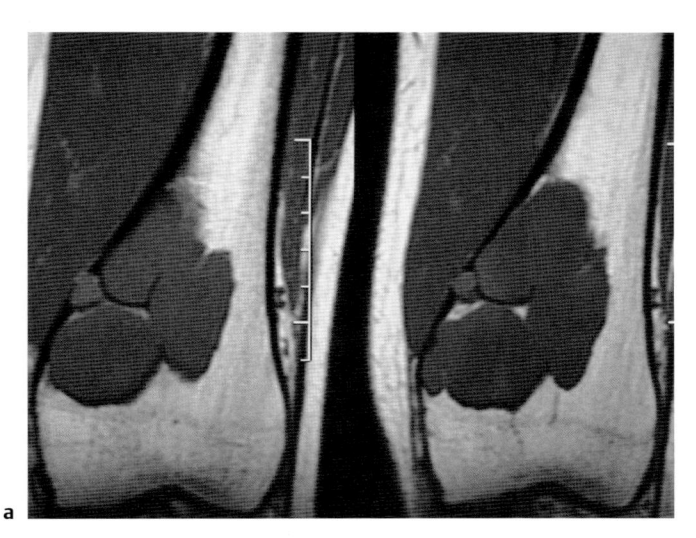

Figure 6.4 a, b A 17-year-old female with a unicameral bone cyst within the distal metadiaphyseal portion of the femur as seen on coronal T1WI (a) and sagittal FS T2WI (b). Cortical thinning and slight expansion are seen.

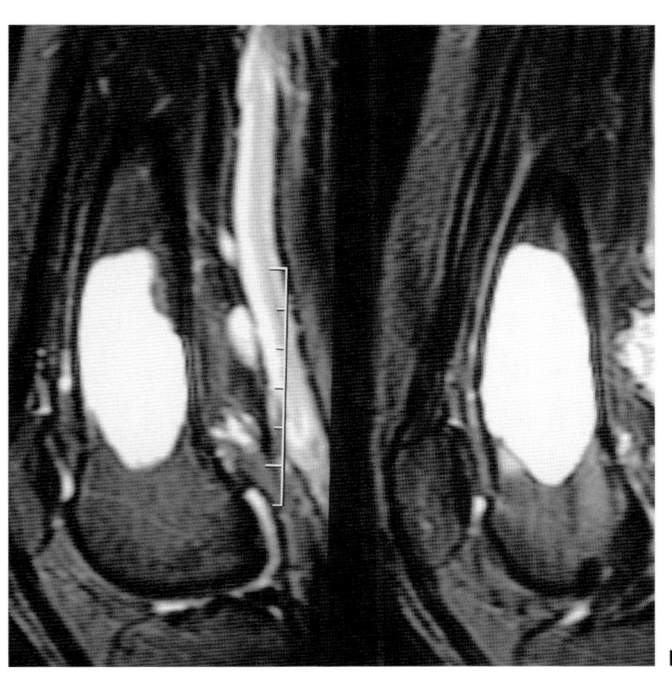

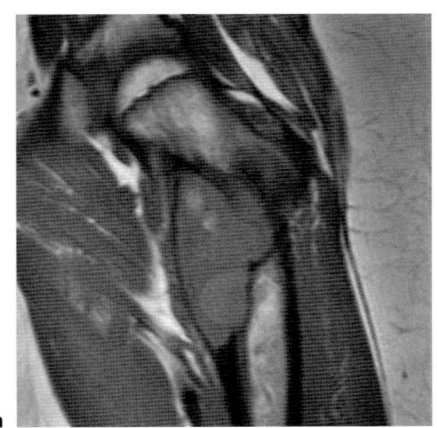

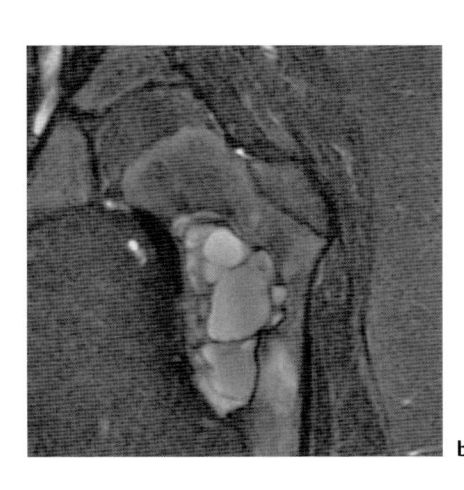

Figure 6.5 a, b An 11-year-old boy with an aneurysmal bone cyst involving the medial proximal shaft of the femur. Coronal T1WI (a) shows an expansile lesion with thinned cortex containing zones with intermediate and high signal. Coronal FS T2WI (b) shows a multi-septated lesion with fluid–fluid levels containing high and low–intermediate signal.

Table 6 (Continued) **Intramedullary lesions associated with expansion of intact cortical margins**

Lesion	MRI Findings	Comments
Giant cell reparative granuloma (solid aneurysmal bone cyst) (Fig. 6.6)	Radiolucent bone lesions on CT, typically occur in the metaphysis and/or diaphysis. Bone expansion may occur with or without intact thin cortical margins. Extraosseous extension of lesions may occur. Lesions can have heterogeneous low, intermediate, and/or high signal on T1WI, PDWI, and T2WI; as well as peripheral rim-like and central Gd-contrast enhancement on FS T1WI.	Giant cell granulomas (also known as solid aneurysmal bone cysts) are reactive granulomatous lesions that have histologic features similar to Brown tumors. Lesions contain multinucleated giant cells adjacent to sites of hemorrhage, and fibroblasts. Osteoid formation adjacent to sites of hemorrhage can be seen. Lesions usually occur in patients less than 30 years, and are most frequently found in the mandible, maxilla, and small bones of the hands and feet. Lesions in long bones have also been referred to as solid variants of aneurysmal bone cysts. **(See Atlas Chapter A 2)**

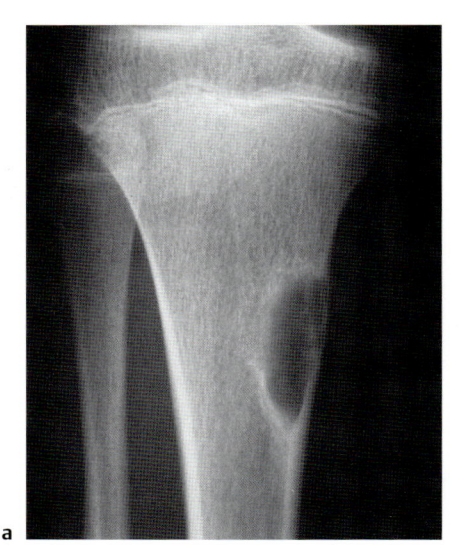

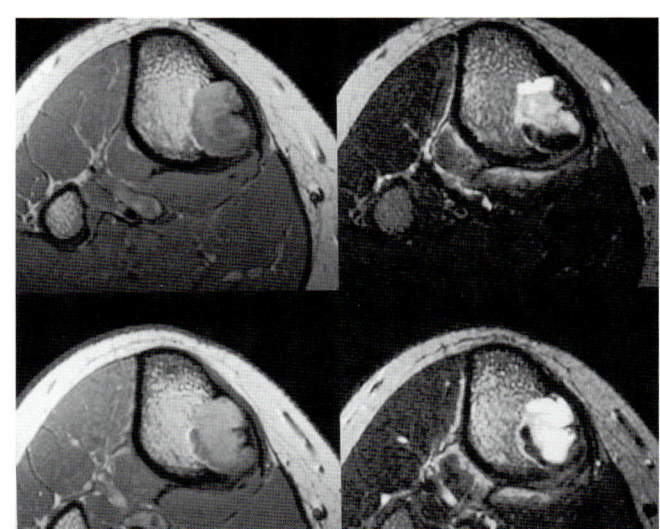

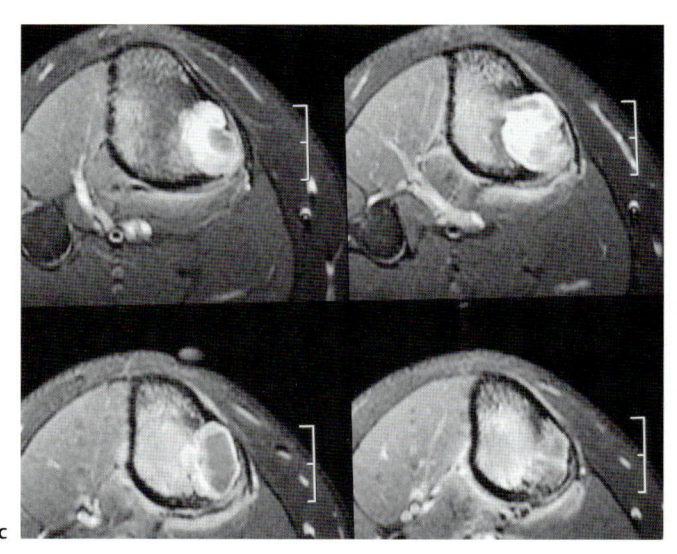

Figure 6.6 a–d A 14-year-old girl with a giant cell reparative granuloma (solid aneurysmal bone cyst) involving the medial portion of the proximal tibial shaft. The AP radiograph (**a**) shows a well-circumscribed radiolucent lesion with thin sclerotic margins, thinning, and expansion of the bone cortex. The lesion has intermediate signal on axial PDWI (**b**, *images on left*) and mixed low, intermediate, and high signal on axial T2WI (**b**, *images on right*). The lesion shows prominent heterogeneous Gd-contrast enhancement on axial (**c**) and coronal (**d**) FS T1WI. Poorly defined contrast enhancement is also seen in the marrow peripheral to the lesion.

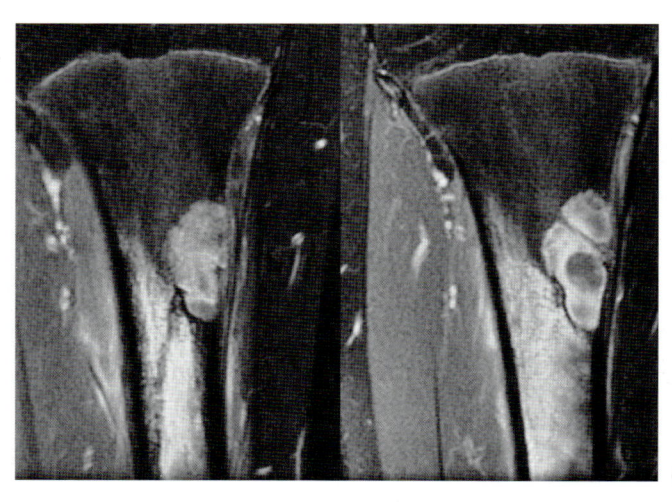

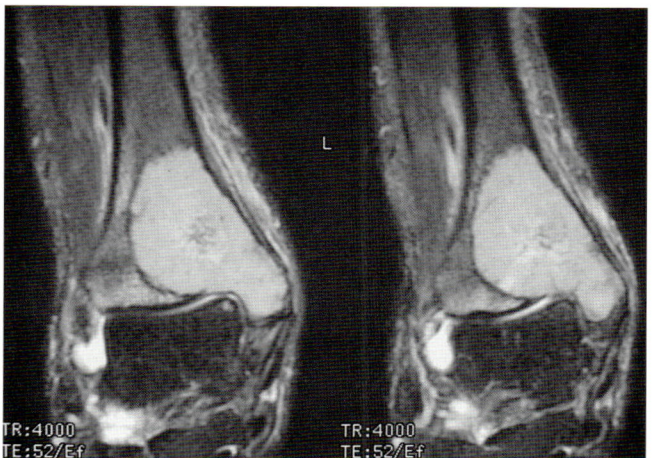

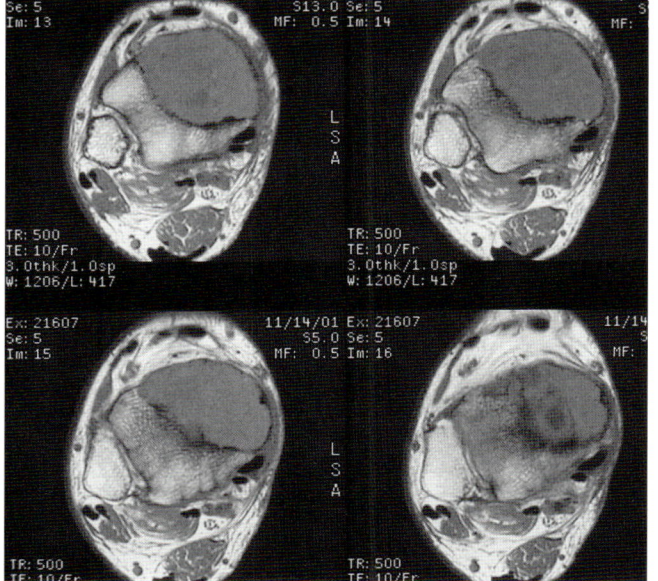

Table 6 (Continued)   Intramedullary lesions associated with expansion of intact cortical margins

Lesion	MRI Findings	Comments
Giant cell tumor of bone (Fig. 6.7)	Lesions may have expanded and thinned cortical margins on radiographs. Lesions may also show cortical disruption and extraosseous extension on MRI. Solid portions of giant cell tumors often have low to intermediate signal on T1WI and PDWI, intermediate to high signal on T2WI, and high signal on FS PDWI and FS T2WI. Signal heterogeneity on T2WI is common. Aneurysmal bone cysts can be seen in 14% of giant cell tumors. Varying degrees of Gd-contrast enhancement can be seen. Peripheral rim-like Gd-contrast enhancement may be seen around cystic zones/aneurysmal bone cysts.	Aggressive tumors composed of neoplastic ovoid mononuclear cells and scattered multinucleated osteoclast-like giant cells (derived from fusion of marrow mononuclear cells). Up to 10% of all giant cell tumors are malignant. Benign giant cell tumors account for ~5 to 9.5% of all bone tumors and up to 23% of benign bone tumors. Occur in patients 4 to 81 years (median = 30 years), 75% occur in patients between the ages of 15 and 45 years. (See Atlas Chapter A 29)

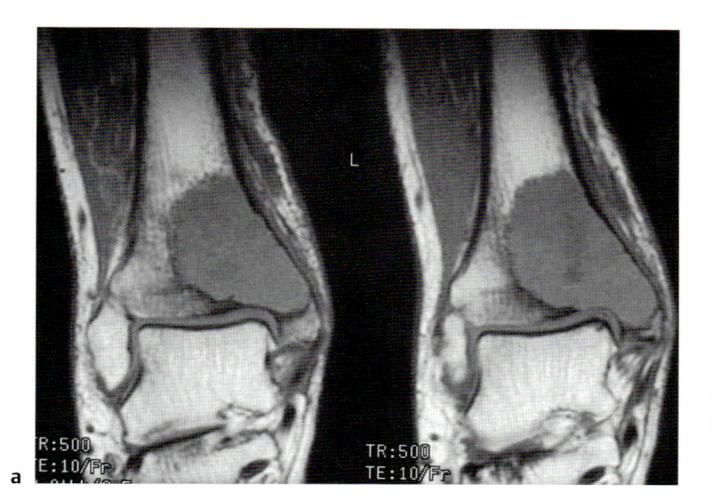

Figure 6.7 a–c   A 61-year-old man with a giant cell tumor involving the distal tibia with thinning and expansion of bone cortex as seen on coronal (**a**) and axial (**c**) T1WI and coronal FS T2WI (**b**).

Lesion	MRI Findings	Comments
Brown tumor	Lesions are usually radiolucent on radiographs and CT. Lesions often have low-intermediate signal on T1WI, intermediate to slightly high signal on T2WI, and typically show Gd-contrast enhancement. Zones of low signal on T2WI may occur from hemosiderin. Expansion of cortical margins can occur with or without cortical disruption/destruction.	Lesions in bone contain multinucleated giant cells, fibrous tissue, blood vessels, and zones of hemorrhage/hemosiderin. Histologic and imaging features are similar to giant cell reparative granulomas. Most often involves ribs, mandible, clavicle, pelvis, craniofacial bones, and vertebrae. Can result from primary hyperparathyroidism (3–7%) (oversecretion of parathyroid hormone [PTH] from parathyroid adenoma associated with hypercalcemia), secondary type (vitamin D deficiency or chronic renal failure with hypocalcemia resulting in secretion of PTH and parathyroid gland hyperplasia) (1–2%), or tertiary type in which the secondary type leads to eventual autonomous elevated PTH secretion from parathyroid gland hyperplasia.
Enchondroma (Fig. 6.8)	Lobulated intramedullary lesions with well-defined borders ranging in size from 3 to 16 cm, mean = 5 cm. Mild endosteal scalloping can be seen. Cortical bone expansion rarely occurs. Lesions usually have low-intermediate signal on T1WI and intermediate signal on PDWI. On T2WI and fat-suppressed T2WI, lesions usually have predominantly high signal with foci and/or bands of low signal representing areas of matrix mineralization and fibrous strands. No zones of abnormal high signal on T2WI are typically seen in the marrow outside the borders of the lesions. Lesions typically show Gd-contrast enhancement in various patterns (peripheral curvilinear lobular, central nodular/septal, and peripheral lobular, or heterogeneous diffuse).	Benign intramedullary lesions composed of hyaline cartilage, represent ~10% of benign bone tumors. Enchondromas can be solitary (88%) or multiple (12%). Ollier disease is a dyschondroplasia involving endochondral-formed bone resulting in multiple enchondromas (enchondromatosis). Metachondromatosis is a combination of enchondromatosis and osteochondromatosis, and is rare. Maffucci disease refers to a syndrome with multiple enchondromas and soft tissue hemangiomas, and is very rare. Patients range in age from 3 to 83 years, median = 35 years, mean = 38 to 40 years, peak in 3rd and 4th decades. **(See Atlas Chapter A 8)**
Chondromyxoid fibroma (Fig. 6.9)	Lesions are often slightly lobulated with low-intermediate signal on T1WI, intermediate signal on PDWI, and heterogeneous predominantly high signal on T2WI. Thin low signal septa within lesions on T2WI are secondary to fibrous strands. Lesions are surrounded by low signal borders representing thin sclerotic reaction. Edema is not typically seen in medullary bone. Lesions show prominent diffuse Gd-contrast enhancement.	Rare benign slow-growing bone lesions that contain chondroid, myxoid, and fibrous components. Chondromyxoid fibromas represent 2–4% of primary benign bone lesions, and <1% of primary bone lesions. Most chondromyxoid fibromas occur between the ages of 1 to 40 years, with a median of 17 years, and peak incidence in the 2nd to 3rd decades. **(See Atlas Chapter A 10)**
Osteoblastoma (Fig. 6.10)	Lesions appear as spheroid or ovoid zone measuring greater than 1.5 to 2 cm located within medullary and/or cortical bone with low-intermediate signal on T1WI; low-intermediate to slightly high signal on PDWI; and low-intermediate and/or high signal on T2WI and FS T2WI. After Gd-contrast administration, osteoblastomas show variable degrees of enhancement. Expansion of thinned cortical margins can be seen as well as thickening of cortical bone and medullary sclerosis. Zones of sclerotic bone reaction adjacent to osteoblastomas typically show low signal on T1W, T2WI, and FS T2WI. Poorly defined zones of marrow signal alteration consisting of low-intermediate signal on T1WI, high signal on T2WI and FS T2WI, and corresponding Gd-contrast enhancement can be seen in the marrow adjacent to osteoblastomas as well as within the extraosseous soft tissues.	Rare benign bone-forming tumors that are histologically related to osteoid osteomas. Osteoblastomas are larger than osteoid osteomas and show progressive enlargement. Account for 3–6% of primary benign bone tumors and <1–2% of all primary bone tumors. Occurs in patients from 1 to 30 years, median = 15 years, mean age = 20 years. Approximately 90% of lesions occur in patients less than 30 years. **(See Atlas Chapter A 61)**

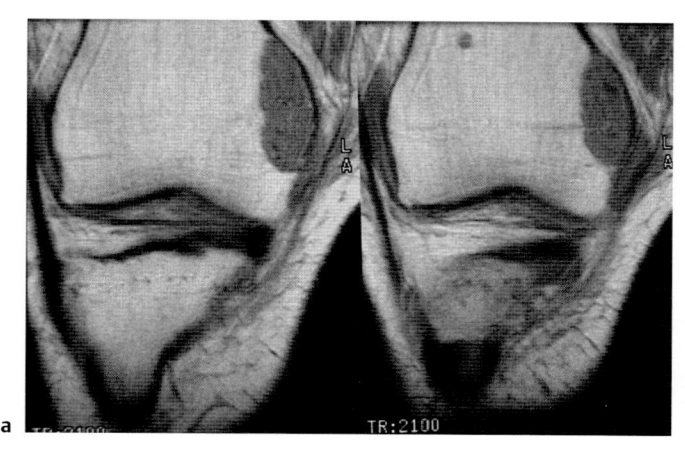

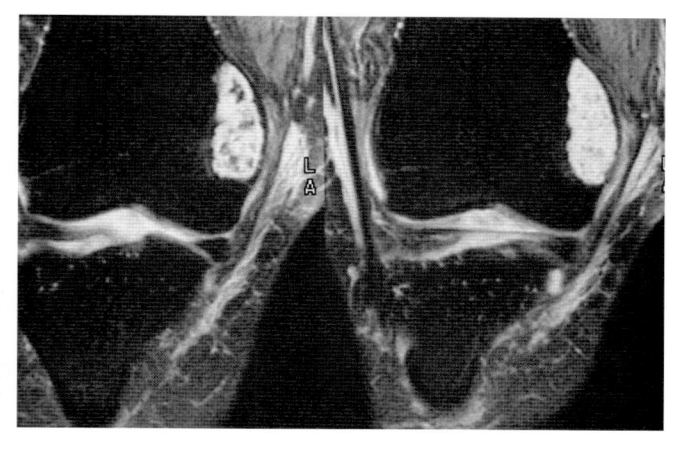

Figure 6.**8 a, b** A 46-year-old woman with an enchondroma in the marrow of the distal medial femur. The circumscribed lesion has intermediate signal on coronal PDWI (**a**) and mostly high signal on coronal FS T2WI (**b**). The lesion is associated with thinning and slight expansion of the adjacent bone cortex.

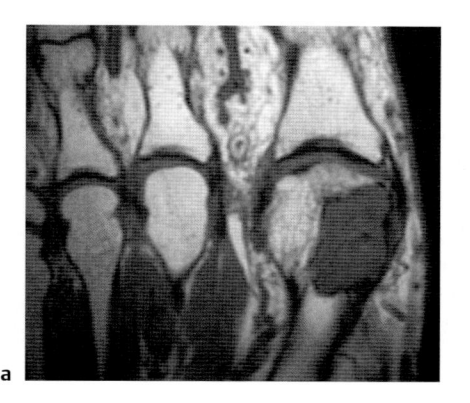

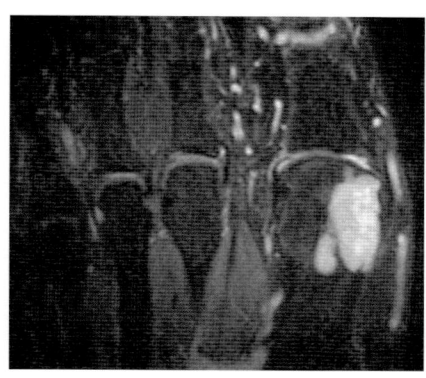

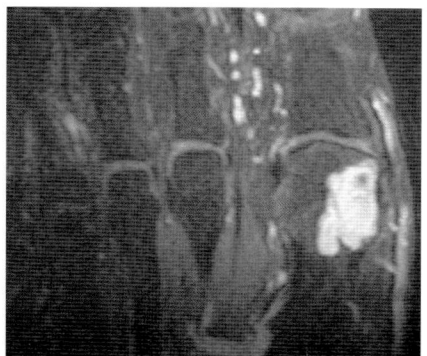

Figure 6.**9 a–c** A 34-year-old man with a chondromyxoid fibroma involving the metatarsal head. The circumscribed lesion has intermediate signal on coronal PDWI (**a**), mostly high signal on coronal FS T2WI (**b**), and shows prominent Gd-contrast enhancement on coronal FS T1WI (**c**). The lesion is associated with thinning and slight expansion of the adjacent bone cortex.

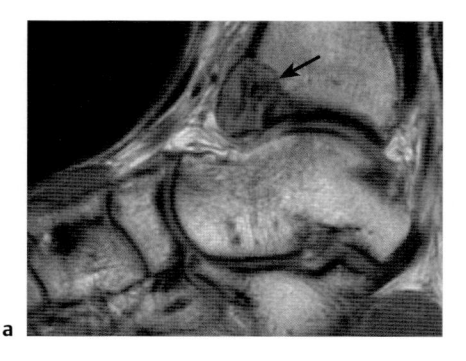

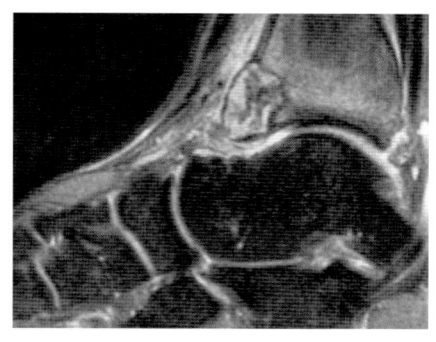

Figure 6.**10 a, b** A 24-year-old man with an osteoblastoma involving the distal tibia. The lesion has heterogeneous low and intermediate signal on sagittal T1WI (**a**) and heterogeneous signal with zones of high and low signal on sagittal FS T2WI (**b**). The tumor causes expansion and irregular thinning of the anterior margin of the distal tibia. Poorly defined zones of high signal on FS T2WI are seen in the marrow and soft tissues adjacent to the lesion.

Table 6 (Continued) Intramedullary lesions associated with expansion of intact cortical margins			
Lesion	MRI Findings	Comments
Hemangioma	Often well-circumscribed lesions that often have intermediate to high signal on T1WI, PDWI, T2WI, and FS T2WI. Hemangiomas usually show Gd-contrast enhancement (mild to prominent). Expansion of cortical margins can occasionally occur with intraosseous hemangiomas.	Benign lesions of bone and soft tissues comprised of capillary, cavernous, and/or malformed venous vessels. Considered to be a hamartomatous disorder, account for 2–4% of benign bone tumors and ~1% of all bone tumors. **(See Atlas Chapter A 34)**
Chondroblastoma (Fig. 6.11)	Tumors often have fine lobular margins, and typically have low-intermediate heterogeneous signal on T1WI, and mixed low, intermediate, and/or high signal on T2WI. Areas of low signal on T2WI are secondary to chondroid matrix mineralization, and/or hemosiderin. Lobular, marginal, or septal Gd-contrast enhancement patterns can be seen. Tumors may have thin margins of low signal on T2WI representing sclerotic borders. Bone expansion can occasionally occur. Zones with high signal on FS T2WI and Gd-contrast enhancement are seen in adjacent marrow.	Benign cartilaginous tumors with chondroblast-like cells and areas of chondroid matrix formation. Account for 5–9% of benign bone lesions and 1–3% of all primary bone tumors, patients range from 10 to 30 years, median = 17 years. **(See Atlas Chapter A 7)**
Ameloblastoma (Fig. 6.12)	Lesions are often radiolucent with associated bone expansion and cortical thinning on CT. Tumors often have circumscribed margins, and can show mixed low, intermediate, and/or high signal on T1WI, T2WI, and FS T2WI. Lesions can show heterogeneous Gd-contrast enhancement.	Ameloblastomas are slow-growing solid and cystic tumors that contain epithelioid cells (basaloid and/or squamous types) associated with regions of spindle cells and fibrous stroma. These tumors occur in the mandible and maxilla and typically lack metastatic potential.
Desmoplastic fibroma (Fig. 6.13)	Lobulated lesions with abrupt zones of transition. Lesions usually have low-intermediate signal on T1WI, intermediate signal on PDWI, heterogeneous intermediate to high signal on T2WI. Lesions may have internal or peripheral zones of low signal on T1WI and T2WI secondary to dense collagenous parts of the lesions and/or foci with high signal on T2WI from cystic zones. Thin curvilinear zones of low signal on T2WI can be seen at the margins of the lesions. Lesions show variable degrees and patterns of Gd-contrast enhancement.	Represent rare intraosseous desmoid tumors that are comprised of benign fibrous tissue with elongated or spindle-shaped cells adjacent to collagen. Account for <1% of primary bone lesions. Occur in patients 1 to 71 years, mean = 20 years, median = 34 years, peak 2nd decade. **(See Atlas Chapter A 16)**
Osteofibrous dysplasia (Fig. 6.14)	Multiple irregular intracortical zones of low-intermediate signal on T1WI, intermediate to slightly high signal on PDWI, and high signal on T2WI and FS T2WI separated by irregular zones of low signal on T1WI and T2WI, the latter representing thickened sclerotic cortical bone. The outer cortical margins can be expanded and thinned. The intracortical lesions usually show prominent Gd-contrast enhancement. Thin juxtacortical/periosteal enhancement may be seen in lesions with thinned and expanded cortical margins. Prominent diffuse high signal on T2WI and marrow enhancement are seen for lesions with acute/subacute pathologic fractures.	Osteofibrous dysplasia represents rare benign fibro-osseous bone lesions that typically involve the cortex of the tibia and/or fibula in children and adolescents. **(See Atlas Chapter A 61)**

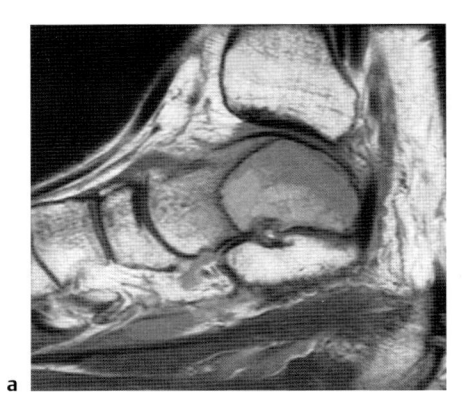

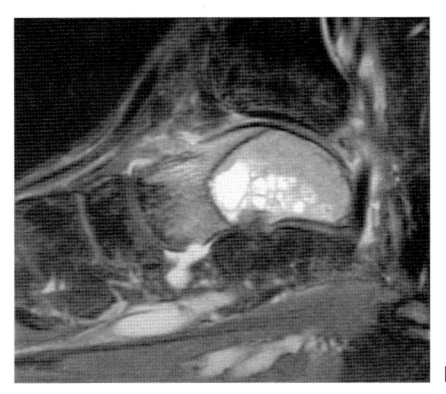

Figure 6.**11 a, b** A 20-year-old man with chondroblastoma in the talus. The lesion has a thin peripheral zone of low signal on sagittal PDWI (**a**) and sagittal FS T2WI (**b**). The lesion has low-intermediate signal on PDWI, and both zones of intermediate and high signal on FS T2WI, as well as in the adjacent marrow. Mild thinning and expansion of the cortex is seen.

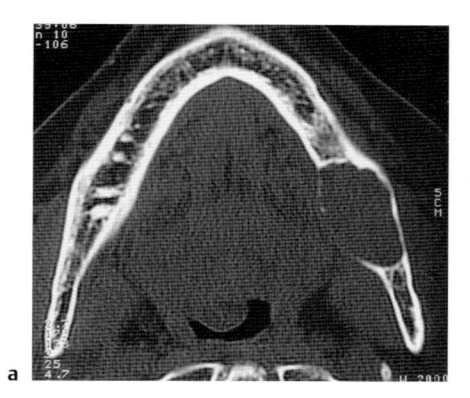

Osteofibrous dysplasia **125**

Figure 6.**12 a, b** A 70-year-old woman with ameloblastoma involving the mandible. The axial CT image (**a**) shows a radiolucent lesion with expansion and thinning of cortical bone. The lesion has mixed low, intermediate, and high signal on axial FS T2WI (**b**).

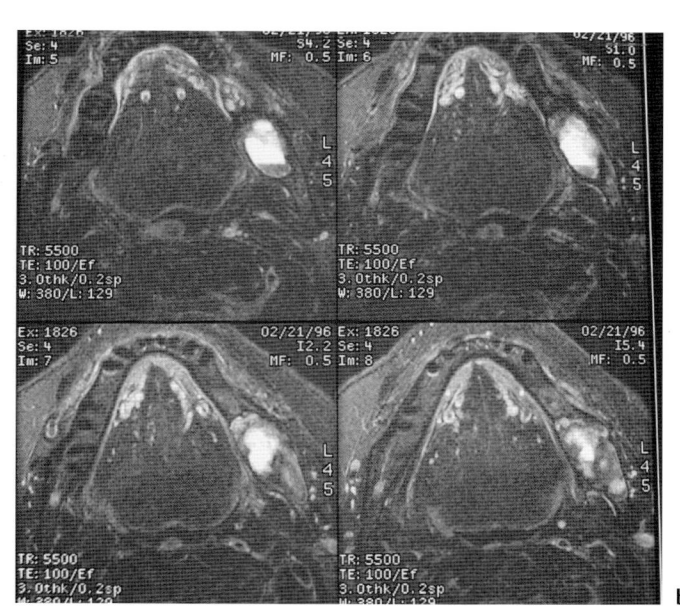

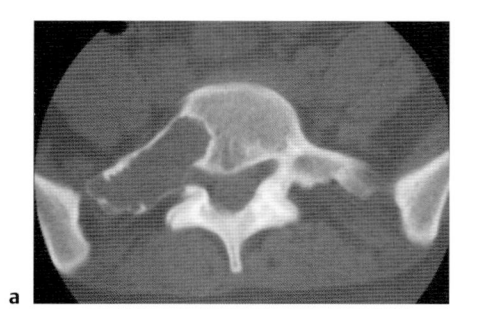

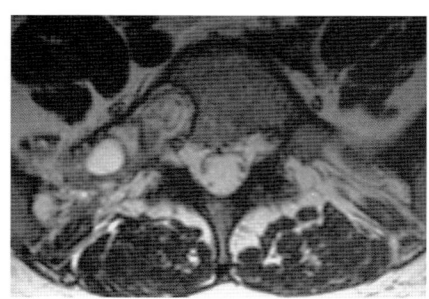

Figure 6.**13 a, b** Desmoplastic fibroma involving the L5 vertebral body, right pedicle, and transverse process. Axial CT image (**a**) shows an expansile radiolucent lesion with a thin peripheral shell of bone. The lesion has mixed signal with zones of intermediate, slightly high, high, and low signal on axial T2WI (**b**).

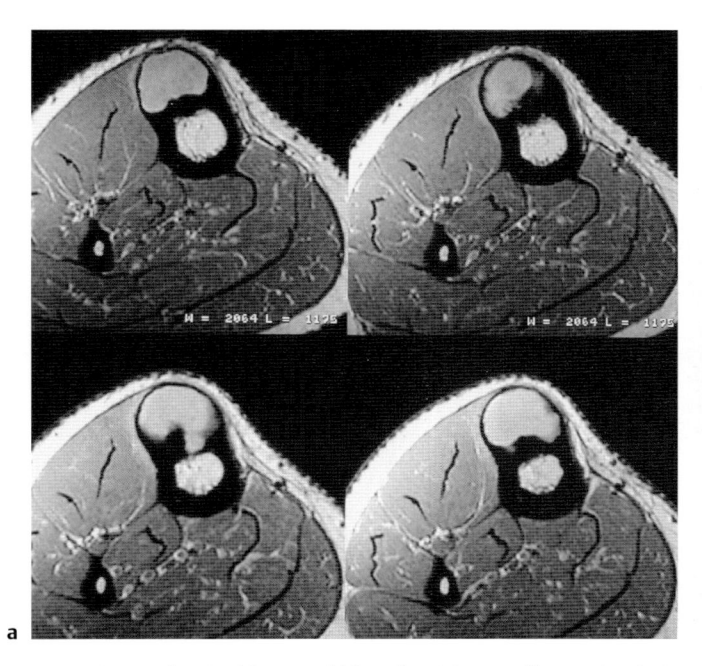

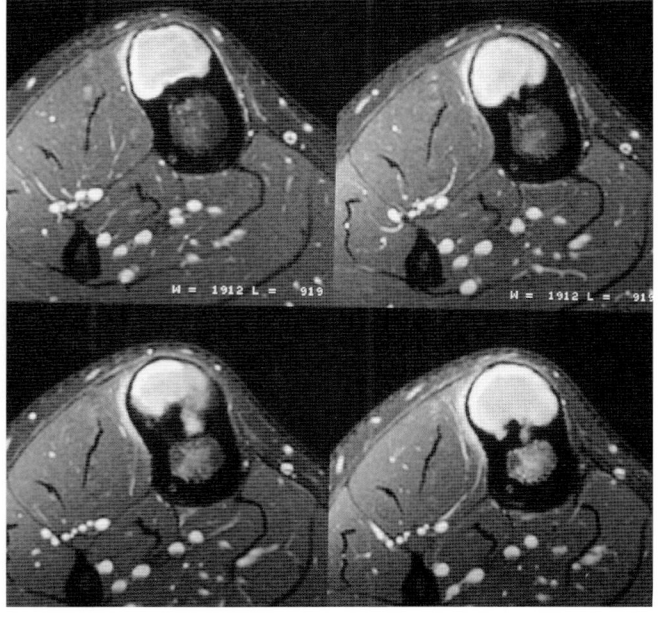

Figure 6.**14 a, b** An 18-year-old female with osteofibrous dysplasia involving the anterior tibial cortex. Intracortical intermediate to slightly high signal is seen in the lesion on axial PDWI (**a**) with corresponding prominent Gd-contrast enhancement on axial FS T1WI (**b**). The outer cortical margin is expanded and markedly thinned.

Table 6 (Continued) Intramedullary lesions associated with expansion of intact cortical margins		
Lesion	MRI Findings	Comments
Gaucher disease (Fig. 6.15)	Diffuse and/or patchy heterogeneous zones with low-intermediate signal on T1WI, and intermediate to slightly high heterogeneous signal on T2WI and FS T2WI.	Rare, heritable metabolic disorder with deficient activity of the lysosomal enzyme-hydrolase β-glucosidase. Results in accumulation of the lipid-glucosylceramide within lysosomes of the monocyte-macrophage system (Gaucher cells) of the bone marrow, liver, and spleen. Marrow infiltration by Gaucher cells often results in zones of ischemia and bone infarction.
Hemophilic pseudotumor	Can appear as expansile radiolucent lesions on radiographs and CT. Lesions usually have mixed low, intermediate, and high signal on T1WI and T2WI, as well as fluid–fluid levels.	Lesions can occur within bone (femur, pelvis, tibia, hand) or soft tissue in 1–2 % of patients with factor VIII or IX deficiency. Enlarging lesions may require surgical resection.
Malignant lesions		
Adamantinoma (Fig. 6.16)	Can appear as a solitary lobulated focus versus multinodular pattern of signal alteration in thickened bone cortex. More than half involve bone cortex and marrow compared with only cortical involvement. Bone cortex can be expanded and thinned. Tumor foci in bone typically have low–intermediate signal on T1WI and PDWI, and slightly high to high signal on T2WI and FS T2WI. Lesions usually show prominent Gd-contrast enhancement. Adamantinomas with a multinodular pattern have enhancing nodules which have high signal on T2WI and FS T2WI separated by zones of low signal from intervening cortical bone.	Rare low-grade malignant bone tumors consisting of epithelial cells surrounded by spindle cells and osteo-fibrous tissue that often involve the shaft of the tibia. Account for <1 % of primary bone tumors. Patients range in age from 3 to 86 years, median = 19 to 25 years, average = 35 years, most common in 3rd and 4th decades. **(See Atlas Chapter A 1)**
Other malignant lesions (Fig. 6.17)	Tumors may have poorly defined or sharp margins; and often have low–intermediate signal on T1WI with heterogeneous intermediate-high signal on T2WI and FS T2WI. Lesions often show prominent heterogeneous Gd-contrast enhancement.	Primary and metastatic tumors may initially show expansion of thinned intact cortical margins followed by eventual extraosseous extension of tumor through zones of cortical destruction. Hemangioendotheliomas and metastases from tumors such as renal cell carcinoma, breast, and lung carcinomas can show this pattern.

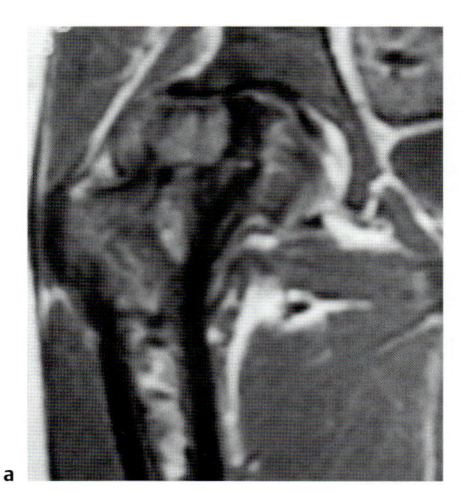

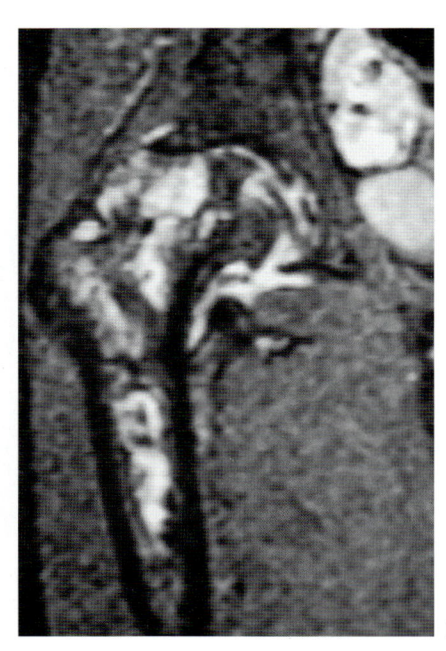

Figure 6.15 a, b A 34-year-old woman with Gaucher disease. Heterogeneous signal is seen in the marrow of the proximal femur on the coronal PDWI (a) and STIR (b), as well as trabecular disruption, and thinning and expansion of cortical bone laterally.

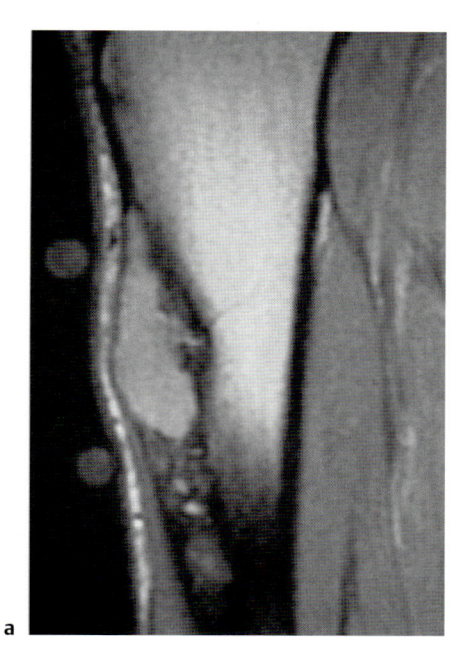

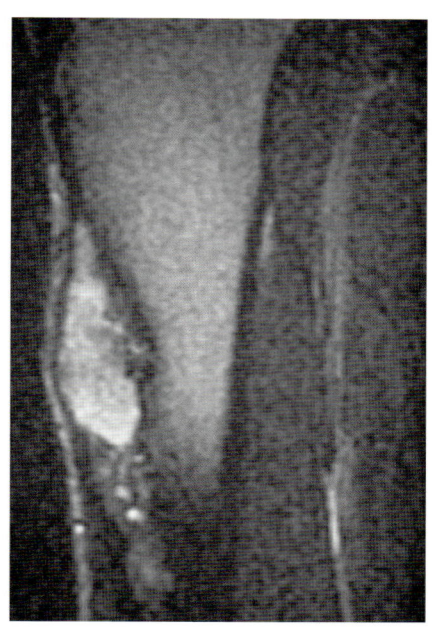

Figure 6.**16 a, b** A 23-year-old woman with an adamantinoma of the tibial diaphysis. The lesion has intermediate signal on sagittal PDWI (**a**) and high signal on sagittal T2WI (**b**). There is thinning and expansion of cortical bone as well as tumor extension toward the marrow.

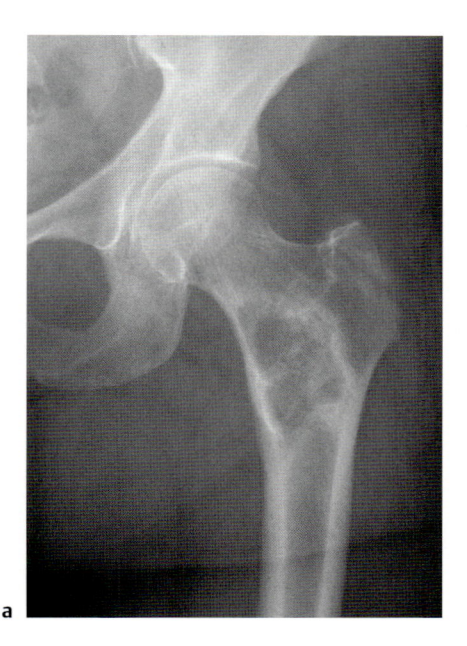

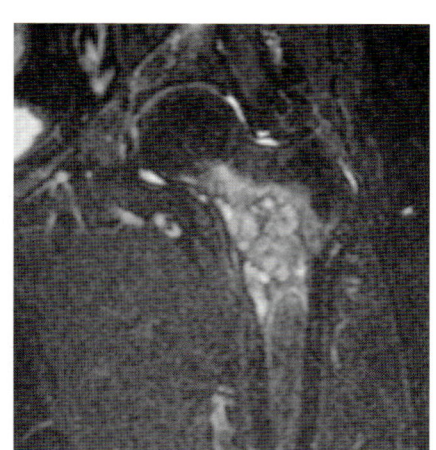

Figure 6.**17 a, b** Metastatic lesion in the proximal femur. The AP radiograph (**a**) shows a radiolucent lesion with partial sclerotic margins and cortical thinning. The coronal FS T2WI (**b**) shows the lesion to have heterogeneous high signal that extends beyond the sclerotic margins and is associated with thinning and slight expansion of bone cortex medially.

References

Ameloblastoma
Asaumi J, Hisatomi M, Yanagi Y, et al. Assessment of ameloblastomas using MRI and dynamic contrast-enhanced MRI. *Eur J Radiol* 2005; 56:25–30.

Cihangiroglu M, Akfirat M, Yildirim H. CT and MRI findings of ameloblastoma in two cases. *Neuroradiology* 2002;44:434–437.

Gaucher Disease
Maas M, Poll LW, Terk MR. Imaging and quantifying skeletal involvement in Gaucher disease. *Brit J Radiol* 2002;75 (Suppl. 1):A13–A24.

Poll LW, Koch JL, vom Dahl S, et al. Magnetic resonance imaging of bone marrow changes in Gaucher disease during enzyme replacement therapy: first German long-term results. *Skeletal Radiol* 2001;30: 496–503.

Roca M, Mota J, Alfonso P, Pocovi M, Giraldo P. S-MRI score: a simple method for assessing bone marrow in Gaucher disease. *Eur J Radiol* 2007;62:132–137.

Wenstrup RJ, Roca-Espiau M, Weinreb NJ, Bembi B. Skeletal aspects of Gaucher disease; a review. *Brit J Radiol* 2002;75(Suppl. 1):A2–A12.

Hemophilic Pseudotumor
Geyskens W, Vanhoenacker FM, Van der Zijden T, Peerlinck K. MR imaging of intra-osseous hemophilic pseudotumor: case report and review of the literature. *JBR-BTR* Nov–Dec 2004;87(6):289–293.

Jaovisidha S, Ryu KN, Hodler J, Schweitzer ME, Sartoris DJ, Resnick D. Hemophilic pseudotumor: spectrum of MR findings. *Skeletal Radiol* 1997;26:468–474.

Park JS, Ryu KN. Hemophilic pseudotumor involving the musculoskeletal system: spectrum of radiologic findings. *AJR* 2004;183:55–61.

Table 7 Intramedullary lesions associated with cortical destruction and extraosseous extension

Lesion	MRI Findings	Comments
Nonmalignant		
Osteomyelitis (Fig. 7.1)	Poorly defined zones with high signal on T2WI and FS T2WI and Gd-contrast enhancement are seen in marrow with associated zones of cortical destruction. Periosteal reaction can be seen as a peripheral rim of high signal on T2WI and FS T2WI and Gd-contrast enhancement on FS T1WI adjacent to the low signal of cortical bone. A subperiosteal abscess with high signal on T2WI and FS T2WI can often be seen elevating a single low signal thin band of periosteum.	Infection of bone which can result from hematogenous spread of microorganisms, trauma-direct inoculation, extension from adjacent tissues, and complications from surgery. *Staphylococcus aureus* and *Streptococcus pyogenes* are the most common bacterial infections involving bone. Osteomyelitis can also result from other bacteria as well as from other organisms such as tuberculosis, fungi, parasites, and viruses. **(See Atlas Chapter A 63)**
Eosinophilic granuloma (Fig. 7.2)	Focal intramedullary lesion(s) associated with trabecular and cortical bone destruction that typically have low-intermediate signal on T1WI and PDWI and heterogeneous slightly high to high signal on T2WI. Poorly defined zones of high signal on T2WI are usually seen in the marrow peripheral to the lesions secondary to inflammatory changes. Extension of lesions from the marrow into adjacent soft tissues through areas of cortical disruption are commonly seen as well as linear periosteal zones of high signal on T2WI. Lesions typically show prominent Gd-contrast enhancement in marrow and in extraosseous soft tissue portions of the lesions.	Benign tumor-like lesions consisting of Langerhans' cells (histiocytes) and variable amounts of lymphocytes, polymorphonuclear cells, and eosinophils. Account for 1% of primary bone lesions, and 8% of tumor-like lesions. Occur in patients with median age = 10 years, average = 13.5 years, peak incidence is between 5 and 10 years, 80–85% occur in patients less than 30 years. **(See Atlas Chapter A 18)**
Sarcoidosis (Fig. 7.3)	Lesions usually appear as intramedullary zones with low to intermediate signal on T1WI and slightly high to high signal on T2WI and FS PDWI and FS T2WI. Erosions and zones of destruction involving adjacent bone cortex can occur with or without extraosseous extension of the granulomatous process. After Gd-contrast administration, lesions typically show moderate to prominent enhancement.	Chronic systemic granulomatous disease of unknown etiology in which noncaseating granulomas occur in various tissues and organs including bone. **(See Atlas Chapter A 71)**

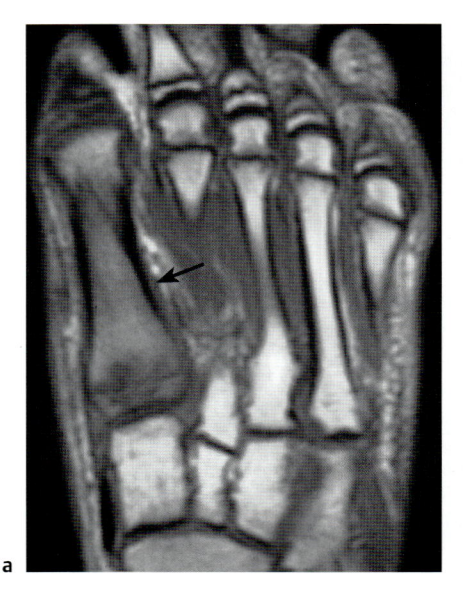

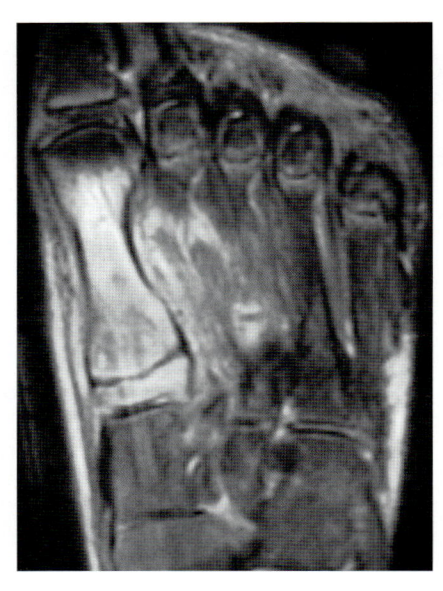

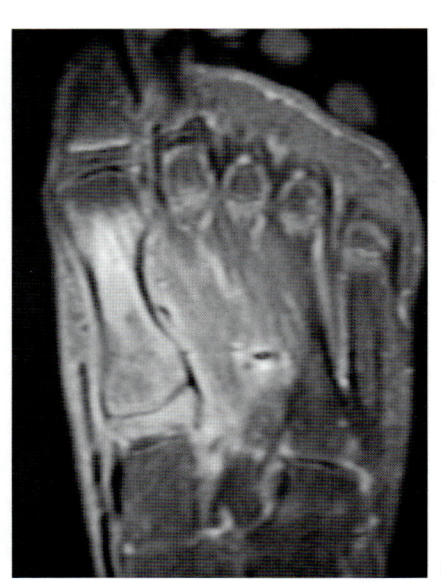

Figure 7.1 a–c A 14-year-old male with osteomyelitis involving the first metatarsal bone. Poorly defined zones of low-intermediate signal on coronal T1WI (**a**), high signal on coronal FS T2WI (**b**) and Gd-contrast enhancement on FS T1WI (**c**) are seen within the marrow as well as zones of cortical disruption and extraosseous extension.

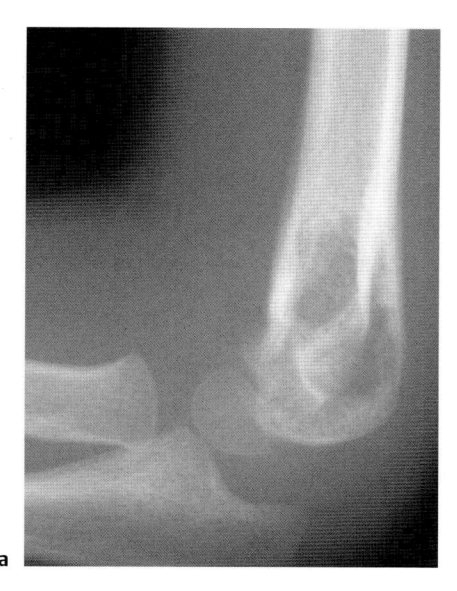

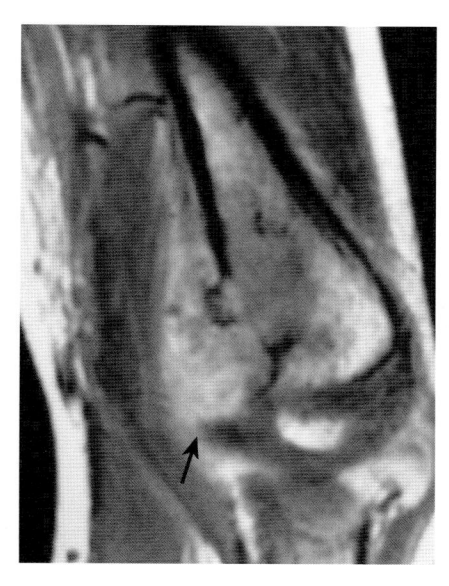

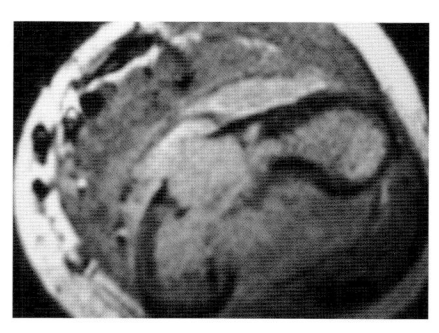

Figure 7.2 a–c A 5-year-old boy with an eosinophilic granuloma involving the distal humerus. Lateral radiograph (a) shows a radiolucent intramedullary lesion associated with a single layer of periosteal reaction. The lesion in the marrow is associated with cortical destruction and extraosseous extension into the adjacent soft tissues as seen on sagittal Gd-contrast enhanced T1WI (b) and axial (c) PDWI.

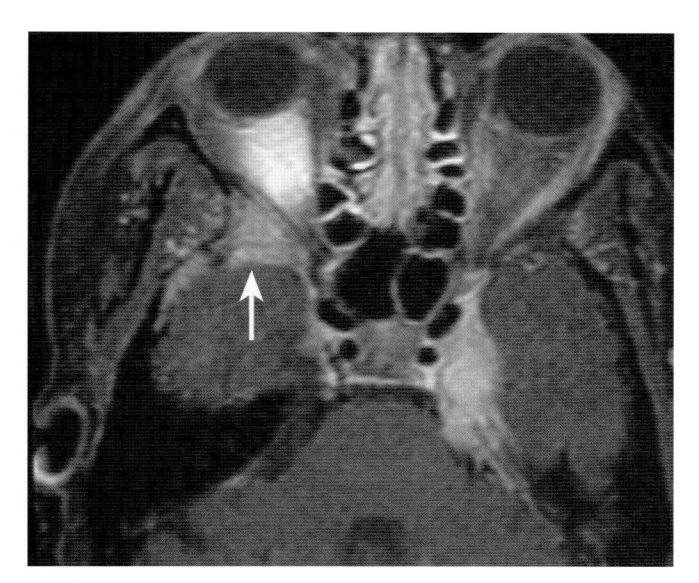

Figure 7.3 A 55-year-old woman with sarcoidosis involving the right sphenoid bone. The lesion in the marrow shows Gd-contrast enhancement as well as erosion of cortical bone and extension into the anterior portion of the right middle cranial fossa on axial FS T1WI. Also seen is abnormal subarachnoid contrast enhancement in the left trigeminal cistern surrounding the left fifth cranial nerve.

Lesion	MRI Findings	Comments
Nonmalignant giant cell tumor (Fig. 7.4)	Usually well-defined lesions with thin low signal margins on T1WI, PDWI, and T2WI. Solid portions of giant cell tumors often have low to intermediate signal on T1WI and PDWI, intermediate to high signal on T2WI, and high signal on FS PDWI and FS T2WI. Signal heterogeneity on T2WI is common. Aneurysmal bone cysts can be seen in 14% of giant cell tumors. Varying degrees of Gd-contrast enhancement can be seen in the lesions, as well as peripheral rim-like enhancement around cystic zones / aneurysmal bone cysts. Poorly defined zones of enhancement and high signal on FS T2WI may also be seen in the marrow peripheral to the lesions secondary to reactive inflammatory changes from elevated tumor prostaglandin levels.	Aggressive tumors composed of neoplastic ovoid mononuclear cells and scattered multinucleated osteoclast-like giant cells (derived from fusion of marrow mononuclear cells). Up to 10% of all giant cell tumors are malignant. Benign giant cell tumors account for ~5 to 9.5% of all bone tumors and up to 23% of benign bone tumors. Occur in patients 4 to 81 years (median = 30 years), 75% occur in patients aged between 15 and 45 years. **(See Atlas Chapter A 29)**
Sickle cell disease with adjacent extramedullary hematopoiesis (Fig. 7.5)	Lesions can have low, intermediate, and/or high signal on T1WI and T2WI depending on the proportions and distribution of fat and red marrow. Lesions may be seen extending from marrow through zones of cortical disruption, or as isolated abnormalities.	Represents proliferation of erythroid precursors outside of medullary bone secondary to physiologic compensation for abnormal medullary hematopoiesis from congenital disorders such as hemoglobinopathies (Sickle cell, Thalassemia, etc.) as well as acquired disorders such as myelofibrosis, leukemia, lymphoma, myeloma, or metastatic carcinoma.
Brown tumor	Lesions are usually radiolucent on radiographs and CT. Lesions often have low-intermediate signal on T1WI, intermediate to slightly high signal on T2WI, and typically show Gd-contrast enhancement. Zones of low signal on T2WI may occur from hemosiderin. Expansion of cortical margins can occur with or without cortical disruption/destruction.	Lesions in bone containing multinucleated giant cells, fibrous tissue, blood vessels, and zones of hemorrhage/hemosiderin. Histologic and imaging features are similar to giant cell reparative granulomas.
Atypical hemangioma (Fig. 7.6)	Rare intraosseous hemangiomas may be associated with cortical disruption and extraosseous extension. Lesions can have low-intermediate signal on T1WI, and usually have high signal on T2WI and FS T2WI. Lesions typically show prominent Gd-contrast enhancement.	Benign hamartomatous lesions of bone and soft tissues comprising capillary, cavernous, and/or malformed venous vessels. Account for 2–4% of benign bone tumors and ~1% of all bone tumors. **(See Atlas Chapter A 34)**

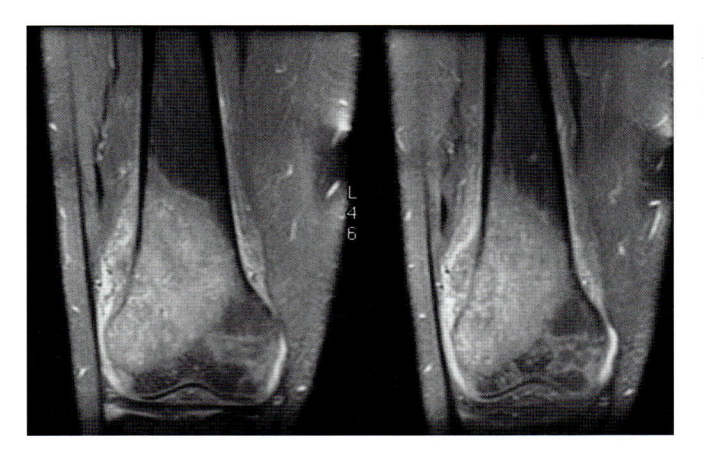

Figure 7.4 A 32-year-old woman with a giant cell tumor in the distal femur associated with cortical destruction and extraosseous extension. The tumor shows Gd-contrast enhancement on the coronal FS T1WI.

Figure 7.**5 a–d** A 56-year-old man with sickle cell disease and extramedullary hematopoiesis. The lesions have a signal comparable to the intraosseous marrow on coronal (**a**) and axial (**c**) T1WI and coronal (**b**) and axial (**d**) T2WI. Small sites of cortical disruption are seen on the axial images.

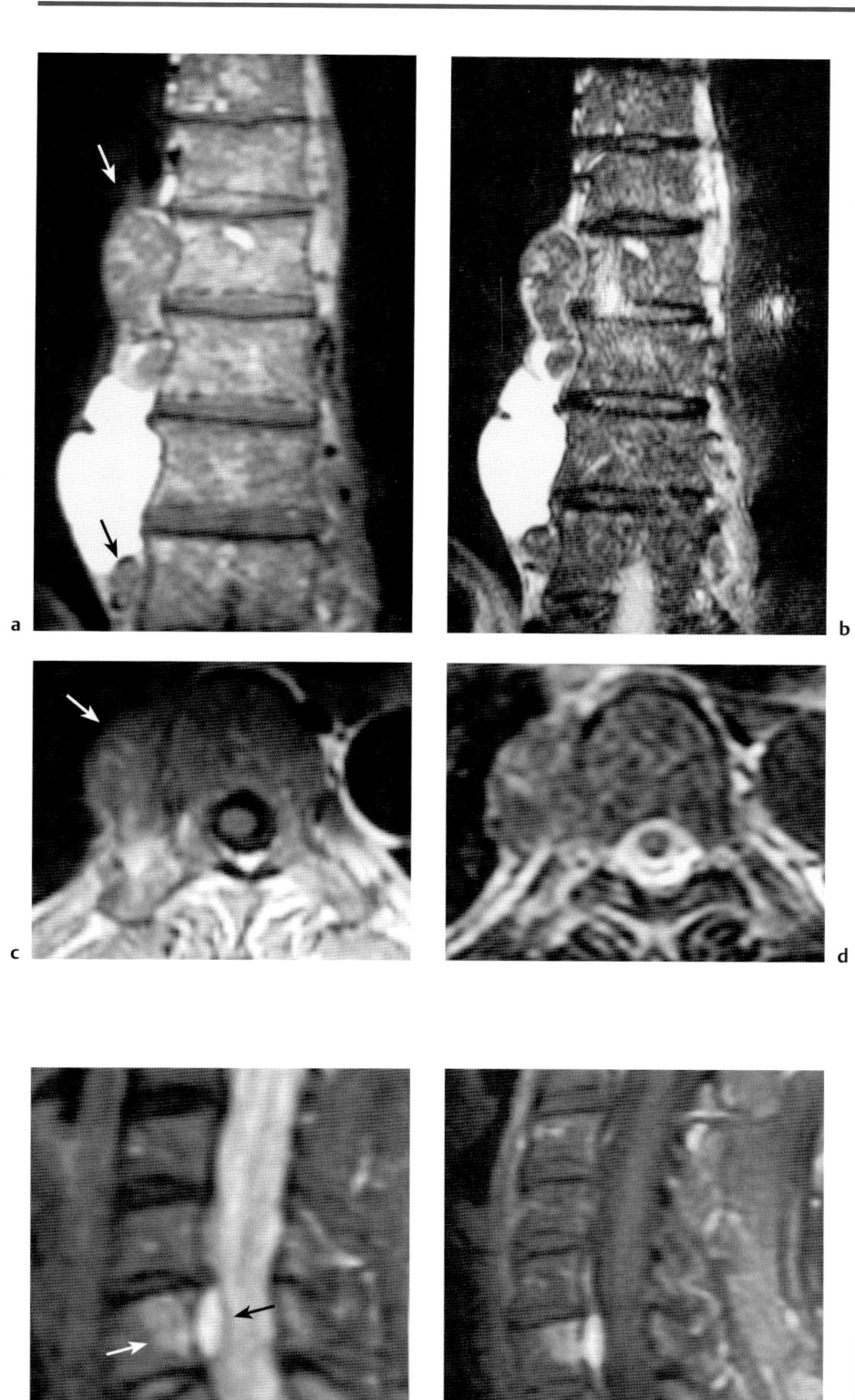

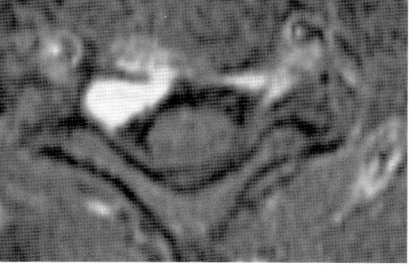

Figure 7.**6 a–c** A 43-year-old woman with an atypical hemangioma involving the posterior right marrow of the C6 vertebra associated with a zone of cortical disruption and extension into the right anterior epidural soft tissues. The lesion has high signal on the sagittal STIR image (**a**) and shows Gd-contrast enhancement on sagittal (**b**) and axial (**c**) FS T1WI.

Table 7 (Continued)   **Intramedullary lesions associated with cortical destruction and extraosseous extension**

Lesion	MRI Findings	Comments
Osteosarcoma (Fig. 7.11)	Destructive intramedullary malignant lesions, low-intermediate signal on T1WI, mixed low, intermediate, high signal on T2WI, usually with matrix mineralization/ossification, low signal on T2WI, typically show Gd-contrast enhancement (usually heterogeneous). Zones of cortical destruction are common, through which tumors extend into the extraosseous soft tissues under an elevated periosteum. Lamellated and/or spiculated zones of bone formation can occur under the periosteal elevation secondary to tumor invasion and perforation of bone cortex. Low signal from spicules of periosteal, reactive, and tumoral bone formation may have a divergent ("sunburst") pattern, perpendicular ("hair on end") pattern, or disorganized or complex appearance. Triangular zones of periosteal elevation (Codman's triangles) can be seen at the borders of zones of cortical destruction and tumor extension.	Malignant tumor comprising proliferating neoplastic spindle-cells that produce osteoid and/or immature tumoral bone, most frequently arising within medullary bone (meta-diaphyseal > metaphyseal > diaphyseal locations). Two age peaks of incidence. The larger peak occurs between the ages of 10 and 20 and accounts for over half of the cases. The second smaller peak occurs in adults over 60 years and accounts for ~10% of the cases. Occurs in children as primary tumors and adults (associated with Paget disease, irradiated bone, chronic osteomyelitis, osteoblastoma, giant cell tumor, fibrous dysplasia). **(See Atlas Chapter A 64)**
Chondrosarcoma (Fig. 7.12)	Intramedullary tumors often have low-intermediate signal on T1WI, intermediate signal on PDWI, and heterogeneous intermediate-high signal on T2WI. Lesions usually show heterogeneous contrast enhancement. Zones of cortical destruction can be seen with extraosseous extension of tumor.	Chondrosarcomas are malignant tumors containing cartilage formed within sarcomatous stroma. Account for 12–21% of malignant bone lesions, 21–26% of primary sarcomas of bone, 5–91 years, mean = 40 years, median = 26–59 years. **(See Atlas Chapter A 11)**
Ewing sarcoma (Fig. 7.13)	Destructive malignant lesions involving marrow, low-intermediate signal on T1WI, mixed low, intermediate, and/or high signal on T2WI and FS T2WI, typically show Gd-contrast enhancement (usually heterogeneous). Extraosseous tumor extension through sites of cortical destruction is commonly seen beneath an elevated periosteum. Thin striated zones of low signal on T2WI can be sometimes seen oriented perpendicular to the long axis of the involved bone under the elevated periosteum representing the "hair on end" appearance of reactive bone formation secondary to the tumor. In long bones, tumors are most often located in the diaphyseal region, followed by the meta-diaphyseal region.	Malignant primitive tumor of bone comprising of undifferentiated small cells with round nuclei. Account for 6–11% of primary malignant bone tumors, 5–7% of primary bone tumors. Usually occur between the ages of 5 and 30, males > females, locally invasive, high metastatic potential. **(See Atlas Chapter A 20)**
Chordoma (Fig. 7.14)	Tumors are often midline in location, often have lobulated or slightly lobulated margins. Lesions can involve marrow with associated destruction of trabecular and cortical bone with extraosseous extension. Chondroid chordomas are either midline or off-midline in location. Chordomas typically have low-intermediate signal on T1WI and heterogeneous predominantly high signal on T2WI. Chordomas typically enhance with Gd-DTPA, often in a heterogeneous pattern.	Rare, locally aggressive, slow-growing low to intermediate malignant tumors derived from ectopic notochordal remnants along the axial skeleton. Chordomas account for 2–4% of primary malignant bone tumors, 1–3% of all primary bone tumors; and <1% of intracranial tumors. Patients range in age from 6 to 84 years, median = 58 years. **(See Atlas Chapter A 12)**

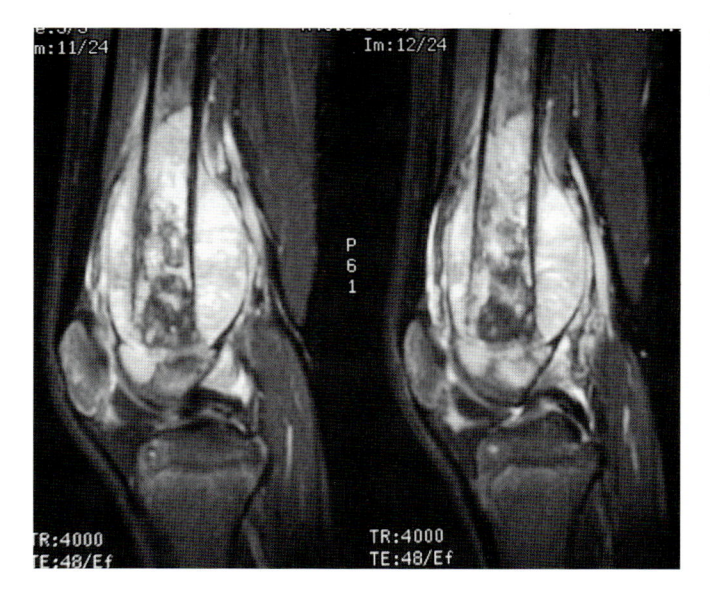

Figure 7.11 A 9-year-old girl with osteosarcoma in the distal femoral marrow associated with cortical destruction and extraosseous extension as seen on the sagittal FS T2WI.

Chordoma 135

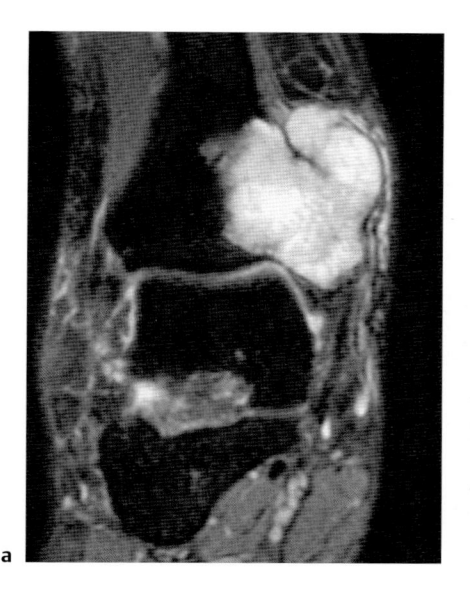

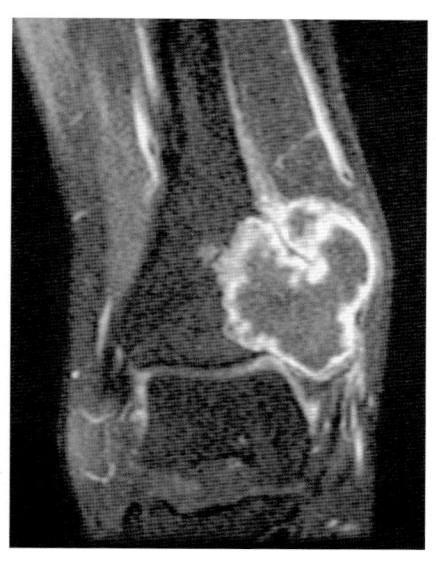

Figure 7.**12 a, b** A 44-year-old woman with a chondrosarcoma in the marrow of the distal tibia associated with cortical destruction and extraosseous extension of tumor. The tumor has high signal on the coronal FS T2WI (**a**) and shows peripheral lobular Gd-contrast enhancement on FS T1WI (**b**).

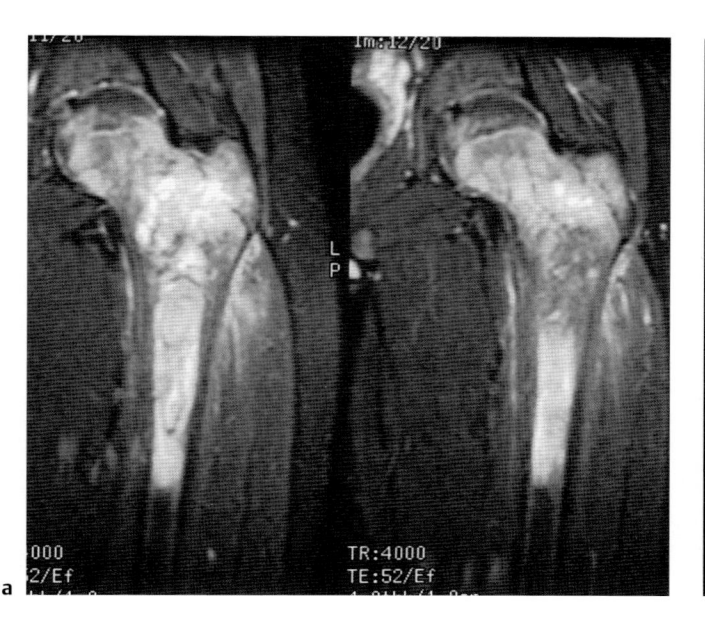

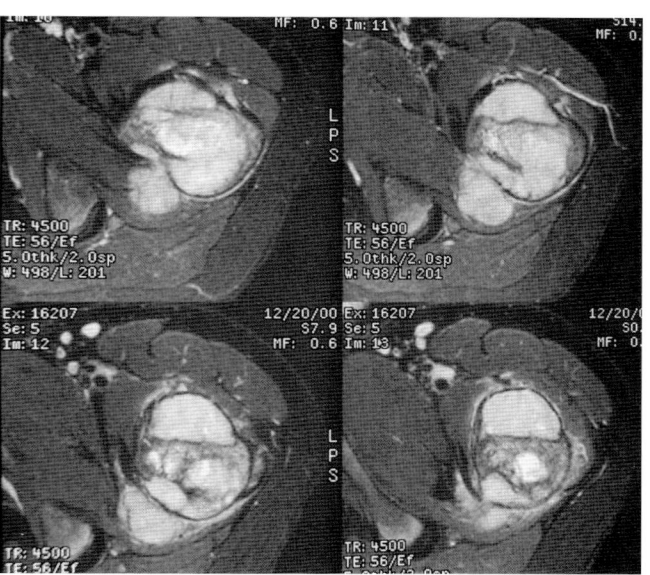

Figure 7.**13 a, b** A 15-year-old male with Ewing sarcoma in the marrow of the proximal femur associated with cortical destruction and extraosseous extension as seen on coronal (**a**) and axial (**b**) FS T2WI.

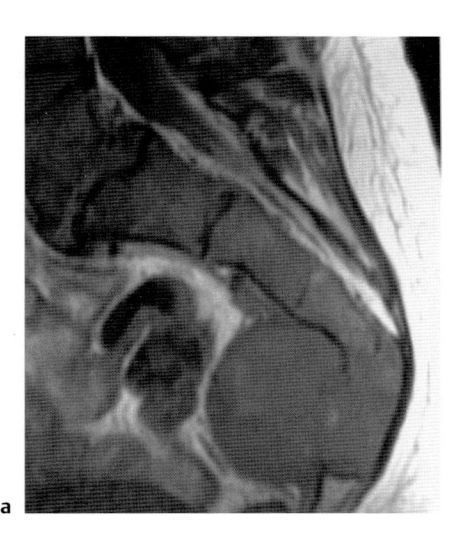

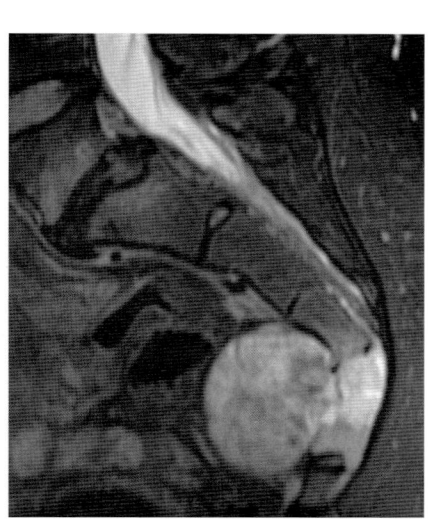

Figure 7.**14 a, b** A 30-year-old woman with a chordoma involving the lower sacrum associated with cortical bone destruction and tumor extension into the adjacent soft tissues. The tumor has mostly intermediate signal on sagittal T1WI (**a**) and heterogeneous mostly high signal on sagittal FS T2WI (**b**).

Table 7 (Continued) **Intramedullary lesions associated with cortical destruction and extraosseous extension**

Lesion	MRI Findings	Comments
Fibrosarcoma (Fig. 7.15)	Intramedullary lesions with irregular margins, with or without associated cortical destruction and/or extraosseous soft tissue masses. Lesions usually have low-intermediate signal on T1WI and PDWI, and heterogeneous intermediate, slightly high, and/or high signal on T2WI. Lesions usually show heterogeneous Gd-contrast enhancement.	Fibrosarcomas are uncommon malignant tumors consisting of bundles of fibroblasts/spindle cells with varying proportions of collagen, lacking other tissue differentiating features such as tumor bone, osteoid, or cartilage. Can be primary lesions (75%) or arise as secondary tumors (25%) associated with prior irradiation, Paget disease, bone infarct, chronic osteomyelitis, fibrous dysplasia, giant cell tumor. Account for 3–5% of primary malignant bone tumors, and 2–4% of all bone tumors, median age = 43 years. **(See Atlas Chapter A 25)**
Malignant fibrous histiocytoma (Fig. 7.16)	Intramedullary lesions with irregular margins and zones of cortical destruction and extraosseous extension. Tumors often have low-intermediate signal on T1WI; low-intermediate signal on PDWI, and heterogeneous intermediate-high signal on T2WI and FS T2WI. Invasion into joints occurs in 30%. May be associated with bone infarcts, bone cysts, chronic osteomyelitis, Paget disease, and other treated primary bone tumors. Lesions usually show heterogeneous Gd-contrast prominent enhancement.	Malignant tumor involving soft tissue and rarely bone derived from undifferentiated mesenchymal cells. Contains cells with limited cellular differentiation such as mixtures of fibroblasts, myofibroblasts, histiocyte-like cells, anaplastic giant cells, and inflammatory cells. Accounts for 1–5% of primary malignant bone tumors and <1–3% of all primary bone tumors, patient ages range from 11 to 80 years, median = 48 years, mean = 55 years. **(See Atlas Chapter A 48)**
Malignant giant cell tumor (Fig. 7.17)	Well-defined lesions with or without thin low signal margins on T1WI and T2WI. Solid portions of giant cell tumors often have low to intermediate signal on T1WI and PDWI, intermediate to high signal on T2WI, and high signal on FS PDWI and FS T2WI. Signal heterogeneity on T2WI is not uncommon. Aneurysmal bone cysts are seen with 14% of giant cell tumors. Lesions show mild to prominent variable and often heterogeneous Gd-contrast enhancement. Poorly defined zones of enhancement and high signal on FS T2WI may occasionally be seen in the adjacent marrow secondary to inflammatory reaction from elevated tumor prostaglandin levels. Cortical destruction and extraosseous tumor extension are frequently seen.	Aggressive tumors composed of neoplastic ovoid mononuclear cells and scattered multinucleated osteoclast-like giant cells. Up to 10% of all giant cell tumors are malignant. Benign giant cell tumors account for ~5 to 9.5% of all bone tumors and up to 23% of benign bone tumors. Malignant giant cell tumors account for 5.8% of all giant cell tumors. 75% occur in patients between the ages of 15 and 45. **(See Atlas Chapter A 29)**
Hemangioendothelioma (Fig. 7.18)	Intramedullary tumors usually with sharp margins that may be slightly lobulated. Lesions often have low–intermediate and/or high signal on T1WI and PDWI, and heterogeneous intermediate–high signal on T2WI and FS T2WI with or without zones of low signal. Lesions can be multifocal. Extraosseous extension of tumor through zones of cortical destruction commonly occur. Lesions often show prominent heterogeneous Gd-contrast enhancement.	Low-grade vasoformative/endothelial malignant neoplasms that are locally aggressive and rarely metastasize compared with the high-grade endothelial tumors such as angiosarcoma. Account for <1% of primary malignant bone tumors. Patients range from 10 to 82 years, median = 36 to 47 years. Patients with multifocal lesions tend to be ~10 years younger on average than those with unifocal tumors. **(See Atlas Chapter A 33)**

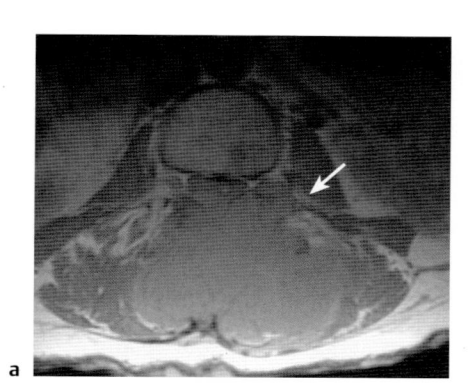

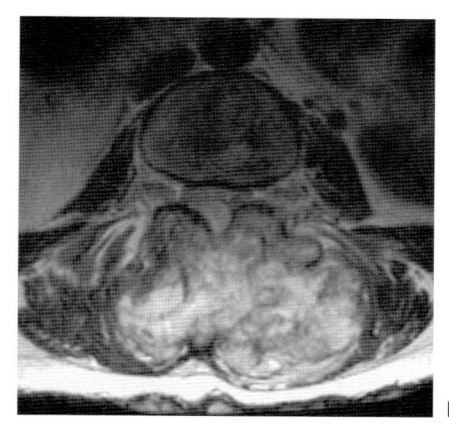

Figure 7.**15 a, b** A 25-year-old man with fibrosarcoma extending from the posterior elements of the L3 vertebra into the adjacent soft tissues through destroyed bone cortex. The tumor has intermediate signal on axial T1WI (**a**) and heterogeneous mostly high signal on axial T2WI (**b**).

Figure 7.**16** A 56-year-old man with a malignant fibrous histiocytoma extending from the posterior elements of the L3 vertebra into the adjacent soft tissues through destroyed bone cortex. The tumor involves the posterior elements of the L3 vertebra. The tumor shows heterogeneous Gd-contrast enhancement on sagittal FS T1WI.

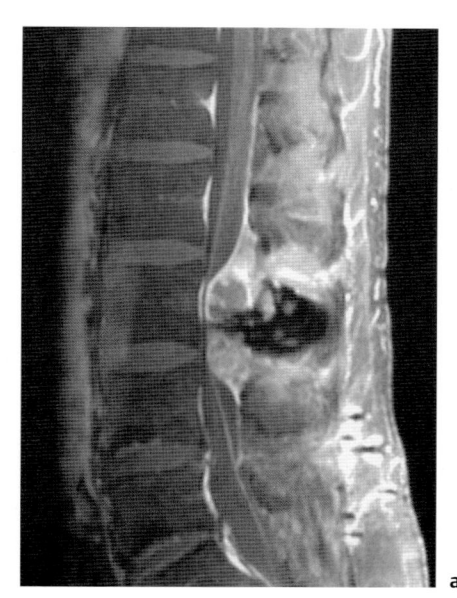

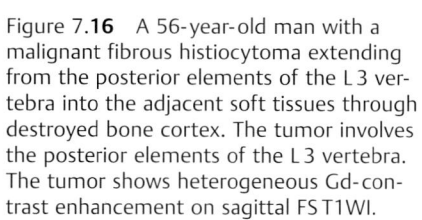

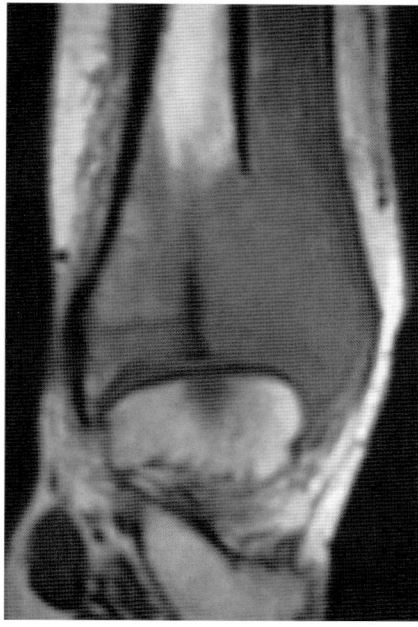

Figure 7.**17 a, b** A 16-year-old male with a malignant giant cell tumor of the distal tibia associated with destruction of cortical bone with extraosseous extension as seen on coronal T1WI (**a**) and FS T2WI (**b**).

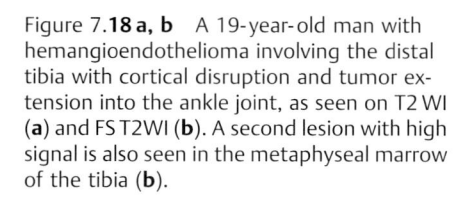

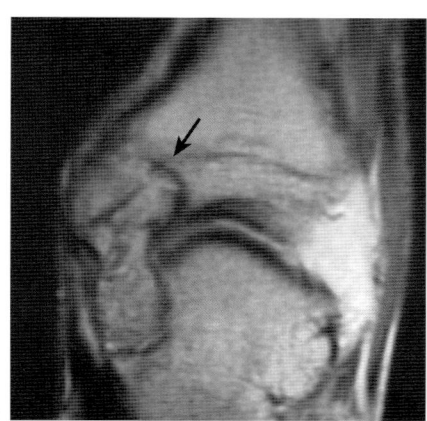

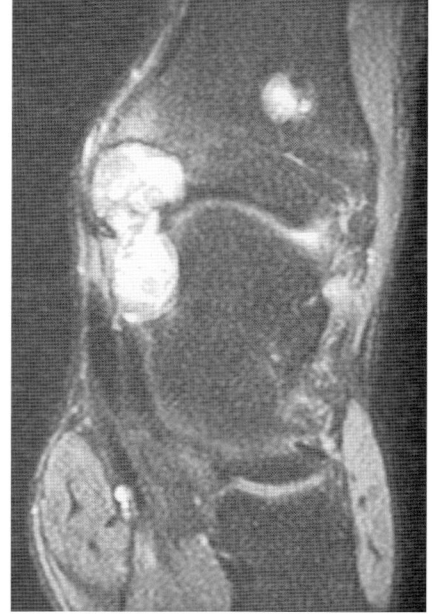

Figure 7.**18 a, b** A 19-year-old man with hemangioendothelioma involving the distal tibia with cortical disruption and tumor extension into the ankle joint, as seen on T2 WI (**a**) and FS T2WI (**b**). A second lesion with high signal is also seen in the metaphyseal marrow of the tibia (**b**).

Table 7 (Continued) **Intramedullary lesions associated with cortical destruction and extraosseous extension**

Lesion	MRI Findings	Comments
Liposarcoma (Fig. 7.19)	Tumors can have intermediate and/or slightly high to high signal on T1WI and T2WI, and show Gd-contrast enhancement.	Malignant mesenchymal tumors containing portions showing differentiation into adipose tissue. Primary liposarcoma in bone is very rare, median = 31 years. **(See Atlas Chapter A 44)**
Paget sarcoma (Fig. 7.20)	Irregular zones of medullary and cortical bone destruction associated with an extraosseous soft tissue mass lesion. The involved marrow typically has low to intermediate signal on T1WI and PDWI, and low to high signal on T2WI. Abnormal Gd-contrast enhancement is seen in the marrow as well as in the extraosseous tumor extension.	Paget disease is the most common bone disease in older adults after osteoporosis. Median age = 66 years. Disordered bone resorption and woven bone formation occurs, resulting in osseous deformity. Associated with < 1 % risk for developing secondary sarcomatous changes. **(See Atlas Chapter A 65)**

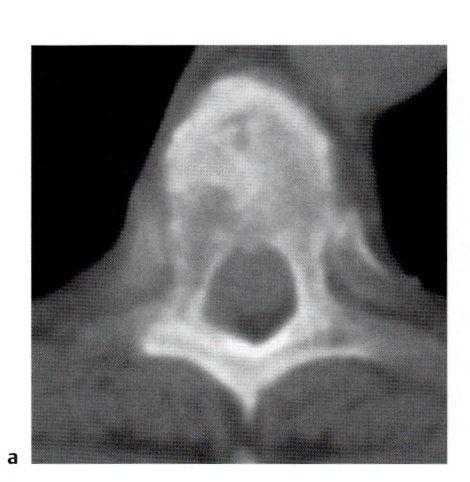

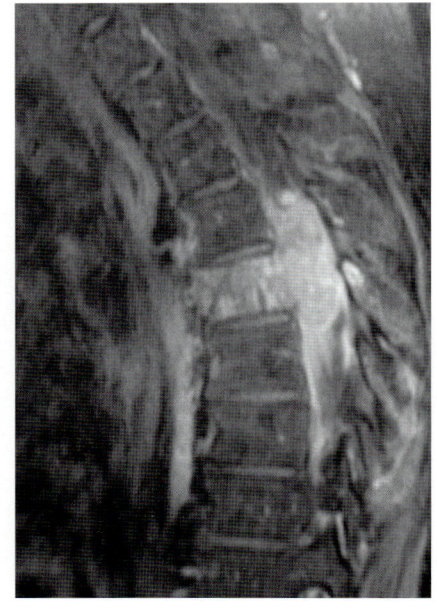

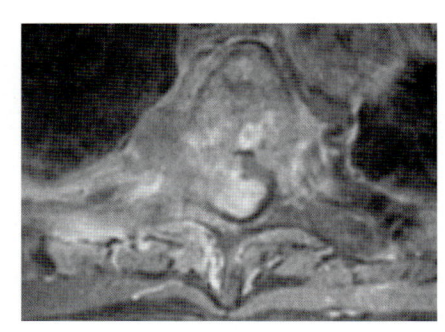

Figure 7.**19 a–c**   An 81-year-old man with an intraosseous liposarcoma involving a thoracic vertebra. Radiolucent and sclerotic changes are seen within the vertebra as well as cortical destruction on axial CT (**a**). The intraosseous tumor shows prominent Gd-contrast enhancement on sagittal (**b**) and axial (**c**) FS T1WI. Also seen is cortical destruction with extraosseous tumor extension and spinal cord compression.

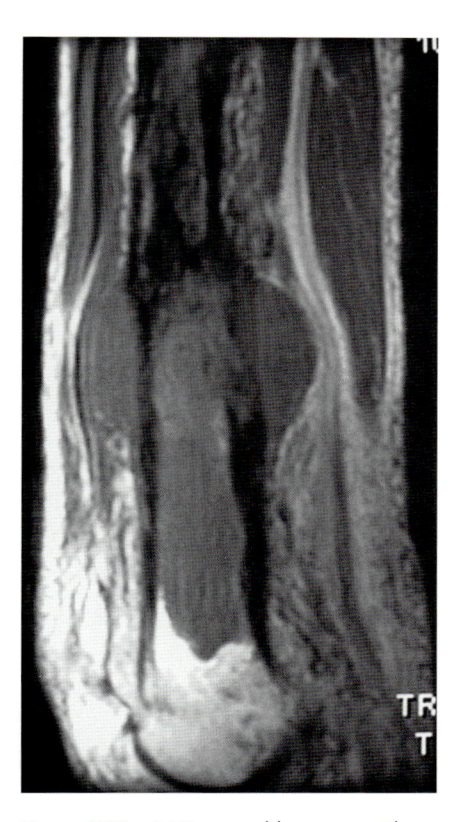

Figure 7.20 A 71-year-old woman with Paget sarcoma extending from the marrow through destroyed bone cortex into the extraosseous soft tissues as seen on sagittal T1WI.

References

Sickle Cell Disease with Extramedullary Hematopoiesis

Castelli R, Graziadei G, Karimi M, Cappellini MD. Intrathoracic masses due to extramedullary hematopoiesis. *Am J Med Sci* 2004;328: 299–303.

Collins WO, Younis RT, Garcia MT. Extramedullary hematopoiesis of the paranasal sinuses in sickle cell disease. *Otolaryngol Head Neck Surg* 2005;132:954–956.

Table 8 Solitary intramedullary lesions with well-circumscribed margins

Lesion	MRI Findings	Comments
Benign		
Hemangioma (Fig. 8.1)	Often well-circumscribed lesions which typically have intermediate to high signal on T1WI, PDWI, T2WI, and FS T2WI. On T1WI, hemangiomas usually have signal equal to or greater than adjacent normal marrow secondary to fatty components. Usually show Gd-contrast enhancement. Pathologic fractures associated with intraosseous hemangiomas usually result in low-intermediate marrow signal on T1WI.	Common benign lesions of bone comprised of capillary, cavernous, and/or malformed venous vessels. Hemangiomas have been considered to be a hamartomatous disorder. Account for 4 % of benign bone tumors and ~1 % of all bone tumors, likely underestimated. Occurs in all ages, median = 33 years. **(See Atlas Chapter A 34)**
Nonossifying fibroma (Fig. 8.2)	Well-circumscribed eccentric intramedullary lesions in the metadiaphyseal regions of long bones that have mixed low-intermediate signal on T1WI, and mixed low, intermediate, and/or high signal on T2WI, PDWI, and FS T2WI. Zones of low signal on T1WI, PDWI, and T2WI can be seen in the central portions of the lesions. Zones with varying thickness of low signal on T1WI, PDWI, and T2WI are seen at the margins of the lesions representing bone sclerosis. Internal septations are commonly seen as zones of low signal on T2WI in these lesions. Lesions can show Gd-contrast enhancement (heterogeneous > homogeneous patterns).	Common benign fibrohistiocytic lesions in the metaphyseal portions of long bones that are comprised of whorls of fibroblastic cells combined with smaller amounts of multinucleated giant cells and xanthomatous cells. Usually asymptomatic, 95 % occur between the ages of 5 and 20, median = 14 years. **(See Atlas Chapter A 26)**

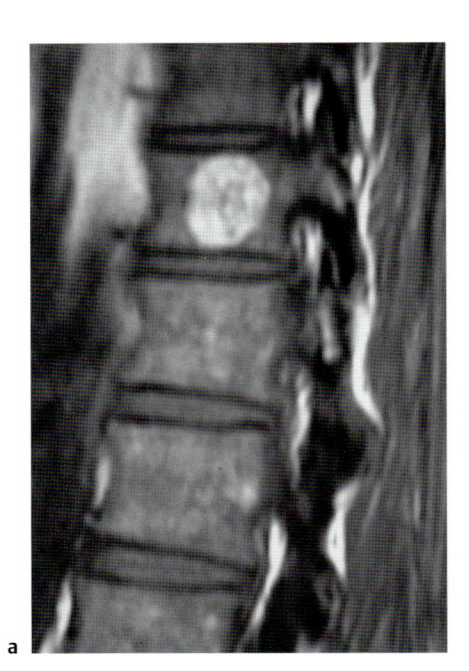

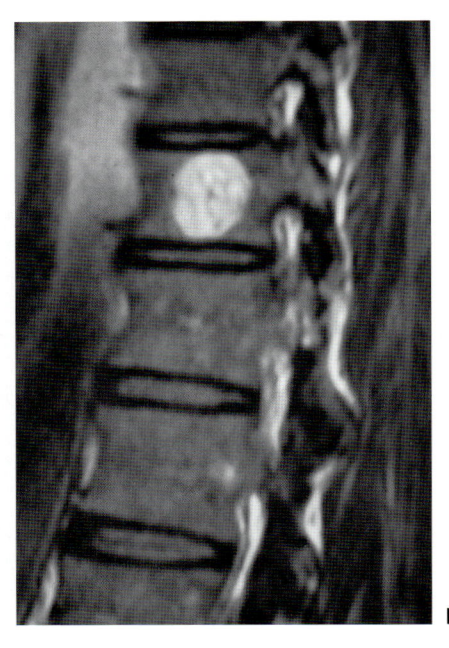

Figure 8.1 a, b Hemangioma within the T12 vertebral body has circumscribed margins and contains high signal on sagittal T1WI (**a**) and T2WI (**b**)

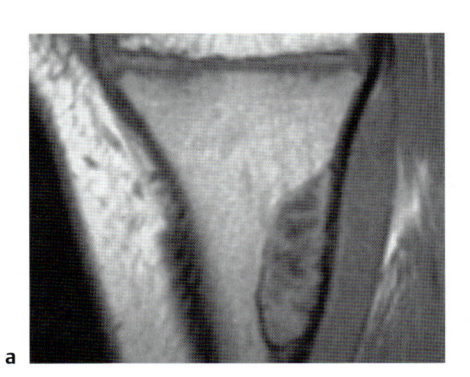

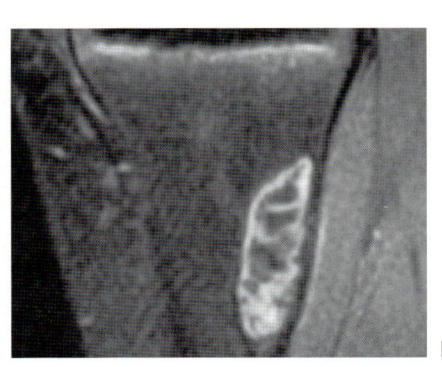

Figure 8.2 a, b Nonossifying fibroma in the dorsal proximal tibia of a 12-year-old girl has heterogeneous low and intermediate signal on sagittal T1WI (**a**) and mixed high and low signal on FS T2WI (**b**)

Table 8 (Continued) Solitary intramedullary lesions with well-circumscribed margins		
Lesion	**MRI Findings**	**Comments**
Enchondroma (Fig. 8.3)	Lobulated intramedullary lesions with well-defined borders, mean size = 5 cm. Lesions usually have low-intermediate signal on T1WI and intermediate signal on PDWI. On T2WI and FS T2WI, lesions usually have predominantly high signal with foci and/or bands of low signal representing areas of matrix mineralization and fibrous strands. Lesions typically show Gd-contrast enhancement in various patterns (peripheral curvilinear lobular, central nodular/septal and peripheral lobular, or heterogeneous diffuse).	Benign intramedullary lesions composed of hyaline cartilage, represent ~10% of benign bone tumors. Enchondromas can be solitary (88%) or multiple (12%). Median age = 35 years, peak in 3rd and 4th decades. **(See Atlas Chapter A 8)**
Fibrous dysplasia (Fig. 8.4)	MRI features depend on the proportions of bony spicules, collagen, fibroblastic spindle cells, hemorrhagic and/or cystic changes, and associated pathologic fracture if present. Lesions are usually well-circumscribed and have low or low-intermediate signal on T1WI and PDWI. On T2WI, lesions have variable mixtures of low, intermediate, and/or high signal often surrounded by a low signal rim of variable thickness. Internal septations and cystic changes are seen in a minority of lesions. Bone expansion with thickened and/or thinned cortex can be seen. Lesions show Gd-contrast enhancement that varies in degree and pattern.	Benign medullary fibro-osseous lesion that can involve a single site (**mono-ostotic**) or multiple locations (**poly-ostotic**). Thought to occur from developmental failure in the normal process of remodeling primitive bone to mature lamellar bone with resultant zone or zones of immature trabeculae within dysplastic fibrous tissue. Accounts for ~10% of benign bone lesions. Patients range in age from <1 to 76 years. 75% occur before age 30 years. **(See Atlas Chapter A 27)**

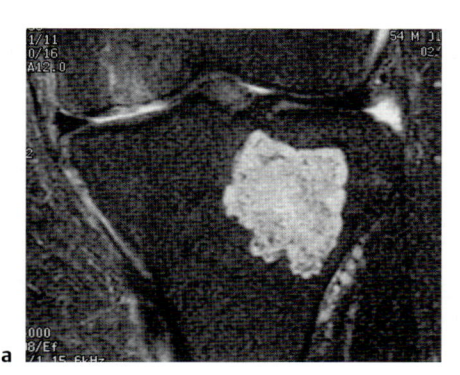

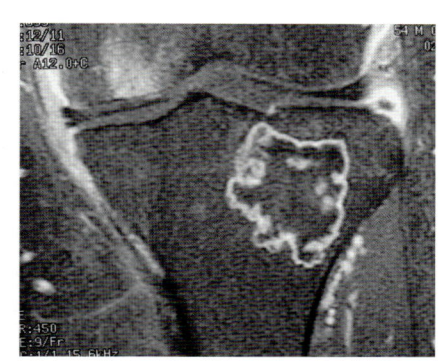

Figure 8.**3 a, b** Enchondroma in a 54-year-old man has slightly lobulated sharp margins. The lesion has high signal on coronal FS T2WI (**a**) and shows thin peripheral Gd-contrast enhancement on FS T1WI (**b**).

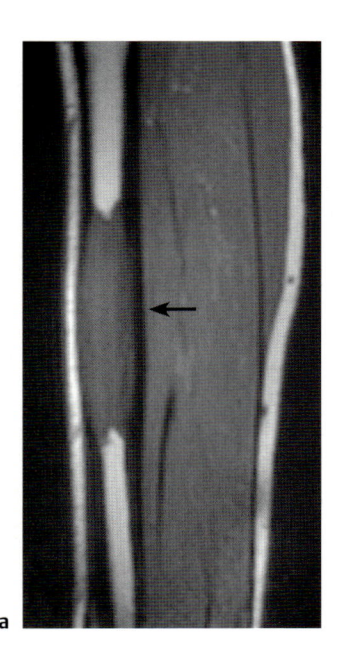

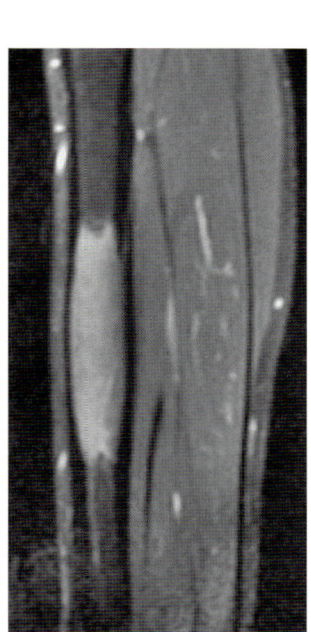

Figure 8.**4 a, b** Fibrous dysplasia in the tibial diaphysis of a 19-year-old man has intermediate signal on sagittal T1WI (**a**) and shows Gd-contrast enhancement on FS T1WI (**b**).

Table 8 (Continued) Solitary intramedullary lesions with well-circumscribed margins

Lesion	MRI Findings	Comments
Liposclerosing myxofibrous tumor (Fig. 8.5)	Lesions have well-defined margins with variable thickness of low signal borders on T1WI and T2WI. Lesions often have low to intermediate signal on T1WI, and intermediate to high signal on T2WI and FS T2WI. Small zones with fat signal may be seen at the periphery of the lesions. Lesions usually lack Gd-contrast enhancement.	Uncommon benign fibro-osseous lesions with mixed histologic features of lipoma, fibroxanthoma, myxoma, fibrous dysplasia, bone cyst, myxofibroma, fat necrosis, and/or ischemic ossification. Most of these lesions occur in the intertrochanteric region of the femur. May represent a variant form of fibrous dysplasia. Patients range from 15 to 69 years, mean = 42 years. **(See Atlas Chapter A 45)**
Unicameral bone cyst (Fig. 8.6)	Unicameral bone cysts (UBCs) often have a peripheral rim of low signal on T1WI and T2WI adjacent to normal medullary bone. UBCs usually contain fluid with low to low-intermediate signal on T1WI, low-intermediate and high signal on T2WI. Fluid–fluid levels may occur. For UBCs without pathologic fracture, thin peripheral Gd-contrast enhancement can be seen at the margins of lesions. UBCs with pathologic fracture can have heterogeneous or homogeneous low-intermediate or slightly high signal on T1WI, and heterogeneous or homogeneous high signal on T2WI and FS T2WI. UBCs complicated by fracture can have internal septations and fluid–fluid levels, as well as irregular peripheral Gd-contrast enhancement at internal septations.	Intramedullary non-neoplastic cavities filled with serous or serosanguineous fluid. Account for 9 % of primary tumor-like lesions of bone. 85 % occur in the first 2 decades, median = 11 years. **(See Atlas Chapter A 3)**
Aneurysmal bone cyst (Fig. 8.7)	ABCs often have a low signal rim on T1WI and T2WI adjacent to normal medullary bone and between extra-osseous soft tissues. Various combinations of low, intermediate, and/or high signal on T1WI, PDWI, and T2WI are usually seen within aneurysmal bone cysts as well as fluid–fluid levels. Variable Gd-contrast enhancement is seen at the margins of lesions as well as involving the internal septae.	Tumor-like expansile bone lesions containing cavernous spaces filled with blood. ABCs can be primary bone lesions (two-thirds) or secondary to other bone lesions/tumors (such as giant cell tumors, chondroblastomas, osteoblastomas, osteosarcomas, chondromyxoid fibromas, nonossifying fibromas, fibrous dysplasia, fibrosarcomas, malignant fibrous histiocytomas, and metastatic disease). Account for ~11 % of primary tumor-like lesions of bone. Patients usually range in age from 1 to 25 years, median = 14 years. **(See Atlas Chapter A 2)**
Giant cell reparative granuloma (Fig. 8.8)	Lesions can have heterogeneous low, intermediate, and/or high signal on T1WI, PDWI, and T2WI as well as peripheral rim-like and central Gd-contrast enhancement on FS T1WI.	Giant cell reparative granulomas are also referred to as solid ABCs. **(See Atlas Chapter A 2)**. Histologic appearance resembles brown tumors.

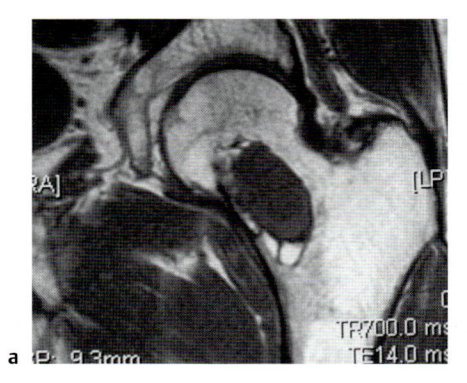

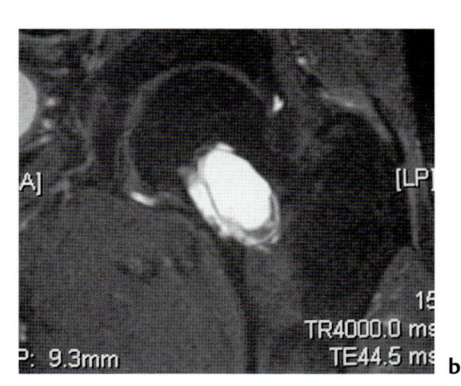

Figure 8.5 a, b Liposclerosing myxofibrous tumor in the femoral neck of a 61-year-old man. The circumscribed lesion has mostly low signal centrally as well as small peripheral zones with a high fat signal on coronal T1WI (**a**), and has mostly high signal on coronal FS T2WI (**b**).

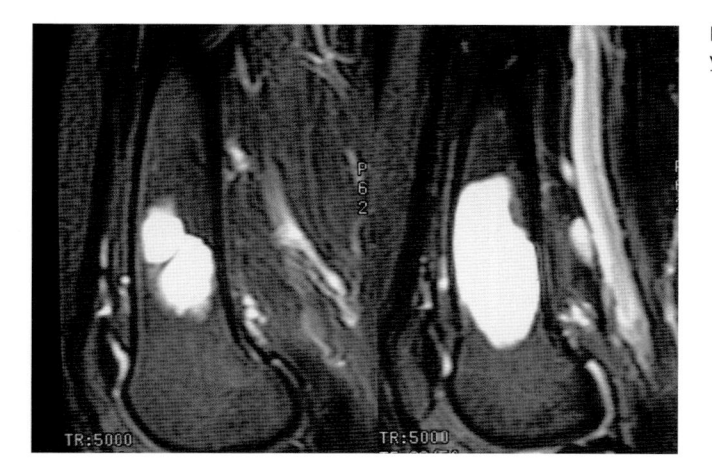

Figure 8.**6** Unicameral bone cyst in the distal femoral shaft of a 17-year-old female has high signal on sagittal FS T2WI.

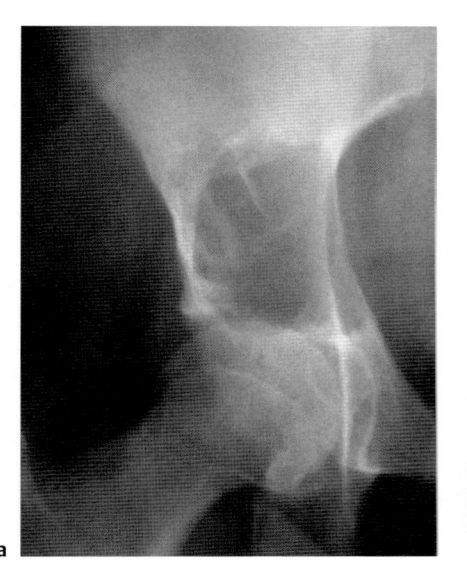

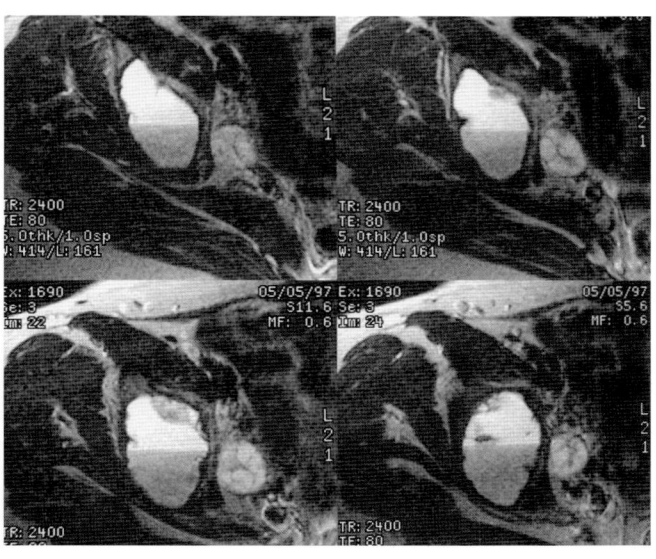

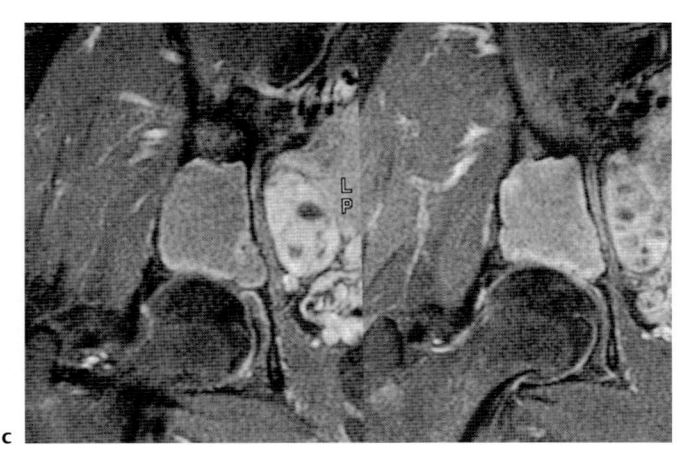

Figure 8.**7 a–c** Aneurysmal bone cyst in a 10-year-old girl is seen as a radiolucent lesion in the right iliac bone on an AP radiograph (**a**). A fluid–fluid level is seen in the lesion on axial T2WI (**b**). A thin zone of peripheral Gd-contrast enhancement is seen on coronal FS T1WI (**c**).

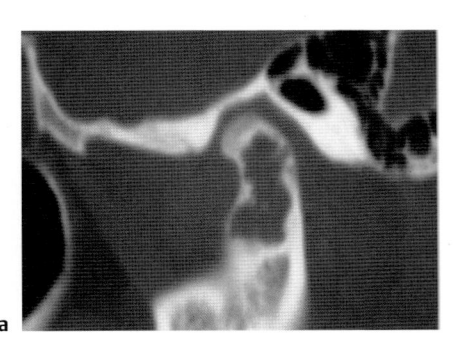

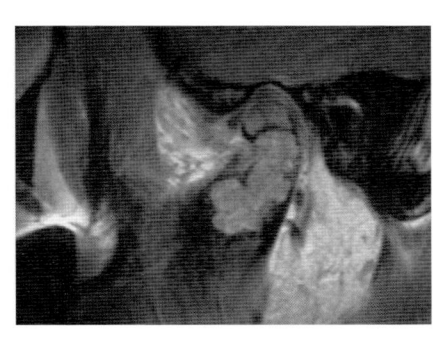

Figure 8.**8 a, b** Giant cell granuloma in a 15-year-old female is seen as a circumscribed radiolucent lesion in the mandible on the sagittal CT image (**a**) that shows Gd-contrast enhancement on sagittal T1WI (**b**).

Table 8 (Continued) **Solitary intramedullary lesions with well-circumscribed margins**

Lesion	MRI Findings	Comments
Intraosseous lipoma (Fig. 8.9)	Lesions can have heterogeneous high, intermediate, and/or low signal on T1WI, PDWI, and T2WI High signal from far is suppressed with FS T1WI, FS T2WI, and STIR. Lesions may show no Gd-contrast enhancement. Peripheral rim-like and central Gd-contrast enhancement may occur occasionally on FS T1WI. Calcifications, when present, usually appear as zones of low signal or signal void.	Uncommon benign hamartomas composed of mature white adipose tissue without cellular atypia. Osseous or chondroid metaplasia with myxoid changes can be associated with lipomas. Account for ~0.1% of bone tumors, likely underreported. (See Atlas Chapter A 43)
Brown tumor	Lesions are usually radiolucent on radiographs and CT. Lesions often have low–intermediate signal on T1WI, intermediate to slightly high signal on T2WI, and typically show Gd-contrast enhancement. Zones of low signal on T2WI may occur from hemosiderin. Expansion of cortical margins can occur with or without cortical disruption/destruction. Lesions may have circumscribed and/or poorly defined margins.	Lesions in bone contain multinucleated giant cells, fibrous tissue, blood vessels, and zones of hemorrhage/hemosiderin. Histologic and imaging features are similar to giant cell reparative granulomas. Most often involves ribs, mandible, clavicle, pelvis, craniofacial bones, and vertebrae. Can result from primary hyperparathyroidism (3–7%) (oversecretion of parathyroid hormone (PTH) from parathyroid adenoma associated with hypercalcemia), secondary type (vitamin D deficiency or chronic renal failure with hypocalcemia resulting in secretion of PTH and parathyroid gland hyperplasia) (1–2%), or tertiary type in which the secondary type leads to eventual autonomous elevated PTH secretion from parathyroid gland hyperplasia.
Geode (Fig. 8.10)	Typically have sharply defined margins and contains low signal on T1WI, low–intermediate signal on PDWI, and homogeneous high signal on T2WI. Poorly defined zones of Gd-contrast enhancement can be seen in the marrow adjacent to the subchondral cysts on FS T1WI.	A geode or subchondral cyst is a cystic lesion located near the end of a long bone where there are changes of degenerative osteoarthropathy. Lesions can result from synovial fluid intrusion and/or bony contusion in the setting of degenerative joint disease. (See Atlas Chapter A 28)
Intraosseous ganglion (Fig. 8.11)	Can have round, oval, or serpiginous configurations with sharply defined margins. These lesions typically contain low signal on T1WI, low-intermediate signal on PDWI, and high signal on T2WI.	Benign cystic lesion usually located at or near the ends of long bones, and is not associated with degenerative osteoarthropathy. Lesions can result from intraosseous extension from a ganglion in the soft tissues or from intraosseous mucoid degeneration, synovial rests, or synovial intrusion. (See Atlas Chapter A 28)
Bone infarct (Fig. 8.12)	A double-line sign (curvilinear adjacent zones of low and high signal on T2WI) is commonly seen at the edges of the infarcts representing the borders of osseous resorption and healing. Irregular Gd-contrast enhancement can be seen from granulation tissue ingrowth.	Zones of ischemic death involving bone trabeculae and marrow which may be idiopathic or result from: trauma, corticosteroid treatment, chemotherapy, radiation treatment, occlusive vascular disease, collagen vascular and other autoimmune diseases, metabolic storage diseases (Gaucher etc.), sickle cell disease, thalassemia, hyperbaric events / Caisson disease, pregnancy, alcohol abuse, pancreatitis, infections, and lymphoproliferative diseases. (See Atlas Chapter A 37)

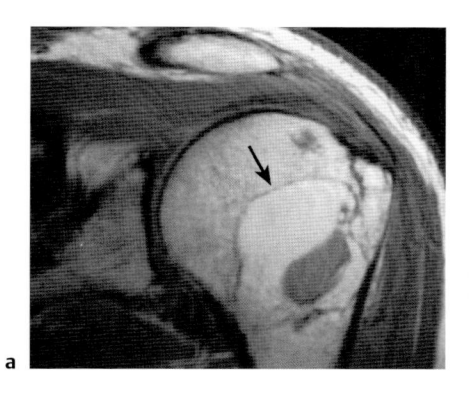

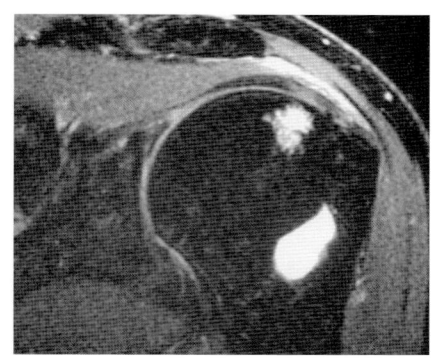

Figure 8.**9 a, b** A 62-year-old man with a lipoma in the proximal humerus. The circumscribed lesion has a thin low signal margin and a signal similar to fat on coronal PDWI (**a**) and FST2WI (**b**). A small zone of cystic degeneration is also seen within the intraosseous lipoma.

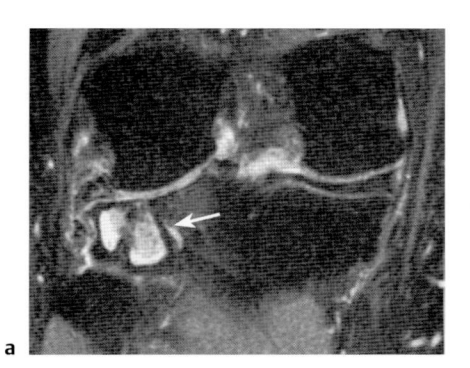

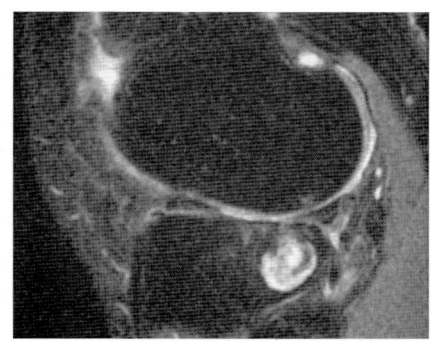

Figure 8.**10 a, b** A 50-year-old man with a degenerative cystic lesion (geode) in the subchondral bone of the lateral proximal tibia related to articular damage. The circumscribed intraosseous lesion has mostly high signal on coronal (**a**) and sagittal (**b**) FS T2WI.

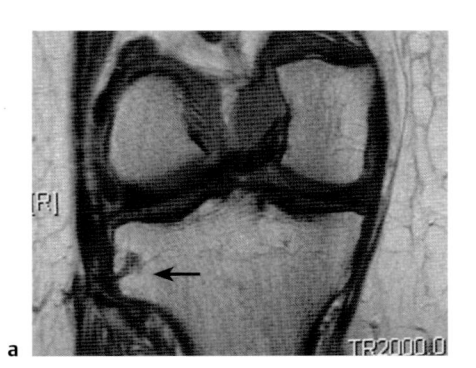

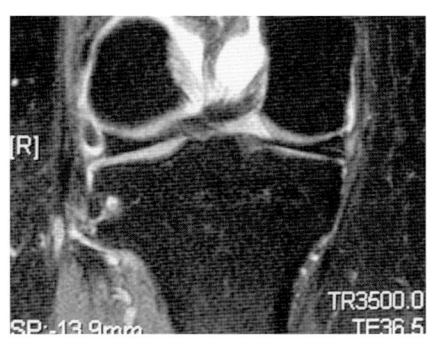

Figure 8.**11 a, b** Intraosseous ganglion within the lateral metaphyseal region of the proximal tibia seen on coronal PDWI (**a**) and coronal FS T2WI (**b**). The lesion has high signal on FS T2WI and is contiguous with an extraosseous ganglion via a small defect in the cortex.

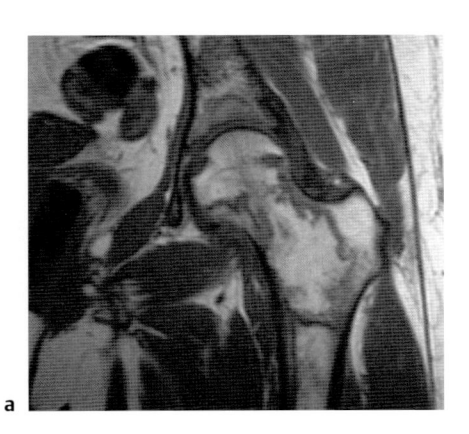

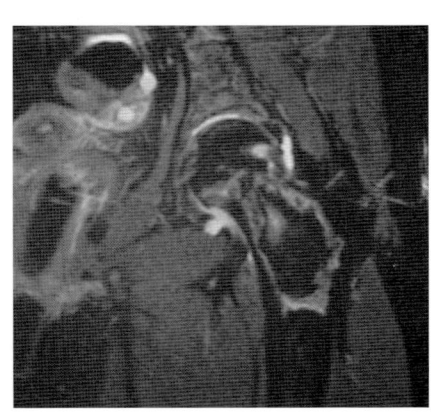

Figure 8.**12 a, b** A 29-year-old woman with a nonacute bone infarct in the femoral neck after chemotherapy for leukemia. The circumscribed lesion has thin margins with intermediate signal on coronal T1WI (**a**) and high signal on coronal FS T2WI (**b**).

Table 8 (Continued)   **Solitary intramedullary lesions with well-circumscribed margins**

Lesion	MRI Findings	Comments
Enostosis/bone island (Fig. 8.13)	Typically appear as well-circumscribed zones of dense bone within marrow with low signal on T1WI, PDWI, T2WI, and FS T2WI. Lesions typically show no Gd-contrast enhancement.	Non-neoplastic intramedullary zones of mature compact bone composed of lamellar bone, considered to be developmental anomalies resulting from localized failure of bone resorption during skeletal maturation. **(See Atlas Chapter A 62)**
Giant cell tumor (Fig. 8.14)	Often well-defined lesions with thin low signal margins on T1WI, PDWI, and T2WI. Solid portions of giant cell tumors often have low to intermediate signal on T1WI and PDWI, intermediate to high signal on T2WI, and high signal on FS PDWI and FS T2WI. Zones of low signal on T2WI may be seen secondary to hemosiderin. Aneurysmal bone cysts can be seen in 14% of giant cell tumors. Areas of cortical thinning, expansion, and/or destruction can occur with extraosseous extension. Tumors show varying degrees of Gd-contrast enhancement.	Aggressive tumors composed of neoplastic mononuclear cells and scattered multinucleated osteoclast-like giant cells. Account for 23% of primary nonmalignant bone tumors, and 5–9% of all primary bone tumors, median age = 30 years. **(See Atlas Chapter A 29)**
Ameloblastoma (Fig. 8.15)	Lesions are often radiolucent with associated bone expansion and cortical thinning on CT. Tumors often have circumscribed margins, and can show mixed low, intermediate, and/or high signal on T1WI, T2WI, and FS T2WI. Lesions can show heterogeneous Gd-contrast enhancement.	Ameloblastomas are slow-growing solid and cystic tumors that contain epithelioid cells (basaloid and/or squamous types) associated with regions of spindle cells and fibrous stroma. These tumors occur in the mandible and maxilla and typically lack metastatic potential.
Hemophilic pseudotumor	Can appear as expansile radiolucent lesions on radiographs and CT. Lesions usually have mixed low, intermediate, and high signal on T1WI and T2WI, as well as fluid–fluid levels.	Lesions can occur within bone (femur, pelvis, tibia, hand) or soft tissue in 1–2% of patients with factor VIII or IX deficiency. Enlarging lesions may require surgical resection.
Desmoplastic fibroma (Fig. 8.16)	Lobulated lesions with abrupt zones of transition. Lesions usually have low-intermediate signal on T1WI, intermediate signal on PDWI, heterogeneous intermediate to high signal on T2WI. Lesions may have internal or peripheral zones of low signal on T1WI and T2WI secondary to dense collagenous parts of the lesions and/or foci with high signal on T2WI from cystic zones. Thin curvilinear zones of low signal on T2WI can be seen at the margins of the lesions. Lesions show variable degrees and patterns of Gd-contrast enhancement.	Rare intraosseous desmoid tumors that comprise benign fibrous tissue with elongated or spindle-shaped cells adjacent to collagen. Account for <1% of primary bone lesions. Mean age = 20 years, median age = 34 years, peak 2nd decade. **(See Atlas Chapter A 16)**
Malignant		
Metastatic tumor (Fig. 8.17)	Single or multiple well-circumscribed or poorly defined infiltrative lesions involving marrow associated with cortical destruction and extraosseous extension. Lesions often have low-intermediate signal on T1WI, low, intermediate, and/or high signal on T2WI and FS T2WI, usually show Gd-contrast enhancement. Cortical destruction and tumor extension into the extraosseous soft tissues can occur. Pathologic fractures can be associated with metastatic lesions involving tubular bones and vertebrae. Periosteal reaction is uncommon.	Metastatic lesions typically occur in the marrow with or without cortical destruction and extraosseous tumor extension. **(See Atlas Chapter A 50)**

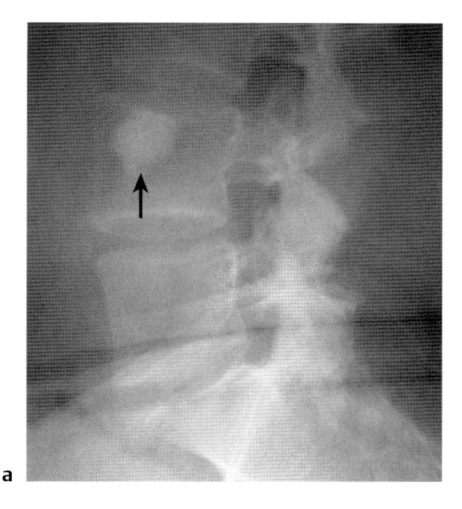

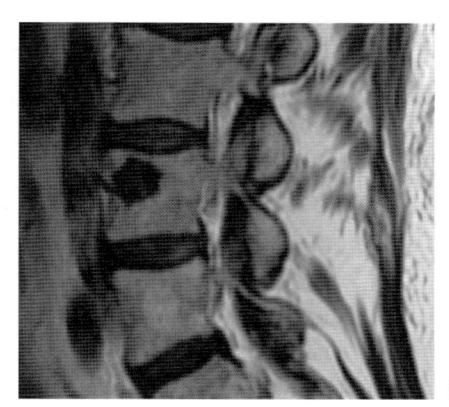

Figure 8.**13 a, b** A 70-year-old woman with a bone island in a lumbar vertebra that has high attenuation on a lateral radiograph (**a**). The circumscribed lesion has low signal on sagittal T2WI (**b**).

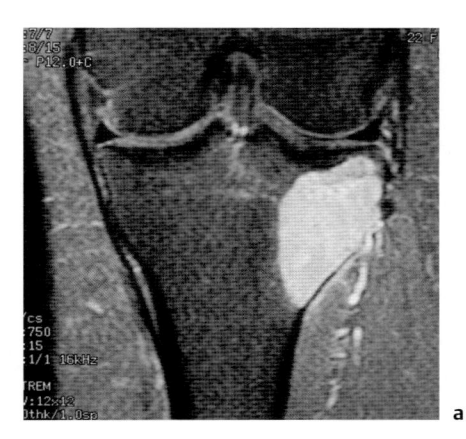

Figure 8.**14** A 22-year-old woman with a giant cell tumor in the proximal tibia that has circumscribed margins and shows Gd-contrast enhancement on coronal FS T1WI.

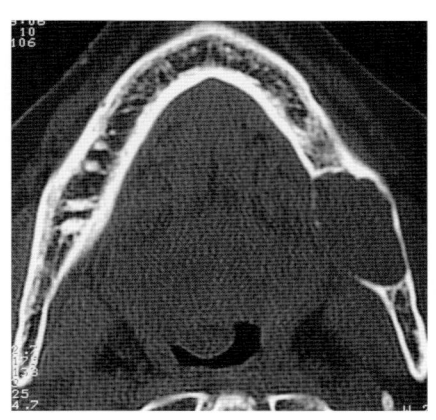

Figure 8.**15 a, b** A 70-year-old woman with an ameloblastoma in the mandible, seen as a radiolucent expansile lesion on axial CT (**a**) that has mostly high signal on axial T2WI (**b**).

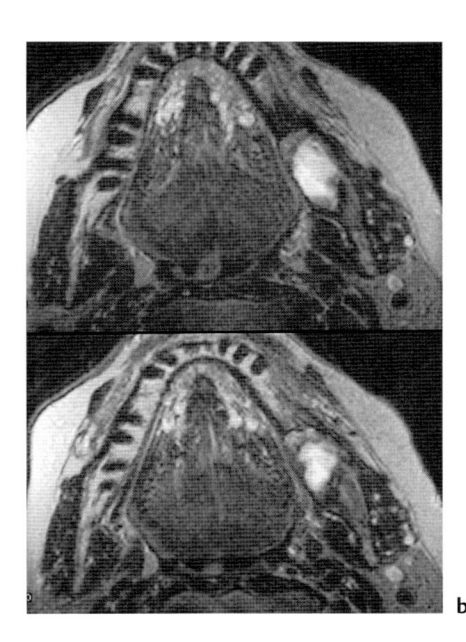

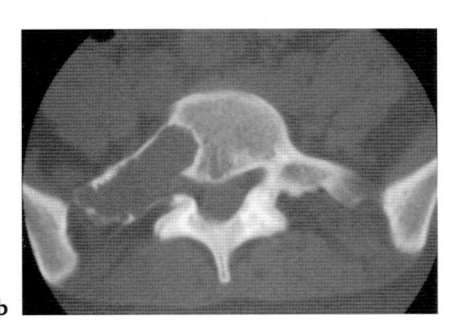

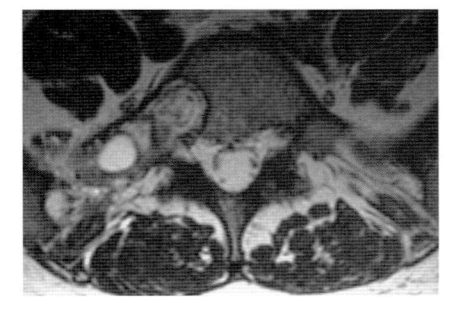

Figure 8.**16 a, b** A 32-year-old woman with a desmoplastic fibroma involving the right lateral portion of the L5 vertebra. The radiolucent lesion has thinned, slightly expanded cortical margins on axial CT (**a**) and has mixed low, intermediate, slightly high, and high signal on axial T2WI (**b**).

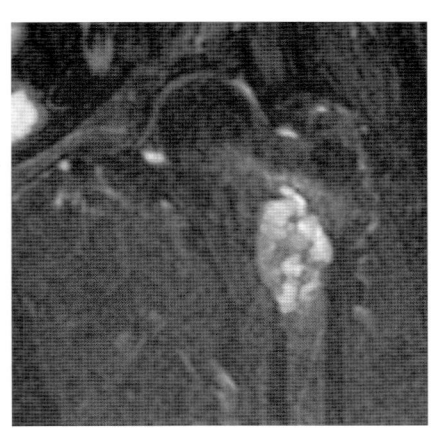

Figure 8.**17** A 56-year-old woman with a metastatic lesion from breast carcinoma involving the proximal shaft of the femur. The lesion has circumscribed margins and contains mixed intermediate and slightly high signal on coronal FS T2WI.

Table 8 (Continued) **Solitary intramedullary lesions with well-circumscribed margins**

Lesion	MRI Findings	Comments
Plasmacytoma (Fig. 8.18)	Well-circumscribed or poorly defined infiltrative lesions involving marrow, low-intermediate signal on T1WI, intermediate-high signal on T2WI and FS T2WI, usually show Gd-contrast enhancement, eventual cortical bone destruction and extraosseous extension.	Malignant tumors comprising proliferating antibody-secreting plasma cells derived from single clones. Most common primary neoplasm of bone in adults, median = 60 years. Most patients are older than 40 years. May have variable destructive or infiltrative changes involving the axial and/or appendicular skeleton. **(See Atlas Chapter A 52)**
Lymphoma (Fig. 8.19)	Non-Hodgkin lymphoma (NHL) and Hodgkin Disease (HD) within bone typically appear as single or multifocal poorly defined or circumscribed intramedullary zones with low-intermediate signal on T1WI, and intermediate, slightly high, and/or high signal on T2WI and high signal on FS T2WI; often show Gd-contrast enhancement. Zones of cortical destruction may occur, associated with extraosseous soft tissue extension.	Lymphoid tumors with neoplastic cells typically within lymphoid tissue (lymph nodes and reticuloendothelial organs). Unlike leukemia, lymphoma usually arises as discrete masses. Lymphomas are subdivided into HD and NHL. Almost all primary lymphomas of bone are B cell NHL. HD, mean age = 32 years. Osseous NHL, median = 35 years. **(See Atlas Chapter A 47)**
Low-grade chondrosarcoma (Fig. 8.20)	Intramedullary tumors often have low-intermediate signal on T1WI, intermediate signal on PDWI, and heterogeneous intermediate-high signal on T2WI. Lesions usually show heterogeneous contrast enhancement.	Malignant tumors containing cartilage formed within sarcomatous stroma. Account for 12–21% of malignant bone lesions, 21–26% of primary sarcomas of bone, mean age = 40 years, median = 26 to 59 years. **(See Atlas Chapter A 11)**
Malignant giant cell tumor	Well-defined lesions with or without thin low signal margins on T1WI and T2WI. Solid portions of giant cell tumors often have low to intermediate signal on T1WI and PDWI, intermediate to high signal on T2WI, and high signal on FS PDWI and FS T2WI. Signal heterogeneity on T2WI is not uncommon. Aneurysmal bone cysts are seen with 14% of giant cell tumors. Lesions show mild to prominent variable and often heterogeneous Gd-contrast enhancement. Cortical destruction and extraosseous tumor extension are frequently seen.	Aggressive tumors composed of neoplastic ovoid mononuclear cells and scattered multinucleated osteoclast-like giant cells. Up to 10% of all giant cell tumors are malignant. Benign giant cell tumors account for ~5 to 9.5% of all bone tumors and up to 23% of benign bone tumors. Malignant giant cell tumors account for 5.8% of all giant cell tumors. 75% occur in patients between the ages of 15 and 45. **(See Atlas Chapter A 29)**

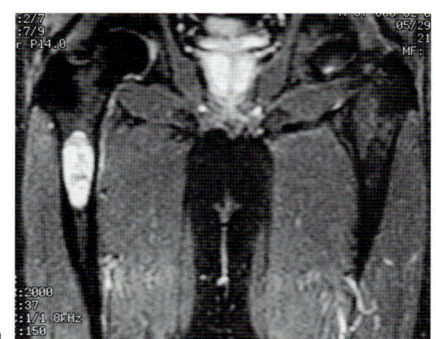

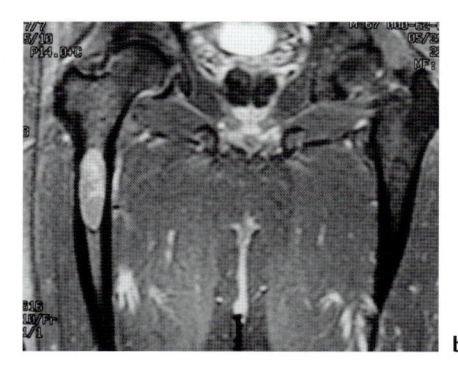

Figure 8.**18 a, b** A 67-year-old man with a plasmacytoma involving the proximal shaft of the femur that has high signal on coronal STIR (**a**). The tumor shows moderate Gd-contrast enhancement on coronal FS T1WI (**b**).

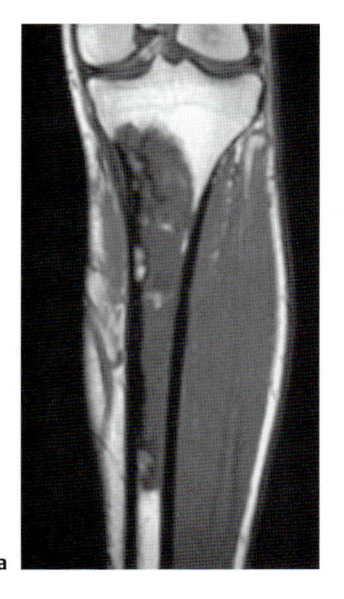

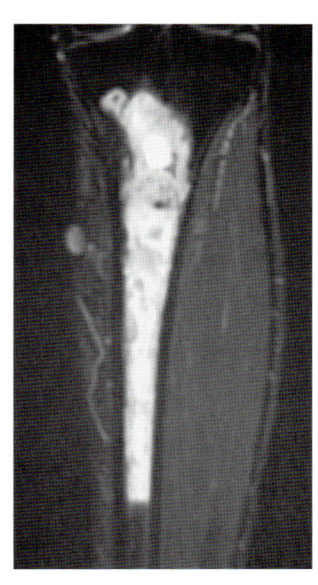

Figure 8.**19 a, b** A 19-year-old man with large cell lymphoma in the marrow of the proximal tibia that has intermediate signal on coronal T1WI (**a**) and high signal on coronal FS T2WI (**b**).

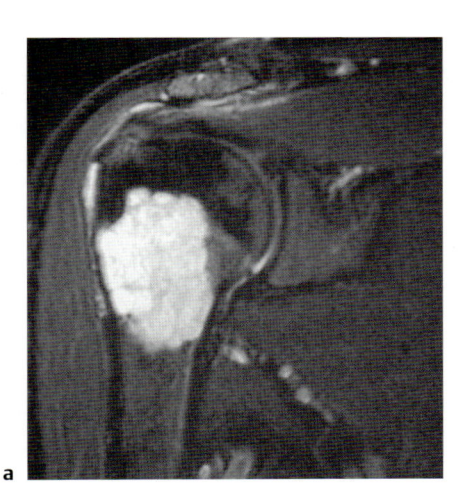

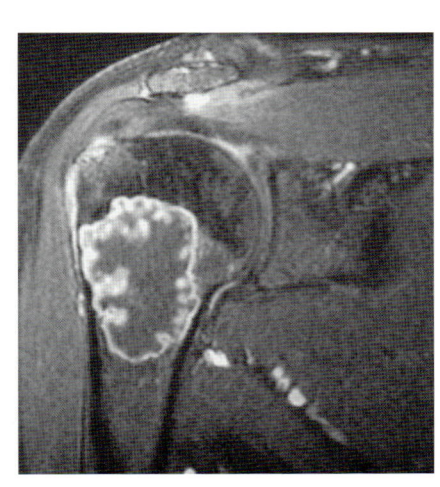

Figure 8.**20 a, b** A 45-year-old woman with a low-grade chondrosarcoma involving the proximal humerus that has high signal on coronal FS T2WI (**a**). The tumor shows peripheral lobular Gd-contrast enhancement on coronal FS T1WI (**b**).

References

Ameloblastoma
Asaumi J, Hisatomi M, Yanagi Y, et al. Assessment of ameloblastomas using MRI and dynamic contrast-enhanced MRI. *Eur J Radiol* 2005;56:25–30.

Cihangiroglu M, Akfirat M, Yildirim H. CT and MRI findings of ameloblastoma in two cases. *Neuroradiology* 2002;44:434–437.

Hemophilic Pseudotumor
Geyskens W, Vanhoenacker FM, Van der Zijden T, Peerlinck K. MR imaging of intra-osseous hemophilic pseudotumor: case report and review of the literature. *JBR-BTR* Nov–Dec 2004;87(6):289–293.

Jaovisidha S, Ryu KN, Hodler J, Schweitzer ME, Sartoris DJ, Resnick D. Hemophilic pseudotumor: spectrum of MR findings. *Skeletal Radiol* 1997;26:468–474.

Park JS, Ryu KN. Hemophilic pseudotumor involving the musculoskeletal system: spectrum of radiologic findings. *AJR* 2004;183:55–61.

Table 9 Solitary intramedullary lesions with poorly defined margins of abnormal marrow signal

Lesion	MRI Findings	Comments
Benign		
Acute and subacute bone ischemia (Figs. 9.1, 9.2)	In the early phases of ischemia, diffuse poorly defined zones of high signal may be seen on FS T2WI, which can overlap the MRI features of transient bone marrow edema. In zones of bone infarction, curvilinear zones of low signal on T1WI and T2WI may occur in marrow from zones of fibrosis. Irregular zones of low signal on T1WI and high signal on T2WI may occur secondary to zones of fluid from edema, ischemia/infarction, or fracture. Zones with high signal on T1WI and T2WI may also occur from hemorrhage in combination with zones of fibrosis and fluid. A double-line sign (curvilinear adjacent zones of low and high signal on T2WI) is often seen at the edges of the infarcts representing the borders of osseous resorption and healing. Irregular Gd-contrast enhancement can be seen from granulation tissue ingrowth.	Bone infarcts are zones of ischemic death involving bone trabeculae and marrow which be idiopathic or result from: trauma, corticosteroid treatment, chemotherapy, radiation treatment, occlusive vascular disease, collagen vascular and other autoimmune diseases, metabolic storage diseases (Gaucher etc.), sickle cell disease, thalassemia, hyperbaric events / Caisson disease, pregnancy, alcohol abuse, pancreatitis, infections, and lymphoproliferative diseases. Osteonecrosis is more common in fatty compared with hematopoietic marrow. **(See Atlas Chapter A 37)**
Transient bone marrow edema; also referred to as: acute bone marrow edema syndromes, transient osteoporosis of the hip, regional migratory osteoporosis (Fig. 9.3)	Poorly defined zones with low-intermediate signal on T1WI and high signal on FS T2WI and STIR are seen in the marrow of the proximal hip (femoral head and neck). The signal abnormalities may spare the subchondral marrow. MRI Findings can be seen within 48 hours from the onset of symptoms. Joint effusions may be present. With dynamic Gd-contrast administration, delayed peak enhancement can be seen with acute bone marrow edema (aBME). With osteonecrosis of the hip, crescentic zones of low signal on T1WI and FS T2WI are seen in the marrow between the necrotic and normal areas. These crescentic zones of low signal on T1WI and FS T2WI are typically absent in aBME.	Acute bone marrow edema (aBME) is an idiopathic spontaneous process with transient edema in bone marrow that is not secondary to trauma, and may or may not be associated with osteoporosis. aBME frequently involves the proximal femur in men between 30 and 50 years, and women in the last trimester of pregnancy. aBME is typically associated with pain and limping disability. Biopsies show active osteoblasts and osteoid seams adjacent to thinned disconnected trabeculae, as well as mild fibrosis, edematous changes, vascular congestion with occasional hemorrhage in marrow without osteonecrosis. With conservative therapy such as analgesics, restricted weight-bearing and antiresortive agents such as bisphosphonates and calcitonin; symptoms resolve in 2 to 9 months. Similar clinical and imaging findings have been reported in other bones, often in juxta-articular locations in the lower extremities, and have been referred to as regional migratory osteoporosis.
Bone contusion (Fig. 9.4)	Contusions usually appear as poorly defined intramedullary zones with low-intermediate signal on T1WI and high signal on FS T2WI, and corresponding Gd-contrast enhancement. Adjacent cortical margins are typically intact.	Also referred to as bone bruises, contusions represent trabecular microfractures without cortical fracture. In the knee, contusions at the lateral femoral condyle and posterolateral proximal tibia are commonly associated with injuries to the anterior cruciate ligament.

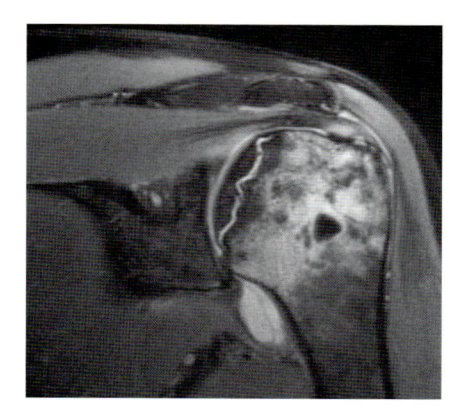

Figure 9.1 A 50-year-old woman with acute ischemia in the proximal humerus superimposed upon prior ischemia as seen on coronal FS PDWI. A poorly defined zone with increased signal is seen in the marrow adjacent to an old bone infarct at the medial aspect of the humeral head.

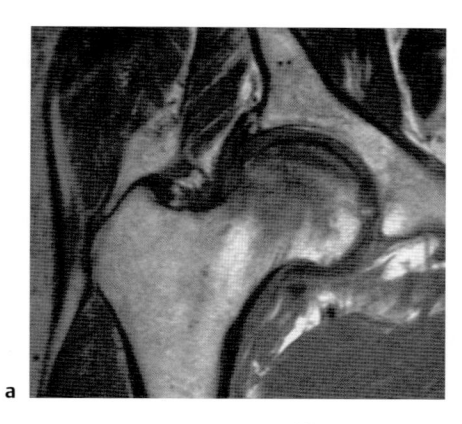

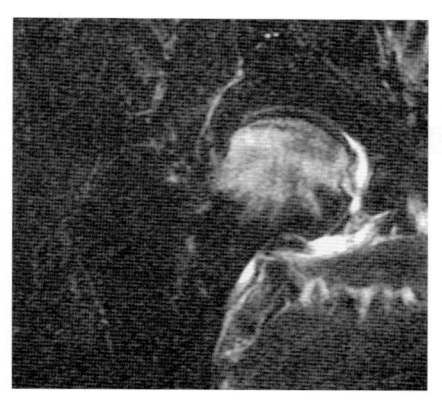

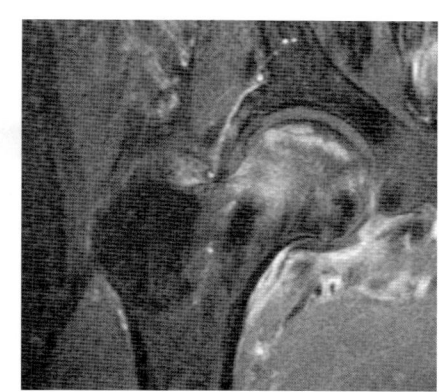

Figure 9.2 a–c A 50-year-old man with acute and subacute ischemia in the proximal femur. A poorly defined zone with low signal on coronal T1WI (**a**), high signal on coronal FS T2WI (**b**), and corresponding abnormal Gd-contrast enhancement on FS T1WI (**c**) is seen in the marrow. A thin linear zone of low signal is also seen in the subchondral marrow representing bone infarction.

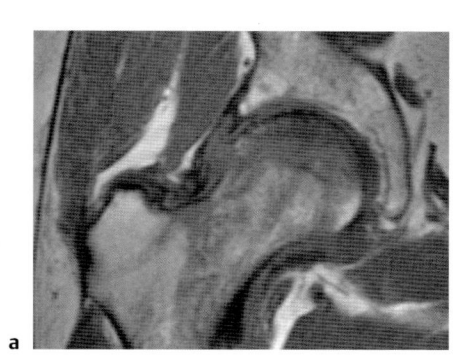

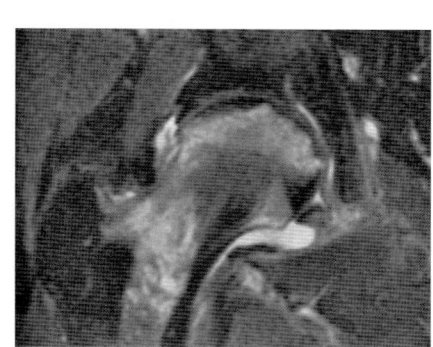

Figure 9.3 a, b A 53-year-old man with acute bone marrow edema in the proximal femur. A poorly defined zone with low-intermediate signal on coronal T1WI (**a**) and high signal on coronal FS T2WI (**b**) is seen in the marrow.

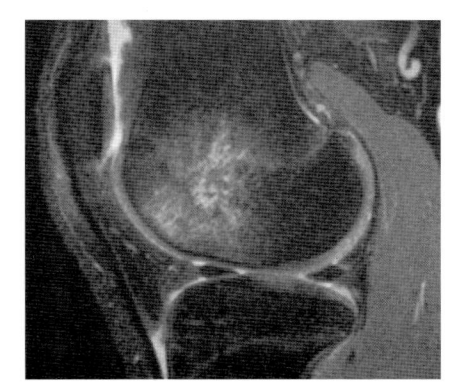

Figure 9.4 Bone contusion in the distal femur is seen as a poorly defined zone with high signal on sagittal FS T2WI.

Table 9 (Continued) Solitary intramedullary lesions with poorly defined margins of abnormal marrow signal		
Lesion	**MRI Findings**	**Comments**
Fracture (Fig. 9.5)	Acute/subacute fractures typically have abnormal marrow signal (usually low signal on T1WI, high signal on T2WI and FS T2WI). Gd-contrast enhancement is typically seen in the postfracture period. Angulated cortical margins and periosteal high signal on FS T2WI can be seen with traumatic fractures. A curvilinear zone of low signal on T2WI and FS T2WI may be seen within the marrow edema in stress fractures.	Fractures can result from trauma, primary bone tumors/lesions, metastatic disease, bone infarcts (steroids, chemotherapy, and radiation treatment), osteoporosis, osteomalacia, metabolic (calcium/phosphate) disorders, vitamin deficiencies, Paget disease, and genetic disorders (osteogenesis imperfecta, etc.)
Osteomyelitis (Fig. 9.6)	In **acute osteomyelitis**, poorly defined zones of low or low-intermediate signal on T1WI; and high signal on T2WI, STIR, and FS T2WI are seen in the marrow. Loss of definition of the low signal line of the cortical margins is often observed on T1WI, T2WI, STIR, and FS T2WI. After Gd-contrast administration, irregular zones of contrast enhancement are seen in the involved marrow on FS T1WI. In the **subacute phase of osteomyelitis**, the pyogenic process becomes more localized. The zone of transition between normal and abnormal bone is sharper and more well-defined in subacute and chronic osteomyelitis than with acute osteomyelitis.	Osteomyelitis is a disorder in which there is infection of bone and commonly the adjacent soft tissues. Can result from hematogenous spread of microorganisms as well as from trauma-direct inoculation, extension from adjacent tissues, and complications from surgery. Bacteria such as *Staphylococcus aureus* and *Streptococcus pyogenes* are the most common infectious organisms. Can also result from other bacteria as well as *Mycobacterium tuberculosis*, fungi, parasites, and viruses. **(See Atlas Chapter A 63)**
Eosinophilic granuloma (Fig. 9.7)	Focal intramedullary lesion associated with trabecular and cortical bone destruction that typically has low-intermediate signal on T1WI and PDWI and heterogeneous slightly high to high signal on T2WI. Poorly defined zones of high signal on T2WI are usually seen in the marrow peripheral to the lesions secondary to inflammatory changes. Extension of lesions from the marrow into adjacent soft tissues through areas of cortical disruption are commonly seen as well as linear periosteal zones of high signal on T2WI. Lesions typically show prominent Gd-contrast enhancement in marrow and in extraosseous soft tissue portions of the lesions.	Benign tumor-like lesions consisting of Langerhans' cells (histiocytes), and variable amounts of lymphocytes, polymorphonuclear cells, and eosinophils. Account for 1 % of primary bone lesions, and 8 % of tumor-like lesions. Occur in patients with median age = 10 years, average = 13.5 years, peak incidence is between 5 and 10 years, 80–85 % occur in patients less than 30 years. **(See Atlas Chapter A 18)**
Sarcoidosis	Lesions usually appear as intramedullary zones with low to intermediate signal on T1WI and slightly high to high signal on T2WI and FS PDWI and FS T2WI. Erosions and zones of destruction of adjacent bone cortex as well as periosseous extension of the granulomatous process can occur. Fine perpendicular lines of low signal on T1WI may be seen extending outward from the region of eroded or destroyed cortex. After Gd-contrast administration, lesions typically show moderate to prominent enhancement.	Chronic systemic granulomatous disease of unknown etiology in which noncaseating granulomas occur in various tissues and organs including bone. **(See Atlas Chapter A 71)**
Chondroblastoma (Fig. 9.8)	Tumors often have fine lobular margins, and typically have low-intermediate heterogeneous signal on T1WI, and mixed low, intermediate, and/or high signal on T2WI. Areas of low signal on T2WI are secondary to chondroid matrix mineralization, and/or hemosiderin. Lobular, marginal, or septal Gd-contrast enhancement patterns can be seen. Poorly defined zones with high signal on T2WI and FS T2WI and corresponding Gd-contrast enhancement are typically seen in the marrow adjacent to the lesions representing inflammatory reaction from prostaglandin synthesis by these tumors.	Benign cartilaginous tumors with chondroblast-like cells and areas of chondroid matrix formation, usually occur in children and adolescents, median = 17 years, mean = 16 years for lesions in long bones, mean = 28 years in other bones. Most cases are diagnosed between the ages of 5 and 25. **(See Atlas Chapter A 7)**

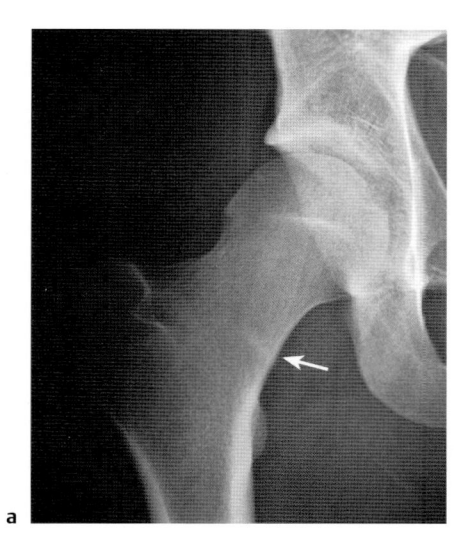

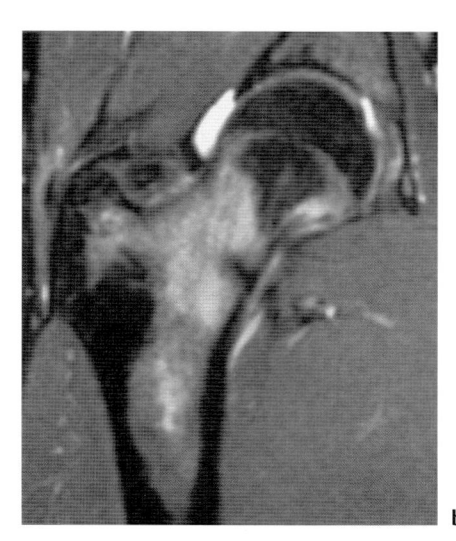

Figure 9.**5 a, b** A 17-year-old male with a fatigue-type stress fracture involving the femoral neck. The AP radiograph (**a**) shows a small linear zone of endosteal sclerosis. A poorly defined zone with high signal is seen in the marrow adjacent to a linear zone of low signal on FS T2WI (**b**), as well as thin periosteal reaction with high signal medially.

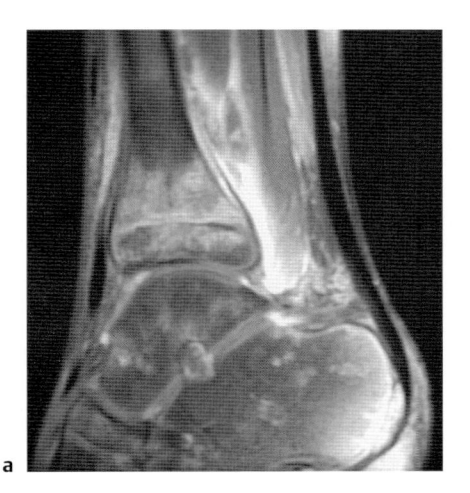

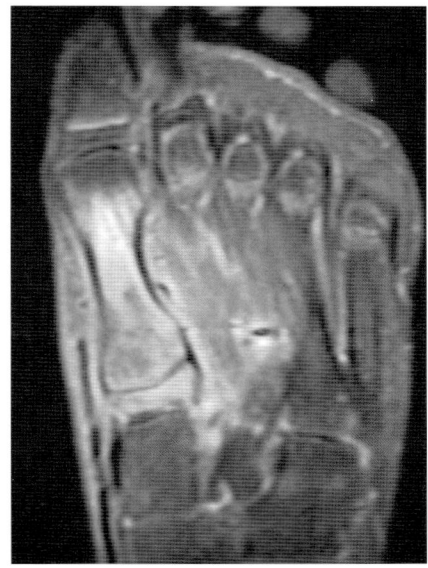

Figure 9.**6 a, b** Pyogenic osteomyelitis seen as poorly defined zones of Gd-contrast enhancement in the marrow of the distal tibia of a 9-year-old girl on FS T1WI (**a**), and involving the first metatarsal marrow of a 14-year-old boy (**b**).

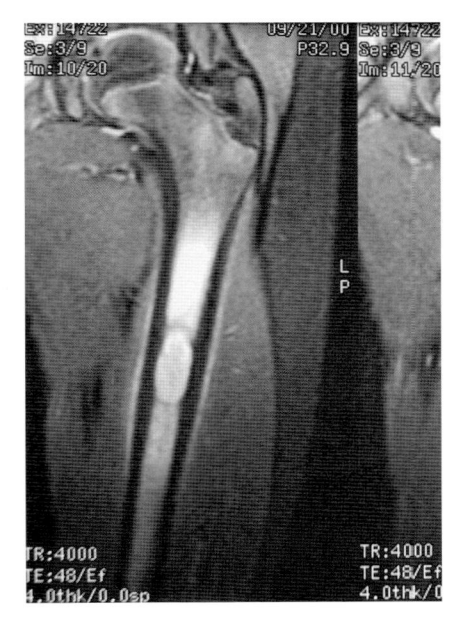

Figure 9.**7** An 18-year-old woman with an eosinophilic granuloma in the marrow of the femur seen as a poorly defined zone with high signal on coronal FS T2WI. Thin periosteal reaction with high signal is also seen.

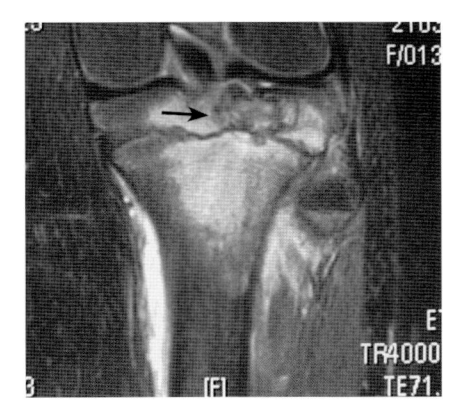

Figure 9.**8** A 13-year-old girl with a chondroblastoma in the epiphysis of the proximal tibia seen as a lesion with thin low signal margins surrounding a central zone with a low, intermediate, slightly high, and high signal on coronal FS T2WI. Poorly defined zones with high signal are seen in the epiphyseal and metaphyseal marrow peripheral to the lesion, as well as periosteal zones with high signal.

Table 9 (Continued) Solitary intramedullary lesions with poorly defined margins of abnormal marrow signal		
Lesion	**MRI Findings**	**Comments**
Giant cell tumor (Fig. 9.9)	Lesions can have thin low signal margins on T1WI, PDWI, and T2WI. Solid portions of giant cell tumors often have low to intermediate signal on T1WI and PDWI, intermediate to high signal on T2WI, and high signal on FS PDWI and FS T2WI. Zones of low signal on T2WI may be seen secondary to hemosiderin. Aneurysmal bone cysts can be seen in 14% of giant cell tumors. Areas of cortical thinning, expansion, and/or destruction can occur with extraosseous extension. Tumors show varying degrees of Gd-contrast enhancement. Poorly defined zones of Gd-contrast enhancement and high signal on FS T2WI may also be seen in the marrow peripheral to the portions of the lesions associated with radiographic evidence of bone destruction, possibly indicating reactive inflammatory and edematous changes associated with elevated tumor prostaglandin levels.	Aggressive tumors composed of neoplastic mononuclear cells and scattered multi-nucleated osteoclast-like giant cells. Account for 23% of primary nonmalignant bone tumors, and 5–9% of all primary bone tumors, median age = 30 years. **(See Atlas Chapter A 29)**
Giant cell reparative granuloma (Fig. 9.10)	Lesions can have heterogeneous low, intermediate, and/or high signal on T1WI, PDWI, and T2WI as well as peripheral rim-like and central Gd-contrast enhancement on FS T1WI. May be surrounded by poorly defined zone of high signal on FS T2WI and Gd-contrast enhancement in the adjacent marrow.	Giant cell reparative granulomas are also referred to as solid aneurysmal bone cysts (ABCs). **(See Atlas Chapter A 2)**. Histologic appearance resembles brown tumors.
Aneurysmal bone cyst (Fig. 9.11)	ABCs often have a low signal rim on T1WI and T2WI adjacent to normal medullary bone, and between extraosseous soft tissues. Various combinations of low, intermediate, and/or high signal on T1WI, PDWI, and T2WI are usually seen within ABCs as well as fluid–fluid levels. Variable Gd-contrast enhancement is seen at the margins of lesions as well as involving the internal septae. Poorly defined zones with increased signal on FS T2WI may be seen in marrow adjacent to these lesions.	Tumor-like expansile bone lesions containing cavernous spaces filled with blood. ABCs can be primary bone lesions (two-thirds) or secondary to other bone lesions/tumors. Account for ~11% of primary tumor-like lesions of bone. Patients usually range in age from 1 to 25 years, median = 14 years. **(See Atlas Chapter A 2)**
Osteoid osteoma (Fig. 9.12)	Intraosseous circumscribed lesions often < 1.5 cm in diameter central zone with low-intermediate signal on T1WI and high signal on T2WI and FS T2WI with prominent Gd-contrast enhancement, surrounded by a peripheral rim of low-intermediate signal on T1WI and T2WI (sclerosis). Lesions usually have poorly defined zones with high signal on T2WI and FS T2WI and Gd-contrast enhancement in the marrow (edema, inflammation) beyond zone of sclerosis or in adjacent soft tissues from prostaglandin synthesis by these lesions.	Benign osseous lesion containing a nidus of vascularized osteoid trabeculae surrounded by osteoblastic sclerosis, usually occurs between ages 5 and 25, males > females. Focal pain and tenderness associated with lesion, often worse at night, relieved with aspirin. **(See Atlas Chapter A 60)**

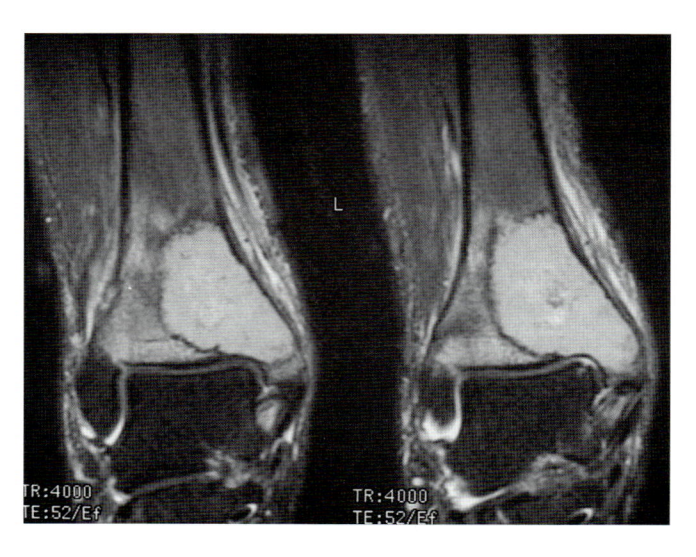

Figure 9.9 A 61-year-old man with a giant cell tumor in the distal medial tibia which has high signal centrally on coronal FS T2WI surrounded by a thin rim of low signal, and a poorly defined peripheral zone of high signal in the marrow.

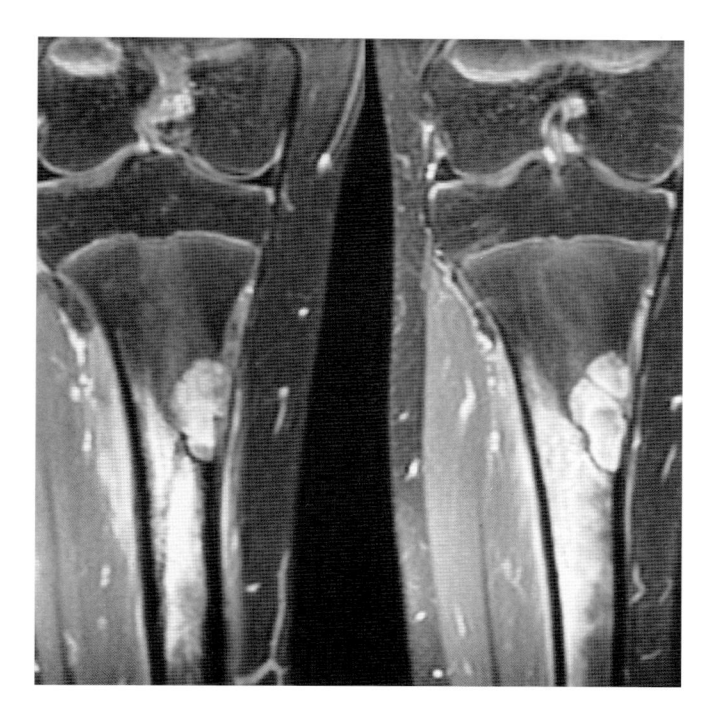

Figure 9.**10** A 14-year-old girl with a giant cell granuloma (solid aneurysmal bone cyst) involving the proximal metadiaphyseal region of the tibia. The lesion shows peripheral rim-like and central Gd-contrast enhancement as well as in the adjacent marrow on coronal FS T1WI.

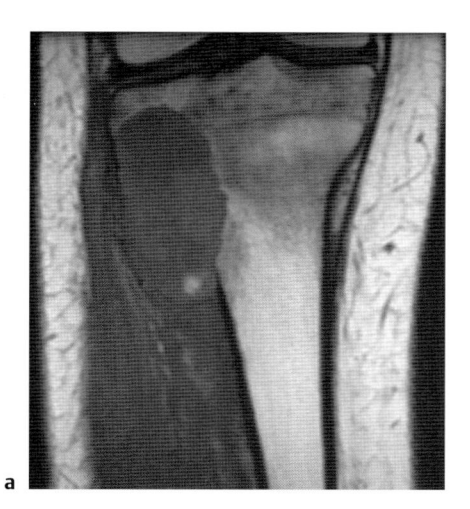

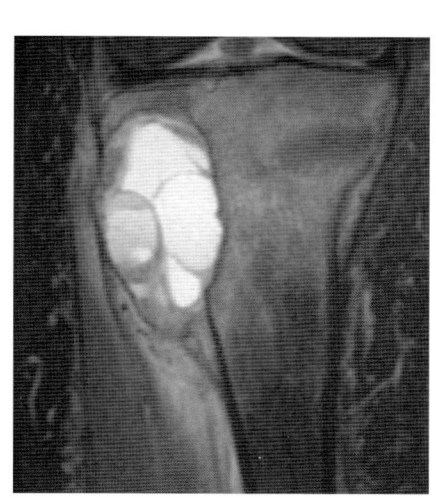

Figure 9.**11 a, b** A 14-year-old girl with an aneurysmal bone cyst in the proximal tibia that has low to intermediate signal as well as a small focus of high signal on coronal T1WI (**a**). The lesion contains multiple fluid-fluid levels on coronal FS T2WI (**b**). Poorly defined zones with increased signal on FS T2WI are also seen in the adjacent marrow.

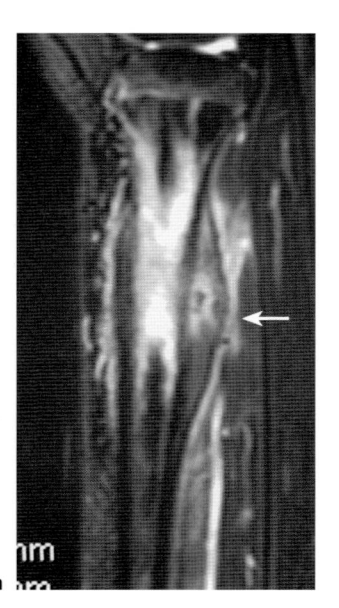

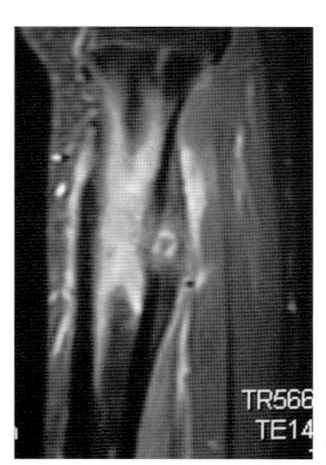

Figure 9.**12 a, b** A 15-year-old female with a subperiosteal osteoid osteoma involving the proximal tibia. The nidus of the lesion has high signal on sagittal FS T2WI (**a**). The small central calcification in the nidus has low signal on FS T2WI. Thickened cortex adjacent to the nidus has low and intermediate-slightly high signal on FS T2WI, and is associated with periosteal reaction with high signal. The nidus shows Gd-contrast enhancement on sagittal (**b**) FS T1WI. Prominent Gd-contrast enhancement is seen at the periosteal reaction, and mild diffuse enhancement is seen in the cortical thickening adjacent to the nidus. Poorly defined zones of high signal on FS T2WI and corresponding Gd-contrast enhancement on FS T1WI are also seen in the marrow adjacent to the lesion.

Table 9 (Continued) Solitary intramedullary lesions with poorly defined margins of abnormal marrow signal		
Lesion	MRI Findings	Comments
Osteoblastoma (Fig. 9.13)	Expansile lesion often >1.5 cm in diameter with low-intermediate signal on T1WI and intermediate-high signal on T2WI and FS T2WI, usually show Gd-contrast enhancement. Lesions usually have poorly defined zones with high signal on T2WI and FS T2WI and Gd-contrast enhancement in the marrow (edema, inflammation) beyond zone of sclerosis or in adjacent soft tissues from prostaglandin synthesis by these lesions.	Rare benign bone neoplasm (2% of bone tumors) usually occurs between 6 and 30 years. (See Atlas Chapter A 61)
Brown tumor	Lesions are usually radiolucent on radiographs and CT. Lesions often have low-intermediate signal on T1WI, intermediate to slightly high signal on T2WI, and typically show Gd-contrast enhancement. Zones of low signal on T2WI may occur from hemosiderin. Expansion of cortical margins can occur with or without cortical disruption/destruction. Lesions may have circumscribed and/or poorly defined margins.	Most often involves ribs, mandible, clavicle, pelvis, craniofacial bones, and vertebrae. Can result from primary hyperparathyroidism (3–7%) (oversecretion of PTH from parathyroid adenoma associated with hypercalcemia), secondary type (vitamin D deficiency or chronic renal failure with hypocalcemia resulting in secretion of PTH and parathyroid gland hyperplasia) (1–2%), or tertiary type in which the secondary type leads to eventual autonomous elevated PTH secretion from parathyroid gland hyperplasia.

Malignant

Metastatic tumor (Fig. 9.14)	Single or multiple well-circumscribed or poorly defined infiltrative lesions involving the marrow associated with cortical destruction and extraosseous extension. Lesions often have low-intermediate signal on T1WI, low, intermediate, and/or high signal on T2WI and FS T2WI, usually show Gd-contrast enhancement. Cortical destruction and tumor extension into the extraosseous soft tissues can occur. Pathologic fractures can be associated with metastatic lesions involving tubular bones and vertebrae. Periosteal reaction is uncommon.	Metastatic lesions typically occur in the marrow with or without cortical destruction and extraosseous tumor extension. (See Atlas Chapter A 50)
Plasmacytoma (Fig. 9.15)	Multiple (myeloma) or single (plasmacytoma) are well-circumscribed or poorly defined infiltrative lesions involving marrow, low-intermediate signal on T1WI, intermediate-high signal on T2WI and FS T2WI, usually show Gd-contrast-enhancement, eventual cortical bone destruction and extraosseous extension.	Malignant tumors comprising proliferating antibody-secreting plasma cells derived from single clones. Most common primary neoplasm of bone in adults, median = 60 years. Most patients are older than 40 years. May have variable destructive or infiltrative changes involving the axial and/or appendicular skeleton. (See Atlas Chapter A 52)
Leukemia	Single or multiple well-circumscribed or poorly defined infiltrative lesions involving marrow; low-intermediate signal on T1WI, intermediate-high signal on T2WI and FS T2WI, often show Gd-contrast enhancement, +/− cortical bone destruction and extraosseous extension.	Lymphoid neoplasms with involvement of bone marrow with tumor cells also in peripheral blood. In children and adolescents, acute lymphoblastic leukemia (ALL) is the most frequent type. In adults, chronic lymphocytic leukemia (CLL; small lymphocytic lymphoma) is the most common type of lymphocytic leukemia. Myelogenous leukemias are neoplasms derived from abnormal myeloid progenitor cells. Acute myelogenous leukemia (AML) occurs in adolescents and young adults, and represents ~20% of childhood leukemia. Chronic myelogenous leukemia (CML) usually affects adults older than 25 years. (See Atlas Chapter A 41)

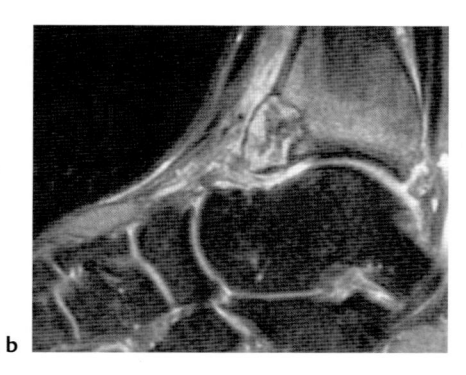

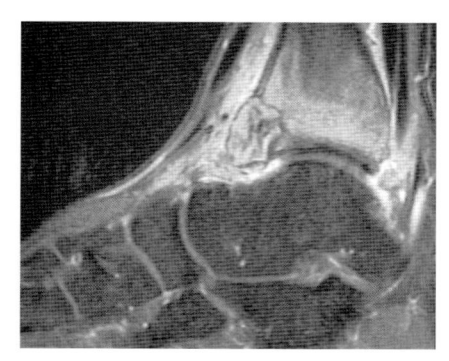

Figure 9.**13 a, b** A 24-year-old man with an osteoblastoma involving the distal tibia that has heterogeneous high and low signal on sagittal FS T2WI (**a**). A thin rim of low signal is seen at the periphery of the tumor and at the border with medullary bone. The tumor causes expansion and irregular thinning of the anterior margin of the distal tibia. The lesion shows prominent heterogeneous Gd-contrast enhancement on sagittal FS T1WI (**b**). Poorly defined zones of high signal on T2WI and corresponding Gd-contrast enhancement are seen in the marrow and soft tissues adjacent to the osteoblastoma.

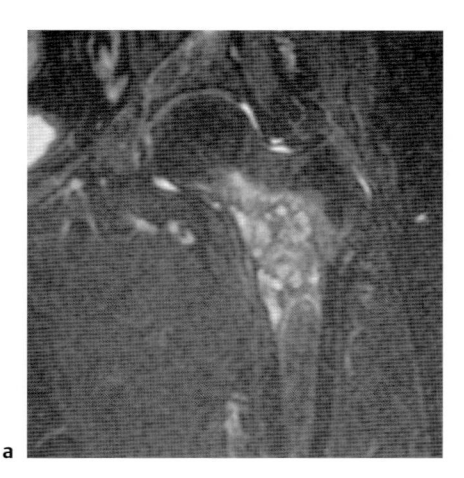

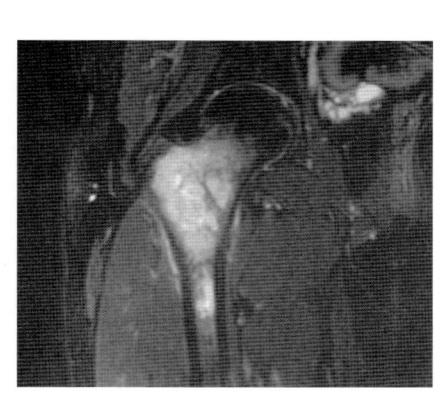

Figure 9.**14 a, b** Metastatic disease in the marrow of the femur seen as poorly defined zones with slightly high to high signal on coronal FS T2WI from breast carcinoma in a 57-year-old woman (**a**) and from seminoma in a 26-year-old man (**b**).

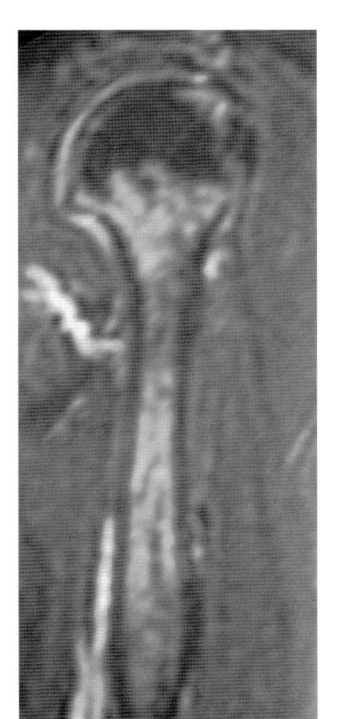

Figure 9.**15** Myeloma involving the humerus seen as a poorly defined zone of high signal in the marrow on sagittal FS T2WI.

Table 9 (Continued) Solitary intramedullary lesions with poorly defined margins of abnormal marrow signal

Lesion	MRI Findings	Comments
Lymphoma (Fig. 9.16)	Non-Hodgkin lymphoma (NHL) and Hodgkin disease (HD) within bone typically appear as single or multifocal poorly defined or circumscribed intramedullary zones with low-intermediate signal on T1WI, and intermediate, slightly high, and/or high signal on T2WI and high signal on FS T2WI; often show Gd-contrast enhancement. Zones of cortical destruction may occur associated with extraosseous soft tissue extension.	Lymphoid tumors with neoplastic cells typically within lymphoid tissue (lymph nodes and reticuloendothelial organs). Unlike leukemia, lymphoma usually arises as discrete masses. Lymphomas are subdivided into HD and NHL. Almost all primary lymphomas of bone are B cell NHL. HD, mean age = 32 years. Osseous NHL, median = 35 years. **(See Atlas Chapter A 47)**
Chondrosarcoma (Fig. 9.17)	Intramedullary tumors often have low-intermediate signal on T1WI, intermediate signal on PDWI, and heterogeneous intermediate-high signal on T2WI. Lesions usually show heterogeneous contrast enhancement.	Malignant tumors containing cartilage formed within sarcomatous stroma. Account for 12–21% of malignant bone lesions, 21–26% of primary sarcomas of bone, mean age = 40 years, median = 26 to 59 years. **(See Atlas Chapter A 11)**
Osteosarcoma (Fig. 9.18)	Destructive intramedullary malignant lesions, low-intermediate signal on T1WI, mixed low, intermediate, high signal on T2WI, usually with matrix mineralization/ossification-low signal on T2WI, typically show Gd-contrast enhancement (usually heterogeneous). May have circumscribed and/or ill-defined margins. Zones of cortical destruction are typically seen, through which tumors extend into the extraosseous soft tissues under an elevated periosteum. Lamellated and/or spiculated zones of bone formation can occur under the periosteal elevation secondary to tumor invasion and perforation of bone cortex. Low signal from spicules of periosteal, reactive, and tumoral bone formation may have a divergent ("sunburst") pattern, perpendicular ("hair on end") pattern, or disorganized or complex appearance. Triangular zones of periosteal elevation (Codman's triangles) can be seen at the borders of zones of cortical destruction and tumor extension.	Malignant tumor comprising proliferating neoplastic spindle cells which produce osteoid and/or immature tumoral bone most frequently arising within medullary bone (metadiaphyseal > metaphyseal > diaphyseal locations). Two age peaks of incidence. The larger peak occurs between the ages of 10 and 20 and accounts for over half of the cases. The second smaller peak occurs in adults over 60 years and accounts for ~10% of the cases. Occurs in children as primary tumors and adults (associated with Paget disease, irradiated bone, chronic osteomyelitis, osteoblastoma, giant cell tumor, fibrous dysplasia. **(See Atlas Chapter A 64)**

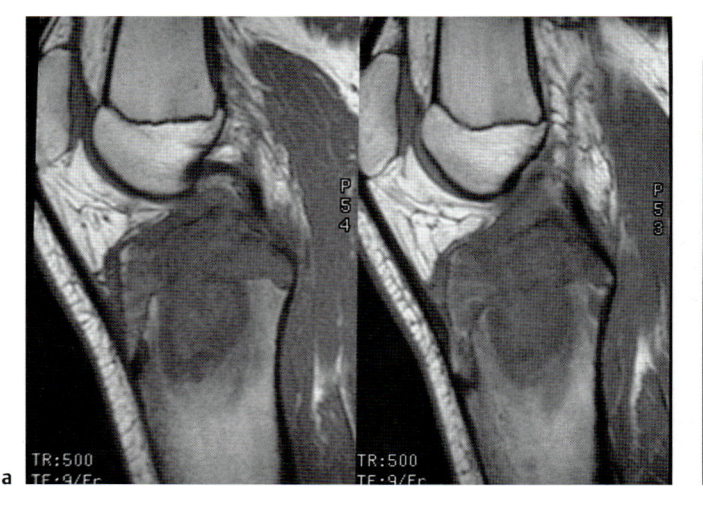

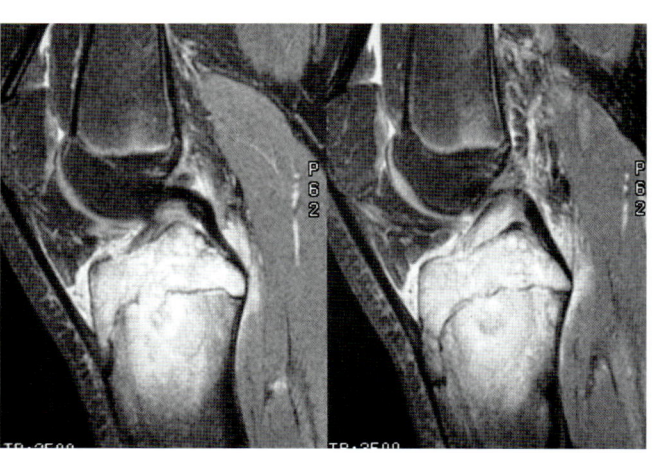

Figure 9.**16 a, b**   A 13-year-old girl with Burkitt lymphoma involving the marrow of the proximal tibia seen as poorly defined zones with low-intermediate signal on sagittal T1WI (**a**) and high signal on FS T2WI (**b**).

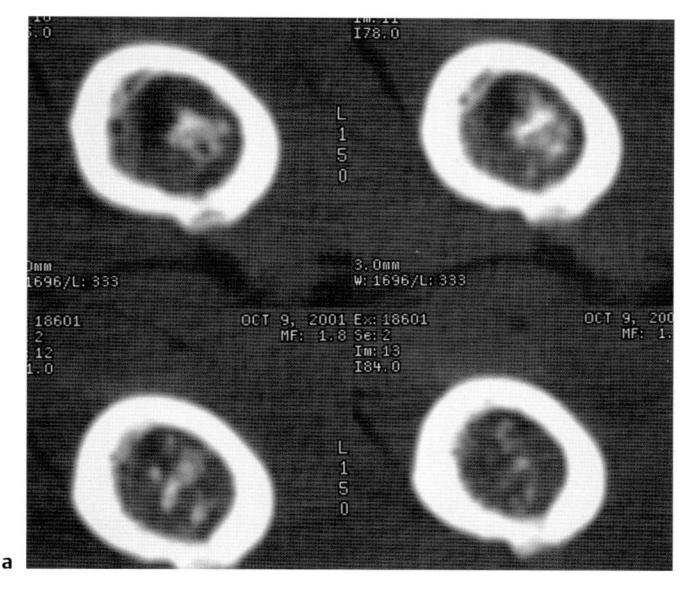

Figure 9.**17 a, b** A 44-year-old woman with a chondrosarcoma in the proximal shaft of the femur that has chondroid mineralization on the axial CT (**a**). The tumor has high signal with poorly defined margins on coronal FS T2WI (**b**).

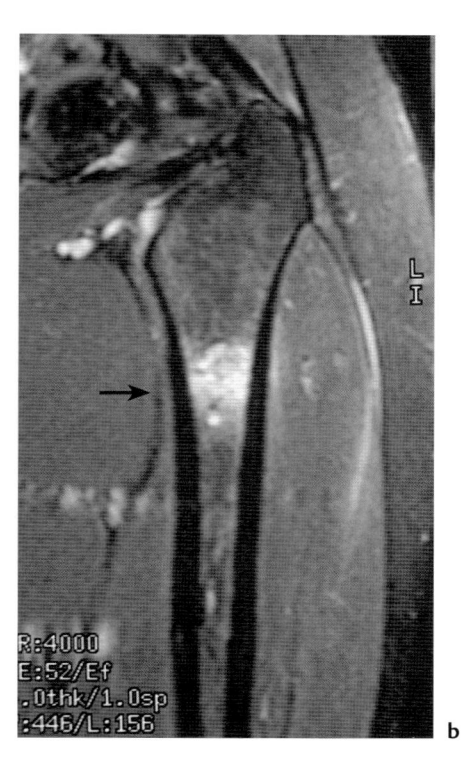

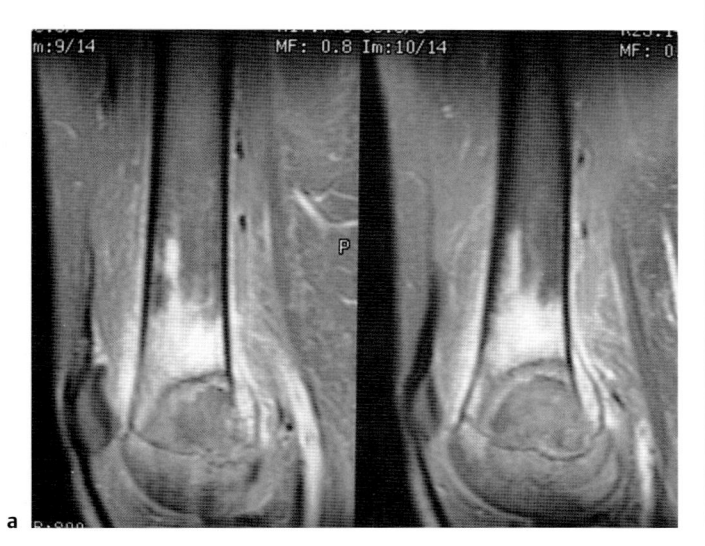

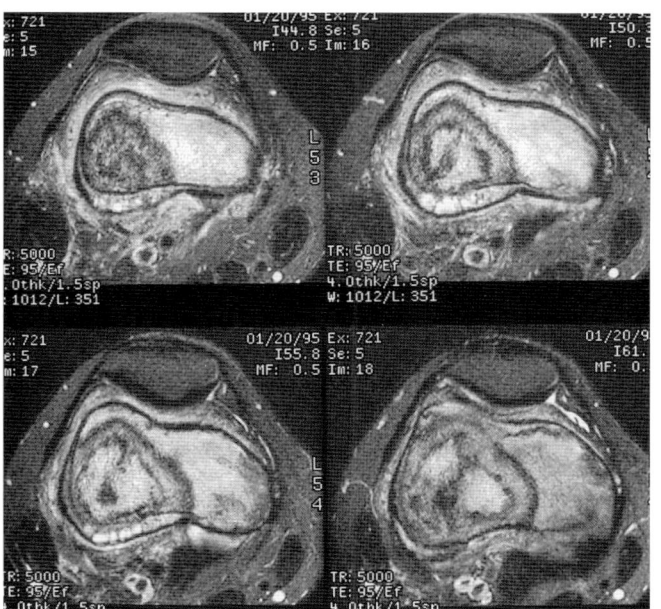

Figure 9.**18 a, b** A 13-year-old girl with an osteosarcoma involving the marrow of the distal epi- and metaphyseal portions of the femur associated with disrupted periosteal elevation, cortical destruction, and extraosseous extension. The tumor has poorly defined margins and shows Gd-contrast enhancement on sagittal FS T1WI (**a**) and has heterogeneous low and high signal on axial FS T2WI (**b**).

Table 9 (Continued) Solitary intramedullary lesions with poorly defined margins of abnormal marrow signal		
Lesion	MRI Findings	Comments
Ewing sarcoma (Fig. 9.19)	Destructive malignant lesions involving marrow, low-intermediate signal on T1WI, mixed low, intermediate, and/or high signal on T2WI and FS T2WI, typically shows Gd-contrast enhancement (usually heterogeneous). Extraosseous tumor extension through sites of cortical destruction is commonly seen beneath an elevated periosteum. Thin striated zones of low signal on T2WI can be sometimes seen oriented perpendicular to the long axis of the involved bone under the elevated periosteum representing the "hair on end" appearance of reactive bone formation secondary to the tumor. In long bones, tumors are most often located in the diaphyseal region, followed by the metadiaphyseal region.	Malignant primitive tumor of bone comprised of undifferentiated small cells with round nuclei. Accounts for 6–11% of primary malignant bone tumors, 5–7% of primary bone tumors. Usually occurs between the ages of 5 and 30, males > females, locally invasive, high metastatic potential. (See Atlas Chapter A 20)
Malignant giant cell tumor (Fig. 9.20)	Well-defined or poorly-marginated lesions with or without thin low signal margins on T1WI and T2WI. Solid portions of giant cell tumors often have low to intermediate signal on T1WI and PDWI, intermediate to high signal on T2WI, and high signal on FS PDWI and FS T2WI. Signal heterogeneity on T2WI is not uncommon. Aneurysmal bone cysts are seen with 14% of giant cell tumors. Lesions show mild to prominent variable and often heterogeneous Gd-contrast enhancement. Cortical destruction and extraosseous tumor extension are frequently seen.	Aggressive tumors composed of neoplastic ovoid mononuclear cells and scattered multinucleated osteoclast-like giant cells. Up to 10% of all giant cell tumors are malignant. Benign giant cell tumors account for ~5 to 9.5% of all bone tumors and up to 23% of benign bone tumors. Malignant giant cell tumors account for 5.8% of all giant cell tumors. 75% occur in patients between the ages of 15 and 45 years. (See Atlas Chapter A 29)
Fibrosarcoma	Intramedullary lesions with irregular margins, with or without associated cortical destruction and/or extraosseous soft tissue masses. Lesions usually have low-intermediate signal on T1WI and PDWI, and heterogeneous intermediate, slightly high, and/or high signal on T2WI. Lesions usually show heterogeneous Gd-contrast enhancement.	Fibrosarcomas are uncommon malignant tumors consisting of bundles of fibroblasts/spindle cells with varying proportions of collagen, lacking other tissue differentiating features such as tumor bone, osteoid, or cartilage. Can be primary lesions (75%) or arise as secondary tumors (25%) associated with prior irradiation, Paget disease, bone infarct, chronic osteomyelitis, fibrous dysplasia, giant cell tumor. Accounts for 3–5% of primary malignant bone tumors, and 2–4% of all bone tumors, median age = 43 years. (See Atlas Chapter A 25)
Malignant fibrous histiocytoma (Fig. 9.21)	Intramedullary lesions with irregular margins and zones of cortical destruction and extraosseous extension. Tumors often have low-intermediate signal on T1WI; low-intermediate signal on PDWI and heterogeneous intermediate-high signal on T2WI and FS T2WI. Invasion into joints occurs in 30%. May be associated with bone infarcts, bone cysts, chronic osteomyelitis, Paget disease, and other treated primary bone tumors. Lesions usually show heterogeneous Gd-contrast prominent enhancement.	Malignant tumor involving soft tissue and rarely bone derived from undifferentiated mesenchymal cells. Contains cells with limited cellular differentiation such as mixtures of fibroblasts, myofibroblasts, histiocyte-like cells, anaplastic giant cells, and inflammatory cells. Accounts for 1–5% of primary malignant bone tumors and <1–3% of all primary bone tumors, patient ages range from 11 to 80 years, median = 48 years, mean = 55 years. (See Atlas Chapter A 48)
Paget sarcoma (Fig. 9.22)	Irregular zones of medullary and cortical bone destruction associated with an extraosseous soft tissue mass lesion. The involved marrow typically has low to intermediate signal on T1WI and PDWI, and low to high signal on T2WI. Abnormal Gd-contrast enhancement is seen in the marrow as well as in the extraosseous tumor extension.	Paget disease is the second most common bone disease in older adults after osteoporosis. Median age = 66 years. Disordered bone resorption and woven bone formation occurs resulting in osseous deformity. Associated with less than 1% risk for developing secondary sarcomatous changes. (See Atlas Chapter A 65)

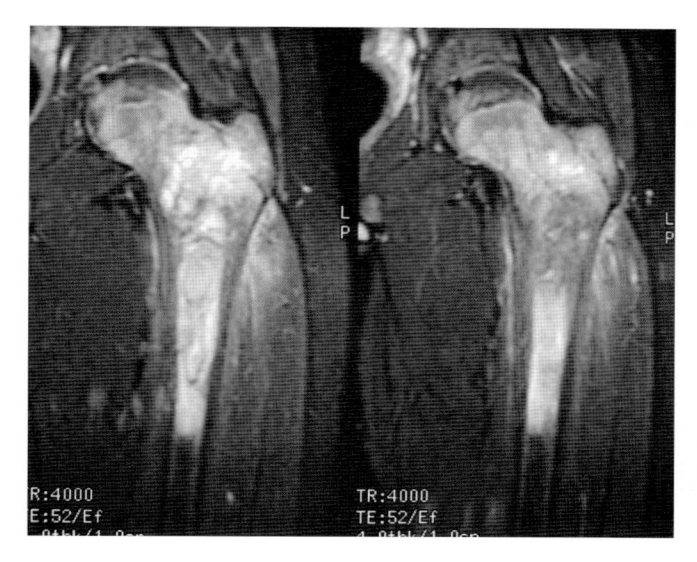

Figure 9.19 A 15-year-old male with Ewing sarcoma in the proximal femur seen as a poorly defined zone with high signal in the marrow on coronal FS T2WI. Cortical disruption and extraosseous tumor extension are also present.

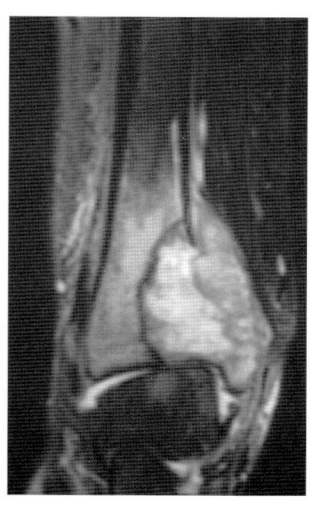

Figure 9.20 A 16-year-old male with a malignant giant cell tumor in the marrow of the distal tibia associated with cortical destruction and extraosseous extension. The intramedullary portion of the tumor has high signal centrally on coronal FS T2WI surrounded by a rim of low signal, and a poorly defined peripheral zone of high signal in the marrow.

a, b

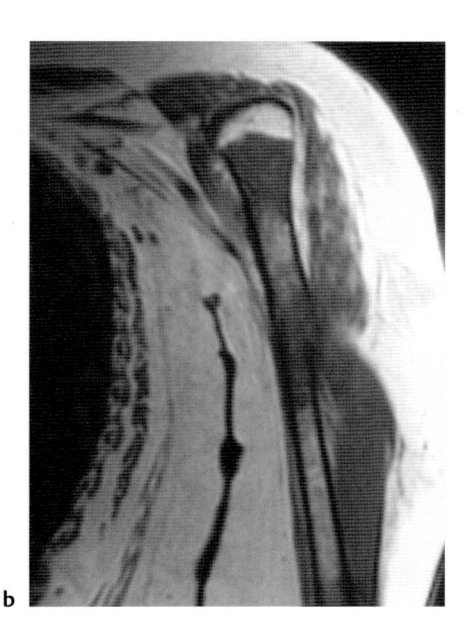

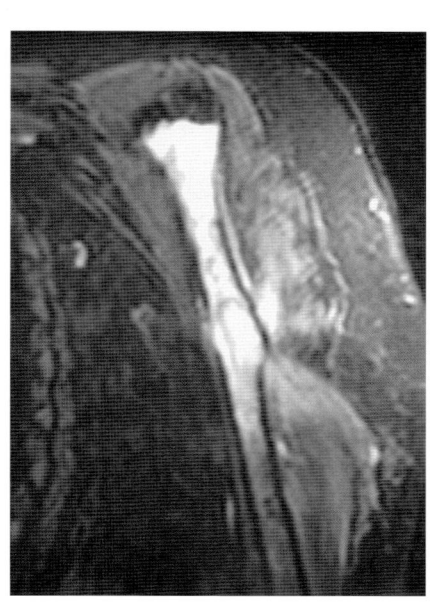

Figure 9.21 a, b A 55-year-old woman with a malignant fibrous histiocytoma involving the humerus seen as a poorly defined lesion in the marrow with low-intermediate signal on coronal T1WI (a) and high signal on coronal FS T2WI (b).

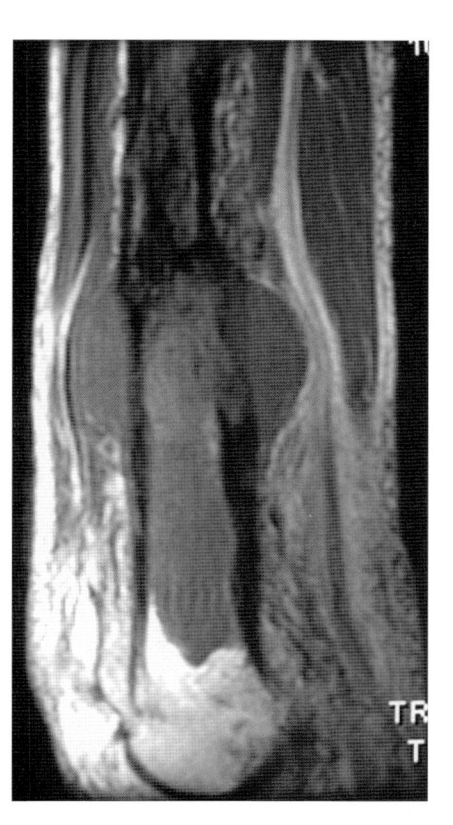

Figure 9.22 A 71-year-old woman with Paget sarcoma involving the marrow of the distal femur associated with cortical destruction and extraosseous extension as seen on sagittal T1WI.

References

Transient Bone Marrow Edema

Balakrishnan A, Schemitsch EH, Pearce D, McKee MD. Distinguishing transient osteoporosis of the hip from avascular necrosis. *Can J Surg* June 2003;46(3):187–192.

Malizos KN, Zibis AH, Dailiana Z, Hantes M, Karahalios T, Karantanas AH. MR imaging findings in transient osteoporosis of the hip. *Eur J Radiol* 2004;50:238–244.

Toms AP, Marshall TJ, Becker E, Donell ST, Lobo-Mueller EM, Barker T. Regional migratory osteoporosis: a review illustrated by five cases. *Clin Radiol* 2005;60:425–438.

Yamamoto T, Kubo T, Hirasawa Y, Noguchi Y, Iwamoto Y, Sueishi K. A clinicopathologic study of transient osteoporosis of the hip. *Skeletal Radiol* 1999;28:621–627.

Intraosseous Calcific Tendinopathy

Flemming DJ, Murphey MD, Shekitka KM, Temple HT, Jelinek JJ, Kransdorf MJ. Osseous involvement in calcific tendonitis: a retrospective review of 50 cases. *AJR* 2003;181:965–972.

Table 10 Solitary intramedullary lesions located near the ends of tubular bones		
Lesion	**MRI Findings**	**Comments**
Benign		
Enchondroma (Figs. 10.1, 10.2)	Lobulated circumscribed intramedullary lesions that usually have low-intermediate signal on T1WI and intermediate signal on PDWI. On T2WI and FS T2WI, lesions usually have predominantly high signal with foci and/or bands of low signal representing areas of matrix mineralization and fibrous strands. Lesions typically show Gd-contrast enhancement in various patterns (peripheral curvilinear lobular, central nodular/septal and peripheral lobular, or heterogeneous diffuse).	Benign intramedullary lesions comprising hyaline cartilage, represent ~10% of benign bone tumors. Enchondromas can be solitary (88%) or multiple (12%). Median age = 35 years, peak in 3rd and 4th decades. **(See Atlas Chapter A 8).**

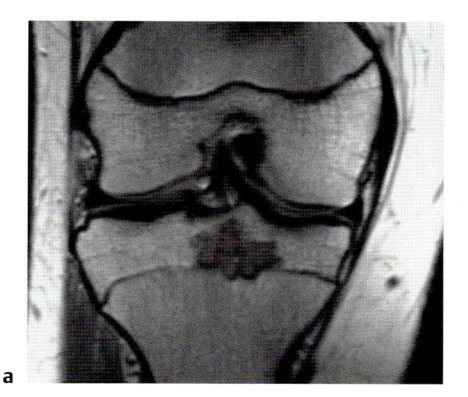

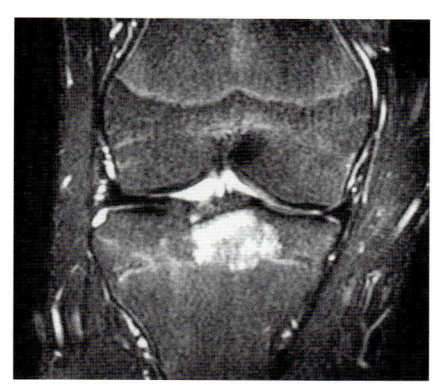

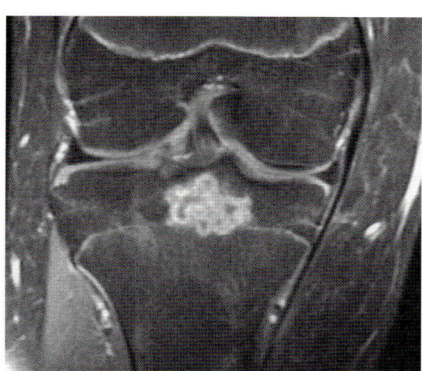

Figure 10.1 a–c A 14-year-old girl with an enchondroma in the epiphysis of the proximal tibia which has low-intermediate signal on coronal T1WI (**a**), and high signal on FS T2WI (**b**). The lesion shows peripheral lobular Gd-contrast enhancement on FS T1WI (**c**).

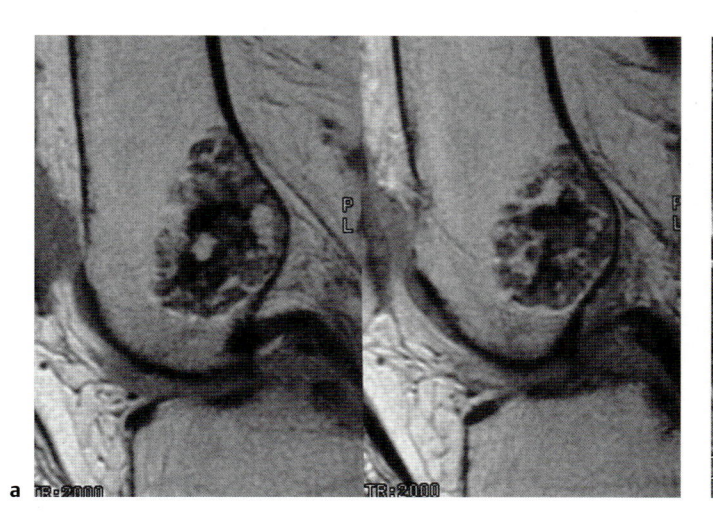

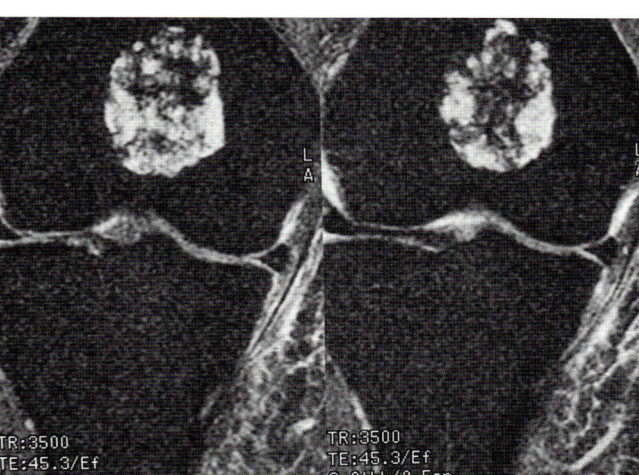

Figure 10.2 a, b A 66-year-old woman with an enchondroma in the marrow of the distal femur that has mixed low, intermediate, and slightly high signal on sagittal PDWI (**a**), and mixed low and high signal on coronal FS T2WI (**b**).

Table 10 (Continued) **Solitary intramedullary lesions located near the ends of tubular bones**

Lesion	MRI Findings	Comments
Giant cell tumor (Fig. 10.3)	Often well-defined lesions with thin low signal margins on T1WI, PDWI, and T2WI. Solid portions of giant cell tumors often have low to intermediate signal on T1WI and PDWI, intermediate to high signal on T2WI, and high signal on FS PDWI and FS T2WI. Zones of low signal on T2WI may be seen secondary to hemosiderin. Aneurysmal bone cysts can be seen in 14% of giant cell tumors. Areas of cortical thinning, expansion, and/or destruction can occur with extraosseous extension. Tumors show varying degrees of Gd-contrast enhancement.	Aggressive tumors composed of neoplastic mononuclear cells and scattered multi-nucleated osteoclast-like giant cells. Account for 23% of primary nonmalignant bone tumors and 5–9% of all primary bone tumors, median age = 30 years. **(See Atlas Chapter A 29)**
Chondroblastoma (Fig. 10.4)	Tumors often have fine lobular margins, and typically have low-intermediate heterogeneous signal on T1WI, and mixed low, intermediate, and/or high signal on T2WI. Areas of low signal on T2WI are secondary to chondroid matrix mineralization, and/or hemosiderin. Lobular, marginal, or septal Gd-contrast enhancement patterns can be seen. Poorly defined zones with high signal on T2WI and FS T2WI and corresponding Gd-contrast enhancement are typically seen in the marrow adjacent to the lesions representing inflammatory reaction from prostaglandin synthesis by these tumors.	Benign cartilaginous tumors with chondroblast-like cells and areas of chondroid matrix formation, usually occur in children and adolescents, median = 17 years, mean = 16 years for lesions in long bones, mean = 28 years in other bones. Most cases are diagnosed between the ages of 5 and 25. **(See Atlas Chapter A 7)**
Chondromyxoid fibroma (Fig. 10.5)	Lesions are often slightly lobulated with low-intermediate signal on T1WI and heterogeneous predominantly high signal on T2WI. MR signal heterogeneity on T2WI is related to the proportions of myxoid, chondroid, and fibrous components within the lesions. Thin low signal septa on T2WI can be seen. Lesions are surrounded by low signal borders representing thin sclerotic reaction. Edema is not typically seen in adjacent medullary bone. Lesions show prominent diffuse Gd contrast enhancement.	Rare, benign, slow-growing bone lesions that contain chondroid, myxoid, and fibrous components. Chondromyxoid fibromas represent 2–4% of primary benign bone lesions, and <1% of primary bone lesions. Most chondromyxoid fibromas occur between the ages of 1 to 40 years, with a median of 17 years, and peak incidence in the 2nd to 3rd decades. **(See Atlas Chapter A 10)**
Osteoblastoma (Fig. 10.6)	Expansile lesion often >1.5 cm in diameter with low-intermediate signal on T1WI and intermediate-high signal on T2WI and FS T2WI, typically shows Gd-contrast enhancement. Lesions usually have poorly defined zones with high signal on T2WI and FS T2WI and Gd-contrast enhancement in the marrow (edema, inflammation) beyond zone of sclerosis or in adjacent soft tissues from prostaglandin synthesis by these lesions.	Rare benign bone neoplasm (2% of bone tumors) usually occurs between the ages 6 and 30 years. **(See Atlas Chapter A 61)**
Intraosseous lipoma (Fig. 10.7)	Lesions can have heterogeneous high, intermediate, and/or low signal on T1WI, PDWI, and T2WI. Fat signal in lesions is suppressed on FS T1WI, FS T2W and STIR. Lesions often show no Gd-contrast enhancement. Peripheral rim-like and central Gd-contrast enhancement may occasionally be seen on FS T1WI.	Uncommon benign hamartomas composed of mature white adipose tissue without cellular atypia. Osseous or chondroid metaplasia with myxoid changes can be associated with lipomas. Account for ~0.1% of bone tumors, likely under-reported. **(See Atlas Chapter A 43)**

Intraosseous lipoma **165**

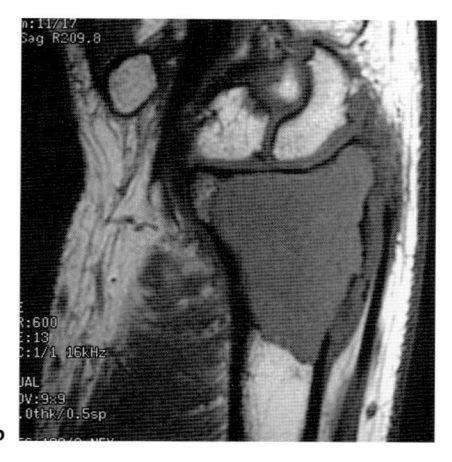

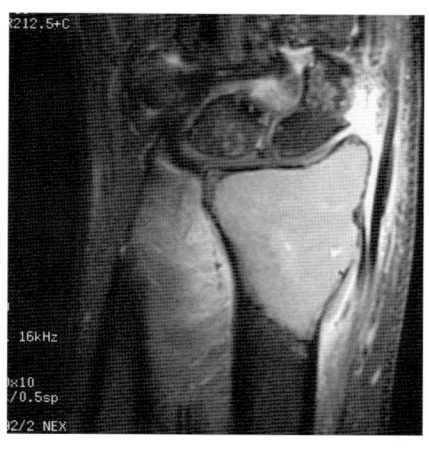

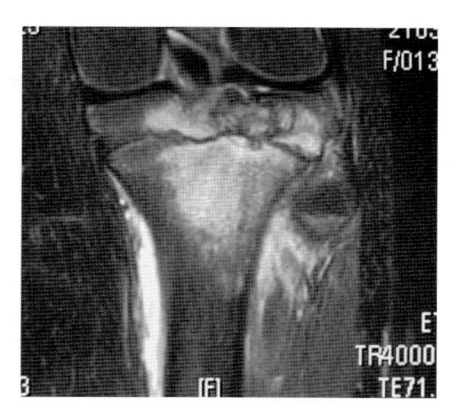

Figure 10.**3 a, b** A 26-year-old woman with a giant cell tumor in the distal radius that has intermediate signal on coronal T1WI (**a**), and shows Gd-contrast enhancement on coronal FS T1WI (**b**)

Figure 10.**4** A 13-year-old girl with a chondroblastoma involving the epiphysis of the proximal tibia. A lesion with mixed low and high signal is seen with thin low signal margins on coronal FS T2WI. Poorly defined zones with high signal are seen in the adjacent marrow.

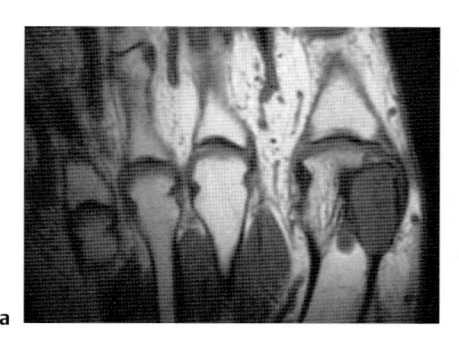

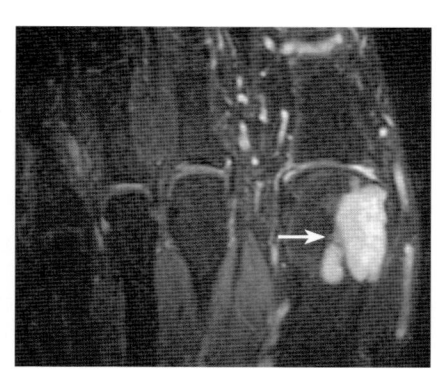

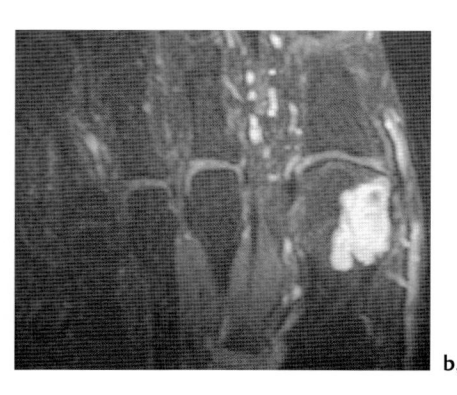

Figure 10.**5 a–c** A 34-year-old man with a chondromyxoid fibroma involving the first metatarsal head. The lesion has circumscribed low signal margins and contains intermediate signal on coronal T1WI (**a**) and high signal on coronal FS T2WI (**b**). The lesion shows Gd-contrast enhancement on coronal FS T1WI (**c**).

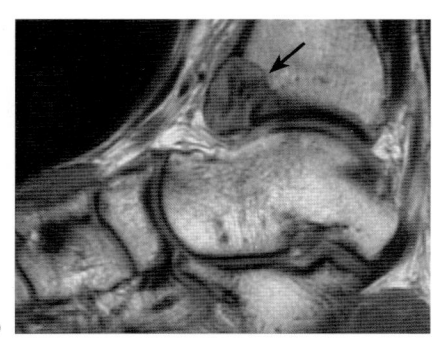

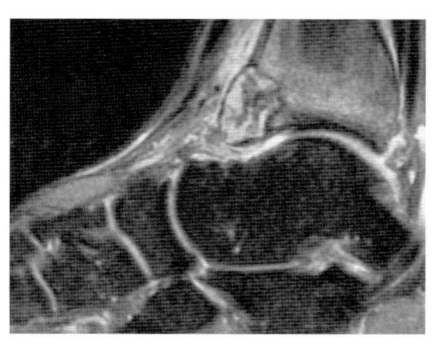

Figure 10.**6 a, b** A 24-year-old man with an osteoblastoma in the distal tibia. The lesion is associated with cortical thinning and expansion, and has low-intermediate signal on sagittal PDWI (**a**), and heterogeneous high and low signal on sagittal FS T2WI (**b**). Poorly defined high signal on FS T2WI is also seen in the marrow adjacent to the lesion.

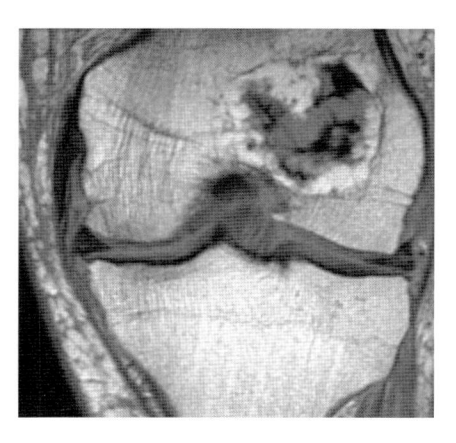

Figure 10.**7** A 74-year-old man with an intraosseous lipoma in the distal portion of the femur that has high signal peripherally surrounding a central zone with intermediate and low signal from cystic degeneration and dystrophic calcifications on PDWI.

Table 10 (Continued) Solitary intramedullary lesions located near the ends of tubular bones

Lesion	MRI Findings	Comments
Geode/subchondral degenerative cyst (Fig. 10.8)	Typically have sharply defined margins and contains low signal on T1WI, low-intermediate signal on PDWI, and homogeneous high signal on T2WI. Poorly defined zones of Gd-contrast enhancement can be seen in the marrow adjacent to the subchondral cysts on FS T1WI.	A geode or subchondral cyst is a cystic lesion located near the end of a long bone where there are changes of degenerative osteoarthropathy. Lesions can result from synovial fluid intrusion and/or bony contusion in the setting of degenerative joint disease. **(See Atlas Chapter A 28)**
Intraosseous ganglion (Fig. 10.9)	Can have round, oval, or serpiginous configurations with sharply defined margins. These lesions typically contain low signal on T1WI, low-intermediate signal on PDWI, and high signal on T2WI.	Benign cystic lesion usually located at or near the ends of long bones, and is not associated with degenerative osteoarthropathy. Lesions can result from intraosseous extension from a ganglion in the soft tissues; or from intraosseous mucoid degeneration, synovial rests, or synovial intrusion. **(See Atlas Chapter A 28)**
Intraosseous extension of inflammatory synovium/pannus (Fig. 10.10)	Hypertrophied synovium can be diffuse, nodular and/or villous, and often has low to intermediate or intermediate signal on T1WI and PDWI, and low to intermediate, intermediate, and/or slightly high to high signal on T2WI. Erosive changes in subchondral bone appear as zones of low signal on T1WI, and high signal on T2WI. Contrast enhancement is often seen within the erosions.	Inflammatory synovitis associated with rheumatoid arthritis can result in progressive destruction of cartilage and cortical bone leading with intraosseous extension and trabecular destruction. Prevalence ranges from 0.3 to 2.1 % of the world population. 80 % of adult patients present between the ages of 35 and 50. Incidence of juvenile rheumatoid arthritis (JRA) ranges from 6 to 19.6 cases per 100,000. Patients with JRA range from 5 to 16 years, mean = 10.2 years. **(See Atlas Chapter A 70)**
Intraosseous calcific tendinopathy (Fig. 10.11)	Zones with slightly high and low signal on T2WI and FS T2WI are seen in tendons with or without erosion of bone cortex. Intramedullary zones with mixed low, intermediate, and/or high signal on T2WI and FS T2WI may be seen in the adjacent marrow.	Degenerative disorder with amorphous calcifications in tendons or bursa associated with erosion of adjacent bone cortex, with or without marrow invasion. Most common in humerus and femur in patients 16 to 82 years, average = 50 years.

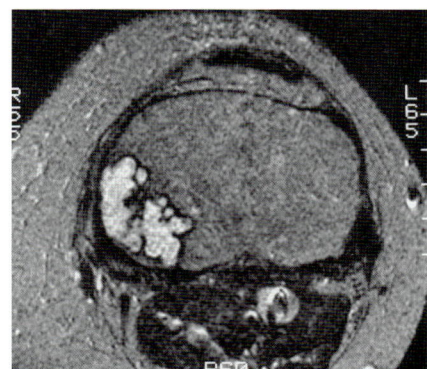

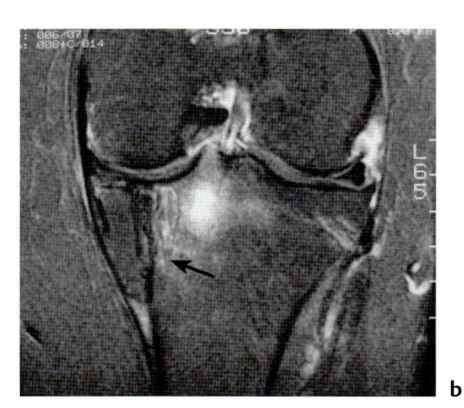

Figure 10.8 a, b Geode or degenerative arthritic subchondral cyst in the proximal medial tibia beneath degenerated disrupted hyaline cartilage that has high signal centrally surrounded by a thin lobulated rim of low signal on axial T2WI (**a**). A poorly-defined zone of Gd-contrast enhancement is seen in the marrow medially on coronal FS T1WI (**b**); may be secondary to chronic pressure effects from the geode as well as reaction to overlying chondral damage.

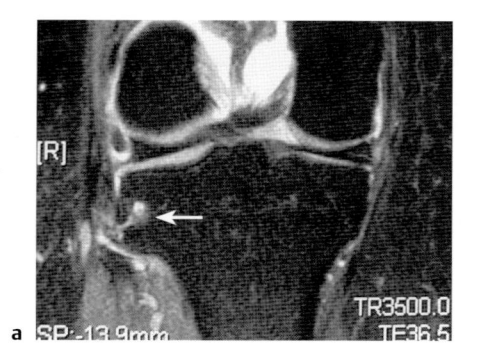

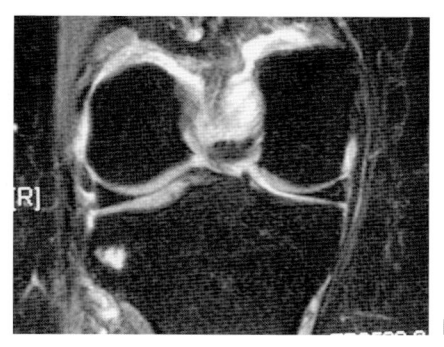

Figure 10.**9 a, b** Juxtacortical ganglion eroding bone cortex resulting in an intraosseous ganglion in the proximal lateral tibia that has high signal and circumscribed margins on coronal FS T2WI (**a**, **b**).

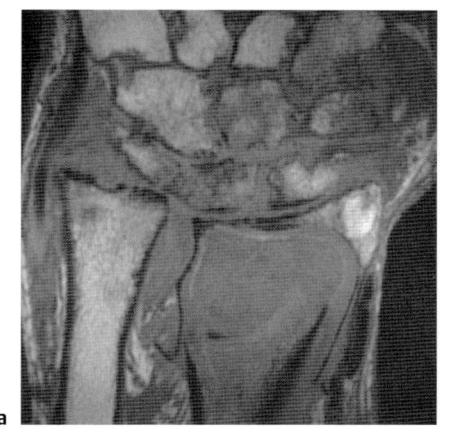

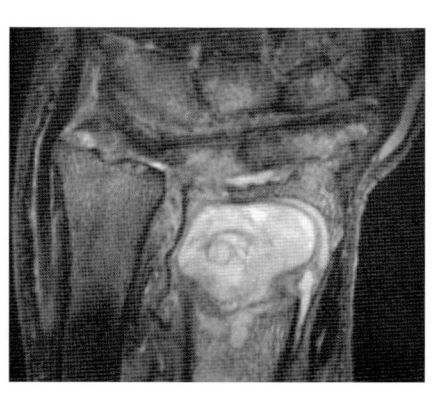

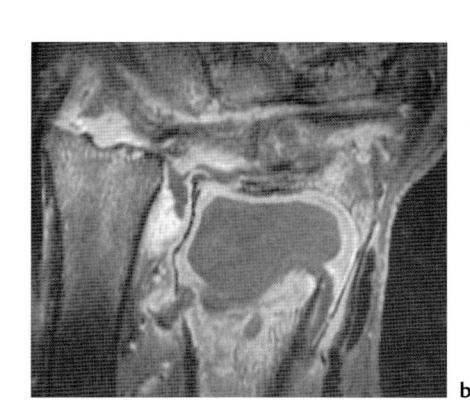

Figure 10.**10 a–c** A 71-year-old man with pannus eroding into the distal radius resulting in destruction of trabecular bone and intraosseous cyst-like lesion. The intraosseous lesion has intermediate signal on coronal T1WI (**a**) and heterogeneous high signal on coronal T2WI (**b**). Gd-contrast enhancement is seen at the margins of the intraosseous lesion on coronal FS T1WI (**c**) as well as in the hypertrophied synovium in the wrist. Also seen is destruction of hyaline cartilage at the carpal bones and distal ulna.

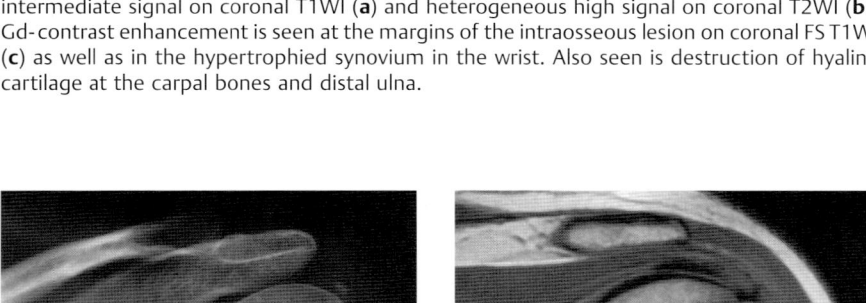

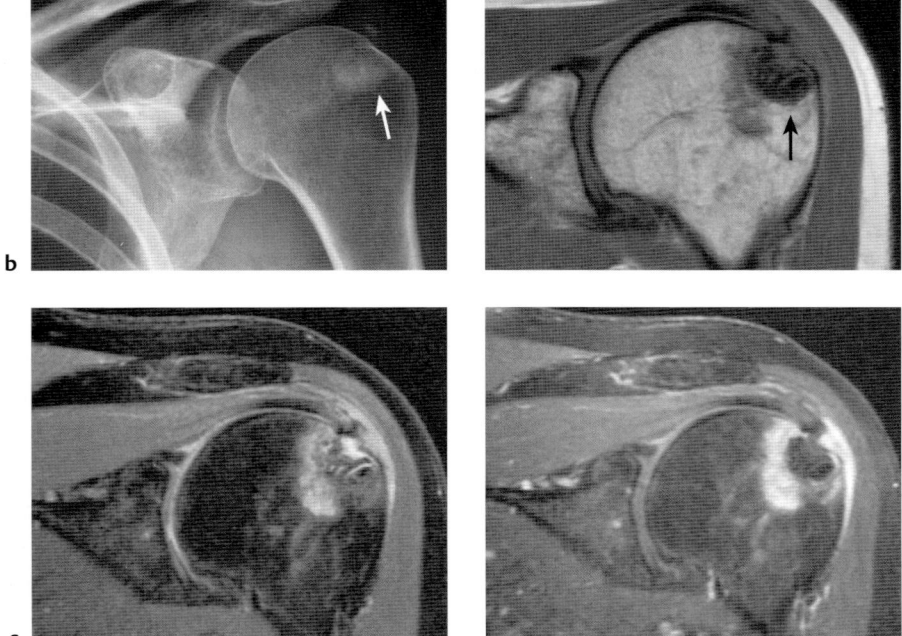

Figure 10.**11 a–d** A 57-year-old woman with intraosseous calcific tendinopathy in the humerus. Calcification is seen in the rotator cuff near the insertion site as well as an intraosseous zone of increased attenuation on the AP radiograph (**a**). Coronal PDWI (**b**) shows a circumscribed intraosseous zone with low and intermediate signal beneath a zone of cortical disruption. The intraosseous lesion has mixed high and low signal on coronal FS T2WI (**c**), as well as a poorly defined zone with high T2 signal in the adjacent marrow. The intraosseous lesion shows marginal Gd-contrast enhancement surrounding the circumscribed lesion, and a poorly defined zone of contrast enhancement is seen in the adjacent bone marrow on FS T1WI (**d**).

Table 10 (Continued)	Solitary intramedullary lesions located near the ends of tubular bones	
Lesion	**MRI Findings**	**Comments**
Fracture (Fig. 10.12)	Acute/subacute fractures typically have abnormal marrow signal (usually low signal on T1WI, high signal on T2WI and FS T2WI). Gd-contrast enhancement is typically seen in the postfracture period. Angulated cortical margins and periosteal high signal on FS T2WI can be seen with traumatic fractures. A curvilinear zone of low signal on T2WI and FS T2WI may be seen within the marrow edema in stress fractures.	Can result from trauma, primary bone tumors/lesions, metastatic disease, bone infarcts (steroids, chemotherapy, and radiation treatment), osteoporosis, osteomalacia, metabolic (calcium/ phosphate) disorders, vitamin deficiencies, Paget disease, and genetic disorders (osteogenesis imperfecta, etc.)
Bone contusion (Fig. 10.13)	Contusions usually appear as poorly defined intramedullary zones with low-intermediate signal on T1WI and high signal on FS T2WI, and corresponding Gd-contrast enhancement. Adjacent cortical margins are typically intact.	Also referred to as bone bruises, contusions represent trabecular microfractures without cortical fracture. In the knee, contusions at the lateral femoral condyle and posterolateral proximal tibia are commonly associated with injuries to the anterior cruciate ligament.
Osteochondritis dissecans (Fig. 10.14)	Subchondral lesions in marrow ranging from 1 to 3 cm with low-intermediate signal on T1WI and T2WI. Small irregular zones with slightly high to high signal may be seen with FS T2WI. A linear zone with high signal on T2WI along the margins can represent tracking of synovial fluid from a defect in the overlying hyaline cartilage, and is associated with an increased risk of fragmentation and separation.	Osteochondrosis in which there is localized necrosis followed by reossification and healing unless there is osteochondral fragmentation and separation. Lesions commonly occur at the lateral surface of the medial femoral condyle, as well as the capitellum, talar dome, and femoral head.
Bone infarct (Fig. 10.15)	A double-line sign (curvilinear adjacent zones of low and high signal on T2WI) is commonly seen at the edges of the infarcts representing the borders of osseous resorption and healing. Irregular Gd-contrast enhancement can be seen from granulation tissue ingrowth.	Zones of ischemic death involving bone trabeculae and marrow which can be idiopathic or result from: trauma, corticosteroid treatment, chemotherapy, radiation treatment, occlusive vascular disease, collagen vascular and other autoimmune diseases, metabolic storage diseases (Gaucher etc.), sickle cell disease, thalassemia, hyperbaric events / Caisson disease, pregnancy, alcohol abuse, pancreatitis, infections, and lymphoproliferative diseases. **(See Atlas Chapter A 37)**
Transient bone marrow edema (Fig. 10.16)	Poorly defined zones with low-intermediate signal on T1WI and high signal on FS T2WI and STIR are seen in the marrow of the proximal hip (femoral head and neck). The signal abnormalities may spare the subchondral marrow. MRI Findings can be seen within 48 hours from the onset of symptoms. Joint effusions may be present. With dynamic Gd-contrast administration, delayed peak enhancement can be seen.	Idiopathic spontaneous process with transient edema in bone marrow that is not secondary to trauma, and may or may not be associated with osteoporosis. Transient bone marrow edema or acute bone marrow edema frequently involves the proximal femur in men between 30 and 50 years, and women in the last trimester of pregnancy.

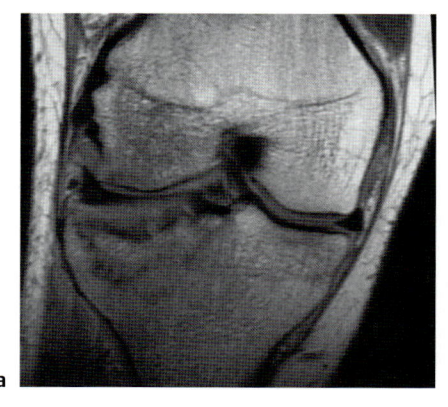

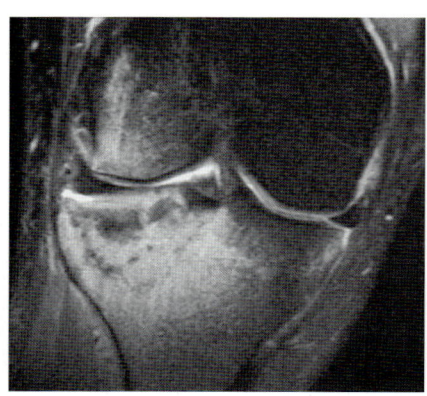

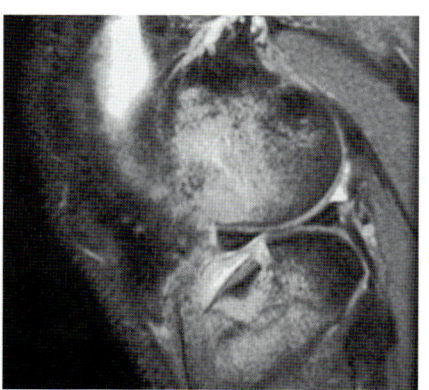

Figure 10.12 a–c   A traumatic fracture of the lateral tibial plateau is seen with subjacent poorly defined zones of low-intermediate signal in the marrow on coronal PDWI (**a**) and high signal on coronal (**b**) and sagittal (**c**) FS T2WI. Also seen is a bone contusion in the marrow of the lateral femoral condyle.

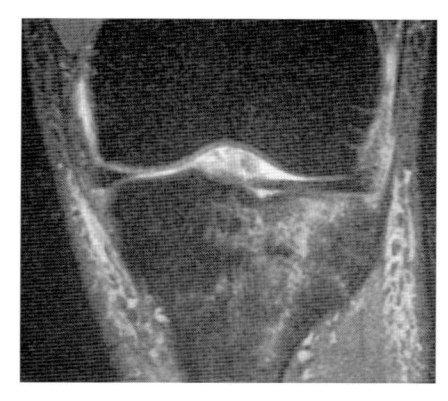

Figure 10.13 A bone contusion is seen as a poorly defined zone with increased signal on coronal FS T2WI in the proximal tibia with intact overlying bone cortex.

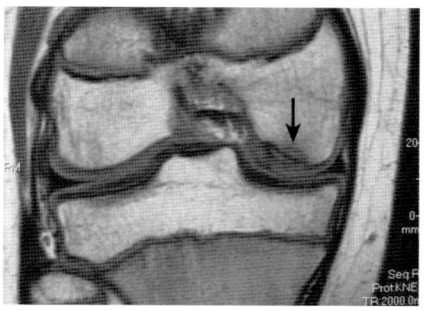

Figure 10.14 a, b Osteochondritis involving the lateral aspect of the medial femoral condyle in a 12-year-old boy that is seen as a poorly defined zone of low-intermediate signal in the subchondral marrow on coronal PDWI (**a**) and high signal on coronal FS T2WI (**b**).

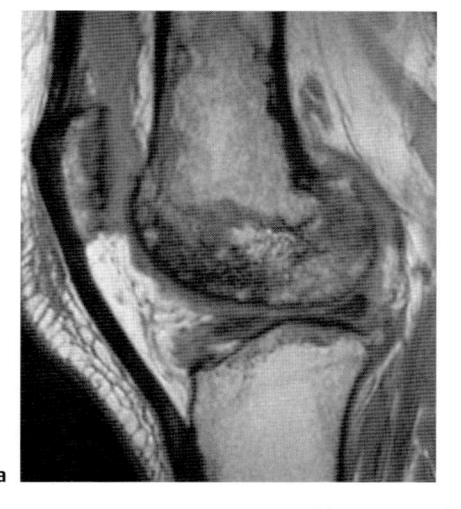

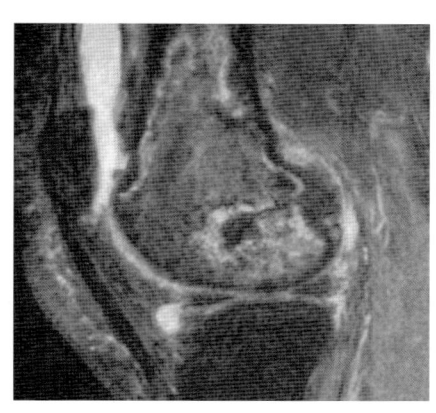

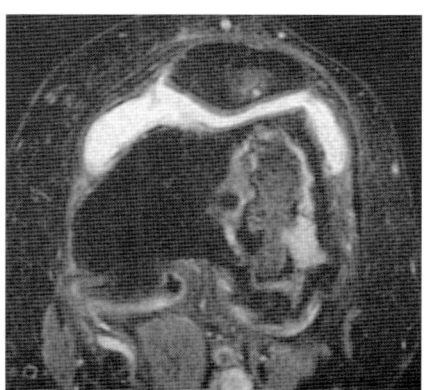

Figure 10.15 a–c A 49-year-old woman with a bone infarct in the distal femur as seen on sagittal PDWI (**a**), and sagittal (**b**) and axial (**c**) FS T2WI.

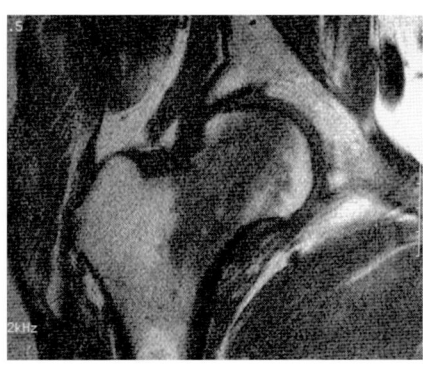

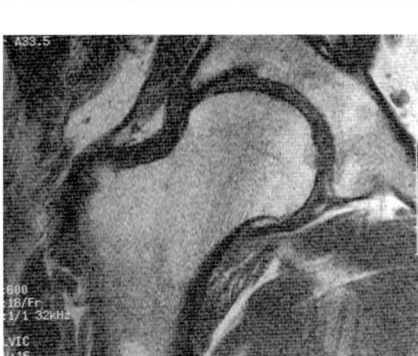

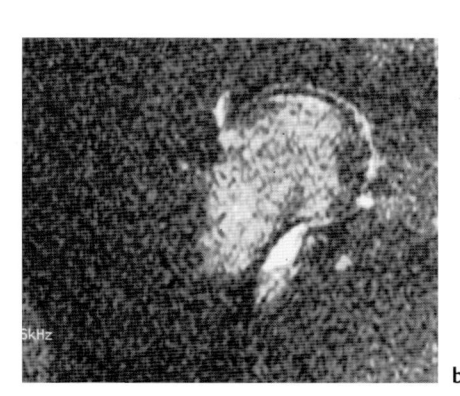

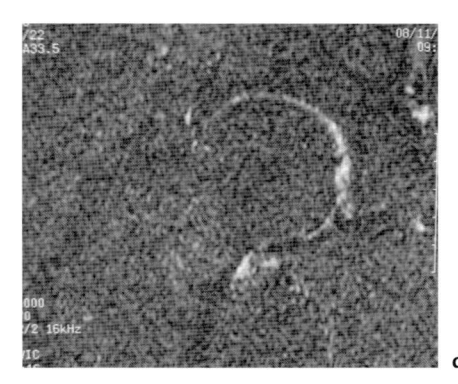

Figure 10.16 a–d A 51-year-old man with hip pain. MRI showing acute bone marrow edema with a poorly defined zone with low-intermediate signal in the marrow of the proximal femur on coronal T1WI (**a**) with corresponding high signal on coronal FS T2WI (**b**). The abnormal marrow signal resolved 2 months later, as seen on coronal T1WI (**c**) and FS T2WI (**d**).

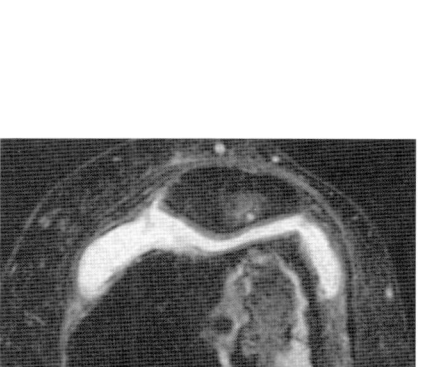

Table 10 (Continued) Solitary intramedullary lesions located near the ends of tubular bones		
Lesion	**MRI Findings**	**Comments**
Osteomyelitis (Fig. 10.17)	In **acute osteomyelitis**, poorly defined zones of low or low-intermediate signal on T1WI; and high signal on T2WI, STIR, and FS T2WI are seen in the marrow. Loss of definition of the low signal line of the cortical margins is often observed on T1WI, T2WI, STIR, and FS T2WI. After Gd-contrast administration, irregular zones of contrast enhancement are seen in the involved marrow on FS T1WI. In the **subacute phase of osteomyelitis**, the pyogenic process becomes more localized. The zone of transition between normal and abnormal bone is sharper and more well-defined in subacute and chronic osteomyelitis than with acute osteomyelitis.	Infection of bone that can result from hematogenous spread of microorganisms as well as from trauma-direct inoculation, extension from adjacent tissues, and complications from surgery. Bacteria such as *Staphylococcus aureus* and *Streptococcus pyogenes* are the most common infectious organisms. Can also result from other bacteria as well as *Mycobacterium tuberculosis*, fungi, parasites, and viruses. **(See Atlas Chapter A 63)**
Eosinophilic granuloma (Fig. 10.18)	Intramedullary lesion associated with trabecular and cortical bone destruction which typically has low-intermediate signal on T1WI and PDWI and heterogeneous slightly high to high signal on T2WI. Poorly defined zones of high signal on T2WI are usually seen in the marrow peripheral to the lesions secondary to inflammatory changes. Extension of lesions from the marrow into adjacent soft tissues through areas of cortical disruption are commonly seen as well as linear periosteal zones of high signal on T2WI. Lesions typically show prominent Gd-contrast enhancement in marrow and in extraosseous soft tissue portions of the lesions.	Benign tumor-like lesions consisting of Langerhans' cells (histiocytes) and variable amounts of lymphocytes, polymorphonuclear cells, and eosinophils. Account for 1% of primary bone lesions and 8% of tumor-like lesions. Occur in patients with median age = 10 years, average = 13.5 years, peak incidence is between 5 and 10 years, 80 to 85% occur in patients less than 30 years. **(See Atlas Chapter A 18)**
Malignant		
Metastatic lesion	Single or multiple well-circumscribed or poorly defined infiltrative lesions involving marrow associated with cortical destruction and extraosseous extension. Lesions often have low-intermediate signal on T1WI, low, intermediate, and/or high signal on T2WI and FS T2WI, usually show Gd-contrast enhancement. Cortical destruction and tumor extension into the extraosseous soft tissues can occur. Pathologic fractures can be associated with metastatic lesions involving tubular bones and vertebrae. Periosteal reaction is uncommon.	Metastatic lesions typically occur in the marrow with or without cortical destruction and extraosseous tumor extension. **(See Atlas Chapter A 50)**
Plasmacytoma (Fig. 10.19)	Well-circumscribed or poorly defined infiltrative lesions involving marrow, low-intermediate signal on T1WI, intermediate-high signal on T2WI and FS T2WI, usually show Gd-contrast-enhancement, eventual cortical bone destruction and extraosseous extension.	Malignant tumors composed of proliferating antibody-secreting plasma cells derived from single clones. Most common primary neoplasm of bone in adults, median = 60 years. Most patients are older than 40 years. May have variable destructive or infiltrative changes involving the axial and/or appendicular skeleton. **(See Atlas Chapter A 52)**

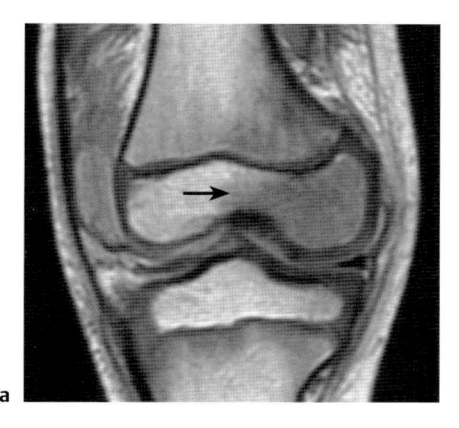

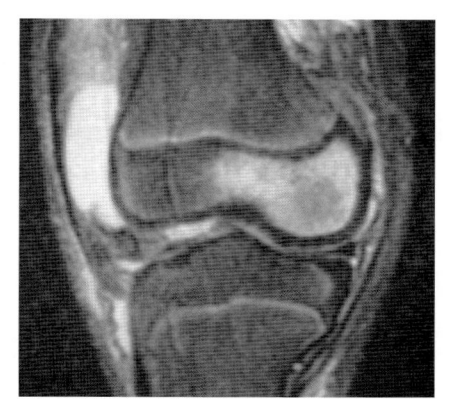

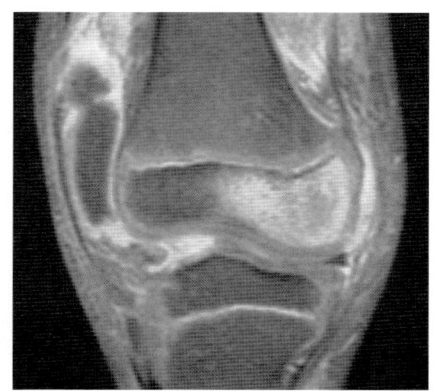

Figure 10.**17 a–c** An 11-year-old boy with septic arthritis and pyogenic osteomyelitis from *Staphylococcus aureus* involving the marrow of the femoral epiphysis. A poorly defined zone of low-intermediate signal is seen in the epiphyseal marrow on coronal T1WI (**a**) with corresponding high signal on coronal FS T2WI (**b**). Abnormal Gd-contrast enhancement is seen in the marrow on coronal FS T1WI (**c**) as well as within the septic joint collection.

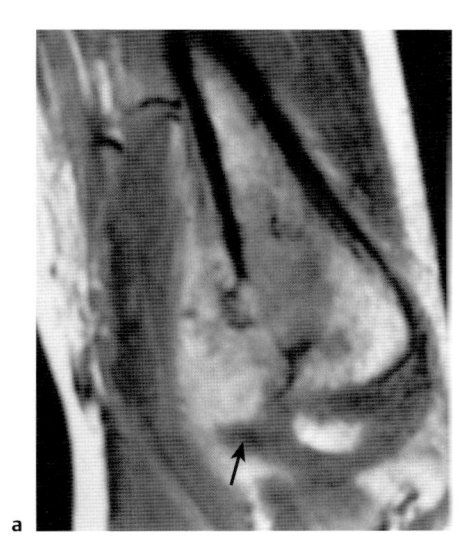

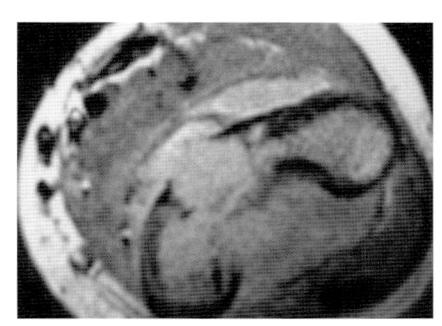

Figure 10.**18 a, b** A 5-year-old male with an eosinophilic granuloma involving the distal humerus. The lesion in the marrow is associated with cortical destruction and extra-osseous extension into the adjacent soft tissues as seen on sagittal Gd-contrast-enhanced T1WI (**a**) and axial PDWI (**b**).

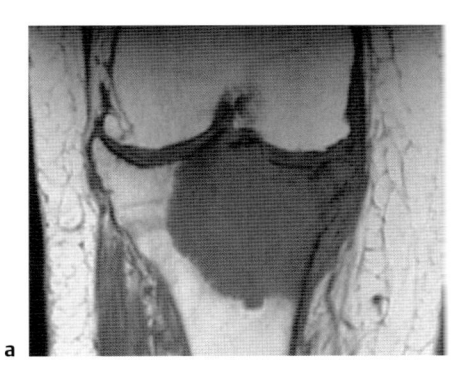

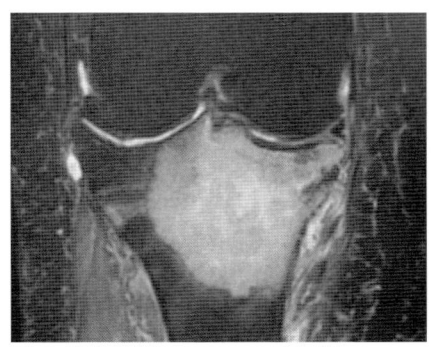

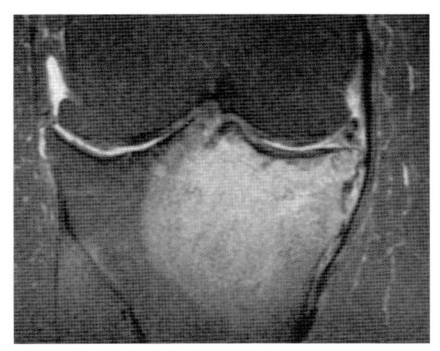

Figure 10.**19 a–c** A 77-year-old woman with myeloma involving the marrow of the proximal tibia that has low-intermediate signal on coronal T1WI (**a**) and high signal on coronal FS T2WI (**b**). The tumor shows Gd-contrast enhancement on FS T1WI (**c**).

Table 10 (Continued) Solitary intramedullary lesions located near the ends of tubular bones

Lesion	MRI Findings	Comments
Lymphoma (Fig. 10.20)	Non-Hodgkin lymphoma (NHL) and Hodgkin disease (HD) within bone typically appears as single or multifocal poorly defined or circumscribed intramedullary zones with low-intermediate signal on T1WI, and intermediate, slightly high, and/or high signal on T2WI and high signal on FS T2WI; often show Gd-contrast enhancement. Zones of cortical destruction may occur associated with extraosseous soft tissue extension.	Lymphoid tumors with neoplastic cells typically within lymphoid tissue (lymph nodes and reticuloendothelial organs). Unlike leukemia, lymphoma usually arises as discrete masses. Lymphomas are subdivided into HD and NHL. Almost all primary lymphomas of bone are B cell NHL. HD, mean age = 32 years. Osseous NHL, median = 35 years. **(See Atlas Chapter A 47)**
Leukemia	Single or multiple well-circumscribed or poorly defined infiltrative lesions involving marrow; low-intermediate signal on T1WI, intermediate-high signal on T2WI and FS T2WI, often shows Gd-contrast enhancement, +/− cortical bone destruction and extraosseous extension.	Malignant lymphoid neoplasms with involvement of bone marrow and with tumor cells also in peripheral blood. **(See Atlas Chapter A 41)**
Chondrosarcoma (Fig. 10.21)	Intramedullary tumors often have low-intermediate signal on T1WI, intermediate signal on PDWI, and heterogeneous intermediate-high signal on T2WI. Lesions usually show heterogeneous contrast enhancement.	Malignant tumors containing cartilage formed within sarcomatous stroma. Account for 12–21% of malignant bone lesions, 21–26% of primary sarcomas of bone, mean age = 40 years, median = 26 to 59 years. Clear cell chondrosarcoma is commonly located near the ends of long bones. **(See Atlas Chapter A 11)**
Osteosarcoma (Fig. 10.22)	Destructive intramedullary malignant lesions, low–intermediate signal on T1WI, mixed low, intermediate, high signal on T2WI, usually with matrix mineralization/ossification-low signal on T2W images, typically show Gd-contrast enhancement (usually heterogeneous). Zones of cortical destruction are typically seen through which tumors extend into the extraosseous soft tissues under an elevated periosteum. Lamellated and/or spiculated zones of bone formation can occur under the periosteal elevation secondary to tumor invasion and perforation of bone cortex.	Malignant tumor comprising proliferating neoplastic spindle cells that produce osteoid and/or immature tumoral bone most frequently arising within medullary bone. Two age peaks of incidence. The larger peak occurs between the ages of 10 and 20 and accounts for over half of the cases. The second smaller peak occurs in adults over 60 years and accounts for ~10% of the cases. **(See Atlas Chapter A 64)**
Ewing sarcoma (Fig. 10.23)	Destructive malignant lesions involving marrow, low-intermediate signal on T1WI, mixed low, intermediate, and/or high signal on T2WI and FS T2WI, typically shows Gd-contrast enhancement (usually heterogeneous). Extraosseous tumor extension through sites of cortical destruction is commonly seen beneath an elevated periosteum. Thin striated zones of low signal on T2WI can be sometimes seen oriented perpendicular to the long axis of the involved bone under the elevated periosteum representing the "hair on end" appearance of reactive bone formation secondary to the tumor. In long bones, tumors are most often located in the diaphyseal region, followed by the metadiaphyseal region.	Malignant primitive tumor of bone comprising undifferentiated small cells with round nuclei. Accounts for 6–11% of primary malignant bone tumors, 5–7% of primary bone tumors. Usually occurs between the ages of 5 and 30, males > females, locally invasive, high metastatic potential. **(See Atlas Chapter A 20)**

Ewing sarcoma **173**

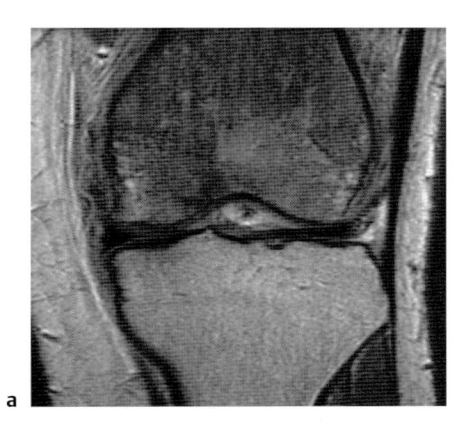

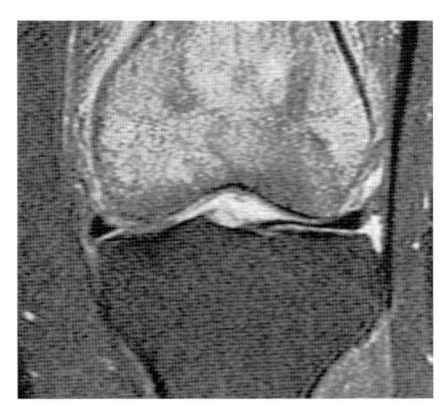

Figure 10.**20 a, b** A 26-year-old man with large cell NHL involving the marrow of the distal femur as seen as diffuse low signal on coronal PDWI (**a**) and high signal on coronal FS T2WI (**b**).

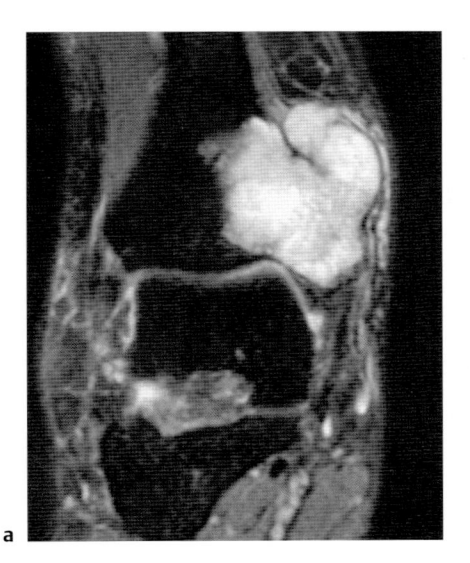

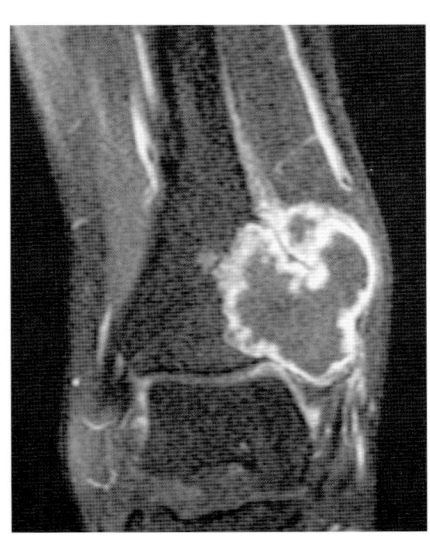

Figure 10.**21 a, b** A 44-year-old woman with a chondrosarcoma in the marrow of the distal tibia associated with cortical destruction and extraosseous extension of tumor. The tumor has high signal on coronal FS T2WI (**a**) and shows peripheral lobular Gd-contrast enhancement on FS T1WI (**b**).

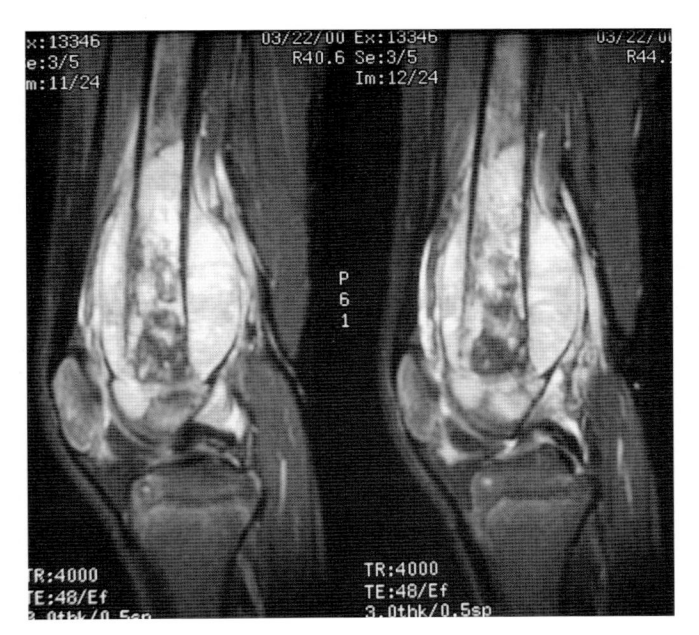

Figure 10.**22** A 9-year-old girl with osteosarcoma in the distal femoral marrow associated with cortical destruction and extraosseous extension as seen on sagittal FS T2WI.

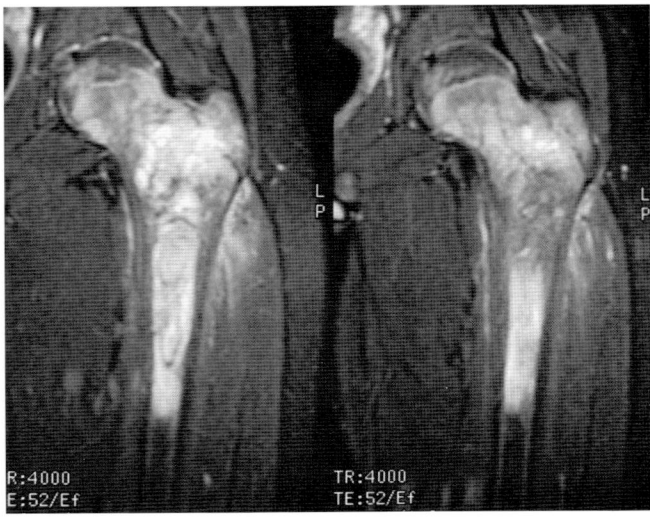

Figure 10.**23** A 15-year-old male with Ewing sarcoma in the marrow of the proximal femur that has high signal on coronal FS T2WI.

Lesion	MRI Findings	Comments
Malignant giant cell tumor (Fig. 10.24)	Well-defined lesions with or without thin low signal margins on T1WI and T2WI. Solid portions of giant cell tumors often have low to intermediate signal on T1WI and PDWI, intermediate to high signal on T2WI, and high signal on FS PDWI and FS T2WI. Signal heterogeneity on T2WI is not uncommon. Aneurysmal bone cysts are seen with 14% of giant cell tumors. Lesions show mild to prominent variable and often heterogeneous Gd-contrast enhancement. Cortical destruction and extraosseous tumor extension are frequently seen.	Aggressive tumors composed of neoplastic ovoid mononuclear cells and scattered multinucleated osteoclast-like giant cells. Up to 10% of all giant cell tumors are malignant. Benign giant cell tumors account for ~5 to 9.5% of all bone tumors and up to 23% of benign bone tumors. Malignant giant cell tumors account for 5.8% of all giant cell tumors. 75% occur between the ages of 15 and 45. **(See Atlas Chapter A 29)**
Fibrosarcoma	Intramedullary lesions with irregular margins, with or without associated cortical destruction and/or extraosseous soft tissue masses. Lesions usually have low-intermediate signal on T1WI and PDWI, and heterogeneous intermediate, slightly high, and/or high signal on T2WI. Lesions usually show heterogeneous Gd-contrast enhancement.	Uncommon malignant tumors consisting of bundles of fibroblasts/spindle cells with varying proportions of collagen, lacking other tissue differentiating features such as tumor bone, osteoid, or cartilage. Can be primary lesions (75%) or arise as secondary tumors (25%) associated with prior irradiation, Paget disease, bone infarct, chronic osteomyelitis, fibrous dysplasia, giant cell tumor. Account for 3–5% of primary malignant bone tumors, and 2–4% of all bone tumors, median age = 43 years. **(See Atlas Chapter A 25)**
Malignant fibrous histiocytoma	Intramedullary lesions with irregular margins and zones of cortical destruction and extraosseous extension. Tumors often have low-intermediate signal on T1WI; low-intermediate signal on PDWI, and heterogeneous intermediate-high signal on T2WI and FS T2WI. Invasion into joints occurs in 30%. May be associated with bone infarcts, bone cysts, chronic osteomyelitis, Paget disease, and other treated primary bone tumors. Lesions usually show heterogeneous Gd-contrast prominent enhancement.	Malignant tumor involving soft tissue and rarely bone derived from undifferentiated mesenchymal cells. Contains cells with limited cellular differentiation such as mixtures of fibroblasts, myofibroblasts, histiocyte-like cells, anaplastic giant cells, and inflammatory cells. Accounts for 1–5% of primary malignant bone tumors and < 1–3% of all primary bone tumors, patient ages range from 11 to 80 years, median = 48 years, mean = 55 years. **(See Atlas Chapter A 48)**
Hemangioendothelioma (Fig. 10.25)	Intramedullary tumors which often have low-intermediate and/or high signal on T1WI, and heterogeneous intermediate-high signal on T2WI and FS T2WI with or without zones of low signal. Cortical expansion with or without extraosseous extension of tumor through zones of cortical destruction can occur. Lesions often show prominent heterogeneous Gd-contrast enhancement.	Low-grade vasoformative/endothelial malignant neoplasms that are locally aggressive and rarely metastasize compared with the high-grade endothelial tumors such as angiosarcoma. Account for less than 1% of primary malignant bone tumors. Patients range from 10 to 82 years, median = 36 to 47 years. Patients with multifocal lesions tend to be ~10 years younger on average than those with unifocal tumors. **(See Atlas Chapter A 33)**

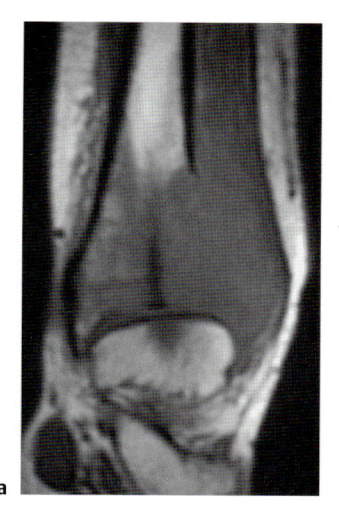

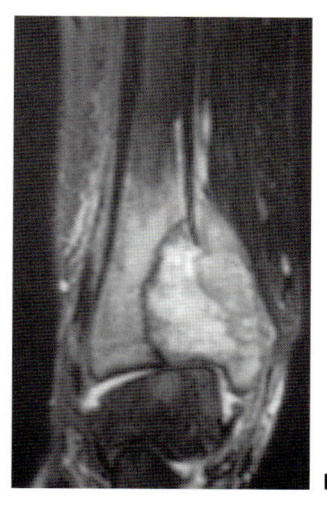

Figure 10.**24** A 16-year-old male with a malignant giant cell tumor of the distal tibia associated with destruction of cortical bone with extraosseous extension as seen on coronal T1WI (**a**) and FS T2WI (**b**).

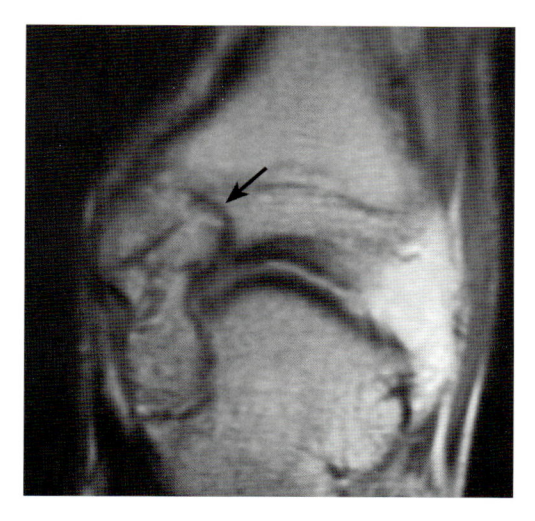

Figure 10.**25** A 19-year-old man with hemangioendothelioma involving the distal tibia with cortical disruption and tumor extension into the ankle joint as seen on coronal T2WI.

References

Fracture

Ahovuo JA, Kiuru MJ, Visuri T. Fatigue stress fractures of the sacrum: diagnosis with MR imaging. *Eur Radiol* March 2004;14(3):500–505. Epub October 24, 2003.

Berger FH, de Jonge MC, Maas M. Stress fractures in the lower extremity. The importance of increasing awareness amongst radiologists. *Eur J Radiol* 2007;62:16–26.

Grangier C, Garcia J, Howarth NR, May M, Rossier P. Role of MRI in the diagnosis of insufficiency fractures of the sacrum and acetabular roof. *Skeletal Radiol* 1997;26:517–524.

Meyers SP, Wiener SN. Magnetic resonance imaging features of fractures using the short tau inversion recovery (STIR) sequence: correlation with radiographic findings. *Skeletal Radiol* 1991;20(7): 499–507.

Pham T, Azulay-Parrado J, Champsaur P, Chagnaud C, Legré V, Lafforgue P. Occult osteoporotic vertebral fractures. Vertebral body fractures without radiologic collapse. *Spine* 2005;30(21):2430–2435.

Takahara K, Kamimura M, Nakagawa H, Hashidate H, Uchiyama S. Radiographic evaluation of vertebral fractures in osteoporotic patients. *J Clin Neurosci* 2007;14:122–126.

Bone Contusion

Boks SS, Vroegindeweij D, Koes BW, Hunink MGM, Bierma-Zeinstra SMA. Follow-up of occult bone lesions detected at MR imaging: systematic review. *Radiology* March 2006;238(3):853–862.

Davies NH, Niall D, King LJ, Lavelle J, Healy JC. Magnetic resonance imaging of bone bruising in the acutely injured knee – short-term outcome. *Clin Radiol* 2004;59:439–445.

Osteochondritis Dissecans

Kijowski R, De Smet AA. MRI findings of osteochondritis dissecans of the capitellum with surgical correlation. *AJR* December 2005;185: 1453–1459.

O'Connor MA, Palaniappan M, Khan N, Bruce CE. Osteochondritis dissecans of the knee in children. *J Bone Joint Surg* March 2002; 84-B(2):258–262.

Sanders TG, Paruchuri NB, Zlatkin MB. MRI of osteochondral defects of the lateral femoral condyle: incidence and pattern of injury after transient lateral dislocation of the patella. *AJR* November 2006;187: 1332–1337.

Schmid MR, Hodler J, Vienne P, Binkert CA, Zanetti M. Bone marrow abnormalities of foot and ankle: STIR versus T1-weighted contrast-enhanced fat-suppressed spin-echo MR imaging. *Radiology* August 2002;224(2):463–469.

Transient Bone Marrow Edema

Balakrishnan A, Schemitsch EH, Pearce D, McKee MD. Distinguishing transient osteoporosis of the hip from avascular necrosis. *Can J Surg* June 2003;46(3):187–192.

Malizos KN, Zibis AH, Dailiana Z, Hantes M, Karahalios T, Karantanas AH. MR imaging findings in transient osteoporosis of the hip. *Eur J Radiol* 2004;50:238–244.

Toms AP, Marshall TJ, Becker E, Donell ST, Lobo-Mueller EM, Barker T. Regional migratory osteoporosis: a review illustrated by five cases. *Clin Radiol* 2005;60:425–438.

Yamamoto T, Kubo T, Hirasawa Y, Noguchi Y, Iwamoto Y, Sueishi K. A clinicopathologic study of transient osteoporosis of the hip. *Skeletal Radiol* 1999;28:621–627.

Table 11 Solitary intramedullary metadiaphyseal lesions

Lesion	MRI Findings	Comments
Benign		
Nonossifying fibroma (Fig. 11.1)	Well-circumscribed eccentric intramedullary lesions in the metadiaphyseal regions of long bones that have mixed low-intermediate signal on T1WI, and mixed low, intermediate, and/or high signal on T2WI, PDWI, and FS T2WI. Zones of low signal on T1WI, PDWI, and T2WI can be seen in the central portions of the lesions. Zones with varying thickness of low signal on T1WI, PDWI, and T2WI are seen at the margins of the lesions representing bone sclerosis. Internal septations are commonly seen as zones of low signal on T2WI in these lesions. Lesions can show Gd-contrast enhancement (heterogeneous > homogeneous patterns).	Common benign fibrohistiocytic lesions in the metaphyseal portions of long bones that are comprised of whorls of fibroblastic cells combined with smaller amounts of multinucleated giant cells and xanthomatous cells. Usually asymptomatic, 95% occur between the ages of 5 and 20, median = 14 years. **(See Atlas Chapter A 26)**
Enchondroma (Fig. 11.2)	Lobulated intramedullary lesions with well-defined borders, mean size = 5 cm. Lesions usually have low-intermediate signal on T1WI and intermediate signal on PDWI. On T2WI and FS T2WI, lesions usually have predominantly high signal with foci and/or bands of low signal representing areas of matrix mineralization and fibrous strands. Lesions typically show Gd-contrast enhancement in various patterns (peripheral curvilinear lobular, central nodular/septal and peripheral lobular, or heterogeneous diffuse).	Benign intramedullary lesions composed of hyaline cartilage, represent ~10% of benign bone tumors. Enchondromas can be solitary (88%) or multiple (12%). Median age = 35 years, peak in 3rd and 4th decades. **(See Atlas Chapter A 8)**
Unicameral bone cyst (Fig. 11.3)	Unicameral bone cysts (UBCs) often have a peripheral rim of low signal on T1WI and T2WI adjacent to normal medullary bone. UBCs usually contain fluid with low to low-intermediate signal on T1WI; low-intermediate; and high signal on T2WI. Fluid–fluid levels may occur. For UBCs without pathologic fracture, thin peripheral Gd-contrast enhancement can be seen at the margins of lesions. UBCs with pathologic fracture can have heterogeneous or homogeneous low-intermediate or slightly high signal on T1WI, and heterogeneous or homogeneous high signal on T2WI and FS T2WI. UBCs complicated by fracture can have internal septations and fluid–fluid levels, as well as irregular peripheral Gd-contrast enhancement and at internal septations.	Intramedullary non-neoplastic cavities filled with serous or serosanguineous fluid. Account for 9% of primary tumor-like lesions of bone. 85% occur in the first 2 decades, median = 11 years. **(See Atlas Chapter A 3)**

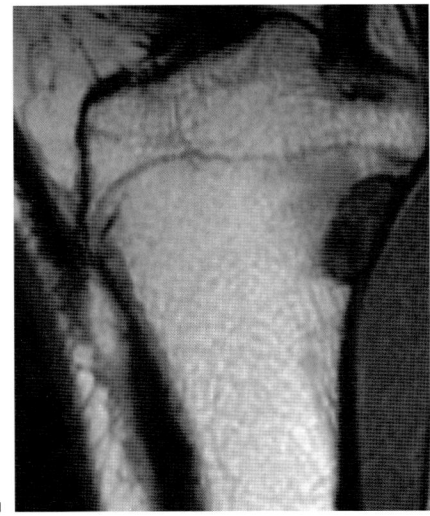

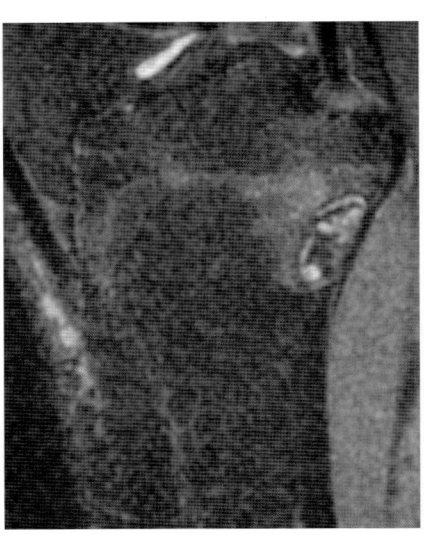

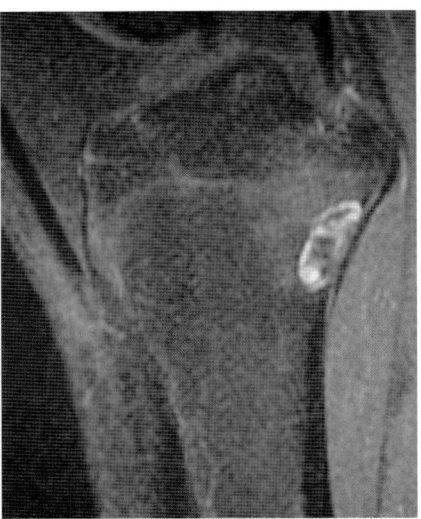

Figure 11.1 a–c A 15-year-old female with a nonossifying fibroma in the dorsal proximal tibia that has a thin peripheral rim of low signal surrounding a central zone with low-intermediate signal on sagittal T1WI (**a**) and mixed low and high signal on FS T2WI (**b**). The lesion shows thin marginal and central Gd-contrast enhancement on sagittal FS T1WI (**c**).

Osteosarcoma **185**

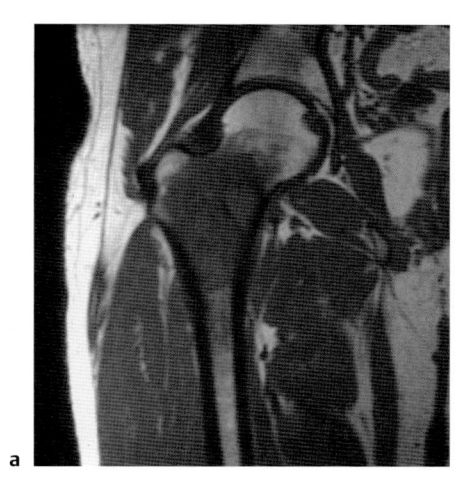

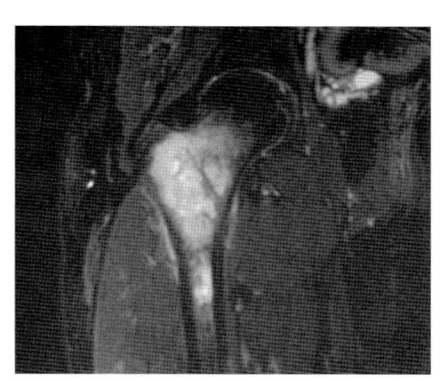

Figure 11.**15 a, b** A 26-year-old man with a metastatic lesion in the metadiaphyseal portion of the proximal femur from seminoma that has low-intermediate signal on coronal T1WI (**a**) and high signal on coronal FS T2WI (**b**). A thin zone of periosteal reaction with high signal on FS T2WI is also seen laterally.

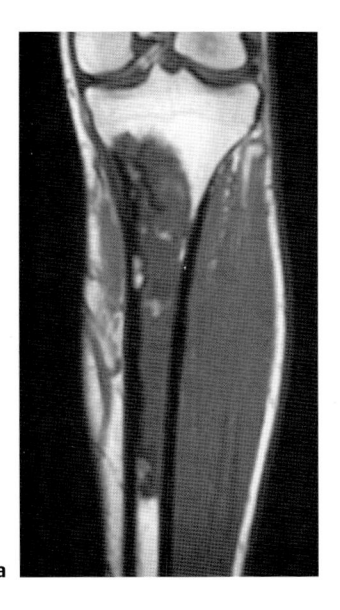

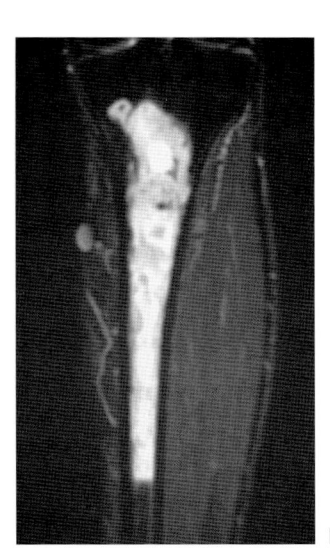

Figure 11.**16 a, b** A 19-year-old man with a large B cell non-Hodgkin lymphoma in the metadiaphyseal marrow of the proximal tibia that has mostly intermediate signal on coronal T1WI (**a**) and high signal on coronal FS T2WI (**b**).

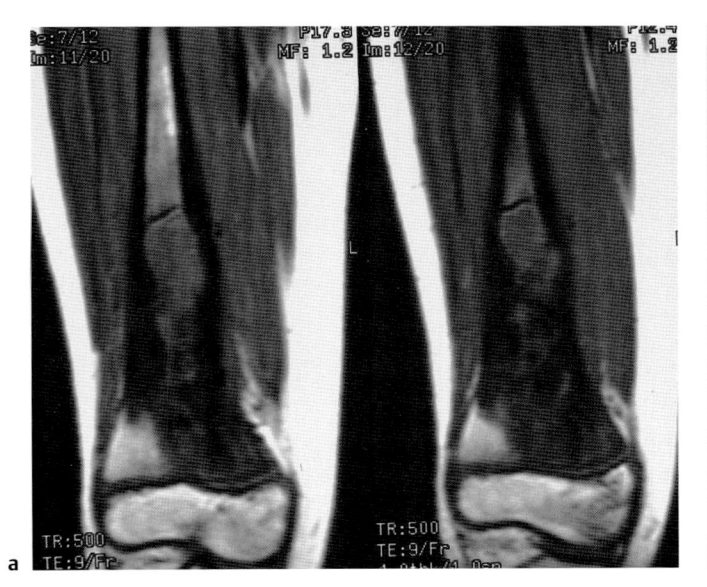

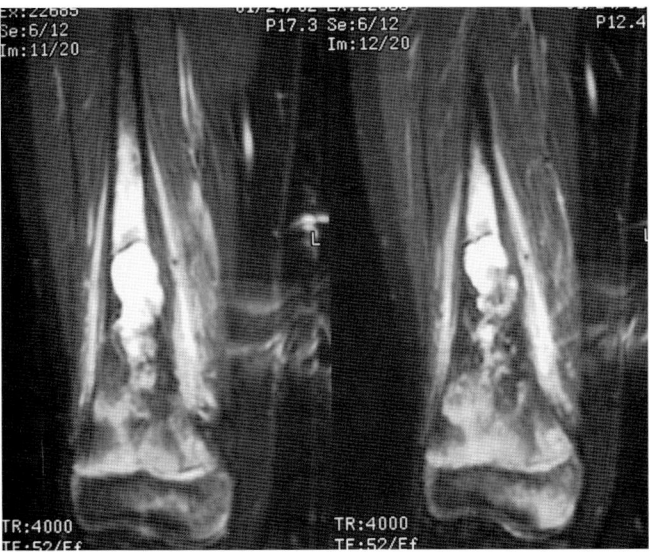

Figure 11.**17 a, b** A 9-year-old boy with a chondroblastic osteosarcoma in the metadiaphyseal marrow of the distal femur that has low and intermediate signal on coronal T1WI (**a**) and heterogeneous high and low signal on coronal FS T2WI (**b**).

Table 11 (Continued) Solitary intramedullary metadiaphyseal lesions		
Lesion	**MRI Findings**	**Comments**
Ewing sarcoma (Fig. 11.18)	Destructive malignant lesions involving marrow, low-intermediate signal on T1WI, mixed low, intermediate, and/or high signal on T2WI and FS T2WI, typically shows Gd-contrast enhancement (usually heterogeneous). Extraosseous tumor extension through sites of cortical destruction is commonly seen beneath an elevated periosteum. Thin striated zones of low signal on T2WI can be sometimes seen oriented perpendicular to the long axis of the involved bone under the elevated periosteum representing the "hair on end" appearance of reactive bone formation secondary to the tumor. In long bones, tumors are most often located in the diaphyseal region, followed by the metadiaphyseal region.	Malignant primitive tumor of bone comprised of undifferentiated small cells with round nuclei. Accounts for 6–11% of primary malignant bone tumors, 5–7% of primary bone tumors. Usually occurs between the ages of 5 and 30, males > females, locally invasive, high metastatic potential. **(See Atlas Chapter A 20)**
Chondrosarcoma (Fig. 11.19)	Intramedullary tumors often have low-intermediate signal on T1WI, intermediate signal on PDWI, and heterogeneous intermediate-high signal on T2WI. Lesions usually show heterogeneous contrast enhancement. Zones of cortical destruction can be seen with extraosseous extension of tumor.	Chondrosarcomas are malignant tumors containing cartilage formed within sarcomatous stroma. Account for 12–21% of malignant bone lesions, 21–26% of primary sarcomas of bone, 5 to 91 years, mean = 40 years, median = 26 to 59 years. **(See Atlas Chapter A 11)**
Fibrosarcoma	Intramedullary lesions with irregular margins, with or without associated cortical destruction and/or extraosseous soft tissue masses. Lesions usually have low-intermediate signal on T1WI and PDWI, and heterogeneous intermediate, slightly high, and/or high signal on T2WI. Lesions usually show heterogeneous Gd-contrast enhancement.	Fibrosarcomas are uncommon malignant tumors consisting of bundles of fibroblasts/spindle cells with varying proportions of collagen, lacking other tissue differentiating features such as tumor bone, osteoid, or cartilage. Can be primary lesions (75%) or arise as secondary tumors (25%) associated with prior irradiation, Paget disease, bone infarct, chronic osteomyelitis, fibrous dysplasia, giant cell tumor. Account for 3–5% of primary malignant bone tumors, and 2–4% of all bone tumors, median age = 43 years. **(See Atlas Chapter A 25)**
Malignant fibrous histiocytoma (Fig. 11.20)	Intramedullary lesions with irregular margins and zones of cortical destruction and extraosseous extension. Tumors often have low-intermediate signal on T1WI, low-intermediate signal on PDWI, and heterogeneous intermediate-high signal on T2WI and FS T2WI. Invasion into joints occurs in 30%. May be associated with bone infarcts, bone cysts, chronic osteomyelitis, Paget disease, and other treated primary bone tumors. Lesions usually show heterogeneous Gd-contrast prominent enhancement.	Malignant tumor involving soft tissue and rarely bone derived from undifferentiated mesenchymal cells. Contains cells with limited cellular differentiation such as mixtures of fibroblasts, myofibroblasts, histiocyte-like cells, anaplastic giant cells, and inflammatory cells. Accounts for 1–5% of primary malignant bone tumors and <1–3% of all primary bone tumors, patient ages range from 11 to 80 years, median = 48 years, mean = 55 years. **(See Atlas Chapter A 48)**

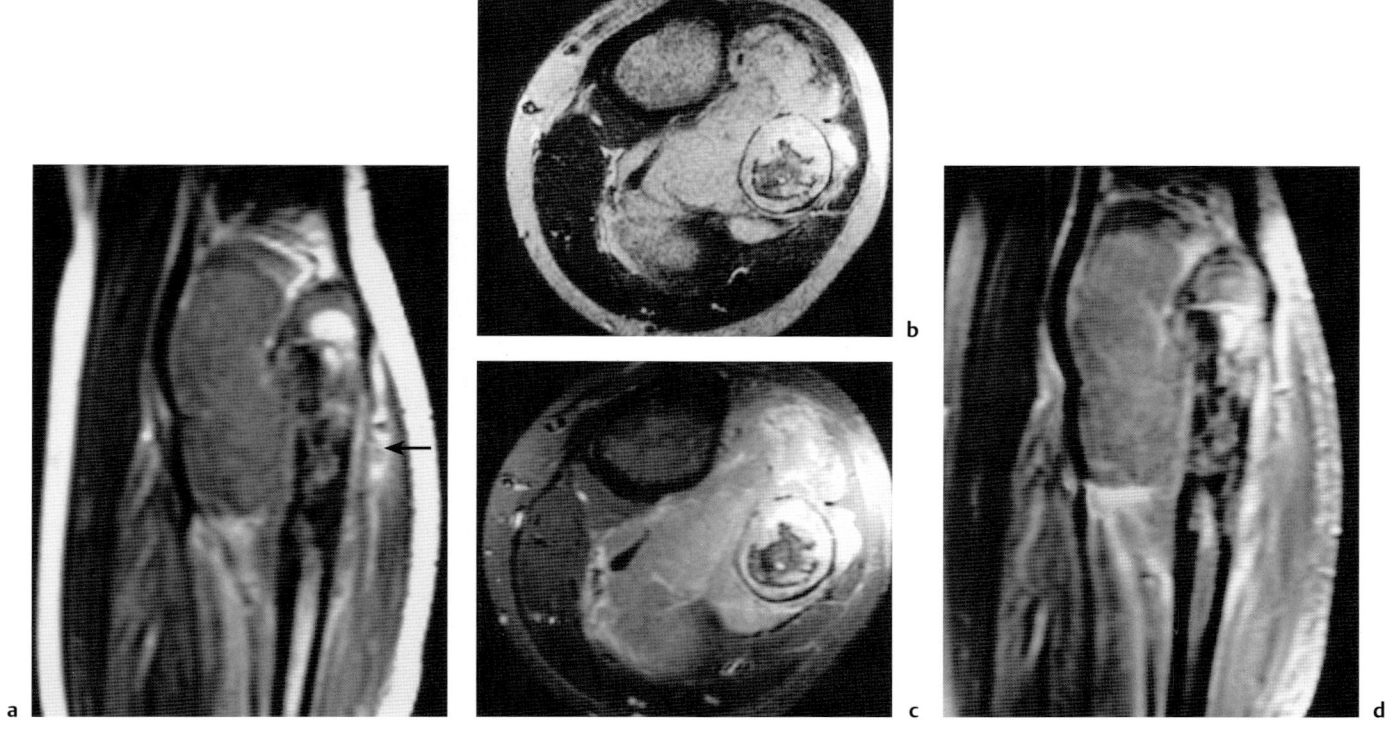

Figure 11.**18a–d** A 9-year-old boy with Ewing sarcoma in the metadiaphyseal portion of the proximal fibula that has intermediate signal on sagittal T1WI (**a**) and high signal in the marrow on axial T2WI (**b**), and has associated cortical destruction, periosteal elevation, and extraosseous tumor extension. The intra- and extraosseous tumor shows prominent Gd-contrast enhancement on axial (**c**) and sagittal (**d**) FS T1WI.

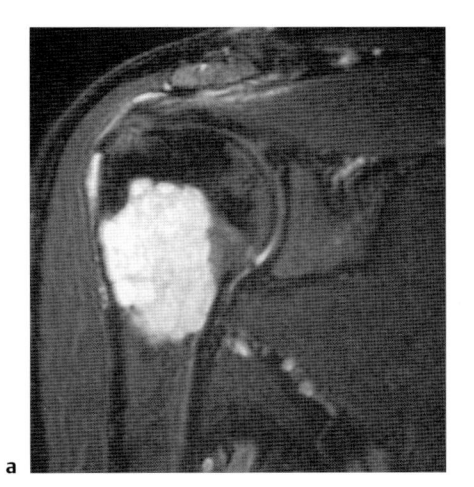

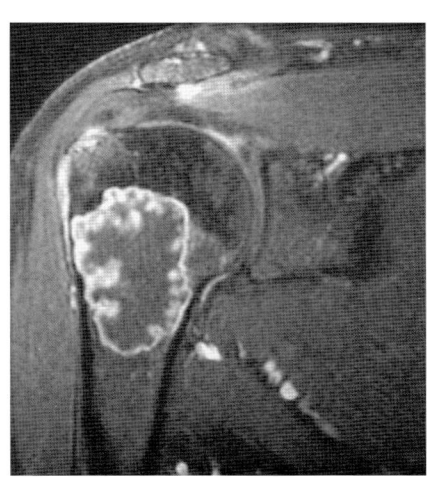

Figure 11.**19a, b** A 45-year-old woman with a low-grade chondrosarcoma in the metadiaphyseal portion of the proximal humerus that has high signal on coronal FS T2WI (**a**). The tumor shows thin peripheral lobular Gd-contrast enhancement on coronal FS T1WI (**b**).

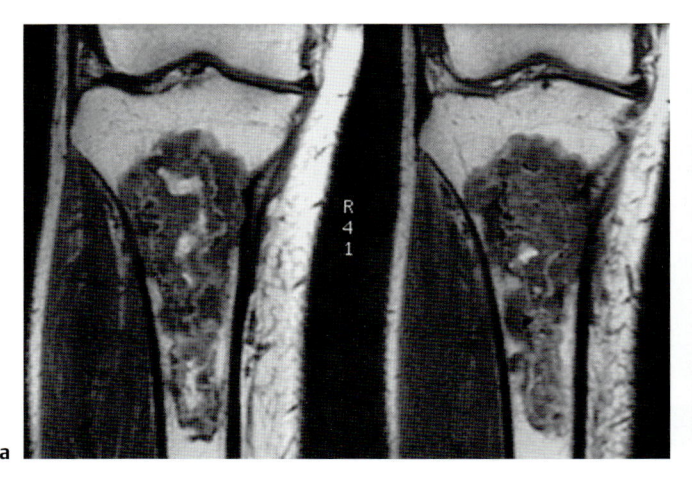

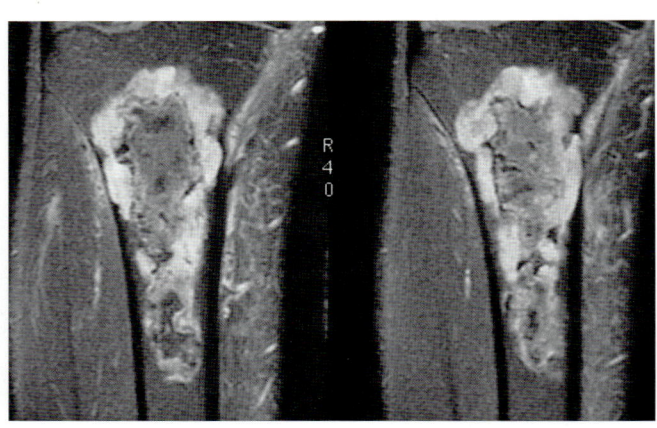

Figure 11.**20 a, b** A 53-year-old man with a malignant fibrous histiocytoma in the metadiaphyseal region of the proximal tibia that arose from a bone infarct. The lesion has low, intermediate, and high signal on coronal T1WI (**a**), and shows heterogeneous Gd-contrast enhancement on coronal FS T1WI (**b**). The lesion is associated with cortical erosions.

References

Stress Fracture

Ahovuo JA, Kiuru MJ, Visuri T. Fatigue stress fractures of the sacrum: diagnosis with MR imaging. *Eur Radiol* March 2004;14(3):500–505. Epub October 24, 2003.

Berger FH, de Jonge MC, Maas M. Stress fractures in the lower extremity. The importance of increasing awareness amongst radiologists. *Eur J Radiol* 2007;62:16–26.

Grangier C, Garcia J, Howarth NR, May M, Rossier P. Role of MRI in the diagnosis of insufficiency fractures of the sacrum and acetabular roof. *Skeletal Radiol* 1997;26:517–524.

Meyers SP, Wiener SN. Magnetic resonance imaging features of fractures using the short tau inversion recovery (STIR) sequence: correlation with radiographic findings. *Skeletal Radiol* 1991;20(7): 499–507.

Table 12	Solitary intramedullary diaphyseal lesions	
Lesion	**MRI Findings**	**Comments**
Benign		
Stress fracture (Fig. 12.1)	Fractures often have associated poorly defined zones of abnormal marrow signal with low signal on T1WI, and high signal on T2WI and FS T2WI. Gd-contrast enhancement is typically seen in the postfracture period. Angulated cortical margins and periosteal high signal on FS T2WI can be seen. A curvilinear zone of low signal on T2WI and FS T2WI may be seen within the marrow edema, which is often perpendicular or oblique to the long axis of the involved bone.	Stress fractures can result from persistent chronic mechanical overload, as well as from osteoporosis or osteomalacia. Primary bone tumors/lesions, metastatic disease, bone infarcts.
Bone infarct (Fig. 12.2)	In the early phases of ischemia, poorly-defined zones with high signal on FS T2WI or STIR are seen in the marrow. Later a double-line sign (curvilinear adjacent zones of low and high signal on T2WI) is commonly seen at the edges of the infarcts representing the borders of osseous resorption and healing. Irregular Gd-contrast enhancement can be seen from granulation tissue in-growth.	Zones of ischemic death involving bone trabeculae and marrow that may be idiopathic or result from: trauma, corticosteroid treatment, chemotherapy, radiation treatment, occlusive vascular disease, collagen vascular and other autoimmune diseases, metabolic storage diseases (Gaucher, etc.), sickle cell disease, thalassemia, hyperbaric events / Caisson disease, pregnancy, alcohol abuse, pancreatitis, infections, and lymphoproliferative diseases. **(See Atlas Chapter A 37)**

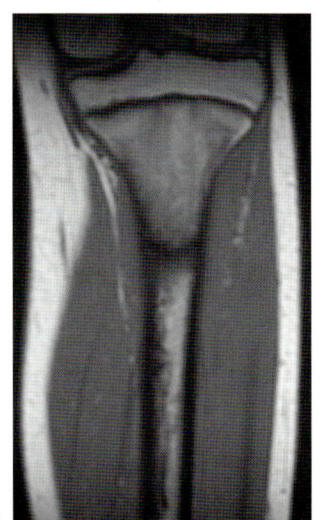

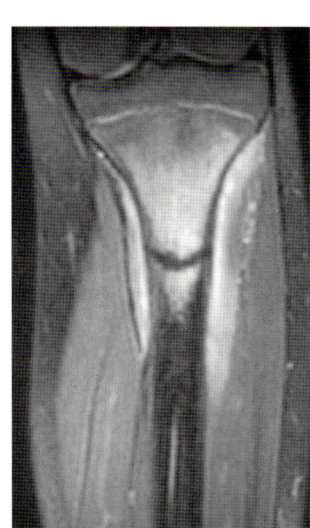

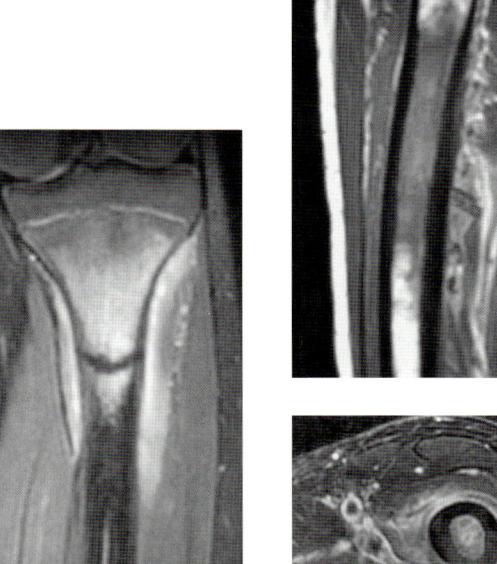

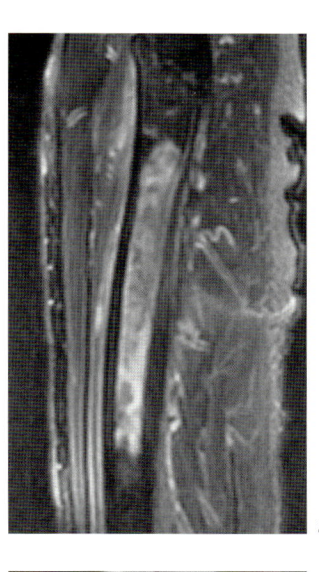

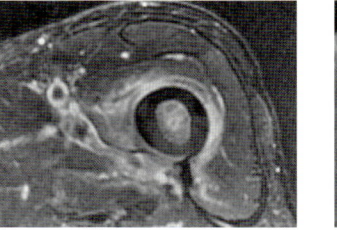

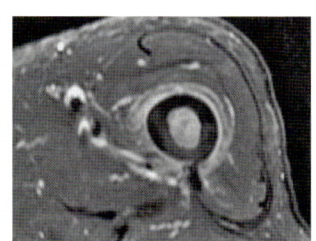

Figure 12.**1 a, b** A 12-year-old girl with a fatigue-type stress fracture in the proximal diaphysis of the tibia. A horizontal linear zone of low signal is seen within the marrow surrounded by a poorly defined zone of low-intermediate signal on coronal T1WI (**a**) and high signal on coronal FS T2WI (**b**). The high signal on FS T2WI from edema extends up into the metaphyseal marrow.

Figure 12.**2 a–d** A 76-year-old man with an acute bone infarct in the diaphysis of the femur that is seen as a poorly defined zone of low-intermediate signal in the marrow on sagittal T1WI (**a**), heterogeneous high signal on sagittal (**b**) and axial (**c**) FS T2WI with elevated thin periosteal reaction with adjacent high signal in the extraosseous soft tissues. The acute infarct shows Gd-contrast enhancement on axial FS T1WI (**d**).

Table 12 (Continued) **Solitary intramedullary diaphyseal lesions**

Lesion	MRI Findings	Comments
Fibrous dysplasia (Fig. 12.3)	MRI features depend on the proportions of bony spicules, collagen, fibroblastic spindle cells, hemorrhagic and/or cystic changes, and associated pathologic fracture if present. Lesions are usually well-circumscribed, and have low or low-intermediate signal on T1WI and PDWI. On T2WI, lesions have variable mixtures of low, intermediate, and/or high signal often surrounded by a low signal rim of variable thickness. Internal septations and cystic changes are seen in a minority of lesions. Bone expansion with thickened and/or thinned cortex can be seen. Lesions show Gd-contrast enhancement that varies in degree and pattern.	Benign medullary fibro-osseous lesion that can involve a single site (**mono-ostotic**) or multiple locations (**poly-ostotic**). Thought to occur from developmental failure in the normal process of remodeling primitive bone to mature lamellar bone with resultant zone or zones of immature trabeculae within dysplastic fibrous tissue. Accounts for ~10% of benign bone lesions. Patients range in age from <1 to 76 years. 75% occur before the age of 30 years. **(See Atlas Chapter A 27)**
Fibroxanthoma	Well-circumscribed eccentric intramedullary lesions in the diaphyseal regions of long bones which have mixed low–intermediate signal on T1WI, and mixed low, intermediate, and/or high signal on T2WI, PDWI, and FS T2WI. Zones of low signal on T1WI, PDWI, and T2WI can be seen in the central portions of the lesions. Zones with varying thickness of low signal on T1WI, PDWI, and T2WI are seen at the margins of the lesions representing bone sclerosis. Internal septations are commonly seen as zones of low signal on T2WI in these lesions. Lesions can show Gd-contrast enhancement (heterogeneous > homogeneous patterns).	Histologically identical to nonossifying fibromas but occur in diaphyseal portions of long bones. Lesions contain whorls of fibroblastic cells combined with smaller amounts of multinucleated giant cells and xanthomatous cells. Patients range in age from 6 to 74 years, 60% of patients are older than 20 years at diagnosis. **(See Atlas Chapter A 26)**
Enchondroma (Fig. 12.4)	Lobulated intramedullary lesions with well-defined borders that usually have low-intermediate signal on T1WI and intermediate signal on PDWI. On T2WI and FS T2WI, lesions usually have predominantly high signal with foci and/or bands of low signal representing areas of matrix mineralization and fibrous strands. No zones of abnormal high signal on T2WI are typically seen in the marrow outside the borders of the lesions. Lesions typically show Gd-contrast enhancement in various patterns (peripheral curvilinear lobular, central nodular/septal and peripheral lobular, or heterogeneous diffuse).	Benign intramedullary lesions composed of hyaline cartilage, represent ~10% of benign bone tumors. Enchondromas can be solitary (88%) or multiple (12%). Ollier disease is a dyschondroplasia involving endochondral-formed bone resulting in multiple enchondromas (enchondromatosis). Metachondromatosis is a combination of enchondromatosis and osteochondromatosis, and is rare. Maffucci disease refers to a syndrome with multiple enchondromas and soft tissue hemangiomas, and is very rare. Patients range in age from 3 to 83 years, median = 35 years, mean = 38 to 40 years, peak in 3rd and 4th decades. **(See Atlas Chapter A 8)**

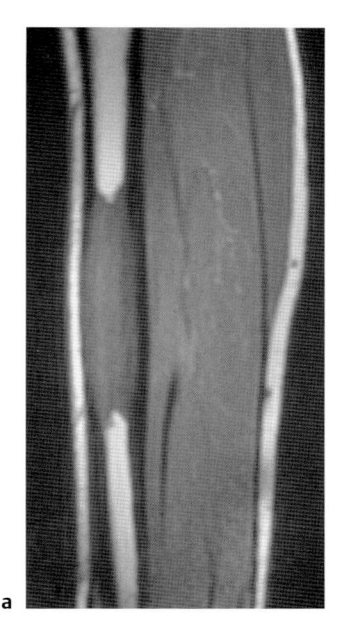

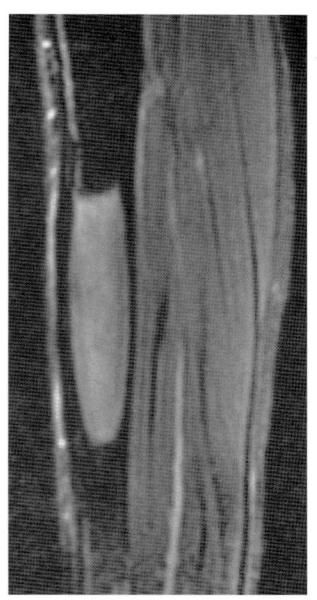

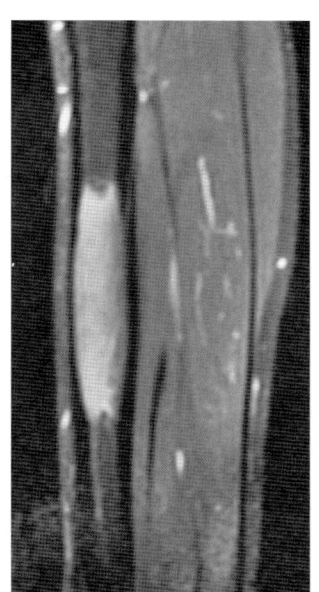

Figure 12.**3 a–c** A 19-year-old man with fibrous dysplasia involving the diaphysis of the tibia. The lesion is associated with slight expansion and thinning of adjacent cortical margins and has low-intermediate signal on sagittal T1WI (**a**), slightly high signal on sagittal FS T2WI (**b**), and Gd-contrast enhancement on sagittal FS T1WI (**c**).

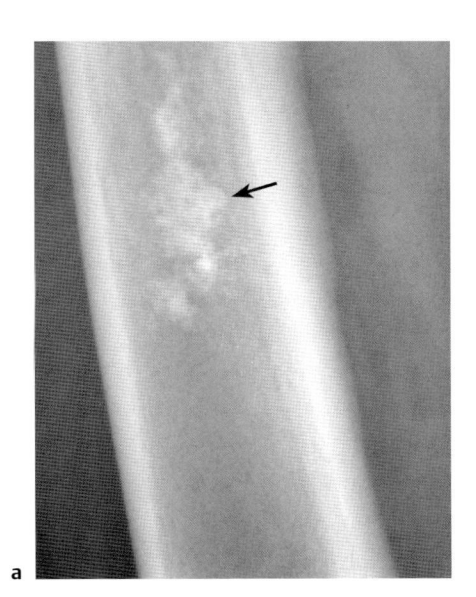

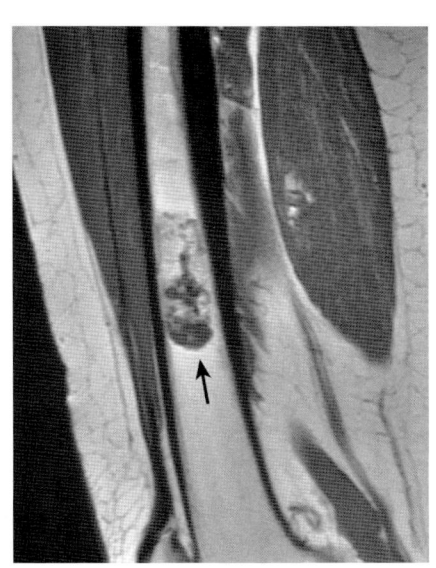

Figure 12.**4 a–d** A 47-year-old woman with an enchondroma in the diaphyseal portion of the femur that contains chondroid matrix mineralization on the lateral radiograph (**a**). The lesion has mixed low-intermediate signal on sagittal T1WI (**b**) and mixed intermediate and high signal on sagittal FS T2WI (**c**). The lesion shows heterogeneous Gd-contrast enhancement on sagittal FS T1WI (**d**).

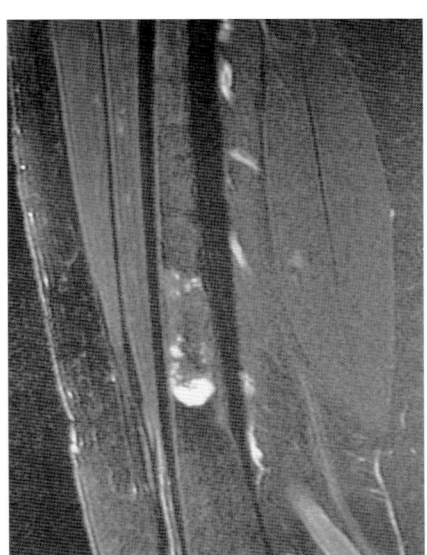

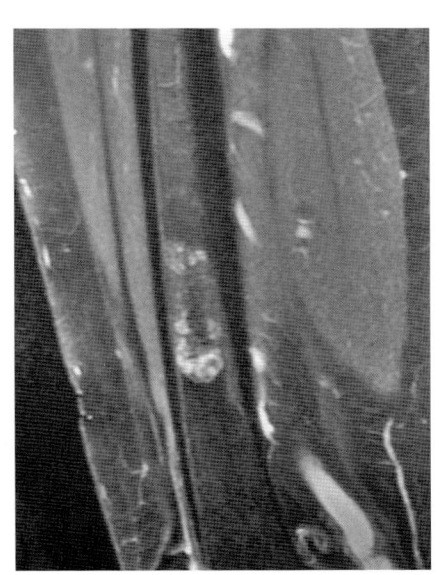

Table 12 (Continued) **Solitary intramedullary diaphyseal lesions**

Lesion	MRI Findings	Comments
Eosinophilic granuloma (Fig. 12.5)	Focal intramedullary lesion(s) associated with trabecular and cortical bone destruction that typically have low-intermediate signal on T1WI and PDWI and heterogeneous slightly high to high signal on T2WI. Poorly defined zones of high signal on T2WI are usually seen in the marrow peripheral to the lesions secondary to inflammatory changes. Extension of lesions from the marrow into adjacent soft tissues through areas of cortical disruption are commonly seen as well as linear periosteal zones of high signal on T2WI. Lesions typically show prominent Gd-contrast enhancement in marrow and in extraosseous soft tissue portions.	Benign tumor-like lesions consisting of Langerhans' cells (histiocytes), and variable amounts of lymphocytes, polymorphonuclear cells, and eosinophils. Account for 1 % of primary bone lesions, and 8 % of tumor-like lesions. Occur in patients with median age = 10 years, average = 13.5 years, peak incidence is between 5 and 10 years, 80–85 % occur in patients less than 30 years. **(See Atlas Chapter A 18)**
Osteomyelitis (Fig. 12.6)	Poorly defined zones with high signal on T2WI and FS T2WI and Gd-contrast enhancement are seen in marrow with associated zones of cortical destruction. Periosteal reaction can be seen as a peripheral rim of high signal on T2WI and FS T2WI and Gd-contrast enhancement on FS T1WI adjacent to the low signal of cortical bone. A subperiosteal abscess with high signal on T2WI and FS T2WI can be often seen elevating a single low signal thin band of periosteum.	Infection of bone that can result from hematogenous spread of microorganisms, trauma-direct inoculation, extension from adjacent tissues, and complications from surgery. *Staphylococcus aureus* and *Streptococcus pyogenes* are the most common bacterial infections involving bone. Osteomyelitis can also result from other bacteria as well as from other organisms such as *Mycobacterium tuberculosis*, fungi, parasites, and viruses. **(See Atlas Chapter A 63)**

Malignant

Metastatic lesion (Fig. 12.7)	Single or multiple well-circumscribed or poorly defined infiltrative lesions involving marrow associated with cortical destruction and extraosseous extension. Lesions often have low-intermediate signal on T1WI, low, intermediate, and/or high signal on T2WI and FS T2WI, usually show Gd-contrast enhancement. Cortical destruction and tumor extension into the extraosseous soft tissues frequently occurs. Pathologic fractures can be associated with metastatic lesions involving tubular bones and vertebrae. Periosteal reaction is uncommon.	Metastatic lesions typically occur in the marrow with or without cortical destruction and extraosseous tumor extension. **(See Atlas Chapter A 50)**

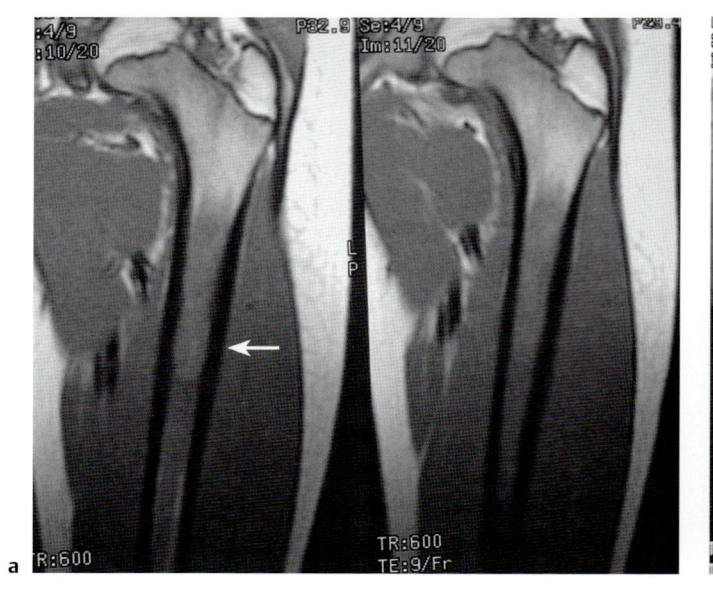

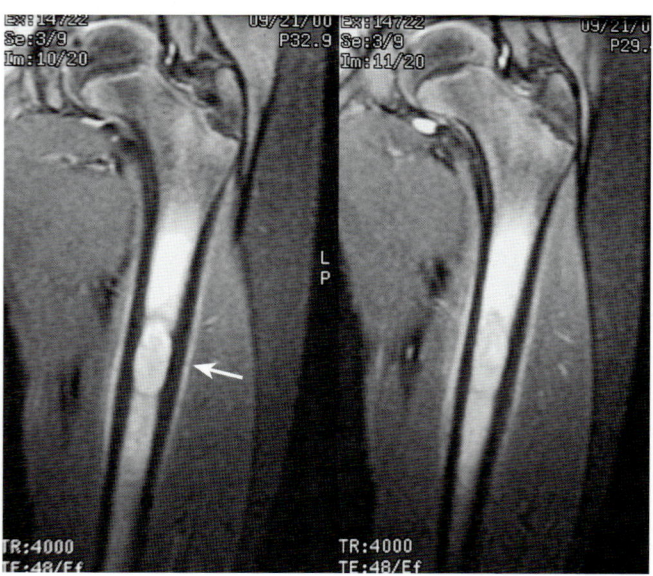

Figure 12.**5 a, b** An 18-year-old woman with an eosinophilic granuloma involving the diaphyseal marrow of the femur, seen as a poorly defined zone of low-intermediate signal on coronal T1WI (**a**). A thin marginal rim of low signal is seen surrounding a central zone of high signal on coronal FS T2WI (**b**), as well as a poorly defined zone of peripheral high signal in the adjacent marrow and thin periosteal reaction with high signal.

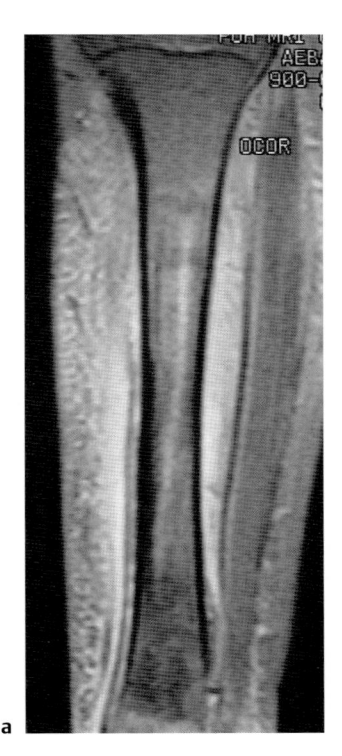

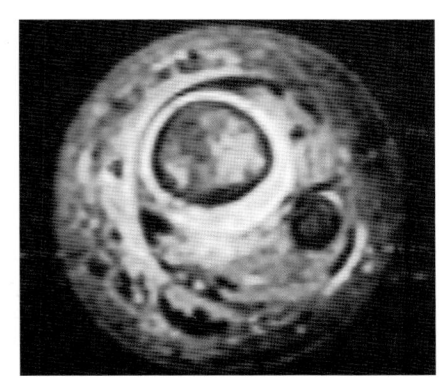

Figure 12.**6 a, b** A 9-year-old girl with pyogenic osteomyelitis involving the diaphysis of the tibia, seen as a poorly defined zone of Gd-contrast enhancement in the marrow associated with periosteal elevation and juxtacortical enhancement on coronal FS T1WI (**a**). Abnormal increased signal is seen in the marrow on axial STIR (**b**) as well as unilayer periosteal elevation surrounded by high signal in the extraosseous soft tissues.

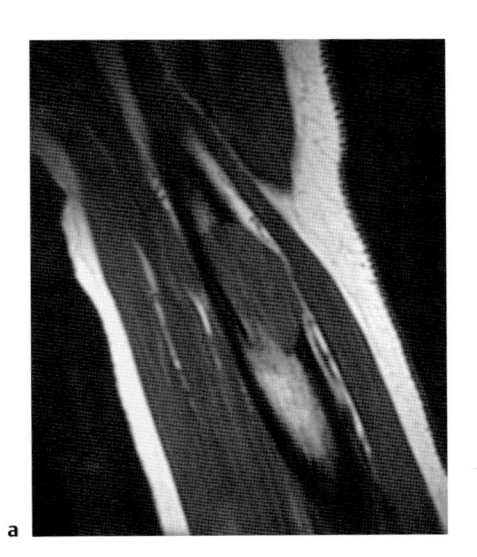

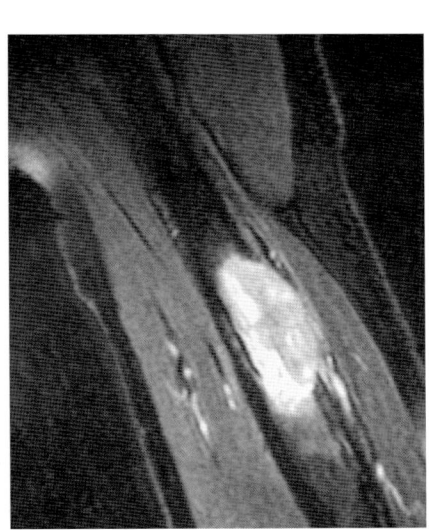

Figure 12.**7 a, b** A 63-year-old woman with metastatic lung carcinoma involving the diaphyseal portion of the humerus. The lesion has intermediate signal on sagittal T1WI (**a**) and high signal on sagittal FS T2WI (**b**). The tumor is seen extending from the marrow into the extraosseous soft tissues through a zone of cortical destruction.

Table 12 (Continued) Solitary intramedullary diaphyseal lesions

Lesion	MRI Findings	Comments
Plasmacytoma/myeloma (Fig. 12.8)	Multiple (myeloma) or single (plasmacytoma) are well-circumscribed or poorly defined diffuse infiltrative lesions involving marrow, low-intermediate signal on T1WI, intermediate-high signal on T2WI and FS T2WI, usually show Gd-contrast-enhancement, eventual cortical bone destruction and extraosseous extension.	Malignant tumors comprising proliferating antibody-secreting plasma cells derived from single clones. Most common primary neoplasm of bone in adults, median = 60 years. Most patients are older than 40 years. May have variable destructive or infiltrative changes involving the axial and/or appendicular skeleton. **(See Atlas Chapter A 52)**
Lymphoma (Fig. 12.9)	Non-Hodgkin lymphoma (NHL) and Hodgkin disease (HD) within bone typically appear as single or multifocal poorly defined or circumscribed intramedullary zones with low-intermediate signal on T1WI, and intermediate, slightly high, and/or high signal on T2WI and high signal on FS T2WI; often show Gd-contrast enhancement. Zones of cortical destruction may occur associated with extraosseous soft tissue extension. HD involving bone with associated sclerosis seen on plain films or CT usually have low signal on T1WI and variable/mixed signal on T2WI. In some cases of NHL, intramedullary tumor may be associated with bulky extraosseous lesions without extensive cortical destruction. High-resolution MRI in these cases shows thin penetrating channels of tumor extending through bone cortex into the extraosseous soft tissues.	Lymphoid tumors with neoplastic cells typically within lymphoid tissue (lymph nodes and reticuloendothelial organs). Unlike leukemia, lymphoma usually arises as discrete masses. Lymphomas are subdivided into HD and non-Hodgkin lymphoma NHL. Almost all primary lymphomas of bone are B cell NHL. HD, mean age = 32 years. Osseous NHL, median = 35 years. **(See Atlas Chapter A 47)**

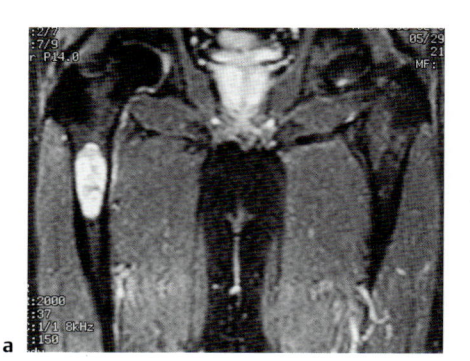

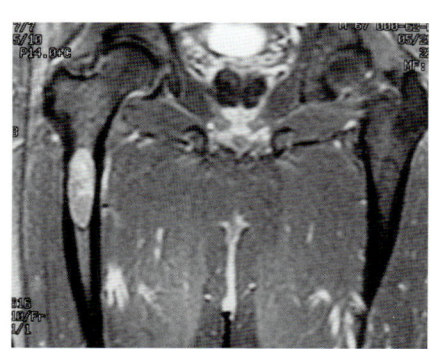

Figure 12.8 a, b Plasmacytoma in the proximal diaphysis of the femur that has high signal on coronal STIR (a) and shows Gd-contrast enhancement on coronal FS T1WI (b).

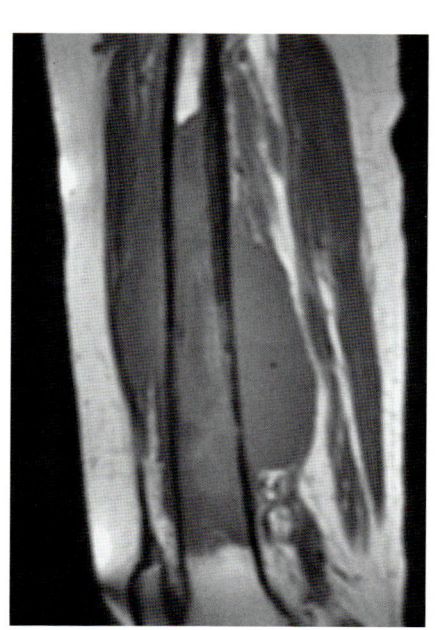

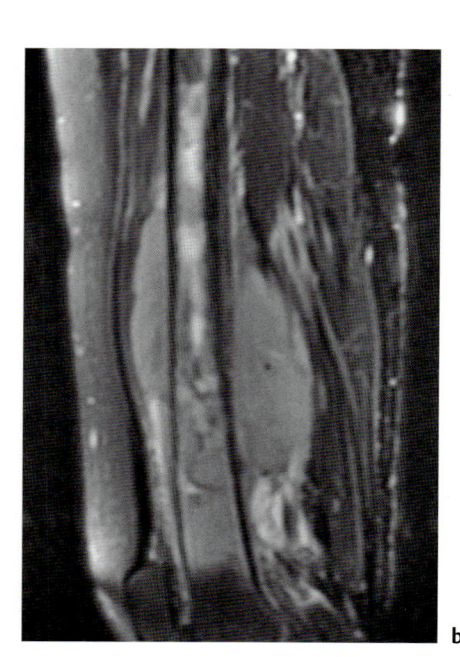

Figure 12.9 a, b A 36-year-old woman with large cell non-Hodgkin lymphoma involving the marrow of the femur that has slightly indistinct margins and shows extensive extraosseous tumor extension relative to the degree of cortical disruption. The tumor has heterogeneous intermediate signal on sagittal T1WI (a) and heterogeneous slightly high and high signal on sagittal FS T2WI (b).

Table 12 (Continued) **Solitary intramedullary diaphyseal lesions**

Lesion	MRI Findings	Comments
Osteosarcoma (Fig. 12.10)	Destructive intramedullary malignant lesions, low-intermediate signal on T1WI, mixed low, intermediate, high signal on T2WI, usually with matrix mineralization/ossification, low signal on T2WI, typically show Gd-contrast enhancement (usually heterogeneous). Zones of cortical destruction are common through which tumors extend into the extraosseous soft tissues under an elevated periosteum. Lamellated and/or spiculated zones of bone formation can occur under the periosteal elevation secondary to tumor invasion and perforation of bone cortex. Low signal from spicules of periosteal, reactive and tumoral bone formation may have a divergent ("sunburst") pattern, perpendicular ("hair on end") pattern, or disorganized or complex appearance. Triangular zones of periosteal elevation (Codman's triangles) can be seen at the borders of zones of cortical destruction and tumor extension.	Malignant tumor comprising proliferating neoplastic spindle cells that produce osteoid and/or immature tumoral bone most frequently arising within medullary bone (metadiaphyseal > metaphyseal > diaphyseal locations). Two age peaks of incidence. The larger peak occurs between the ages of 10 and 20 and accounts for over half of the cases. The second smaller peak occurs in adults over 60 years and accounts for ~10% of the cases. Occurs in children as primary tumors and adults (associated with Paget disease, irradiated bone, chronic osteomyelitis, osteoblastoma, giant cell tumor, fibrous dysplasia). **(See Atlas Chapter A 64)**

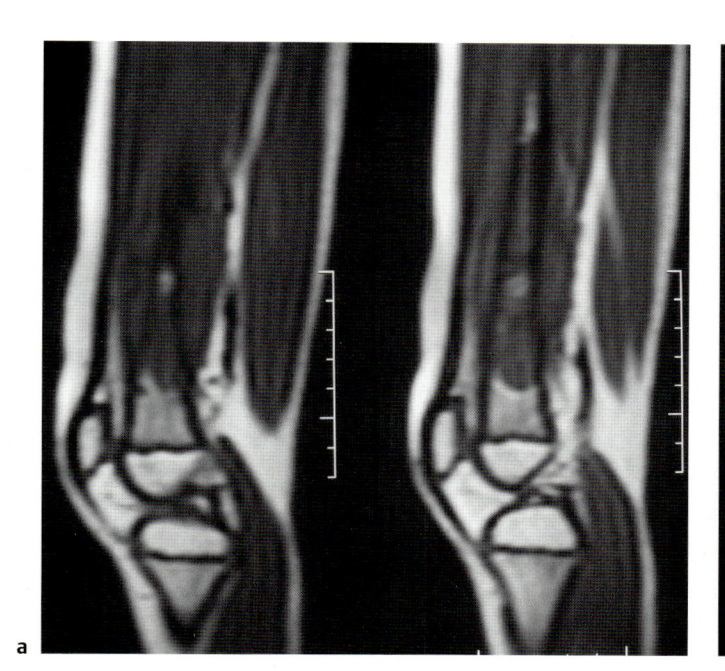

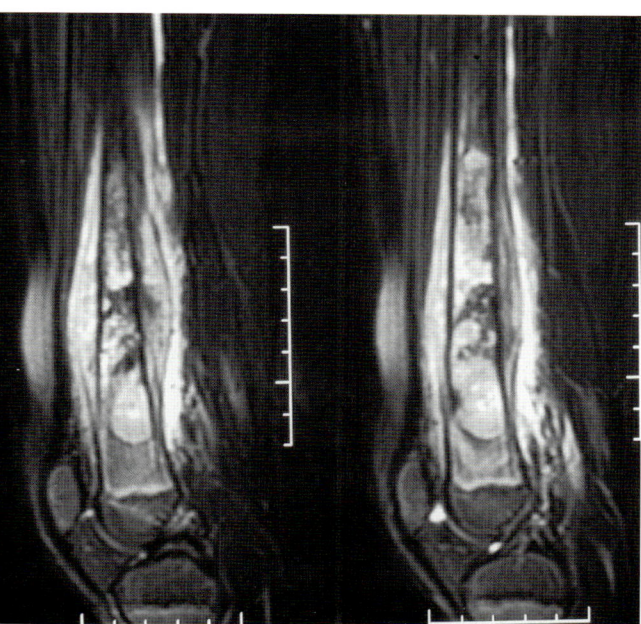

Figure 12.**10 a, b**   A 6-year-old girl with an osteosarcoma in the marrow of the distal femur that has low-intermediate signal on sagittal T1WI (**a**) and high signal on sagittal FS T2WI (**b**). The tumor is associated with cortical destruction, periosteal elevation, and extraosseous extension.

Table 12 (Continued) **Solitary intramedullary diaphyseal lesions**

Lesion	MRI Findings	Comments
Ewing sarcoma (Fig. 12.11)	Destructive malignant lesions involving marrow, low-intermediate signal on T1WI, mixed low, intermediate, and/or high signal on T2WI and FS T2WI, typically shows Gd-contrast enhancement (usually heterogeneous). Extraosseous tumor extension through sites of cortical destruction is commonly seen beneath an elevated periosteum. Thin striated zones of low signal on T2WI can be sometimes seen oriented perpendicular to the long axis of the involved bone under the elevated periosteum representing the "hair on end" appearance of reactive bone formation secondary to the tumor. In long bones, tumors are most often located in the diaphyseal region, followed by the metadiaphyseal region.	Malignant primitive tumor of bone comprising undifferentiated small cells with round nuclei. Accounts for 6–11% of primary malignant bone tumors, 5–7% of primary bone tumors. Usually occurs between the ages of 5 and 30, males > females, locally invasive, high metastatic potential. **(See Atlas Chapter A 20)**
Chondrosarcoma (Fig. 12.12)	Intramedullary tumors often have low-intermediate signal on T1WI, intermediate signal on PDWI, and heterogeneous intermediate-high signal on T2WI. Lesions usually show heterogeneous contrast enhancement. Zones of cortical destruction can be seen with extraosseous extension of tumor.	Chondrosarcomas are malignant tumors containing cartilage formed within sarcomatous stroma. Account for 12–21% of malignant bone lesions, 21–26% of primary sarcomas of bone, 5 to 91 years, mean = 40 years, median = 26 to 59 years. **(See Atlas Chapter A 11)**
Fibrosarcoma	Intramedullary lesions with irregular margins, with or without associated cortical destruction and/or extraosseous soft tissue masses. Lesions usually have low-intermediate signal on T1WI and PDWI, and heterogeneous intermediate, slightly high, and/or high signal on T2WI. Lesions usually show heterogeneous Gd-contrast enhancement.	Fibrosarcomas are uncommon malignant tumors consisting of bundles of fibroblasts/spindle cells with varying proportions of collagen, lacking other tissue differentiating features such as tumor bone, osteoid, or cartilage. Can be primary lesions (75%) or arise as secondary tumors (25%) associated with prior irradiation, Paget disease, bone infarct, chronic osteomyelitis, fibrous dysplasia, giant cell tumor. Account for 3–5% of primary malignant bone tumors, and 2–4% of all bone tumors, median age = 43 years. **(See Atlas Chapter A 25)**
Malignant fibrous histiocytoma	Intramedullary lesions with irregular margins with zones of cortical destruction and extraosseous extension. Tumors often have low-intermediate signal on T1WI; low-intermediate signal on PDWI, and heterogeneous intermediate-high signal on T2WI and FS T2WI. Invasion into joints occurs in 30%. May be associated with bone infarcts, bone cysts, chronic osteomyelitis, Paget disease, and other treated primary bone tumors. Lesions usually show heterogeneous Gd-contrast prominent enhancement.	Malignant tumor involving soft tissue and rarely bone derived from undifferentiated mesenchymal cells. Contains cells with limited cellular differentiation such as mixtures of fibroblasts, myofibroblasts, histiocyte-like cells, anaplastic giant cells, and inflammatory cells. Accounts for 1–5% of primary malignant bone tumors and <1–3% of all primary bone tumors, patient ages range from 11 to 80 years, median = 48 years, mean = 55 years. **(See Atlas Chapter A 48)**
Paget sarcoma (Fig. 12.13)	Irregular zones of medullary and cortical bone destruction associated with an extraosseous soft tissue mass lesion. The involved marrow typically has low to intermediate signal on T1WI and PDWI, and low to high signal on T2WI. Abnormal Gd-contrast enhancement is seen in the marrow as well as in the extraosseous tumor extension.	Paget disease is most common bone disease in older adults after osteoporosis. Median age = 66 years. Disordered bone resorption and woven bone formation occurs resulting in osseous deformity. Associated with less than 1% risk for developing secondary sarcomatous changes. **(See Atlas Chapter A 65)**

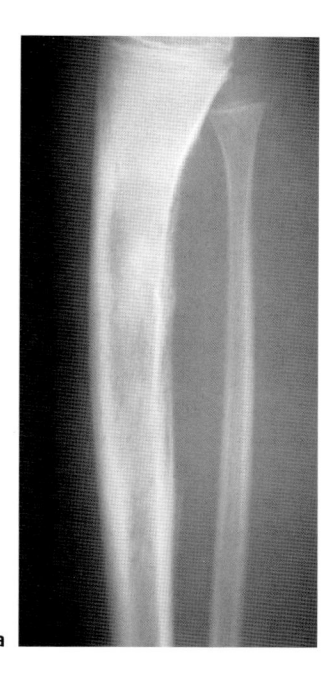

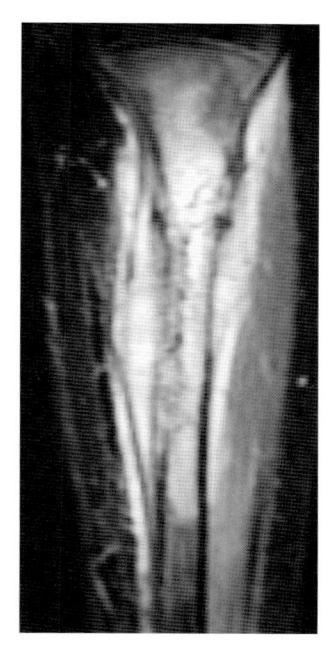

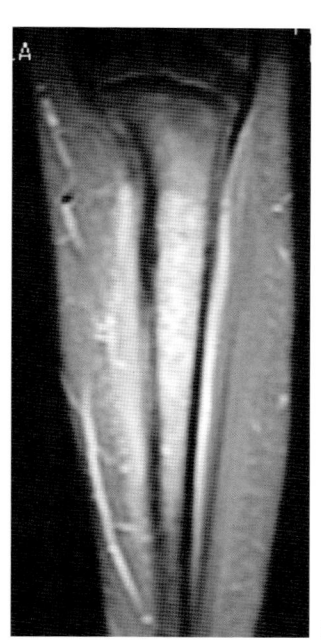

Figure 12.**11 a–c** An 11-year-old boy with Ewing sarcoma involving the shaft of the proximal tibia. The tumor has permeative radiolucent intramedullary changes, zones of cortical destruction, periosteal elevation, and a Codman's triangle inferiorly on the oblique radiograph (**a**). The intramedullary tumor has high signal on coronal FS T2WI (**b**) and shows Gd-contrast enhancement on coronal FS T1WI (**c**). The tumor is associated with cortical destruction, periosteal elevation, and extraosseous extension.

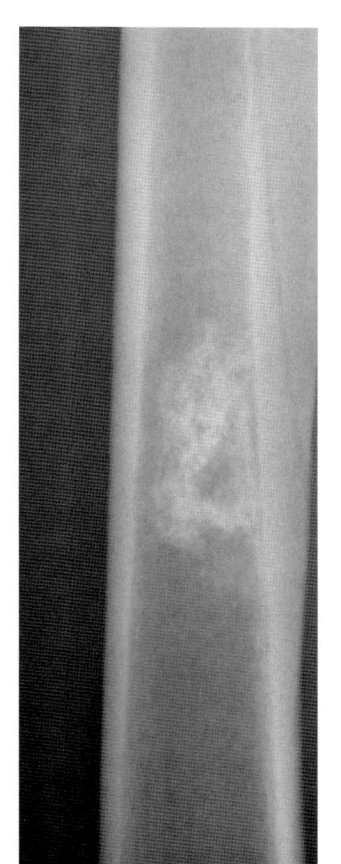

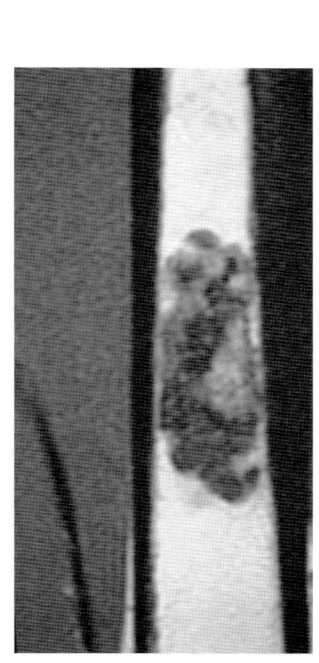

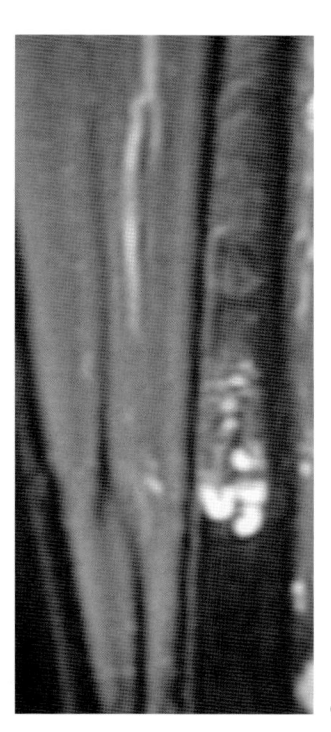

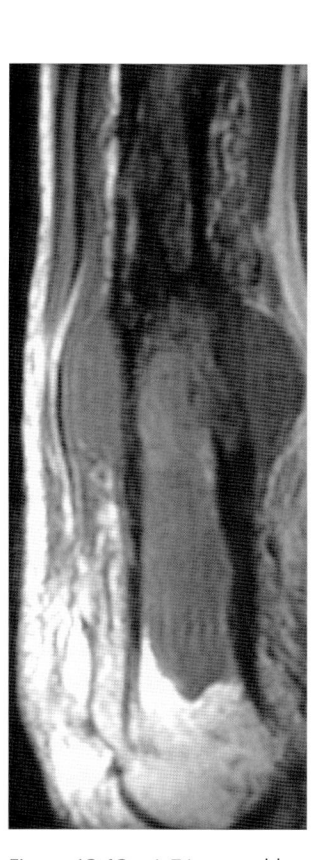

Figure 12.**12 a–c** A 39-year-old man with a chondrosarcoma in the marrow of the distal tibial shaft that has chondroid matrix mineralization on a lateral radiograph (**a**). The tumor has mixed low and intermediate signal on sagittal T1WI (**b**) and heterogeneous slightly high and high signal on FS T2WI (**c**).

Figure 12.**13** A 71-year-old woman with Paget sarcoma involving the marrow of the distal femur associated with cortical destruction and extraosseous extension as seen on sagittal T1WI.

References

Stress Fracture

Ahovuo JA, Kiuru MJ, Visuri T. Fatigue stress fractures of the sacrum: diagnosis with MR imaging. *Eur Radiol* March 2004;14(3):500–505. Epub October 24, 2003.

Berger FH, de Jonge MC, Maas M. Stress fractures in the lower extremity. The importance of increasing awareness amongst radiologists. *Eur J Radiol* 2007;62:16–26.

Grangier C, Garcia J, Howarth NR, May M, Rossier P. Role of MRI in the diagnosis of insufficiency fractures of the sacrum and acetabular roof. *Skeletal Radiol* 1997;26:517–524.

Meyers SP, Wiener SN. Magnetic resonance imaging features of fractures using the short tau inversion recovery (STIR) sequence: correlation with radiographic findings. *Skeletal Radiol* 1991;20(7):499–507.

Table 13 Osseous tumors and tumorlike lesions at the hands and feet

Tumor/tumorlike Lesion	MRI Findings	Comments
Benign		
Enchondroma (Figs. 13.1, 13.2)	Lobulated intramedullary lesions with well-defined borders that usually have low-intermediate signal on T1WI and intermediate signal on PDWI. On T2WI and FS T2WI, lesions usually have predominantly high signal. Lesions typically show Gd-contrast enhancement in various patterns (peripheral curvilinear lobular, central nodular/septal and peripheral lobular, or heterogeneous diffuse).	Benign intramedullary lesions composed of hyaline cartilage, represent ~10% of benign bone tumors. Enchondromas can be solitary (88%) or multiple (12%). Ollier disease is a dyschondroplasia involving endochondral-formed bone resulting in multiple enchondromas (enchondromatosis). Maffucci disease refers to a syndrome with multiple enchondromas and soft tissue hemangiomas, and is very rare. Median age = 35 years, peak in 3rd and 4th decades. **(See Atlas Chapter A 8)**

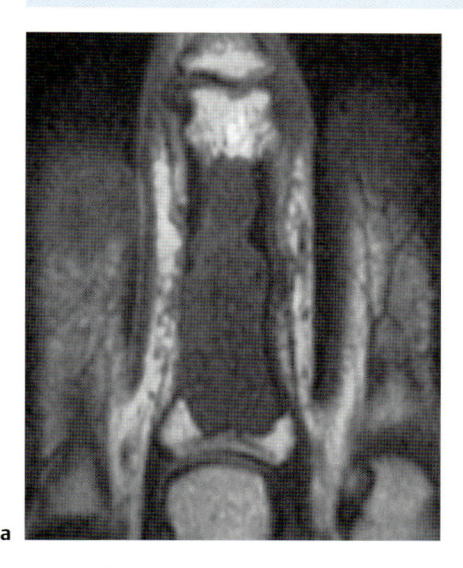

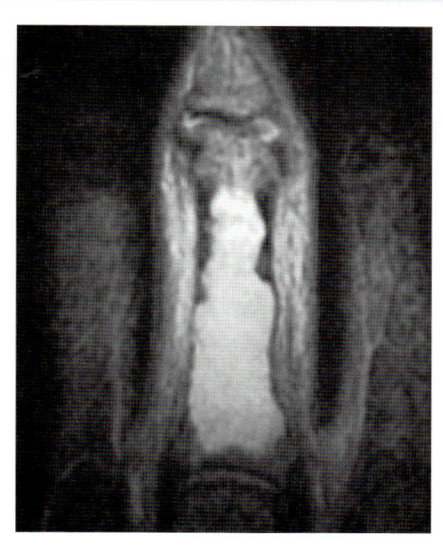

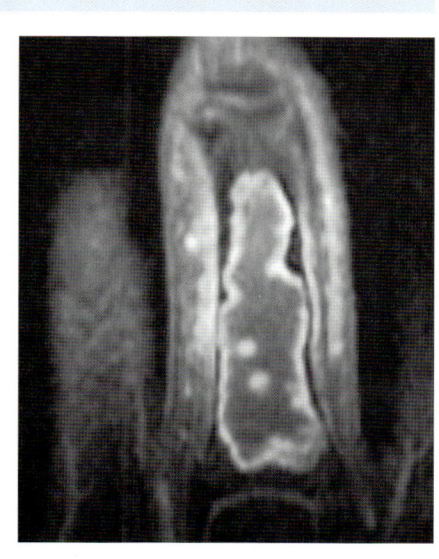

Figure 13.1 a–c A 39-year-old woman with an enchondroma in a proximal phalanx that has intermediate signal on coronal T1WI (**a**) and high signal on coronal FS T2WI (**b**). The lesion shows thin peripheral and central nodular Gd-contrast enhancement on coronal FS T1WI (**c**). The lesion is associated with thinning and slight expansion of adjacent cortical bone.

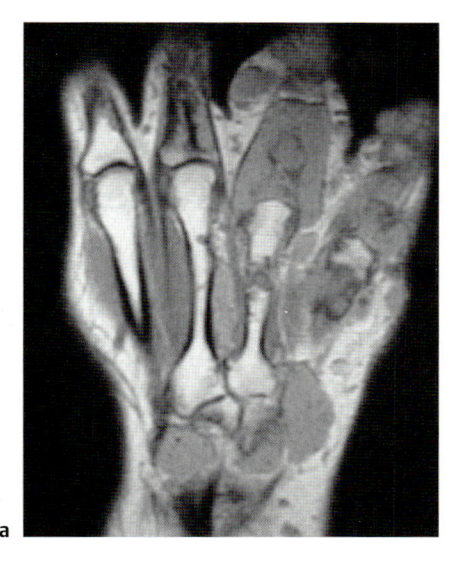

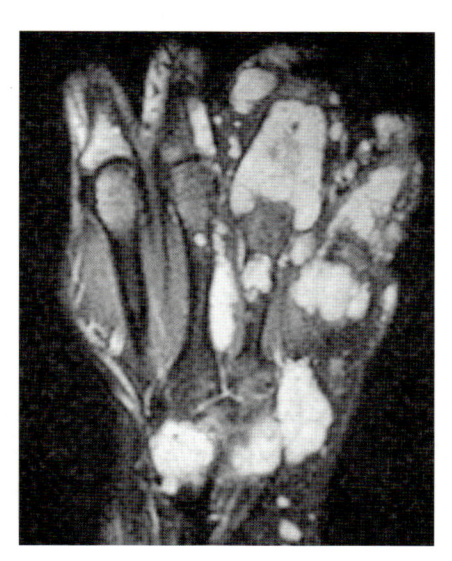

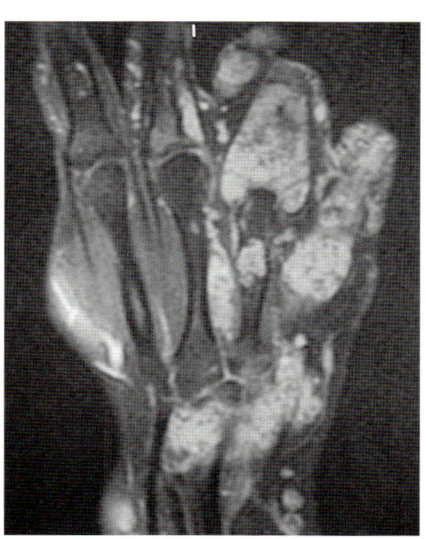

Figure 13.2 a–c A 20-year-old woman with Maffucci disease with multiple enchondromas within bones of the hand that have intermediate signal on coronal T1WI (**a**) and high signal on coronal FS T2WI (**b**). The enchondromas and soft tissue hemangiomas show Gd-contrast enhancement on coronal FS T1WI (**c**).

Table 13 (Continued) Osseous tumors and tumorlike lesions at the hands and feet		
Tumor/tumorlike Lesion	MRI Findings	Comments
Osteochondroma (Fig. 13.3)	Circumscribed protruding lesion arising from outer cortex with a central zone with intermediate signal on T1WI and T2WI similar to marrow surrounded by a peripheral outer zone of low signal on T1WI and T2WI, over which a cartilaginous cap is usually present in children and young adults. Increased malignant potential when cartilaginous cap is > 2 cm thick.	Benign cartilaginous tumors arising from defect at periphery of growth plate during bone formation with resultant bone outgrowth covered by a cartilaginous cap. Usually benign lesions unless associated with pain and increasing size of cartilaginous cap. Osteochondromas are common lesions, accounting for 14–35 % of primary bone tumors. Occur with median age of 20 years, up to 75 % of patients are less than 20 years. **(See Atlas Chapter A 58)**
Bizarre parosteal osteochondromatous proliferation (Fig. 13.4)	Smooth and/or lobulated calcified and/or ossified lesions often with a broad base or stalk of attachment to an intact outer cortical surface of bone. Remodeling of adjacent bone cortex can occur. Typically does not invade adjacent extraosseous soft tissues.	Lesions adjacent to or attached to the outer periosteal surface of bone consisting of disorganized conglomerations of bone with short trabeculae, cartilage containing enlarged dysmorphic binucleate chondrocytes, spindle cells, fibrous tissue, and/or myxoid regions. Commonly occurs in the hands and feet (70 %), less commonly in long bones. Peak age = 4th decade. May represent a type of heterotopic ossification vs. benign tumor. Can be cured by surgical excision although local recurrence is common.
Juxtacortical chondroma	Lesions are located at the bone surface and are usually lobulated with low-intermediate signal on T1WI which is hypo- or isointense relative to muscle. Lesions usually have heterogeneous predominantly high signal on T2WI. Lesions are surrounded by low signal borders on T2WI representing thin sclerotic reaction. Areas of low signal on T2WI are secondary to matrix mineralization. Edema is not typically seen in nearby medullary bone. Lesions often show a peripheral pattern of Gd-contrast enhancement.	Benign protuberant hyaline cartilaginous tumors that arise from the periosteum and superficial to bone cortex. Juxtacortical chondromas account for < 1 % of bone lesions. Occur with median age of 26 years. **(See Atlas Chapter A 9)**
Osteoblastoma (Fig. 13.5)	Expansile radiolucent lesions often greater than 1.5 cm in diameter with or without matrix mineralization and peripheral bone sclerosis seen on radiographs and CT. Lesions often have low-intermediate signal on T1WI and intermediate-high signal on T2WI and FS T2WI, usually show Gd-contrast enhancement. Lesions usually have poorly defined zones with high signal on T2WI and FS T2WI and Gd-contrast enhancement in the marrow (edema, inflammation) beyond zone of sclerosis or in adjacent soft tissues from prostaglandin synthesis by these lesions.	Rare benign bone neoplasm (2 % of bone tumors) usually occurs between the ages 6 and 30 years. **(See Atlas Chapter A 61)**
Osteoid osteoma (Fig. 13.6)	Typically shows dense fusiform thickening of the cortex that has low to intermediate signal on T1WI, PDWI, T2WI, and FS T2WI. Within the thickened cortex, a spheroid or ovoid zone (nidus) measuring < 1.5 cm is seen. The nidus can have irregular, distinct, or indistinct margins relative to the adjacent region of cortical thickening. The nidus can have low-intermediate signal on T1WI, and low-intermediate or high signal on T2WI and FS T2WI. Calcifications in the nidus can be seen as low signal on T2WI. After Gd-contrast administration, variable degrees of enhancement are seen at the nidus.	Benign osteoblastic lesion with a circumscribed nidus < 1.5 cm and usually surrounded by reactive bone formation. These lesions are usually painful and have limited growth potential. Osteoid osteoma accounts for 11–13 % of primary benign bone tumors. Occurs in patients 6 to 30 years, median = 17 years. Approximately 75 % occur in patients less than 25 years. **(See Atlas Chapter A 60)**

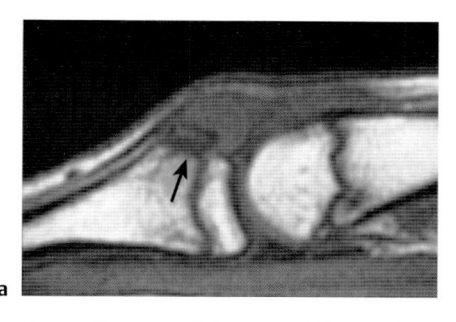

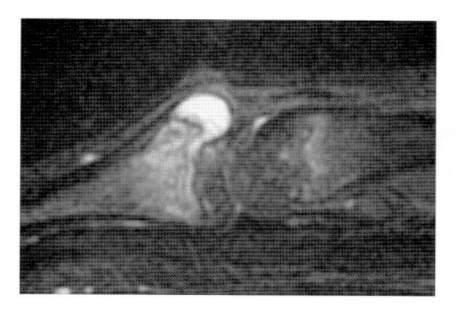

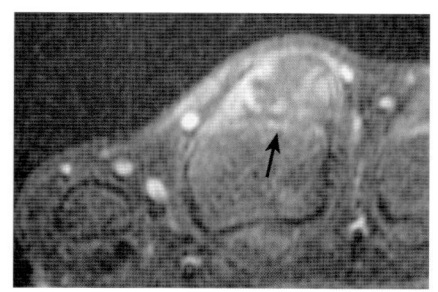

Figure 13.**3 a–c**   A 14-year-old boy with an osteochondroma involving the proximal metaphyseal surface of a phalanx that has intermediate signal on sagittal T1WI (**a**) and high signal on sagittal FS T2WI (**b**). The lesion shows thin peripheral Gd-contrast enhancement on axial FS T1WI (**c**).

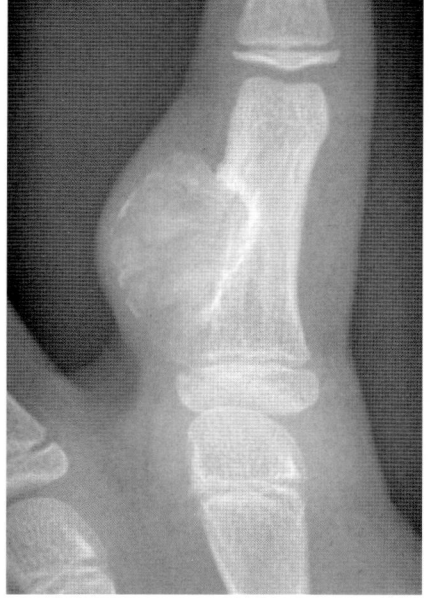

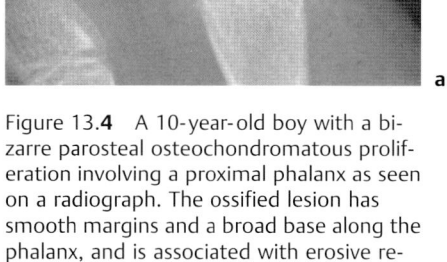

Figure 13.**4**   A 10-year-old boy with a bizarre parosteal osteochondromatous proliferation involving a proximal phalanx as seen on a radiograph. The ossified lesion has smooth margins and a broad base along the phalanx, and is associated with erosive remodeling of the adjacent cortical bone.

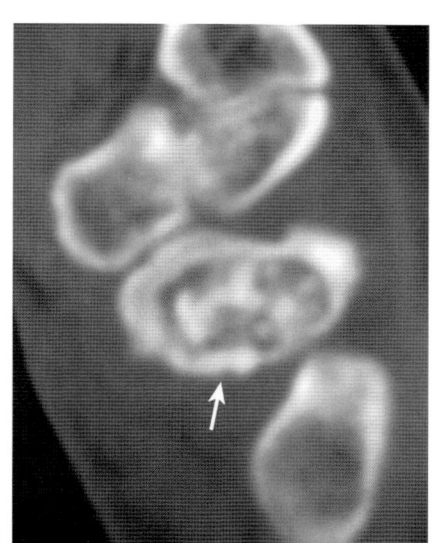

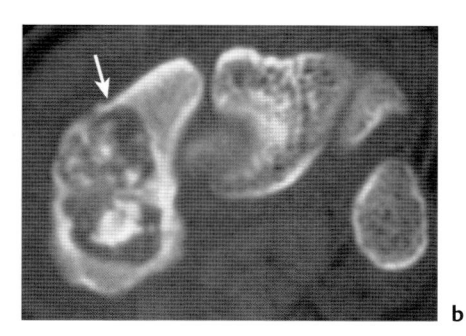

Figure 13.**5 a, b**   A 16-year-old male with an osteoblastoma within the scaphoid bone in the wrist, seen as a radiolucent lesion containing mineralized matrix on sagittal (**a**) and axial (**b**) CT.

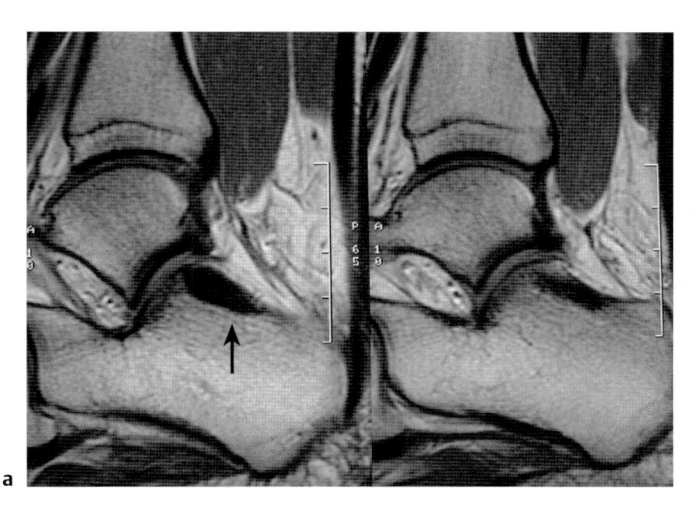

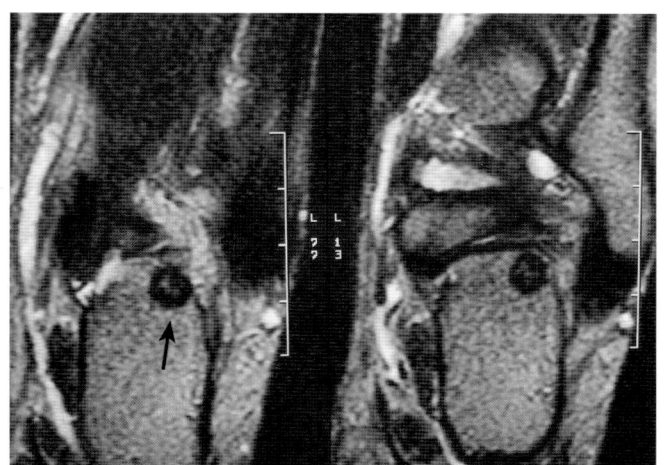

Figure 13.**6 a, b**   An 18-year-old woman with an osteoid osteoma in the calcaneus. The lesion has low signal on sagittal PDWI (**a**) and low signal peripheral to a central area of intermediate signal on axial T2WI (**b**).

Table 13 (Continued) Osseous tumors and tumorlike lesions at the hands and feet

Tumor/tumorlike Lesion	MRI Findings	Comments
Chondromyxoid fibroma (Fig. 13.7)	Lesions are often slightly lobulated with low-intermediate signal on T1WI, and heterogeneous predominantly high signal on T2WI secondary to myxoid and hyaline chondroid components with high water content. MR signal heterogeneity on T2WI is related to the proportions of myxoid, chondroid, and fibrous components within the lesions. Thin low signal septa within lesions on T2WI are secondary to fibrous strands. Lesions are surrounded by low signal borders representing thin sclerotic reaction. Lesions show prominent diffuse Gd-contrast enhancement.	Rare, benign, slow-growing bone lesions that contain chondroid, myxoid, and fibrous components. Chondromyxoid fibromas represent 2–4% of primary benign bone lesions, and <1% of primary bone lesions. Most chondromyxoid fibromas occur between the ages of 1 and 40 years, with a median of 17 years, and peak incidence in the 2nd to 3rd decades. **(See Atlas Chapter A 10)**
Lipoma (Fig. 13.8)	Lesions can have heterogeneous high, intermediate, and/or low signal on T1WI, PDWI, and T2WI. Fat signal of lesions is suppressed on FS T1WI, FS T2WI, and STIR. Lesions usually show no Gd-contrast enhancement. Peripheral rim-like and central Gd-contrast enhancement on FS T1WI may occassionally occur.	Uncommon benign hamartomas composed of mature white adipose tissue without cellular atypia. Osseous or chondroid metaplasia with myxoid changes can be associated with lipomas. Account for ~0.1% of bone tumors, likely under-reported. **(See Atlas Chapter A 43)**
Enostosis/bone island	Typically appear as well-circumscribed zones of dense bone with low signal on T1WI, PDWI, T2WI, and FS T2WI. No infiltration into the adjacent soft tissues is seen by osteomas. Zones of bone destruction or associated soft tissue mass lesions are not associated with osteomas. Periosteal reaction is not associated with osteomas except in cases with coincidental antecedent trauma.	Benign primary bone lesion composed of dense lamellar, woven and/or compact cortical bone usually located at the surface of bone. Multiple osteomas usually occur in Gardner syndrome, which is an autosomal dominant disorder that is associated with intestinal polyposis, fibromas, and desmoid tumors. Accounts for <1% of primary benign bone tumors. Occurs in patients 16 to 74 years, most frequent in 6th decade. **(See Atlas Chapter A 62)**
Aneurysmal bone cyst (Fig. 13.9)	Aneurysmal bone cysts (ABCs) often have a low signal rim on T1WI and T2WI adjacent to normal medullary bone, and between extraosseous soft tissues. Various combinations of low, intermediate, and/or high signal on T1WI, PDWI, and T2WI are usually seen within aneurysmal bone cysts as well as fluid–fluid levels. Variable Gd-contrast enhancement is seen at the margins of lesions as well as involving the internal septae.	Tumor-like expansile bone lesions containing cavernous spaces filled with blood. ABCs can be primary bone lesions (two-thirds) or secondary to other bone lesions/tumors (such as giant cell tumors, chondroblastomas, osteoblastomas, osteosarcomas. chondromyxoid fibromas, nonossifying fibromas, fibrous dysplasia, fibrosarcomas, malignant fibrous histiocytomas, and metastatic disease). Account for ~11% of primary tumor-like lesions of bone. Patients usually range in age from 1 to 25 years, median = 14 years. **(See Atlas Chapter A 2)**
Giant cell reparative granuloma (Fig. 13.10)	Lesions can have heterogeneous low, intermediate, and/or high signal on T1WI, PDWI, and T2WI; as well as peripheral rim-like and central Gd-contrast enhancement on FS T1WI.	Giant cell reparative granulomas are also referred to as solid ABCs. **(See Atlas Chapter A 2)**. Histologic appearance resembles brown tumors.

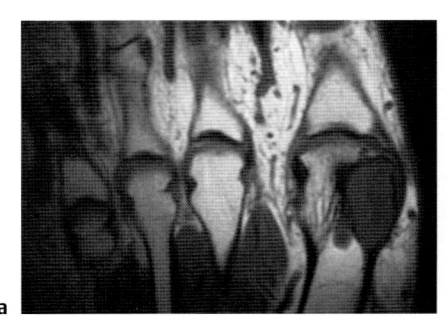

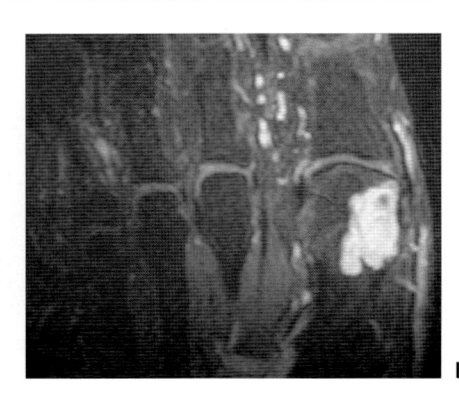

Figure 13.7 a, b A 34-year-old man with chondromyxoid fibroma in the distal first metatarsal bone. The lesion has low-intermediate signal on coronal T1WI (a) and heterogeneous high signal on FS T2WI (b).

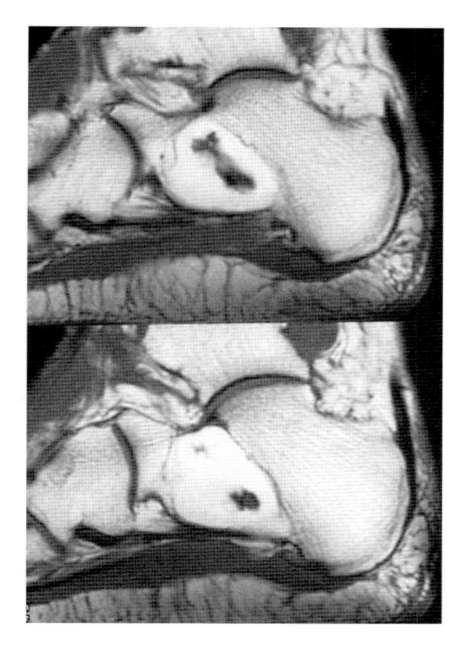

Figure 13.**8** A 47-year-old woman with an intraosseous lipoma in the calcaneus that has thin low signal margins and mostly high signal on sagittal T1WI as well as several small zones of intermediate signal from cystic degeneration.

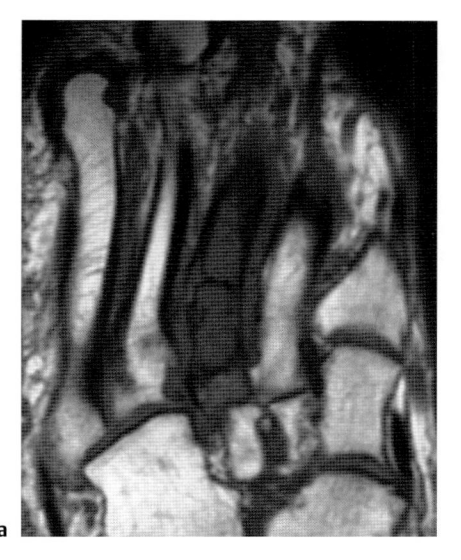

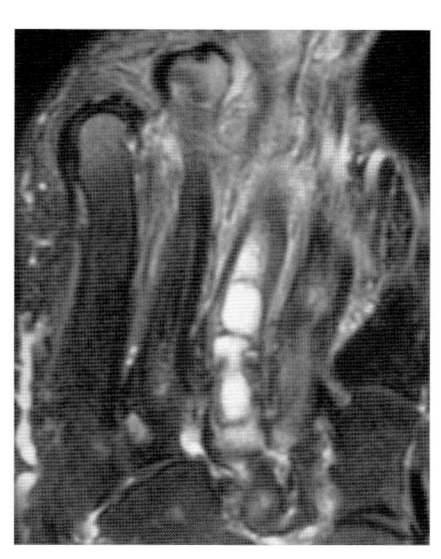

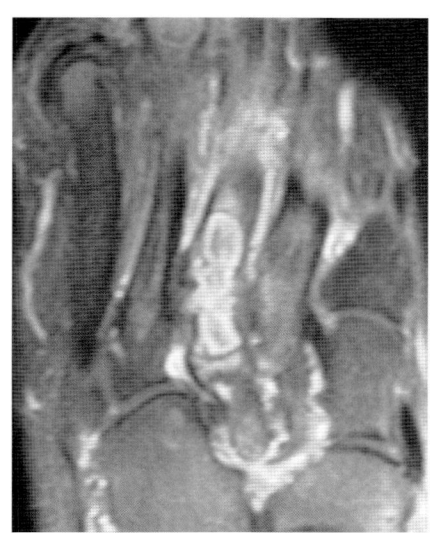

a b, c

Figure 13.**9 a–c** A 48-year-old man with an aneurysmal bone cyst in the proximal portion of the third metatarsal bone that has low-intermediate signal on coronal T1WI (**a**) and mostly high signal on coronal FS T2WI (**b**). The lesion shows thin, mostly peripheral Gd-contrast enhancement on coronal FS T1WI (**c**). Also seen are slight expansion and thinning of the adjacent cortical margins, and poorly defined zones of increased signal on FS T2WI and Gd-contrast enhancement in the adjacent bone marrow.

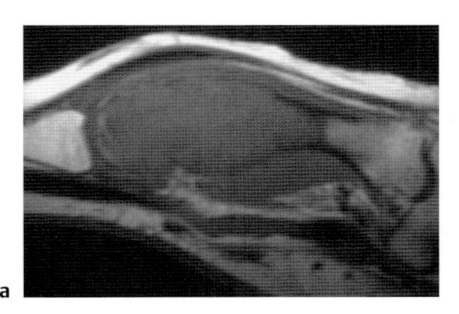

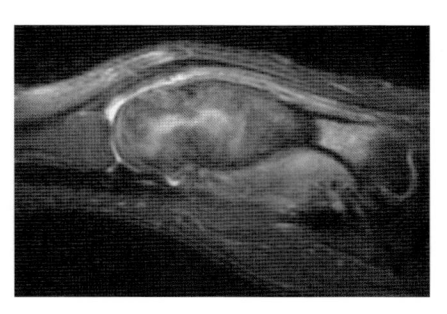

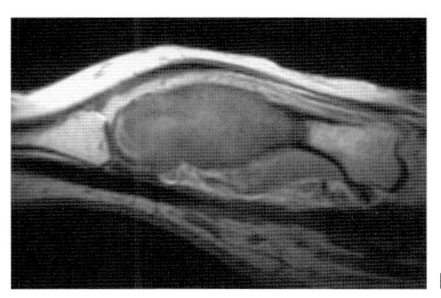

a b, c

Figure 13.**10 a–c** A 39-year-old woman with a giant cell granuloma involving a metacarpal bone. The intramedullary lesion expands and thins bone cortex, and has intermediate signal on sagittal T1WI (**a**), heterogeneous low, intermediate, slightly high, and high signal on sagittal FS T2WI (**b**). The lesion shows Gd-contrast enhancement on sagittal T1WI (**c**).

Table 13 (Continued) Osseous tumors and tumorlike lesions at the hands and feet

Tumor/tumorlike Lesion	MRI Findings	Comments
Unicameral bone cyst (Fig. 13.11)	Unicameral bone cysts (UBCs) often have a peripheral rim of low signal on T1WI and T2WI adjacent to normal medullary bone. Usually contain fluid with low to low-intermediate signal on T1WI, low-intermediate and high signal on T2WI. Fluid–fluid levels may occur. For UBCs without pathologic fracture, thin peripheral Gd-contrast enhancement can be seen at the margins of lesions. UBCs with pathologic fracture can have heterogeneous or homogeneous low-intermediate or slightly high signal on T1WI, and heterogeneous or homogeneous high signal on T2WI and FS T2WI. UBCs complicated by fracture can have internal septations and fluid–fluid levels, as well as irregular peripheral Gd-contrast enhancement at internal septations.	Intramedullary non-neoplastic cavities filled with serous or serosanguineous fluid. Account for 9% of primary tumor-like lesions of bone. 85% occur in the first 2 decades, median = 11 years. **(See Atlas Chapter A 3)**
Chondroblastoma (Fig. 13.12)	Tumors often have fine lobular margins, and typically have low-intermediate heterogeneous signal on T1WI, and mixed low, intermediate, and/or high signal on T2WI. Lobular, marginal septal or diffuse Gd-contrast enhancement patterns can be seen. Poorly defined zones with high signal on T2WI and FS T2WI and corresponding Gd-contrast enhancement are typically seen in the marrow adjacent to the lesions representing inflammatory reaction from prostaglandin synthesis by these tumors.	Benign cartilaginous tumors with chondroblast-like cells and areas of chondroid matrix formation, usually occur in children and adolescents, median = 17 years, mean = 16 years for lesions in long bones, mean = 28 years in other bones. Most cases are diagnosed between the ages of 5 and 25. **(See Atlas Chapter A 7)**
Hemangioma	Often well-circumscribed lesions that typically have intermediate to high signal on T1WI, PDWI, T2WI, and FS T2WI. On T1WI, hemangiomas usually have signal equal to or greater than adjacent normal marrow secondary to fatty components. Usually show Gd-contrast enhancement. Pathologic fractures associated with intraosseous hemangiomas usually result in low-intermediate marrow signal on T1WI.	Benign lesions of bone comprising capillary, cavernous, and/or malformed venous vessels. Considered to be a hamartomatous disorder. Account for 4% of benign bone tumors and ~1% of all bone tumors, likely underestimated. Occur in all ages, median = 33 years. **(See Atlas Chapter A 34)**
Glomus body tumor (Fig. 13.13)	Glomus body tumors are well-circumscribed ovoid lesions measuring < 1 cm and are often located under the nail beds at the distal phalanges of fingers and toes. Glomus body tumors often have low-intermediate signal on T1WI and PDWI, although may be hypointense or hyperintense on T1WI relative to the adjacent dermis layers. Glomus tumors usually have high signal T2WI and FS T2WI, and typically show Gd-contrast enhancement.	Benign mesenchymal hamartomas derived from the neuromyoarterial apparatus (glomus bodies) that regulate arteriolar blood flow to the skin, and are normally present throughout the reticular dermis throughout the body. Glomus bodies occur in large numbers under the nail beds of the fingers and toes. **(See Atlas Chapter A 31)**
Giant cell tumor (Fig. 13.14)	Often well-defined lesions with thin low signal margins on T1WI, PDWI, and T2WI. Solid portions of giant cell tumors often have low to intermediate signal on T1WI and PDWI, intermediate to high signal on T2WI, and high signal on FS PDWI and FS T2WI. Zones of low signal on T2WI may be seen secondary to hemosiderin. Aneurysmal bone cysts can be seen in 14% of giant cell tumors. Areas of cortical thinning, expansion, and/or destruction can occur with extraosseous extension. Tumors show varying degrees of Gd-contrast enhancement.	Aggressive tumors composed of neoplastic mononuclear cells and scattered multinucleated osteoclast-like giant cells. Account for 23% of primary nonmalignant bone tumors, and 5–9% of all primary bone tumors, median age = 30 years. **(See Atlas Chapter A 29)**

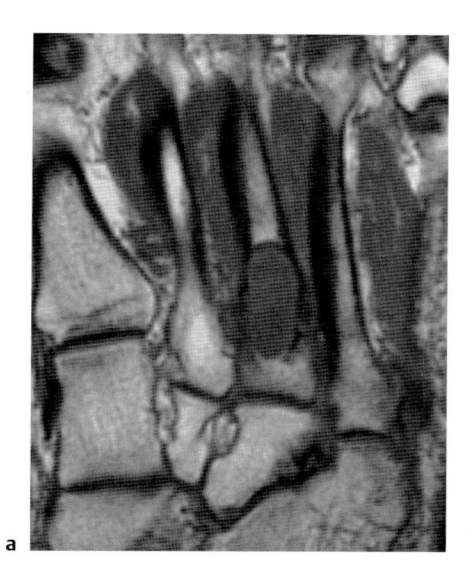

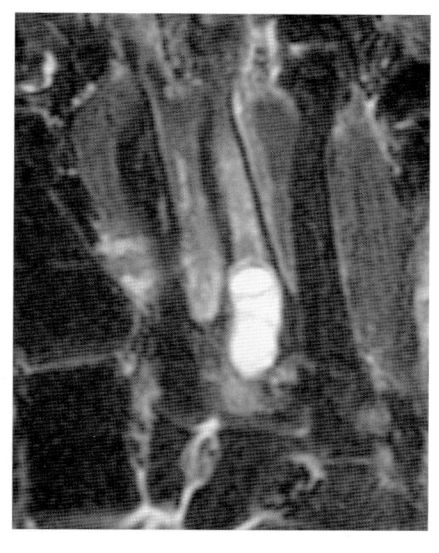

Figure 13.**11 a, b** A 60-year-old woman with a unicameral bone cyst in the proximal portion of a metatarsal bone. The lesion has low-intermediate signal on coronal T1WI (**a**) and mostly high signal on coronal FS T2WI (**b**). Also seen are poorly defined zones of slightly increased signal on FS T2 W in the adjacent bone marrow.

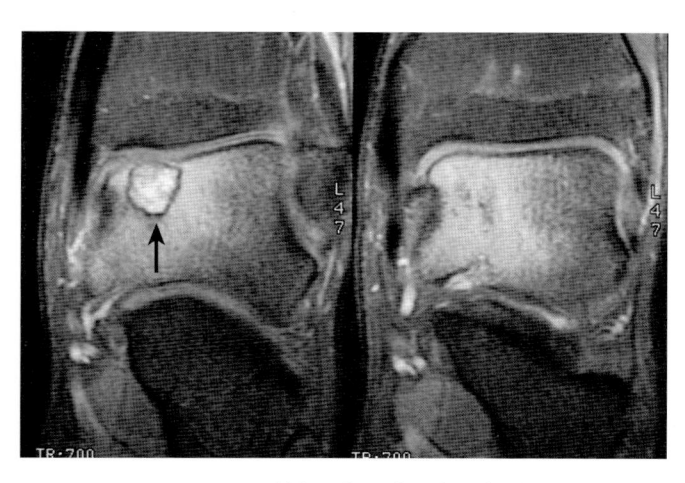

Figure 13.**12** A 15-year-old female with a chondroblastoma involving the talus. The lesion shows prominent Gd-contrast centrally surrounded by a thin rim of low signal on coronal FS T1WI. Poorly defined zones of contrast enhancement are also seen in the marrow adjacent to the lesion.

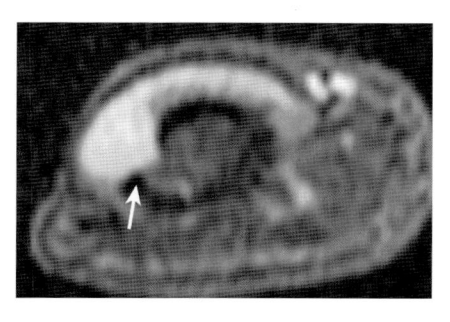

Figure 13.**13** A 24-year-old woman with a glomus tumor under the nail bed laterally associated with erosion of the adjacent cortex of the distal phalanx. The lesion shows prominent Gd-contrast enhancement on coronal FS T1WI.

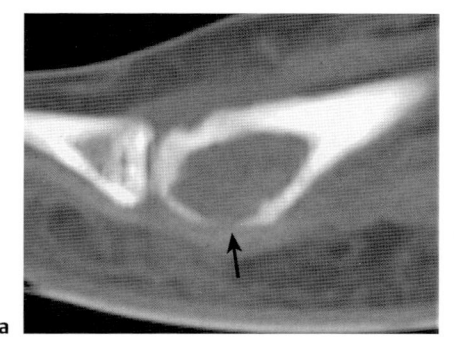

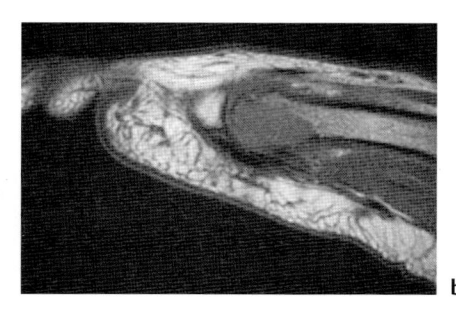

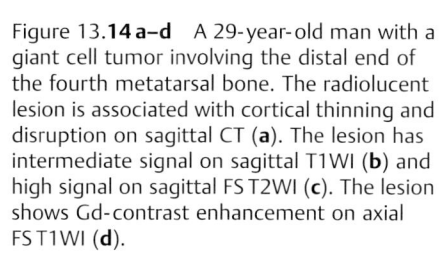

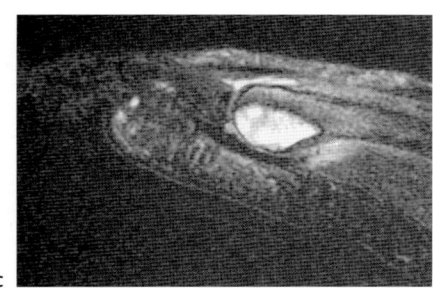

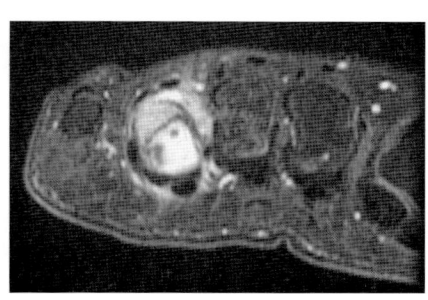

Figure 13.**14 a–d** A 29-year-old man with a giant cell tumor involving the distal end of the fourth metatarsal bone. The radiolucent lesion is associated with cortical thinning and disruption on sagittal CT (**a**). The lesion has intermediate signal on sagittal T1WI (**b**) and high signal on sagittal FS T2WI (**c**). The lesion shows Gd-contrast enhancement on axial FS T1WI (**d**).

Table 13 (Continued)　　Osseous tumors and tumorlike lesions at the hands and feet

Tumor/tumorlike Lesion	MRI Findings	Comments
Fibrous dysplasia (Fig. 13.15)	MRI features depend on the proportions of bony spicules, collagen, fibroblastic spindle cells, hemorrhagic and/or cystic changes, and associated pathologic fracture if present. Lesions are usually well-circumscribed, and have low or low-intermediate signal on T1WI and PDWI. On T2WI, lesions have variable mixtures of low, intermediate, and/or high signal often surrounded by a low signal rim of variable thickness. Internal septations and cystic changes are seen in a minority of lesions. Bone expansion with thickened and/or thinned cortex can be seen. Lesions show Gd-contrast enhancement that varies in degree and pattern.	Benign medullary fibro-osseous lesion that can involve a single site (**mono-ostotic**) or multiple locations (**poly-ostotic**). Thought to occur from developmental failure in the normal process of remodeling primitive bone to mature lamellar bone with resultant zone or zones of immature trabeculae within dysplastic fibrous tissue. Accounts for ~10% of benign bone lesions. Patients range in age from <1 to 76 years. 75% occur before the age of 30 years. **(See Atlas Chapter A 27)**
Osteomyelitis (Fig. 13.16)	In **acute osteomyelitis**, poorly defined zones of low or low-intermediate signal on T1WI and high signal on T2WI, STIR, and FS T2WI are seen in the marrow. Loss of definition of the low signal line of the cortical margins is often observed on T1WI, T2WI, STIR, and FS T2WI. After Gd-contrast administration, irregular zones of contrast enhancement are seen in the involved marrow on FS T1WI. In the **subacute phase of osteomyelitis**, the pyogenic process becomes more localized. The zone of transition between normal and abnormal bone is sharper and more well-defined in subacute and chronic osteomyelitis than with acute osteomyelitis.	Osteomyelitis is a disorder in which there is infection of bone and commonly the adjacent soft tissues. Can result from hematogenous spread of microorganisms as well as from trauma-direct inoculation, extension from adjacent tissues, and complications from surgery. Bacteria such as *Staphylococcus aureus* and *Streptococcus pyogenes* are the most common infectious organisms. Can also result from other bacteria as well as *Mycobacterium tuberculosis*, fungi, parasites, and viruses. **(See Atlas Chapter A 63)**
Eosinophilic granuloma	Focal intramedullary lesion associated with trabecular and cortical bone destruction that typically has low-intermediate signal on T1WI and PDWI and heterogeneous slightly high to high signal on T2WI. Poorly defined zones of high signal on T2WI are usually seen in the marrow peripheral to the lesions secondary to inflammatory changes. Extension of lesions from the marrow into adjacent soft tissues through areas of cortical disruption are commonly seen as well as linear periosteal zones of high signal on T2WI. Lesions typically show prominent Gd-contrast enhancement in marrow and in extraosseous soft tissue portions of the lesions.	Benign tumor-like lesions consisting of Langerhans' cells (histiocytes), and variable amounts of lymphocytes, polymorphonuclear cells, and eosinophils. Account for 1% of primary bone lesions and 8% of tumor-like lesions. Occur in patients with median age = 10 years, average = 13.5 years, peak incidence is between 5 and 10 years, 80 to 85% occur in patients less than 30 years. **(See Atlas Chapter A 18)**
Sarcoidosis	Lesions usually appear as intramedullary zones with low to intermediate signal on T1WI and slightly high to high signal on T2WI and FS PDWI and FS T2WI. Erosions and zones of destruction of adjacent bone cortex as well as periosseous extension of the granulomatous process can occur. Fine perpendicular lines of low signal on T1WI may be seen extending outward from the region of eroded or destroyed cortex representing collagen separating periosseous extension of granulomas. After Gd-contrast administration, lesions typically show moderate to prominent enhancement.	Chronic systemic granulomatous disease of unknown etiology in which noncaseating granulomas occur in various tissues and organs including bone. **(See Atlas Chapter A 71)**
Gout (Fig. 13.17)	Tophi have variable sizes and shapes, and have low-intermediate signal on T1WI, FS T2WI, and T2WI. Zones of high signal on T2WI can also be seen in tophi. Erosions of bone, synovial pannus, joint effusion, bone marrow, and soft tissue edema can be seen with MRI. Tophi may show heterogeneous, diffuse, or peripheral/marginal Gd-contrast enhancement patterns.	Gout is an inflammatory disease involving synovium resulting from deposition of monosodium urate crystals and occurs when the serum urate level exceeds its solubility in various tissues and body fluid. **(See Atlas Chapter A 32)**

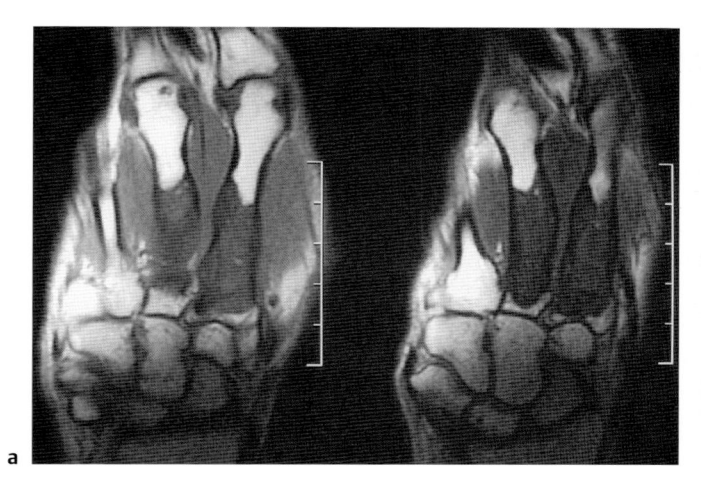

Figure 13.**15 a, b** Polyostotic fibrous dysplasia involving two adjacent metacarpal bones. The intramedullary lesions have low-intermediate signal on coronal T1WI (**a**), and mostly high signal on axial T2WI (**b**). Slight cortical thickening and expansion are also seen.

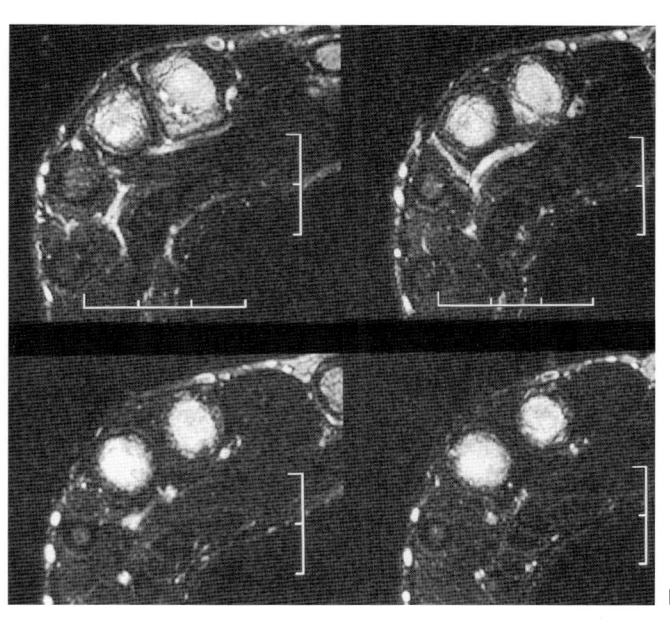

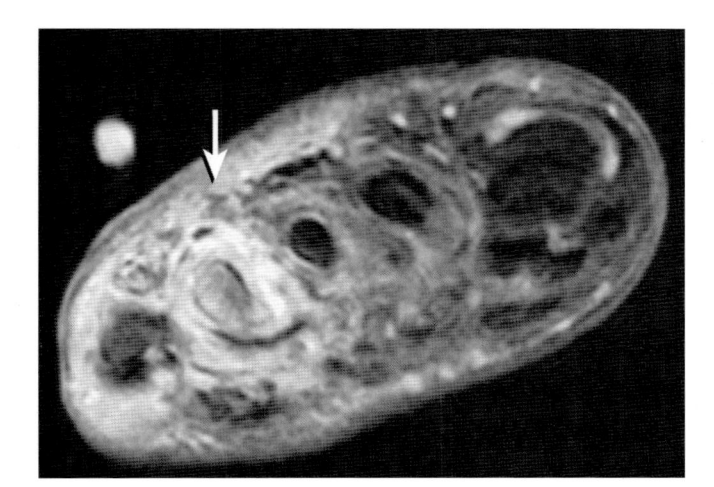

Figure 13.**16** A 54-year-old woman with pyogenic osteomyelitis involving the fourth metatarsal bone with abnormal high signal in the marrow and adjacent soft tissues on coronal FS T2WI.

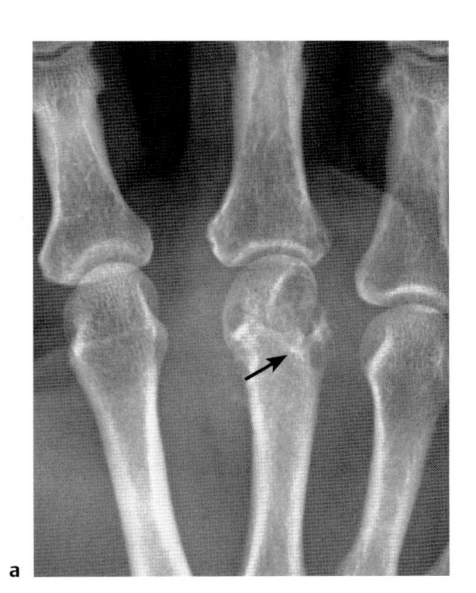

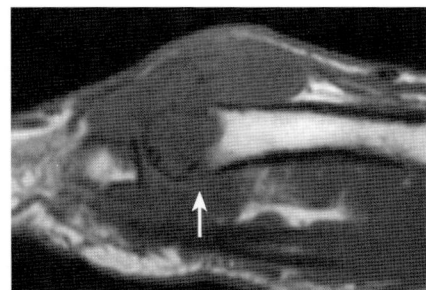

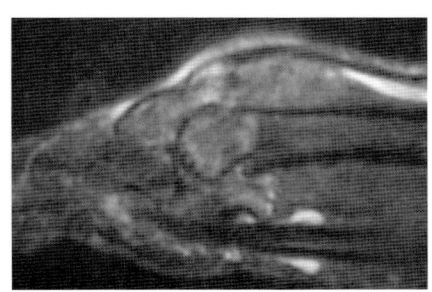

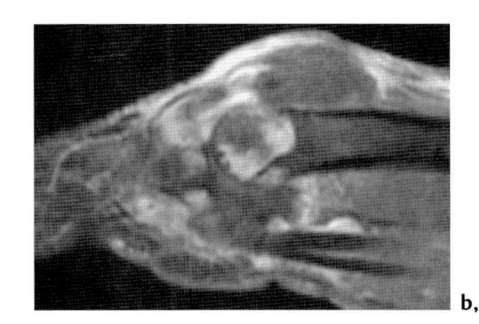

Figure 13.**17 a–d** A 53-year-old man with gout involving the metatarsal–phalangeal joint with bone erosions seen on a radiograph (**a**). MRI shows a soft tissue lesion (tophus) with intermediate signal on sagittal T1WI (**b**), and heterogeneous intermediate, slightly high, and high signal on FS T2WI (**c**). The lesion erodes cortical bone and extends into the marrow of the metatarsal head. Only peripheral irregular Gd-contrast enhancement is seen with the intraosseous and extraosseous lesions on sagittal FS T1WI (**d**).

Table 13 (Continued)   Osseous tumors and tumorlike lesions at the hands and feet

Tumor/tumorlike Lesion	MRI Findings	Comments
Bone infarct (Fig. 13.18)	A double-line sign (curvilinear adjacent zones of low and high signal on T2WI) is commonly seen at the edges of the infarcts representing the borders of osseous resorption and healing. Irregular Gd-contrast enhancement can be seen from granulation tissue ingrowth.	Zones of ischemic death involving bone trabeculae and marrow that may be idiopathic or result from: trauma, corticosteroid treatment, chemotherapy, radiation treatment, occlusive vascular disease, collagen vascular and other autoimmune diseases, metabolic storage diseases (Gaucher, etc.), sickle cell disease, thalassemia, hyperbaric events / Caisson disease, pregnancy, alcohol abuse, pancreatitis, infections, and lymphoproliferative diseases. **(See Atlas Chapter A 37)**
Malignant		
Metastatic lesion	Single or multiple well-circumscribed or poorly defined infiltrative lesions involving marrow associated with cortical destruction and extraosseous extension. Lesions often have low-intermediate signal on T1WI, low, intermediate, and/or high signal on T2WI and FS T2WI, and usually show Gd-contrast enhancement. Cortical destruction and tumor extension into the extraosseous soft tissues can occur. Pathologic fractures can be associated with metastatic lesions involving tubular bones and vertebrae. Periosteal reaction is uncommon.	Metastatic lesions typically occur in the marrow with or without cortical destruction and extraosseous tumor extension. **(See Atlas Chapter A 50)**
Plasmacytoma/myeloma	Well-circumscribed or poorly defined infiltrative lesions involving marrow, low-intermediate signal on T1WI, intermediate-high signal on T2WI and FS T2WI, usually show Gd-contrast enhancement, eventual cortical bone destruction and extraosseous extension.	Malignant tumors comprised of proliferating antibody-secreting plasma cells derived from single clones. Most common primary neoplasm of bone in adults, median = 60 years. Most patients are older than 40 years. May have variable destructive or infiltrative changes involving the axial and/or appendicular skeleton. **(See Atlas Chapter A 52)**

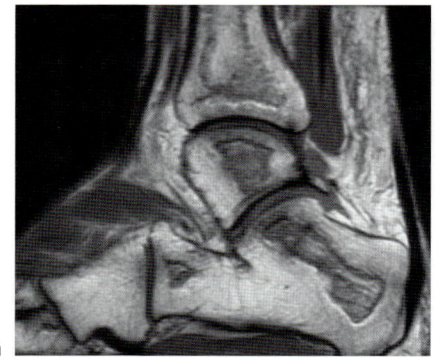

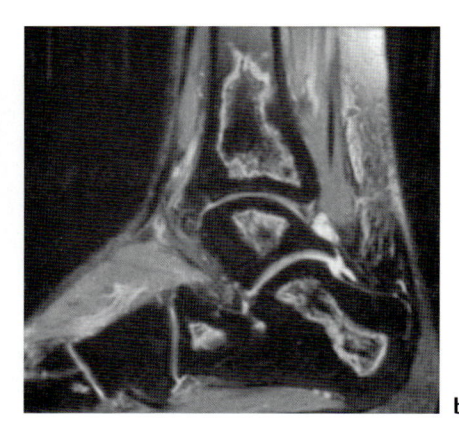

Figure 13.**18 a, b**   A 36-year-old man with sickle cell trait and bone infarcts in the distal tibia, talus, and calcaneus as seen on sagittal T1WI (**a**) and sagittal FS T2WI (**b**).

Table 13 (Continued)   Osseous tumors and tumorlike lesions at the hands and feet

Tumor/tumorlike Lesion	MRI Findings	Comments
Chondrosarcoma (Fig. 13.19)	Intramedullary tumors often have low-intermediate signal on T1WI, intermediate signal on PDWI, and heterogeneous intermediate-high signal on T2WI. Lesions usually show heterogeneous contrast enhancement.	Malignant tumors containing cartilage formed within sarcomatous stroma. Account for 12–21% of malignant bone lesions, 21–26% of primary sarcomas of bone, mean age =40 years, median =26 to 59 years. **(See Atlas Chapter A 11)**
Osteosarcoma	Destructive intramedullary malignant lesions, low-intermediate signal on T1WI, mixed low, intermediate, high signal on T2WI, usually with matrix mineralization/ossification-low signal on T2WI, usually show Gd-contrast enhancement. Zones of cortical destruction are typically seen through which tumors extend into the extraosseous soft tissues. Low signal from spicules of periosteal, reactive, and tumoral bone formation may be seen.	Malignant tumor comprising proliferating neoplastic spindle cells that produce osteoid and/or immature tumoral bone, most frequently arising within medullary bone. Two age peaks of incidence. The larger peak occurs between the ages of 10 and 20 and accounts for over half of the cases. The second smaller peak occurs in adults over 60 years and accounts for ~10% of the cases. Occurs in children as primary tumors and adults (associated with Paget disease, irradiated bone, chronic osteomyelitis, osteoblastoma, giant cell tumor, fibrous dysplasia. **(See Atlas Chapter A 64)**
Ewing sarcoma	Destructive malignant lesions involving marrow, low-intermediate signal on T1WI, mixed low, intermediate, and/or high signal on T2WI and FS T2WI, usually shows Gd-contrast enhancement (usually heterogeneous). Extraosseous tumor extension through sites of cortical destruction is commonly seen. Thin striated zones of low signal on T2WI can be sometimes seen oriented perpendicular to the long axis of the involved bone under the elevated periosteum representing the "hair on end" appearance of reactive bone formation secondary to the tumor.	Malignant primitive tumor of bone comprised of undifferentiated small cells with round nuclei. Accounts for 6–11% of primary malignant bone tumors, 5–7% of primary bone tumors. Usually occurs between the ages of 5 and 30, males > females, locally invasive, high metastatic potential. **(See Atlas Chapter A 20)**

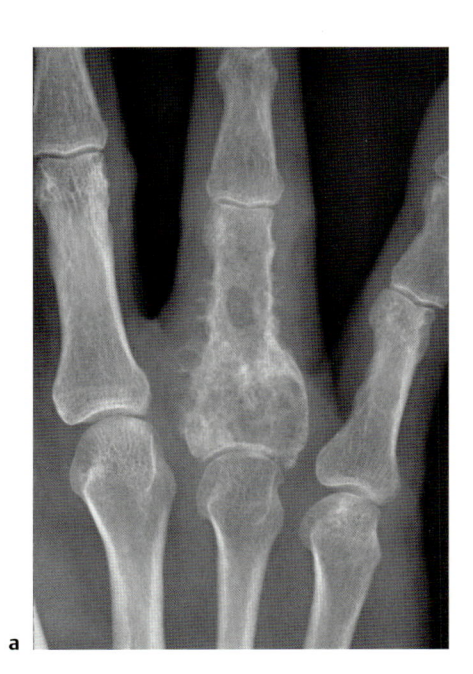

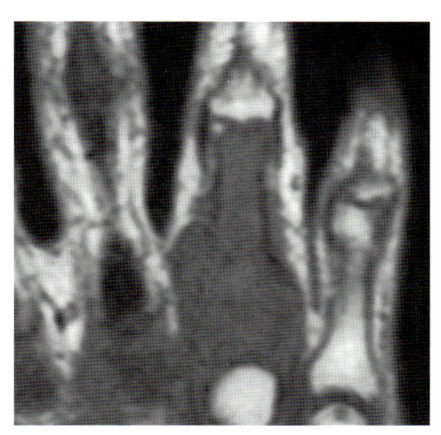

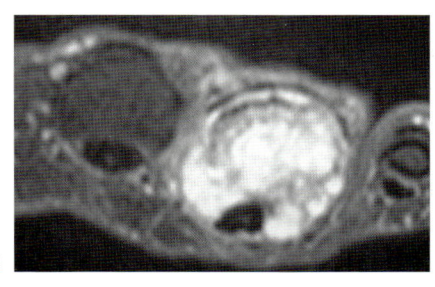

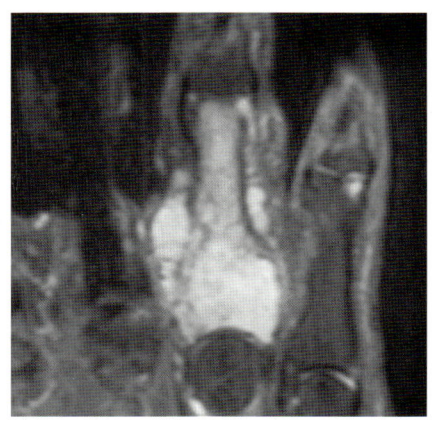

Figure 13.**19 a–d**   A 56-year-old man with a chondrosarcoma involving a metacarpal bone. The radiograph (**a**) shows an intramedullary lesion with chondroid matrix and cortical destruction. The lesion has intermediate signal on coronal T1WI (**b**) and high signal on coronal FS T2WI (**c**). The tumor shows Gd-contrast enhancement on axial FS T1WI (**d**). Cortical destruction and extraosseous tumor extension is seen with MRI.

References

Bizarre Parosteal Osteochondromatous Proliferation

Ambramovici L, Steiner GC. Bizarre parosteal osteochondromatous proliferation (Nora's Lesion): a retrospective study of 12 cases, 2 arising in long bones. *Hum Pathol* 2002;33:1205–1210.

Michelsen H, Abramovici L, Steiner G, Posner MA. Bizarre parosteal osteochondromatous proliferation (Nora's Lesion) in the hand. *J Hand Surg* May 2004;29A(3):520–525.

Orui H, Ishikawa A, Tsuchiya T, Ogino T. Magnetic resonance imaging characteristics of bizarre parosteal osteochondromatous proliferation of the hand: a case report. *J Hand Surg* November 2002;27A(6):1104–1108.

Torreggiani WC, Munk PL, Al-Ismail K, et al. MR imaging features of bizarre parosteal osteochondromatous proliferation of bone (Nora's Lesion). *Eur J Radiol* 2001;40:224–231.

Table 14 Diffuse, multiple, poorly defined and/or multifocal zones of abnormal marrow signal

Disorder	MRI Findings	Comments
Nonmalignant		
Red marrow reconversion (Figs. 14.1, 14.2, 14.3)	Involved marrow has slightly to moderately decreased signal relative to fat on T1WI and PDWI, isointense signal relative to muscle and slightly increased signal relative to fat on FS T2WI.	Hyperplasia of normal marrow elements at sites that were previously composed mostly of yellow marrow. May be seen in obese middle-aged patients, tobacco smokers, marathon runners, and those living in high altitudes.

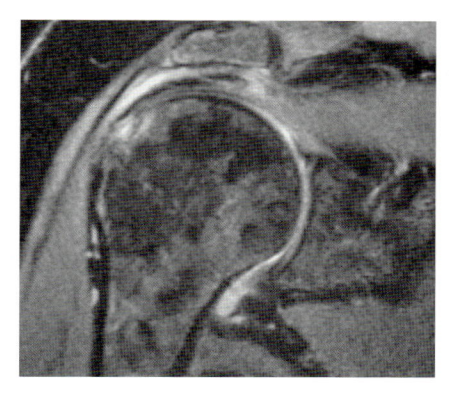

Figure 14.1 A 48-year-old woman with red marrow reconversion in the proximal humerus seen as irregular zones with isointense signal relative to muscle and slightly increased signal relative to fat on coronal FS T2WI.

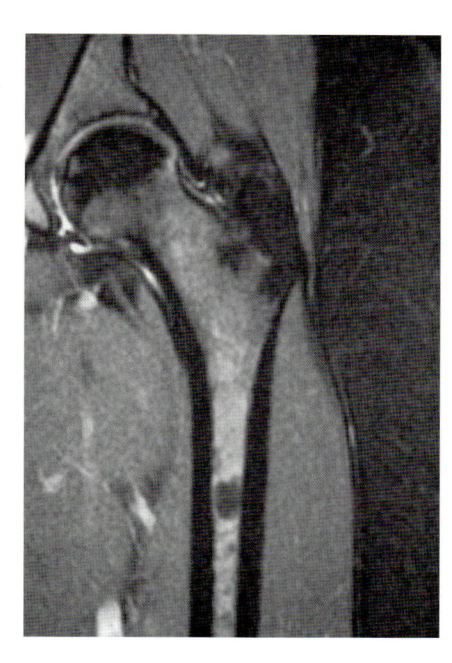

Figure 14.2 A 40-year-old woman with red marrow reconversion in the metadiaphyseal marrow of the femur as seen on coronal FS T2WI.

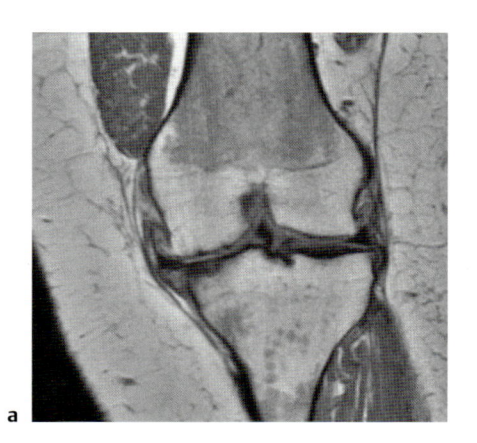

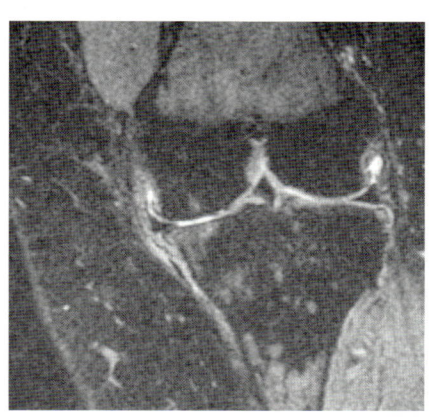

Figure 14.3 a, b A 36-year-old woman with red marrow reconversion in the metadiaphyseal marrow of the distal femur and proximal tibia as seen on coronal PDWI (**a**) and coronal FS T2WI (**b**).

Table 14 (Continued) Diffuse, multiple, poorly defined and/or multifocal zones of abnormal marrow signal

Disorder	MRI Findings	Comments
Inherited anemias (sickle cell anemia, thalassemia, sideroblastic anemia) (Figs. 14.4–14.7)	Involved marrow has slightly to moderately decreased signal relative to fat on T1WI and T2WI, isointense to slightly hyperintense signal relative to muscle and increased signal relative to fat on FS T2WI.	Inherited anemias result in hyperplasia of normal marrow elements. Sickle cell disease is the most common hemoglobinopathy in which abnormal hemoglobin S is combined with itself, or other hemoglobin types such as C, D, E, or thalassemia. Hemoglobin SS, SC, and S-thalassemia have the most sickling of erythrocytes. In addition to marrow hyperplasia seen in sickle cell disease, bone infarcts and extramedullary hematopoiesis can also occur. β-thalassemia is a disorder in which there is deficient synthesis of β chains of hemoglobin resulting in excess α chains in erythrocytes and erythrocytes causing dysfunctional hematopoiesis and hemolysis. The decrease in β chains can be severe as in the major type (homozygous), moderate in the intermediate type (heterozygous), or mild in the minor type (heterozygous).

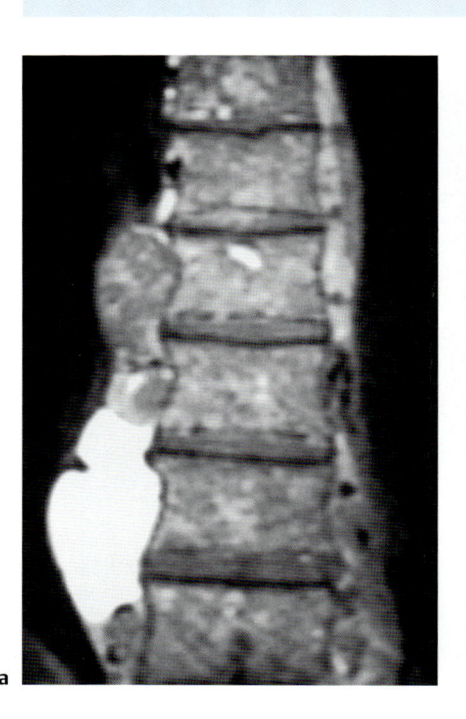

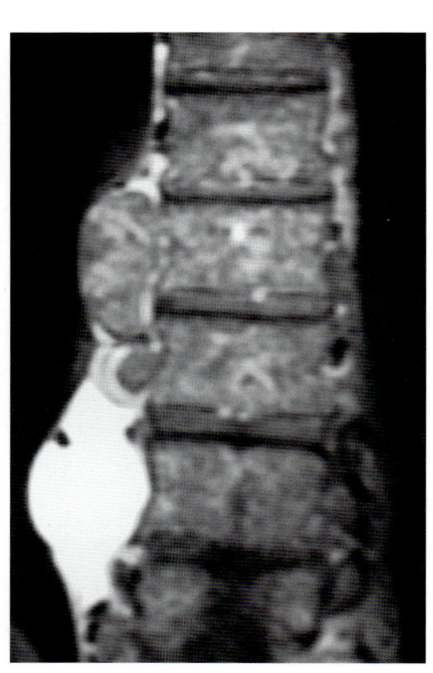

Figure 14.**4 a, b** A 54-year-old man with sickle cell disease and extramedullary hematopoiesis. The marrow has heterogeneous mixed low-intermediate signal and slightly high signal on coronal T1WI (**a**) and coronal T2WI (**b**) that is hypointense to fat.

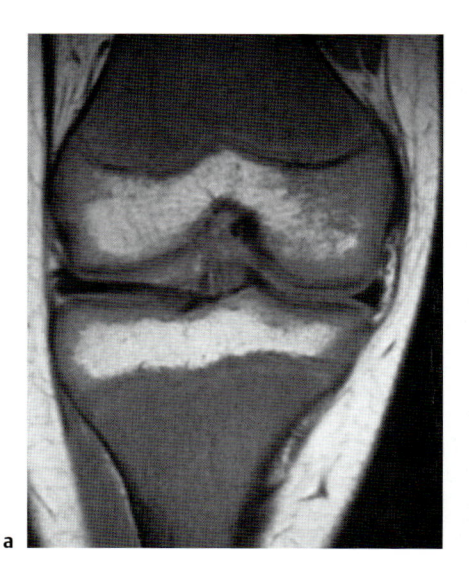

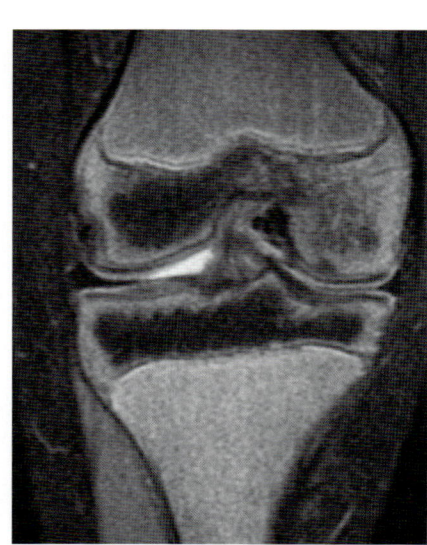

Figure 14.**5 a, b** A 14-year-old girl with sickle cell disease with marrow signal alteration in the metaphyseal regions of the knee, and to a lesser extent within epiphyseal marrow. Marrow signal is low-intermediate on coronal T1WI (**a**) and hypointense relative to fat. The marrow signal is slightly high on coronal FS T2WI (**b**), which is hyperintense relative to fat and muscle.

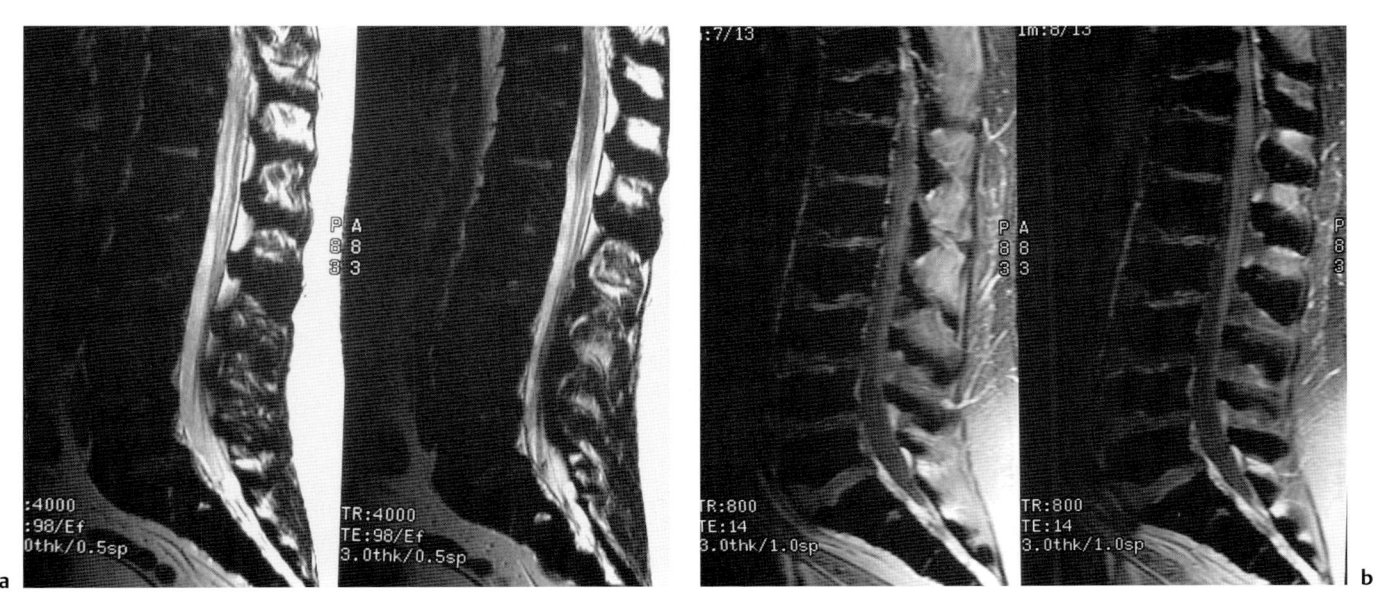

Figure 14.**6 a, b** A 22-year-old man with β thalassemia major. Marrow signal is low on sagittal T2WI (**a**) and post-Gd-contrast FS T1WI (**b**) secondary to iron overload.

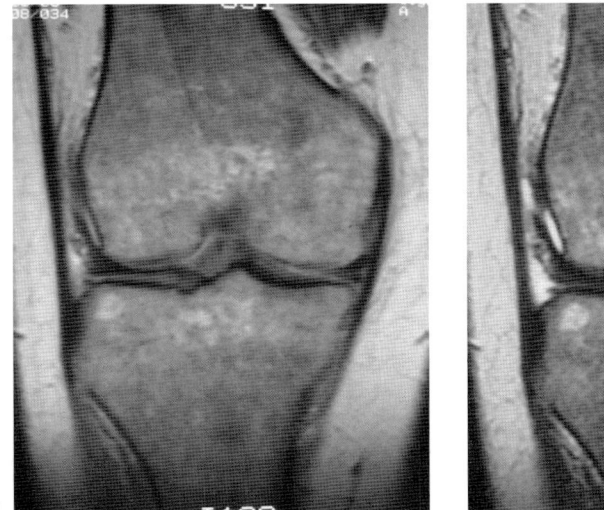

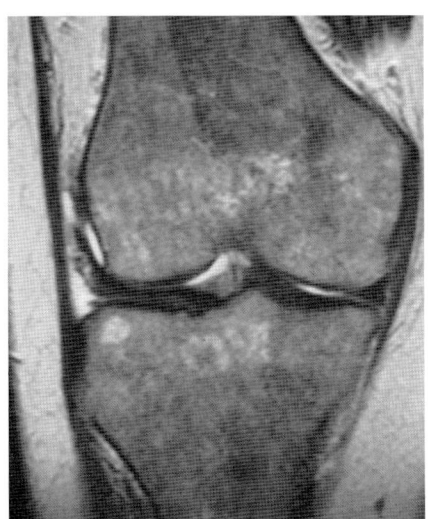

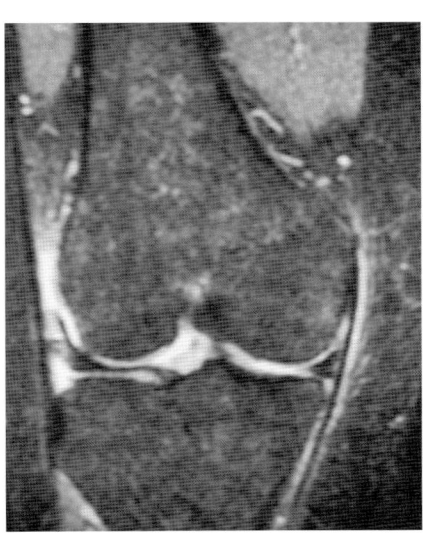

Figure 14.**7 a–c** A 49-year-old woman with β thalassemia minor. The marrow has heterogeneous mixed low-intermediate signal on coronal PDWI (**a**) and coronal T2WI (**b**), which is hypointense relative to fat, and slightly high signal on coronal FS T2WI (**c**), which is hyperintense relative to fat.

Table 14 (Continued) Diffuse, multiple, poorly defined and/or multifocal zones of abnormal marrow signal

Disorder	MRI Findings	Comments
Marrow hyperplasia from exogenous erythropoietin (Fig. 14.8)	Involved marrow has slightly to moderately decreased signal relative to fat on T1WI and T2WI; isointense signal relative to muscle and slightly increased signal relative to fat on FS T2WI.	Exogenous source (medication) of erythropoietin used for treatment of anemia.
Granulocyte/macrophage colony stimulating factor (G/M-CSF) (Fig. 14.9)	Use of these medications induces red marrow reconversion, which occurs more commonly in a diffuse pattern compared with focal sites. Involved marrow has slightly decreased signal relative to fat on T1WI and T2WI; isointense signal relative to muscle and slightly increased signal relative to fat on FS T2WI.	G-CSF is used as an adjunct for chemotherapy to minimize or correct treatment-related neutropenia by regulating the proliferation and differentiation of hematopoietic progenitor cells.
Hemochromatosis and iron deposition from multiple transfusions (Fig. 14.10)	Involved marrow has low signal on T1WI, PDWI, and T2WI.	Hemochromatosis is an iron storage disorder with abnormal increased deposition of iron in various tissues. Hemochromatosis can be a primary autosomal recessive disorder in which there is increased intestinal absorption of iron resulting in a 10 to 50-fold increase in total body iron. The primary disorder is associated with a gene on chromosome 6, and occurs with an incidence of 3–5 per 1000. Usually presents in adults, and occasionally in children. Secondary hemochromatosis occurs from iron overload from transfusions for sickle cell disease and thalassemia, alcoholic liver disease, and excessive dietary iron.

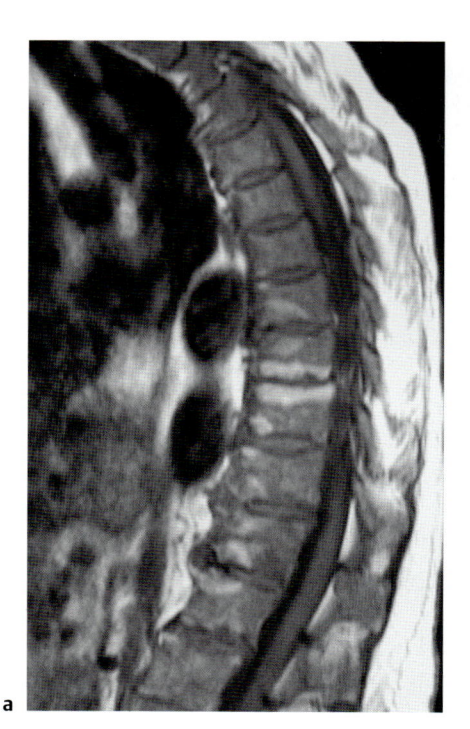

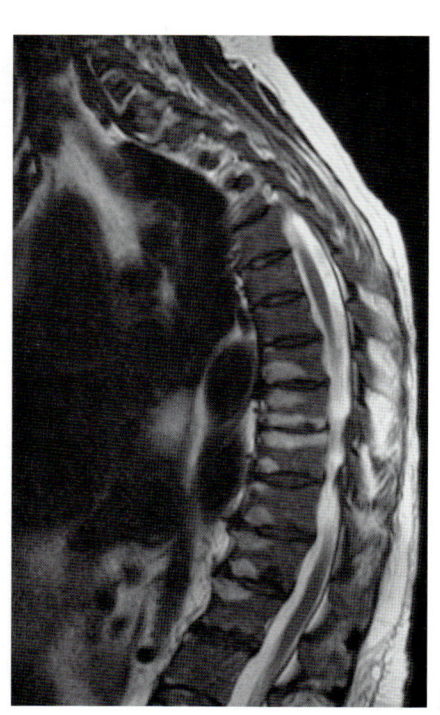

Figure 14.8 a, b   A 60-year-old woman treated with exogenous erythropoietin for anemia. Marrow has slightly to moderately decreased signal relative to fat on sagittal T1WI (**a**) and sagittal (**b**) T2WI.

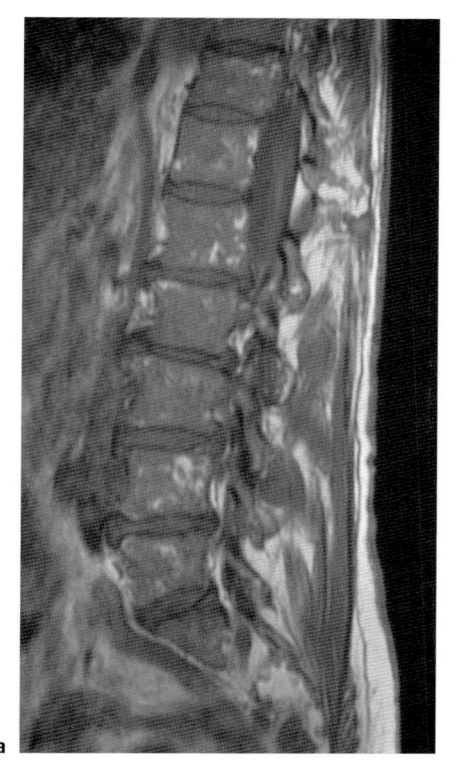

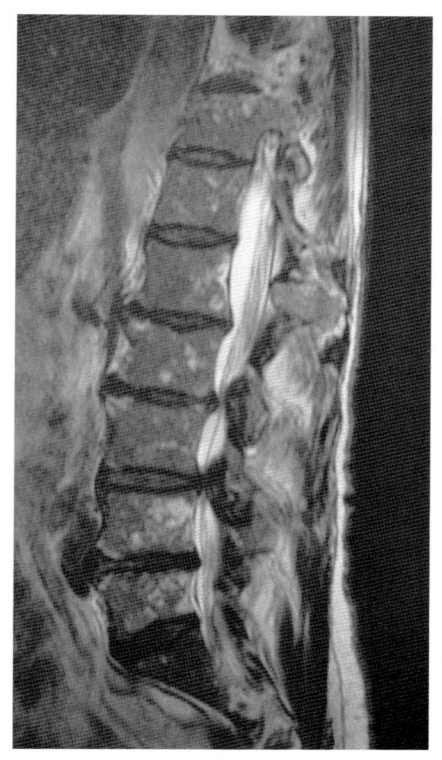

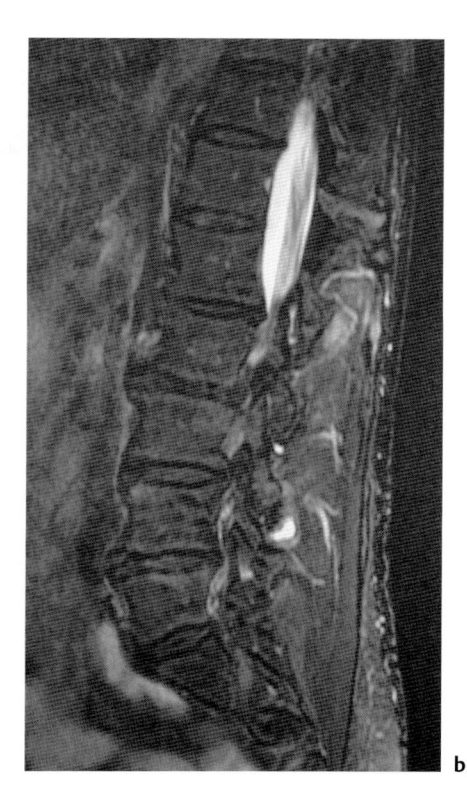

Figure 14.**9 a–c** A 79-year-old woman with neutropenia treated with granulocyte colony stimulating factor. Marrow has heterogeneous slightly to moderately decreased signal relative to fat on sagittal T1WI (**a**) and sagittal T2WI (**b**). Marrow signal is minimally increased relative to fat on FS T2WI (**c**).

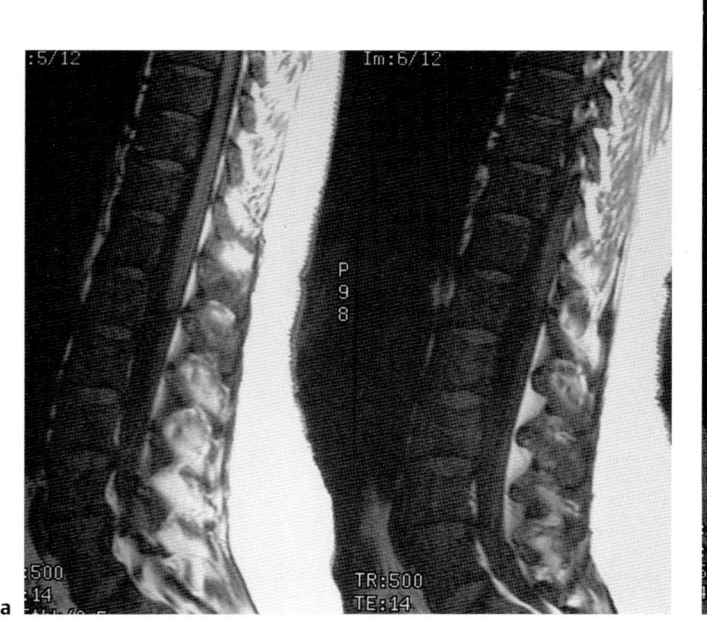

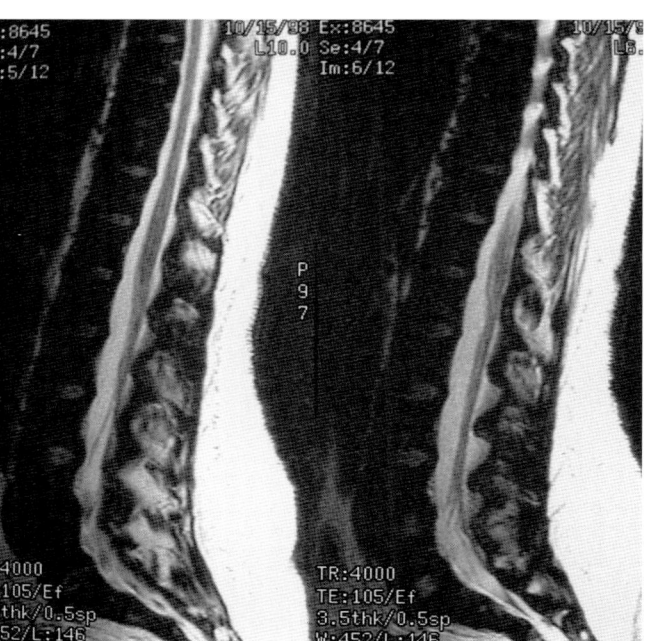

Figure 14.**10 a, b** Iron overload in a patient with sickle cell disease from multiple transfusions. Marrow signal is low on sagittal T1WI (**a**) and T2WI (**b**).

Table 14 (Continued) Diffuse, multiple, poorly defined and/or multifocal zones of abnormal marrow signal		
Disorder	**MRI Findings**	**Comments**
Paget disease	In the initial phases, thickening of the involved cortex is seen, which has low to intermediate signal on T1WI and PDWI and often has various combinations of low, intermediate, slightly high, and/or high signal on T2WI and FS T2WI. Irregular Gd-contrast enhancement can be seen in the thickened cortex. Marrow signal during the initial phases of Paget disease can be within normal limits, or slightly increased in a V-shape on FS T2WI secondary to fibrovascular tissue replacement of normal marrow, and/or dilated blood vessels with slow flow. In the late or inactive phases of the disease, findings include osseous expansion, cortical thickening, decreased diameter of the medullary canal, and coarsened trabeculae along stress lines. Zones of cortical thickening usually have low signal on T1WI and T2WI. Thick linear intramedullary zones of low signal on T1WI and T2WI can be seen secondary to thickened bone trabeculae. Marrow in late or inactive phases of Paget disease can: 1) have signal similar to normal marrow, 2) contain focal areas of fat signal, 3) have low signal on T1WI and T2WI secondary to regions of sclerosis, 4) have areas of high signal on FS T2WI from edema or persistent fibrovascular tissue, or 5) have various combinations of the aforementioned.	Paget disease is a chronic skeletal disease in which there is disordered bone resorption and woven bone formation resulting in osseous deformity. A paramyxovirus may be an etiologic agent for Paget disease. Can be poly-ostotic in up to 66% of patients. Paget disease is associated with a risk of less than 1% for developing secondary sarcomatous changes. **(See Atlas Chapter A 65)**
Renal osteodystrophy (Fig. 14.11)	Zones of low signal on T1WI and T2WI corresponding to regions of bone sclerosis are seen. In the spine, bands of low signal on T1WI and T2WI can be seen at bands of sclerosis that occur parallel to endplates (*rugger jersey vertebrae*).	Osteoblastic and osteoclastic changes can occur in bone as a result of chronic end-stage renal disease, secondary hyperparathyroidism (hyperplasia of parathyroid glands), and osteomalacia (abnormal vitamin D metabolism). Can result in pathologic fracture. Unlike secondary hyperparathyroidism, diffuse or patchy bone sclerosis infrequently occurs.

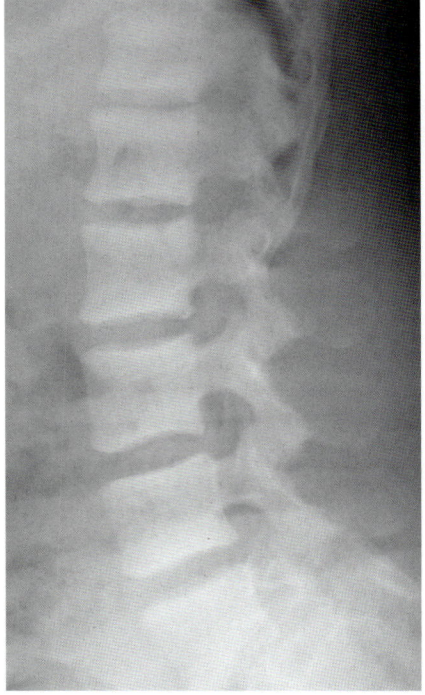

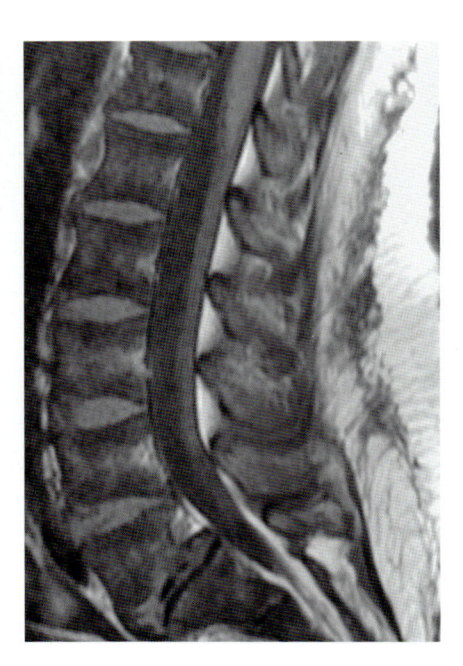

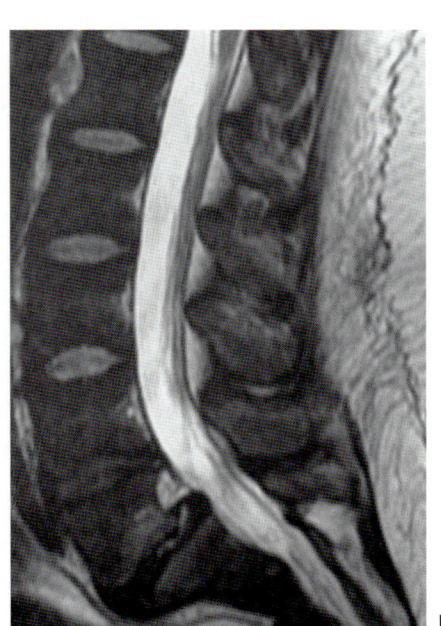

Figure 14.11 a–c A 34-year-old woman with renal osteodystrophy. Lateral radiograph (**a**) shows bands of sclerosis parallel to end plates (*rugger jersey vertebrae*). Zones of low signal on sagittal T1WI (**b**) and T2WI (**c**) correspond to regions of bone sclerosis.

Table 14 (Continued)	Diffuse, multiple, poorly defined and/or multifocal zones of abnormal marrow signal	
Disorder	**MRI Findings**	**Comments**
Hypoparathyroidism	Localized or generalized osteosclerosis can be seen in bone on radiographs and CT, with corresponding low signal on T1WI and T2WI.	Deficiency in functional parathyroid hormone formation (surgical excision, radiation, trauma, autoimmune disease) results in hypocalcemia and generalized or localized osteosclerosis.
Pseudohypoparathyroidism	Bone density can be normal or diffusely increased or decreased as seen on radiographs. Other features include premature physeal plate closure resulting in short stature, calvarial thickening, shortening of the 1st, 4th, and 5th metacarpal bones, soft tissue calcifications, and ossification of the posterior longitudinal ligament.	Heritable disorder with end-organ resistance to parathyroid hormone resulting in hypocalcemia, hyperphosphatemia with deposition of calcium in soft tissues and basal ganglia in the brain. More common in females, X-linked dominant trait.
Pseudo-pseudohypo-parathyroidism	Imaging findings similar to pseudohypoparathyroidism.	Similar clinical and imaging features to pseudohypoparathyroidism except patients are normocalcemic.
Osteitis condensans (Fig. 14.12)	Zones of subchondral osteosclerosis usually have corresponding zones of low signal on T1WI and T2WI. In addition, small irregular zones of slightly high signal may be seen in the marrow on FS T2WI, as well as mild irregular Gd-contrast enhancement.	Unilateral or asymmetric or symmetric bilateral osteosclerotic process in the subchondral marrow adjacent to the sacroiliac joints (iliac bone more pronounced than the sacral marrow) and/or pubic symphysis, usually occurs in women and is often associated with pregnancy. The subchondral bone is usually well defined, and the sacroiliac joint is typically intact. Findings may persist or regress.

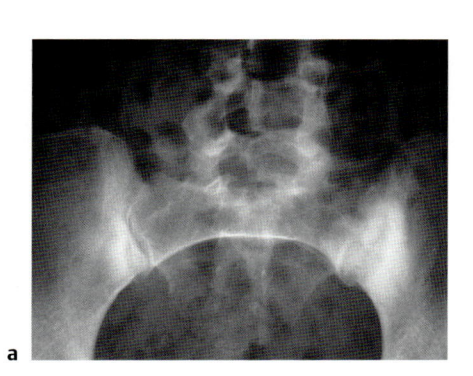

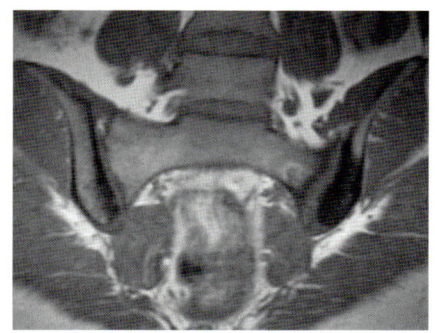

Figure 14.12 a–d A 35-year-old woman with osteitis condensans ilii at both sacroiliac joints. Zones of subchondral osteosclerosis are seen on the AP radiograph (**a**) at both sacroiliac joints. They have corresponding zones of mostly low signal on coronal T1WI (**b**) and FS T2WI (**c**). Small irregular zones of slightly high signal are seen in the subchondral marrow on FS T2WI (**c**) and show mild irregular Gd-contrast enhancement on coronal FS T1WI (**d**).

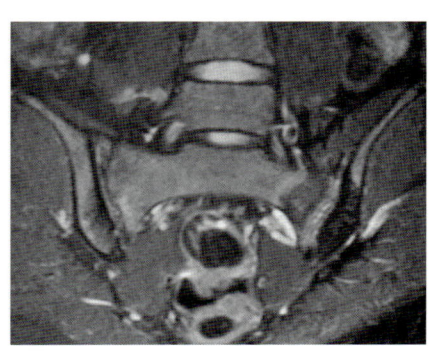

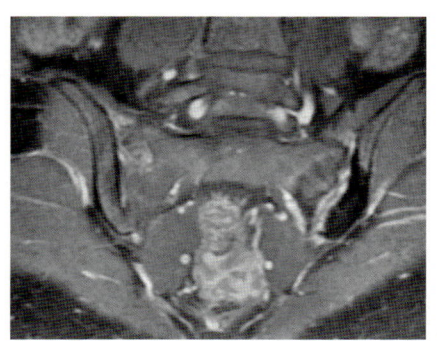

Table 14 (Continued) Diffuse, multiple, poorly defined and/or multifocal zones of abnormal marrow signal		
Disorder	**MRI Findings**	**Comments**
Bilateral sacroiliitis (Fig. 14.13)	Asymmetric or symmetric poorly defined zones with high signal on T2WI and FS T2WI and corresponding Gd-contrast enhancement in the subchondral marrow of the iliac and sacral bones adjacent to the sacroiliac joints.	Commonly occurs in ankylosing spondylitis, which is an autoimmune inflammatory disorder associated with HLA-B27 that frequently involves both sacroiliac joints in most patients, as well as the hips in 35% of patients.
Bilateral sacral insufficiency fractures (Fig. 14.14)	Asymmetric or symmetric poorly defined zones with low signal on T1WI, high signal on T2WI and FS T2WI, and corresponding Gd-contrast enhancement are seen in the marrow of both sacral ala within which may be serpiginous curvilinear zones of low signal. No zones with abnormal signal are typically seen in the iliac bones or sacroiliac joints.	Axial forces to sacral bone can result in insufficiency-type stress fractures in osteopenic bone in older patients or from osteomalacia, or fatigue-type stress fractures in athletes (runners, gymnasts, etc.). May be associated with pubic bone fractures. Patients can have point tenderness, pain with weight bearing and movement.
Bone infarction (Fig. 14.15)	In the early phases of ischemia, diffuse poorly defined zones of high signal may be seen on FS T2WI that can overlap the MRI features of transient painful bone marrow edema. In zones of bone infarction, curvilinear zones of low signal on T1WI and T2WI representing zones of fibrosis are usually seen in the marrow. In addition to the above findings, irregular zones of low signal on T1WI and high signal on T2WI and FS T2WI may be seen in the marrow representing zones of fluid from edema, ischemia/infarction, or fracture if present. Irregular zones with high signal on T1WI and T2WI can occasionally be seen resulting from hemorrhage in combination with zones of fibrosis and fluid. A double-line sign (curvilinear adjacent zones of low and high signal on T2WI) is often seen at the edges of the infarcts representing the borders of osseous resorption and healing. After Gd-contrast administration, irregular enhancement can be seen from granulation tissue ingrowth.	Bone infarcts are zones of ischemic death involving bone trabeculae and marrow, which may be idiopathic or result from: trauma, corticosteroid treatment, chemotherapy, radiation treatment, occlusive vascular disease, collagen vascular and other autoimmune diseases, metabolic storage diseases (Gaucher etc.), sickle cell disease, thalassemia, hyperbaric events / Caisson disease, pregnancy, alcohol abuse, pancreatitis, infections, and lymphoproliferative diseases. Osteonecrosis is more common in fatty compared with hematopoietic marrow. Avascular necrosis involving specific bones may have names such as: Legg–Calvé–Perthes disease (femoral head), Kienbock disease (lunate), Preiser disease (scaphoid), Kohler disease (tarsal navicular), Freiberg infarction (metatarsal head), Panner disease (capitulum of humerus), and Thiemann disease (phalanges of hand). **(See Atlas Chapter A 37)**
Reflex sympathetic dystrophy (also referred to as Sudek atrophy, algodystrophy. complex regional pain syndromes type I)	Poorly defined zones with increased signal on FS T2WI may be seen in the bone marrow of one or more bones in some cases during the warm phase of RSD, but signal abnormalities are typically absent in the dystrophic cold phases of this disorder. Findings of increased signal on FS T2WI may also occur in the adjacent soft tissues in some cases.	Syndromes in which there are clinical findings such as abnormal sensation (continuing pain in the absence of external stimuli, hyperesthesia), and altered vasomotor (skin temperature asymmetry, skin color asymmetry) and autonomic function (edema, sweating changes or sweating asymmetry). In Chronic regional pain syndrome type 1 (RSD), no nerve damage can be detected. RSD can occur in a limb after fracture or other injury, or in immobilized limbs of patients who have had cerebral infarcts. Chronic regional pain syndrome type 2 (causalgia) differs from type 1 (RSD) in that the former is associated with nerve damage detectable with electromyography.

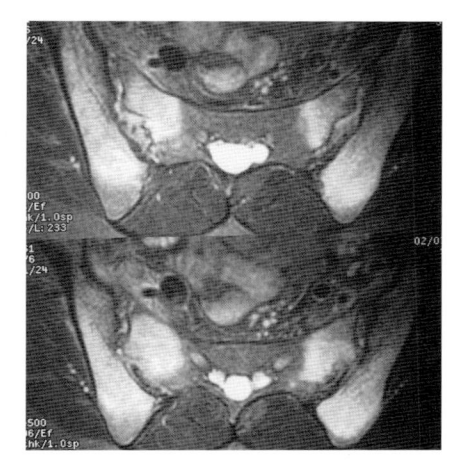

Figure 14.**13** A 35-year-old woman with bilateral sacroiliitis seen as symmetric poorly defined zones with high signal on axial FS T2WI. Zones with high signal are also seen in the sacroiliac joints.

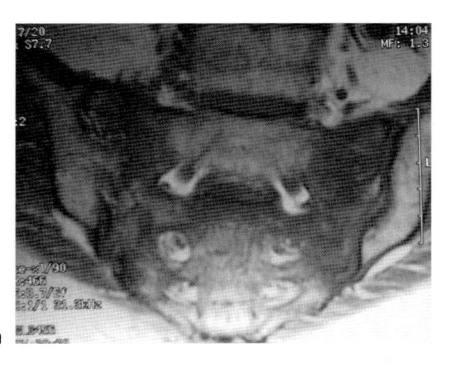

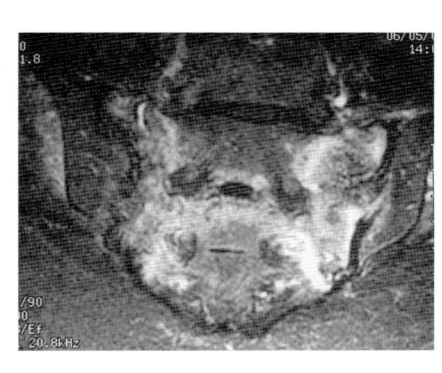

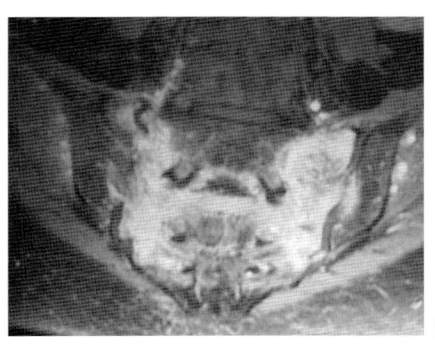

Figure 14.**14 a–c** An 85-year-old woman with bilateral sacral insufficiency fractures that have poorly defined zones of abnormal marrow signal consisting of low signal on coronal T1WI (**a**) and high signal on FS T2WI (**b**), with corresponding Gd-contrast enhancement on coronal FS T1WI (**c**). Serpiginous thin curvilinear zones of low signal are also seen at the fracture sites on FS T2WI.

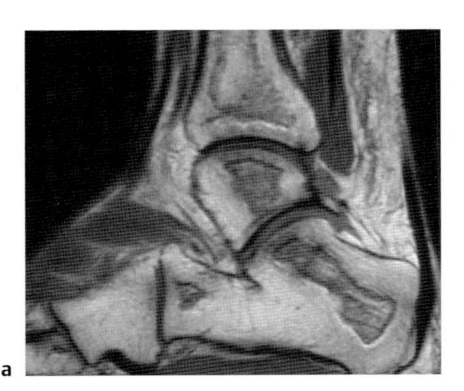

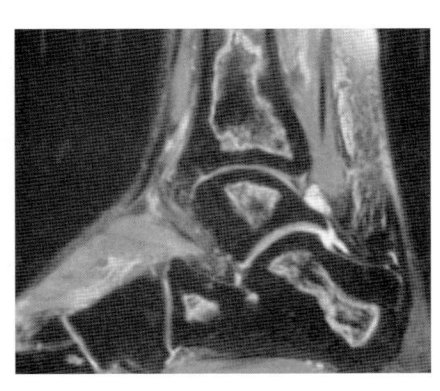

Figure 14.**15 a, b** A 36-year-old man with bone infarcts in the distal tibia, talus, and calcaneus bones seen as serpiginous zones of low signal on sagittal PDWI (**a**) and high signal on FS T2WI (**b**).

Table 14 (Continued) Diffuse, multiple, poorly defined and/or multifocal zones of abnormal marrow signal		
Disorder	**MRI Findings**	**Comments**
Serous atrophy of marrow from malnutrition (Figs. 14.16, 14.17)	Depending on the severity of the malnutrition, involved marrow can have low-intermediate signal on T1WI and high signal on T2WI and FS T2WI. No Gd-contrast enhancement is usually seen. The marrow signal abnormalities may be localized or diffuse.	In emaciated patients from various causes (malnutrition, malabsorption, anorexia nervosa/bulimia, chronic renal insufficiency, HIV infection, and cancer), decreases in adipose tissue progressively occurs in bone marrow and subcutaneous tissue followed by orbital fat. With progression of malnutrition, serous atrophy occurs in marrow in which there is accumulation of extracellular matrix containing hyaluronic acid associated with adipose and hematopoietic cell atrophy. The degree and extent of serous atrophy in marrow are related to body mass index and hemoglobin concentration. The lower limbs are frequent sites of serous atrophy, often being more prominent distally than proximally.
Gaucher disease (Fig. 14.18)	Diffuse and/or patchy heterogeneous zones with low-intermediate signal on T1WI and heterogeneous intermediate to high signal on T2WI and FS T2WI.	Rare, heritable metabolic disorder with deficient activity of the lysosomal enzyme-hydrolase β-glucosidase. Results in accumulation of the lipid-glucosylceramide within lysosomes of the monocyte-macrophage system (Gaucher cells) of the bone marrow, liver, and spleen. Marrow infiltration by Gaucher cells often results in zones of ischemia and bone infarction.
Glycogen storage disease type 1B	Myeloid hyperplasia present in this disorder results in inhomogeneous decreased signal of marrow on T1WI compared with fat, and inhomogeneous hyperintense signal on FS T2WI or STIR.	Disorder affecting children and young adults in which there is deficiency of functional microsomal glucose-6-phosphatase activity causing impairment of glycogenolysis and gluconeogenesis. As a result. Patients suffer from postprandial and fasting hypoglycemia, increased production of lactic acid, uric acid, and triglycerides. Patients have increased susceptibility to bacterial infections secondary to chronic neutropenia, abnormal myeloid maturation, and dysfunction of circulating neutrophils and monocytes. Patients are often treated with G-CSF for neutropenia.
Glycogen storage disease type 1A	Marrow in this disorder is typically fatty.	Disorder affecting children and young adults in which there is deficiency of functional microsomal glucose-6-phosphatase activity causing impairment of glycogenolysis and gluconeogenesis. As a result, patients suffer from postprandial and fasting hypoglycemia, increased production of lactic acid, uric acid, and triglycerides. Unlike Glycogen storage disease type 1B, patients do not have increased susceptibility to bacterial infections.
Osteopetrosis (Fig. 14.19)	Radiographs show diffuse and/or band-like zones of osteosclerosis that appear as zones of low signal on T1WI and T2WI.	Osteopetrosis consists of four types (precocious type: autosomal recessive form that is usually lethal; delayed type: autosomal dominant form described by Albers-Schönberg that can be asymptomatic until there is a pathologic fracture or anemia; intermediate recessive type in which patients have short stature, hepatomegaly, and anemia; and tubular acidosis autosomal recessive form in which cerebral calcifications occur as well as renal tubular acidosis, mental retardation, muscle weakness, and hypotonia.

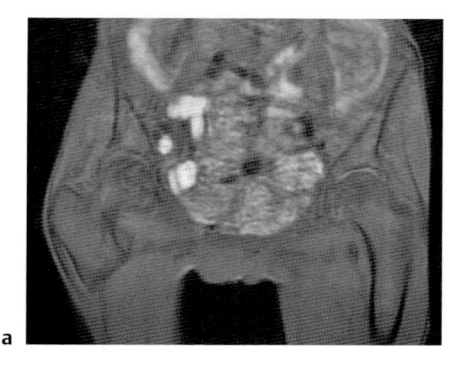

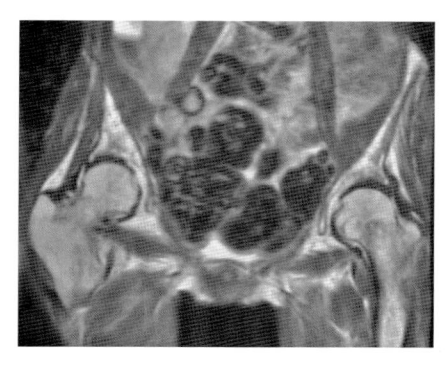

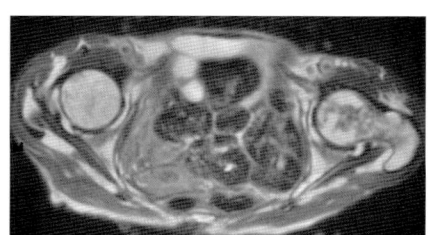

Figure 14.**16 a–c** A 66-year-old woman with malabsorption syndrome and cachexia with extensive diffuse serous atrophy of marrow seen as loss of normal fat signal in the soft tissues and marrow on coronal (**a**) T1WI. Diffuse abnormal high signal is seen in the marrow on coronal (**b**) and axial (**c**) T2WI.

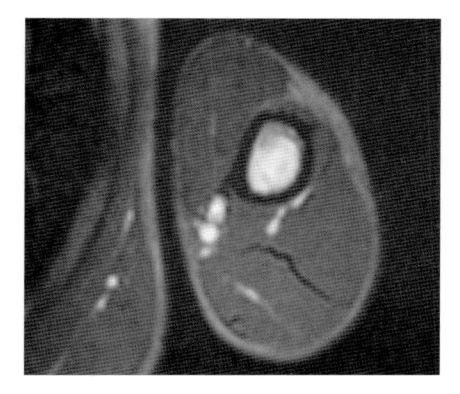

Figure 14.**17** A 16-year-old male with anorexia and serous atrophy involving the marrow of the humerus seen as high signal on axial FS T2WI. Note diminished subcutaneous fat.

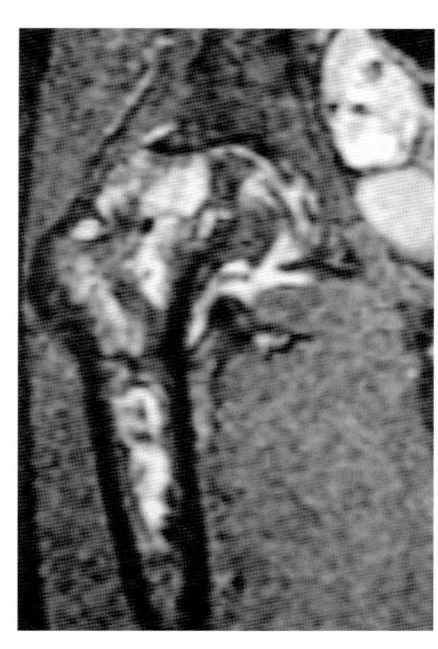

Figure 14.**18** A 34-year-old woman with Gaucher disease with diffuse and patchy heterogeneous zones with intermediate to high signal in the marrow on coronal STIR.

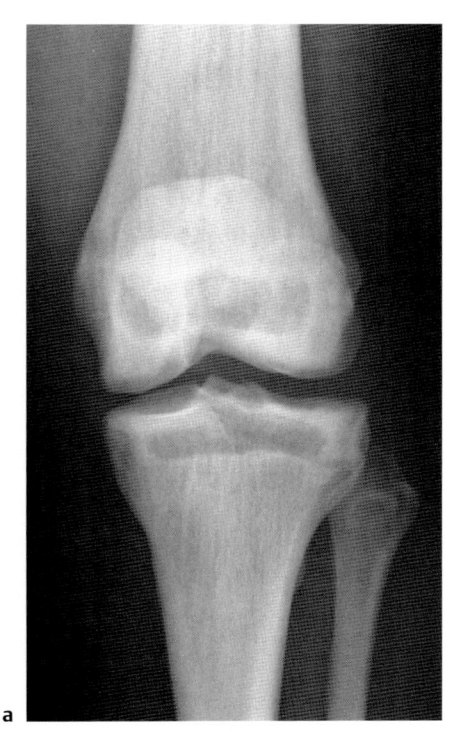

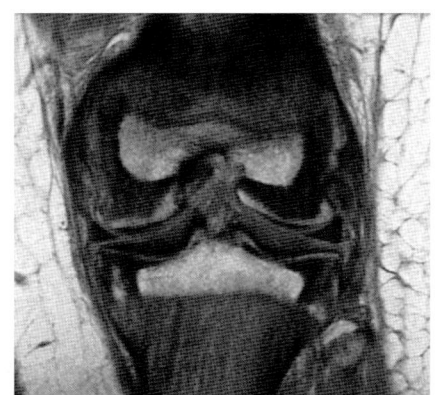

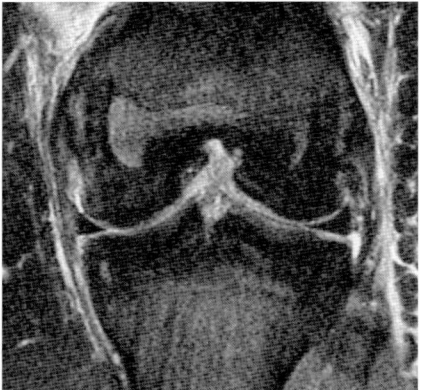

Figure 14.**19 a–c** A 28-year-old woman with osteopetrosis. The AP (**a**) radiograph shows diffuse osteosclerosis that appears as zones with low signal on coronal (**b**) T1WI and FS T2WI (**c**).

Table 14 (Continued) Diffuse, multiple, poorly defined and/or multifocal zones of abnormal marrow signal		
Disorder	MRI Findings	Comments
Hypervitamosis A and D	Hyperostosis and cortical thickening may be seen involving tubular bones of children on plain films and CT.	Intoxication of vitamins A and D can lead to hyperostosis in children from cortical thickening from increased periosteal bone formation.
Fluorosis	Often seen as dense diffuse osteosclerosis associated with osteophytes involving the spine, thorax, and pelvis. Limited osseous changes are seen in tubular bones of the extremities and the skull. MRI can show corresponding low signal in the spine on T1WI and T2WI.	Disease caused by excessive intake of fluoride via water containing more than 4 ppm. Fluorosis is associated with increased ossification and sclerosis of bone, as well as the posterior longitudinal ligament with resultant myelopathy. Hypertrophy of joints and bones can occur with osteoarthropathy.
Osteomyelitis (Fig. 14.20)	In **acute osteomyelitis**, poorly defined zones of low or low-intermediate signal on T1WI; and high signal on T2WI, STIR, and FS T2WI are seen in the marrow. A wide zone of transition between normal bone and edematous and infected bone is typically seen in acute osteomyelitis. Loss of definition of the low signal line of the cortical margins is often observed on T1WI, T2WI, STIR, and FS T2WI. After Gd-contrast administration, irregular zones of contrast enhancement are seen in the involved marrow on FS T1WI.	Osteomyelitis is a disorder in which there is infection of bone and commonly the adjacent soft tissues. Can result from hematogenous spread of microorganisms as well as from trauma-direct inoculation, extension from adjacent tissues, and complications from surgery. Bacteria such as *Staphylococcus aureus* and *Streptococcus pyogenes* are the most common infectious organisms. Can also result from other bacteria as well as *Mycobacterium tuberculosis*, fungi, parasites, and viruses. **(See Atlas Chapter A 63)**
Eosinophilic granuloma (Langerhans cell histiocytosis)	Focal intramedullary lesion(s) associated with trabecular and cortical bone destruction that typically have low-intermediate signal on T1WI and PDWI and heterogeneous slightly high to high signal on T2WI. Poorly defined zones of high signal on T2WI are usually seen in the marrow peripheral to the lesions secondary to inflammatory changes. Extension of lesions from the marrow into adjacent soft tissues through areas of cortical disruption are commonly seen as well as linear periosteal zones of high signal on T2WI. Lesions typically show prominent Gd-contrast enhancement in marrow and in extraosseous soft tissue portions of the lesions.	Benign tumor-like lesions consisting of Langerhans cells (histiocytes), and variable amounts of lymphocytes, polymorphonuclear cells, and eosinophils. Account for 1% of primary bone lesions, and 8% of tumor-like lesions. Occur in patients with median age = 10 years, average = 13.5 years, peak incidence is between 5 and 10 years, 80–85% occur in patients less than 30 years. Multifocal subtypes (Letterer–Siwe disease and Hand–Schüller–Christian disease) account for 30% of cases. **(See Atlas Chapter A 18)**
Sarcoidosis (Fig. 14.21)	In **small bones**, lesions usually appear as intramedullary zones with low to intermediate signal on T1WI and slightly high to high signal on T2WI, FS PDWI, and FS T2WI. After Gd-contrast administration, lesions typically show moderate to prominent enhancement. In **long bones and axial skeleton**, sarcoid lesions are often multiple with variable sizes or solitary within marrow. Zones of cortical destruction associated with intramedullary lesions are uncommon, unlike with sarcoid involving small bones. Lesions can have circumscribed and/or indistinct margins within marrow. Irregular confluent or patchy zones as well as a diffuse stippled pattern of signal alteration in marrow have also been described for skeletal sarcoid lesions. Lesions usually have low to intermediate signal on T1WI and PDWI, and often have slightly high to high signal on T2WI and FS T2WI. Occasional lesions may also have low or intermediate signal on T2WI. Focal areas with MRI signal similar to fat are seen in some lesions in long bones. Lesions with low signal on T2WI correspond to plain film and CT findings of osteosclerosis. After Gd-contrast administration, variable enhancement can be seen.	Sarcoidosis is a chronic systemic granulomatous disease of unknown etiology in which noncaseating granulomas occur in various tissues and organs. Sarcoidosis appears to be related to an abnormal or exaggerated T helper-induced cellular immune response to antigens or self-antigens resulting in the collection of large numbers of activated T cells in the affected tissue. Bones of the hands and feet are common sites of involvement, but any bone can be affected. **(See Atlas Chapter A 71)**

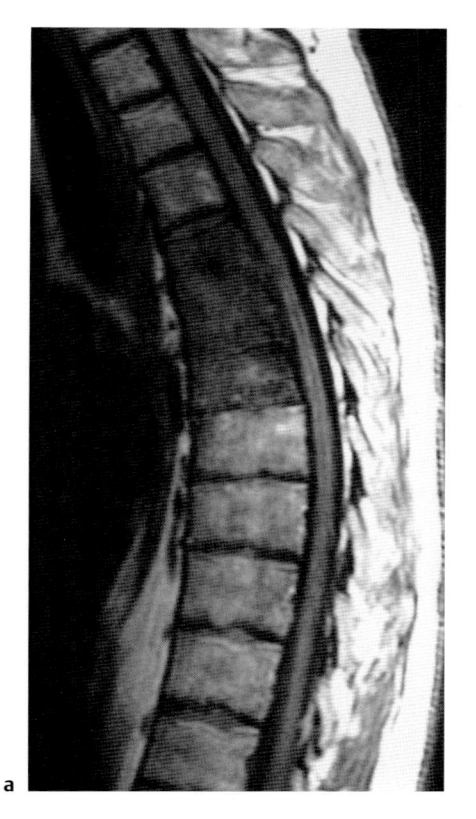

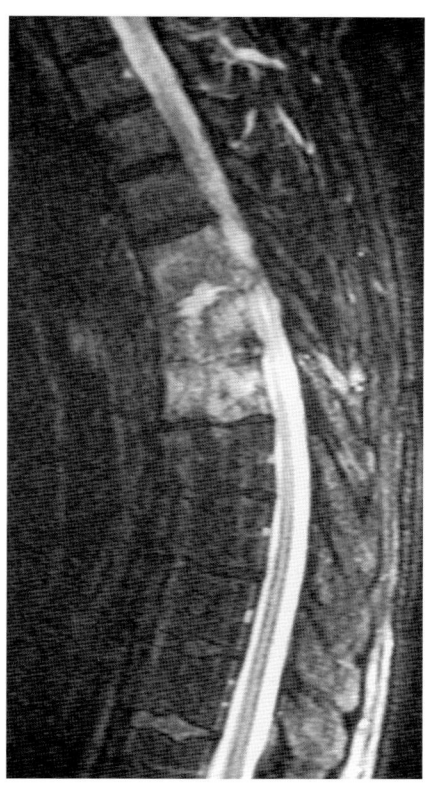

Figure 14.**20 a, b**   Coccidioidal osteomyelitis involving three adjacent thoracic vertebrae and intervening disks seen as poorly defined zones of low-intermediate signal on sagittal T1WI (**a**) and high signal on FS T2WI (**b**) in the marrow and disks. Loss of definition of the low signal line of the vertebral end plates is seen on T1WI and FS T2WI.

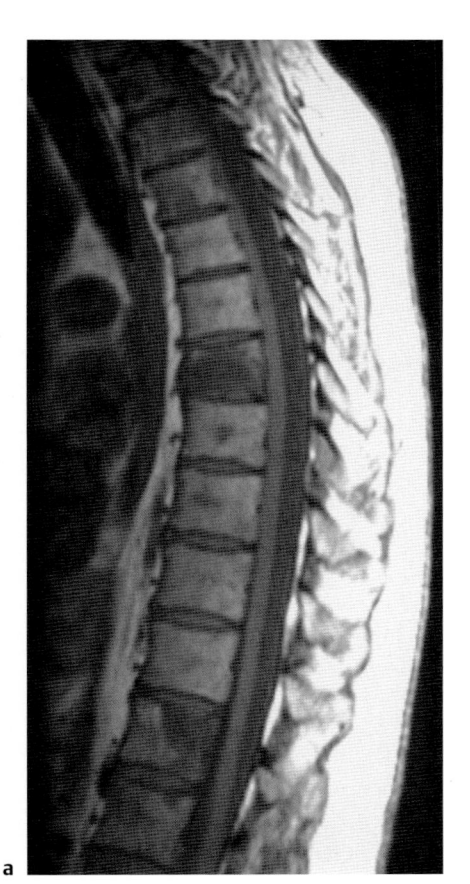

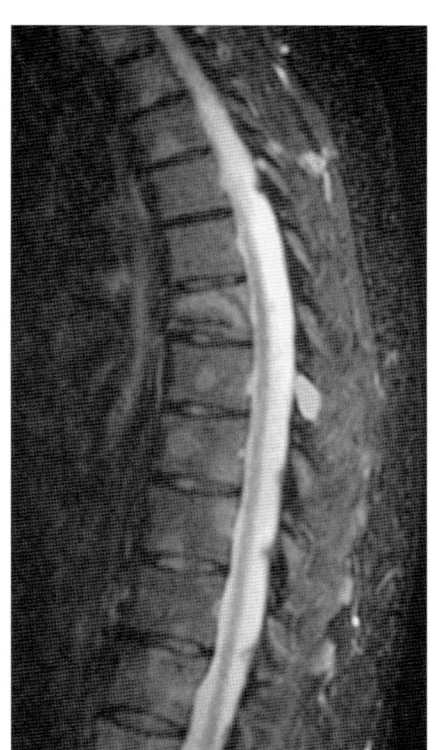

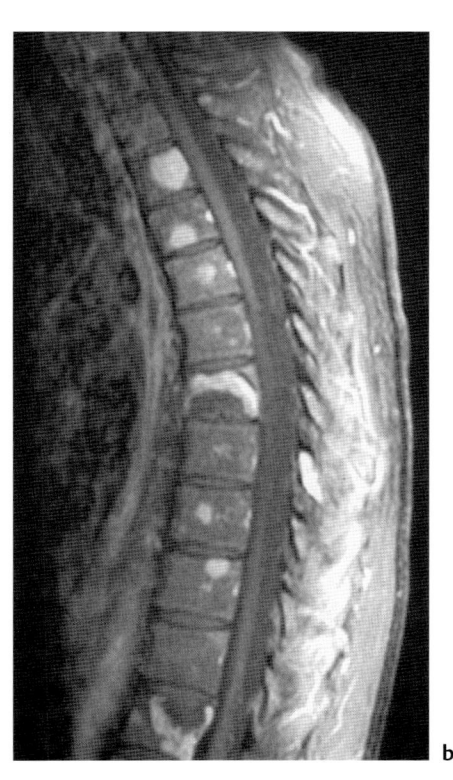

Figure 14.**21 a–c**   A 50-year-old man with sarcoidosis and multiple intraosseous spinal lesions that have low-intermediate signal on sagittal T1WI (**a**) and slightly high signal on sagittal FS T2WI (**b**). The lesions show prominent Gd-contrast enhancement on sagittal FS T1WI (**c**).

Table 14 (Continued) Diffuse, multiple, poorly defined and/or multifocal zones of abnormal marrow signal

Disorder	MRI Findings	Comments
Erdheim–Chester disease (Fig. 14.22)	Lesions can appear as irregular zones with low and/or intermediate signal on T1WI and PDWI, and mixed low, intermediate, and/or high signal on T2WI and FS T2WI within marrow. Zones of cortical destruction with or without extraosseous lesion extension may be seen occasionally with lesions in long bones. After Gd-contrast administration, heterogeneous enhancement may be seen in the involved marrow and zones of extraosseous extension if present.	Erdheim–Chester disease is a rare multisystem non-Langerhans cell histiocytic disorder of unknown etiology that usually affects adults. Collections of foamy macrophages can be seen within various tissues and organs of the musculoskeletal, pulmonary, cardiac, gastrointestinal, and central nervous systems. **(See Atlas Chapter A 19)**
Radiation injury (Fig. 14.23)	Involved marrow has a signal similar to fat. Bone infarcts may be present.	Radiation treatment or exposure typically converts red marrow to yellow due to damage to myeloid and erythroid producing cells.
Multiple enchondromatosis (Ollier disease, metachondromatosis, and Maffucci syndrome (Figs. 14.24, 14.25)	Lobulated intramedullary lesions with well-defined borders with mean size = 5 cm. Mild endosteal scalloping can be seen. Lesions usually have low-intermediate signal on T1WI and intermediate signal on PDWI. On T2WI and FS T2WI, lesions usually have predominantly high signal with foci and/or bands of low signal representing areas of matrix mineralization and fibrous strands. No zones of abnormal high signal on T2WI are typically seen in the marrow outside the borders of the lesions. Lesions typically show Gd-contrast enhancement in various patterns.	**Ollier disease** results from anomalies of endochondral bone formation with multiple enchondromas located predominantly or only in limbs on one side. Short and long tubular bones of the limbs are primarily affected. Median age = 12 years. **Metachondromatosis** is a rare disorder that includes the combination of enchondromatosis and osteochondromatosis. **Maffucci syndrome** is a very rare disease that occurs in children and adults with simultaneous occurrence of multiple enchondromas and soft tissue cutaneous or visceral hemangiomas. **(See Atlas Chapter A 8)**

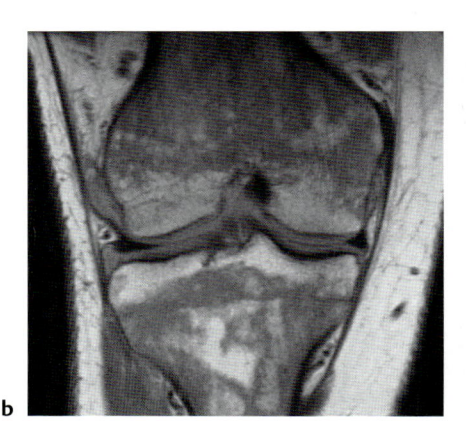

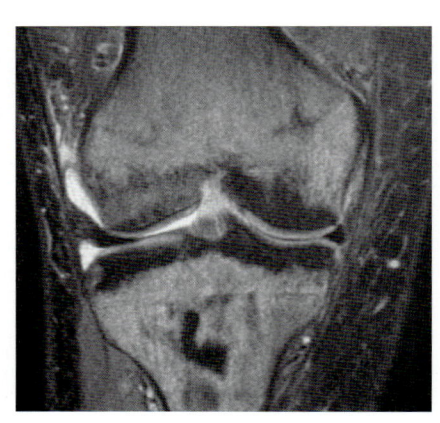

Figure 14.22 a, b A 39-year-old man with Erdheim–Chester disease with bone marrow involvement. Irregular zones with intermediate signal on coronal PDWI (a) and slightly high signal on coronal FS T2WI (b) are seen within the marrow in the epiphyseal, metaphyseal, and metadiaphyseal regions.

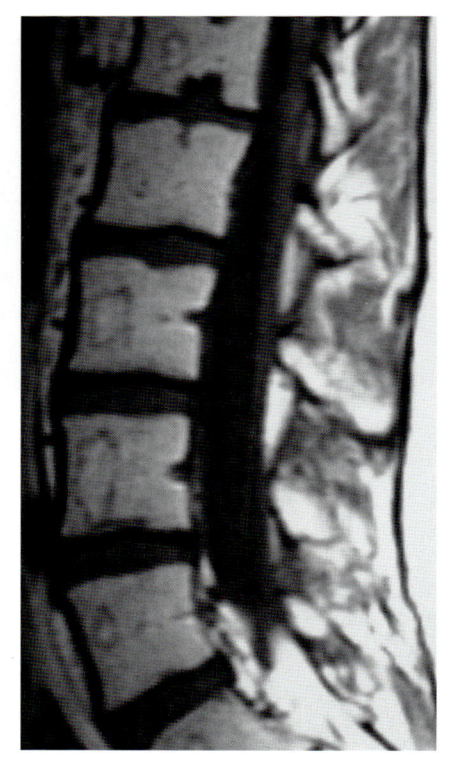

Figure 14.23 A 21-year-old woman who has been treated with craniospinal radiation for medulloblastoma shows fatty marrow as well as multiple bone infarcts on sagittal T1WI.

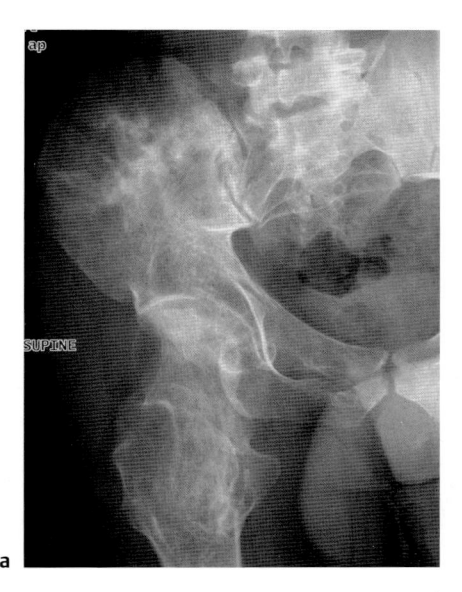

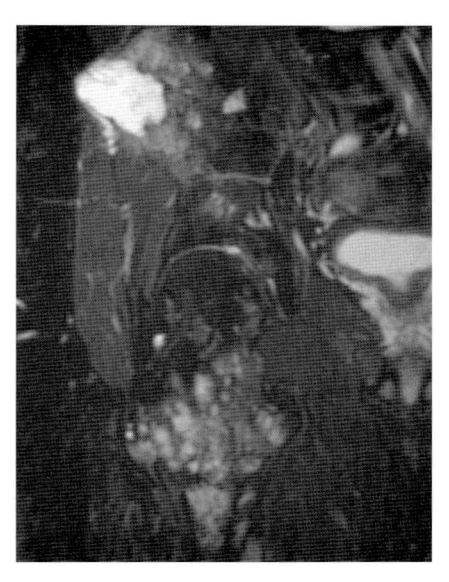

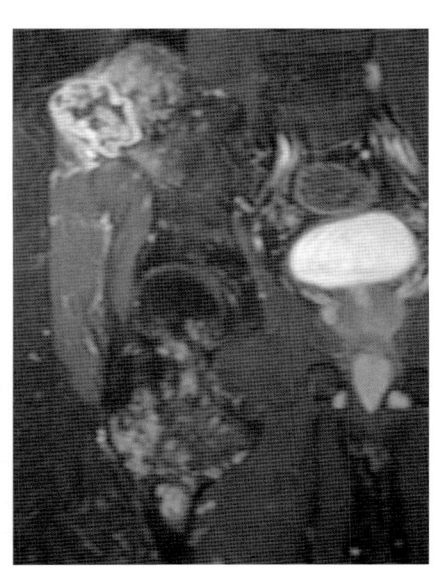

Figure 14.**24 a–c** A 29-year-old man with Ollier disease. The AP radiograph (**a**) shows multiple enchondromas involving the iliac bone, ischium, pubic bone, and femur. The lesions show high signal on coronal FS T2WI (**b**). The lesions show nodular and lobulated peripheral Gd-contrast enhancement on coronal FS T1WI (**c**).

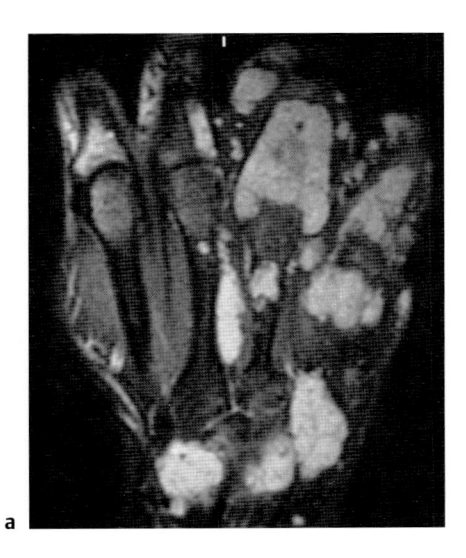

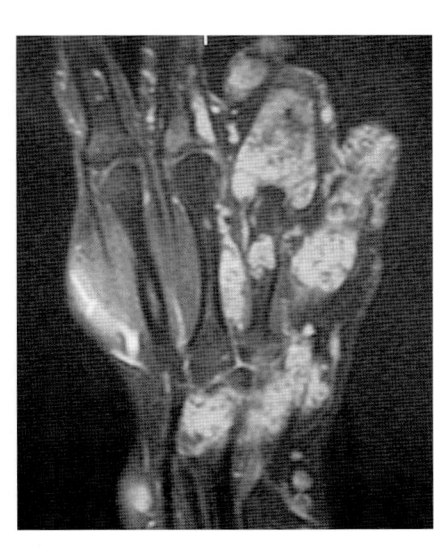

Figure 14.**25 a, b** A 20-year-old woman with Maffucci syndrome who has multiple intraosseous enchondromas and soft tissue hemangiomas involving the wrist and hand. The intra- and extraosseous lesions have high signal on coronal FS T2WI (**a**). Some of the intraosseous lesions are associated with cortical expansion. The lesions show prominent Gd-contrast enhancement on coronal FS T1WI (**b**).

Table 14 (Continued) Diffuse, multiple, poorly defined and/or multifocal zones of abnormal marrow signal

Disorder	MRI Findings	Comments
Poly-ostotic fibrous dysplasia (Fig. 14.26)	MRI features depend on the proportions of bony spicules, collagen, fibroblastic spindle cells, hemorrhagic and/or cystic changes, and pathologic fracture if present. Lesions are usually well-circumscribed and have low or low-intermediate signal on T1WI and PDWI. On T2WI, lesions have variable mixtures of low, intermediate, and/or high signal often surrounded by a low signal rim of variable thickness. Internal septations and cystic changes are seen in a minority of lesions. Bone expansion is commonly seen. All or portions of the lesions can show Gd-contrast enhancement that varies from mild to marked in degree.	Benign medullary fibro-osseous lesion of bone that can occur as a solitary lesion (**mono-ostotic type**) (80–85%); or as multiple lesions (**poly-ostotic fibrous dysplasia** type). Results from developmental failure in the normal process of remodeling primitive bone to mature lamellar bone with resultant zone or zones of immature trabeculae within dysplastic fibrous tissue. Lesions do not mineralize normally with predisposition to pathologic fracture. **(See Atlas Chapter A 27)**
Osteopoikilosis (Fig. 14.27)	Multiple foci with low signal comparable to cortical bone are seen on all pulse sequences within marrow	**Osteopoikilosis (osteopathia condensans disseminata or spotted bone disease)** is a sclerosing bone dysplasia in which numerous small round or oval radiodense foci are seen in medullary bone giving the appearance of multiple bone islands. **(See Atlas Chapter A 62)**

Figure 14.26 a–d An 8-year-old girl with McCune–Albright syndrome of polyostotic fibrous dysplasia. Axial CT image (**a**) shows multiple lesions involving the calvaria and sphenoid bone that have an expansile "ground glass" appearance. The lesions have low signal on axial T2WI (**b**) and coronal T1WI (**c**). The lesions shows Gd-contrast enhancement on coronal T1WI (**d**).

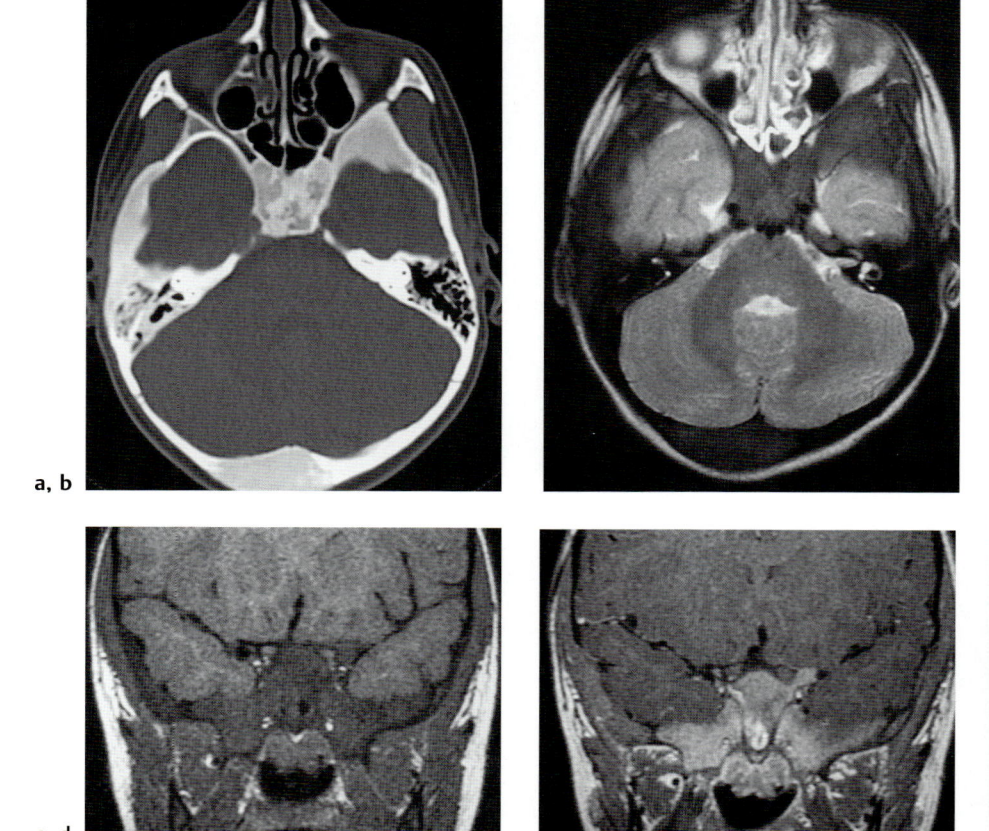

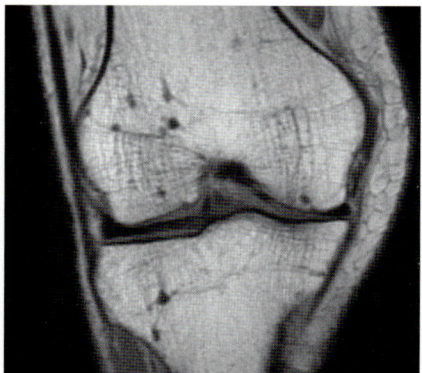

Figure 14.27 A 41-year-old woman with osteopoikilosis seen as multiple foci with low signal in the marrow of the distal femur and proximal tibia, on coronal T1WI.

Metastatic disease

Table 14 (Continued) Diffuse, multiple, poorly defined and/or multifocal zones of abnormal marrow signal

Disorder	MRI Findings	Comments
Malignant		
Metastatic disease (Figs. 14.28, 14.29)	Metastatic tumor within bone often appears as intramedullary zones with low-intermediate signal on T1WI, low-intermediate to slightly high signal on PDWI, and slightly high to high signal on T2WI and FS T2WI. Sclerotic lesions often have low signal on T1WI and mixed low, intermediate, and/or high signal on T2WI. Metastatic spinal lesions may be focal or involve most of a vertebra. In tubular bones, metastatic lesions are usually intramedullary with frequent cortical destruction and tumor extension into the extraosseous soft tissues. Metastatic skeletal lesions usually show varying degrees of Gd-contrast enhancement.	Metastatic lesions represent proliferating neoplastic cells that are located in sites or organs separated or distant from their origins. Metastatic lesions can disseminate hematogenously via arteries or veins, along CSF pathways, along surgical tracts, and along lymphatic structures. Metastatic carcinoma is the most frequent malignant tumor involving bone. In adults, metastatic lesions to bone occur most frequently from carcinomas of the lung, breast, prostate, kidney, thyroid, as well as from sarcomas. Primary malignancies of the lung, breast, and prostate account for 80% of bone metastases. **(See Atlas Chapter A 50)**

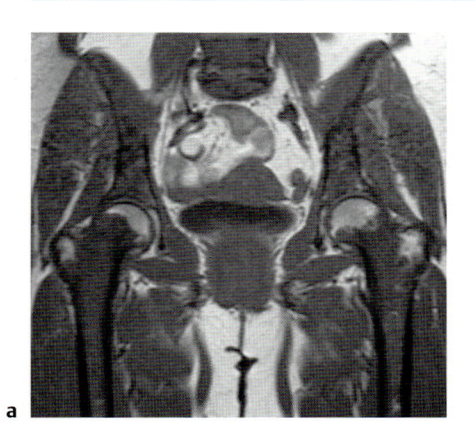

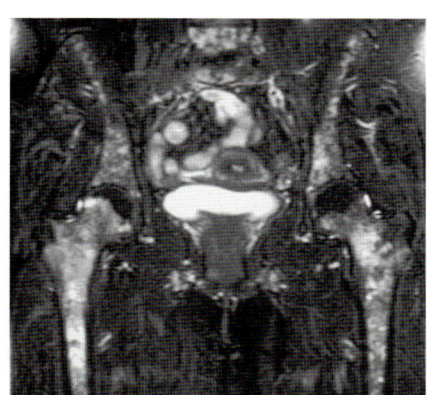

Figure 14.**28 a, b** A 53-year-old woman with metastatic breast carcinoma involving the marrow of spine, pelvis, and femur seen as poorly defined zones with low-intermediate signal on coronal T1WI (**a**) and high signal on coronal STIR (**b**).

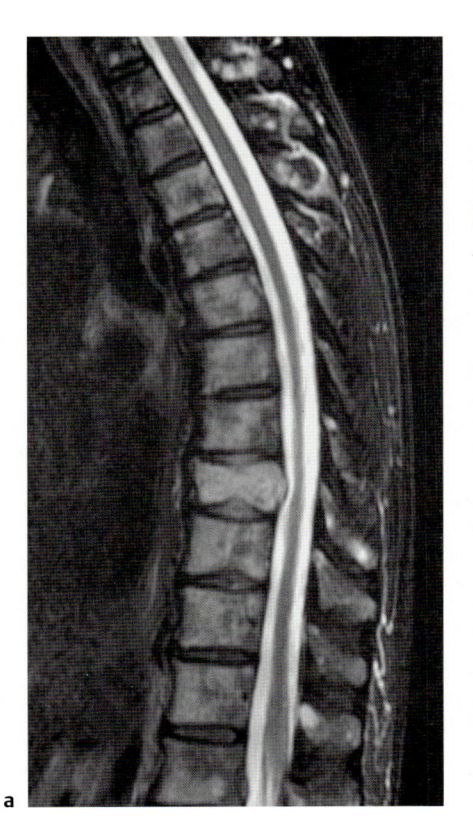

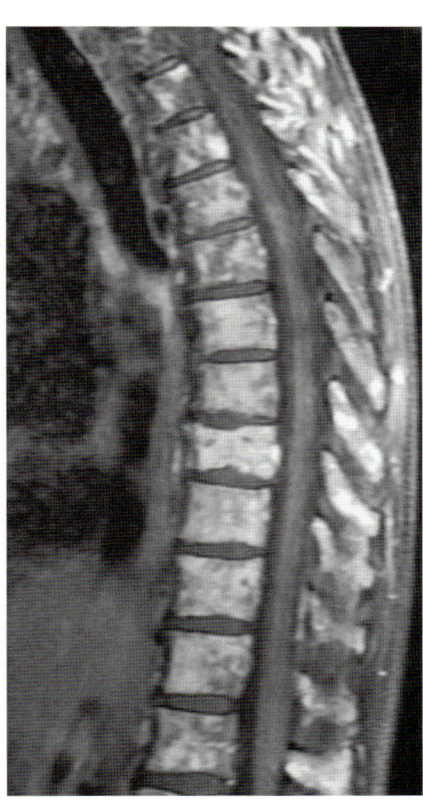

Figure 14.**29** A 63-year-old woman with extensive diffuse metastatic breast carcinoma involving the marrow of the spine seen as poorly defined zones with high signal on sagittal FS T2WI (**a**) and Gd-contrast enhancement on FS T1WI (**b**).

Table 14 (Continued) Diffuse, multiple, poorly defined and/or multifocal zones of abnormal marrow signal

Disorder	MRI Findings	Comments
Multiple myeloma (Fig. 14.30)	Multiple myeloma typically appears as multiple intramedullary zones with low-intermediate signal on T1WI and PDWI, intermediate, slightly high to high signal on T2WI, and slightly high to high signal on FS T2WI. FS T2WI is important for detecting myeloma because intermediate and high signal heterogeneity on T1WI from red and yellow marrow, respectively, can be seen in normal vertebral marrow in elderly patients. Intramedullary lesions and corresponding signal abnormalities may be diffuse, focal with poorly defined or distinct margins, and/or in an extensive variegated pattern. Multifocal lesions can be seen in long bones. Zones of cortical destruction may occur associated with extraosseous soft tissue lesions. Lesions usually show Gd-contrast enhancement.	Multiple myelomas are malignant tumors comprising proliferating antibody-secreting plasma cells derived from single clones. Multiple myeloma is primarily located in bone marrow. A solitary myeloma or plasmacytoma is an infrequent variant in which a neoplastic mass of plasma cells occurs at a single site of bone or soft tissues. **(See Atlas Chapter A 52)**
Non-Hodgkin lymphoma (Fig. 14.31)	Non-Hodgkin lymphoma (NHL) within bone typically appears as intramedullary zones with low-intermediate signal on T1WI and PDWI, slightly high to high signal on T2WI, and high signal on FS T2WI. Zones of low signal on T1WI and T2WI may be secondary to fibrosis. Zones of cortical destruction may occur associated with extraosseous soft tissue lesions. NHL typically shows Gd-contrast enhancement. Destruction of cortical and medullary bone may also occur from invasion from adjacent extraosseous NHL.	Lymphoma represents a group of lymphoid tumors whose neoplastic cells typically arise within lymphoid tissue (lymph nodes and reticuloendothelial organs). Unlike leukemia, lymphoma usually arises as discrete masses. Almost all primary lymphomas of bone are B cell NHL. NHL frequently originates at extranodal sites and spreads in an unpredictable pattern. **(See Atlas Chapter A 47)**
Hodgkin lymphoma (Fig. 14.32)	Hodgkin disease (HD) within bone typically appears as intramedullary zones with low-intermediate signal on T1WI, and intermediate, slightly high, and/or high signal on T2WI and high signal on FS T2WI. Intramedullary lesions may have poorly defined or distinct margins. Multifocal lesions can be seen in long bones and vertebrae. Zones of cortical destruction may occur associated with extraosseous soft tissue lesions. Most lesions show Gd-contrast enhancement. HD involving bone with associated sclerosis seen on plain films or CT usually has low signal on T1WI and variable/mixed signal on T2WI. Destruction of cortical and medullary bone may also occur from invasion from adjacent extraosseous lymphadenopathy from HD.	Lymphoma represents a group of lymphoid tumors whose neoplastic cells typically arise within lymphoid tissue (lymph nodes and reticuloendothelial organs). Unlike leukemia, lymphoma usually arises as discrete masses. HD typically arises in lymph nodes and often spreads along nodal chains. **(See Atlas Chapter A 47)**

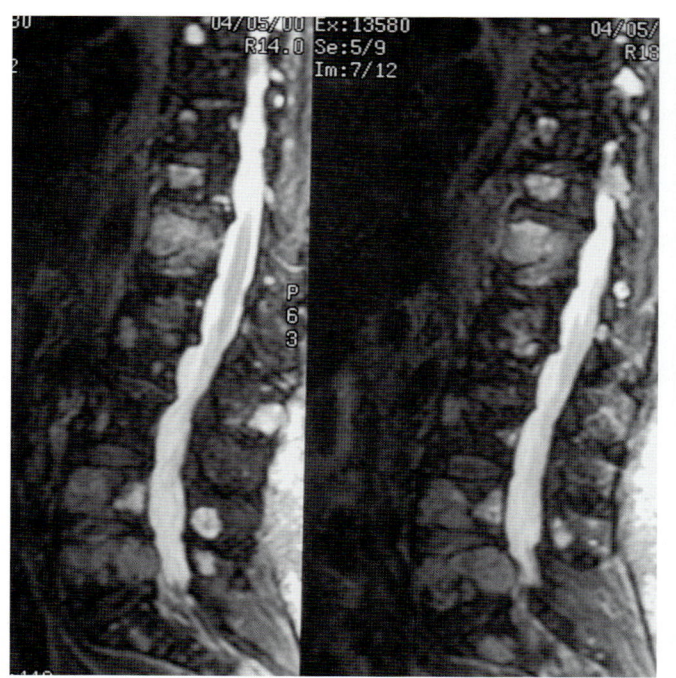

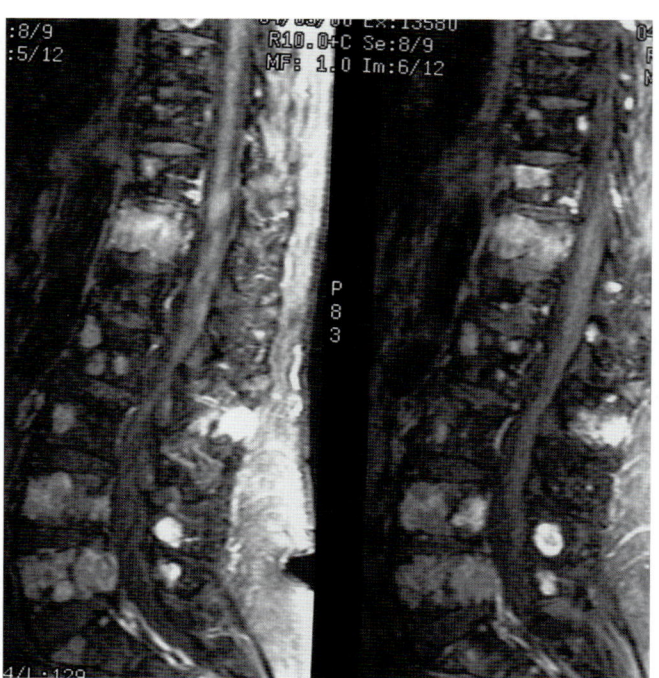

Figure 14.**30 a, b** Multiple myeloma seen as numerous lesions in the vertebral marrow with high signal on sagittal FS T2WI (**a**) and Gd-contrast enhancement on FS T1WI (**b**).

Hodgkin lymphoma **229**

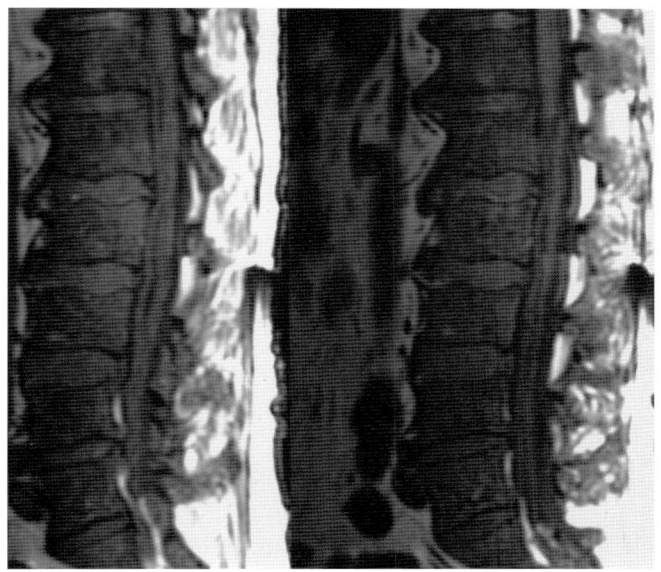

Figure 14.**31 a–c** NHL involving vertebral marrow as well as within the lumbar subarachnoid space. Diffuse low-intermediate signal on sagittal T1WI (**a**) is seen throughout the marrow. Heterogeneous mostly low signal is seen in the marrow on sagittal T2WI (**b**). Heterogeneous Gd-contrast enhancement is seen throughout the marrow as well as within the thecal sac on sagittal FS T1WI (**c**).

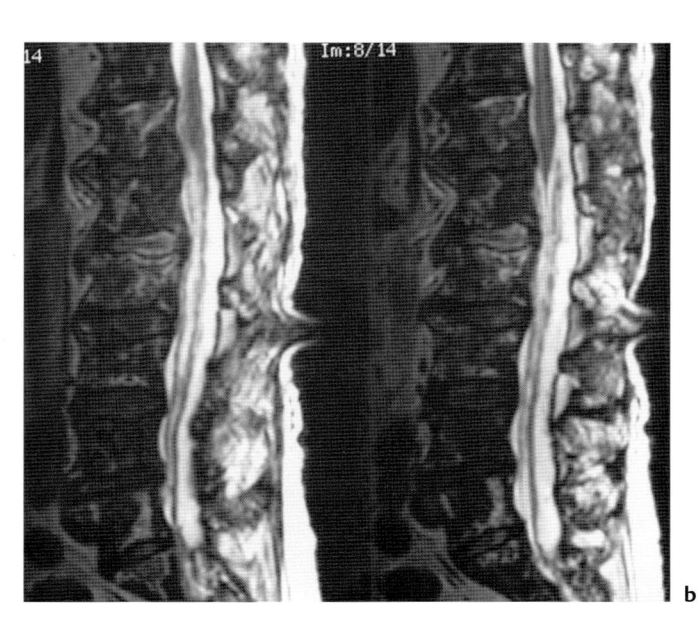

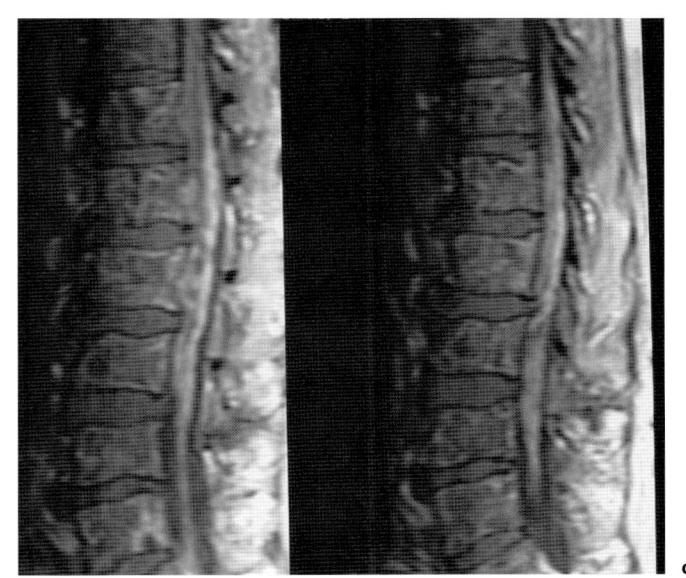

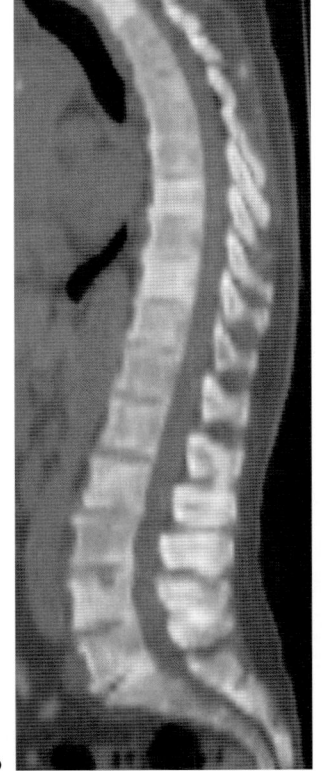

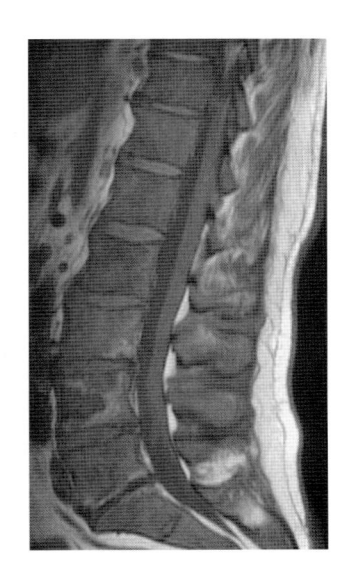

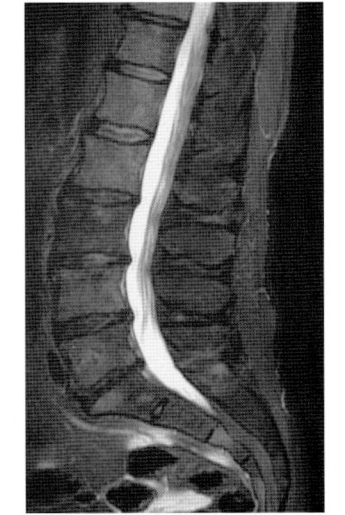

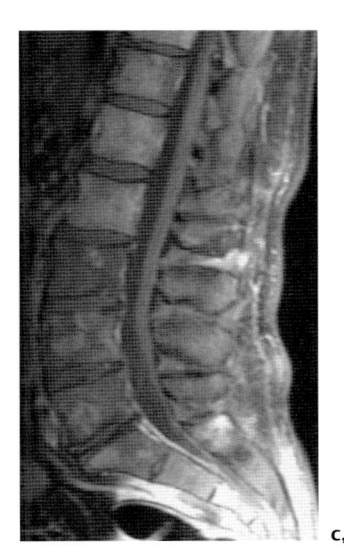

Figure 14.**32 a–d** A 46-year-old man with Hodgkin lymphoma with osteosclerotic lesions involving many thoracic and lumbar vertebrae on sagittal reconstructed CT (**a**). Multiple poorly defined lesions in the marrow have low-intermediate signal on sagittal T1WI (**b**), slightly high signal on sagittal FS T2WI (**c**), and mild-moderate Gd-contrast enhancement on sagittal FS T1WI (**d**).

Table 14 (Continued) Diffuse, multiple, poorly defined and/or multifocal zones of abnormal marrow signal

Disorder	MRI Findings	Comments
Leukemia (Figs. 14.33–14.36)	Acute lymphoblastic leukemia (ALL), chronic lymphocytic leukemia (CLL), acute myelogenous leukemia (AML), and chronic myelogenous leukemia (CML) infiltration in marrow can appear as diffuse or poorly defined zones of low-intermediate signal on T1WI and PDWI, intermediate-slightly high to high signal on FS T2WI. Focal or geographic regions with similar signal alteration can also be seen. After Gd-contrast administration, ALL, CLL, AML, and CML may show Gd-contrast enhancement on T1WI and FS T1WI. Note should be made that Gd-contrast enhancement may be seen in normal vertebral marrow in children less than 7 years.	Lymphoid neoplasms that have widespread involvement of the bone marrow as well as tumor cells in peripheral blood. ALL is the most frequent type in children and adolescents. In adults, CLL is the most common type. Myelogenous leukemias represent neoplasms derived from abnormal myeloid progenitor cells that, if normal, would form erythrocytes, monocytes, granulocytes, and platelets. AML usually occurs in adolescents and young adults, and accounts for ~20% of childhood leukemia. CML occurs in adults older than 25 years. **(See Atlas Chapter A 41)**
Myelodysplastic syndromes (Fig. 14.37)	Marrow signal on FS T2WI and STIR can be isointense or hyperintense to muscle depending on the degree of cellular hyperplasia in the marrow and stage of the disease. Can progress to myelofibrosis and myelosclerosis.	Myelodysplastic syndromes (MDS) are clonal hematopoietic stem cell diseases associated with dysplasias of myeloid cell lines resulting in decreased functional hematopoiesis. Myeloblasts can occur up to 20% in MDS. Progressive marrow failure occurs in MDS as well as eventual progression to acute myeloid leukemia. Usually occurs in older adults over the age of 60 years, incidence up to 30 per million. MDS includes chronic myelomonocytic leukemia, atypical chronic myeloid leukemia, juvenile myelomonocytic leukemia, and myelodysplastic/myeloproliferative disease.

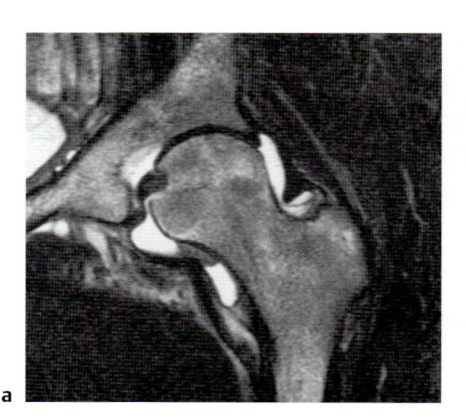

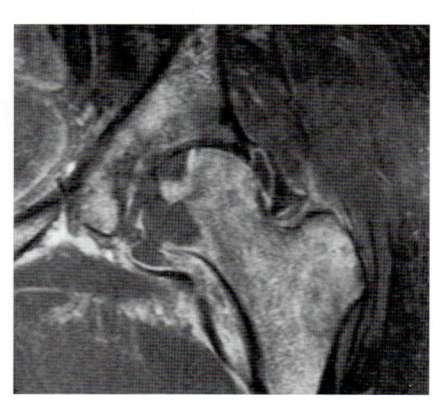

Figure 14.33 a, b   A 16-year-old male with ALL involving the femur and bony pelvis. Leukemic infiltration in the marrow of the pelvis and femur has heterogeneous slightly high signal on coronal FS T2WI (**a**) and Gd-contrast enhancement on coronal FS T1WI (**b**). Zones with no Gd-contrast enhancement in the femoral head represent sites of bone marrow ischemia/infarction.

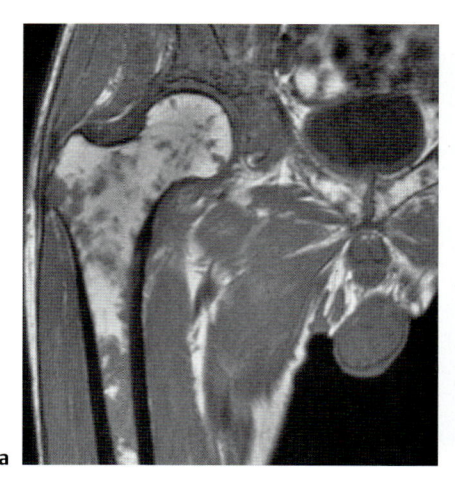

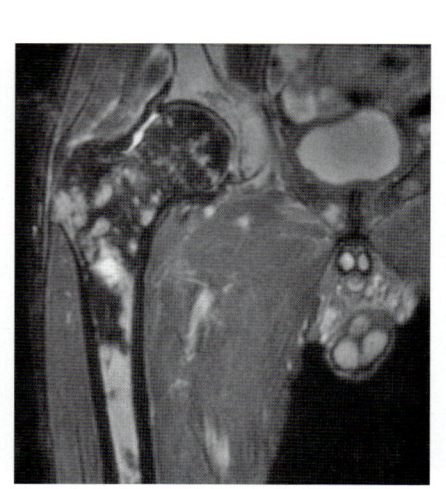

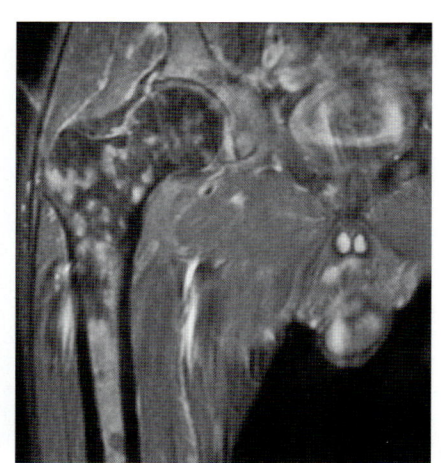

Figure 14.34 a–c   CLL involving the marrow of a 61-year-old man. Leukemic deposits are seen as irregular zones with low-intermediate signal on coronal T1WI (**a**) and slightly high or high signal on coronal FS T2WI (**b**). Lesions show Gd-contrast enhancement on coronal FS T1WI (**c**).

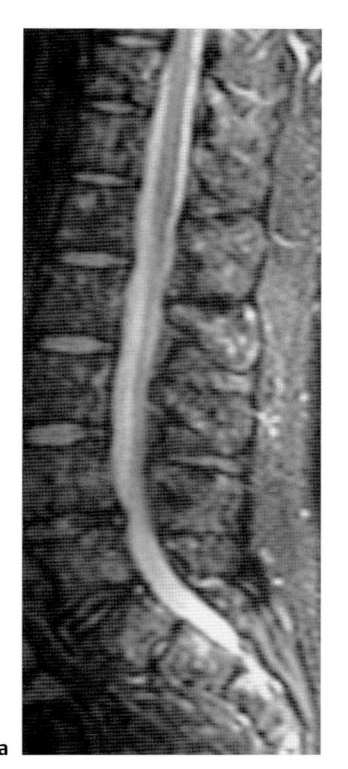

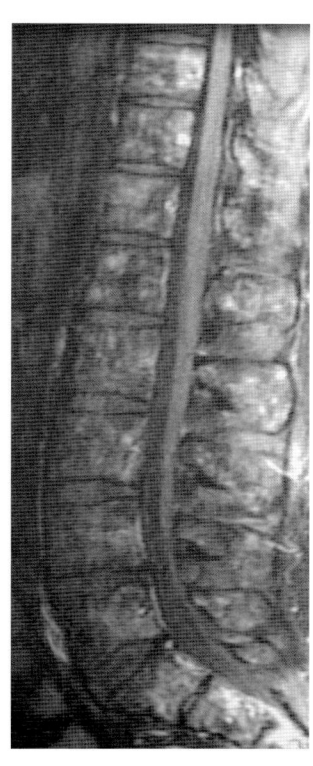

Figure 14.**35 a, b** A 28-year-old man with AML involving the marrow of the spine. The leukemic deposits have heterogeneous intermediate and slightly high signal on sagittal FS T2WI (**a**), and mild heterogeneous Gd-contrast enhancement on sagittal FS T1WI (**b**).

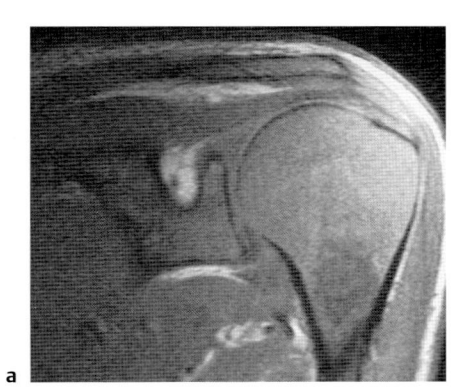

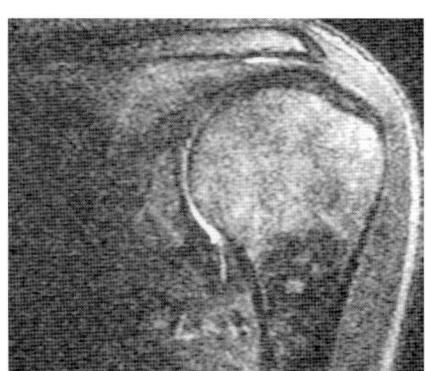

Figure 14.**36 a, b** A 39-year-old man with CML involving the marrow of the humerus and scapula. The leukemic deposits have heterogeneous low-intermediate signal on coronal PDWI (**a**) and heterogeneous high signal on coronal FS T2WI (**b**).

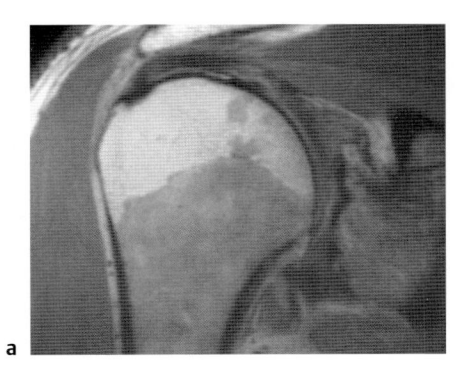

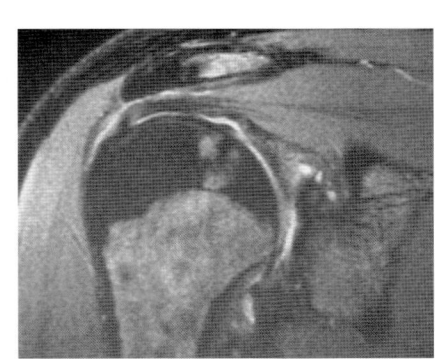

Figure 14.**37 a, b** A 45-year-old man with chronic myelodysplastic syndrome with metaphyseal marrow signal that is hypointense to fat on coronal PDWI (**a**) and hyperintense relative to fat on coronal FS T2WI (**b**).

Table 14 (Continued) Diffuse, multiple, poorly defined and/or multifocal zones of abnormal marrow signal

Disorder	MRI Findings	Comments
Chronic myeloproliferative disease (Fig. 14.38)	Involved bone marrow often has low or low-intermediate signal on T1WI and slightly high signal on T2WI and FS T2WI. CPMDs typically have an insidious onset, but can progress to myelofibrosis, myelosclerosis, and acute leukemia.	Chronic myeloproliferative diseases (CMPDs) represent bone marrow disorders in which there is proliferation of one or more hematopoietic stem cells (granulocytic, erythrocytic, and/or megakaryocytic). Unlike myelodysplastic syndromes, there is relatively normal maturation of the blood cells and platelets along with increased numbers of the cells from the derivatives of the abnormal clonal proliferations in CMPD. Incidence of CMPD is 90 per million, usually involves adults older than 40 years. Percent of marrow blasts is less than 10%. CMPD includes polycythemia vera (PCV), chronic idiopathic myelofibrosis, essential thrombocytopenia, chronic eosinophilic leukemia, chronic neutrophilic leukemia, and chronic early phases of myelogenous leukemia (Philadelphia chromosome t(9;22)(q34;q11), BCR/ABL positive). PCV occurs in up to 13 per million per year, and results from proliferation of a clonal hematopoietic stem cell lacking the normal regulatory mechanism for erythropoiesis. Other myeloid clonal proliferations can occur concurrently. PCV occurs in two phases. The initial phase is followed by a postpolycythemic phase that is associated with anemia and cytopenia, myelofibrosis, and potential development of acute leukemia.
Waldenstrom macroglobulinemia (lymphoplasmacytic lymphoma) (Fig. 14.39)	Marrow may have no associated abnormal signal or have irregular and/or diffuse findings similar to red marrow reconversion. Signal changes in the marrow may become more prominent as well as Gd-contrast enhancement with increasing lymphoplasmacytoid infiltration of bone marrow.	Waldenstrom macroglobulinemia, also referred to as Lymphoplasmacytic lymphoma, is a rare neoplasm of plasmacytoid lymphocytes, plasma cells and small B lymphocytes that usually involves bone marrow, spleen, and lymph nodes. Typically associated with a serum monoclonal IgM protein in concentrations >3 g/dl, often with hyperviscosity and cryoglobulinemia. Occurs in older adults, mean age = 63 years. Median survival is ~5 years.
Mastocytosis	Radiographs and CT can show indistinctly marginated sclerotic lesions, radiolucent zones, or mixed sclerotic and radiolucent lesions in medullary bone. Sclerotic lesions usually have low signal on T1WI and T2WI, whereas radiolucent lesions may have intermediate, slightly high to high signal on T2WI and FS T2WI. Marrow signal abnormalities also include varying degrees of nonfatty homogeneous or heterogeneous zones of low signal on T1WI and intermediate, slightly high, and/or high signal on FS T2WI or STIR. In some cases, marrow signal may be normal or have intermediate signal on T1WI and FS T2WI or STIR.	Heterogeneous uncommon disorders with pathologic accumulation of mast cells in various tissues (age ranges from 1st to 7th decades, mean in 4th decade) and can be classified into four clinical categories. Category 1 is the most common and includes 1A which involves the skin (cutaneous mastocytosis or urticaria pigmentosa), and 1B or systemic mastocytosis with mast cells occurring in various tissues (bone marrow, spleen, gastrointestinal tract, and lymph nodes). Category 1 usually has a favorable prognosis. Category II includes mastocytosis associated with a myeloproliferative or myelodysplastic disorder. Prognosis depends on the associated degree of myelodysplasia. Category III (lymphadenopathic mastocytosis with eosinophilia or aggressive mastocytosis) is associated with a poor prognosis related to large mast cell burdens. Category IV results from mast cell leukemia and has a very poor prognosis.

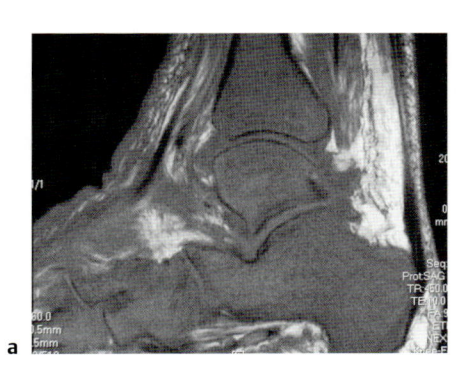

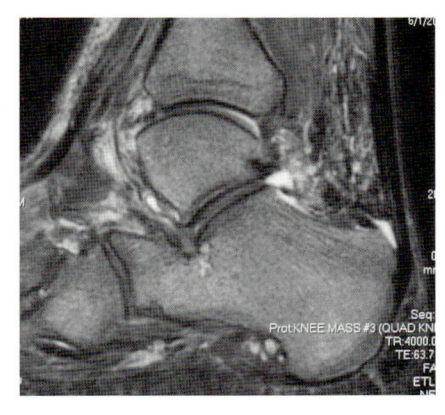

Figure 14.**38 a, b** A 49-year-old man with polycythemia rubra with diffuse low-intermediate signal in the marrow on sagittal T1WI (**a**) and slightly high signal on sagittal T2WI (**b**) that is slightly hyperintense relative to muscle.

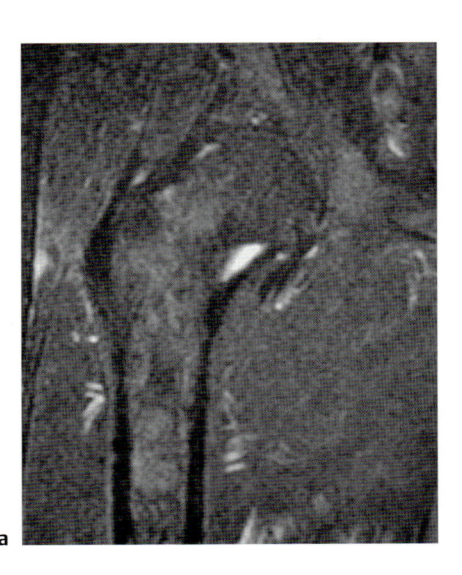

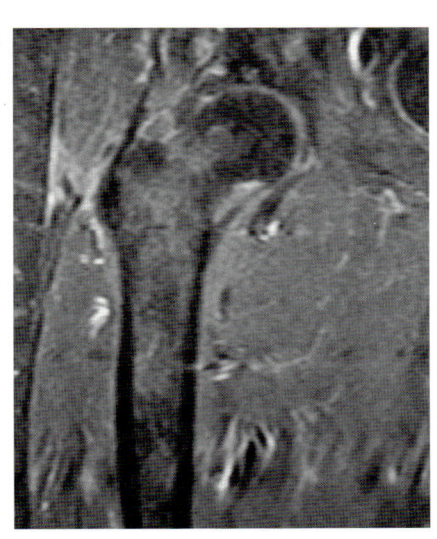

Figure 14.**39** A 61-year-old man with Waldenstrom macroglobulinemia with irregular zones of intermediate signal in the metadiaphyseal marrow on coronal FS T2WI (**a**) and post-Gd-contrast FS T1WI (**b**).

References

Red Marrow Reconversion

Barnewolt CE, Shapiro F, Jaramillo D. Normal gadolinium-enhanced MR images of the developing appendicular skeleton: Part 1. Cartilaginous epiphysis and physis. *AJR* July 1997;169:183–189.

Dwek JR, Shapiro F, Laor T, Barnewolt CE, Jaramillo D. Normal gadolinium-enhanced MR images of the developing appendicular skeleton: Part 2. Epiphyseal and metaphyseal marrow. *AJR* July 1997; 169:191–196.

Moore SG, Dawson KL. Red and yellow marrow in the femur: age-related changes in appearance at MR imaging. *Radiology* 1990;175: 219–223.

Waitches G, Zawin JK, Poznanski AK. Sequence and rate of bone marrow conversion in the femora of children as seen on MR imaging: are accepted standards accurate? *AJR* June 1994;162(6):1399–1406.

Inherited Anemias

Aydmgoz Ü, Oto A, Cila A. Spinal cord compression due to epidural extramedullary hematopoiesis in thalassaemia: MRI. *Neuroradiology* 1997;39:870–872.

Lorand-Metze I, Santiago GF, Lima CSP, Zanardi VA, Torriani M. Magnetic resonance imaging of femoral marrow cellularity in hypocellular haemopoietic disorders. *Clin Radiol* 2001;56:107–110.

Niggemann P, Krings T, Hans F, Thron A. Fifteen-year follow-up of a patient with β thalassaemia and extramedullary hematopoietic tissue compressing the spinal cord. *Neuroradiology* 2005;47:263–266.

Salehi SA, Koski T, Ondra SL. Spinal cord compression in β-thalassemia: case report and review of the literature. *Spinal Cord* 2004;42: 117–123.

States LJ. Imaging of metabolic bone disease and marrow disorders in children. *Radiol Clin N Am* July 2001;39(4):749–772.

Tan TC, Tsao J, Cheung FC. Extramedullary haemopoiesis in thalassemia intermedia presenting as paraplegia. *J Clin Neurosci* 2002;9(6): 721–725.

Tyler PA, Madani G, Chaudhuri R, Wilson LF, Dick EA. The radiological appearances of thalassaemia. *Clin Radiol* 2006;61:40–52.

Marrow Hyperplasia from Exogenous Erythropoietin

Biljanovic-Paunovic L, Djukanovic, Lezaic V, Stojanovic N, Marisavljevic D, Pavlovic-Kentera V. In vivo effects of recombinant human erythropoietin on bone marrow hematopoiesis in patients with chronic renal failure. *Eur J Med Res* 1998;16:564–570.

Horina JH, Schmid CR, Roob JM, et al. Bone marrow changes following treatment of renal anemia with erythropoietin. *Kidney Int* 1991; 40:917–922.

Jensen KE, Stenver D, Jensen M, et al. Magnetic resonance imaging of bone marrow following treatment with recombinant human erythropoietin in patients with end-stage renal disease. *Int J Artif Organs* 1990;13:477–481.

Granulocyte/Macrophage Colony Stimulating Factor

Altehoefer C, Bertz H, Ghanem NA, Langer M. Extent and time course of morphologic changes of bone marrow induced by granulocyte-colony stimulating factor as assessed by magnetic resonance imaging of healthy blood cell donors. *J Mag Reson Imaging* 2001;14:141–146.

Chabanova E, Johnsen HE, Knudsen LM, et al. Magnetic resonance investigation of bone marrow following priming and stem cell mobilization. *J Magn Reson Imaging* 2006;24:1364–1370.

Ciray I, Lindman H, Astrom GKO, Wanders A, Bergh J, Ahlstrom HK. Effect of granulocyte colony-stimulating factor (G-CSF)-supported chemotherapy on MR imaging of normal red bone marrow in breast cancer patients with focal bone metastases. *Acta Radiologica* 2003;44:472–484.

Hartman RP, Sundaram M, Okuno SH, Sim FH. Effect of granulocyte-stimulating factors on marrow of adult patients with musculoskeletal malignancies: incidence and MRI findings. *AJR* 2004;183:645–653.

Hemochromatosis/Iron Overload

Emy PY, Levin TL, Sheth SS, Ruzal-Shapiro C, Garvin J, Berdon WE. Iron overload in reticuloendothelial systems of pediatric oncology patients who have undergone transfusions: MR observations. *AJR* April 1997;168(4):1011–1015.

Kornreich L, Horev G, Yaniv I, Stein J, Grunebaum M, Zaizov R. Iron overload following bone marrow transplantation in children: MR findings. *Pediatr Radiol* 1997;27:869–872.

Levin TL, Sheth SS, Hurlet A, et al. MR marrow signs of iron overload in transfusion-dependent patients with sickle cell disease. *Pediatr Radiol* 1995;25(8):614–619.

Renal Osteodystrophy

Al-Gahtany M, Cusimano M, Singer W, Bilbao J, Kovacs K, Marotta T. Brown tumors of the skull base. Case report and review of the literature. *J Neurosurg* February 2003;98:417–420.

Davies AM, Evans N, Mangham DC, Grimer RJ. MR imaging of brown tumor with fluid–fluid levels: a report of three cases. *Eur Radiol* 2001;11(8):1445–1449.

Mustonen AOT, Kiuru MJ, Stahls A, Bohling T, Kivioja A, Koskinen SK. Radicular lower extremity pain as the first symptom of primary hyperparathyroidism. *Skeletal Radiol* 2004;33:467–472.

Hypoparathyroidism, Pseudo-, Pseudo-Pseudo-Hypoparathyroidism

Koch CA. Rapid increase in bone mineral density in a child with osteoporosis and autoimmune hypoparathyroidism treated with PTH 1–34. *Exp Clin Endocrinol Diabetes* 2001;109(6):350–354.

Rastogi R, Beauchamp NJ, Ladenson PW. Calcification of the basal ganglia in chronic hypoparathyroidism. *J Clin Endrocrin Metab* April 2003;88(4):1476–1477.

Resnick D. Parathyroid disorders and renal osteodystrophy. In: Resnick D, ed. *Diagnosis of Bone and Joint Disorders*, 4th ed. Philadelphia, Pa: W.B. Saunders; 2002:3:2043–2111.

van Oostenbrugge RJ, Herpers MJ, de Kruijk JR. Spinal cord compression caused by unusual location and extension of ossified ligamenta flava in a Caucasian male: a case report and literature review. *Spine* March 1, 1999;24(5):486–488.

Xiong L, Zeng QY, Jinkins JR. CT and MRI characteristics of ossification of the ligamenta flava in the thoracic spine. *Eur Radiol* 2001;11(9):1798–1802.

Yamamoto Y, Noto Y, Saito M, Ichizen H, Kida H. Spinal cord compression by heterotopic ossification associated with pseudohypoparathyroidism. *J Int Med Res* Nov–Dec 1997;25(6):364–368.

Osteitis Condensans

Clarke DP, Higgins JN, Valentine AR, Black C. Magnetic resonance imaging of osteitis condensans ilii. *Brit J Rheumatol* June 1994; 33(6): 599–600.

Major NM, Helms CA. Pelvic stress injuries: the relationship between osteitis pubis (symphysis pubis stress injury) and sacroiliac abnormalities in athletes. *Skeletal Radiol* 1997;26:711–717.

Olivieri I, Ferri S, Barozzi L. Osteitis condensans ilii. *Brit J Rheumatol* March 1996;35(3):295–297.

Bilateral Sacroiliitis

Bredella MA, Steinbach LS, Morgan S, Ward M, Davis JC. MRI of the sacroiliac joints in patients with moderate to severe ankylosing spondylitis. *AJR* December 2006;187:1420–1426.

Bennett DL, Ohashi K, El-Khoury GY. Spondyloarthropathies: ankylosing spondylitis and psoriatic arthritis. *Radiol Clin North Am* January 2004;42(1):121–134.

Heuft-Dorenbosch L, Landewé R, Weijers R, et al. Combining information obtained from magnetic resonance imaging and conventional radiographs to detect sacroiliitis in patients with recent onset inflammatory back pain. *Ann Rheum Dis* 2006;65:804–808.

Levine DS, Forbat SM, Saifuddin A. MRI of the axial skeletal manifestations of ankylosing spondylitis. *Clin Radiol* 2004;59:400–413.

Oostveen J, Prevo R, den Boer J, van de Laar M. Early detection of sacroiliitis on magnetic resonance imaging and subsequent development of sacroiliitis on plain radiography. A prospective, longitudinal study. *J Rheumatol* September 1999;26(9):1953–1958.

Puhakka KB, Jurik AG, Egund N, et al. Imaging of sacroiliitis in early seronegative spondylarthropathy. Assessment of abnormalities by MR in comparison with radiography and CT. *Acta Radiologica* 2003; 44:218–229.

Sacral Insufficiency Fractures

Ahovuo JA, Kiuru MJ, Visuri T. Fatigue stress fractures of the sacrum: diagnosis with MR imaging. *Eur Radiol* March 2004;14(3):500–505. Epub October 24, 2003.

Grangier C, Garcia J, Howarth NR, May M, Rossier P. Role of MRI in the diagnosis of insufficiency fractures of the sacrum and acetabular roof. *Skeletal Radiol* 1997;26:517–524.

Reflex Sympathetic Dystrophy

Bennett DS, Brookoff D. Complex regional pain syndromes (reflex sympathetic dystrophy and causalgia) and spinal cord stimulation. *Pain Med* May–Jun 2006;7(Suppl 1):64–96.

Crozier F, Champsaur P, Pham T, et al. Magnetic resonance imaging in reflex sympathetic dystrophy syndrome of the foot. *Joint Bone Spine* 2003;70:503–508.

Lechevalier D, Banal F, Damiano J, Imbert I, Magnin J. Correspondence. Reflex sympathetic dystrophy of the foot: MRI with fat suppression is essential (letter with the drafting). *Joint Bone Spine* 2004;71:446–447.

Quisel A, Gill JM, Witherell P. Complex regional pain syndrome: which treatments show promise? *J Fam Pract* July 2005;54(7):599–603.

Quisel A, Gill JM, Witherell P. Complex regional pain syndrome underdiagnosed. *J Fam Pract* June 2005;54(6):524–532.

Sintzoff S, Sintzoff S Jr, Stallenberg B, Matos C. Imaging in reflex sympathetic dystrophy. *Hand Clin* August 1997;13(3):431–442.

Serous Atrophy of Marrow

Kuwashima S, Nishimura G, Yamato M, Fujioka M. Magnetic resonance imaging of clival marrow in patients with anorexia nervosa. *Acta Paediatr Jpn* 1996;38(2):114–117.

Okamoto K, Ito J, Ishikawa K, Sakai K, Tokiguchi S. Change in signal intensity on MRI of fat in the head of markedly emaciated patients. *Neuroradiology* 2001;43:134–138.

Vande Berg BC, Malghem J, Devuyst, O, Malgague BE, Lambert MJ. Anorexia nervosa: correlation between MR appearance of bone marrow and severity of disease. *Radiology* 1994;193:859–864.

Vande Berg BC, Malghem J, Lecouvet FE, Lambert M, Malgague BE. Distribution of serouslike bone marrow changes in the lower limbs of patients with anorexia nervosa: predominant involvement of the distal lower extremities. *AJR* 1996;166:621–625.

Gaucher Disease

Hermann G, Pastores GM, Abdelwahab IF, Lorberboym AM. Gaucher disease: assessment of skeletal involvement and therapeutic responses to enzyme replacement. *Skeletal Radiol* 1997;26:687–696.

Maas M, Poll LW, Terk MR. Imaging and quantifying skeletal involvement in Gaucher disease. *Brit J Radiol* 2002;75 (Suppl. 1):A13–A24.

Poll LW, Koch JL, vom Dahl S, et al. Magnetic resonance imaging of bone marrow changes in Gaucher disease during enzyme replacement therapy: first German long-term results. *Skeletal Radiol* 2001;30:496–503.

Roca M, Mota J, Alfonso P, Pocovi M, Giraldo P. S-MRI score: a simple method for assessing bone marrow in Gaucher disease. *Eur J Radiol* 2007;62:132–137.

Wenstrup RJ, Roca-Espiau M, Weinreb NJ, Bembi B. Skeletal aspects of Gaucher disease; a review. *Brit J Radiol* 2002;75(Suppl. 1):A2–A12.

Glycogen Storage Disease

Scherer A, Engelbrecht V, Neises G, et al. MR imaging of bone marrow in glycogen storage disease type 1B in children and young adults. *AJR* 2001;177:421–425.

Osteopetrosis

Cure JK, Key LL, Goultra DP, VanTassel P. Cranial MR imaging of osteopetrosis. *AJNR* 2000;21:1110–1115.

Elster AD, Theros EG, Key LL, Chen MYM. Cranial imaging in autosomal recessive osteopetrosis. Part I. Facial bones and calvarium. *Radiology* 1992;183:129–135.

Tolar J, Teitelbaum SL, Orchard PJ. Osteopetrosis. *N Engl J Med* 2004; 351:2839–2849.

Hypervitaminosis A and D

Lips P. Hypervitaminosis A and fractures. *N Engl J Med* 2003;384: 347–349.

Jiang YB, Wang YZ, Zhao J, et al. Bone remodeling in hypervitaminosis D 3. Radiologic-microangiographic-pathologic correlations. *Invest Radiol* 1991;26:213–219.

Resnick D. Hypervitaminosis and hypovitaminosis. In: Resnick D, ed. *Diagnosis of Bone and Joint Disorders,* 4th ed. Philadelphia, Pa: W.B. Saunders; 2002:4:3456–3464.

Romero JB, Schreiber A, Von Hochstetter AR, Wagenhauser FJ, Michel BA, Theiler R. Hyperostotic and destructive osteoarthritis in a patient with vitamin A intoxication syndrome: a case report. *Bull Hosp Jt Dis* 1996;54:169–174.

Fluorosis

Haettich B, Lebreton C, Prier A, Kaplan G. Magnetic resonance imaging of fluorosis and stress fractures due to fluoride. *Rev Rhum Mal Osteoartic* November 1991;58(11):803–808.

Muthukumar N. Ossification of the ligamentum flavum as a result of fluorosis causing myelopathy: report of two cases. *Neurosurgery* March 2005;56(3):622.

Reddy DR, Srikanth RD, Misra M. Fluorosis. *Surg Neurol* 1998;49: 635–636.

Myelodysplastic Syndromes

Kusumoto S, Jinnai I, Matsuda A, et al. Bone marrow patterns in patients with aplastic anemia and myelodysplastic syndrome: observations with magnetic resonance imaging. *Eur J Haematol* September 1997;59(3):155–161.

Moulopoulos LA, Dimopoulos MA. Magnetic resonance imaging of the bone marrow in hematologic malignancies. *Blood* 1997;90(6): 2127–2147.

Olipitz W, Beham-Schmid C, Aigner R, et al. Acute myelofibrosis: multifocal bone marrow infiltration detected by scintigraphy and magnetic resonance imaging. *Ann Hematol* 2000;79:275–278.

Takagi S, Tanaka O, Origasa H, Miura Y. Prognostic significance of magnetic resonance imaging of femoral marrow in patients with myelodysplastic syndromes. *J Clin Oncol* January 1999;17(1): 277–283.

Vardiman JW. Myelodysplastic/myeloproliferative diseases: introduction. In: Jaffe ES, Harris NL, Sein H, Vardiman JW, eds. *World Health Organization Classification of Tumors. Pathology and Genetics of Tumors of Hematopoietic and Lymphoid Tissues.* Lyon, France: IARC Press; 2001:47–48.

Chronic Myeloproliferative Disease

Amano Y, Onda M, Amano M, Kumazaki T. Magnetic resonance imaging of myelofibrosis stir and gadolinium-enhanced MR images. *Clin Imag* July/August 1997;21(4):264–268.

Bock O, Loch G, Schade U, et al. Osteosclerosis in advanced chronic idiopathic myelofibrosis is associated with endothelial overexpression of osteoprotegerin. *Brit J Haematol* 2005;130:76–82.

Diamond T, Smith A, Schnier R, Manoharan A. Syndrome of myelofibrosis and osteosclerosis: a series of case reports and review of the literature. *Bone* March 2002;30(3):498–501.

Moulopoulos LA, Dimopoulos MA. Magnetic resonance imaging of the bone marrow in hematologic malignancies. *Blood* 1997;90(6): 2127–2147.

Sale GE, Deeg HJ, Porter BA. Regression of myelofibrosis and osteosclerosis following hematopoietic cell transplantation assessed by magnetic resonance imaging and histologic grading. *Biol Blood Marrow Transplant* 2006;12:1285–1294.

Sideris P, Tassiopoulos S, Sakellaropoulos N, et al. Unusual radiological findings in a case of myelofibrosis secondary to polycythemia vera. *Ann Hematol* 2006;85:555–556.

Thiele J, Pierre R, Imbert M, Vardiman JW, Brunning RD, Flandrin G. Chronic idiopathic myelofibrosis. In: Jaffe ES, Harris NL, Sein H, Vardiman JW, eds. *World Health Organization Classification of Tumors. Pathology and Genetics of Tumors of Hematopoietic and Lymphoid Tissues.* Lyon, France: IARC Press; 2001:35–38.

Waldenstrom Macroglobulinemia

Berger F, Isaacson PG, Piris MA, Harris NL. Lymphoplasmacytic lymphoma/Waldenstrom macroglobulinemia. In: Jaffe ES, Harris NL, Sein H, Vardiman JW, eds. *World Health Organization Classification of Tumors. Pathology and Genetics of Tumors of Hematopoietic and Lymphoid Tissues.* Lyon, France: IARC Press; 2001:132–34.

Moulopoulos LA, Dimopoulos MA. Magnetic resonance imaging of the bone marrow in hematologic malignancies. *Blood* 1997;90(6): 2127–2147.

Mastocytosis

Arias M, Villalba C, Requena I, Vazquez-Veiga H, Sesar A, Pereiro I. Acute spinal epidural hematoma and systemic mastocytosis. *Spine* April 15, 2004;29(8):E161–3.

Avila NA, Ling A, Metcalfe DD, Worobec AS. Mastocytosis: magnetic resonance imaging patterns of marrow disease. *Skeletal Radiol* 1998;27:119–126.

Boncoraglio GB, Brucato A, Carriero MR, et al. Systemic mastocytosis: a potential neurologic emergency. *Neurology* July 2005;65:332–333.

Myers B, Grimley C, Jones SG, Clark D, Kerslake R. Skin, bone marrow and magnetic resonance imaging appearances in systemic mastocytosis. *Brit J Haematol* 2003;122:876.

Roca M, Mota J, Giraldo P, Garcia Erce JA. Systemic mastocytosis: MRI of bone marrow involvement. *Eur Radiol* 1999;9(6):1094–1097.

Siegel S, Sadler MA, Yook C, Chang V, Miller J. Systemic mastocytosis with involvement of the pelvis: a radiographic and clinicopathologic study – a case study. *Clin Imag* 1999;23:245–248.

Valent P., Horny HP, Li CY, et al. Mastocytosis. In: Jaffe ES, Harris NL, Sein H, Vardiman JW, eds. *World Health Organization Classification of Tumors. Pathology and Genetics of Tumors of Hematopoietic and Lymphoid Tissues.* Lyon, France: IARC Press; 2001:293–302.

Table 15 Lesions that contain cartilage

Lesion	MRI Findings	Comments
Benign		
Osteochondroma (Fig. 15.1)	Circumscribed protruding lesion arising from outer cortex with a central zone with intermediate signal on T1WI and T2WI similar to marrow surrounded by a peripheral outer zone of low signal on T1WI and T2WI images over which, a cartilaginous cap is usually present in children and young adults. Increased malignant potential when cartilaginous cap is > 2 cm thick.	Benign cartilaginous tumors arising from defect at periphery of growth plate during bone formation with resultant bone outgrowth covered by a cartilaginous cap. Usually benign lesions unless associated with pain and increasing size of cartilaginous cap. Osteochondromas are common lesions, accounting for 14–35 % of primary bone tumors. Occur with median age of 20 years, up to 75 % of patients are less than 20 years. **(See Atlas Chapter A 58)**
Enchondroma (Fig. 15.2)	Lobulated intramedullary lesions with well-defined borders ranging in size from 3 cm to 16 cm, mean = 5 cm. Mild endosteal scalloping can be seen. Cortical bone expansion rarely occurs. Lesions usually have low-intermediate signal on T1WI and intermediate signal on PDWI. On T2WI and FS T2WI, lesions usually have predominantly high signal with foci and/or bands of low signal representing areas of matrix mineralization and fibrous strands. No zones of abnormal high signal on T2WI are typically seen in the marrow outside the borders of the lesions. Lesions typically show Gd-contrast enhancement in various patterns (peripheral curvilinear lobular, central nodular/septal and peripheral lobular, or heterogeneous diffuse).	Benign intramedullary lesions composed of hyaline cartilage, represent ~10 % of benign bone tumors. Enchondromas can be solitary (88 %) or multiple (12 %). Ollier disease is a dyschondroplasia involving endochondral-formed bone resulting in multiple enchondromas (enchondromatosis). Metachondromatosis is a combination of enchondromatosis and osteochondromatosis, and is rare. Maffucci disease refers to a syndrome with multiple enchondromas and soft tissue hemangiomas and is very rare. Patients range in age from 3 to 83 years, median = 35 years, mean = 38 to 40 years, peak in 3rd and 4th decades. **(See Atlas Chapter A 8)**
Juxtacortical chondroma (Fig. 15.3)	Lesions are located at the bone surface and are usually lobulated with low-intermediate signal on T1WI, which is hypo- or isointense relative to muscle. Lesions usually have heterogeneous predominantly high signal on T2WI. Lesions are surrounded by low-signal borders on T2WI representing thin sclerotic reaction. Areas of low signal on T2WI are secondary to matrix mineralization. Edema is not typically seen in nearby medullary bone. Lesions often show a peripheral pattern of Gd-contrast enhancement.	Benign protuberant hyaline cartilaginous tumors that arise from the periosteum and superficial to bone cortex. Juxtacortical chondromas account for < 1 % of bone lesions. Occur with median age of 26 years. **(See Atlas Chapter A 9)**
Chondroblastoma (Fig. 15.4)	Tumors often have fine lobular margins and typically have low-intermediate heterogeneous signal on T1WI, and mixed low, intermediate, and/or high signal on T2WI. Areas of low signal on T2WI are secondary to chondroid matrix mineralization and/or hemosiderin. Lobular, marginal or septal Gd-contrast enhancement patterns can be seen. Poorly defined zones with high signal on T2WI and FS T2WI and corresponding Gd-contrast enhancement are typically seen in the marrow adjacent to the lesions representing inflammatory reaction from prostaglandin synthesis by these tumors.	Benign cartilaginous tumors with chondroblast-like cells and areas of chondroid matrix formation, usually occur in children and adolescents, median = 17 years, mean = 16 years for lesions in long bones, mean = 28 years in other bones. Most cases are diagnosed between the ages of 5 and 25. **(See Atlas Chapter A 7)**

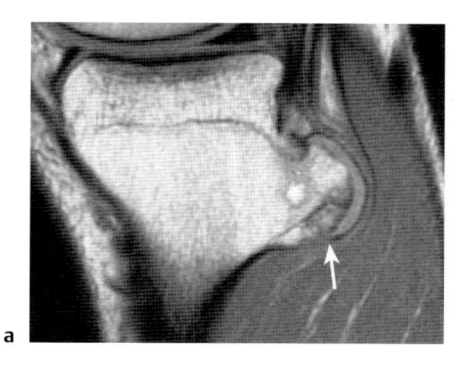

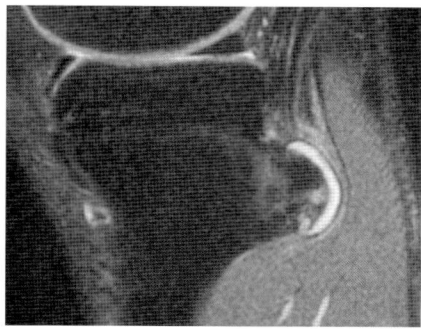

Figure 15.**1 a, b** A 14-year-old boy with an osteochondroma at the proximal dorsal surface of the tibia as seen on sagittal PDWI (**a**) and FS T2WI (**b**).

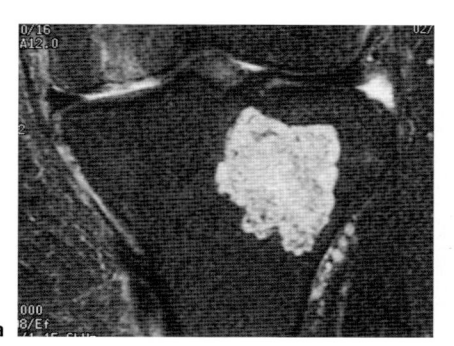

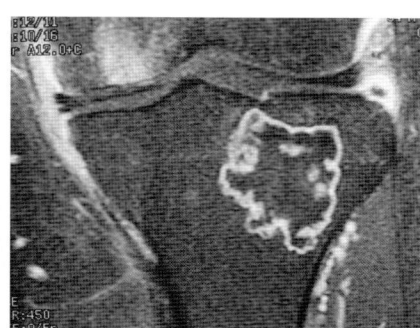

Figure 15.**2 a, b** A 54-year-old man with an enchondroma in the marrow of the proximal tibia that has mostly high signal on coronal FS T2WI (**a**) and thin peripheral lobulated Gd-contrast enhancement on FS T1WI (**b**).

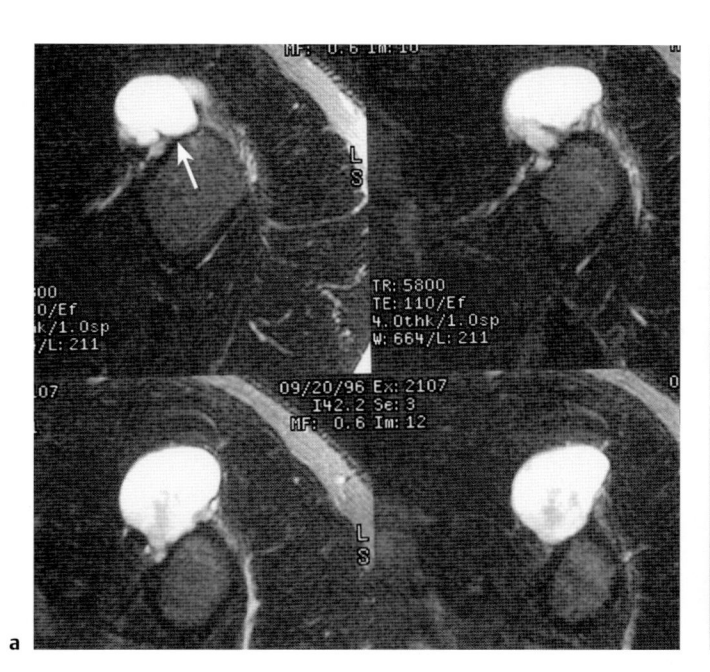

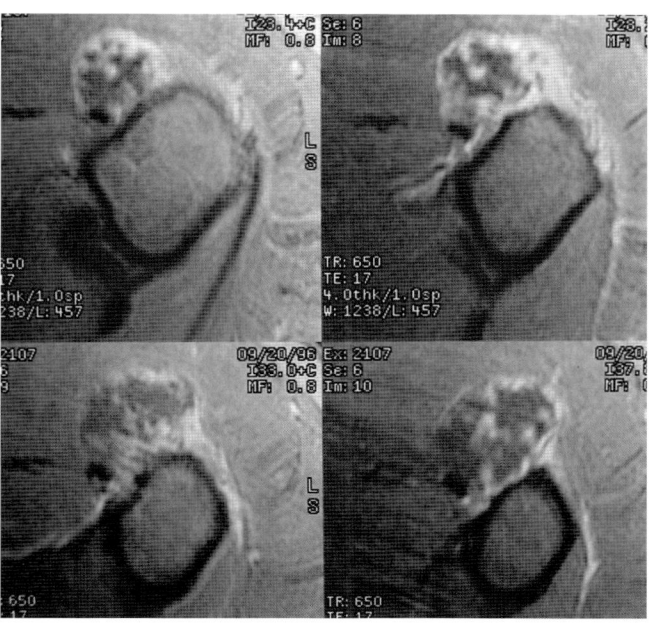

Figure 15.**3 a, b** A 28-year-old man with a juxtacortical/periosteal chondroma involving the proximal humerus. The lesion has high signal on axial FS T2WI (**a**) and shows nodular and lobulated peripheral Gd-contrast enhancement on axial FS T1WI (**b**).

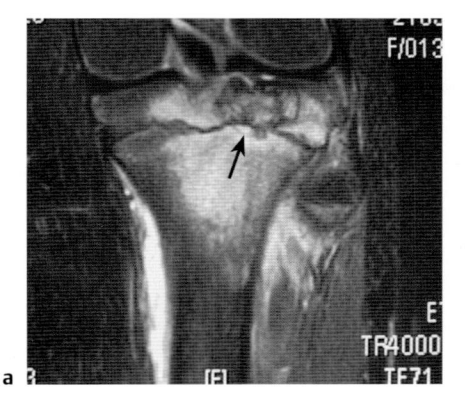

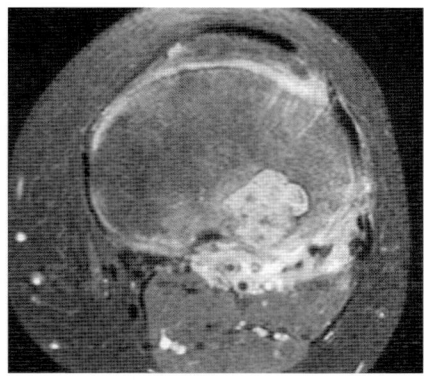

Figure 15.**4 a, b** A 13-year-old girl with a chondroblastoma in the epiphysis of the proximal tibia that has slightly lobulated margins. The lesion has high signal on coronal FS T2WI (**a**) as well as in the adjacent marrow. The lesion shows Gd-contrast enhancement on axial FS T1WI (**b**) as well as poorly defined enhancement in the adjacent marrow.

Table 15 (Continued) **Lesions that contain cartilage**

Lesion	MRI Findings	Comments
Chondromyxoid fibroma (Fig. 15.5)	Lesions are often slightly lobulated with low-intermediate signal on T1WI, intermediate signal on PDWI, and heterogeneous predominantly high signal on T2WI secondary to myxoid and hyaline chondroid components with high water content. MR signal heterogeneity on T2WI is related to the proportions of myxoid, chondroid, and fibrous components within the lesions. Thin low signal septa within lesions on T2WI are secondary to fibrous strands. Lesions are surrounded by low-signal borders representing thin sclerotic reaction. Edema is not typically seen in medullary bone. Lesions show prominent diffuse Gd-contrast enhancement.	Rare, benign, slow-growing bone lesions that contain chondroid, myxoid, and fibrous components. Chondromyxoid fibromas represent 2–4% of primary benign bone lesions, and <1% of primary bone lesions. Most chondromyxoid fibromas occur between the ages of 1 and 40 years, with a median of 17 years, and peak incidence in the 2nd to 3rd decades. **(See Atlas Chapter A 10)**
Synovial chondroma, chondromatosis/osteochondroma, osteochondromatosis (Figs. 15.6, 15.7)	MRI features depend on the relative proportions of cartilage, calcified cartilage, and mineralized osseous tissue within the lesions. Calcifications result in low signal on T1WI, PDWI, T2WI, and FS T2WI. Synovial osteochondromas with ossification can have peripheral low signal on T1WI and T2WI surrounding a central region with fat/marrow signal. Noncalcified portions of the lesions typically have low to intermediate signal on T1WI, intermediate signal on PDWI, and slightly high to high signal on T2WI and FS T2WI. Low signal septae on T2WI can be seen within the lesions. Synovial chondromas/osteochondromas can show irregular, thin-peripheral and/or septal Gd-contrast enhancement.	**Primary synovial chondromatosis** is a benign disorder resulting from nodular metaplastic cartilaginous proliferation in synovium of joints. The cartilaginous nodules can become detached forming intra-articular loose bodies. Metaplasia of connective tissue into cartilage can also occur in bursae and in tendon sheaths. **Secondary synovial chondromatosis** is associated with joint disorders (degenerative osteoarthrosis, avascular necrosis, osteonecrosis, osteochondritis dissecans, trauma/osteochondral fractures). In the secondary type, osteocartilaginous loose bodies arise from avulsion of hyaline cartilage into the joint, which can enlarge via nutrients supplied from synovial fluid. Solitary lesions can occur in both primary and secondary disorders and are referred to as synovial chondromas. Synovial chondromas with osseous metaplasia are referred to as **primary or secondary synovial osteochondromas** Account for <1% of benign soft tissue tumors. Occur most frequently between the ages of 25 to 65 years, mean = 44 years. **(See Atlas Chapter A 73)**

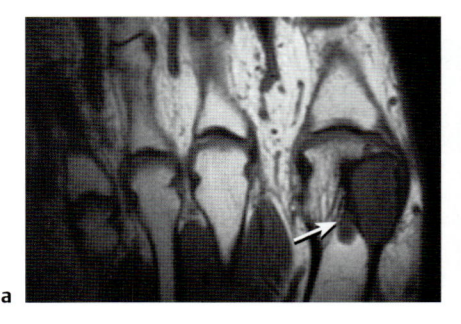

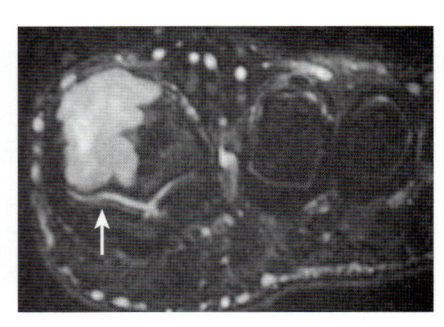

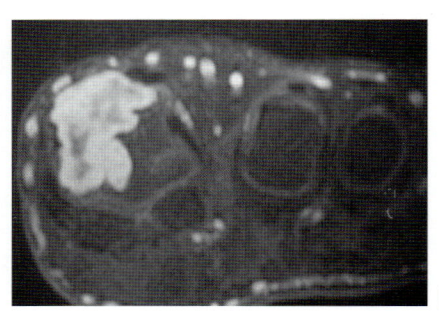

Figure 15.**5 a–c** A 34-year-old man with chondromyxoid fibroma in the distal first metatarsal bone that has low-intermediate signal on coronal T1WI (**a**) and heterogeneous high signal on axial FS T2WI (**b**). The lesion shows Gd-contrast enhancement on axial FS T1WI (**c**).

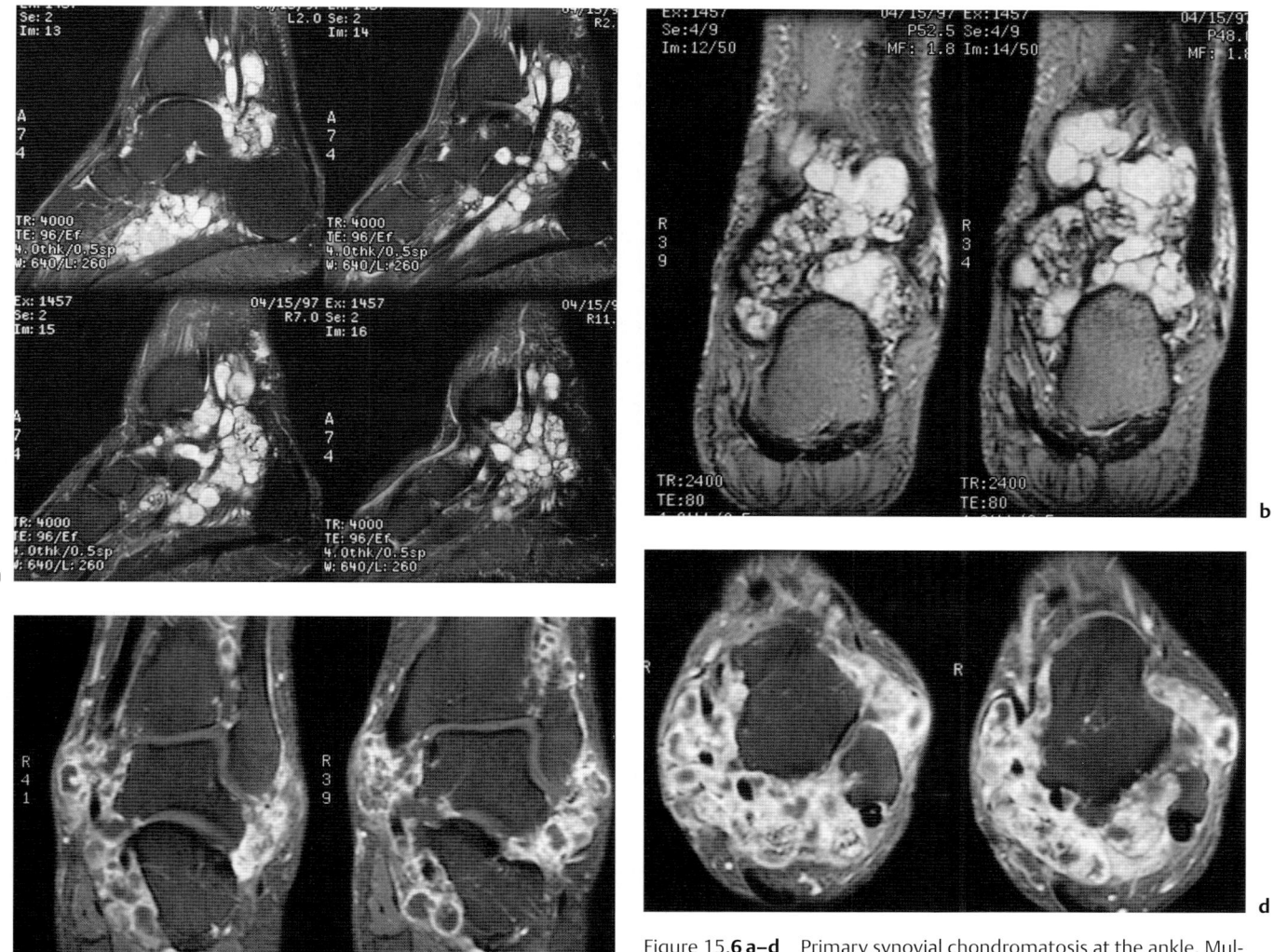

Figure 15.**6 a–d** Primary synovial chondromatosis at the ankle. Multiple lobulated zones are seen at the ankle joint and tendon sheaths that have high signal on sagittal FS T2WI (**a**) and coronal T2WI (**b**). Lesions show irregular peripheral-lobular and septal patterns of Gd-contrast enhancement on coronal (**c**) and axial (**d**) FS T1WI.

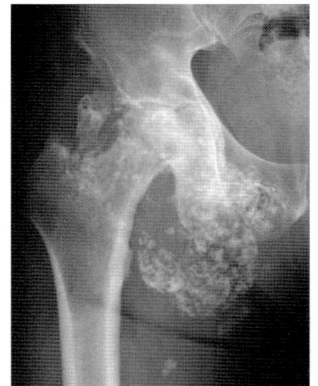

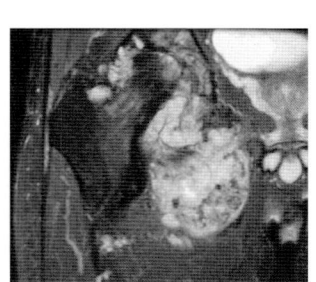

Figure 15.**7 a–c** A 51-year-old man with extensive primary synovial osteochondromatosis at the right hip. The AP radiograph (**a**) shows multiple nodules with chondroid-type calcifications within the hip joint with secondary osteoarthritic changes. Noncalcified portions of the lesion have high signal on coronal FS T2WI (**b**). Low signal septa on T2WI and multiple foci with low signal correspond to calcified cartilage nodules. The lesion shows irregular peripheral-lobular and septal patterns of Gd-contrast enhancement on coronal FS T1WI (**c, d**).

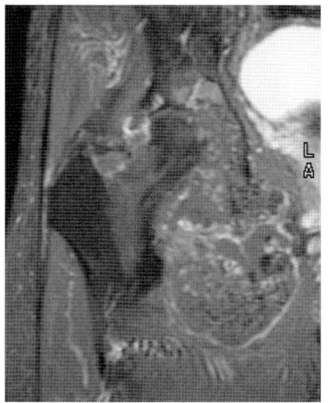

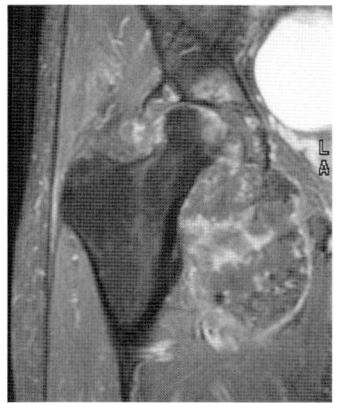

Table 15 (Continued) Lesions that contain cartilage		
Lesion	**MRI Findings**	**Comments**
Chondroid lipoma (Fig. 15.8)	Chondroid lipomas are much less common than the classic benign lipomas. Lesions can show irregular zones of nonfatty signal on T1WI and T2WI resulting from chondroid zones, calcifications, and thick septa which may or may not show Gd-contrast enhancement. Most atypical lipomas contain more than 75% fat, whereas liposarcomas often have less than 75% fat. Distinguishing between atypical lipomas and low grade liposarcomas with MRI, however, can be difficult and challenging.	Osseous or chondroid metaplasia with myxoid changes can be associated with lipomas. These **atypical lipomas** have been labeled as **chondroid lipomas**, **osteolipomas**, or **benign mesenchymomas** Chondroid lipomas are benign adipose tumors that contain mature fat, lipoblasts, and chondroid matrix. **(See Atlas Chapter A 43)**
Malignant		
Conventional chondrosarcoma (Figs. 15.9, 15.10)	Lesions usually have low-intermediate signal on T1WI, intermediate signal on PDWI, and heterogeneous predominantly high signal on T2WI. Zones of low signal on T2WI can occur from matrix mineralization and/or fibrous tissue. Lesions often have lobulated margins, with or without internal septations. Peritumoral high signal on T2WI in marrow and periosteal soft tissues may be seen associated with chondrosarcomas, and typically not with enchondromas. Chondrosarcomas usually show Gd-contrast enhancement in patterns ranging from lobulated peripheral and/or septal, or homogeneous versus heterogeneous depending on the degree of matrix mineralization and/or necrosis. MRI can readily show sites of cortical destruction and extension of tumor into the adjacent soft tissues.	Malignant tumors containing cartilage formed within sarcomatous stroma. Can contain areas of calcification/mineralization, myxoid material, and/or ossification. Primary chondrosarcomas (62–86%) represent lesions occurring without pre-existent lesions, whereas secondary chondrosarcomas arise from formerly benign cartilaginous lesions (enchondroma, osteochondroma, etc.) or other lesions (Paget disease, fibrous dysplasia, prior irradiation, repetitive trauma). Account for 12–21% of malignant bone lesions, 21–26% of primary sarcomas of bone, 9–14% of all bone tumors. Mean age = 40 years, median age = 26 to 59 years. **(See Atlas Chapter A 11)**

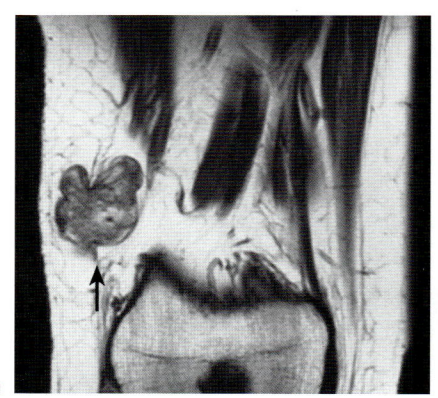

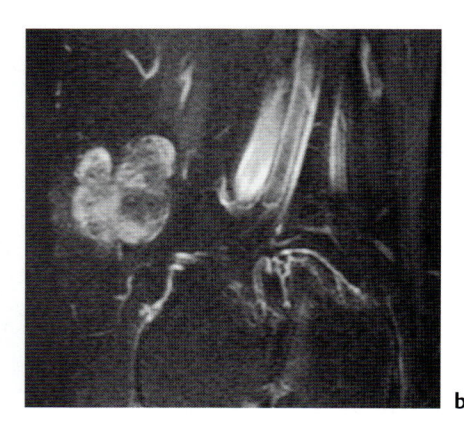

Figure 15.**8 a, b** A 57-year-old woman with a chondroid/myxoid lipoma in the soft tissues of the distal lateral thigh. The lesion has lobulated well-defined margins, and has heterogeneous low, intermediate, and high signal on coronal T1WI (**a**) and coronal FS T2WI (**b**).

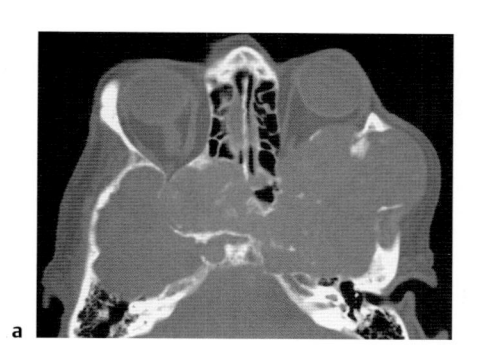

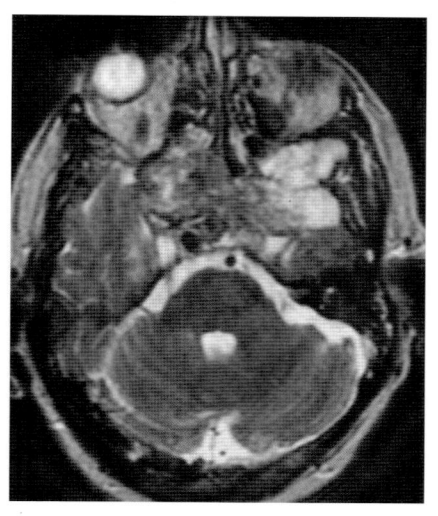

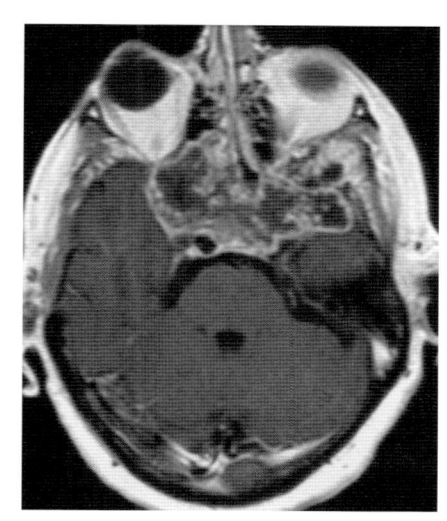

Figure 15.**9 a–c** An 81-year-old woman with a large low-grade conventional chondrosarcoma involving the sphenoid bone with extension into both middle cranial fossae. The tumor contains chondroid mineralization and is associated with extensive destruction and remodeling of bone as seen on axial CT (**a**). The tumor has heterogeneous intermediate high and low signal on axial T2WI (**b**) and shows peripheral lobular and central nodular Gd-contrast enhancement on axial T1WI (**c**).

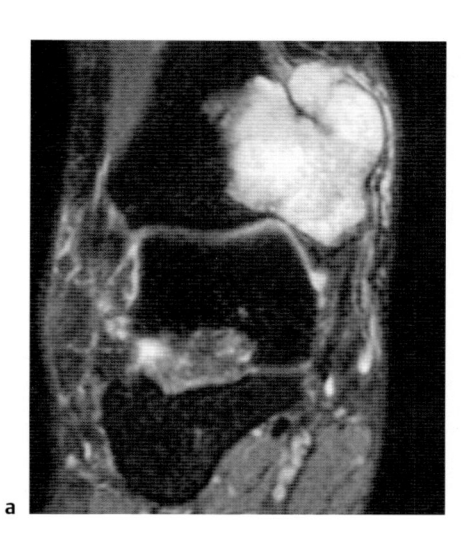

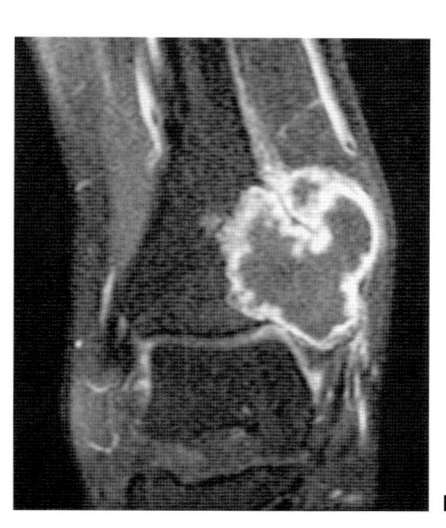

Figure 15.**10 a, b** A 44-year-old woman with a grade 2 conventional chondrosarcoma involving the distal tibia. The tumor has mostly high signal on coronal FS T2WI (**a**) and extends into the adjacent soft tissues through a zone of cortical destruction. The tumor shows irregular peripheral lobular Gd-contrast enhancement on coronal FS T1WI (**b**).

Table 15 (Continued) **Lesions that contain cartilage**

Lesion	MRI Findings	Comments
Myxoid chondrosarcoma (Figs. 15.11. 15.12)	These tumors can arise in bone or soft tissues. In soft tissues, tumors often have lobulated margins and range in size from 4 to 7 cm. Lesions usually have low-intermediate signal on T1WI and PDWI, and predominantly high signal on T2WI. Hemorrhagic foci in myxoid chondrosarcomas can show intermediate to high signal on T1WI and T2WI. Myxoid chondrosarcomas show heterogeneous Gd-contrast enhancement.	Patients range in age from 6 to 89 years, median = 52 years, mean = 49 years. Considered low-grade tumors, and are also known as chordoid sarcoma. Tumors can contain abundant myxoid/mucoid stroma with strands and/or foci of cells with small hyperchromatic nuclei and moderate cytoplasm containing glycogen granules. Well-differentiated cartilage cells are also seen. Areas of hemorrhage and cysts often seen in extraosseous tumors. Matrix mineralization/calcification is rarely seen. Typically, minimal or no mitotic activity is seen in tissue samples. These tumors often arise in soft tissues of the extremities (thigh most common), and rarely in bone.
Dedifferentiated chondrosarcoma (Fig. 15.13)	Tumors usually have low-intermediate signal on T1WI and PDWI, heterogeneous predominantly high signal on T2WI. Zones of low signal on T2WI are related to the presence and degree of matrix mineralization and/or fibrous tissue. Lesions often have irregular poorly defined margins and associated cortical destruction. Lesions usually show heterogeneous contrast-enhancement. MRI can readily show sites of extension of the lesion into the adjacent soft tissues.	Occurs as both primary and secondary chondrosarcomas in patients ranging in age from 29 to 85 years, with the average between 50 and 60 years. Tumors have mixtures of high-grade spindle cells and low-grade or high-grade malignant cartilage cells. **(See Atlas Chapter A 11)**
Clear cell chondrosarcoma	Lesions usually are seen near the ends of long bones +/− extension into metaphyseal and diaphyseal regions. Smaller lesions may be well circumscribed, larger lesions may have associated cortical disruption and extension into adjacent soft tissues. Lesions typically have low-intermediate signal on T1WI and heterogeneous intermediate-high signal on T2WI. Lesions usually show prominent Gd-contrast enhancement.	These slow-growing tumors have been referred to as "malignant chondroblastoma." Patients range in age from 14 to 84 years, mean = 37 years, peak in 4th and 5th decades. Occur two to three times more frequently in males compared with females. Tumor cells have clear cytoplasm with centrally positioned nuclei with few mitotic figures. Multinucleated osteoclast-like giant cells may also be seen. Tumor matrix and/or zones with histology similar to conventional chondrosarcoma are often present. Tumor cartilage may be calcified/ossified. **(See Atlas Chapter A 11)**
Periosteal chondrosarcoma (also referred to as juxtacortical chondrosarcoma) (Fig. 15.14)	Tumors vary in size from 4 to 11 cm. Bone cortex is either thinned or thickened but not destroyed. Lesions occasionally involve medullary bone. Tumors have low-intermediate signal on T1WI, intermediate signal on PDWI, and heterogeneous intermediate-high signal on T2WI. Tumors show heterogeneous Gd-contrast enhancement.	Low-grade tumors that account for 1–2% of chondrosarcomas. Tumors occur on the surface of bones and are often large (> 5 cm). Typically have histologic features similar to conventional chondrosarcomas.

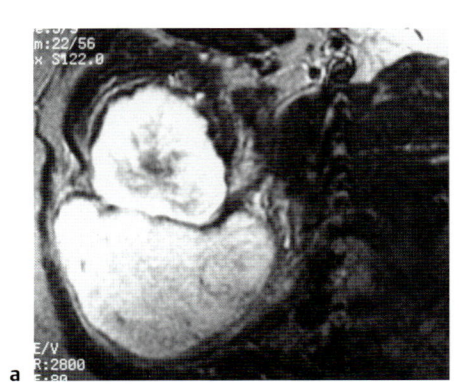

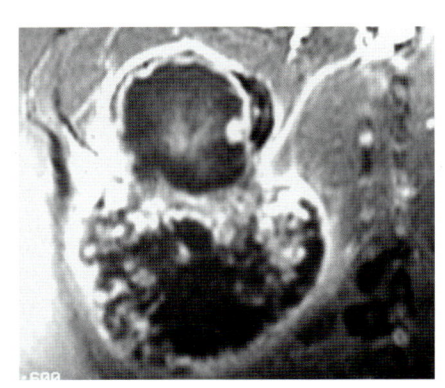

Figure 15.**11 a, b** A 34-year-old man with a high-grade myxoid chondrosarcoma involving the proximal femur with cortical destruction and extraosseous extension of tumor dorsally. The lesion has irregular circumscribed margins and contains high signal on axial T2WI (**a**). The tumor shows lobulated irregular peripheral Gd-contrast enhancement on axial FS T1WI (**b**).

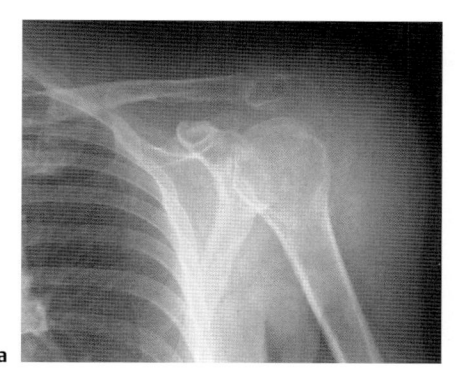

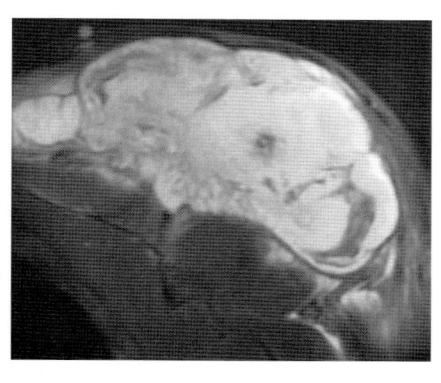

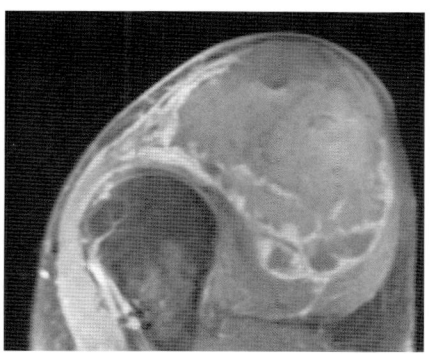

Periosteal chondrosarcoma (also referred to asjuxtacortical chondrosarcoma) **243**

Figure 15.**12 a–c** A 63-year-old man with an extraosseous myxoid chondrosarcoma involving the soft tissues at the left shoulder. The radiograph (**a**) shows chondroid mineralization associated with the tumor. The large tumor has mostly high signal on coronal FS T2WI (**b**) as well as irregular zones of low signal. The tumor shows lobulated irregular peripheral Gd-contrast enhancement on sagittal FS T1WI (**c**).

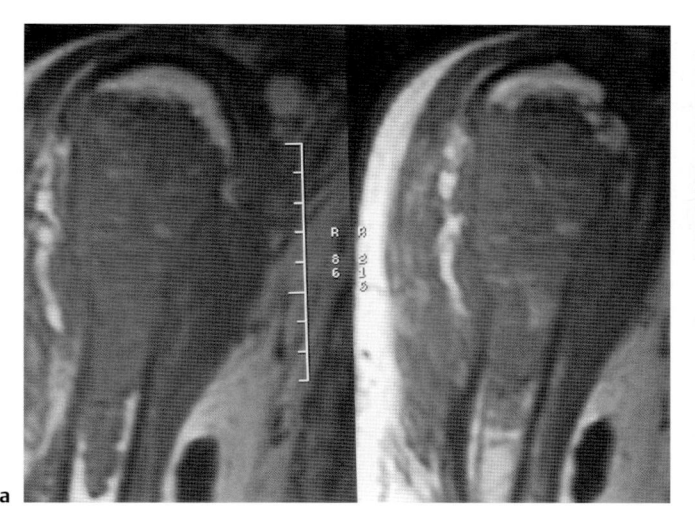

Figure 15.**13 a, b** An 88-year-old man with a dedifferentiated chondrosarcoma involving the proximal humerus that has low-intermediate signal on sagittal T1WI (**a**). The lesion shows prominent heterogeneous Gd-contrast enhancement on axial FS T1WI (**b**) that extends through disrupted cortex.

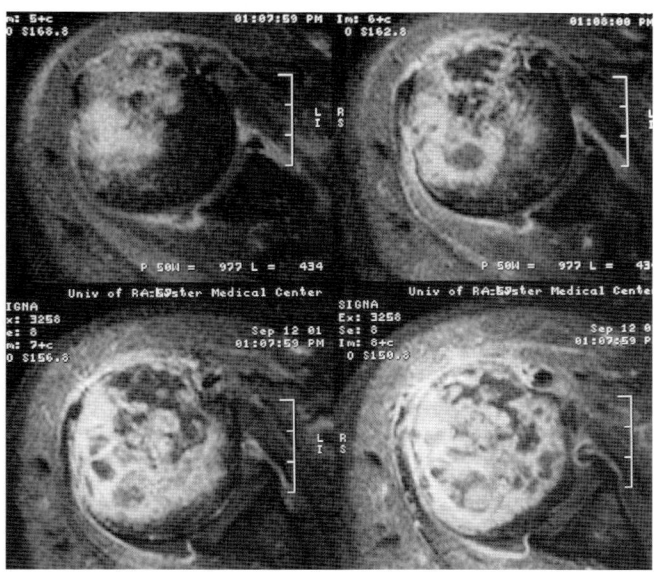

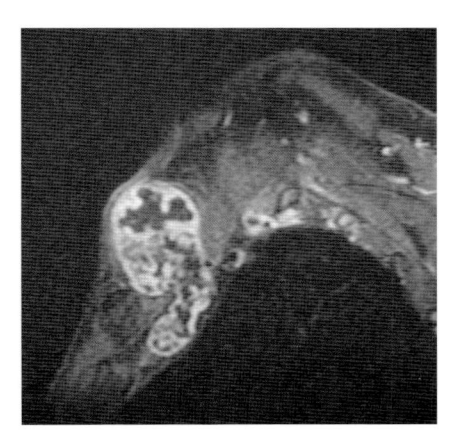

Figure 15.**14** A 40-year-old man with a low-grade periosteal chondrosarcoma along the cortical surface of the clavicle. The lesion has circumscribed margins and shows irregular peripheral and central lobular Gd-contrast enhancement on sagittal FS T1WI.

Table 15 (Continued) Lesions that contain cartilage

	MRI Findings	Comments
Mesenchymal chondrosarcoma (Fig. 15.15)	These tumors can arise in bone or soft tissue. Tumors in bone are usually destructive lesions commonly associated with extraosseous soft tissue masses. Lesions have low-intermediate signal on T1WI, intermediate signal on PDWI, and heterogeneous intermediate-high or slightly high signal on T2WI. Foci of low signal on T1WI and T2WI can be seen secondary to chondroid matrix mineralization. Lesions typically show heterogeneous Gd-contrast enhancement.	Patients range in age from 5 to 74 years, with peak occurrences in the 2nd and 3rd decades. Tumors contain undifferentiated small cells with oval nuclei associated with an extracellular reticulin network. Small to large foci of cartilage are seen in the lesions, with or without reactive osteoid and bone formation. This type can also arise in soft tissues. **(See Atlas Chapter A 11)**
Secondary chondrosarcoma from osteochondroma (Fig. 15.16)	MRI can demonstrate the thickness of cartilaginous caps of osteochondromas as well as erosive and/or destructive bone changes involving osteochondromas. Cartilage cap thickness exceeding 2 cm is associated with malignant degeneration of osteochondromas into secondary chondrosarcomas. Lesions have low-intermediate signal on T1WI, intermediate signal on PDWI, and heterogeneous intermediate-high signal on T2WI. Lesions show heterogeneous contrast enhancement, with or without Gd-contrast enhancement in adjacent soft tissues.	Peripheral chondrosarcomas refer to secondary chondrosarcomas that arise from osteochondromas, and usually have histologic features similar to a conventional intraosseous chondrosarcomas. **(See Atlas Chapter A 11)**
Chondroblastic osteosarcoma (Fig. 15.17)	Tumors usually have low-intermediate signal on T1WI. Tumors can have variable MRI signal on T2WI, and FS T2WI depending upon the relative proportions of calcified/mineralized osteoid, chondroid, fibroid, hemorrhagic, and necrotic components. Zones of necrosis typically have high signal on T2WI, whereas mineralized zones usually have low signal on T2WI. Zones of cortical destruction are often seen through which tumors extend into the extraosseous soft tissues. Zones of low signal from spicules of periosteal, reactive, and tumoral bone formation may be seen under an elevated periosteum. Tumors typically show prominent Gd-contrast enhancement in nonmineralized/calcified portions of the tumors.	Chondroblastic osteosarcomas account for 25% of osteosarcomas. These tumors contain chondroid zones with malignant spindle-shaped cells. Endochondral ossification and metaplastic bone formation are commonly seen.
Periosteal osteosarcoma (Fig. 15.18)	Often involves the diaphyseal regions with associated cortical thickening seen as low signal on T1WI and T2WI. Tumors can have a broad base along the outer cortex with tumor seen extending outward toward the adjacent soft tissues. Cortical thickening associated with these tumors is often thinner or eroded at the center or base of the protruding mass. Periosteal reaction, seen as linear zones of low signal on T1WI and T2WI, can be associated with these tumors, as well as Codman's triangles. Can involve 50% or more of the bone circumference. Tumors often have low-intermediate signal on T1WI, heterogeneous slightly high to high signal on T2WI and FS T2WI, and show Gd-contrast enhancement. Tumor extension into the marrow is uncommon, and when present is usually seen associated with a zone of cortical destruction.	Histologic features are often similar to moderately differentiated chondroblastic osteosarcoma. Tumors are often covered by periosteum associated with immature cells. Tumors consist of lobules of malignant-appearing cartilage separated and surrounded by malignant spindle-shaped cells within an osteoid matrix. Endochondral ossification can be seen in the central portions of the chondroid lobules. Tumor may extend into Haversian canals and bone marrow. Occurs in patients aged from 11 to 57 years, median = 17 to 24 years.

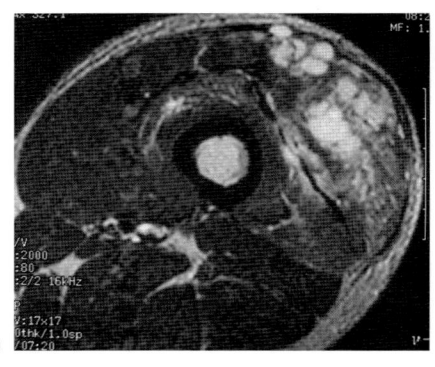

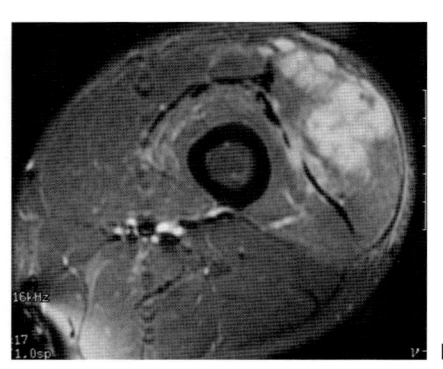

Figure 15.**15 a, b** An 18-year-old man with an extraosseous mesenchymal chondrosarcoma involving the vastus lateralis and adjacent soft tissues in the distal thigh. The tumor has poorly defined margins and has heterogeneous mostly high signal on axial T2WI (**a**). The tumor shows irregular Gd-contrast enhancement on axial FS T1WI (**b**).

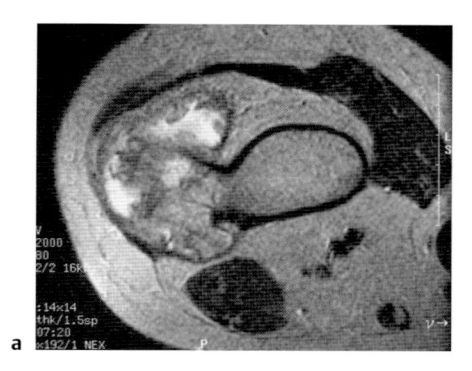

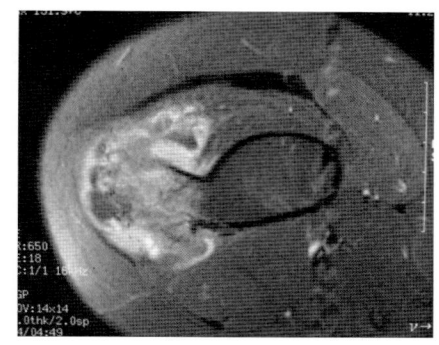

Figure 15.**16 a, b**   An 18-year-old woman with a secondary low-grade chondrosarcoma arising from an osteochondroma at the distal femur. The thickened cartilaginous cap of the tumor has irregular margins and contains heterogeneous slightly high and high signal with small foci of low signal on axial T2WI (**a**). Zones of cortical destruction are seen at the osteochondroma adjacent to the malignant cartilaginous cap. The lesion shows irregular heterogeneous Gd-contrast enhancement on axial FS T1WI (**b**).

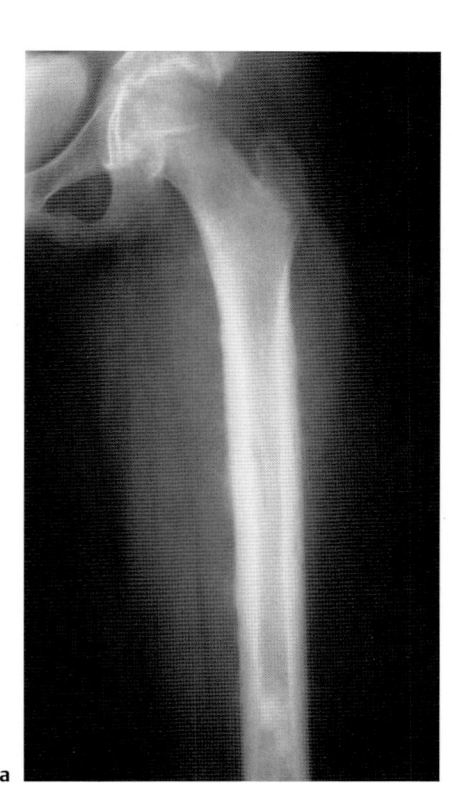

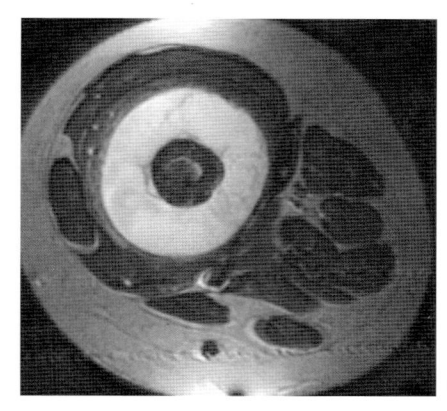

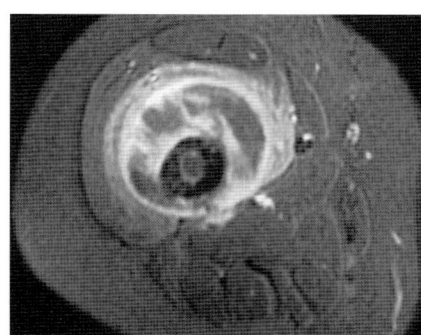

Figure 15.**17 a–c**   A 10-year-old female with a chondroblastic osteosarcoma involving the proximal diaphysis of the femur. The AP radiograph (**a**) shows osteoid matrix mineralization from intramedullary tumor associated with interrupted perpendicular, lamellated periosteal reaction, and a Codman's triangle at the upper border of tumor extension. The intramedullary tumor has mostly low signal on axial T2WI (**b**), whereas the circumferential extraosseous tumor has mostly high signal. Irregular thin strands of low signal are seen in the extraosseous tumor representing perpendicular periosteal reaction. Irregular Gd-contrast enhancement is seen mostly in the extraosseous tumor on axial FS T1WI (**c**).

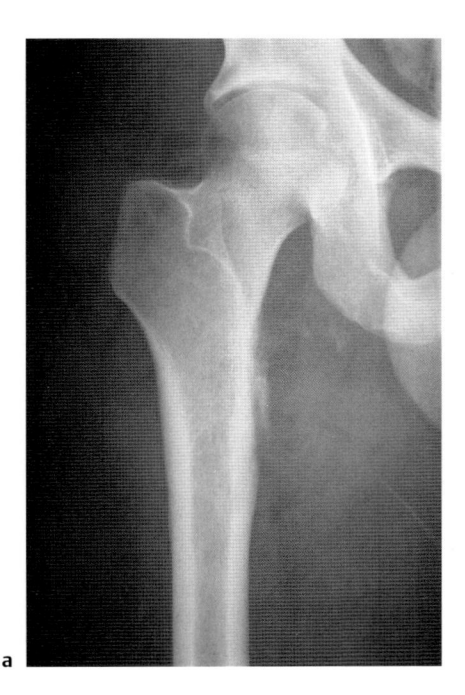

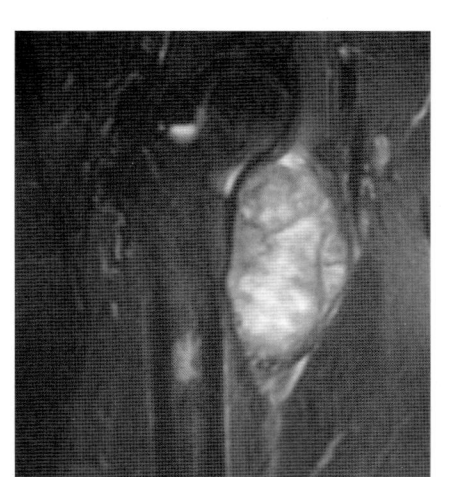

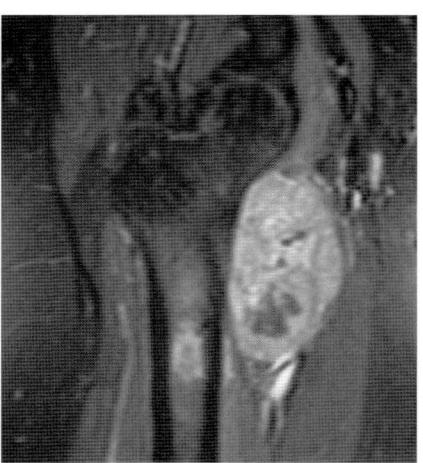

Figure 15.**18 a–c**   A 26-year-old man with a periosteal osteosarcoma involving the anteromedial surface of the proximal femur. The AP radiograph (**a**) shows an extraosseous tumor containing mineralized matrix as well as interrupted lamellated periosteal reaction adjacent to the femur. The tumor has mixed intermediate, slightly high, and high signal on coronal FS T2WI (**b**) and shows heterogeneous Gd-contrast enhancement on coronal FS T1WI (**c**).

Table 15 (Continued) Lesions that contain cartilage		
Lesion	**MRI Findings**	**Comments**
Chondroid chordoma	Chondroid chordomas are either midline or off-midline in location, and typically have low-intermediate signal on T1WI and heterogeneous predominantly high signal on T2WI. Typically show Gd-contrast enhancement. Lesions can displace and encase blood vessels, and extend into adjacent structures such as the cavernous sinus, sella, nasopharynx, and hypoglossal canal.	Rare, locally aggressive, slow-growing malignant tumors derived from ectopic notochordal remnants along the axial skeleton. Chondroid chordomas (5–15% of chordomas) show both chordomatous and chondromatous differentiation. Average survival for chondroid chordomas (16 years) is greater than conventional chordomas (4 years). Morbidity and mortality are usually secondary to local recurrence and extension. Distant metastasis is uncommon. **(See Atlas Chapter A 12)**

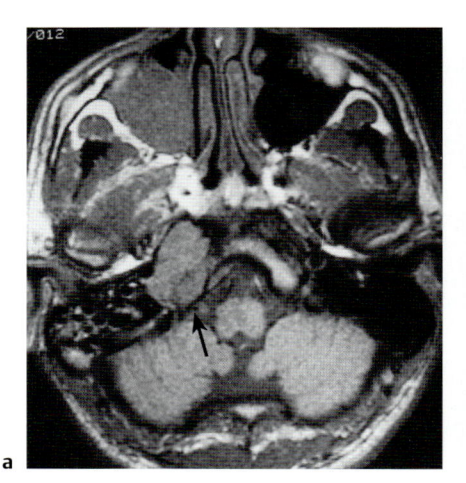

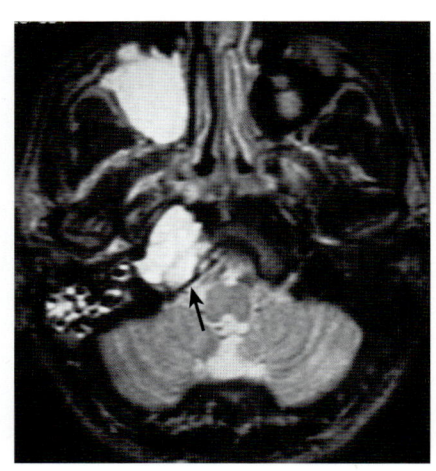

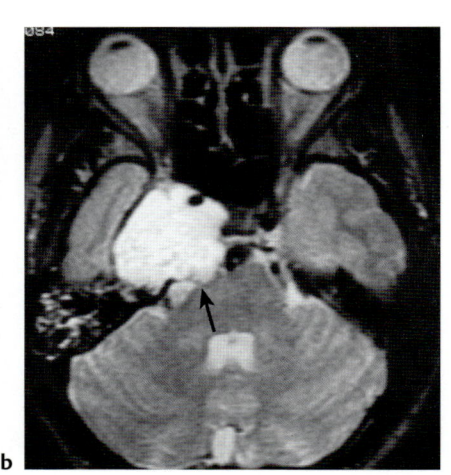

Figure 15.**19 a–c** A 21-year-old man with chondroid chordoma at the right petro-occipital synchondrosis. The lesion is associated with bone destruction and extraosseous extension, and has intermediate signal on axial T1WI (**a**) and high signal on axial T2WI (**b**, **c**).

Table 16 Tumors and tumorlike lesions within joints

Lesion	MRI Findings	Comments
Benign		
Synovial osteochondroma/ osteochondromatosis (Figs. 16.1, 16.2)	MRI features of osteochondromatosis are dependent on the relative proportions of cartilage, calcified cartilage, and mineralized osseous tissue within the lesions. Calcifications result in low signal on T1WI, PDWI, T2WI, and FS T2WI. Lesions with extensive calcification can have signal voids. Mature ossifications can have peripheral low signal on T1WI and T2WI surrounding a central region with fat signal. Noncalcified portions of the lesions can have low to intermediate signal on T1WI, intermediate signal on PDWI, and slightly high to high signal on T2WI and FS T2WI. Lesions can show irregular, thin-peripheral and/or septal enhancement.	**Primary synovial osteochondromatosis** is a benign disorder that results from cartilaginous and osseous metaplastic proliferation in synovium of joints. The osteocartilaginous nodules can become detached forming intra-articular loose bodies. **Secondary synovial osteochondromatosis** occurs from avulsion of osteochondral fragments into the joint, forming loose bodies that can enlarge via nutrient supply from synovial fluid. **(See Atlas Chapter A 73)**

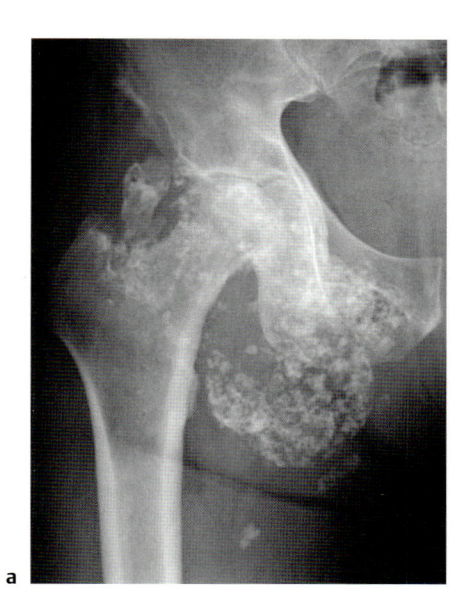

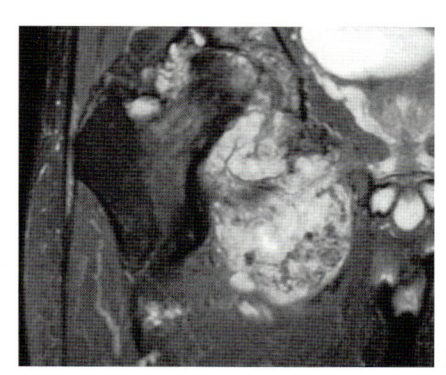

Figure 16.1 a, b A 51-year-old man with extensive primary synovial osteochondromatosis at the right hip. The AP radiograph (**a**) shows multiple nodules with chondroid-type calcifications within the hip joint with associated osteoarthritic changes. Noncalcified portions of the lesion have high signal on coronal FS T2WI (**b**). Low signal septa on T2WI are seen within the lesion. Multiple foci of low signal and signal void on FS T2WI correspond to calcified cartilage nodules seen on the radiograph.

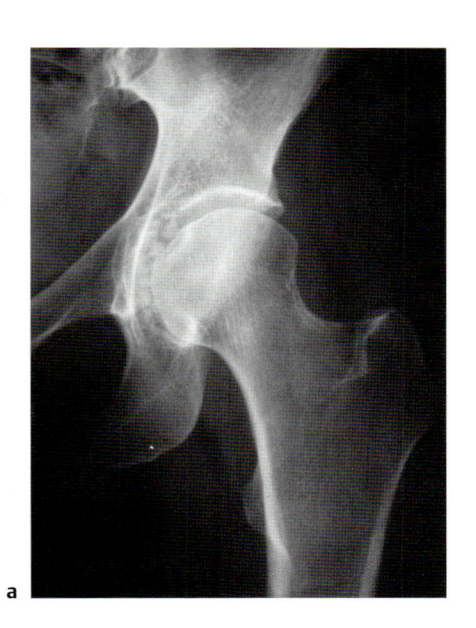

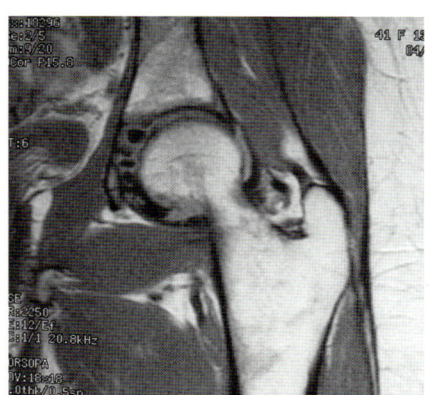

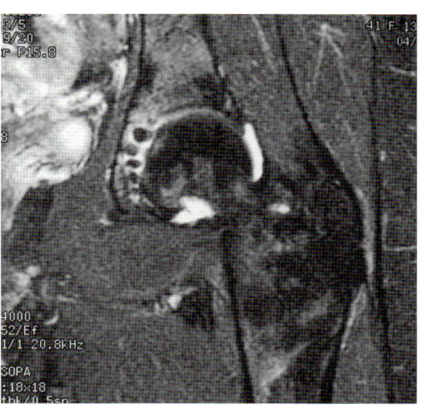

Figure 16.2 a–c A 41-year-old woman with secondary synovial osteochondromatosis at the left hip. The AP radiograph (**a**) shows multiple calcified nodules within the medial portion of the left hip joint. Foci of low signal on coronal T1WI (**b**) and coronal FS T2WI (**c**) are seen within the medial portion of the hip joint, which correspond to calcified cartilage nodules.

Table 16 (Continued)   Tumors and tumorlike lesions within joints

Lesion	MRI Findings	Comments
Synovial chondroma/ chondromatosis (Figs. 16.3, 16.4)	Synovial chondromas are typically radiolucent and have low to intermediate signal on T1WI (that is iso- or hyperintense relative to muscle), intermediate signal on PDWI, and slightly high to high signal on T2WI and FS T2WI. Low signal septae on T2WI can be seen within the lesions. Synovial chondromas can show irregular, thin-peripheral and/or septal Gd-contrast enhancement.	**Primary synovial chondromatosis** accounts for < 1 % of benign soft tissue tumors and is a disorder that results from cartilaginous metaplastic proliferation in synovium of joints. Usually occurs in patients from 25 to 65 years, mean = 44 years. The cartilaginous nodules can become detached forming intra-articular loose bodies. Metaplasia of connective tissue into cartilage can also occur in bursae and in tendon sheaths. **Secondary synovial chondromatosis** occurs from avulsion of hyaline cartilage into the joint, forming loose bodies that can enlarge via nutrient supply from synovial fluid. **(See Atlas Chapter A 73)**
Pigmented villonodular synovitis (Fig. 16.5)	Often appears as irregular, multinodular, and/or diffuse thickening of synovium. Occasionally occurs as single nodular intra-articular lesions. Lesions often have low or low-intermediate signal on T1WI, PDWI, and T2WI. Areas of low signal on T2WI and T2*WI are secondary to hemosiderin in Pigmented villonodular synovitis (PVNS). Areas of slightly high to high signal on T2WI and FS T2WI can also occur from edema and/or inflammatory reaction. Joint effusions are usually present, rarely with fluid–fluid levels. PVNS can show Gd-contrast enhancement in irregular heterogeneous and/or homogeneous patterns.	Benign intra-articular lesions of proliferative synovium (tendon sheaths, joints, and bursae) containing zones of recent or remote hemorrhage. PVNS has similar histopathologic features with giant cell tumors of the tendon sheath/nodular synovitis; although PVNS lesions have frond-like or villous growth patterns and contain large amounts of hemosiderin. Accounts for < 1 % of benign and all soft tissue tumors. Patients range in age from 9 to 74 years, mean = 38 years, median age = 32 years. **(See Atlas Chapter A 67)**
Nodular synovitis (also referred to as giant cell tumors of the tendon sheath and soft tissue) (Fig. 16.6)	Lesions can be ovoid or multilobulated and usually have low-intermediate or intermediate signal on T1WI and PDWI that is often similar to or less than muscle. On T2WI and FS T2WI, lesions can have mixed intermediate and/or high signal. Small zones of low signal on T2WI can represent small sites of hemosiderin deposition. Lesions often show Gd-contrast enhancement in either homogeneous or heterogeneous pattern. Erosions of adjacent bone can be seen with some lesions.	Benign proliferative lesions of synovium (tendon sheaths, joints, and bursae). Can occur as localized nodular lesions attached to tendon sheaths outside of joints (hands, feet) or within joints (infrapatellar portion of knee joint); or as a diffuse form near/outside of large joints such as the knees, ankles, etc. Nodular synovitis accounts for 4 % of benign soft tissue tumors and 2 % of all soft tissue tumors. Occurs in patients aged from 6 to 71 years, mean = 39 to 46 years, peak ages in 3rd to 4th decades. **(See Atlas Chapter A 30)**

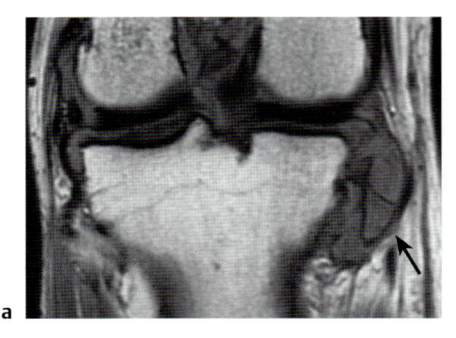

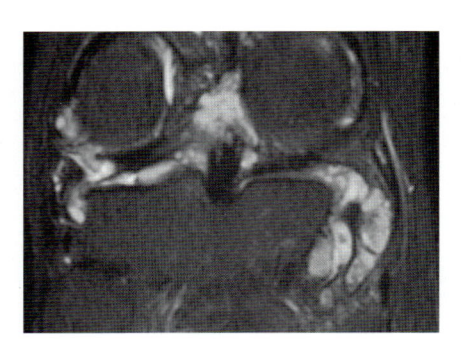

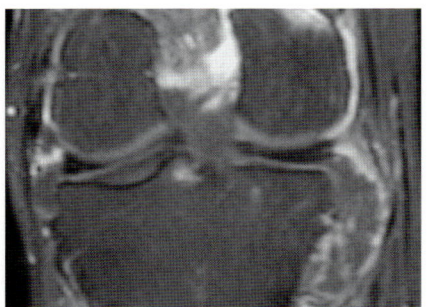

Figure 16.3 a–c   A 37-year-old woman with primary synovial chondromatosis at the knee. Multiple lobulated zones are seen that have intermediate signal on coronal PDWI (**a**) and high signal on coronal FS T2WI (**b**). The lobules have thin margins of low signal. The lesions show irregular peripheral-lobular and septal patterns of Gd-contrast enhancement on coronal FS T1WI (**c**). No mineralized zones were seen on the radiographs (not shown).

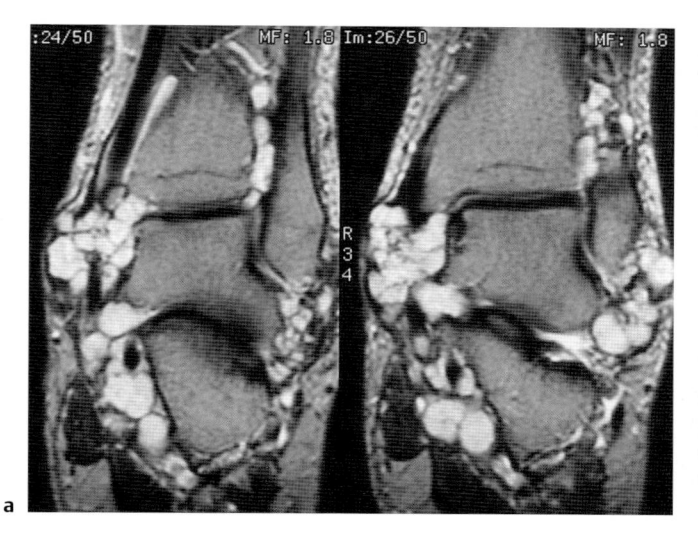

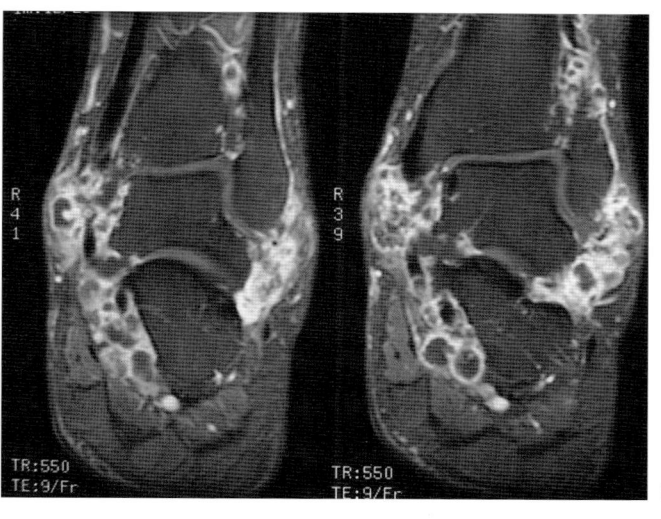

Figure 16.**4 a, b** A 57-year-old man with primary synovial chondromatosis at the ankle. Multiple lobulated zones are seen at the ankle joint and tendon sheaths that have high signal on coronal T2WI (**a**). The lobules have thin margins of low signal on T2WI. The lesion shows irregular peripheral-lobular and septal patterns of Gd-contrast enhancement on coronal FS T1WI (**b**). No mineralized zones were seen on the radiographs (not shown).

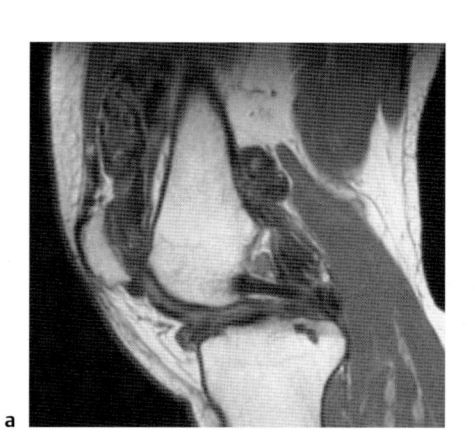

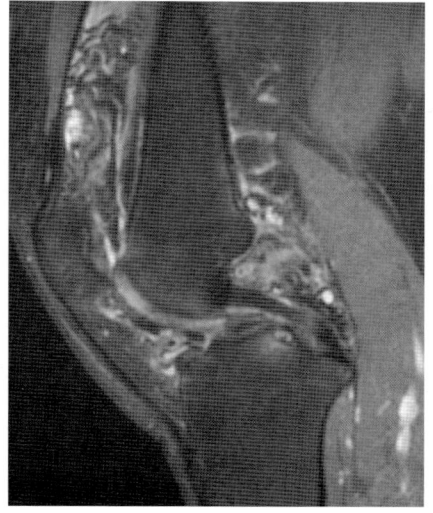

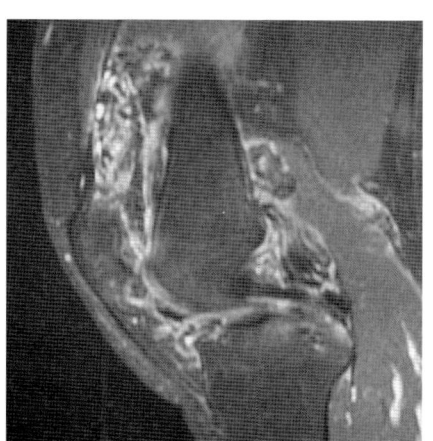

Figure 16.**5 a–c** A 36-year-old woman with PVNS involving the knee. Poorly defined and ovoid zones with heterogeneous intermediate and low signal on sagittal T1WI (**a**), and heterogeneous intermediate, slightly high, and low signal on sagittal FS T2WI (**b**) are seen in the anterior and posterior portions of the knee joint. Heterogeneous Gd-contrast enhancement of the lesions is seen on sagittal FS T1WI (**c**).

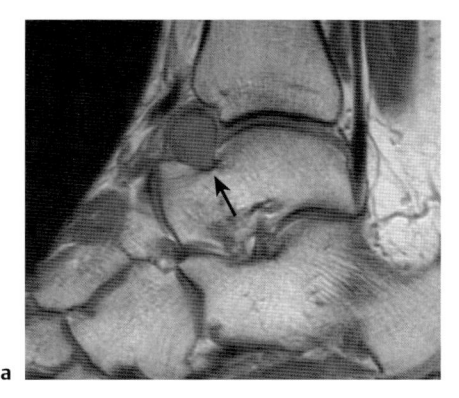

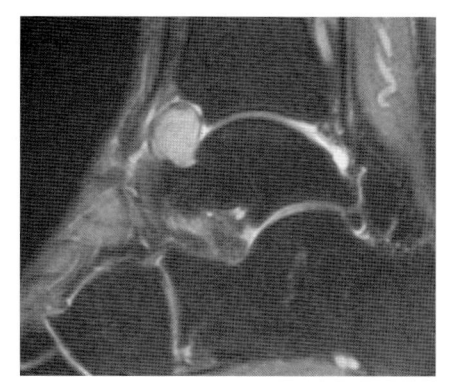

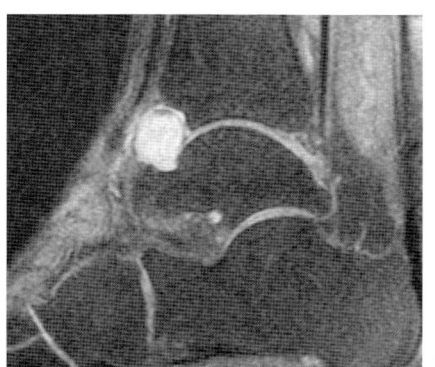

Figure 16.**6 a–c** A 68-year-old woman with a giant cell tumor of the tendon sheath/nodular synovitis at the ankle. An ovoid lesion with well-defined margins is seen that has mostly intermediate signal on sagittal T1WI (**a**) and high signal on sagittal FS T2WI (**b**). The lesion shows prominent Gd-contrast enhancement on sagittal FS T1WI (**c**).

Table 16 (Continued) **Tumors and tumorlike lesions within joints**

Lesion	MRI Findings	Comments
Rheumatoid arthritis (Figs. 16.7, 16.8. 16.9)	Hypertrophied synovium seen with rheumatoid arthritis can be diffuse, nodular, and/or villous, and usually has low to intermediate or intermediate signal on T1WI and PDWI. On T2WI, hypertrophied synovium can have low to intermediate, intermediate, and/or slightly high to high signal that is typically lower than joint fluid. Signal heterogeneity of hypertrophied synovium on T2WI can result from variable amounts of fibrin, hemosiderin, and fibrosis. Chronic fibrotic nonvascular synovium usually has low signal on T1WI and T2WI. Hypertrophied synovium can show prominent homogeneous or variable heterogeneous Gd-contrast enhancement. Joint effusions can be seen. Zones of erosion and/or destruction of hyaline cartilage and subchondral bone, meniscal damage; bursal and joint fluid collections containing "rice bodies," other extra-articular cysts; intraosseous cystic-like areas, joint effusion, and rheumatoid nodules can eventually occur.	Chronic multisystem disease of unknown etiology with persistent inflammatory synovitis involving peripheral joints in a symmetric distribution. Can result in progressive destruction of cartilage and bone leading to joint dysfunction. Affects ~1% of the world population. Eighty percent of adult patients present between the ages of 35 and 50 years. In patients with juvenile rheumatoid arthritis, patients range from 5 to 16 years, mean = 10.2 years. **(See Atlas Chapter A 70)**
Gout/tophi (Fig. 16.10)	Tophi have variable sizes and shapes, and often have low-intermediate signal on T1WI, FS T2WI, and T2WI. Zones of high signal on T2WI can be seen secondary to regions with increased hydration and proteinaceous zones associated with the deposits of urate crystals. Erosions of bone, synovial pannus, joint effusion, bone marrow and soft tissue edema can be seen with MRI. Tophi may be associated with heterogeneous, diffuse, or peripheral/marginal Gd-contrast enhancement patterns. Contrast enhancement seen with tophi is likely secondary to the hypervascular granulation tissue and reactive inflammatory cells in the synovium and/or adjacent soft tissues.	Inflammatory disease involving synovium resulting from deposition of monosodium urate crystals when serum urate levels exceed its solubility (7 mg/dL in men and 6 mg/dL in women) in various tissues and body fluids. Can be a primary disorder (inherited metabolic defects in purine metabolism or abnormal renal tubular secretion of urate) or secondary disorder (alcohol and medications; thiazide diuretics, salicylates, cyclosporin) that results from diminished renal excretion of uric acid salts, or from increased metabolic turnover of nucleic acids associated with malignancy, chemotherapy, endocrine, vascular, and/or myeloproliferative diseases. Prevalence of gout ranges from 0.5 to 2.8% of men and 0.1 to 0.6% of women in the United States. Accounts for 5% of arthritis cases. Usually occurs in middle-aged and elderly patients. **(See Atlas Chapter A 32)**

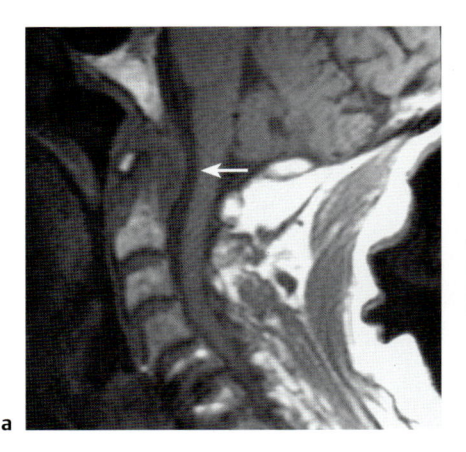

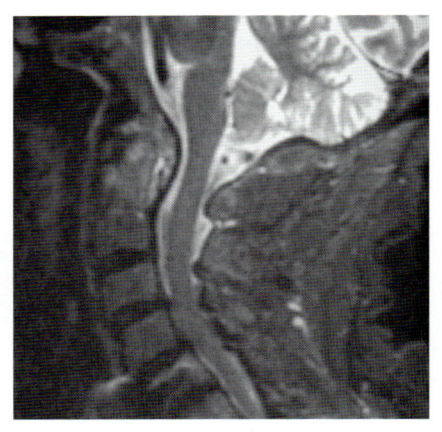

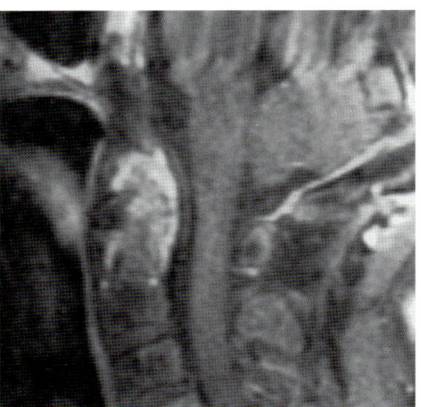

Figure 16.**7 a–c** A 72-year-old woman with pannus from rheumatoid arthritis at the upper dens and atlas. The low signal line of bone cortex at the upper dens is markedly thinned and eroded on sagittal T1WI (**a**) and sagittal FS T2WI (**b**). The pannus and adjacent marrow have low-intermediate signal on T1WI and heterogeneous intermediate to slightly high signal on FS T2WI. The pannus and adjacent marrow show Gd-contrast enhancement on sagittal FS T1WI (**c**).

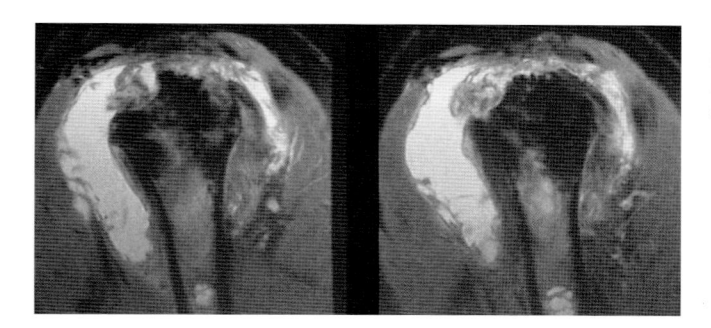

Gout/tophi 251

Figure 16.8 Rheumatoid arthritis involving the shoulder with pannus formation associated with erosions into the humeral head. Pannus has mixed intermediate, slightly high, high, and low signal on sagittal FS T2WI. A large effusion with high signal is also seen.

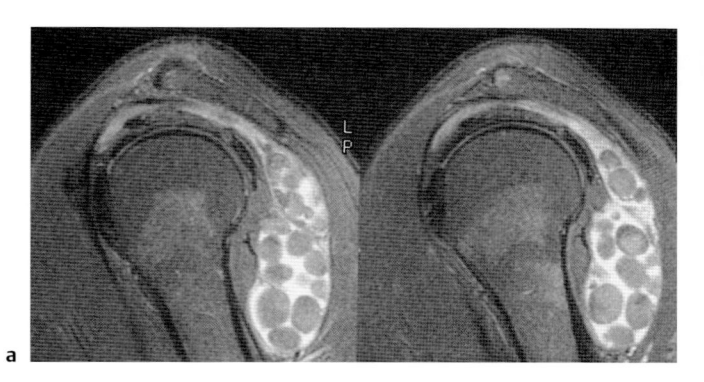

Figure 16.9 a, b A 56-year-old woman with rheumatoid arthritis involving the bursa of the shoulder with hypertrophied synovium appearing as "rice bodies." The ovoid and spheroid zones of synovial proliferation have intermediate signal on sagittal (a) and coronal (b) FS T2WI and are located within a large effusion in the subdeltoid bursa.

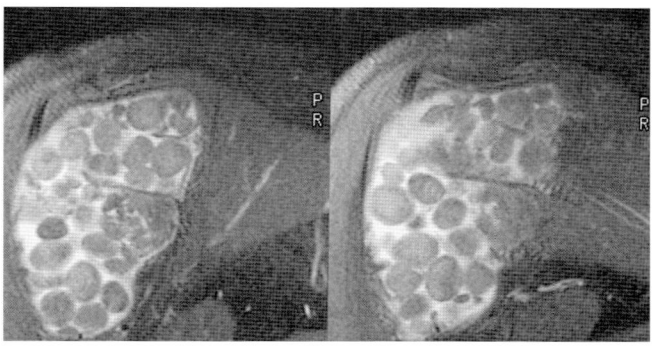

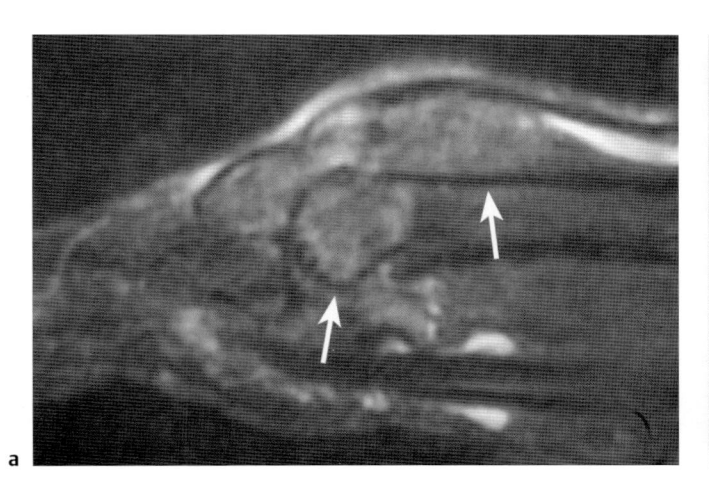

Figure 16.10 a, b A 53-year-old man with gout involving a metatarsal-phalangeal joint. Bone erosions are seen associated with soft tissue lesions (tophus) with heterogeneous intermediate, slightly high, and high signal on FS T2WI (a). Only peripheral irregular Gd-contrast enhancement is seen with the intraosseous and extraosseous gout lesions on sagittal FS T1WI (b).

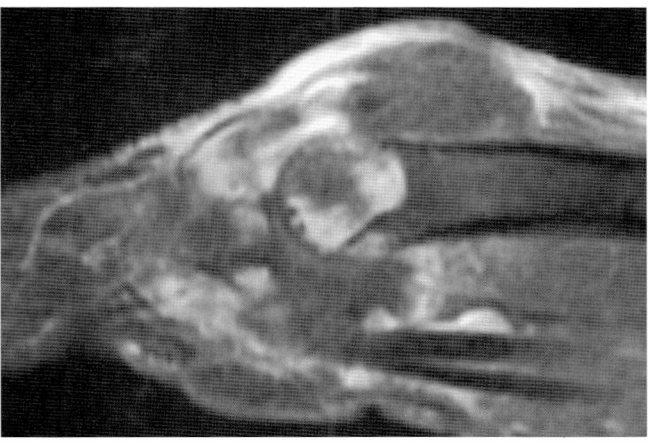

Table 16 (Continued) **Tumors and tumorlike lesions within joints**

Lesion	MRI Findings	Comments
Calcium pyrophosphate dihydrate deposition disease (Fig. 16.11)	Radiographs and CT show chondrocalcinosis, which is typically difficult to visualize with MRI except at the C1-odontoid articulation. At C1–C2, hypertrophy of synovium may occur that can have low-intermediate signal on T1WI and T2WI. Small zones of low signal may correspond to calcifications seen with CT.	Calcium pyrophosphate dihydrate deposition (CPPD) disease is a common disorder in older adults in which there is deposition of CPPD crystals resulting in calcifications of hyaline and fibrocartilage, and is associated with cartilage degeneration, subchondral cysts, and osteophyte formation. Symptomatic CPPD is referred to as pseudogout because of overlapping clinical features with gout. Usually occurs in the knee, hip, shoulder, elbow, and wrist, and rarely at the odontoid-C1 articulation.
Eosinophilic granuloma (Fig. 16.12)	Intramedullary lesions associated with trabecular and cortical bone destruction that typically have low-intermediate signal on T1WI and PDWI and heterogeneous slightly high to high signal on T2WI. Poorly defined zones of high signal on T2WI are usually seen in the marrow peripheral to the lesions secondary to inflammatory changes. Extension of lesions from the marrow into adjacent soft tissues through areas of cortical disruption are commonly seen as well as linear periosteal zones of high signal on T2WI. Lesions typically show prominent Gd-contrast enhancement in marrow and in extraosseous soft tissue portions of the lesions.	Benign tumorlike lesions consisting of Langerhans cells (histiocytes), and variable amounts of lymphocytes, polymorphonuclear cells, and eosinophils. Account for 1% of primary bone lesions, and 8% of tumorlike lesions. Occur in patients with median age = 10 years, average = 13.5 years, peak incidence is between 5 and 10 years, 80–85% occur in patients less than 30 years. **(See Atlas Chapter A 18)**
Fracture and hemarthrosis (Fig. 16.13)	Fluid–fluid levels and debris can be seen with zones of mixed low, intermediate, and/or high signal on T1WI and T2WI within joints.	Fractures involving articular surfaces of bone can result in loose osteochondral fragments, marrow fat, hemorrhage, and inflammatory reaction within joints.
Synovial hemangioma (Fig. 16.14)	Lesions can have well-circumscribed margins with or without lobulation. Usually have low-intermediate signal or heterogeneous low-intermediate and high signal on T1WI and PDWI. The high-signal regions on T1WI and PDWI can range from thin linear zones to thick irregular zones, and are most often secondary to fat and occasionally from slow-flowing blood within these lesions. On T2WI, hemangiomas usually have distinct margins with or without lobulation, and slightly high to high signal. On FS T2WI, hemangiomas typically have high signal except for zones of fat within the lesions. Lesions usually show prominent Gd-contrast enhancement. Prominent adjacent veins may be seen.	Benign hamartomatous lesions comprised of capillary, cavernous, and/or malformed venous vessels with varying amounts of mature adipose tissue. **(See Atlas Chapter A 34)**

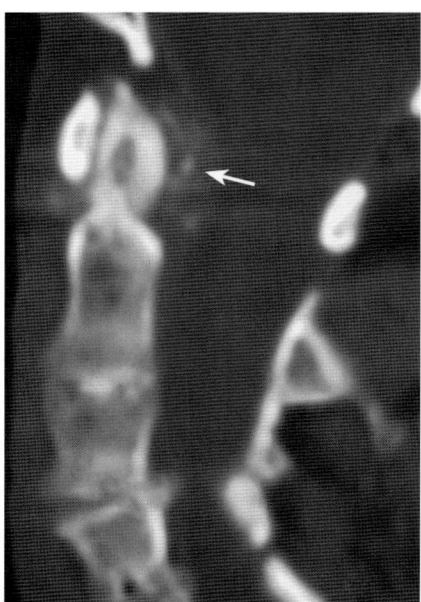

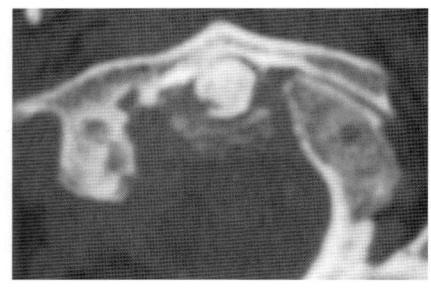

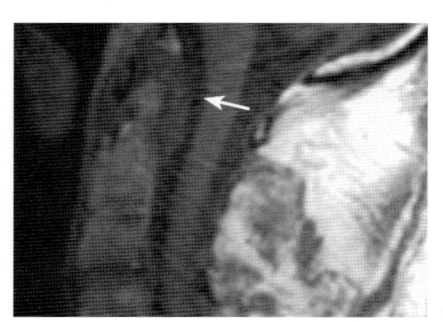

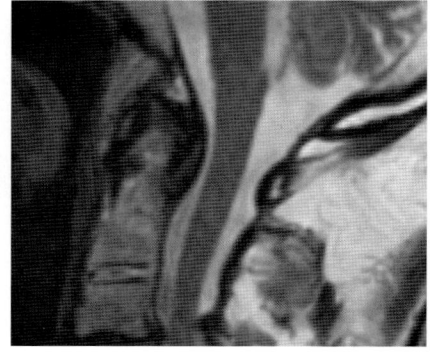

Figure 16.11 a–d An 80-year-old man with CPPD at the C1–C2 articulation. Sagittal (**a**) and axial (**b**) CT images show mineralization within hypertrophied synovium. The hypertrophied synovium has low-intermediate signal on sagittal T1WI (**c**) and T2WI (**d**).

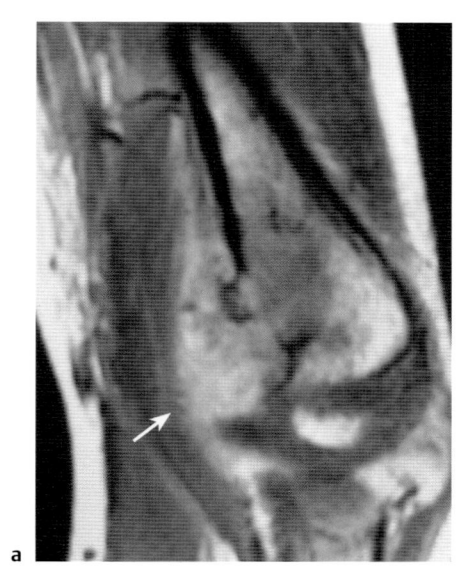

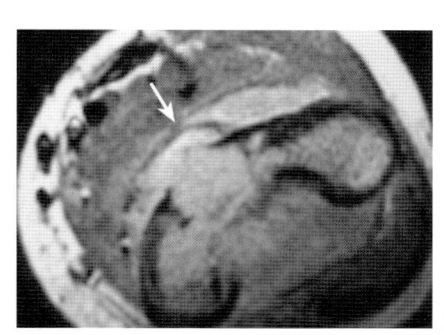

Figure 16.**12 a, b** A 5-year-old boy with an eosinophilic granuloma involving the distal humerus. The lesion in the marrow is associated with cortical destruction and extra-osseous extension into the adjacent soft tissues and elbow joint as seen on sagittal Gd-contrast enhanced T1WI (**a**) and axial PDWI (**b**).

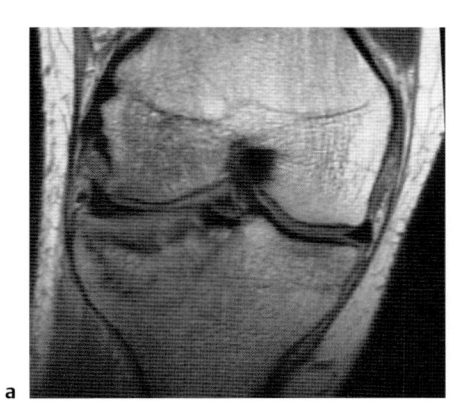

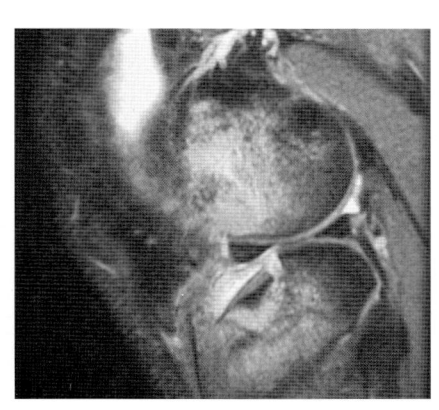

Figure 16.**13 a, b** A traumatic fracture of the lateral tibial plateau is seen with subjacent poorly defined zones of low-intermediate signal in the marrow on coronal PDWI (**a**) and high signal on sagittal FS T2WI (**b**). Also seen is a bone contusion in the marrow of the lateral femoral condyle.

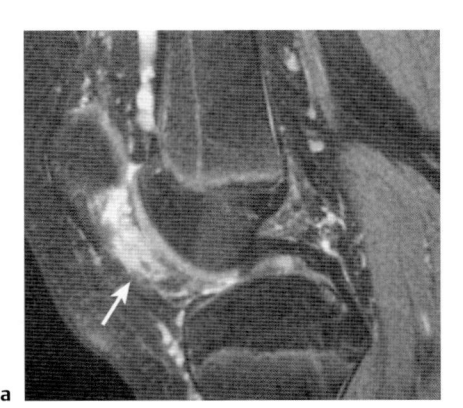

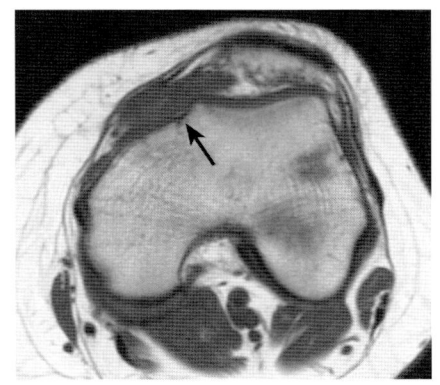

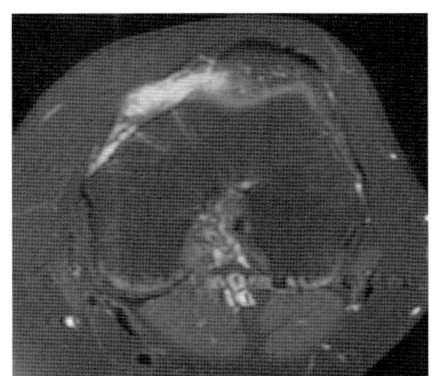

Figure 16.**14 a–c** A 13-year-old girl with a synovial hemangioma in the knee. The lesion has high signal on sagittal FS T2WI (**a**). Multiple enlarged veins are seen adjacent to the hemangioma. The hemangioma has intermediate signal on axial T1WI (**b**) and shows prominent Gd-contrast enhancement on axial FS T1WI (**c**).

Table 16 (Continued) Tumors and tumorlike lesions within joints		
Lesion	MRI Findings	Comments
Lipoma arborescens (Fig. 16.15)	Appears as multiple nodular or frond-like deposits with fat signal within hypertrophied synovium, often associated with a joint effusion.	Disorder with multiple villous or frond-like zones of fatty deposition in synovium within a joint, tendon sheath, and/or bursa. Most frequently involves the knee. May be idiopathic, or occur in the setting of degenerative arthritis, collagen vascular disorders, or trauma. Occurs in patients aged from 9 to 66 years. **(See Atlas Chapter A 43)**
Intra-articular lipoma (Fig. 16.16)	Lesions usually have circumscribed margins and have MRI signal comparable to subcutaneous fat on T1WI, PDWI, T2WI, and FS T2WI. Often do not show Gd-contrast enhancement except for minimal to mild enhancement along the thin nonfatty septa.	Common benign hamartomas composed of mature white adipose tissue without cellular atypia. Most common soft tissue tumor, representing 10% of all soft tissue tumors and 16% of benign soft tissue tumors. **(See Atlas Chapter A 43)**
Giant cell tumor of bone with joint extension (Fig. 16.17)	Intraosseous lesions near the ends of long bones that often have low to intermediate signal on T1WI and PDWI, intermediate to high signal on T2WI, and high signal on FS PDWI and FS T2WI. Aneurysmal bone cysts can be seen in 14% of giant cell tumors, resulting in cystic zones with variable signal and fluid–fluid levels. Lesions frequently have areas of cortical destruction with extraosseous extension, including into joints. Tumors show mild to prominent Gd-contrast enhancement.	Aggressive tumors composed of neoplastic ovoid mononuclear cells and scattered multinucleated osteoclast-like giant cells. Account for ~5 to 9.5% of all bone tumors and up to 23% of benign bone tumors. Malignant giant cell tumors account for 5.8% of all giant cell tumors. Occur in patients aged from 4 to 81 years, median = 30 years, mean = 33 years. **(See Atlas Chapter A 29)**
Chondroblastoma (Fig. 16.18)	Lesions typically involve the physeal plate, adjacent epiphysis, and metaphysis. Lesions often have fine lobular margins, and typically have low-intermediate heterogeneous signal on T1WI and mixed low, intermediate, and/or high signal on T2WI. Areas of low signal on T2WI are secondary to chondroid matrix mineralization, and/or hemosiderin. Lesions can show marginal or septal Gd-contrast enhancement patterns. Cortical disruption and extraosseous extension into joints is uncommon. Perilesional zones with high signal on T2WI and Gd-contrast enhancement are commonly seen in bone marrow as well as periosteal location indicating reactive hyperemia and/or edema.	Benign cartilaginous tumors with chondroblast-like cells and areas of chondroid matrix formation usually involving the epiphysis. Usually present before cessation of endochondral bone growth. Account for 5–9% of benign bone lesions, 1–3% of all bone lesions. Occur in patients with median age = 17 years, mean age = 16 years for lesions in long bones, mean age = 28 years in other bones. **(See Atlas Chapter A 7)**
Malignant		
Intra-articular extension from metastatic tumor involving bone	Intramedullary lesions with low-intermediate signal on T1WI; low-intermediate to slightly high signal on PDWI; slightly high to high signal on T2WI and FS T2WI. Sclerotic lesions often have low signal on T1WI; and mixed low, intermediate, and/or high signal on T2WI. Tumors frequently cause cortical destruction with extension into the extraosseous soft tissues, including joints. Most lesions show Gd-contrast enhancement.	Proliferating neoplastic cells that are located in sites or organs separated or distant from their origins. Intraosseous metastatic lesions can have associated bone destruction and extraosseous extension, including into joints. **(See Atlas Chapter A 50)**
Intra-articular extension from myeloma (Fig. 16.19)	Appear as multiple or single intramedullary zones with low-intermediate signal on T1WI and PDWI; and intermediate, slightly high to high signal on T2WI and slightly high to high signal on FS T2WI. Intramedullary lesions and corresponding signal abnormalities may be diffuse, focal with poorly defined or distinct margins, and/or in an extensive variegated pattern. Lesions usually show Gd-contrast enhancement. Tumors frequently cause cortical destruction with extension into the extraosseous soft tissues, including joints.	Malignant tumors comprised of proliferating antibody-secreting plasma cells derived from single clones within bone marrow. Plasma cells normally account for <5% of the cells in bone marrow. Most common primary neoplasm of bone in adults, accounts for 44% of primary malignant bone tumors and 34% of all primary bone tumors. Occurs in patients aged from 16 to 80 years, median = 60 years. Most patients are older than 40 years. **(See Atlas Chapter A 52)**

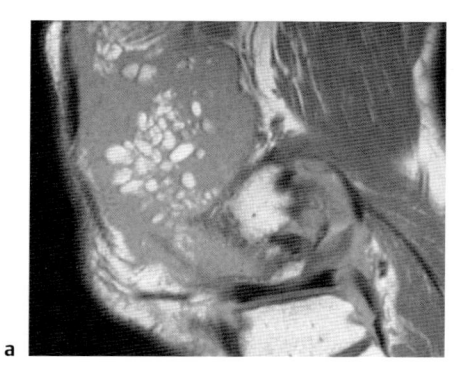

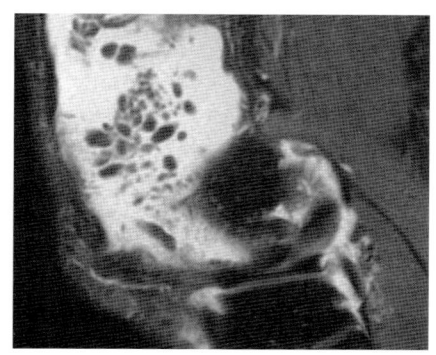

Figure 16.**15 a, b** A 37-year-old man with lipoma arborescens at the knee. Multiple nodular and frond-like/villous deposits with fat signal are seen within hypertrophied synovium on sagittal PDWI (**a**). The fat signal is suppressed on sagittal FS T2WI (**b**). The hypertrophied fatty synovium is seen within a large joint effusion.

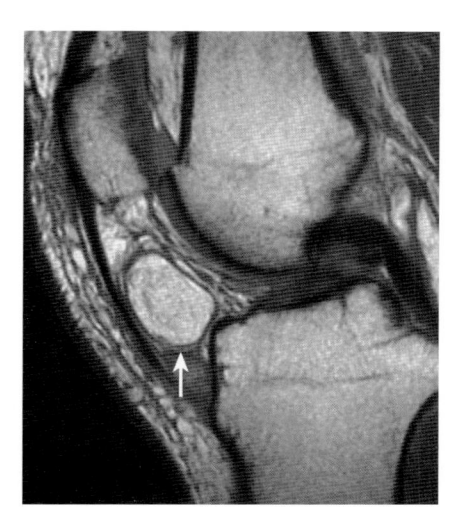

Figure 16.**16** A 56-year-old man with a lipoma in Hoffa's fat pad that has high signal on sagittal T1WI.

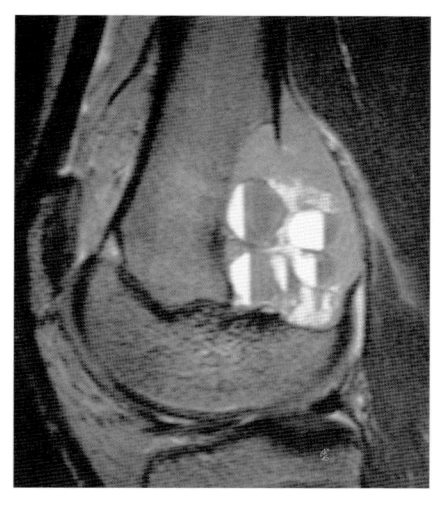

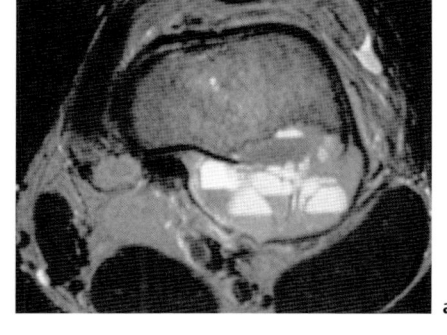

Figure 16.**17 a, b** A 17-year-old male with a giant cell tumor involving the distal metaphyseal portion of the femur associated with a secondary aneurysmal bone cyst. The tumor has mixed intermediate and high signal on sagittal (**a**) and axial (**b**) T2WI. Multiple fluid–fluid levels are seen at the aneurysmal cyst associated with the tumor within bone and at the extraosseous portion which extends through disrupted cortex dorsally into the knee joint.

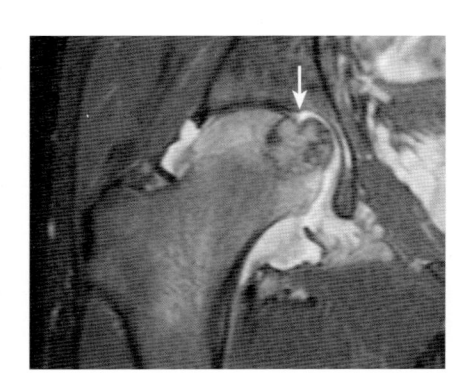

Figure 16.**18** A 17-year-old male with chondroblastoma in the proximal femur. The lesion is located mostly in the epiphysis, but also involves the physeal plate and a small portion of the metaphysis. The lesion has expanded and thinned the medial margin of the femoral head with resultant extension into the hip joint. The lesion has slightly lobulated margins, and has slightly high signal on coronal FS T2WI as well as in the adjacent marrow. A joint effusion is also present.

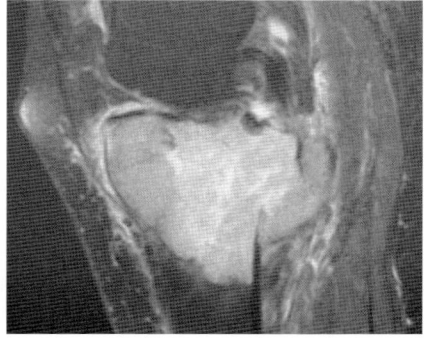

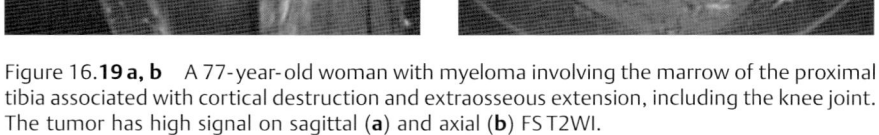

Figure 16.**19 a, b** A 77-year-old woman with myeloma involving the marrow of the proximal tibia associated with cortical destruction and extraosseous extension, including the knee joint. The tumor has high signal on sagittal (**a**) and axial (**b**) FS T2WI.

Table 16 (Continued)   Tumors and tumorlike lesions within joints

Lesion	MRI Findings	Comments
Intra-articular extension from lymphoma involving bone (Fig. 16.20)	Appear as multiple or single intramedullary zones with low-intermediate signal on T1WI and PDWI; and intermediate, slightly high to high signal on T2WI and slightly high to high signal on FS T2WI. Intramedullary lesions and corresponding signal abnormalities may be diffuse, focal with poorly defined or distinct margins, and/or in an extensive variegated pattern. Lesions usually show Gd-contrast enhancement. Tumors frequently cause cortical destruction with extension into the extraosseous soft tissues, including joints.	Lymphoma represents a group of lymphoid tumors whose neoplastic cells typically arise within lymphoid tissue (lymph nodes and reticuloendothelial organs). Unlike leukemia, lymphoma usually arises as discrete masses. Almost all primary lymphomas of bone are B cell non-Hodgkin lymphomas (NHL). NHL frequently originates at extranodal sites and spreads in an unpredictable pattern. **(See Atlas Chapter A 47)**
Intra-articular extension from leukemia	Leukemic infiltration in marrow can appear as diffuse or poorly defined zones of low-intermediate signal on T1WI and PDWI, intermediate-slightly high to high signal on FS T2WI. Focal or geographic regions with similar signal alteration can also be seen. After Gd-contrast administration, leukemia can show Gd-contrast enhancement on T1WI and FS T1WI. It should be noted that Gd-contrast enhancement may be seen in normal vertebral marrow in children less than 7 years. Tumors can cause cortical destruction with extension into the extraosseous soft tissues, including joints.	Lymphoid neoplasms that have widespread involvement of the bone marrow as well as tumor cells in peripheral blood. Acute lymphoblastic leukemia (ALL) is the most frequent type in children and adolescents. In adults, chronic lymphocytic leukemia (CLL) is the most common type. Myelogenous leukemias represent neoplasms derived from abnormal myeloid progenitor cells that, if normal, would form erythrocytes, monocytes, granulocytes, and platelets. Acute myelogenous leukemia (AML) usually occurs in adolescents and young adults and accounts for ~20% of childhood leukemia. Chronic myelogenous leukemia (CML) occurs in adults older than 25 years. **(See Atlas Chapter A 41)**
Intra-articular extension from primary malignant bone tumors (Figs. 16.21, 16.22)	Appear as intramedullary zones with low-intermediate signal on T1WI; and intermediate, slightly high to high signal on T2WI and slightly high to high signal on FS T2WI. Lesions usually show Gd-contrast enhancement. Tumors frequently cause cortical destruction with extension into the extraosseous soft tissues, including joints.	Primary sarcomas involving bone (osteosarcoma, chondrosarcoma, fibrosarcoma, etc.) can cause cortical destruction with extraosseous extension of tumor, including into joints.
Synovial chondrosarcoma	Lesions usually have low-intermediate signal on T1WI and heterogeneous predominantly high signal on T2WI. Zones of low signal on T2WI are related to the presence and degree of matrix mineralization and/or fibrous tissue. Lesions often have lobulated margins, with or without internal septations. Tumors usually show contrast enhancement in patterns ranging from lobulated peripheral and/or septal, or homogeneous versus heterogeneous depending on the degree of matrix mineralization and/or necrosis.	Chondrosarcomas rarely arise within synovium. **(See Atlas Chapter A 11).**

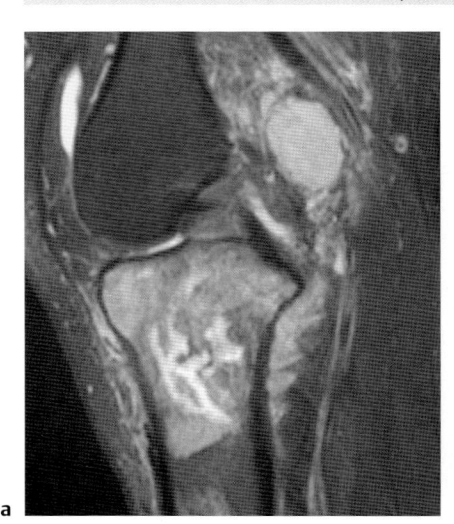

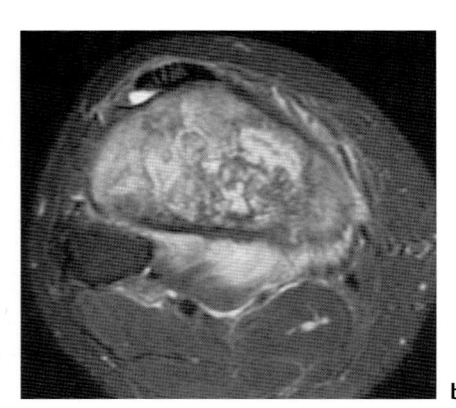

Figure 16.**20 a, b**   A 32-year-old woman with large B cell NHL involving the marrow of the proximal tibia associated with cortical destruction and extraosseous extension into the knee joint. The lymphoma has heterogeneous high signal on sagittal (**a**) and axial (**b**) FS T2WI. A nodular lymphoma lesion is also seen dorsal and superior to the posterior cruciate ligament.

a, b

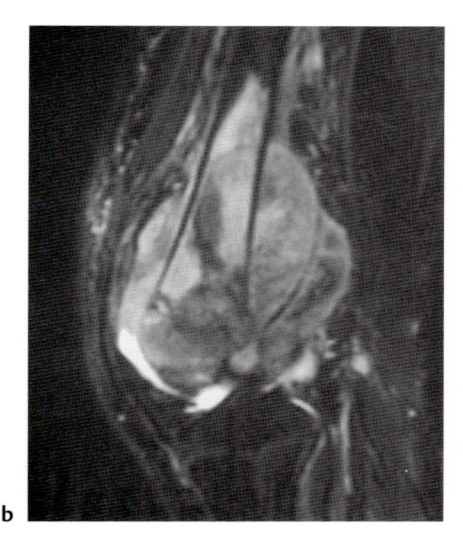

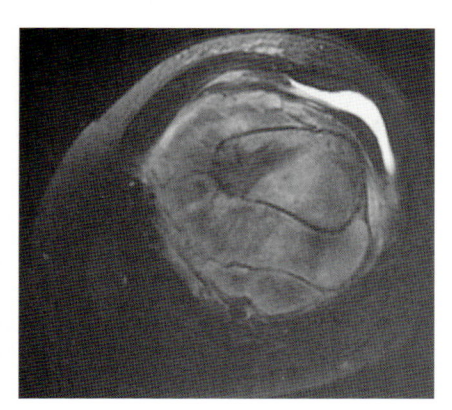

Figure 16.**21 a, b** Primary osteosarcoma in the distal metaphysis and epiphysis of the femur that extends from the marrow into adjacent extraosseous tissues and knee joint via multiple zones of cortical disruption. The intramedullary and extraosseous tumor has heterogeneous slightly high, intermediate, and low signal on sagittal (**a**) and axial (**b**) FS T2WI. Irregular amorphous, divergent, and perpendicular bands and strands of low signal are seen in the extraosseous tumor representing tumor-induced bone formation/periosteal reaction. A thin slightly irregular zone of low signal on T1WI is seen at portions of the peripheral border of the extraosseous tumor representing a partially intact elevated periosteum.

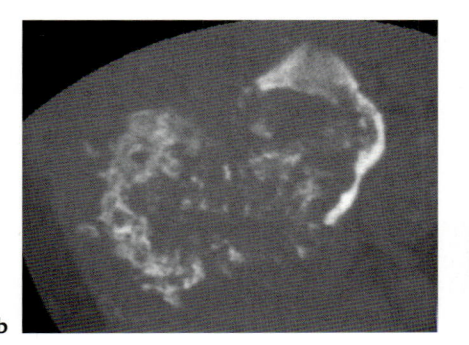

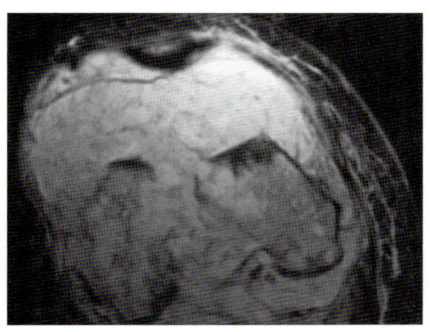

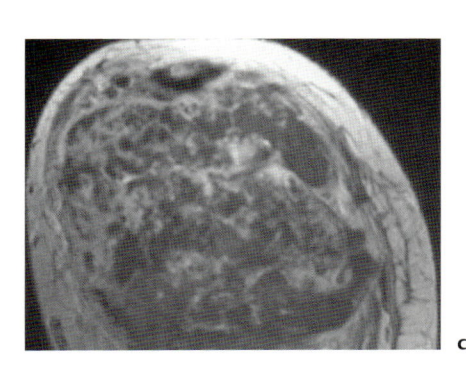

a, b   c

Figure 16.**22 a–c** A 60-year-old woman with a dedifferentiated chondrosarcoma involving the distal femur. Axial CT image (**a**) shows a radiolucent lesion with chondroid matrix mineralization and associated zones of cortical destruction. The tumor has heterogeneous high signal on axial (**b**) FS T2WI. Extensive cortical destruction is seen with tumor extension from the marrow into the knee joint and adjacent soft tissues. The lesion shows irregular heterogeneous Gd-contrast enhancement on axial T1WI (**c**).

References

Calcium Pyrophosphate Deposition Disease
Abreu M, Johnson K, Chung CB, et al. Calcification in calcium pyrophosphate dehydrate (CPPD) crystalline deposits in the knee: anatomic, radiographic, MR imaging, and histologic study in cadavers. *Skeletal Radiol* 2004;33:392–398.
Lin SH, Hsieh ET, Wu TY, Chang CW. Cervical myelopathy induced by pseudogout in ligamentum flavum and retro-odontoid mass: a case report. *Spinal Cord* 2006;44:692–694.
Mahmud T, Basu D, Dyson PHP. Crystal arthropathy of the lumbar spine – a series of six cases and a review of the literature. *J Bone Joint Surg* April 2005;87-B(4):513–517.

| Table 17 | Solitary tumors and tumorlike lesions of the soft tissues located mostly deep to the subcutaneous fat |

Lesion	MRI Findings	Comments
Neoplastic-malignant		
Malignant fibrous histiocytoma (Fig. 17.1)	Tumors have poorly defined and or circumscribed margins, and often have low-intermediate signal on T1WI and heterogeneous intermediate-high signal on T2WI and FS T2WI. Tumors show heterogeneous, often prominent Gd-contrast, enhancement.	Malignant tumors involving soft tissue and rarely bone that are presumed to derive from undifferentiated mesenchymal cells. The World Health Organization (WHO) now uses the term undifferentiated pleomorphic sarcoma for malignant fibrous histiocytoma (MFH). **(See Atlas Chapter A 48)**
Fibrosarcoma/myxofibrosarcoma (Fig. 17.2)	Tumors can have slightly irregular margins, with or without associated destruction and invasion of adjacent bone. High-grade fibrosarcomas may have an infiltrative pattern with respect to adjacent soft tissues. Lesions usually have low-intermediate signal on T1WI, intermediate to slightly high signal on PDWI, and heterogeneous intermediate-high signal on T2WI. Margins of lesions may be indistinct on T2WI for high-grade lesions. Zones with high signal on T2WI can be seen in myxoid regions of myxofibrosarcoma. For sclerosing epithelioid fibrosarcoma, zones of low signal on T1WI and T2WI can be seen from regions of decreased cellularity and dense collagen deposition in these neoplasms. Tumors usually show heterogeneous Gd-contrast enhancement. Enhancing margins may be indistinct for high-grade lesions.	Uncommon malignant tumors consisting of bundles of fibroblasts/spindle cells with varying proportions of collagen, lacking other tissue differentiating features such as tumor bone, osteoid, or cartilage. Infantile fibrosarcoma accounts for <1% of all malignant soft tissue tumors and 12% of soft tissue tumors in infants, and occurs in young patients with mean age = 2 years. Adult fibrosarcomas account for 4% of malignant soft tissue tumors, mean age of patients = 41 years. Variants of fibrosarcoma include: myxofibrosarcoma, low-grade fibromyxoid sarcoma, and sclerosing epithelioid fibrosarcoma. **(See Chapters A 25 and A 48)**

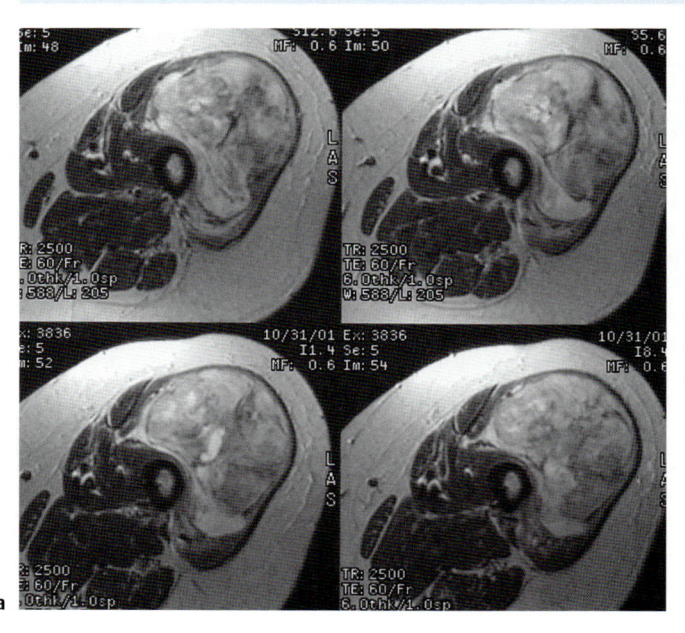

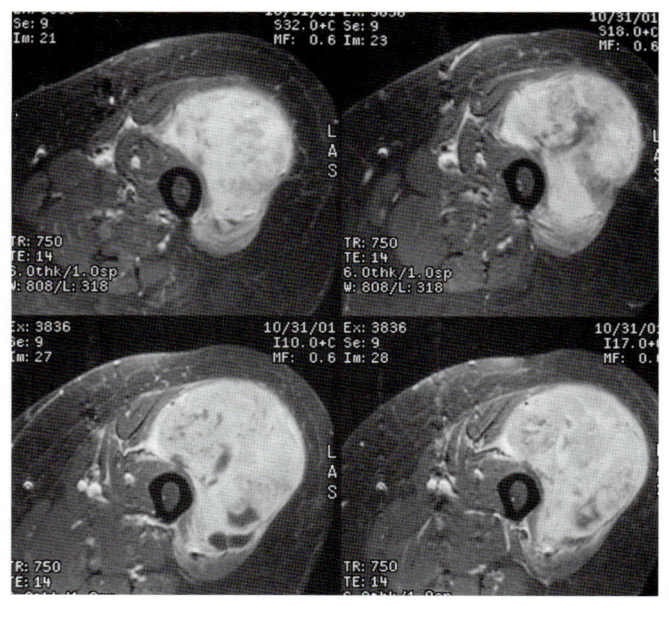

Figure 17.1 a, b A 66-year-old woman a malignant fibrous histiocytoma involving the vastus lateralis muscle of the proximal thigh. The tumor has heterogeneous slightly high and high signal on axial T2WI (**a**) and shows irregular prominent Gd-contrast enhancement as well as several nonenhancing zones of necrosis on axial FS T1WI (**b**).

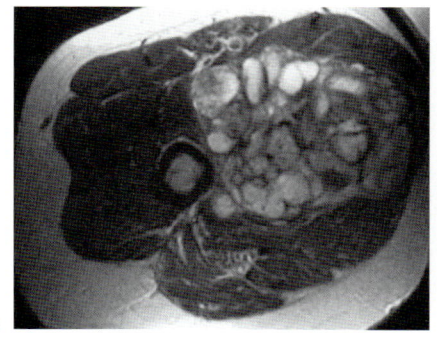

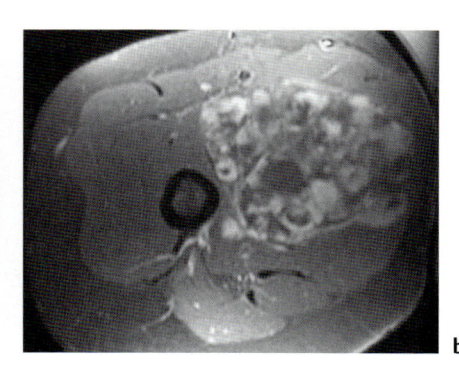

Figure 17.2 a, b A 37-year-old man with a myxofibrosarcoma involving the adductor muscles in the proximal thigh, showing mixed zones of low, intermediate, and high signal on axial T2WI (**a**). The tumor shows prominent heterogeneous Gd-contrast enhancement on axial FS T1WI (**b**).

Table 17 (Continued) Solitary tumors and tumorlike lesions of the soft tissues located mostly deep to the subcutaneous fat

Lesion	MRI Findings	Comments
Liposarcoma, well differentiated (Fig. 17.3)	Tumors contain up to 75 % overall fat signal, and contain thick nonadipose septae, and/or nodular nonadipose zones. The nonadipose zones can have low-intermediate signal on T1WI and PDWI; and low, intermediate, and/or high signal on T2WI. Nonadipose tumor portions show variable degrees of Gd-contrast enhancement.	Malignant mesenchymal tumors containing portions showing differentiation into adipose tissue. Compared with benign lipomas, these tumors have thicker and more numerous fibrous septae containing fibroblastic spindle cells, atypical cells and vacuolated lipoblasts surrounding various-sized lobules of fat. Fat cells have nuclear atypia, and hyperchromatic stromal cells are seen in fibrous septa. Account for 40–54 % of liposarcomas. Occur in patients 39 to 77 years, mean = 50 years (See Atlas Chapter A 44)
Myxoid liposarcoma (Fig. 17.4)	Tumors usually have mostly low signal on T1WI, and may contain small zones of high fat signal in lacy, amorphous, and/or linear configurations. Most myxoid liposarcomas contain less than 25 % fat. Some myxoid liposarcomas do not contain fatty zones. Tumors can have heterogeneous or homogeneous high signal on PDWI, T2WI, and some have a multi-loculated pattern. Low signal septa may be present on T2WI. Tumors usually show Gd-contrast enhancement in varying degrees and patterns, or rarely none at all.	Composed of proliferating stellate and/or fusiform lipoblasts in varying stages of differentiation, signet cells containing lipids, variable myxoid matrix, and plexiform capillary network. Mitotic activity is usually low. Osseous, cartilaginous, and/or leiomyomatous metaplasia may occur in these tumors. Fat content in these myxoid liposarcomas is usually < 10 –25 % of tumor volume. Account for 23 % of liposarcomas. Occur in patients 18 to 67 years, mean = 42 years. (See Atlas Chapter A 44)

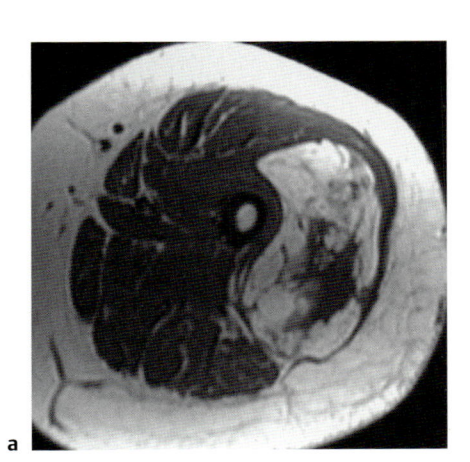

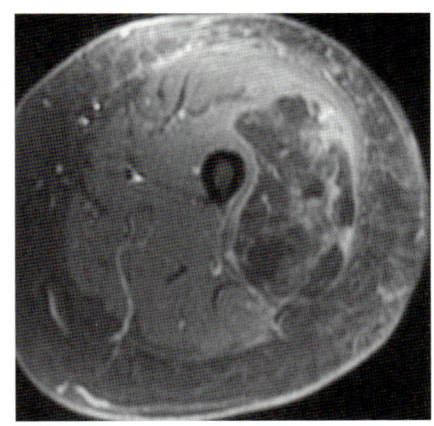

Figure 17.3 a, b A 57-year-old woman with a well-differentiated low-grade liposarcoma involving the vastus lateralis muscle of the thigh. The tumor has high fat signal on axial T1WI (a) as well as zones with low-intermediate signal. The nonfatty portions of the tumor show Gd-contrast enhancement on axial FS T1WI (b).

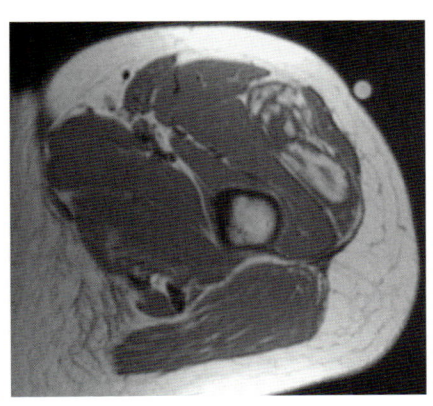

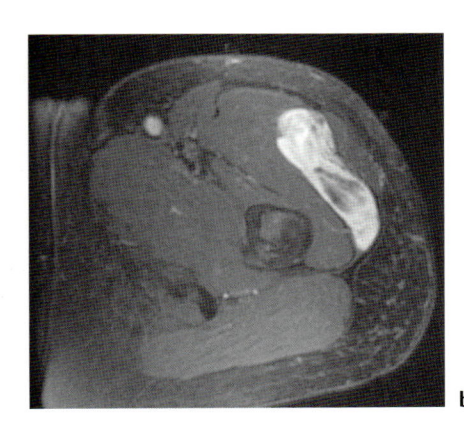

Figure 17.4 a, b A 13-year-old female with a myxoid liposarcoma involving the vastus lateralis muscle in the upper thigh. This tumor has circumscribed margins and contains both low-intermediate signal and high signal on axial T1WI (a). Some of the zones with high signal on T1WI secondary to fat are suppressed on axial FS T2WI (b) whereas most of the tumor has high signal from the myxoid components.

Table 17 (Continued) Solitary tumors and tumorlike lesions of the soft tissues located mostly deep to the subcutaneous fat

Lesion	MRI Findings	Comments
Pleomorphic liposarcoma (Fig. 17.5)	Tumors often have relatively well-defined margins, and have heterogeneous/mixed low, intermediate, and/or high signal on T1WI, PDWI, and T2WI. Less than 26% of the tumor volumes have fat signal. Tumors usually show prominent Gd-contrast enhancement in a heterogeneous pattern.	Tumors contain lipogenic and nonlipogenic zones that have features similar to malignant fibrous histiocytoma, round cell liposarcoma, and/or epithelioid carcinoma. Tumors have prominent cellular pleomorphism with malignant pleomorphic lipoblasts, pleomorphic spindle cells, and occasional giant cells. Mitoses are common. Variable degrees of necrosis are seen. Most tumors have infiltrative borders microscopically. Account for 5–7% of liposarcomas. Occur in patients 41 to 78 years, mean = 60 years **(See Atlas Chapter A 44)**
Round cell liposarcoma	Tumors can have relatively well-defined margins (72%) or poorly defined margins (28%), and have heterogeneous/mixed low, intermediate, and/or high signal on T1WI, PDWI, and T2WI. Most round cell liposarcomas contain <26% fat. Tumors usually show prominent Gd-contrast enhancement (61%) in a heterogeneous pattern that may be globular or nodular.	Contain round small cells with single naked round or slightly oval nuclei, scarce cytoplasm containing vacuoles with minimal intracellular lipid. Tumor cells have low mitotic activity and occur within a myxoid matrix. Have been considered to represent poorly differentiated myxoid liposarcomas. Account for 6% of liposarcomas. Occur in patients 30 to 64 years, mean = 43 years. **(See Atlas Chapter A 44)**
Dedifferentiated liposarcoma (Fig. 17.6)	Tumors can contain portions with features of a well-differentiated liposarcoma as well as a focal nonlipomatous mass. Frequently occur in the retroperitoneum and can be large (mean = 19.3 cm). Tumors can have circumscribed, and/or irregular/poorly defined margins. Tumors often have heterogeneous/mixed low, intermediate, and/or high signal on T1WI, PDWI, and T2WI. Hemorrhage and necrosis can be seen in the nonlipomatous portions. Tumors often show prominent Gd-contrast enhancement in nonlipomatous portions in a heterogeneous or homogeneous pattern.	Occur most frequently in the retroperitoneum and often contain both well-differentiated and poorly differentiated zones. The poorly differentiated component is usually a high-grade sarcoma. Account for 10% of liposarcomas. Occur in patients 42 to 78 years, mean = 63 years **(See Atlas Chapter A 44)**
Metastatic disease (Fig. 17.7)	Tumors can occur as lymphadenopathy or as focal lesions. Lesions have low-intermediate signal on T1WI; and intermediate to slightly high signal or high signal on T2WI and FS T2WI. Variability in MRI signal characteristics may be related to differing histologic features of the metastatic lesions. Tumors can show variable degrees of Gd-contrast enhancement.	Metastatic lesions are proliferating neoplastic cells that are located in sites or organs separated or distant from their origins. **(See Atlas Chapter A 50)**
Myeloma	Lesions usually have low-intermediate signal on T1WI and slightly high to high signal on T2WI and high signal on FS T2WI. Extraosseous tumors can occur from extension from intraosseous lesions, or from within the soft tissues. Lesions may have poorly defined or distinct margins. Most lesions show Gd-contrast enhancement. Zones of high signal on T2WI peripheral to the Gd-contrast enhancing portion of the lesion may represent zones of tumor invasion or perilesional edema.	Malignant tumors comprising proliferating antibody-secreting plasma cells derived from single clones. Usually occur in bone and occasionally in soft tissue. **(See Atlas Chapter A 52)**
Lymphoma (Fig. 17.8)	Lymphadenopathy from Hodgkin lymphoma (HL) and lesions of non-Hodgkin lymphoma (NHL) have low-intermediate signal on T1WI and intermediate to slightly high signal on T2WI. Variability in MRI signal may be related to differing histologic features (such as the degree of fibrosis) for the subtypes of HL. After Gd-contrast administration, HL and NHL can show variable Gd-contrast enhancement.	Lymphomas are tumors in which neoplastic cells arise within lymphoid tissue. HL usually occurs in lymph nodes and spreads along nodal chains, whereas NHL frequently originates at extranodal sites and spreads in an unpredictable pattern. Mycosis fungoides is a T-cell lymphoma that involves the skin. **(See Atlas Chapter A 47)**

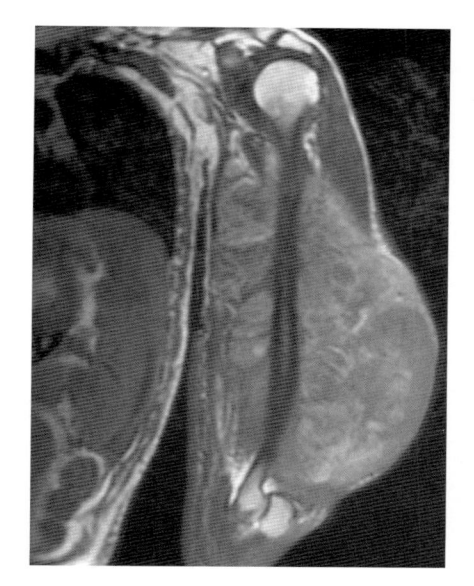

Figure 17.5 A 43-year-old man with a large high-grade pleomorphic liposarcoma involving the left arm that has heterogeneous intermediate and slightly high signal on coronal T1WI.

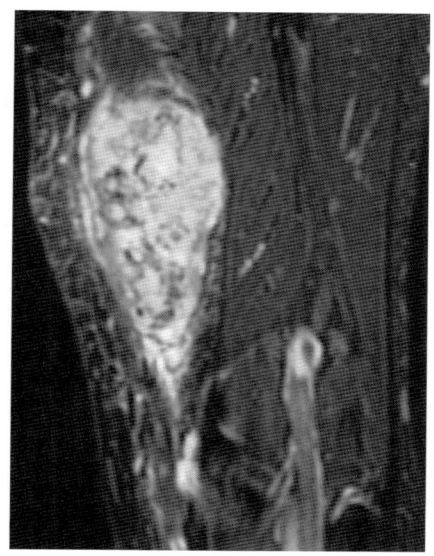

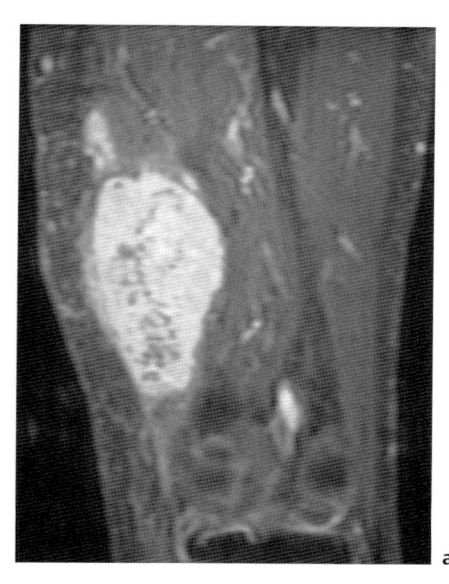

Figure 17.6 a, b A 71-year-old woman with a dedifferentiated liposarcoma in the distal thigh. A large mass lesion involving the soft tissues of the medial thigh that has circumscribed margins and contains mostly high signal on coronal (a) FS T2WI as well as small zones with low signal. The tumor shows prominent slightly heterogeneous Gd-contrast enhancement on coronal FS T1WI (b).

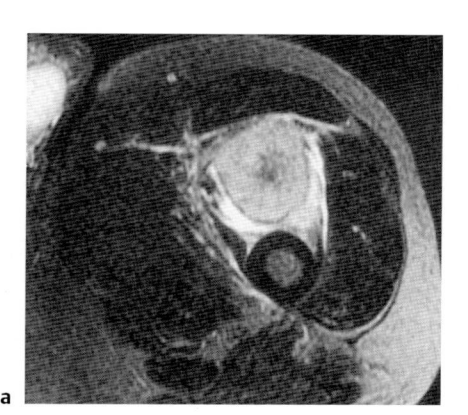

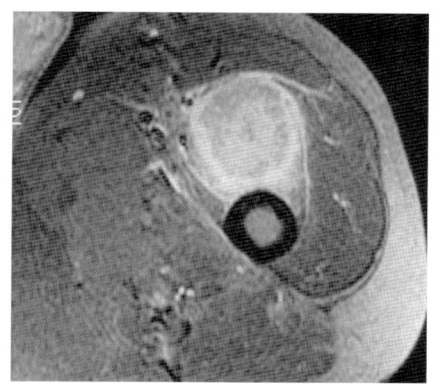

Figure 17.7 a, b A 51-year-old man with a metastatic lesion from lung carcinoma involving the vastus intermedius muscle of the upper thigh, showing high signal on axial T2WI (a). The tumor shows prominent Gd-contrast enhancement on axial FS T1WI (b).

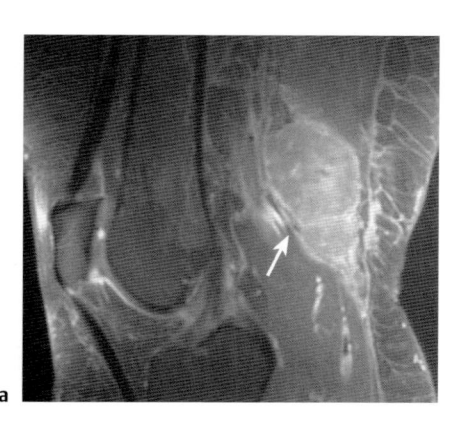

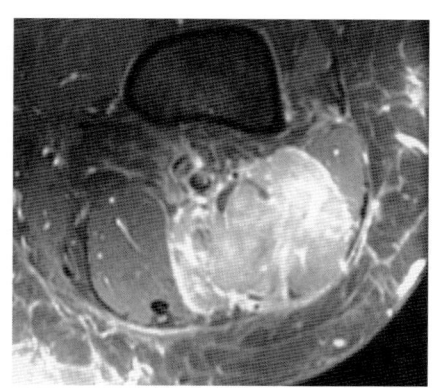

Figure 17.8 a, b A 51-year-old woman with diffuse large B cell NHL involving the posterior soft tissues at the distal thigh, showing slightly heterogeneous Gd-contrast enhancement on sagittal (a) and axial (b) FS T1WI.

Table 17 (Continued)   Solitary tumors and tumorlike lesions of the soft tissues located mostly deep to the subcutaneous fat

Lesion	MRI Findings	Comments
Leukemia (Fig. 17.9)	Appear as single or multiple well-circumscribed or poorly defined infiltrative lesions; low-intermediate signal on T1WI, intermediate-high signal on T2WI and FS T2WI, often shows Gd-contrast enhancement, +/− cortical bone destruction and extraosseous extension from lesions in marrow.	Malignant lymphoid neoplasms with involvement of bone marrow with tumor cells also in peripheral blood and in soft tissues. (See Atlas Chapter A 41)
Synovial cell sarcoma (Fig. 17.10)	Tumors are often ovoid and/or lobulated lesions that often have low-intermediate signal on T1WI and heterogeneous signal (various combinations of intermediate, slightly high, high, and/or low signal) on T2WI. Multiloculated cystic zones are present in 77 %. Calcifications may occur in up to 30 %. Tumors show various patterns of Gd-contrast enhancement.	Mesenchymal tumors comprised of spindle cells and cells with varying degrees of epithelial differentiation. Account for 5 % of primary malignant soft tissue tumors. Occur in patients 14 to 58 years, mean = 32 years. (See Atlas Chapter A 75)
Malignant peripheral nerve sheath tumor (Fig. 17.11)	These lesions usually have heterogeneous signal on T1WI and T2WI; as well as heterogeneous Gd-contrast enhancement because of necrosis and hemorrhage. Some malignant peripheral nerve sheath tumors (MPNSTs) are similar in appearance to benign nerve sheath tumors.	MPNSTs are malignant tumors of the peripheral nerve sheath that contain mixtures of packed hyperchromatic spindle cells with elongated nuclei and slightly eosinophilic cytoplasm, mitotic figures and zones of necrosis. Approximately 50 % of MPNSTs occur in patients with neurofibromatosis type 1 (NF1), followed by de novo evolution from peripheral nerves. Malignant peripheral nerve sheath tumors infrequently arise from schwannomas, ganglioneuroblastomas/ganglioneuromas, and pheochromocytomas. (See Atlas Chapter A 56)
Clear cell sarcoma (also referred to as melanoma of soft parts) (Fig. 17.12)	Tumors can have well defined or irregular margins, and usually have low-intermediate signal on T1WI; and intermediate to slightly high or high signal on T2WI and FS T2WI. Tumors usually show Gd-contrast enhancement. Erosion into bone can occur.	Rare malignant tumors with melanocytic differentiation (immunoreactive to S 100 protein, HMB45) that occur in patients between 10 and 50 years. Usually occur in the deep soft tissues involving aponeuroses and tendons.
Leiomyosarcoma (Fig. 17.13)	Lesions may have well-defined or irregular margins, and often have intermediate signal on T1WI and PDWI, which can be hyperintense relative to muscle, and intermediate to slightly high or high signal on T2WI and FS T2WI. Large lesions often have zones of necrosis or cystic change that have low signal on T1WI and high signal on T2WI. Solid portions of the lesions usually show Gd-contrast enhancement.	Malignant mesodermal tumors associated with smooth muscle differentiation that can arise de novo or occur after radiation treatment. Account for 8 % of primary malignant soft tissue tumors and 3 % of all primary soft tissue tumors. Patients range in age from 35 to 79 years, mean = 58 years. (See Atlas Chapter A 40)

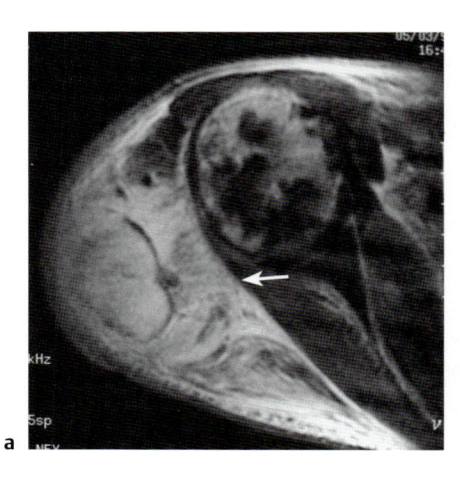

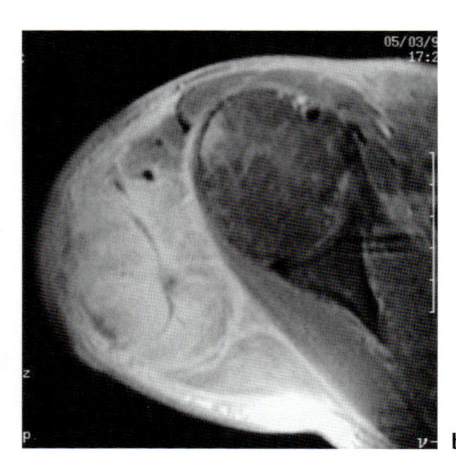

Figure 17.9 a, b   A 69-year-old man with acute myelogenous leukemia involving the soft tissues at the right shoulder and right humerus. Leukemic involvement in the soft tissues has slightly high signal on axial FS T2WI (**a**) and irregular indistinct margins. Leukemic tissue in the marrow of the humerus has heterogeneous slightly high signal on axial FS T2WI. The leukemic tissue in marrow shows minimal Gd-contrast enhancement, whereas the leukemic involvement in the extraosseous soft tissues shows prominent Gd-contrast enhancement on axial FS T1WI (**b**).

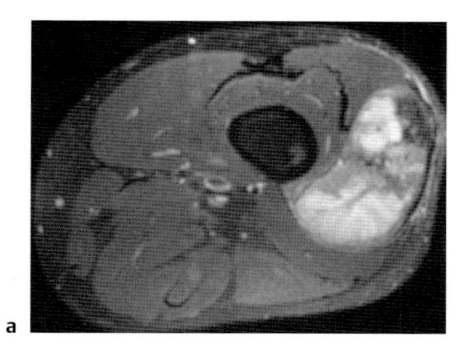

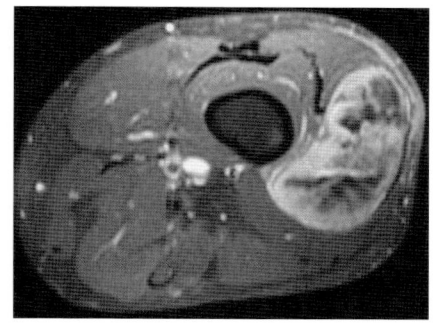

Figure 17.**10 a, b** A 59-year-old man with a synovial sarcoma in the lateral lower thigh involving the vastus lateralis muscle, showing heterogeneous mostly high signal with zones of low and intermediate signal on axial FS T2WI (**a**). The tumor shows prominent heterogeneous Gd-contrast enhancement on axial FS T1WI (**b**).

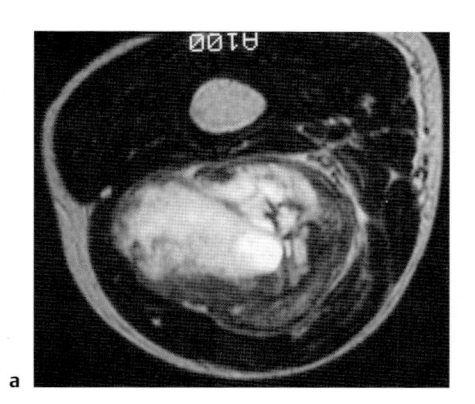

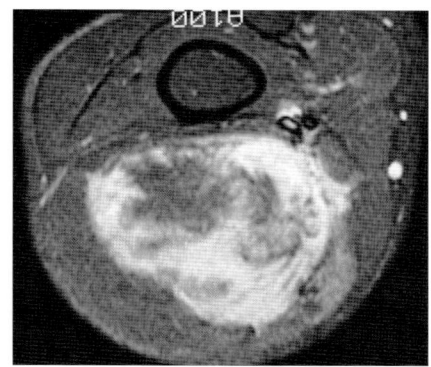

Figure 17.**11 a, b** Malignant peripheral nerve sheath tumor in the posterior soft tissues of the thigh in a 19-year-old man with NF1 and multiple neurofibromas in both thighs. A large lesion is seen in the right thigh that has mixed high, low, and intermediate signal on axial T2WI (**a**). The tumor shows heterogeneous irregular Gd-contrast enhancement on axial FS T1WI (**b**).

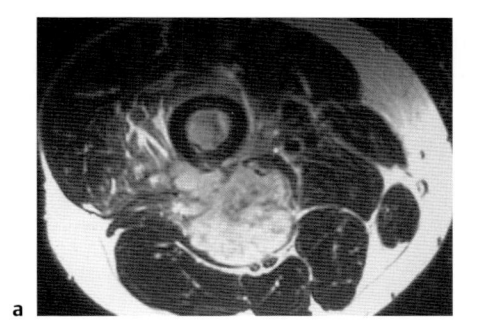

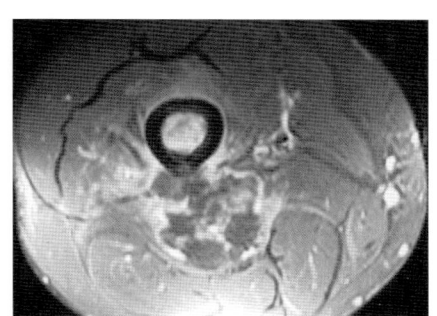

Figure 17.**12 a, b** A 52-year-old man with clear cell sarcoma involving the muscles of the thigh that has mostly high signal on axial T2WI (**a**). The tumor shows heterogeneous Gd-contrast enhancement on axial FS T1WI (**b**). The tumor erodes adjacent cortical bone and extends into the marrow.

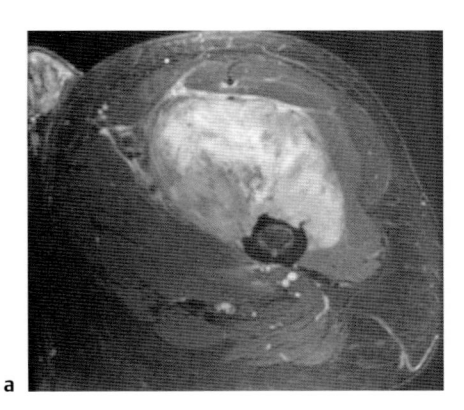

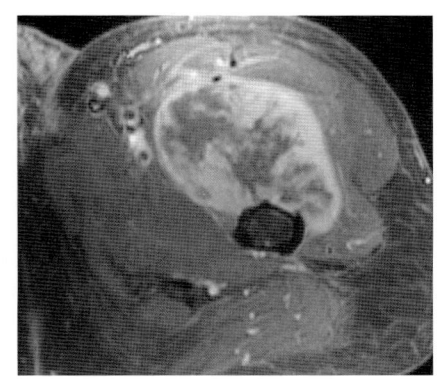

Figure 17.**13 a, b** A 55-year-old man with a leiomyosarcoma involving the muscles of the thigh that has heterogeneous mostly high signal on axial FS T2WI (**a**) as well as small zones of low signal. The tumor shows mostly prominent Gd-contrast enhancement except at several sites of necrosis on axial FS T1WI (**b**). Erosion of the outer cortical margin of the femur by the tumor is present.

Table 17 (Continued)   **Solitary tumors and tumorlike lesions of the soft tissues located mostly deep to the subcutaneous fat**

Lesion	MRI Findings	Comments
Rhabdomyosarcoma (Fig. 17.14)	Tumors can have circumscribed and/or poorly defined margins, and typically have low-intermediate signal on T1WI and heterogeneous signal (various combinations of intermediate, slightly high, and/or high signal) on T2WI and FS T2WI. Tumors show variable degrees of Gd-contrast enhancement.	Malignant mesenchymal tumors with rhabdomyoblastic differentiation that occur primarily in soft tissue. Account for 2% of primary malignant soft tissue tumors and <1% of all primary soft tissue tumors. Account for 19% of soft tissue sarcomas in children. **(See Atlas Chapter A 69)**
Hemangioendothelioma	Tumors have lobulated well-defined or irregular margins, and have intermediate signal on T1WI, and heterogeneous predominantly high signal on T2WI with or without internal low signal septations. Flow voids may be seen with the lesions. Tumors show heterogeneous Gd-contrast enhancement.	Low-grade malignant neoplasms composed of vasoformative/endothelial elements that occur in soft tissues and bone. These tumors are locally aggressive and rarely metastasize, compared with the high-grade endothelial tumors such as angiosarcoma. Account for <1% of malignant and all soft tissue tumors. Patients range in age from 17 to 60 years, mean = 40 years. **(See Atlas Chapter A 33)**
Hemangiopericytoma (Fig. 17.15)	Usually have well-defined margins, often have low-intermediate signal on T1WI, intermediate or slightly high-high signal on T2WI, and heterogeneous high signal on FS T2WI. On T2WI, lesions may contain tubular signal voids centrally or peripherally likely representing tumor vessels. Can contain hemorrhagic zones with corresponding MR signal alteration. Typically show Gd-contrast enhancement.	Rare malignant tumors of presumed pericytic origin that contain various shaped pericytic cells (oval, round, spindle-like) and adjacent irregular branching vascular spaces lined by endothelial cells. Usually occur in soft tissues and less frequently in bone. Account for <1% of primary tumors in the soft tissues. Most tumors, 90–95%, occur in adults, and 5–10% occur in children. **(See Atlas Chapter A 35).**
Angiosarcoma (Fig. 17.16)	Tumors have low-intermediate signal on T1WI, mixed low, intermediate, and/or high signal on T2WI, and show prominent Gd-contrast enhancement in a homogeneous or heterogeneous pattern.	Malignant tumors composed of neoplastic blood vessels in bone and/or soft tissues. These tumors can be associated with Paget disease, radiation treatment, bone infarcts, knee and hip prostheses, synthetic vessel grafts, prior trauma or surgery, osteomyelitis, and hereditary disorders (NF1, Maffucci disease, achondroplasia). Represent <1% of malignant bone tumors. Account for 2% of malignant soft tissue tumors. Patients range in age from 5 to 97 years, mean = 49 years (8, 9, 11). **(See Atlas Chapter A 6)**
Extraosseous osteosarcoma (Fig. 17.17)	Tumors have irregular poorly defined or slightly well-circumscribed margins and heterogeneous signal on most MRI pulse sequences. Various combinations of low, intermediate, and/or high signal on T1WI, T2WI, and FS T2WI can be seen depending on the presence and extent of hemorrhage and/or necrosis within the lesions. On T2WI and FS T2WI, tumors often have heterogeneous predominantly high signal. Fluid–fluid levels may be present at sites of hemorrhage or necrosis. Peripheral nonenhancing high signal on T2WI may be present and represent zones of edema and/or tumor invasion within adjacent tissues. Tumors often show heterogeneous patterns of Gd-contrast enhancement.	Malignant tumor comprised of proliferating neoplastic spindle cells that produce osteoid and/or immature tumoral bone. Osteosarcoma most commonly occurs within bone and less frequently on the external surface of bone. Rarely, osteogenic sarcomas can also occur as extraskeletal primary lesions in the soft tissues. **(See Atlas Chapter A 64)**

Extraosseous osteosarcoma **265**

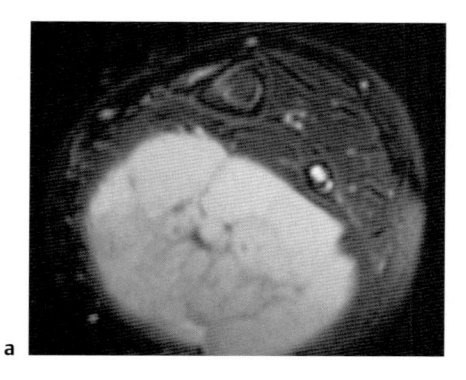

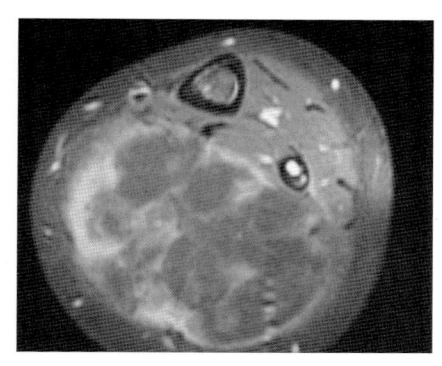

Figure 17.**14a, b** A 2.5-year-old girl with an embryonal rhabdomyosarcoma involving the posterior calf. The tumor has mostly high signal with strands of low signal on axial FS T2WI (**a**). The tumor shows heterogeneous irregular peripheral and central Gd-contrast enhancement on axial FS T1WI (**b**). The tumor is associated with signal alteration of the adjacent fibula.

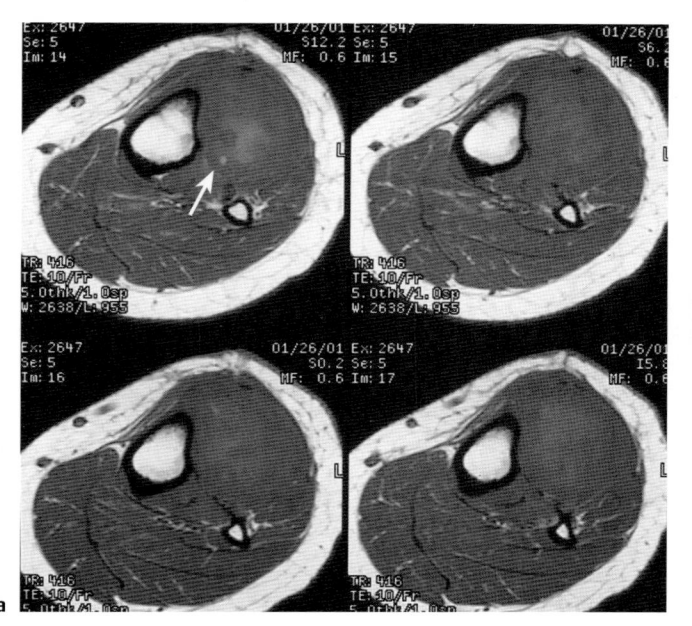

Figure 17.**15a, b** A 29-year-old woman with a hemangiopericytoma involving the tibialis anterior, tibialis posterior, extensor digitorum longus, and popliteus muscles. The tumor has mostly intermediate signal on axial (**a**) T1WI as well as several zones of high signal at sites of hemorrhage. The tumor has mixed intermediate and mostly high signal on axial FS T2WI (**b**) as well as foci and curvilinear zones of low signal.

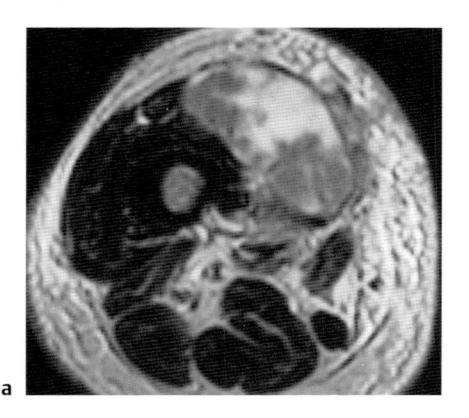

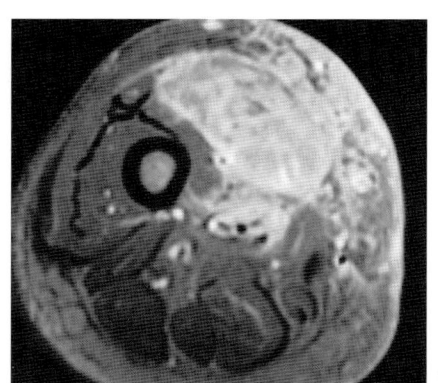

Figure 17.**16a, b** A 74-year-old man with an angiosarcoma in the medial anterior thigh involving the vastus medialis muscle. The tumor has mixed low, intermediate, and/or high signal on axial T2WI (**a**) and shows prominent Gd-contrast enhancement on FS T1WI (**b**).

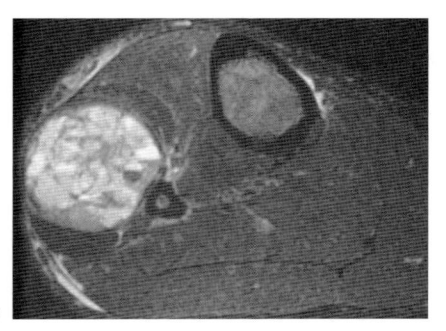

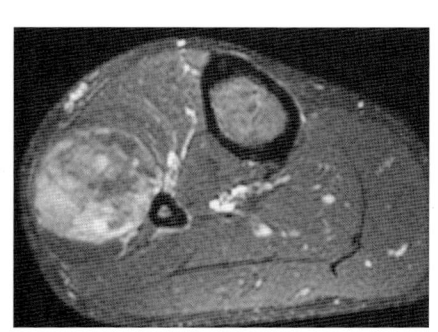

Figure 17.**17a, b** A 32-year-old man with an extraosseous osteosarcoma involving the extensor digitorum longus muscle and peroneus longus and brevis muscles of the proximal lateral leg. The tumor has heterogeneous mostly high signal on axial FS T2WI (**a**) as well as septa with low signal and fluid–fluid levels with high and low signal. Fluid–fluid levels represent sites of hemorrhage within the tumor. The tumor shows heterogeneous Gd-contrast enhancement on axial FS T1WI (**b**).

Table 17 (Continued) Solitary tumors and tumorlike lesions of the soft tissues located mostly deep to the subcutaneous fat

Lesion	MRI Findings	Comments
Extraosseous Ewing sarcoma (Fig. 17.18)	Tumors usually have low-intermediate signal on T1WI, and heterogeneous slightly high to high signal on T2WI and FS T2WI. Tumors often show prominent irregular Gd-contrast enhancement.	Malignant primitive tumors of bone and occasionally soft tissue that are comprised of undifferentiated small cells with round nuclei. (See Atlas Chapter A 20)
Extraosseous chondrosarcoma (Fig. 17.19)	Tumors have low-intermediate signal on T1WI, intermediate signal on PDWI, and heterogeneous intermediate, slightly high and/or high signal on T2WI. Foci of low signal on T1WI and T2WI can be seen secondary to chondroid matrix mineralization. Lesions typically show heterogeneous Gd-contrast enhancement.	Malignant tumors containing cartilage formed within sarcomatous stroma, with or without areas of calcification/mineralization, myxoid material, and/or ossification. (See Atlas Chapter A 11)

Neoplastic-benign

Lesion	MRI Findings	Comments
Lipoma (Fig. 17.20)	Often have circumscribed margins and have MRI signal comparable to subcutaneous fat on T1WI, PDWI, T2WI, and FS T2WI. Often do not show Gd-contrast enhancement except for minimal to mild enhancement along the thin nonfatty septa.	Common benign hamartomas composed of mature white adipose tissue without cellular atypia. Most common soft tissue tumor, representing 10% of all soft tissue tumors and 16% of benign soft tissue tumors. (See Atlas Chapter A 43)
Lipomatosis (Fig. 17.21)	Infiltrating adipose tissue or multiple lobules of fat can be seen in muscles, fascial planes, and/or subcutaneous fat.	Diffuse proliferation of mature adipose tissue. Can occur as several types. The diffuse type typically occurs in the soft tissues of an extremity or trunk in children with or without associated osseous hypertrophy. Multiple symmetric lipomatosis (Madelung disease) usually occurs in the neck, trunk, and pelvis of adult men (peak incidence in the 5th decade). Shoulder girdle lipomatosis usually occurs in women and involves the muscles at one shoulder and adjacent chest wall. Adiposis dolorosa (Dercum syndrome) usually occurs in obese postmenopausal women who have multiple painful fatty lesions in the extremities or trunk.
Atypical lipoma (Fig. 17.22)	Atypical lipomas may contain cystic/necrotic zones, calcifications, thick septa, and/or nodular zones that may or may not show Gd-contrast enhancement. Most atypical lipomas contain >75% fat, whereas liposarcomas often have <75% fat. Distinguishing between atypical lipomas and low-grade liposarcomas with MRI can be difficult and challenging.	Atypical lipomas account for up to 31% of lipomas. Lesions contain zones with osseous, chondroid, or fibrous metaplasia with myxoid changes. Atypical lipomas have been labeled as chondroid lipomas, osteolipomas, or benign mesenchymomas. Chondroid lipomas contain mature fat, lipoblasts, and chondroid matrix. Spindle cell and pleomorphic lipomas are variants that have varying proportions of mature fat cells, spindle cells, collagen, and multinucleated giant cells. Lipomas with high content of fibrous tissue have been labeled as fibrolipomas. (See Atlas Chapter A 43)

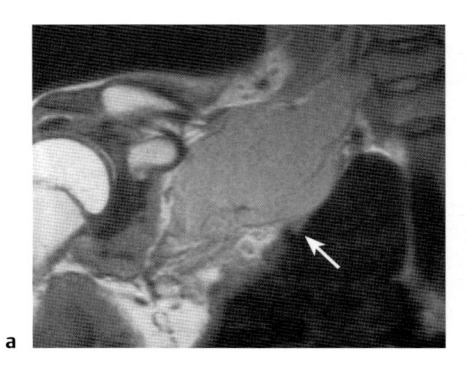

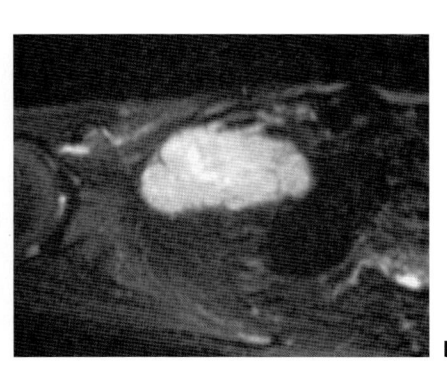

Figure 17.**18 a, b** An 11-year-old girl with an extraosseous Ewing sarcoma in the soft tissues adjacent to the right clavicle. The tumor has intermediate signal on coronal PDWI (**a**) and high signal on axial FS T2WI (**b**).

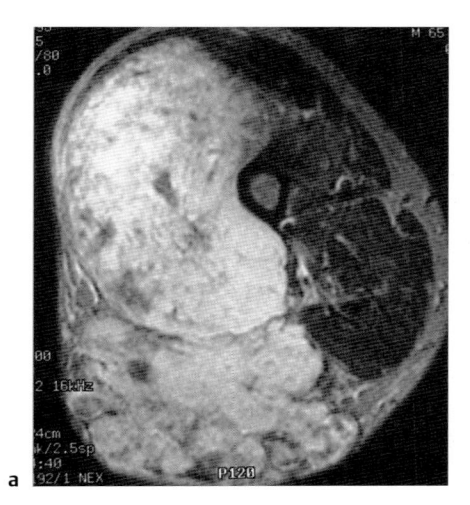

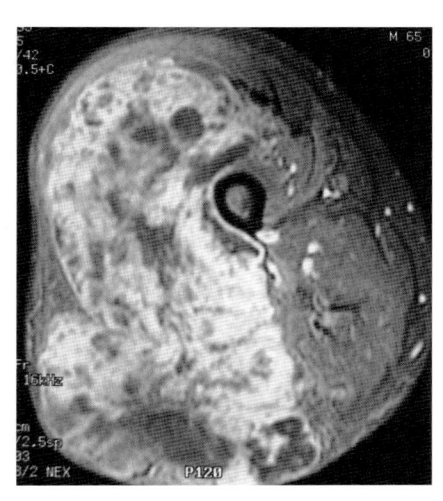

Figure 17.**19 a, b** A 65-year-old man with an extraosseous myxoid chondrosarcoma in the distal thigh that has circumscribed margins and contains heterogeneous mostly high signal with small foci of low signal on axial T2WI (**a**). The lesion shows prominent irregular heterogeneous Gd-contrast enhancement on axial FS T1WI (**b**).

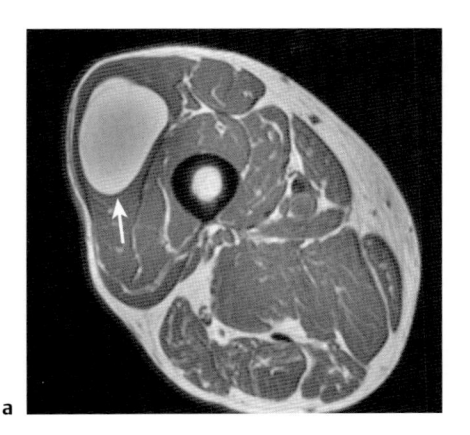

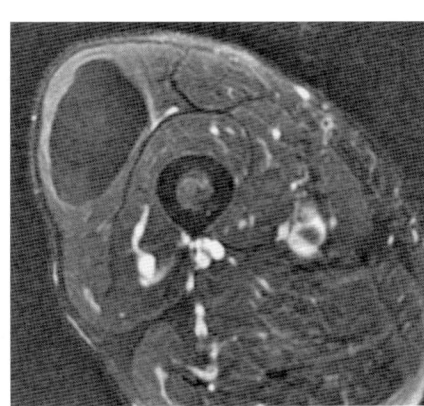

Figure 17.**20 a, b** A 71-year-old woman with an intramuscular lipoma in the thigh. The lipoma has high signal on axial T1WI (**a**). The fat signal of the lipoma is suppressed on axial FS T2WI (**b**).

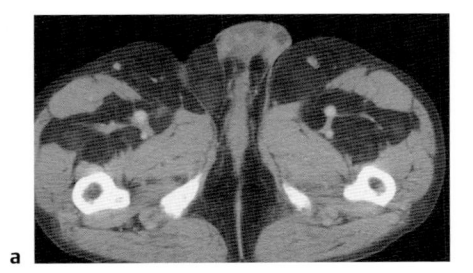

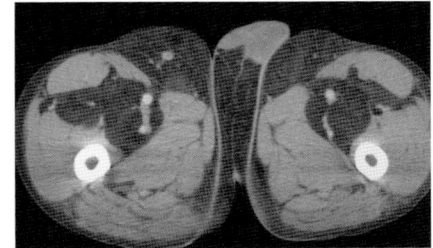

Figure 17.**21 a, b** A 42-year-old man with bilateral symmetric lipomatosis involving the inguinal regions, subcutaneous and intermuscular soft tissues of both proximal thighs. Multiple fatty lobules are seen with thin peripheral nonfatty septa on axial CT images (**a, b**). Poorly defined zones with attenuation slightly higher than fat are also seen in the fatty lobules.

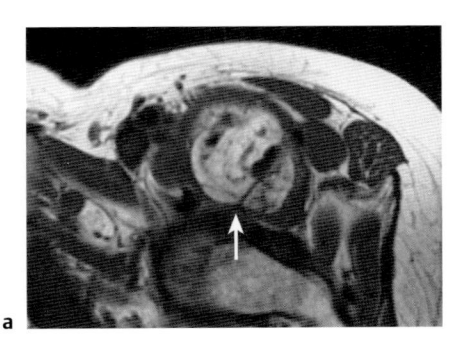

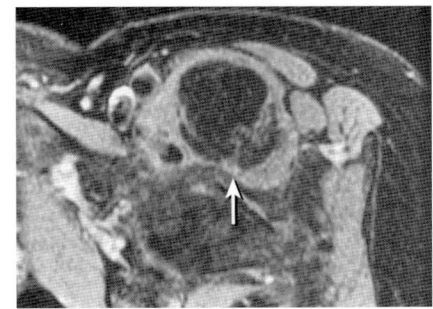

Figure 17.**22 a, b** A 55-year-old woman with an atypical lipoma/osteolipoma involving the iliopsoas muscle ventral to the proximal femur The lesion contains mostly fat signal on axial T1WI (**a**) as well as curvilinear and small nodular zones of low signal. The signal of the fatty portions of the lesion is suppressed on axial FS T2WI (**b**), whereas several of the small nonfatty portions show intermediate to high signal.

Table 17 (Continued) Solitary tumors and tumorlike lesions of the soft tissues located mostly deep to the subcutaneous fat

Lesion	MRI Findings	Comments
Hibernoma (Fig. 17.23)	Well-defined lesions that often have intermediate to high signal on T1WI (hypo- or isointense relative to fat), and slightly high signal on T2WI. Lesions can have slightly hyperintense signal relative to fat on FS T2WI and STIR. Internal septations, and/or branching-serpentine slow-flow vascular channels may be seen on T1WI and T2WI. Lesions can show Gd-contrast enhancement within branching vascular channels.	Rare benign lesions derived from brown adipose tissue intermixed with white adipose tissue. Account for <2% of fatty tumors. Occur in patients aged from 2 to over 75 years, mean = 32 to 38 years. **(See Atlas Chapter A 43)**
Lipoblastoma (Fig. 17.24)	Lesions often have mixed low, intermediate, and high signal on T1WI, T2WI, and FS T2WI. Lesions often show heterogeneous Gd-contrast enhancement.	Rare benign mesenchymal tumors that contain embryonal fat. Account for <1% of benign soft tissue tumors. Occur in patients from less than 1 to 10 years, mean = 4 years. **(See Atlas Chapter A 42)**
Hemangioma (Fig. 17.25)	Hemangiomas have circumscribed margins with or without lobulations, and have low-intermediate signal or heterogeneous low-intermediate and high signal on T1WI and PDWI; and high signal on T2WI. On FS T2WI, hemangiomas typically have high signal except for zones of fat within the lesions. Zones of hemorrhage can sometimes be present in hemangiomas as well as phleboliths. Hemangiomas usually show prominent Gd-contrast enhancement.	Benign hamartomatous lesions of bone and soft tissues comprised of capillary, cavernous, and/or malformed venous vessels. **(See Atlas Chapter A 34)**
Lymphangioma (Figs. 273–275 in Atlas section)	Can be circumscribed lesions or occur in infiltrative pattern with extension within and between muscles. Often contain single or multiple cystic zones that have predominantly low signal on T1WI and high signal on T2WI and FS T2WI. Fluid–fluid levels and zones with high signal on T1WI and variable signal on T2WI may result from cysts containing hemorrhage, high protein concentration, and/or necrotic debris. Septa between the cystic zones can vary in thickness and Gd-contrast enhancement, and usually have low signal on T1WI and low to intermediate signal on T2WI and FS T2WI. Nodular zones within the lesions can have variable degrees of Gd-contrast enhancement.	Benign vascular tumors that typically occur in soft tissue and only rarely in bone that result from abnormal proliferation of lymphatic vessels. Lesions are composed of endothelium-lined lymphatic channels interspersed within connective tissue stroma. Account for <1% of benign soft tissue tumors, 5.6% of all benign lesions of infancy and childhood. Can occur in association with Turner syndrome and Proteus syndrome. Patients usually range in age from 1 to 50 years, mean = 19 years. Can be congenital, with ~50% present at birth. Approximately 85% are detected by age 2. **(See Atlas Chapter A 46)**
Nodular fasciitis (Fig. 17.26)	Lesions can have mildly irregular or stellate borders. Lesions usually have intermediate signal on T1WI and PDWI; and homogeneous or mildly heterogeneous high signal on T2WI and FS T2WI. Surrounding edema is occasionally seen. Older lesions with high fibrous content may have intermediate signal on T2WI. Lesions can show homogeneous or peripheral rim-like patterns of Gd-contrast enhancement.	Benign reactive lesion comprised of proliferating fibroblasts, usually occur in the subcutaneous tissue or muscle. Account for 11% of benign soft tissue tumors and 7% of all soft tissue tumors. Patients range from 11 to 51 years, mean = 31 years. **(See Atlas Chapter A 21)**

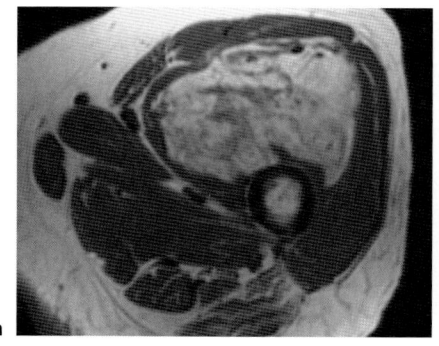

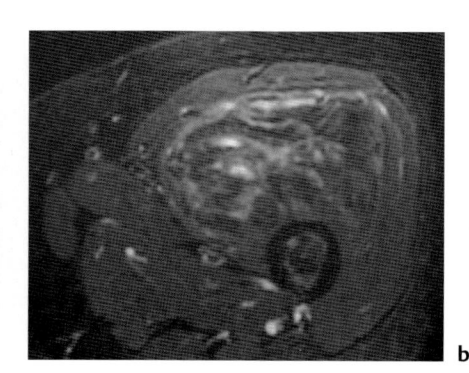

Figure 17.**23 a, b** A 71-year-old woman with a hibernoma involving the vastus muscles of the proximal thigh. The lesion has well-defined margins and contains mostly fat signal on axial T1WI (**a**) as well as curvilinear and small nodular zones of low signal. The signal of the fatty portions of the lesion is suppressed on axial FS T2WI (**b**), whereas nonfatty portions show intermediate to high signal on FS T2WI.

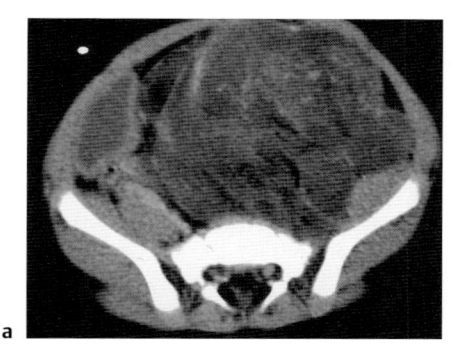

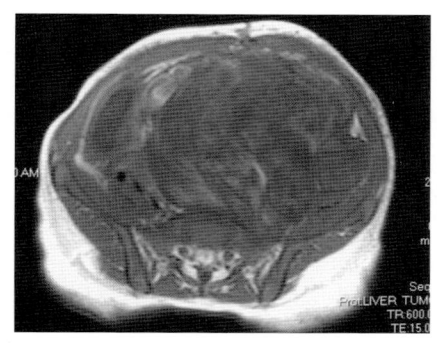

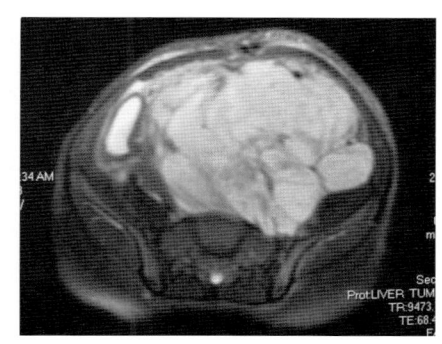

Figure 17.**24 a–c** A 1.5-year-old boy with a large intra-abdominal and pelvic lipoblastoma that has heterogeneous attenuation with zones of soft tissue, fluid, and fat attenuation on axial CT (**a**). The lesion has mixed low-intermediate, intermediate, and high signal on axial T1WI (**b**) and heterogeneous mostly high signal with thin strands of low signal on axial FS T2WI (**c**).

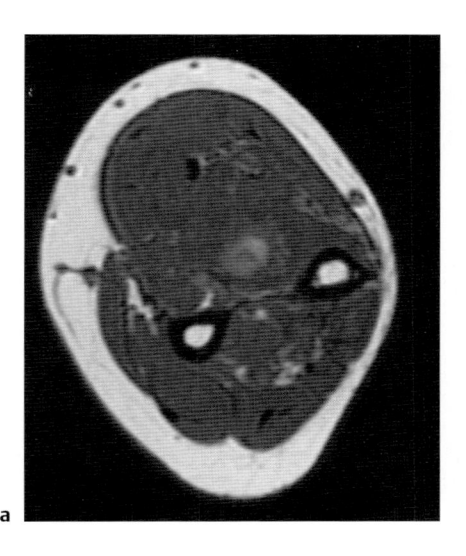

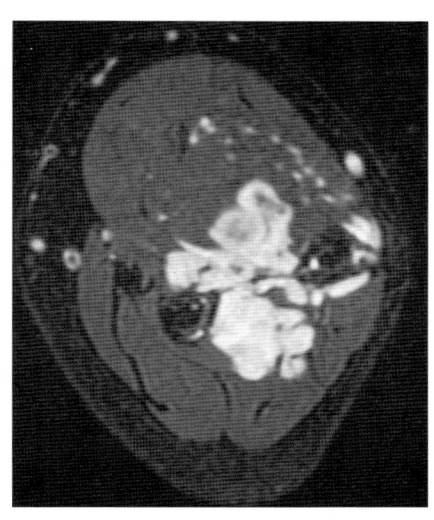

Figure 17.**25 a, b** A 14-year-old female with a hemangioma in the soft tissues of the forearm that has mostly intermediate signal on axial T1WI (**a**) and contains a zone of high signal from an area of hemorrhage. The lesion has mostly high signal on axial FS T2WI (**b**). Several prominent veins are also seen.

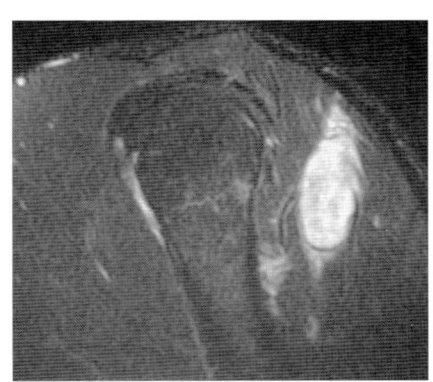

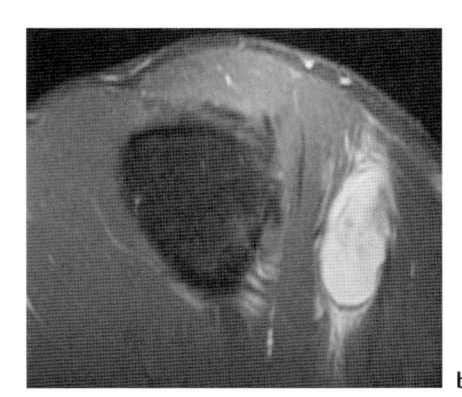

Figure 17.**26 a, b** A 43-year-old man with intramuscular nodular fasciitis involving the deltoid muscle at the left shoulder. The lesion has high signal on sagittal FS T2WI (**a**) that is surrounded by a thin rim of low signal and poorly defined zones of high signal in the adjacent soft tissues. The lesion shows prominent Gd-contrast enhancement on sagittal FS T1WI (**b**).

Table 17 (Continued) Solitary tumors and tumorlike lesions of the soft tissues located mostly deep to the subcutaneous fat

Lesion	MRI Findings	Comments
Nerve sheath tumor (schwannoma, neurofibroma) (Figs. 17.27–17.29)	**Localized neurofibromas and Schwannomas** are circumscribed ovoid or fusiform lesions with low-intermediate signal on T1WI, intermediate signal on PDWI, and intermediate to high signal on T2WI and FS T2WI. Lesions typically show moderate to prominent Gd-contrast enhancement. Multiple neurofibromas and schwannomas are frequently seen with NF1 and NF2, respectively. Neurofibromas can occur in various soft tissues. **Plexiform neurofibromas** appear as curvilinear and multinodular lesions involving multiple nerve branches. They have low to intermediate signal on T1WI and intermediate, slightly high to high signal on T2WI and FS T2WI with or without bands or strands of low signal. Lesions usually show Gd-contrast enhancement.	Benign nerve sheath tumors include schwannomas and neurofibromas. Schwannomas are benign encapsulated tumors that contain differentiated neoplastic Schwann cells. Neurofibromas contain mixtures of Schwann cells, perineural-like cells, and interlacing fascicles of fibroblasts associated with abundant collagen. Unlike schwannomas, neurofibromas lack Antoni A and B regions and cannot be separated pathologically from the underlying nerve. Neurofibromas can be localized lesions, or occur as diffuse or plexiform lesions. Multiple neurofibromas are typically seen with NF1. Multiple schwannomas are typically seen with NF2. **(See Atlas Chapters A 56, A 72)**
Neurothekeoma (Fig. 17.30)	Occurs as circumscribed lesions with low-intermediate signal on T1WI, high signal on T2WI, and heterogeneous Gd-contrast enhancement.	Neurothekeoma, also referred to as nerve sheath myxoma, is considered to be a neurofibroma with prominent myxoid matrix separated into lobules by fibrous connective tissue. **(See Atlas Chapter A 56)**
Paraganglioma (Fig. 17.31)	Paragangliomas are circumscribed ovoid or fusiform lesions with low-intermediate signal on T1WI and PDWI, and intermediate to high signal on T2WI and FS T2WI. Multiple tortuous and/or punctate zones of signal void or low signal on PDWI, T2WI, and FS T2WI can be seen within tumors as a "salt and pepper" pattern. Lesions typically show moderate to prominent Gd-contrast enhancement.	Extra-adrenal paragangliomas are benign encapsulated neuroendocrine tumors that arise from neural crest cells associated with autonomic ganglia (paraganglia) throughout the body. In the superficial soft tissues, paragangliomas can occur at the carotid body in the neck or near the vagus nerve. Patients range from 24 to 70 years, mean = 47 years. **(See Atlas Chapter A 66)**
Solitary fibrous tumor (Fig. 17.32)	SFTs often have circumscribed margins. Often have low to intermediate signal on T1WI and PDWI, low, intermediate, and/or slightly high signal on T2WI, and heterogeneous slightly high to high signal on FS T2WI. Usually show Gd-contrast enhancement.	Rare benign spindle-cell mesenchymal neoplasms that occur in a wide range of anatomic sites including the extremities. Tumors typically show a hemangiopericytoma-like branching vascular pattern and resemble pleural SFTs. Account for <2% of soft tissue tumors. Median patient age from 50 to 60 years. **(See Atlas Chapter A 24)**

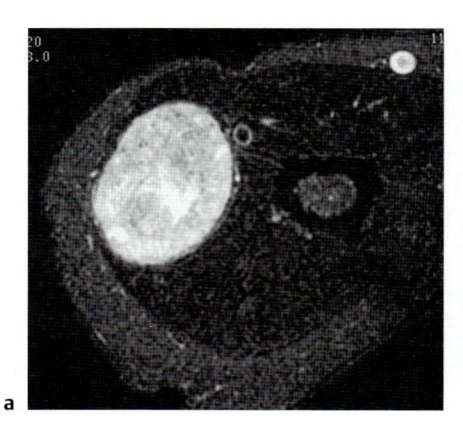

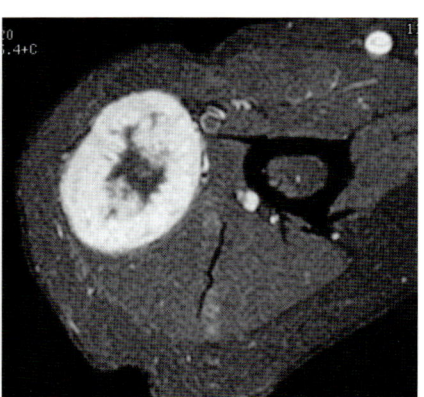

Figure 17.**27 a, b** A 61-year-old woman with an intramuscular schwannoma in the arm that has high signal on axial T2WI (**a**) and shows heterogeneous Gd-contrast enhancement on axial FS T1WI (**b**).

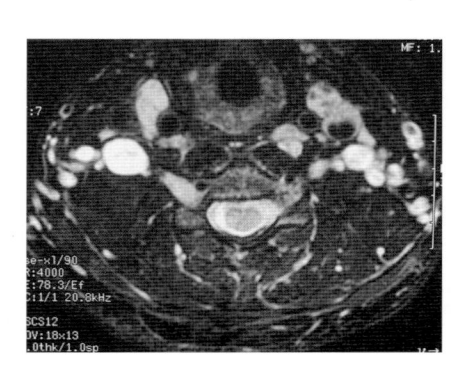

Figure 17.**28** A 22-year-old man with NF1 with multiple neurofibromas in the soft tissues in the neck, showing high signal on axial FS T2WI.

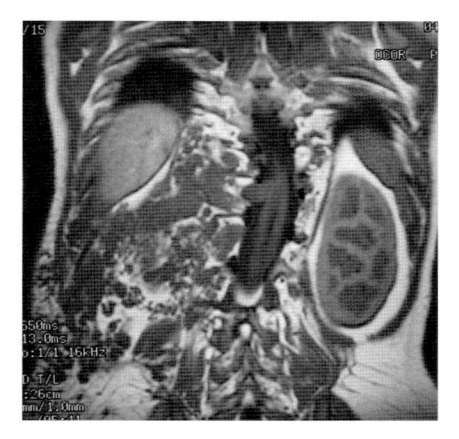

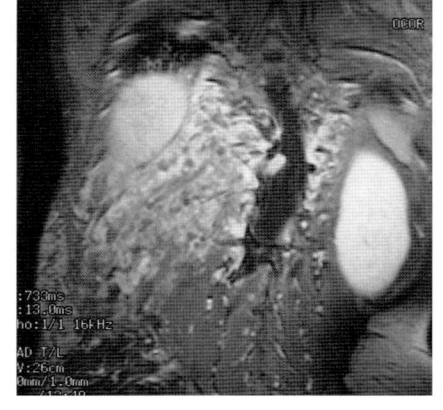

Figure 17.**29 a, b** A 2-year-old girl with NF1 and a plexiform neurofibroma posterior and medial to the right kidney with extension into the spinal canal. The tumor appears as curvilinear and multinodular zones with intermediate signal on coronal T1WI (**a**) and heterogeneous Gd-contrast enhancement on coronal FS T1WI (**b**).

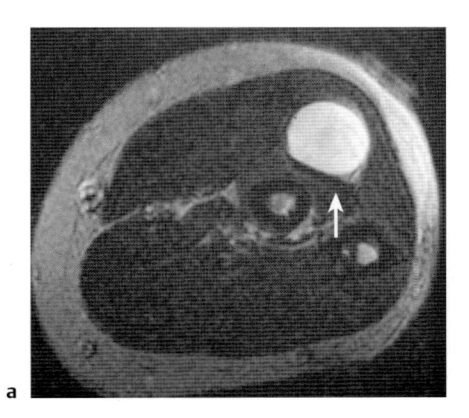

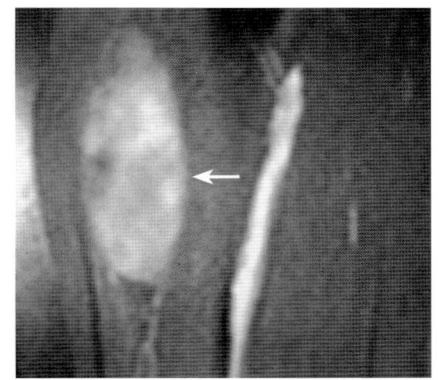

Figure 17.**30 a, b** A 38-year-old man with a neurothekeoma involving the flexor digitorum superficialis muscle of the proximal forearm. The lesion has high signal on axial T2WI (**a**) and shows moderate heterogeneous Gd-contrast enhancement on sagittal FS T1WI (**b**).

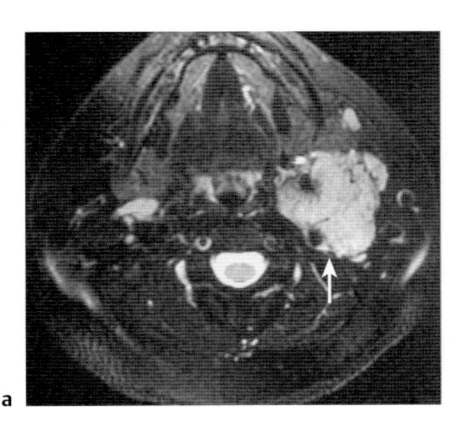

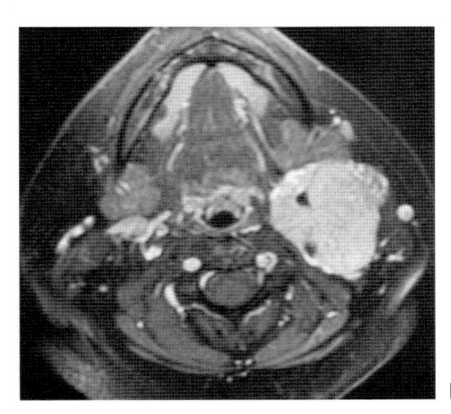

Figure 17.**31 a, b** A 27-year-old woman with a paraganglioma (carotid body tumor) at the left common carotid artery bifurcation. The lesion has heterogenous mostly high signal on axial FS T2WI (**a**) and shows prominent Gd-contrast enhancement on axial FS T1WI (**b**). The tumor splays the proximal external carotid artery from the internal carotid artery.

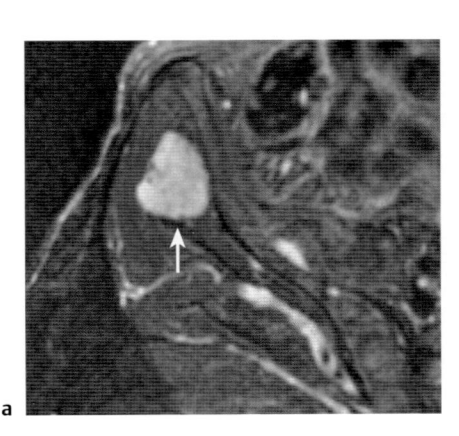

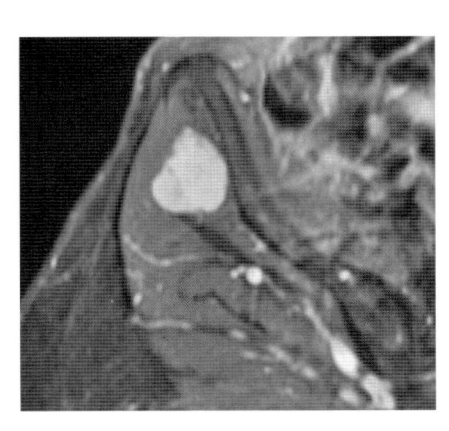

Figure 17.**32 a, b** An 81-year-old man with a solitary fibrous tumor involving the gluteus minimus muscle. The lesion has circumscribed margins, high signal on axial FS T2WI (**a**), and shows Gd-contrast enhancement on axial FS T1WI (**b**).

Table 17 (Continued)   Solitary tumors and tumorlike lesions of the soft tissues located mostly deep to the subcutaneous fat

Lesion	MRI Findings	Comments
Desmoid tumor (Fig. 17.33)	Lesions can have distinct and/or poorly defined margins, homogeneous or heterogeneous low-intermediate signal on T1WI, and variable intermediate-high signal on T2WI, +/− zones of low signal. Myxoid zones in the lesions can have high signal on T1WI and T2WI. Tumors with high cellularity tend to show higher signal on T2WI than lesions with larger proportions of collagen. Lesions show variable degrees and patterns (heterogeneous versus homogenous) of Gd-contrast enhancement. Pattern or degree of Gd-contrast enhancement by desmoids does not enable prediction of rate of tumor recurrence.	Desmoid tumors or fibromatosis represent a group of soft tissue lesions comprised of benign fibrous tissue with elongated or spindle-shaped cells adjacent to collagen. **(See Atlas Chapter A 16)**
Myxoma (Fig. 17.34)	Lesions usually have low or low-intermediate signal on T1WI and PDWI, and high signal on T2WI and FS T2WI. Myxomas can have heterogeneous mild or moderate degrees of enhancement in noncystic portions.	Benign lesions that contain fibroblasts (spindle cells) and abundant mucoid material (glycosaminoglycans, other mucopolysaccharides). Account for 3% of benign soft tissue tumors/lesions and 2% of all soft tissue tumors/lesions. Occur in adults aged from 24 to 74 years, mean = 52 years. **(See Atlas Chapter A 54)**
Tumorlike lesions		
Ganglion cyst (Fig. 17.35)	Ganglia are sharply defined lesions with low signal on T1WI, low-intermediate signal on PDWI, and homogeneous high signal on T2WI. Some ganglia may have intermediate signal on T1WI secondary to elevated proteinaceous or fibrous content. Low signal septa on T2WI can be seen. Peripheral rim-like Gd-contrast enhancement can be seen as well as complete lack of enhancement.	Ganglia are juxta-articular benign myxoid lesions that arise from degeneration of peri-articular connective tissue, prior trauma, or prior inflammation. Ganglia may be derived from tendons, tendon sheaths, joint capsules, bursae, or ligaments. **(See Atlas Chapter A 28)**
Hematoma/seroma (Fig. 17.36)	Acute hematomas (< 3–7 days) have mostly intermediate signal similar to muscle on T1WI and mixed low-intermediate and/or high signal relative to muscle on PDWI, T2WI, and FS T2WI. Poorly defined zones of high signal on PDWI, T2WI, and FS T2WI may also be seen peripheral to the hematoma representing adjacent edema. Subacute hematomas (1 week to 3 months) have high and/or intermediate signal on T1WI, and high signal on FS T1WI, PDWI, T2WI, and FS T2WI. Peripheral and central zones of low signal on PDWI, T2WI, and FS T2WI can be seen in mid to late subacute hematomas secondary to the presence of hemosiderin from breakdown of blood cells and oxidation/metabolism of hemoglobin. Mild peripheral Gd-contrast may be seen Chronic hematomas (> 3 months) usually have high signal on T1WI, PDWI, T2WI, and FS T2WI. A thick peripheral rim of low signal on T2WI from hemosiderin is often seen with chronic hematomas. Chronic hematomas often evolve eventually into zones with low-intermediate signal on T1WI and T2WI secondary to fibrosis and residual hemosiderin.	Hematomas are extravascular collections of red and white blood cells that can result from trauma, surgery, coagulopathy (hemophilia, thrombocytopenia, medications/coumadin/heparin, and sepsis). **(See Atlas Chapter A 36)**

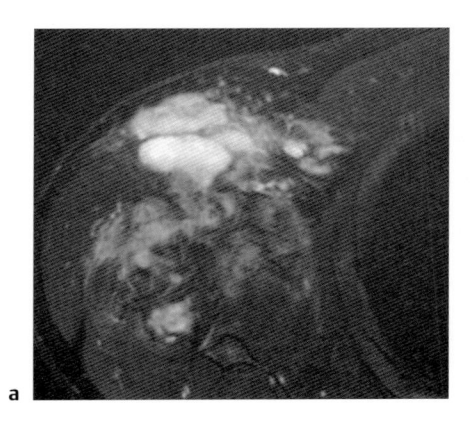

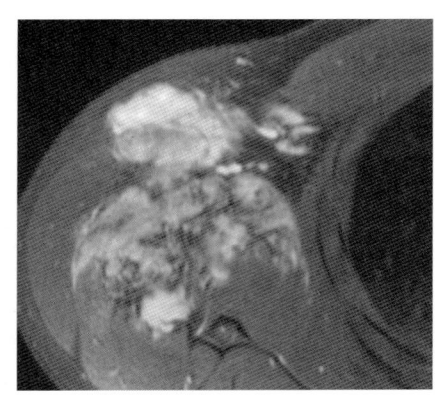

Figure 17.**33 a, b** A 32-year-old man with aggressive fibromatosis involving the soft tissues in the right axilla. MRI shows a lobulated lesion with indistinct margins that has slightly high and high signal on axial FS T2WI (**a**). Foci and thin curvilinear zones of low signal are also seen. The lesion shows prominent heterogeneous Gd-contrast enhancement on axial FS T1WI (**b**).

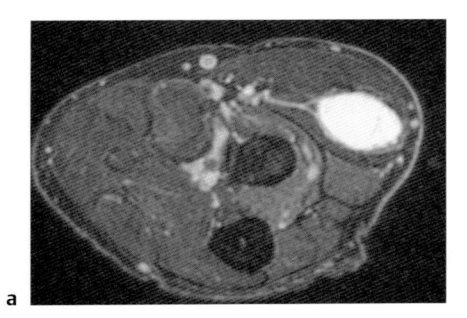

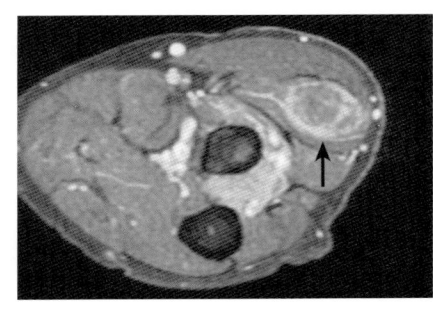

Figure 17.**34 a, b** A 77-year-old man with an intramuscular myxoma involving the extensor carpi radialis longus and brevis muscles of the proximal forearm. The lesion has high signal on axial FS T2WI (**a**) and shows mild irregular Gd-contrast enhancement on axial FS T1WI (**b**).

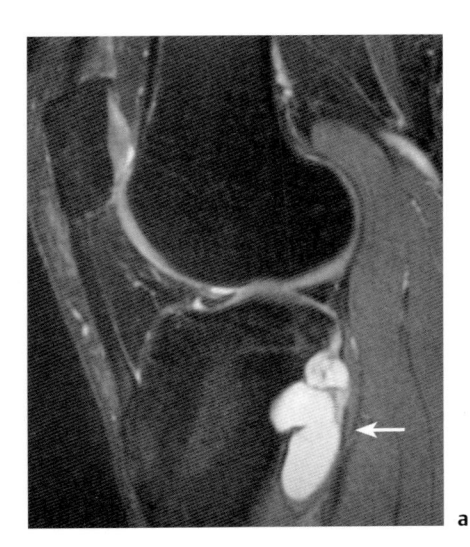

Figure 17.**35** Periosteal ganglion along the posterolateral proximal tibia of a 30-year-old man. The lesion has sharply defined margins, and has high signal on sagittal FS T2WI. The lesion causes erosion and concave deformity of the tibial cortex.

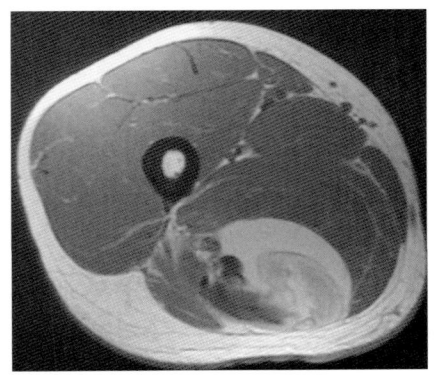

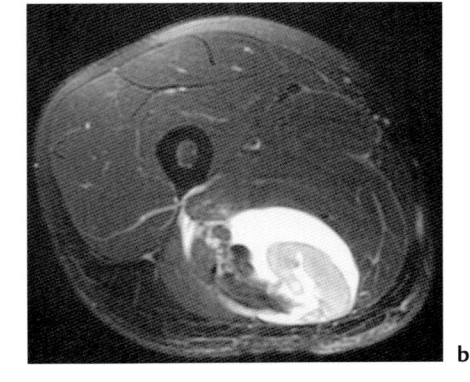

Figure 17.**36 a, b** Subacute intramuscular hematoma involving the semitendinosus muscle in the upper thigh. The hematoma has heterogeneous slightly high, intermediate, and low signal on axial PDWI (**a**), and heterogeneous high, slightly high, and low signal on axial FS T2WI (**b**).

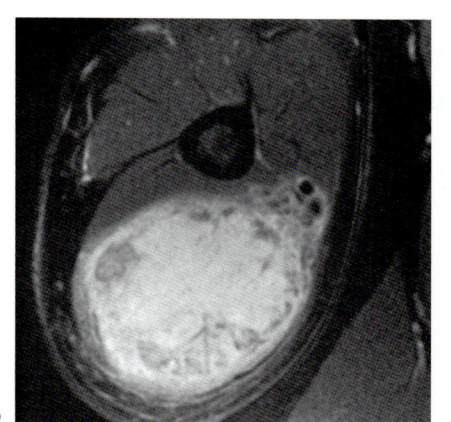

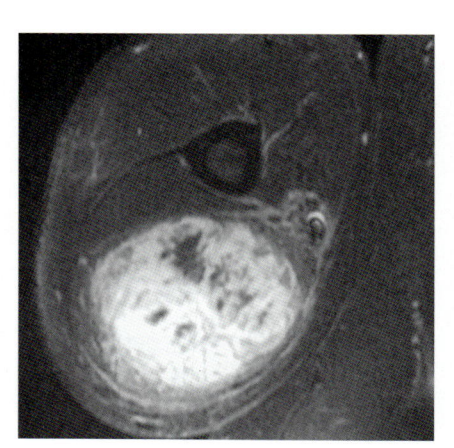

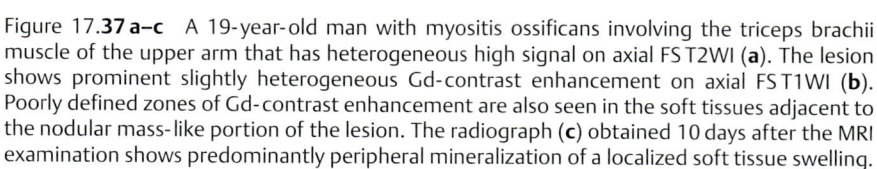

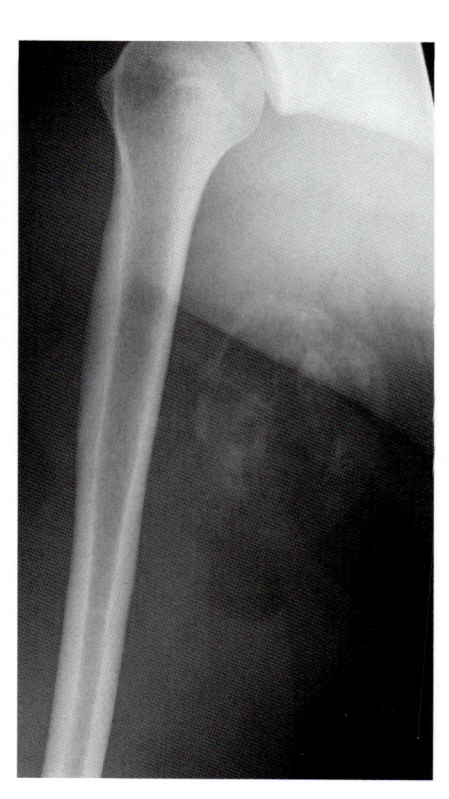

Table 17 (Continued) Solitary tumors and tumorlike lesions of the soft tissues located mostly deep to the subcutaneous fat

Lesion	MRI Findings	Comments
Heterotopic ossification (Fig. 17.37)	MRI features vary depending on the age, location, and degree of mineralization/ossification. Lesions <2 weeks have localized mass effect with poorly defined margins, heterogeneous low-intermediate or slightly high signal on T1WI, and heterogeneous slightly high to high signal on T2WI and FS T2WI. Poorly defined zones of high signal on T2WI may be seen in the adjacent soft tissues. After 2 weeks, curvilinear and/or amorphous zones of low signal on T2WI and FS T2WI can be seen at the peripheral portions of the subacute lesions resulting from mineralization/ossification. Subsequent progressive centripetal mineralization/ossification appears as irregular zones of low signal on T2WI with heterogeneous Gd-contrast enhancement. Old lesions have well-defined margins, and variable low signal on T1WI, PDWI, and T2WI depending on the degree of mineralization/ossification, fibrosis, and hemosiderin deposition. Zones of high signal on T1WI and T2WI may occur from fatty marrow metaplasia. Gd-contrast enhancement in old mature lesions is often minimal or absent.	Heterotopic ossification or myositis ossificans are non-neoplastic reparative extraosseous lesions that are comprised of reactive hypercellular fibrous tissue, cartilage, and/or bone. These lesions can arise secondary to trauma (myositis ossificans circumscripta, ossifying hematoma), although may also occur without a history of prior injury (pseudomalignant osseous tumor of the soft tissues). **(See Atlas Chapter A 53)**

Figure 17.37 a–c A 19-year-old man with myositis ossificans involving the triceps brachii muscle of the upper arm that has heterogeneous high signal on axial FS T2WI (**a**). The lesion shows prominent slightly heterogeneous Gd-contrast enhancement on axial FS T1WI (**b**). Poorly defined zones of Gd-contrast enhancement are also seen in the soft tissues adjacent to the nodular mass-like portion of the lesion. The radiograph (**c**) obtained 10 days after the MRI examination shows predominantly peripheral mineralization of a localized soft tissue swelling.

Table 17 (Continued) Solitary tumors and tumorlike lesions of the soft tissues located mostly deep to the subcutaneous fat

Lesion	MRI Findings	Comments
Tumoral calcinosis (Fig. 17.38)	Radiographs and CT show lobular and/or multiloculated opacities that may contain radiolucent strands secondary to fibrous septae and calcium fluid levels. Erosion of bone adjacent to the tumoral calcinosis can occur. Lesions have variable signal on MRI with mixed low and intermediate signal on T1WI, and mixed low, intermediate, and/or high signal on T2WI. Gd-contrast may occur in septae or surrounding the lesions secondary to inflammatory reaction.	Rare metabolic disorder related to abnormal phosphate metabolism with elevated levels of 1,25-dihydroxyvitamin D resulting in hyperphosphatemia with precipitation of calcium salts in juxta-articular soft tissues. Common locations include the soft tissues near bursae at the hips, shoulders, elbows, buttocks, and scapula. Can be hereditary in up to 33% as autosomal dominant with variable penetrance. Lesions consist of deposits of hydroxyapatite with or without fibrous septae, macrophages and chronic inflammatory cells, and multinucleated giant cells.
Amyloidoma	Lesions in soft tissue can have low-intermediate signal on T1WI, and intermediate to slightly high signal on T2WI. Lesions can show Gd-contrast enhancement.	Uncommon disease in which various tissues (including bone, muscle, tendons, tendon sheaths, ligaments, and synovium) are infiltrated with extracellular eosinophilic material composed of insoluble proteins with β-pleated sheet configurations (amyloid protein). Amyloidomas are single sites of involvement. Amyloidosis can be a primary disorder associated with an immunologic dyscrasia or secondary to a chronic inflammatory disease.
Aneurysm	Saccular aneurysms are focal well-circumscribed structures contiguous with arteries. Signal voids are usually seen where there is fast blood flow in nonthrombosed portions of the aneurysms. Variable mixed signal on T1WI and T2WI can be seen in thrombosed portions of the aneurysms.	Focal or diffuse zones of arterial dilatation that are associated with wall abnormalities and increased risk of rupture. Focal aneurysms are also referred to as saccular aneurysms that typically occur at arterial branch points. Giant aneurysms are saccular aneurysms that measure >2.5 cm in diameter.

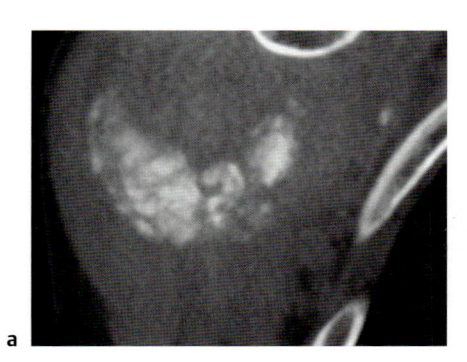

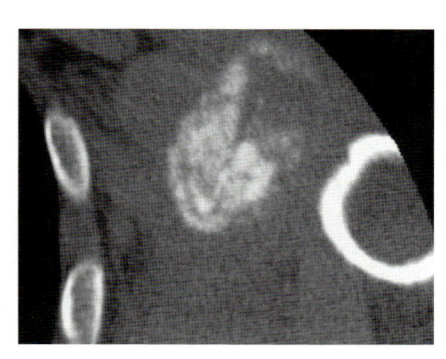

Figure 17.38 a, b   Oblique sagittal (a) and axial (b) CT images show amorphous opacities in the soft tissues at the shoulder and axillary region in a 76-year-old man.

Table 17 (Continued)	Solitary tumors and tumorlike lesions of the soft tissues located mostly deep to the subcutaneous fat	
Lesion	MRI Findings	Comments
Inflammatory		
Abscess/myositis (Fig. 17.39)	Deep infections and myositis typically show poorly defined zones of decreased signal on T1WI, and slightly high to high signal on T2WI and FS T2WI with corresponding Gd-contrast enhancement. Progression to abscess formation occurs with circumscribed zones that have low signal on T1WI and high signal on T2WI (with or without an air–fluid level) that are surrounded by a rim of low signal on T2WI. Rim-like Gd-contrast enhancement is usually seen. Peripherally, a poorly defined zone of high signal may be seen secondary to edema and/or inflammation.	Infection of muscles (myositis) and deep soft tissues from bacteria, fungi, and mycobacteria can eventually progress to liquefaction with necrosis (abscess formation) enclosed by a pseudocapsule surrounded by zones of edema and inflammatory reaction.
Parasitic infection (Fig. 17.40)	Parasitic infections can vary from cystic-appearing lesions to poorly marginated or circumscribed solid lesions depending on the infectious organism and stage of its life cycle.	Parasitic infections can occur in soft tissues in endemic regions or in immunocompromised patients.
Sarcoid (Fig. 17.41)	Sarcoid granulomas can occur in subcutaneous fat and may be associated with superficial adenopathy. Lesions are often nodular with low to intermediate signal on T1WI, and intermediate to high signal on T2WI. Lesions usually show Gd-contrast enhancement. Sarcoid can also involve muscles as discrete or poorly-defined lesions.	Chronic systemic granulomatous disease of unknown etiology in which noncaseating granulomas occur in various tissues and organs. Common sites of involvement include the lungs, lymph nodes, liver, spleen, skin, and eyes. **(See Atlas Chapter A 71)**
Giant cell reaction to foreign body	Lesions usually occur in soft tissue and often have low-intermediate signal on T1WI, and low, intermediate, and/or high signal on T2WI. Lesions can show Gd-contrast enhancement. Sites of bone erosion and/or destruction may be seen particularly with penetrating trauma. The MRI signal of the foreign body varies based on its composition.	Reactive granulomatous lesions can form adjacent to foreign bodies, and may simulate neoplasm.
Gout	Tophi have variable sizes and shapes, and have low-intermediate signal on T1WI, FS T2WI, and T2WI. Zones of high signal on T2WI can also be seen in tophi. Erosions of bone, synovial pannus, joint effusion, bone marrow, and soft tissue edema can be seen with MRI. Tophi may show heterogeneous, diffuse, or peripheral/marginal Gd-contrast enhancement patterns.	Gout is an inflammatory disease involving synovium resulting from deposition of monosodium urate crystals and occurs when the serum urate level exceeds its solubility in various tissues and body fluid. **(See Atlas Chapter A 32)**
Rheumatoid arthritis (Fig. 17.42)	MRI can show diffuse and/or localized zones of synovial hypertrophy; soft tissue swelling; zones of erosion and/or destruction of hyaline cartilage, menisci/fibrocartilage, subchondral bone, tendons, ligaments; bursal fluid collections containing "rice bodies", other extra-articular cysts; intraosseous cystic-like areas, joint effusion, and rheumatoid nodules. With tendon and ligament involvement, abnormal increased signal is seen on PDWI and T2WI. Tendons and ligaments may be thickened from partial tearing or thinned. Tenosynovitis is usually seen with fluid and hypertrophied synovium within tendon sheaths.	Chronic multi-system disease of unknown etiology in which there is a persistent inflammatory synovitis that typically involves peripheral joints in a symmetric distribution. The inflammatory synovitis can result in progressive destruction of cartilage and bone leading to joint dysfunction. **(See Atlas Chapter A 70)**

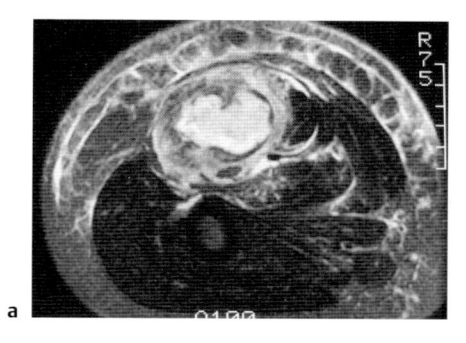

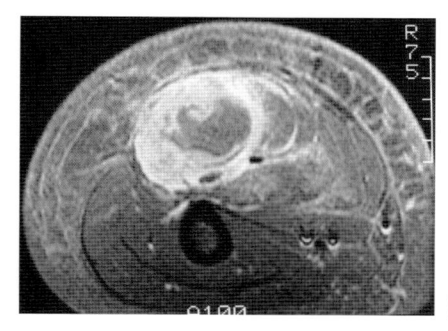

Figure 17.**39 a, b** A 15-year-old male with myositis and abscess involving the anterior thigh muscles seen as a poorly defined zone with slightly high to high signal surrounding a circumscribed central zone (abscess) with high signal on axial T2WI (**a**). Irregular peripheral Gd-contrast enhancement is seen in the soft tissues surrounding the abscess on axial FS T1WI (**b**).

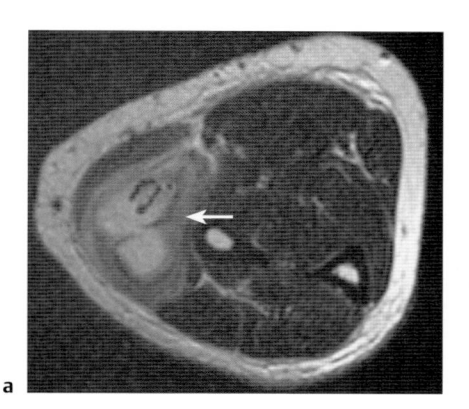

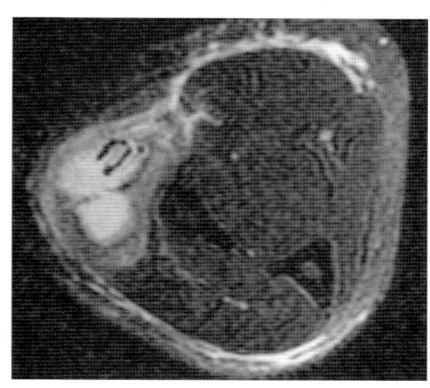

Figure 17.**40 a, b** A 34-year-old woman with intramuscular infection from cysticercosis in the forearm. A curvilinear zone with low signal representing the senescent parasite is surrounded by an abscess and solid inflammatory reaction with slightly high signal and high signal on axial T2WI (**a**) and high signal on axial FS T2WI (**b**).

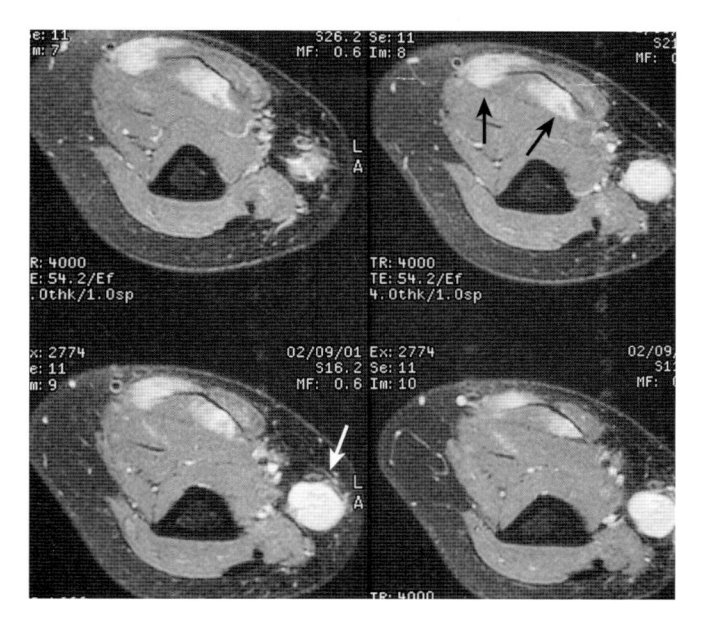

Figure 17.**41** A 49-year-old woman with sarcoid granulomas in the subcutaneous fat and within the biceps brachii muscle at the distal arm. The intramuscular lesions have slightly irregular margins and have high signal on axial FS T2WI.

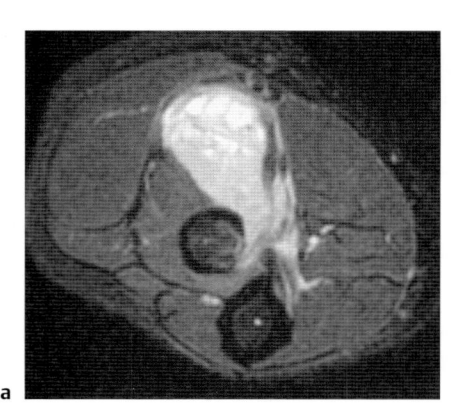

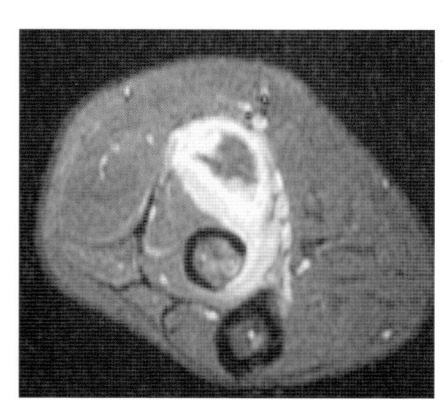

Figure 17.**42 a, b** A 37-year-old woman with an inflammatory lesion from rheumatoid arthritis involving the antecubital bursa and biceps brachii muscle and tendon. The lesion has heterogeneous high signal on axial FS T2WI (**a**) and shows heterogeneous Gd-contrast enhancement on axial FS T1WI (**b**). The lesion causes erosion of the cortex of the adjacent radius.

Table 17 (Continued) Solitary tumors and tumorlike lesions of the soft tissues located mostly deep to the subcutaneous fat		
Lesion	MRI Findings	Comments
Dermatomyositis (Fig. 17.43)	In acute and subacute phases, poorly defined zones of high signal on T2WI are seen in muscles, subcutaneous fat, and fascia secondary to ischemic or infarcted muscle resulting from vasculitis. Zones of low signal on T2WI can result from calcifications seen on radiographs and CT scans. "Milk of calcium" collections may occur which have variable signal on T1WI and T2WI depending on the relative proportions of fluid and fluid–calcium levels. Poorly defined zones of Gd-contrast enhancement can be seen in muscles, fascia, and/or subcutaneous fat if there is active inflammation and/or ischemia infarction. Muscle atrophy with fatty infiltration can be seen in the chronic phases	Nonsuppurative autoimmune systemic vasculopathy involving muscle fibers, skin, and blood vessels. Can be associated with other connective tissue diseases such as scleroderma, and mixed connective tissue disease. Incidence: 2–8 per million, prevalence: 4–60 per million. Juvenile dermatomyositis occurs in children between 2 and 15 years. Adult dermatomyositis occurs with peak incidence in 5th decade. (See Atlas Chapter A 14).

Other

Giant cell tumor of the tendon sheath (Fig. 17.44)	Lesions usually have well-defined margins and are often adjacent to a tendon/tendon sheath. Lesions have low-intermediate or intermediate signal on T1WI and PDWI, and mixed low, intermediate and/or high signal on T2WI and FS T2WI. Zones of low signal on T2WI often correspond to sites of hemosiderin deposition. Lesions often show Gd-contrast enhancement in either a homogeneous or heterogeneous pattern.	Giant cell tumors of the tendon sheath and pigmented villonodular synovitis represent benign proliferative lesions of synovium (tendon sheaths, joints, and bursae). Giant cell tumors of the tendon sheaths can occur as localized nodular lesions attached to tendon sheaths outside of joints (hands, feet) or within joints (infrapatellar portion of knee joint), or as a nodular or diffuse form near/outside of large joints such as the knee, ankles, etc. (See Atlas Chapter A 30)
Fibroma of the tendon sheath	Lesions are ovoid or fusiform and well-circumscribed, and are located adjacent to tendons of the fingers, hands, wrists, feet, and other locations. Lesions usually have low-intermediate signal on T1WI. On T2WI, lesions can have a slightly heterogeneous low-intermediate signal in half, intermediate signal in a third, or mixed low and intermediate signal and/or high signal in the remainder. Lesions can show diffuse or peripheral Gd-contrast enhancement.	Fibromas of the tendon sheath are benign, small fibrous nodules involving tendons and tendon sheaths of the fingers, hands, wrists, or feet. (See Atlas Chapter A 23)
Xanthoma	Xanthomas in tendons often appear as zones of fusiform enlargement with diffuse heterogeneous signal. Xanthomas usually contain multiple longitudinally oriented linear zones or striations with intermediate signal on T1WI and PDWI, and intermediate to slightly high signal on T2WI and FS T2WI interspersed among bands of low signal within the enlarged tendons. On axial images, xanthomas often have a stippled or reticulated pattern on T1WI and T2WI resulting from collagen bundles with low signal surrounded by higher signal from lipid deposits, foamy histiocytes, and inflammatory reaction.	Xanthomas are localized accumulations of lipids within normal structures such as tendons, skin, and bone. Considered reactive lesions and are not true neoplasms. Often occur in the setting of types I, II, and III hyperlipoproteinemia. (See Atlas Chapter A 77)

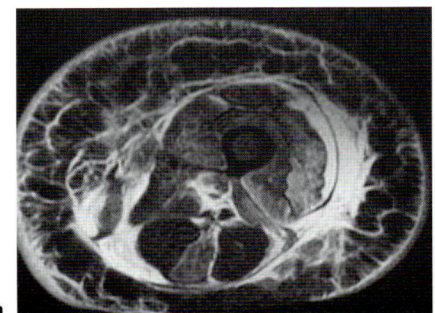

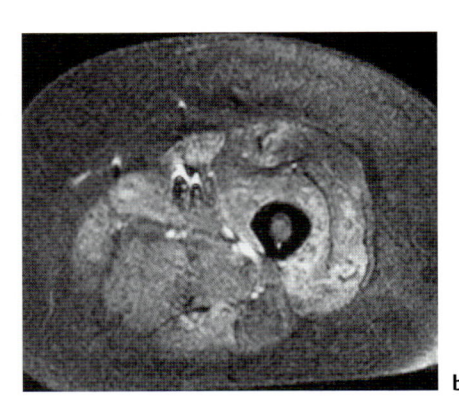

Figure 17.43 a, b A 78-year-old woman with dermatomyositis involving the thigh. Poorly defined zones of abnormal high signal on FS T2WI (a) and abnormal Gd-contrast enhancement on FS T1WI (b) are seen in the thigh muscles secondary to active inflammation. Zones of abnormal high signal on axial FS T2WI are also seen in the subcutaneous fat.

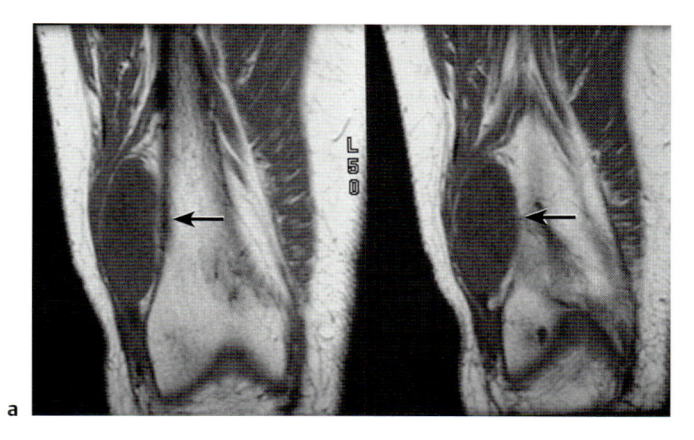

Figure 17.**44 a, b** A 60-year-old woman with a giant cell tumor of the tendon sheath/nodular synovitis at the knee. An ovoid lesion with well-defined margins is seen adjacent to the iliotibial band. The lesion has low-intermediate signal on coronal T1WI (**a**) and shows prominent Gd-contrast enhancement on axial FS T1WI (**b**).

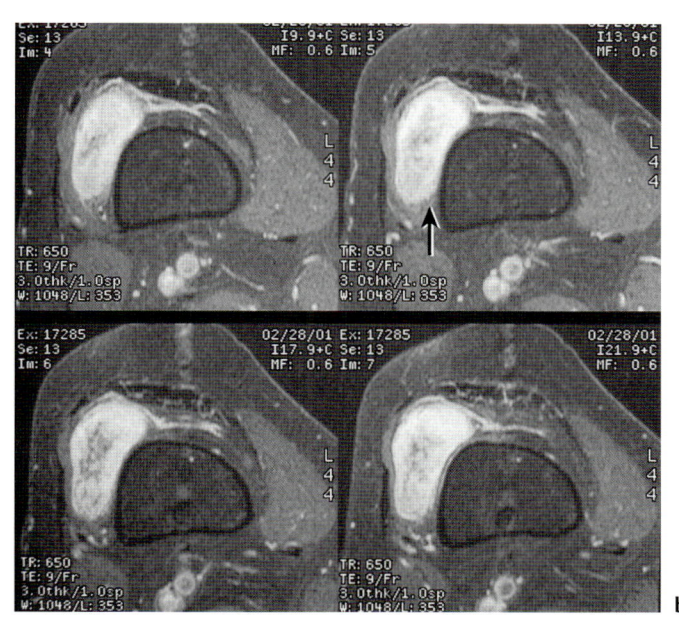

References

Clear Cell Sarcoma
De Beuckeleer LH, De Schepper AM, Vandevenne JE, et al. MR imaging of clear cell sarcoma (malignant melanoma of the soft parts): a multicenter correlative MRI-pathology study of 21 cases and literature review. *Skeletal Radiol* 2000;29:187–195.

Lipomatosis
Amine B, Leguilchard F, Benhamou CL. Dercum's disease (adiposis dolorosa): a new case report. *Joint Bone Spine* 2004;71:147–149.
Drevelegas A, Pilavaki M, Chourmouzi D. Lipomatous tumors of soft tissue: MR appearance with histological correlation. *Eur J Radiol* 2004;50:257–267.
Haloi AK, Ditchfield M, Penington A, Phillips R. Facial infiltrative lipomatosis. *Pediatr Radiol* 2006;36:1159–1162.
Klein FA, Smith MJ, Kasenetz I. Pelvic lipomatosis: 35-year experience. *J Urol* May 1988;139(5):998–1001.
Murphy MD, Carroll JF, Flemming DJ, Pope TL, Gannon FH, Kransdorf MJ. Benign musculoskeletal lipomatous lesions. *RadioGraphics* September–October 2004;24(5):1433–1466.
Sener RN. Epidural, paraspinal, and subcutaneous lipomatosis. *Pediatr Radiol* 2003;33:655–657.
Torigian DA, Siegelman ES. CT findings of pelvic lipomatosis of nerve. *AJR* March 2005;184:94–96.

Tumoral Calcinosis
Durant DM, Riley LH, III, Burger PC, McCarthy EF. Tumoral calcinosis of the spine. A study of 21 cases. *Spine* 2001;26(15):1673–1679.
Martinez S, Vogler JB, III, Harrelson JM, Lyles KW. Imaging of tumoral calcinosis: new observations. *Radiology* January 1990;174(1):215–222.
Olsen KM, Chew FS. Tumoral calcinosis: pearls, polemics, and alternative possibilities. *RadioGraphics* May–June 2006;26(3):871–885.
Şenol U, Karaali K, Çevikol C, Dinçer A. MR imaging findings of recurrent tumoral calcinosis. *J Clin Imag* 2000;24:154–156.

Table 18 Tumors and tumorlike lesions of the superficial soft tissues including subcutaneous fat

Lesion	MRI Findings	Comments
Neoplastic-malignant		
Dermatofibrosarcoma and dermatofibrosarcoma protuberans (Fig. 18.1)	Dermatofibrosarcoma (DFS) are small lesions with circumscribed and/or poorly defined margins involving the skin and/or subcutaneous adipose tissue. Tumors can have low-intermediate signal on T1WI, and intermediate to high signal on T2WI and FS T2WI. DFS show variable degrees of Gd-contrast enhancement. dermatofibrosarcoma protuberans (DFSP) are usually circumscribed lesions in the skin and subcutaneous adipose tissues that can measure up to 25 cm. Ten percent of DFSP have poorly defined margins. DFSP tumors have low-intermediate signal on T1WI, intermediate, slightly high, and/or high signal on T2WI. DFSP show heterogeneous or homogeneous Gd-contrast enhancement.	DFS and DFSP are dermal tumors containing malignant fibroblastic cells with spindle-shaped nuclei. **(See Atlas Chapter A 13)**
Malignant fibrous histiocytoma (Fig. 18.2)	Tumors have poorly defined and or circumscribed margins, and often have low-intermediate signal on T1WI and heterogeneous intermediate-high signal on T2WI and FS T2WI. Tumors show heterogeneous often prominent enhancement.	Malignant tumors involving soft tissue and rarely bone that are presumed to derive from undifferentiated mesenchymal cells. The World Health Organization (WHO) now uses the term undifferentiated pleomorphic sarcoma. **(See Atlas Chapter A 48)**
Liposarcoma (Fig. 18.3)	**Well-differentiated liposarcomas** contain up to 75% overall fat signal, and contain thick nonadipose septae and/or nodular nonadipose zones. The nonadipose zones can have low-intermediate signal on T1WI and PDWI; and low, intermediate, and/or high signal on T2WI. Nonadipose tumor portions show variable degrees of Gd-contrast enhancement. **Myxoid liposarcomas:** These tumors usually contain myxoid material with low signal on T1WI, heterogeneous or homogeneous high signal on T2WI. Tumors may or may not contain fat seen with MRI. Tumors show variable degrees of Gd-contrast enhancement. **Pleomorphic, round cell and dedifferentiated liposarcomas** often have heterogeneous/mixed low, intermediate, and/or high signal on T1WI and T2WI. Less than 26% of pleomorphic liposarcomas have fat signal. Tumors show variable degrees of Gd-contrast enhancement.	Malignant mesenchymal tumors containing portions showing differentiation into adipose tissue. Liposarcomas represent ~14% of malignant soft tissue tumors and 6% of all soft tissue tumors. **(See Atlas Chapter A 44)**
Metastatic disease (Fig. 18.4)	Tumors can occur as lymphadenopathy or as focal lesions. Lesions have low-intermediate signal on T1WI and intermediate to slightly high signal or high signal on T2WI and FS T2WI. Variability in MRI signal characteristics may be related to differing histologic features of the metastatic lesions. Tumors can show variable degrees of Gd-contrast enhancement.	Metastatic lesions are proliferating neoplastic cells that are located in sites or organs separated or distant from their origins. **(See Atlas Chapter A 50)**

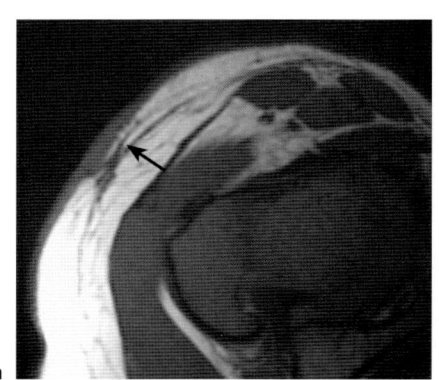

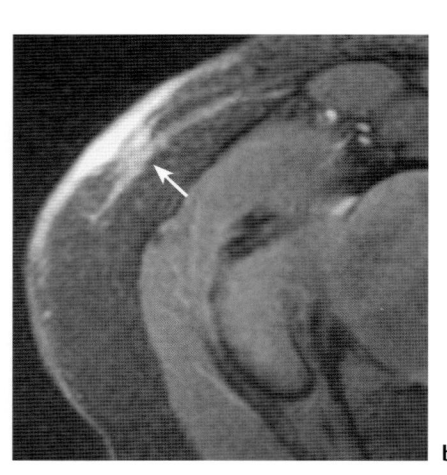

Figure 18.**1 a, b** A 2-year-old boy with a dermatofibrosarcoma in the upper thigh. The lesion is associated with skin thickening, as well as a poorly defined zone of intermediate signal on axial T1WI (**a**) in the subcutaneous fat that shows Gd-contrast enhancement on FS T1WI (**b**).

Metastatic disease 281

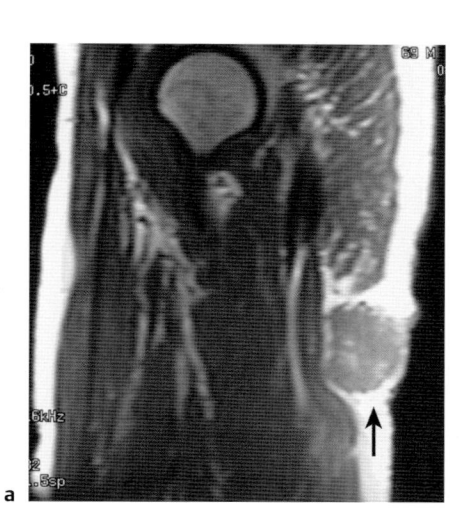

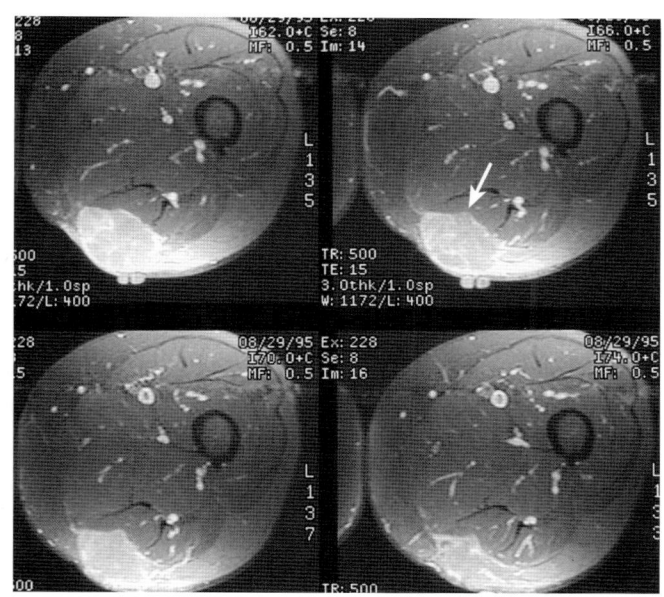

Figure 18.2 a, b A 69-year-old man with a malignant fibrous histiocytoma involving the subcutaneous fat of the posterior thigh. The tumor has intermediate signal on sagittal (a) T1WI and shows slightly heterogeneous Gd-contrast enhancement on axial FS T1WI (b).

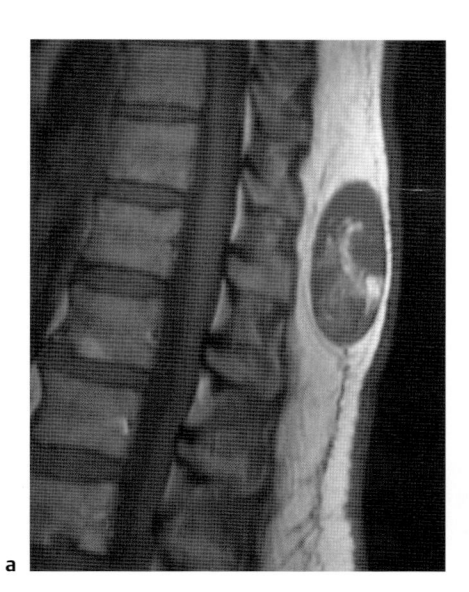

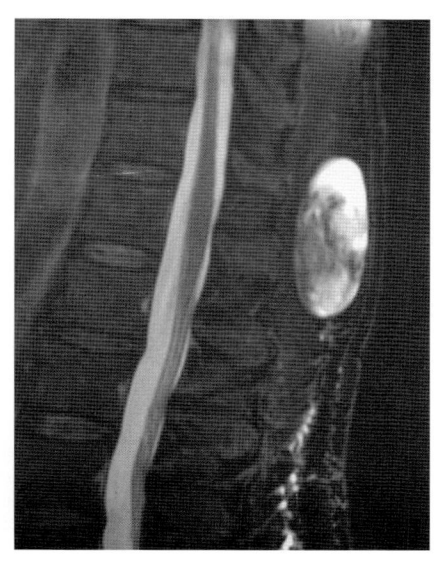

Figure 18.3 a, b A 65-year-old man with a myxoid liposarcoma involving the dorsal subcutaneous fat in the lumbar region. The tumor contains mixed intermediate and high fat signal on sagittal T1WI (a). Myxoid portions of the tumor have high signal on FS T2WI (b). The signal from the small zones of fat is suppressed on sagittal FS T2WI.

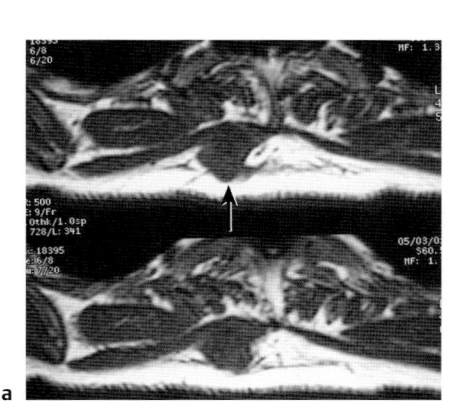

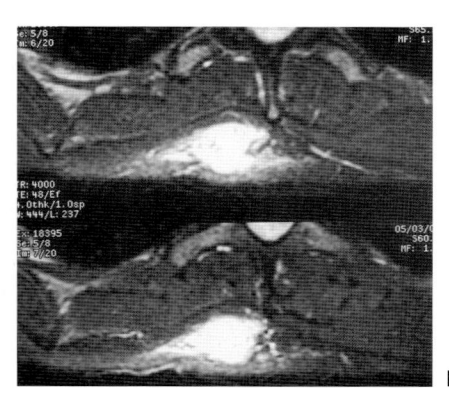

Figure 18.4 a, b Metastatic lesion from lung carcinoma involving the deep subcutaneous fat of the upper dorsal back. The tumor has low-intermediate signal on axial (a) T1WI, and high signal on axial (b) FS T2WI.

Table 18 (Continued)　Tumors and tumorlike lesions of the superficial soft tissues including subcutaneous fat

Lesion	MRI Findings	Comments
Lymphoma (Figs. 18.5, 18.6)	Lymphadenopathy from Hodgkin lymphoma (HL) and lesions of non-Hodgkin lymphoma (NHL) have low-intermediate signal on T1WI and intermediate to slightly high or high signal on T2WI. Variability in MRI signal may be related to differing histologic features (such as the degree of fibrosis) for the subtypes of HL. After Gd-contrast administration, HL and NHL can show variable Gd-contrast enhancement.	Lymphomas are tumors in which neoplastic cells arise within lymphoid tissue. HL usually occurs in lymph nodes and spreads along nodal chains, whereas NHL frequently originates at extranodal sites and spreads in an unpredictable pattern. Mycosis fungoides is a T cell lymphoma that involves the skin. **(See Atlas Chapter A 47)**
Leukemia cutis	Lesions with circumscribed or poorly defined margins with low-intermediate signal on T1WI, intermediate to high signal on T2WI, variable degrees of Gd-contrast enhancement.	Collections of leukemic cells in the epidermis, dermis, and/or subcutaneous fat, associated with poor prognosis. **(See Atlas Chapter A 41)**
Melanoma	Tumors can have low-intermediate signal on T1WI, or slightly high signal on T1WI. Tumors can have low, intermediate, or high signal on T2WI and FS T2WI. Slightly high signal on T1WI and low-intermediate signal on T2WI in melanoma can occur secondary to the presence of melanin (which has T1 and T2 shortening effects). Tumors usually show Gd-contrast enhancement.	Malignant tumors of melanocytes that frequently occur in the skin, and less frequently in the eye and mucosal surfaces. Melanomas can metastasize to brain, bone, cutaneous and subcutaneous tissues.
Squamous cell sarcoma (Fig. 18.7)	Tumors can have irregular margins, and often have low-intermediate signal on T1WI and PDWI, and intermediate to slightly high signal on T2WI and FS T2WI. Tumors can show Gd-contrast enhancement.	Common tumors occurring on sun-exposed sites in older adults. Tumor cells have hyperchromatic and large nuclei, and can break through the basement membrane invading adjacent tissue.
Synovial cell sarcoma (Fig. 18.8)	Tumors are often ovoid and/or lobulated lesions that often have low-intermediate signal on T1WI, and heterogeneous signal (various combinations of intermediate, slightly high, high, and/or low signal) on T2WI. Multiloculated cystic zones are present in 77 %. Calcifications may occur in up to 30 %. Tumors show various patterns of Gd-contrast enhancement.	Mesenchymal tumors comprised of spindle cells and cells with varying degrees of epithelial differentiation. Account for 5 % of primary malignant soft tissue tumors. **(See Atlas Chapter A 75)**

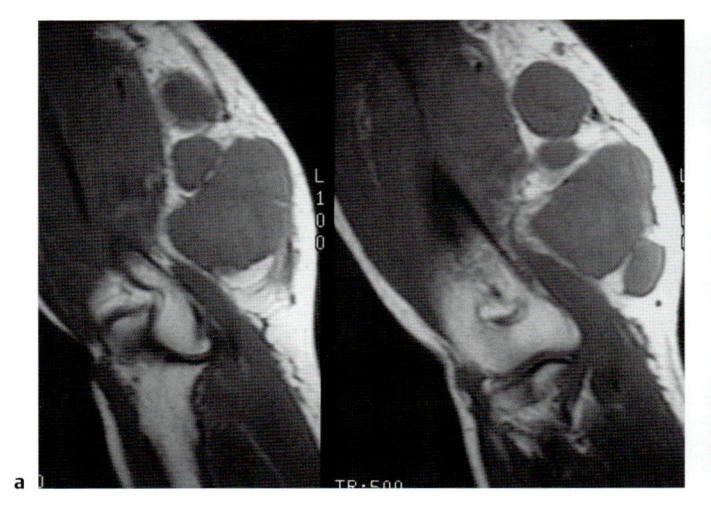

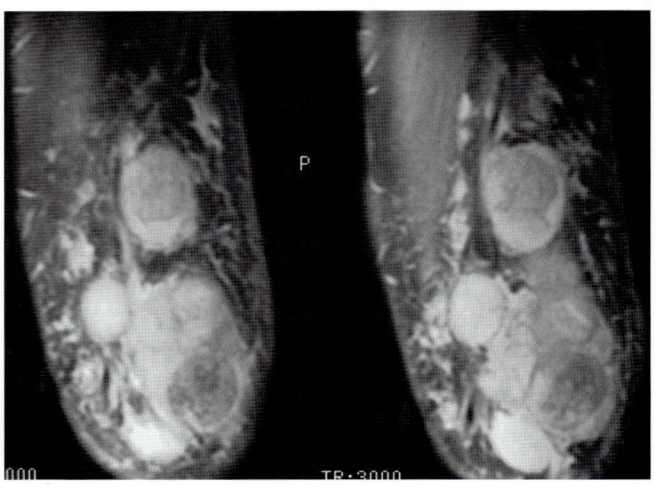

Figure 18.**5 a, b**　A 66-year-old man with diffuse large cell NHL involving the subcutaneous fat, biceps brachii muscle, medial head of the triceps muscle, and neurovascular bundle in the elbow region. Multiple nodular lesions with intermediate signal on coronal T1WI (**a**) are seen which have heterogeneous high signal on coronal FS T2WI (**b**).

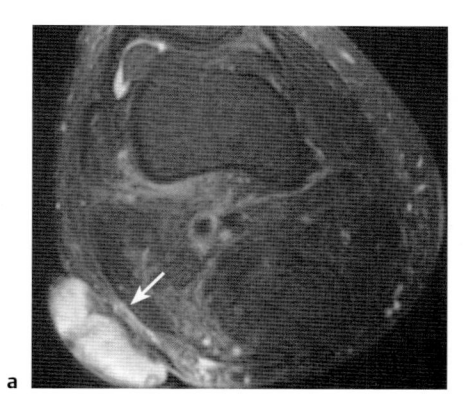

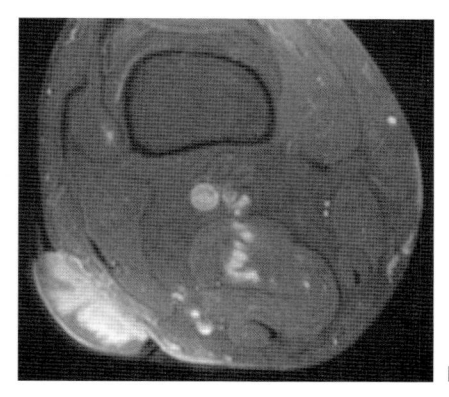

Figure 18.**6 a, b**   A 62-year-old man with T cell lymphoma (mycosis fungoides) involving the skin. The nodular lesion involves the epidermis and has heterogeneous high signal on axial (**a**) FS T2WI and shows heterogeneous Gd-contrast enhancement on axial (**b**) FS T1WI.

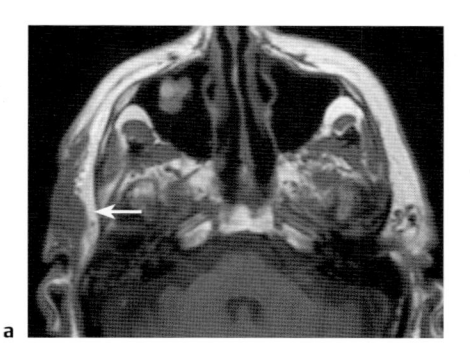

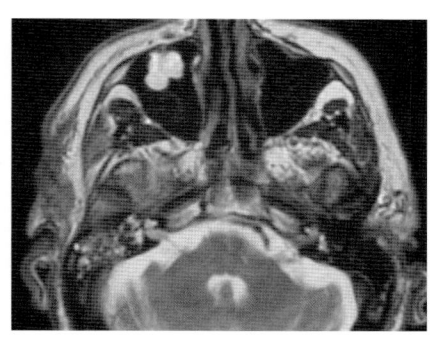

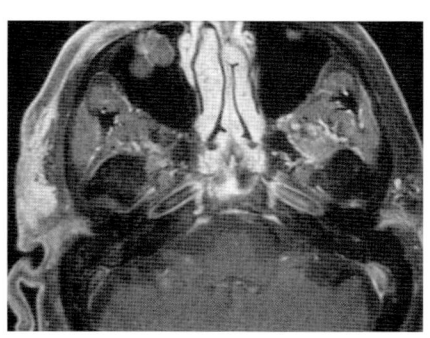

Figure 18.**7 a–c**   An 80-year-old man with squamous cell carcinoma involving the right side of the face. The tumor has irregular margins, and has intermediate signal on axial T1WI (**a**) and axial T2WI (**b**). The tumor shows Gd-contrast enhancement on axial FS T1WI (**c**).

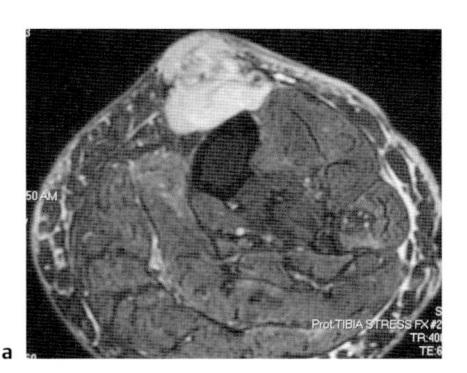

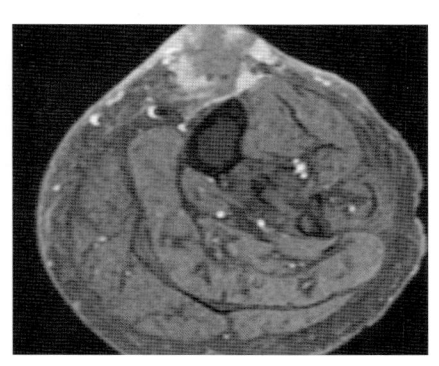

Figure 18.**8 a, b**   An 82-year-old woman with a synovial sarcoma involving the subcutaneous fat of the anterior leg. The tumor has high signal on axial (**a**) FS T2WI and shows heterogeneous Gd-contrast enhancement on axial FS T1WI (**b**).

Table 18 (Continued) **Tumors and tumorlike lesions of the superficial soft tissues including subcutaneous fat**

Lesion	MRI Findings	Comments
Malignant peripheral nerve sheath tumor (Fig. 18.9)	These lesions usually have heterogeneous signal on T1WI and T2WI; as well as heterogeneous Gd-contrast enhancement because of necrosis and hemorrhage. Some malignant peripheral nerve sheath tumors (MPNSTs) are similar in appearance to benign nerve sheath tumors.	MPNSTs are malignant tumors of the peripheral nerve sheath containing mixtures of packed hyperchromatic spindle cells with elongated nuclei and slightly eosinophilic cytoplasm, mitotic figures and zones of necrosis. Approximately 50 % of MPNSTs occur in patients with neurofibromatosis type 1 (NF1), followed by de novo evolution from peripheral nerves. MPNSTs infrequently arise from schwannomas, ganglioneuroblastomas/ganglioneuromas, and pheochromocytomas. **(See Atlas Chapter A 56)**
Leiomyosarcoma (Fig. 18.10)	Lesions may have well-defined or irregular margins and usually have low-intermediate signal on T1WI and PDWI; and intermediate to slightly high or high signal on T2WI and FS T2WI. Large lesions often have zones of necrosis or cystic change that have low signal on T1WI and high signal on T2WI. Solid portions of the lesions usually show Gd-contrast enhancement.	Malignant mesodermal tumors associated with smooth muscle differentiation. Can arise de novo or occur after radiation treatment. **(See Atlas Chapter A 40)**
Rhabdomyosarcoma (Fig. 18.11)	Tumors can have circumscribed and/or poorly defined margins, and typically have low-intermediate signal on T1WI and heterogeneous signal (various combinations of intermediate, slightly high, and/or high signal) on T2WI and FS T2WI. Tumors show variable degrees of Gd-contrast enhancement.	Malignant mesenchymal tumors with rhabdomyoblastic differentiation; occur primarily in soft tissue. **(See Atlas Chapter A 69)**
Hemangioendothelioma (Fig. 18.12)	Tumors have lobulated well-defined or irregular margins, and have intermediate signal on T1WI and heterogeneous predominantly high signal on T2WI with or without internal low signal septations. Flow voids may be seen with the lesions. Tumors show heterogeneous Gd-contrast enhancement.	Low-grade malignant neoplasms composed of vasoformative/endothelial elements that occur in soft tissues and bone. These tumors are locally aggressive and rarely metastasize, compared with high-grade endothelial tumors such as angiosarcoma. **(See Atlas Chapter A 33)**
Angiosarcoma	Tumors have low-intermediate signal on T1WI, mixed low, intermediate, and/or high signal on T2WI, and show prominent Gd-contrast enhancement in a homogeneous or heterogeneous pattern.	Malignant tumors composed of neoplastic blood vessels in bone and/or soft tissues. These tumors can be associated with Paget disease, radiation treatment, bone infarcts, knee and hip prostheses, synthetic vessel grafts, prior trauma or surgery, osteomyelitis, and hereditary disorders (NF1, Maffucci disease, achondroplasia). **(See Atlas Chapter A 6)**

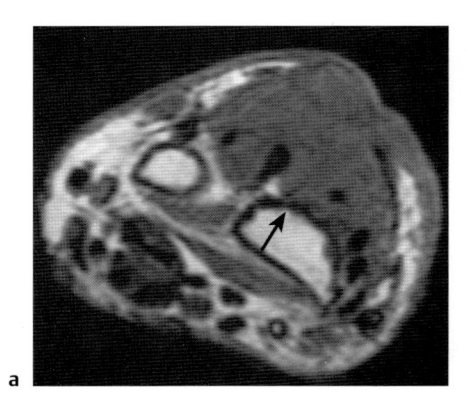

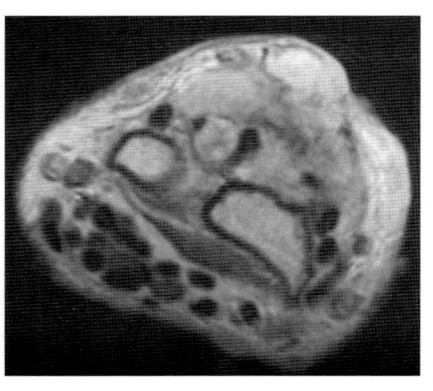

Figure 18.**9 a, b** MPNST in the soft tissues of the wrist in a patient with NF1. The tumor has poorly defined margins and envelops multiple extensor tendons. The tumor has low-intermediate signal on coronal T1WI (**a**) and shows heterogeneous Gd-contrast enhancement on axial T1WI (**b**).

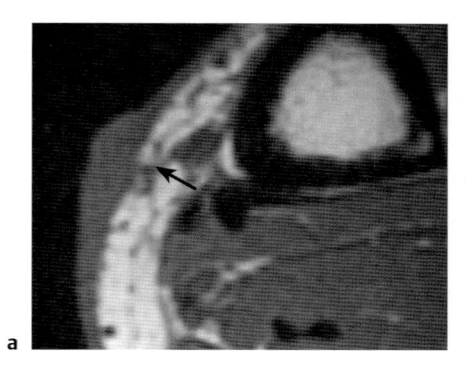

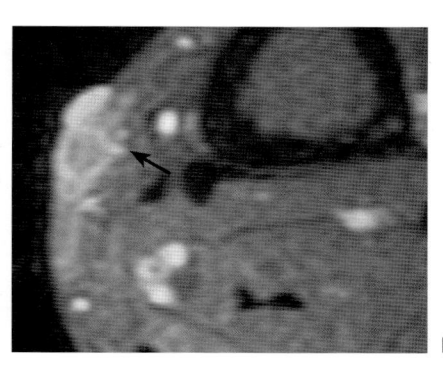

Figure 18.**10 a, b** A 72-year-old man with a leiomyosarcoma involving the dermis with extension into subcutaneous fat. The tumor has intermediate signal on axial T1WI (**a**) and shows heterogeneous Gd-contrast enhancement on axial FS T1WI (**b**).

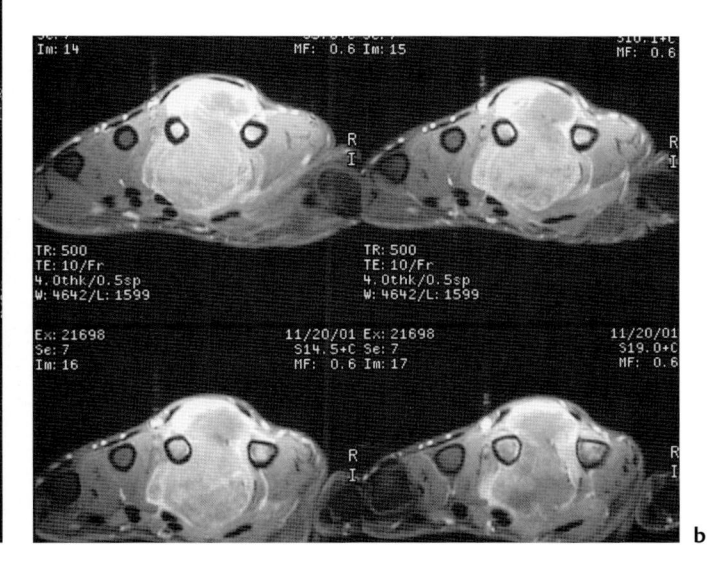

Figure 18.**11 a, b** A 23-year-old man with an alveolar rhabdomyosarcoma involving the soft tissues between the second and third metacarpal bones. The tumor has high signal on coronal FS T2WI (**a**) and shows heterogeneous Gd-contrast enhancement on coronal FS T1WI (**b**).

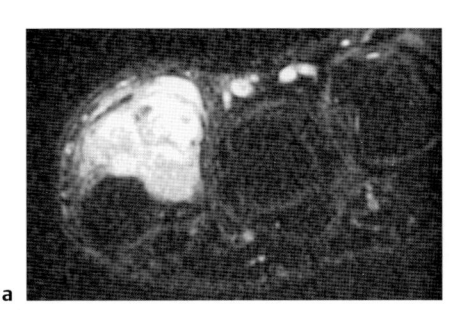

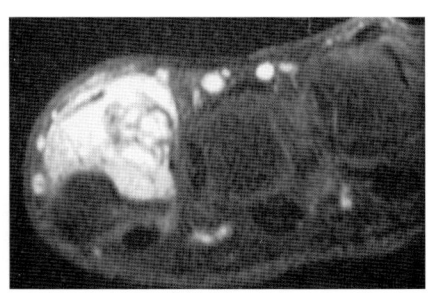

Figure 18.**12 a, b** A 36-year-old man with a hemangioendothelioma involving the dorsal soft tissues of the foot. The tumor has high signal on coronal FS T2WI (**a**) and shows prominent Gd-contrast enhancement on coronal FS T1WI (**b**).

Lesion	MRI Findings	Comments
Extraosseous osteosarcoma (Fig. 18.13)	Tumors have irregular poorly defined or slightly well-circumscribed margins and heterogeneous signal on most MRI pulse sequences. Various combinations of low, intermediate, and/or high signal on T1WI, T2WI, and FS T2WI can be seen depending on the presence and extent of hemorrhage and/or necrosis within the lesions. On T2WI and FS T2WI, tumors often have heterogeneous predominantly high signal. Fluid–fluid levels may be present at sites of hemorrhage or necrosis. Peripheral nonenhancing high signal on T2WI may be present and represent zones of edema and/or tumor invasion within adjacent tissues. Tumors often show heterogeneous patterns of Gd-contrast enhancement.	Malignant tumor comprised of proliferating neoplastic spindle cells that produce osteoid and/or immature tumoral bone. Osteosarcoma most commonly occurs within bone and less frequently on the external surface of bone. Rarely, osteogenic sarcomas can also occur as extraskeletal primary lesions in the soft tissues. **(See Atlas Chapter A 64)**
Extraosseous Ewing Sarcoma	Tumors usually have low-intermediate signal on T1WI and heterogeneous slightly high to high signal on T2WI and FS T2WI. Tumors often show prominent irregular Gd-contrast enhancement.	Malignant primitive tumors of bone and occasionally soft tissue that contain undifferentiated small cells with round nuclei. **(See Atlas Chapter A 20)**
Extraosseous chondrosarcoma (Fig. 18.14)	Tumors have low-intermediate signal on T1WI, intermediate signal on PDWI, and heterogeneous intermediate-high or slightly high signal on T2WI. Foci of low signal on T1WI and T2WI can be seen secondary to chondroid matrix mineralization. Lesions typically show heterogeneous Gd-contrast enhancement.	Malignant tumors containing cartilage formed within sarcomatous stroma, with or without areas of calcification/mineralization, myxoid material and/or ossification. **(See Atlas Chapter A 11)**
Merkel cell tumor (Fig. 18.15)	Tumors can have circumscribed margins, and have low-intermediate signal on T1WI and PDWI, and slightly high to high signal on T2WI. Zones of necrosis with high signal on T2WI may occur within the tumors. Tumors can show Gd-contrast enhancement.	Tumors are rare primary malignant neuroendocrine neoplasms involving the skin and dermis, typically occurring in adults over 60 years. Small round tumor cells contain neurosecretory cytoplasmic granules and are thought to have neural crest origins.
Kaposi Sarcoma (Fig. 18.16)	Tumors can appear as lesions with circumscribed or irregular margins that commonly involve the skin and superficial soft tissues. Tumors often have low to intermediate signal on T1WI and slightly high to high signal on T2WI and FS T2WI. Tumors usually show moderate to marked Gd-contrast enhancement.	Endothelial tumor that is associated with human herpes virus 8 (HHV-8) infections. These tumors are locally invasive and often are located in the cutaneous tissues, mucosa, lymph nodes, and/or visceral organs. **(See Atlas Chapter A 38)**

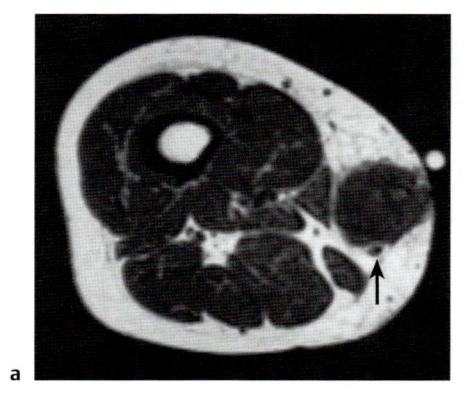

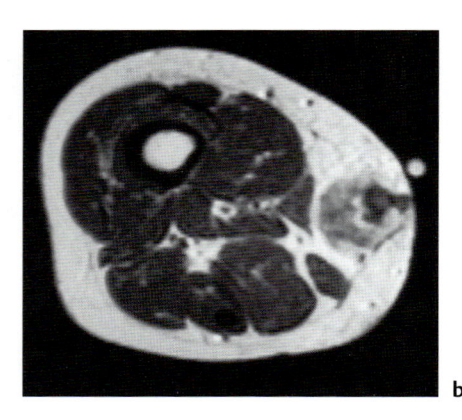

Figure 18.13 a, b A 47-year-old woman with an extraosseous osteosarcoma in the subcutaneous fat of the medial thigh. The tumor has low signal on axial T1WI (**a**) and shows heterogeneous Gd-contrast enhancement on axial T1WI (**b**).

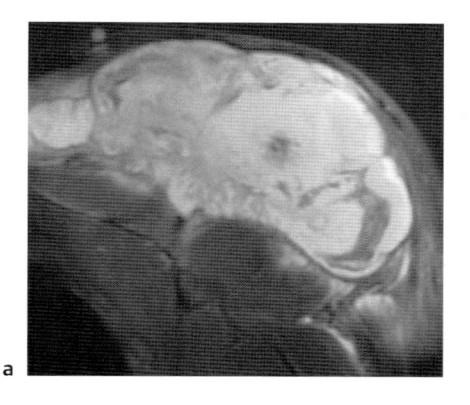

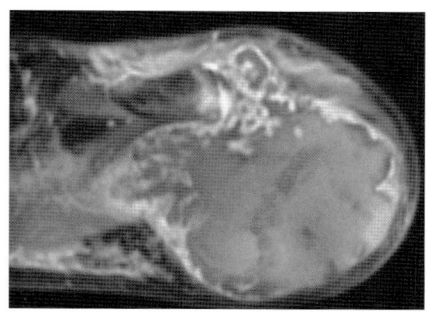

Figure 18.**14 a, b** A 63-year-old man with an extraosseous myxoid chondrosarcoma involving the soft tissues at the left shoulder. The tumor has mostly high signal on coronal FS T2WI (**a**) as well as irregular zones of low signal. The tumor shows lobulated irregular peripheral Gd-contrast enhancement on axial FS T1WI (**b**).

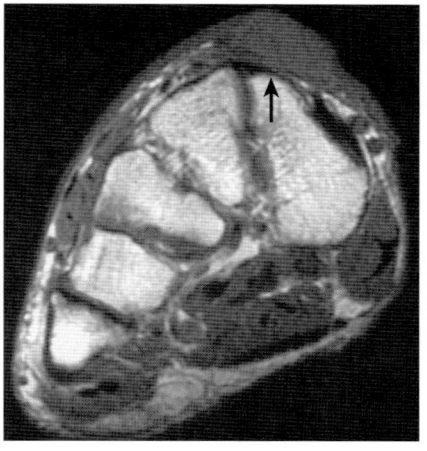

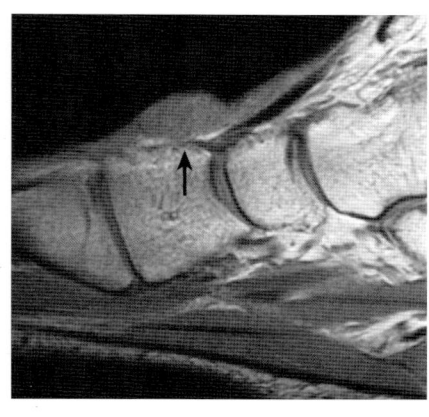

Figure 18.**15 a–d** A 72-year-old man with a Merkel cell tumor involving the dorsal superficial soft tissues of the foot. The tumor has low-intermediate signal on coronal T1WI (**a**) and intermediate signal on sagittal PDWI (**b**) and sagittal T2WI (**c**). The tumor shows moderate Gd-contrast enhancement on sagittal FS T1WI (**d**).

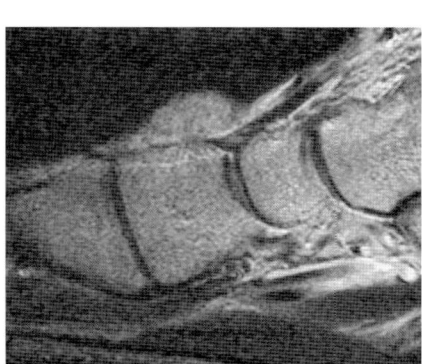

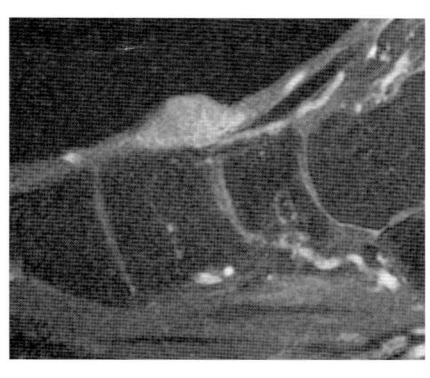

Figure 18.**16** A 70-year-old man with Kaposi sarcoma involving the superficial soft tissues of the foot. The small tumor has high signal on coronal FS T2WI.

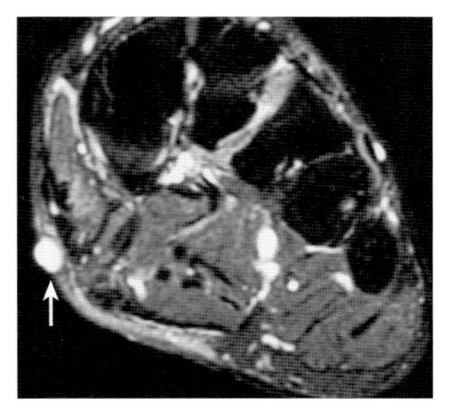

Table 18 (Continued) Tumors and tumorlike lesions of the superficial soft tissues including subcutaneous fat		
Lesion	**MRI Findings**	**Comments**
Epithelioid sarcoma (Fig. 18.17)	Tumors can appear as lesions with circumscribed or irregular margins that commonly involve the skin and superficial soft tissues. Tumors often have low to intermediate signal on T1WI; and mixed low intermediate and/or high signal on T2WI and FS T2WI. Tumors can be solid or can have single or multiple fluid-filled portions with or without hemorrhage or associated inflammatory reaction. Solid portions of tumors can show Gd-contrast enhancement. Marginal Gd-contrast enhancement can be seen at cystic zones.	These sarcomas are firm, slow-growing, aggressive tumors that involve the superficial soft tissues as well as tendons and tendon sheaths. Tumors contain mixtures of eosinophilic epithelioid and spindle cells with nuclear atypia, and occur in young adults (median age = 29 years, female/male ratio 2:1). Recurrence rate of 80% at 10 years, and 5 and 10 year survival rates ranging from 50 to 80%.
Myoepithelial carcinoma (Fig. 18.18)	Tumors can appear as lesions with circumscribed or irregular margins that commonly involve the subcutis and adjacent superficial soft tissues. Tumors often have low to intermediate signal on T1WI; and slightly high to high signal on T2WI and FS T2WI. Tumors usually show Gd-contrast enhancement.	Myoepitheliomas and mixed tumors (*pleomorphic adenomas and carcinomas*) are tumors that usually occur in salivary glands, but can rarely occur in other soft tissues such as the subcutis or deeper soft tissues. Extrasalivary tumors occur in patients with a mean age of 38 years, with near equal gender frequency. Tumors contain epithelioid, ovoid, and/or spindle cells. Unlike benign myoepithelial tumors, malignant tumors have cellular atypia, nuclear pleomorphism, increased mitotic activity, coarse chromatin, and prominent nucleoli. Tumors are typically immunoreactive to keratins (AE1/AE3, PAN-K), and S-100 protein.
Neoplastic-benign		
Lipoblastoma (Fig. 18.19)	Lesions often have mixed low, intermediate, and high signal on T1WI, T2WI, and FS T2WI. Lesions often show heterogeneous Gd-contrast enhancement.	Rare benign mesenchymal tumors that contain embryonal fat. Typically occur in infancy and early childhood. **(See Atlas Chapter A 42)**
Lipoma (Fig. 18.20)	Lipomas in subcutaneous fat often have circumscribed margins and have MRI signal comparable to subcutaneous fat on T1WI, PDWI, T2WI, and FS T2WI. Nonencapsulated superficial lipomas have also been described. Lipomas often show mostly no Gd-contrast enhancement except for minimal to mild enhancement along thin nonfatty septa.	Common benign hamartomas composed of mature white adipose tissue without cellular atypia. Lipomas are the most common soft tissue tumor, representing 10% of all soft tissue tumors and 16% of benign soft tissue tumors. **(See Atlas Chapter A 43)**

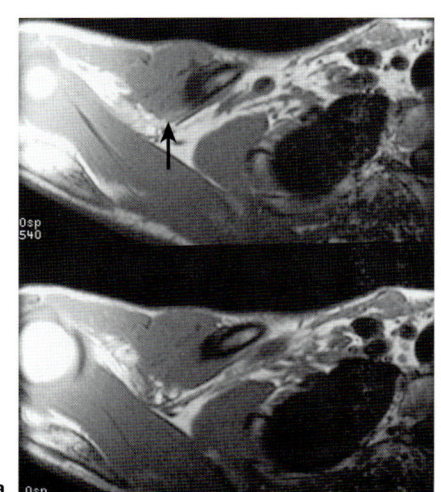

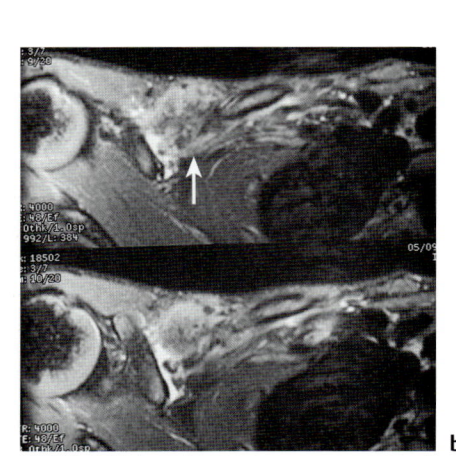

Figure 18.**17 a, b** A 14-year-old boy with an epithelioid sarcoma in the superficial soft tissues adjacent to the right clavicle. The tumor has intermediate signal on axial T1WI (**a**) and mixed intermediate and slightly high signal on axial FS T2WI (**b**).

Lipoma 289

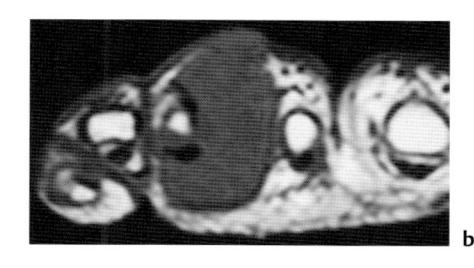

Figure 18.**18 a–e** A 63-year-old man with a myoepithelial carcinoma involving the superficial and subcutaneous tissue between the toes. The tumor has high signal on sagittal (**a**) and axial (**b**) FS T2WI, and intermediate signal on axial T1WI (**c**). The tumor shows Gd-contrast enhancement on axial T1WI (**d**) and axial FS T1WI (**e**).

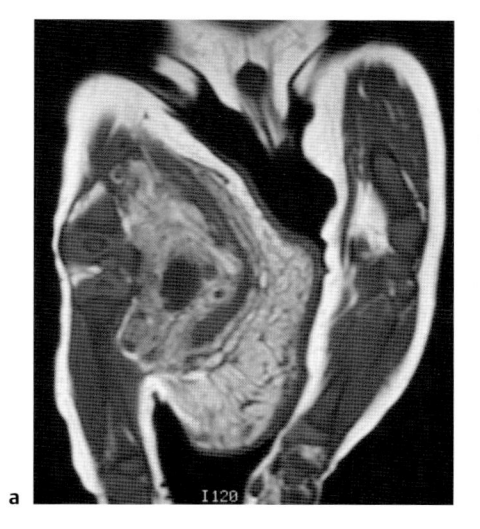

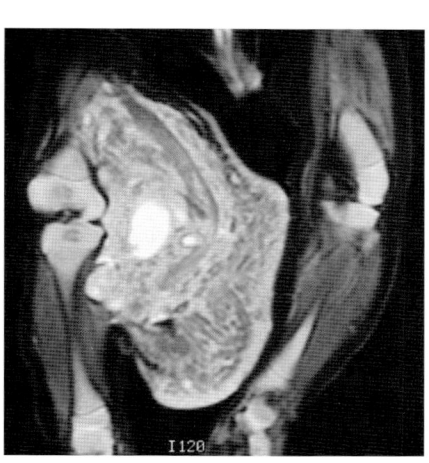

Figure 18.**19 a, b** A 3-month-old boy with a large lipoblastoma that infiltrates the subcutaneous soft tissues and muscles of the thigh. The lesion contains signal approximating that of fat on coronal T1WI (**a**). Many of the fatty zones have signal slightly lower than subcutaneous fat on T1WI as well as higher signal on coronal STIR (**b**). Intralesional bands, septa, and/or nodular zones are seen with low-intermediate signal on T1WI and intermediate-slightly high and high signal on STIR.

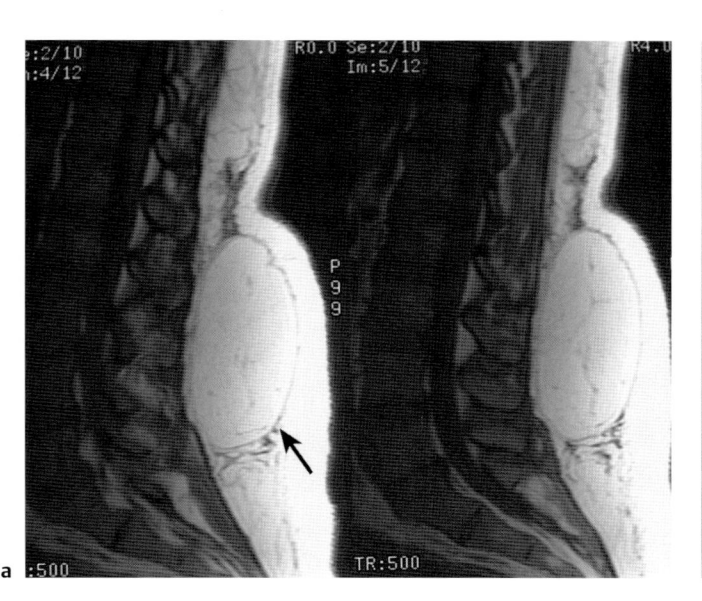

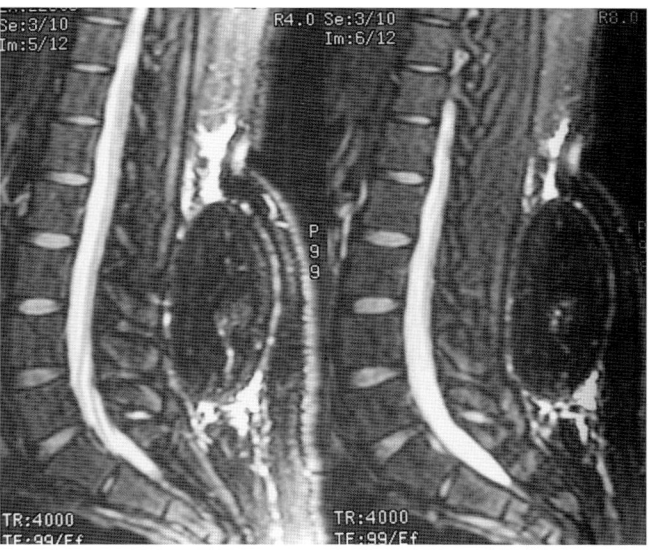

Figure 18.**20 a, b** A 28-year-old woman with a lipoma in the dorsal subcutaneous fat superficial to the lumbar spine. The lipoma has high signal on sagittal T1WI (**a**). The lipoma has a thin capsule of low signal. The signal of the lipoma is suppressed on sagittal FS T2WI (**b**).

Table 18 (Continued) Tumors and tumorlike lesions of the superficial soft tissues including subcutaneous fat		
Lesion	MRI Findings	Comments
Hemangioma (Fig. 18.21)	Hemangiomas have circumscribed margins with or without lobulations, and have low-intermediate signal or heterogeneous low-intermediate and high signal on T1WI and PDWI; and high signal on T2WI. On FS T2WI, hemangiomas typically have high signal except for zones of fat within the lesions. Zones of hemorrhage can sometimes be present in hemangiomas as well as phleboliths. Hemangiomas usually show prominent Gd-contrast enhancement.	Benign hamartomatous lesions of bone and soft tissues composed of capillary, cavernous, and/or malformed venous vessels. (See Atlas Chapter A 34)
Lymphangioma (Fig. 272 in Atlas section)	Can be circumscribed lesions or occur in infiltrative pattern with extension within and between muscles. Often contain single or multiple cystic zones that have predominantly low signal on T1WI and high signal on T2WI and FS T2WI. Fluid–fluid levels and zones with high signal on T1WI and variable signal on T2WI may result from cysts containing hemorrhage, high protein concentration, and/or necrotic debris. Septa between the cystic zones can vary in thickness and Gd-contrast enhancement, and usually have low signal on T1WI and low to intermediate signal on T2WI and FS T2WI. Nodular zones within the lesions can have variable degrees of Gd-contrast enhancement.	Benign vascular tumors that typically occur in soft tissue and only rarely in bone. They result from abnormal proliferation of lymphatic vessels. Lesions are composed of endothelium-lined lymphatic channels interspersed within connective tissue stroma. Account for less than 1% of benign soft tissue tumors, 5.6% of all benign lesions of infancy and childhood. Can occur in association with Turner syndrome and Proteus syndrome. Patients usually range in age from 1 to 50 years, mean = 19 years. Can be congenital, with ~50% present at birth. Approximately 85% are detected by age 2 (See Atlas Chapter A 46).
Nodular fasciitis (Atlas Figs. 109, 110)	Lesions can have mildly irregular or stellate borders. They usually have intermediate signal on T1WI and PDWI and homogeneous or mildly heterogeneous high signal on T2WI and FS T2WI. Surrounding edema is occasionally seen. Older lesions with high fibrous content may have intermediate signal on T2WI. Lesions can show homogeneous or peripheral rim-like patterns of Gd-contrast enhancement.	Benign reactive lesion comprised of proliferating fibroblasts, usually occurring in the subcutaneous tissue or muscle in young adults. (See Atlas Chapter A 21)

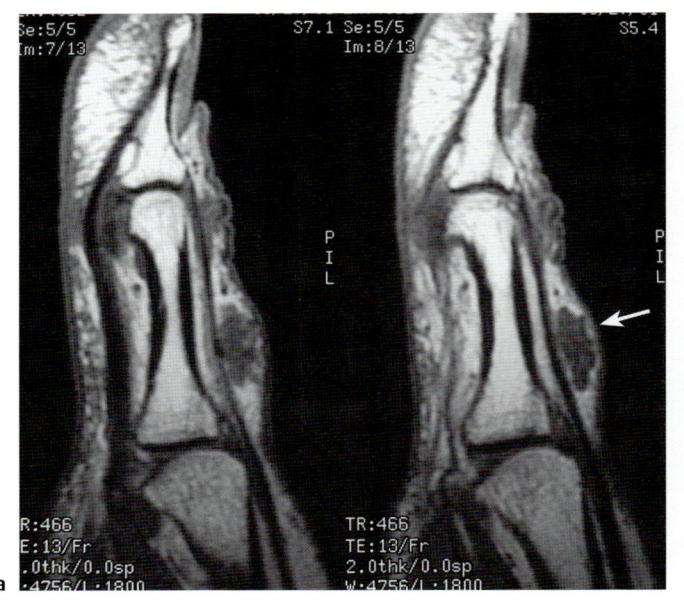

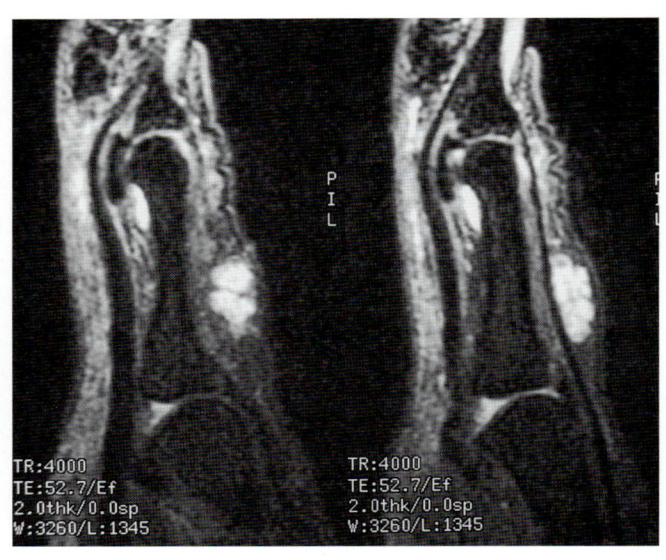

Figure 18.21 a, b A 44-year-old woman with a hemangioma in the dorsal soft tissues of a finger. The hemangioma has circumscribed slightly lobulated margins, and has intermediate signal on sagittal T1WI (a) and high signal on sagittal FS T2WI (b).

Table 18 (Continued)	Tumors and tumorlike lesions of the superficial soft tissues including subcutaneous fat	
Lesion	**MRI Findings**	**Comments**
Nerve sheath tumor (schwannoma, neurofibroma)	**Localized neurofibromas (Figs. 18.22, 18.23) and schwannomas (Fig. 18.24)** are circumscribed ovoid or fusiform lesions with low-intermediate signal on T1WI, intermediate signal on PDWI, and intermediate to high signal on T2WI and FS T2WI. Lesions typically show moderate to prominent Gd-contrast enhancement. Multiple neurofibromas and schwannomas are frequently seen with neurofibromatosis type 1 and 2 (NF1 and NF2), respectively. Neurofibromas can occur in various soft tissues including the skin. **Plexiform neurofibromas (Fig. 18.25)** usually appear as curvilinear and multinodular lesions involving multiple nerve branches. They have low to intermediate signal on T1WI and intermediate, slightly high to high signal on T2WI and FS T2WI with or without bands or strands of low signal. Lesions usually show Gd-contrast enhancement.	Benign nerve sheath tumors include schwannomas and neurofibromas. Schwannomas are benign encapsulated tumors that contain differentiated neoplastic Schwann cells. Neurofibromas are benign tumors of the peripheral nerve sheath that contain mixtures of Schwann cells, perineural-like cells, and interlacing fascicles of fibroblasts associated with abundant collagen. Unlike schwannomas, neurofibromas lack Antoni A and B regions and cannot be separated pathologically from the underlying nerve. Neurofibromas can be localized lesions, or occur as diffuse or plexiform lesions. The presence of multiple neurofibromas is a typical feature of NF1. Multiple schwannomas typically occur in patients with NF2. **(See Atlas Chapters A 56, A 72)**
Paraganglioma	Paragangliomas are circumscribed ovoid or fusiform lesions with low-intermediate signal on T1WI and PDWI, and intermediate to high signal on T2WI and FS T2WI. Multiple tortuous and/or punctate zones of signal void or low signal on PDWI, T2WI, and FS T2WI can be seen within tumors as a "salt and pepper" pattern. Lesions typically show moderate to prominent Gd-contrast enhancement.	Extra-adrenal paragangliomas are benign encapsulated neuroendocrine tumors that arise from neural crest cells associated with autonomic ganglia (paraganglia) throughout the body. In the superficial soft tissues, paragangliomas can occur at the carotid body in the neck or near the vagus nerve. **(See Atlas Chapter A 66)**
Granular cell tumor (Fig. 18.26)	Tumors can have circumscribed and/or irregular margins, and contain low-intermediate signal on T1WI and PDWI, and intemediate, slightly high to high signal on T2WI and FS T2WI. Tumors can also have low-intermediate signal on T2WI. Tumors can show prominent Gd-contrast enhancement.	Rare benign schwannian neoplasms that contain cells with diffuse granular cytoplasm and are immunoreactive to S-100, but not to HMB-45. Tumors are often located in the dermis/subcutis, and occasionally within muscle. Occur more commonly in females compared with males, adults over 30 years old.
Glomus body tumor (Fig. 18.27)	Glomus body tumors are well-circumscribed ovoid lesions measuring less than 1 cm and are often located under the nail beds at the distal phalanges of fingers and toes. Glomus body tumors often have low-intermediate signal on T1WI and PDWI, although may be hypointense or hyperintense on T1WI relative to the adjacent dermis layers. Glomus tumors usually have high signal T2WI and FS T2WI, and typically show Gd-contrast enhancement.	Benign mesenchymal hamartomas derived from the neuromyoarterial apparatus (glomus bodies) that regulate arteriolar blood flow to the skin and are normally present in the reticular dermis throughout the body. Glomus bodies occur in large numbers under the nail beds of the fingers and toes. **(See Atlas Chapter A 31)**
Leiomyoma (Fig. 18.28)	Lesions may have well-defined or irregular margins, and have low–intermediate signal on T1WI and intermediate to slightly high or high signal on T2WI and FS T2WI. Lesions usually show moderate to marked Gd-contrast enhancement.	Benign spindle cell tumors composed of mature smooth muscle bundles. Ninety-five percent of leiomyomas involve the female genitourinary tract, and 3 % occur in the skin with the remainder in the gastrointestinal tract, bladder, and other sites. Cutaneous leiomyomas (leiomyoma cutis) arise from the pilar arrector muscles of the skin, or from the network of muscle fibers in the deep dermis. Angioleiomyomas are tumors that contain mixtures of vascular channels and smooth muscle cells. **(See Atlas Chapter A 39)**
Desmoid tumor (Fig. 18.29)	Lesions can have distinct and/or poorly defined margins, homogeneous or heterogeneous low-intermediate signal on T1WI, and variable intermediate-high signal on T2WI, +/– zones of low signal. Myxoid zones in the lesions can have high signal on T1WI and T2WI. Tumors with high cellularity tend to show higher signal on T2WI than lesions with larger proportions of collagen. Lesions show variable degrees and patterns (heterogeneous versus homogenous) of Gd-contrast enhancement. Pattern or degree of Gd-contrast enhancement by desmoids does not enable prediction of rate of tumor recurrence.	Desmoid tumors or fibromatosis represent a group of soft tissue lesions composed of benign fibrous tissue with elongated or spindle-shaped cells adjacent to collagen. **(See Atlas Chapter A 16)**

292 Table 18 Tumors and tumorlike lesions of the superficial soft tissues including subcutaneous fat

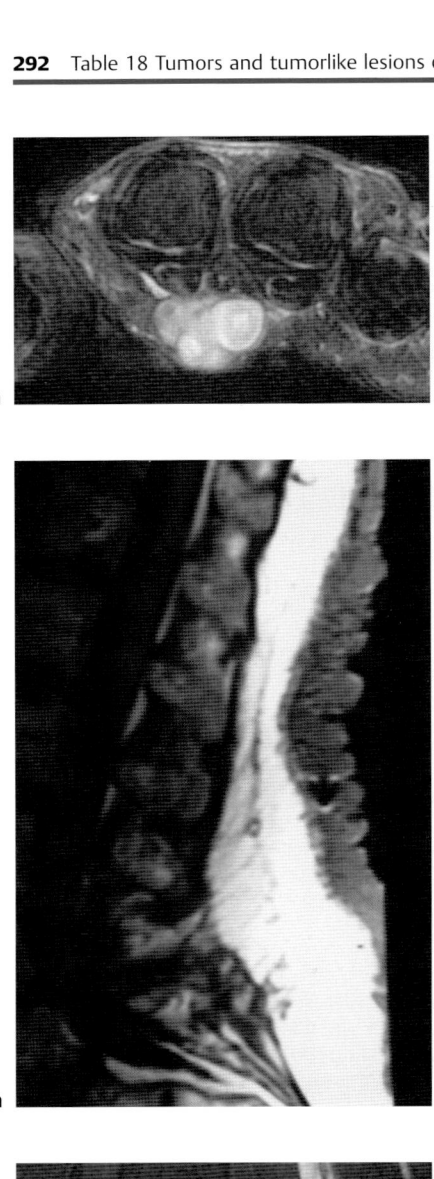

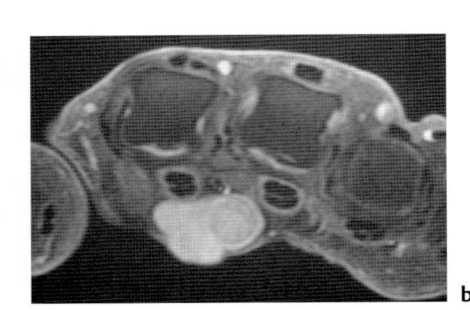

Figure 18.**22 a, b** An 81-year-old woman with a neurofibroma involving the soft tissues ventral to the metacarpophalangeal joint in the hand. The lesion has high signal on axial FS T2WI (**a**) and shows slightly heterogeneous Gd-contrast enhancement on axial FS T1WI (**b**).

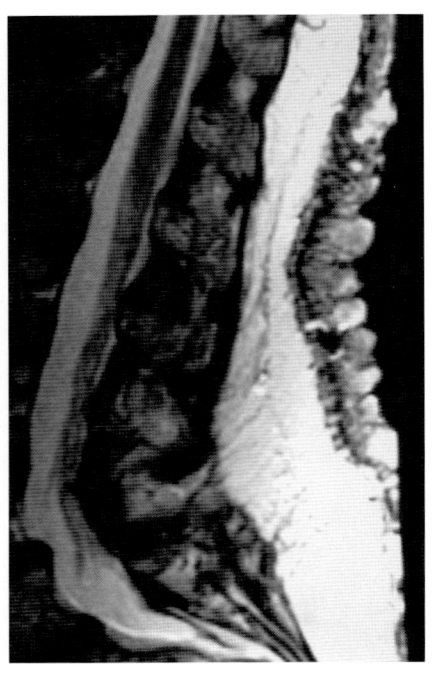

Figure 18.**23 a, b** A 68-year-old woman with NF1 and multiple cutaneous neurofibromas that have intermediate signal on sagittal T1WI (**a**) and mixed intermediate to high signal on sagittal T2WI (**b**).

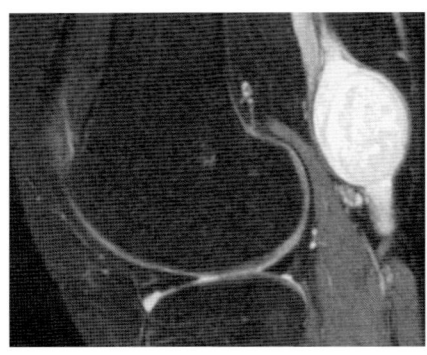

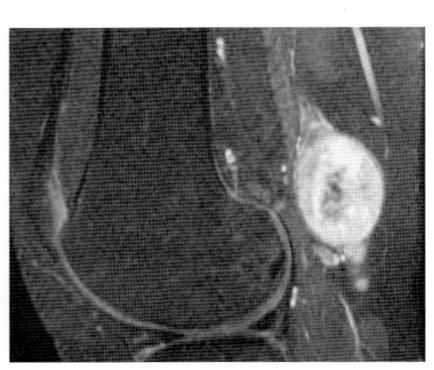

Figure 18.**24 a, b** A 17-year-old woman with a schwannoma involving the tibial nerve at the dorsal knee. The lesion has high signal on sagittal FS T2WI (**a**) and shows prominent Gd-contrast enhancement on sagittal FS T1WI (**b**).

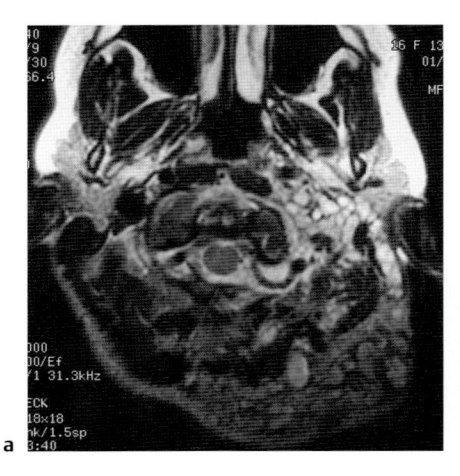

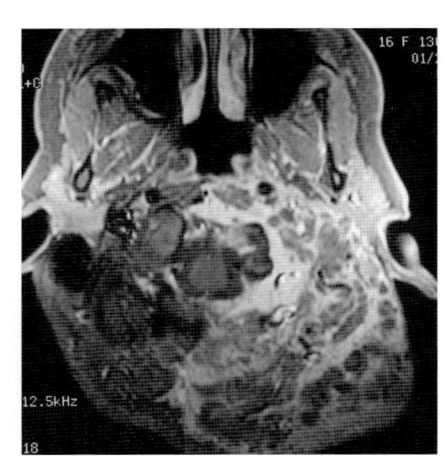

Figure 18.**25 a, b** A 16-year-old female with a plexiform neurofibroma involving the posterior scalp and skull. The lesion appears as curvilinear and multinodular zones with intermediate, slightly high to high signal separated by curvilinear zones of low signal on axial T2WI (**a**). The plexiform neurofibroma shows heterogeneous Gd-contrast enhancement on axial FS T1WI (**b**).

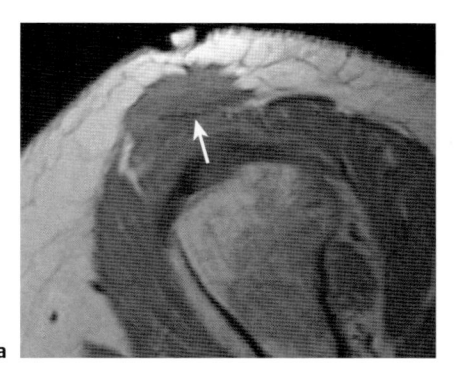

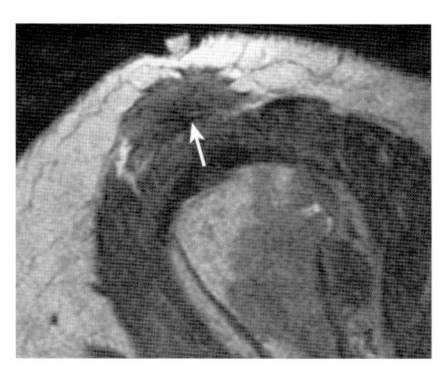

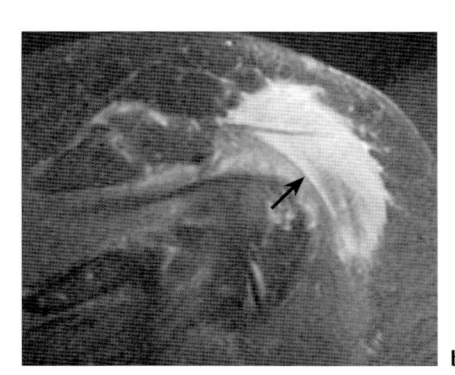

Figure 18.**26 a–c** A 56-year-old woman with a granular cell tumor involving the subcutaneous fat and superficial portion of the deltoid muscle. The tumor has irregular margins and contains low-intermediate signal on sagittal PDWI (**a**) and T2WI (**b**). The tumor shows prominent Gd-contrast enhancement on coronal FS T1WI (**c**).

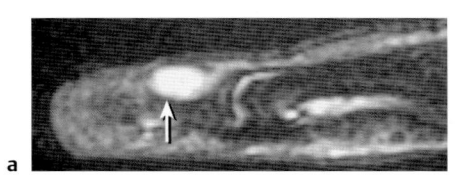

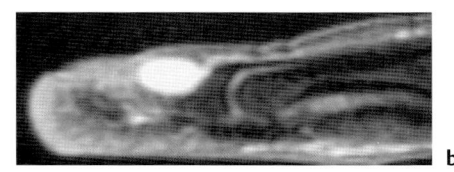

Figure 18.**27 a, b** Glomus tumor in a subungual location of a finger in a 43-year-old woman. The lesion has high signal on sagittal FS T2WI (**a**) and shows prominent Gd-contrast enhancement on sagittal FS T1WI (**b**).

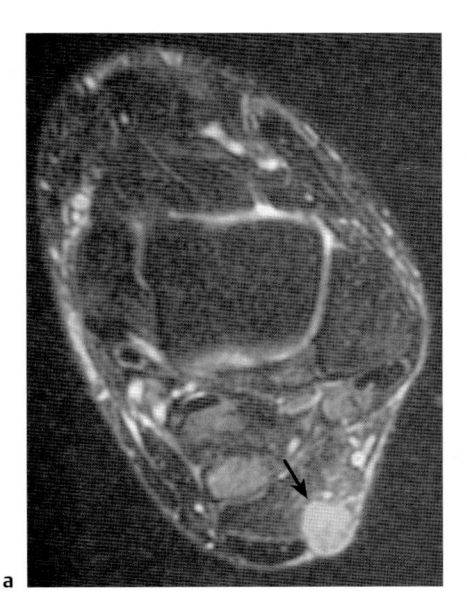

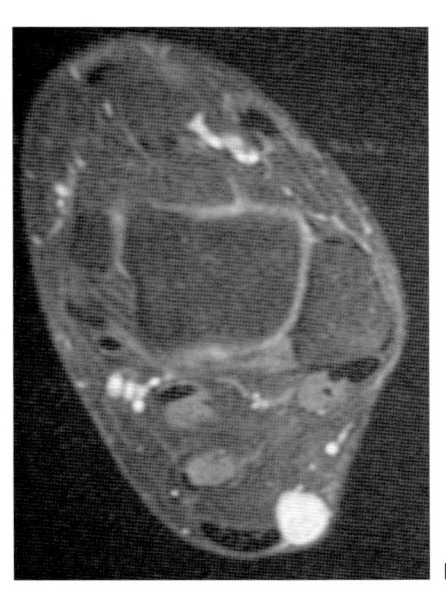

Figure 18.**28 a, b** A 60-year-old woman with a leiomyoma in the subcutaneous fat in the ankle region. The lesion has slightly high to high signal on axial FS T2WI (**a**) and shows prominent Gd-contrast enhancement on axial FS T1WI (**b**).

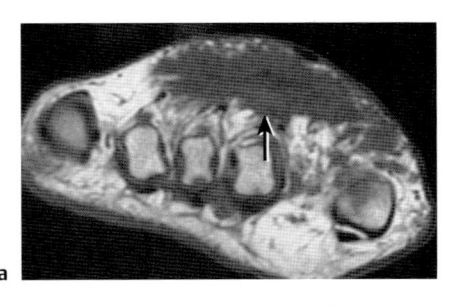

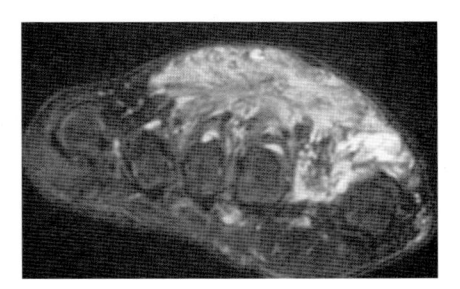

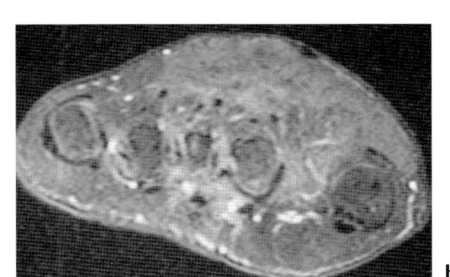

Figure 18.**29 a–c** A 16-year-old male with aggressive fibromatosis (desmoid tumor) involving the dorsal subcutaneous soft tissues of the foot. The lesion has irregular margins and infiltrates adjacent tissue. The lesion has intermediate signal on coronal T1WI (**a**) and heterogeneous high signal on coronal FS T2WI (**b**), and shows only minimal Gd-contrast enhancement on coronal FS T1WI (**c**).

Table 18 (Continued) Tumors and tumorlike lesions of the superficial soft tissues including subcutaneous fat		
Lesion	**MRI Findings**	**Comments**
Myxoma (Atlas Figs. 349–351)	Lesions usually have low or low-intermediate signal on T1WI and PDWI and high signal on T2WI and FS T2WI. Myxomas can have heterogeneous mild or moderate degrees of enhancement in noncystic portions.	Benign lesions containing fibroblasts (spindle cells) and abundant mucoid material (glycosaminoglycans, other mucopolysaccharides). (See Atlas Chapter A 54)
Angiomatoid fibrous histiocytoma (Fig. 18.30)	Tumors can appear as multinodular lesions in the superficial soft tissues with heterogeneous low-intermediate signal on T1WI and PDWI, and heterogeneous high signal on T2WI. Fluid–fluid levels may be seen secondary to hemorrhage. Thin septa with low signal on T2WI may be seen between the multiple nodular zones with high signal. Tumors can show prominent heterogeneous Gd-contrast enhancement.	Low-grade fibrohistiocytic neoplasms that are often located in the deep dermis and subcutis. (See Atlas Chapter A 5)
Pleomorphic hyalinizing angiectatic tumor (Fig. 18.31)	Tumors in the superficial soft tissues can have lobulated and/or irregular/indistinct margins, and have low to intermediate signal on T1WI and PDWI, and slightly high to high signal on T2WI and FS T2WI. Linear or curvilinear zones of low signal on T2WI and FS T2WI can be seen within these tumors. Tumors can show prominent Gd-contrast enhancement.	Pleomorphic hyalinizing angiectatic tumors (PHATs) are rare nonmetastasizing tumors. They contain a spindle cell neoplastic stroma lacking mitotic activity that surrounds aggregates of thin-walled ectatic vessels lined with fibrin. More than 50% involve the subcutaneous tissues of the lower extremity. (See Atlas Chapter A 68)
Tumorlike lesions		
Ganglion cyst (Fig. 18.32)	Ganglia are sharply defined lesions with low signal on T1WI, low-intermediate signal on PDWI, and homogeneous high signal on T2WI. Some ganglia may have intermediate signal on T1WI secondary to elevated proteinaceous or fibrous content. Low signal septa on T2WI can be seen. Peripheral rim-like Gd-contrast enhancement can be seen as well as complete lack of enhancement.	Ganglia are juxta-articular benign myxoid lesions that arise from degeneration of peri-articular connective tissue, prior trauma, or prior inflammation. Ganglia may be derived from tendons, tendon sheaths, joint capsules, bursae, or ligaments. (See Atlas Chapter A 28)
Sebaceous cyst (Figs. 18.33, 18.34)	Lesions usually occur in the subcutaneous fat and have circumscribed margins. Cyst contents often have low-intermediate signal on T1WI, and variable low, intermediate, and/or high signal on T2WI and FS T2WI. Lesions typically do not show Gd-contrast enhancement.	Sebaceous glands are holocrine glands that occur mostly on the face and scalp. These glands shed cells into the excretory stream whose sebum contents include squalene, triglycerides, and wax esters.

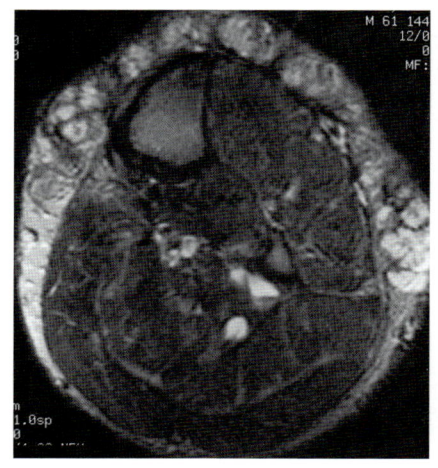

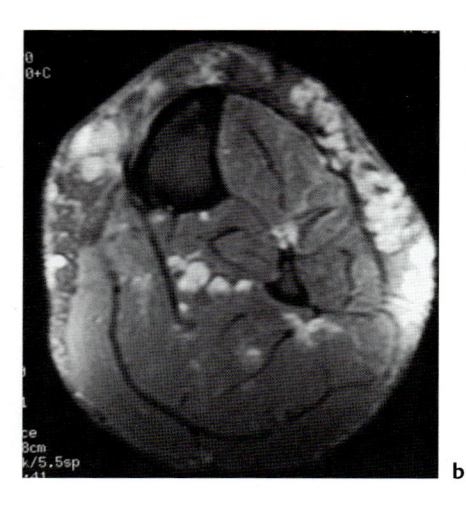

Figure 18.**30 a, b** A 61-year-old man with an angiomatoid fibrous histiocytoma in the subcutaneous fat of the leg. The multinodular lesions in the subcutaneous fat have heterogeneous high signal on axial T2WI (**a**) and show Gd-contrast enhancement on axial FS T1WI (**b**).

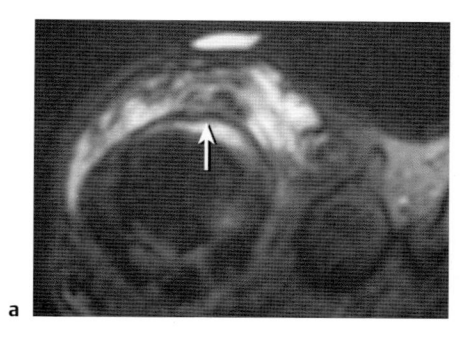

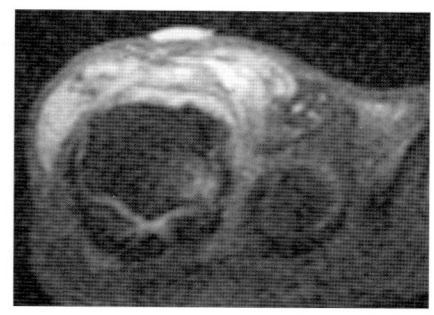

Figure 18.**31 a, b** A 42-year-old woman with a pleomorphic hyalinizing angiectatic tumor involving the dorsal superficial soft tissues of the foot. The tumor has heterogeneous slightly high and high signal on coronal FS T2WI (**a**). Linear and curvilinear zones of low signal on FS T2WI are seen in the lesion. The tumor shows prominent Gd-contrast enhancement on coronal FS T1WI (**b**).

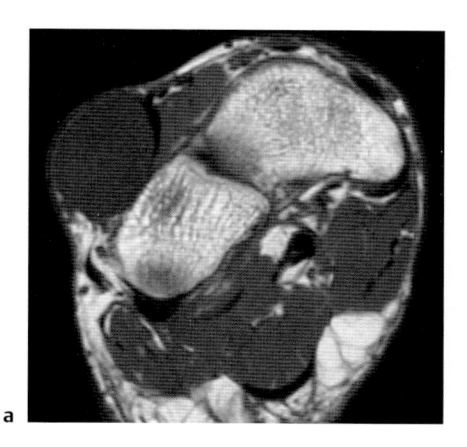

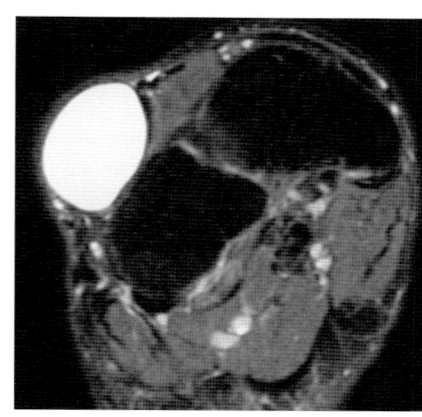

Figure 18.**32 a, b** Ganglion in the dorsal soft tissues of the foot. The lesion has sharply defined margins and has low signal on coronal T1WI (**a**) and high signal on coronal FS T2WI (**b**).

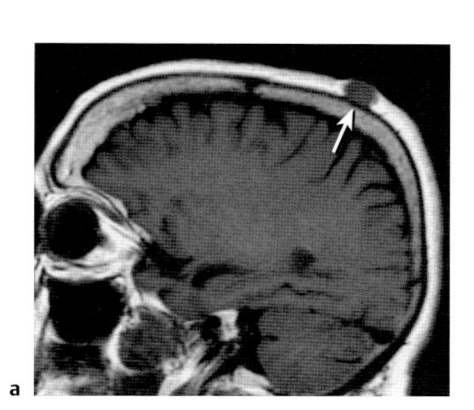

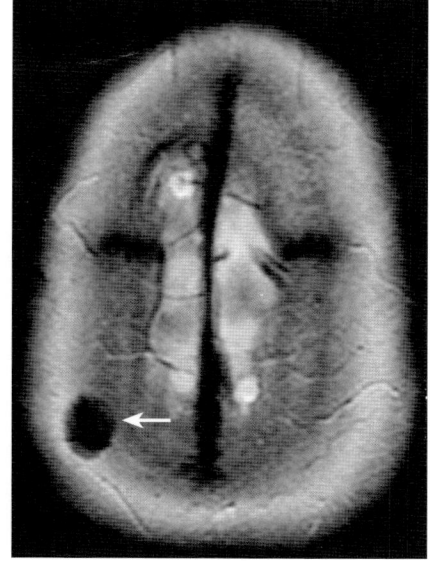

Figure 18.**33 a, b** Sebaceous cyst in the subcutaneous fat of the scalp that has intermediate signal on sagittal T1WI (**a**) and low signal on axial T2WI (**b**).

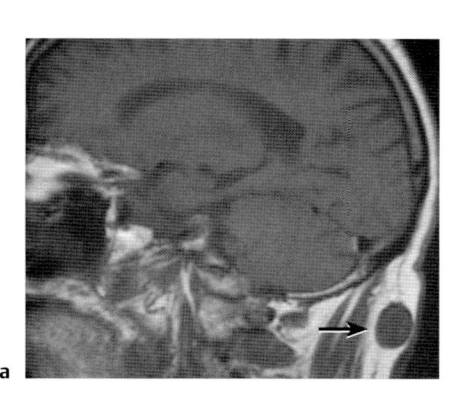

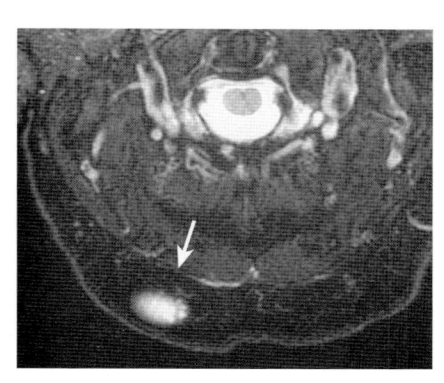

Figure 18.**34 a, b** Sebaceous cyst in the subcutaneous fat of the scalp that has intermediate signal on sagittal T1WI (**a**) and high signal on axial FS T2WI (**b**).

Table 18 (Continued) Tumors and tumorlike lesions of the superficial soft tissues including subcutaneous fat		
Lesion	MRI Findings	Comments
Epidermoid (Fig. 18.35)	Epidermoids are circumscribed lesions with or without lobulated margins, and usually have low signal or low-intermediate signal on T1WI and high signal on T2WI and FS T2WI that may approximate CSF. Lesions occasionally contain foci of high signal on T1WI Epidermoids may show minimal peripheral Gd-contrast enhancement, but no enhancement is typically seen centrally.	Epidermoids are ectoderm-lined inclusion cysts that contain only squamous epithelium. Epidermoids often slowly enlarge, but are not considered to be neoplasms. **(See Atlas Chapter A 15)**
Dermoid	Dermoid cysts are circumscribed lesions with walls with low signal on T1WI and T2WI. The contents of dermoid cysts can have low, intermediate, and/or high signal on T1WI and T2WI **(Atlas Figs. 73–76)** Dermoids may show Gd-contrast enhancement at the wall margins, but not centrally.	Dermoids are ectoderm-lined inclusion cysts that contain hair, sebaceous and sweat glands, and squamous epithelium. Dermoids slowly enlarge, although are not considered to be neoplasms. **(See Atlas Chapter A 15)**
Hematoma/seroma	Acute hematomas (<3–7 days) have mostly intermediate signal similar to muscle on T1WI and mixed low-intermediate and/or high signal relative to muscle on PDWI, T2WI, and FS T2WI. Poorly defined zones of high signal on PDWI, T2WI, and FS T2WI may also be seen peripheral to the hematoma representing adjacent edema. Subacute hematomas (1 week to 3 months) have high and/or intermediate signal on T1WI, and high signal on FS T1WI, PDWI, T2WI, and FS T2WI **(Fig. 18.36)** Peripheral and central zones of low signal on PDWI, T2WI, and FS T2WI can be seen in mid to late subacute hematomas secondary to the presence of hemosiderin from breakdown of blood cells and oxidation/metabolism of hemoglobin. Mild peripheral Gd-contrast may be seen **(Fig. 18.37)** Chronic hematomas (> 3 months) usually have high signal on T1WI, PDWI, T2WI, and FS T2WI. A thick peripheral rim of low signal on T2WI from hemosiderin is often seen with chronic hematomas. Chronic hematomas often evolve eventually into zones with low-intermediate signal on T1WI and T2WI secondary to fibrosis and residual hemosiderin.	Hematomas are extravascular collections of red and white blood cells. They can result from trauma, surgery or coagulopathy (hemophilia, thrombocytopenia, medications/coumadin/heparin, and sepsis). **(See Atlas Chapter A 36)**
Morel-Lavallee lesion (Atlas Fig. 202)	Circumscribed collection in the subcutaneous fat often with low to intermediate signal on T1WI, and high signal on T2WI. A thin or slightly thick rim of low signal on T2WI is often present.	High-velocity injury to the superficial soft tissues in which there is internal degloving or separation of the skin and subcutis from the fascia resulting in a collection filled with fluid and debris. Most often occurs in the pelvic subcutaneous fat. **(See Atlas Chapter A 36)**
Heterotopic ossification (Fig. 18.38)	The MRI features vary depending on the age, location, and degree of mineralization/ossification. Lesions <2 weeks have localized mass effect with poorly defined margins, heterogeneous low-intermediate or slightly high signal on T1WI, and heterogeneous slightly high to high signal on T2WI and FS T2WI. Poorly defined zones of high signal on T2WI may be seen in the adjacent soft tissues. After 2 weeks, curvilinear and/or amorphous zones of low signal on T2WI and FS T2WI can be seen at the peripheral portions of the subacute lesions resulting from mineralization/ossification. Subsequent progressive centripetal mineralization/ossification appears as irregular zones of low signal on T2WI. During this process, heterogeneous Gd-contrast enhancement is typically seen. Old lesions usually have well-defined margins, and have variable low signal on T1WI, PDWI, and T2WI depending on the degree of mineralization/ossification, fibrosis, and hemosiderin deposition. Zones of high signal on T1WI and T2WI may occur from fatty marrow metaplasia. Gd-contrast enhancement in old mature lesions is often minimal or absent.	Heterotopic ossification or myositis ossificans are non-neoplastic reparative extra-osseous lesions that are composed of reactive hypercellular fibrous tissue, cartilage, and/or bone. These lesions can arise secondary to trauma (myositis ossificans circumscripta, ossifying hematoma), though may also occur without a history of prior injury (pseudomalignant osseous tumor of the soft tissues). **(See Atlas Chapter A 53)**

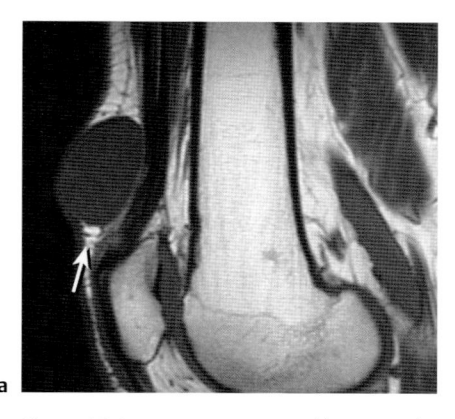

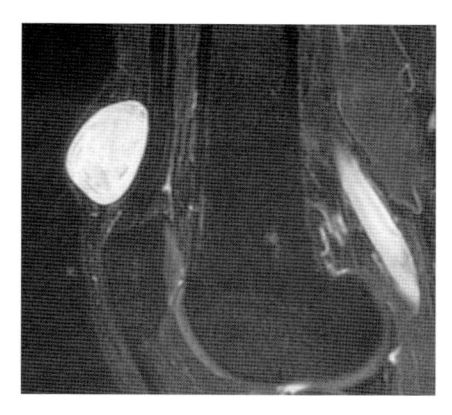

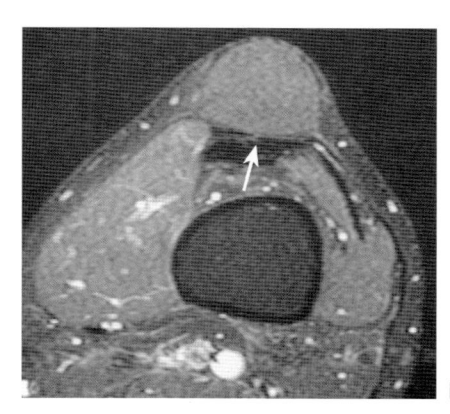

Figure 18.**35 a–c** A 25-year-old man with an epidermoid involving the anterior soft tissues at the knee. The lesion has low-intermediate signal on sagittal PDWI (**a**) and high signal on sagittal FS T2WI (**b**). The lesion shows no Gd-contrast enhancement on axial FS T1WI (**c**).

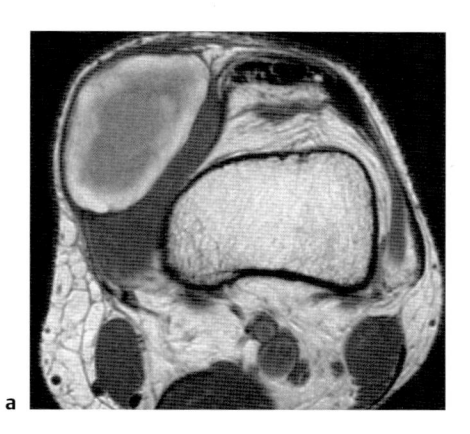

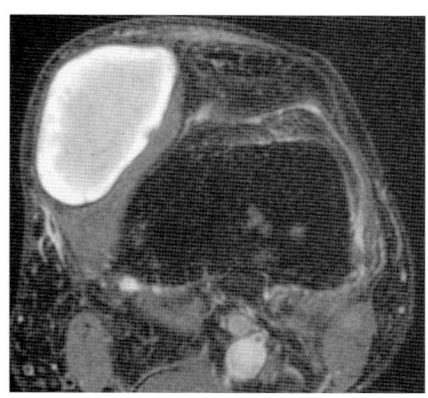

Figure 18.**36 a, b** A 40-year-old woman with a hematoma in the soft tissues at the medial knee. The tumor has mixed high and intermediate signal on axial PDWI (**a**) and high and slightly high signal on axial FS T2WI (**b**). The hematoma is surrounded by a rim of low signal on PDWI and FS T2WI.

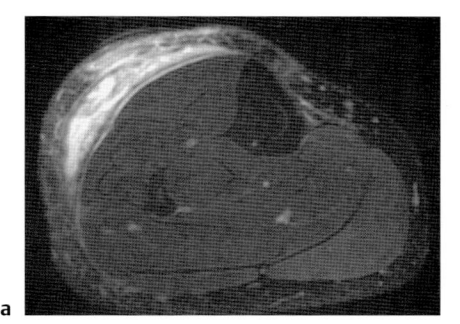

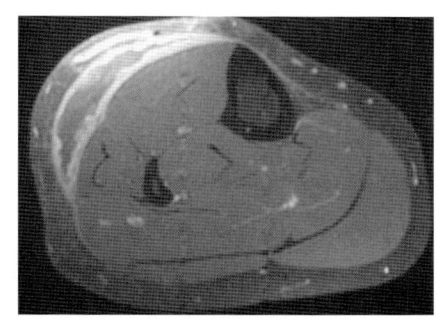

Figure 18.**37 a, b** A 14-year-old girl with a subacute hematoma in the subcutaneous fat of the medial leg. The tumor has heterogeneous high and slightly high signal on axial FS T2WI (**a**). The hematoma has intermediate signal centrally and shows irregular peripheral zones of Gd-contrast enhancement on axial FS T1WI (**b**).

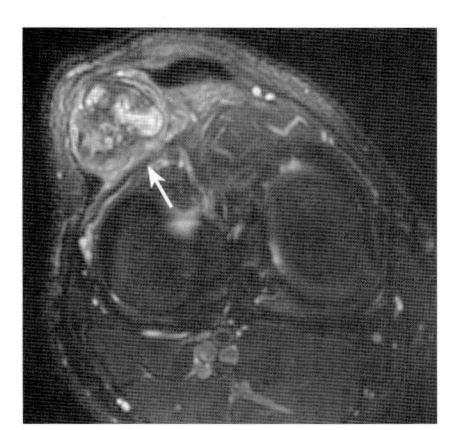

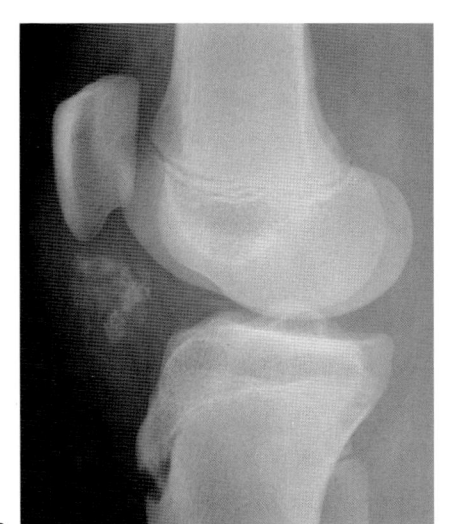

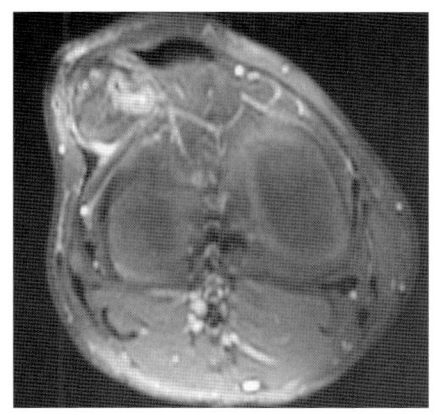

Figure 18.**38 a–c** A 15-year-old male with myositis ossificans involving the soft tissues anterior to the distal femur and lateral to the patellar tendon. Lateral radiograph (**a**) shows amorphous mineralization in the infrapatellar soft tissues. The lesion has heterogeneous high, intermediate, and low signal on axial FS T2WI (**b**). The lesion shows heterogeneous Gd-contrast enhancement on axial FS T1WI (**c**).

Table 18 (Continued) Tumors and tumorlike lesions of the superficial soft tissues including subcutaneous fat		
Lesion	MRI Findings	Comments
Amyloidoma	Lesions in soft tissue can have low-intermediate signal on T1WI, and intermediate to slightly high signal on T2WI. Lesions can show Gd-contrast enhancement.	Uncommon disease in which various tissues (including bone, muscle, tendons, tendon sheaths, ligaments, and synovium) are infiltrated with extracellular eosinophilic material composed of insoluble proteins with β-pleated sheet configurations (amyloid protein). Amyloidomas are single sites of involvement. Amyloidosis can be a primary disorder associated with an immunologic dyscrasia or secondary to a chronic inflammatory disease.
Aneurysm (Figs. 18.39, 18.40)	Saccular aneurysms are focal well-circumscribed structures contiguous with arteries. Signal voids are usually seen where there is fast blood flow in nonthrombosed portions of the aneurysms. Variable mixed signal on T1WI and T2WI can be seen in thrombosed portions of the aneurysms.	Aneurysms are focal or diffuse zones of arterial dilatation that are associated with wall abnormalities and increased risk of rupture. Focal aneurysms are also referred to as saccular aneurysms; they typically occur at arterial branch points. Giant aneurysms are saccular aneurysms that measure >2.5 cm in diameter.
Hypothenar hammer injury (Fig. 18.41)	Thrombosis of the distal ulnar artery can be seen as lack of intraluminal signal void. The thrombosed vessel can have intermediate to high signal on T1WI, and heterogeneous high signal on FS T2WI.	Thrombosis of the superficial branch of the distal ulnar artery can occur from trauma as it travels along the hypothenar muscles after exiting from Guyon canal. Emboli into the superficial palmar arch can result in symptoms.
Inflammatory		
Abscess (Fig. 18.42)	Lesions usually contain a circumscribed portion that has low signal on T1WI and high signal on T2WI (with or without an air–fluid level) that is surrounded by a rim of low signal on T2WI. Rim-like Gd-contrast enhancement is usually seen. Peripherally, a poorly defined zone of high signal may be seen secondary to edema and/or inflammation.	Abscesses are inflammatory lesions that are formed when liquefaction and necrosis occurs at sites of infection, are often enclosed by a pseudocapsule and surrounded by zones of edema and inflammatory reaction. Infectious organisms commonly include bacteria and fungi.

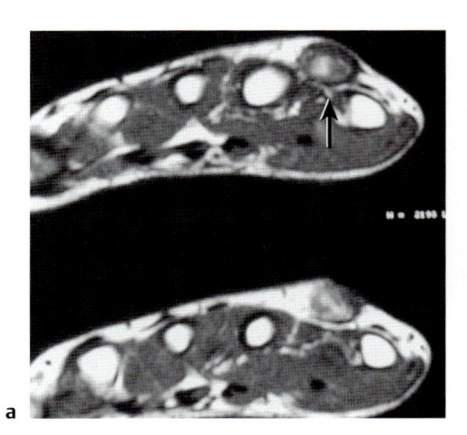

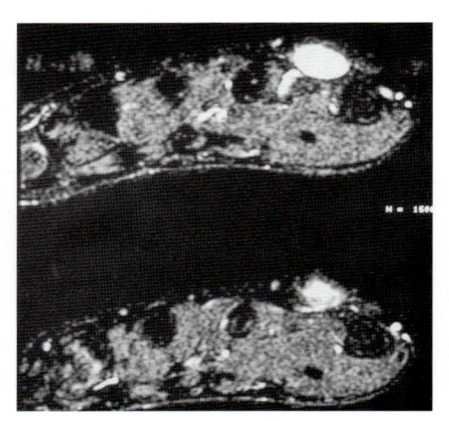

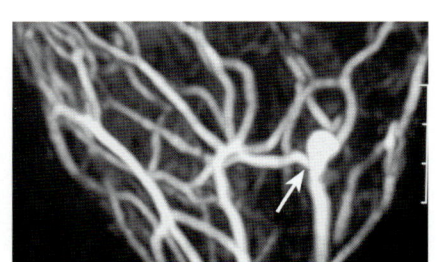

Figure 18.39 a–c Aneurysm of the radial artery has mixed intermediate and high signal on axial PDWI (**a**) and high signal on axial FS T2WI (**b**). The aneurysm is seen on the 3 D time-of-flight MRA (**c**).

Abscess 299

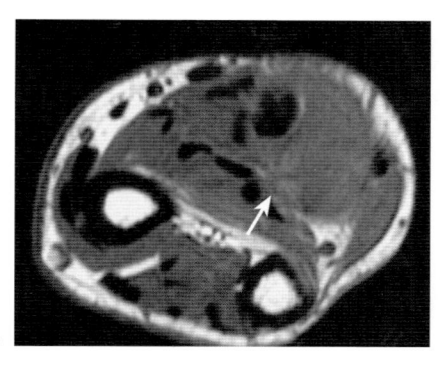

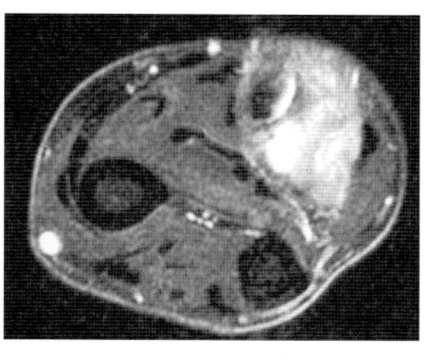

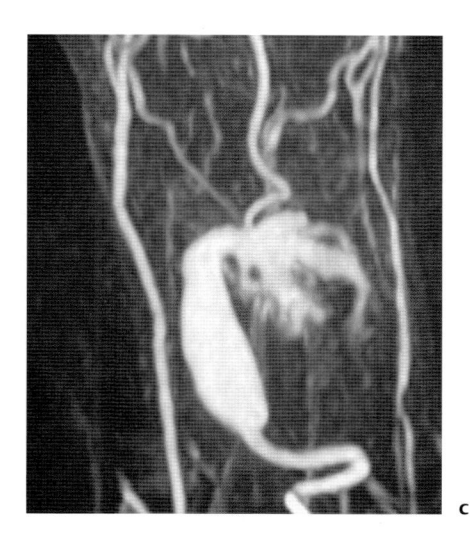

Figure 18.**40 a–c** A large aneurysm of the ulnar artery is seen. The aneurysm has a flow void on axial T1WI (**a**) and FS T2WI (**b**) representing a patent channel adjacent to thrombus that has intermediate signal on T1WI and heterogeneous high signal on FS T2WI. The aneurysm is seen on the 3D time-of-flight MRA (**c**).

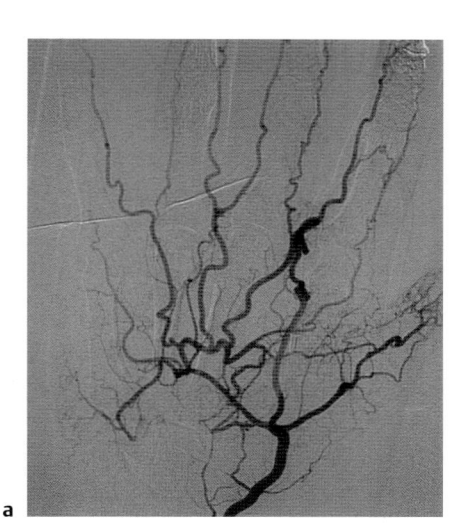

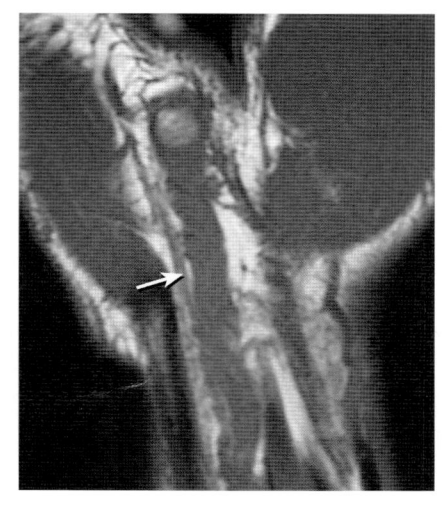

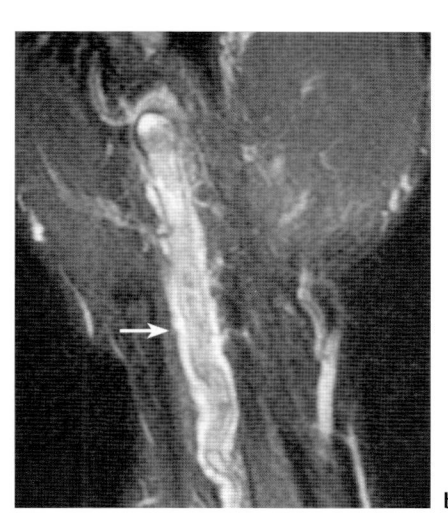

Figure 18.**41 a–d** Hypothenar hammer injury in a 46-year-old man resulting in thrombosis of the ulnar artery. The arteriogram (**a**) shows occlusion of the ulnar artery and patency of the radial artery. The occluded ulnar artery contains intermediate and high signal on coronal T1WI (**b**) and heterogeneous mostly high signal on coronal (**c**) and axial (**d**) FS T2WI.

Figure 18.**42** A 75-year-old man with an abscess in the superficial soft tissues at the elbow. The abscess has irregular peripheral margins of Gd-contrast enhancement surrounding nonenhancing fluid/pus on sagittal FS T1WI.

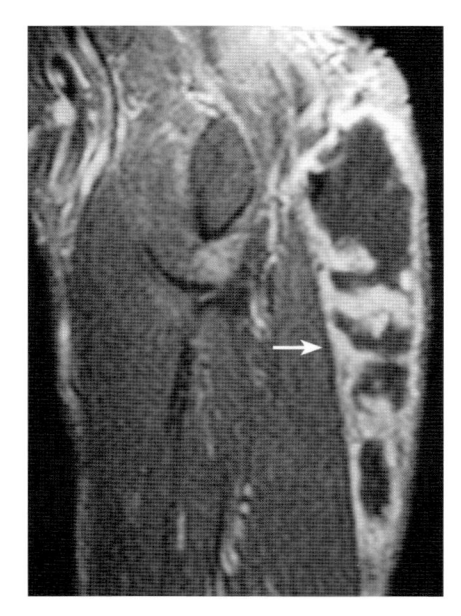

Table 18 (Continued) Tumors and tumorlike lesions of the superficial soft tissues including subcutaneous fat

Lesion	MRI Findings	Comments
Cat-scratch disease (Fig. 18.43)	Single or multiple enlarged lymph nodes are often seen, as well as localized granulomatous lesions. Lesions often occur in the epitrochlear and axillary regions, have low-intermediate signal on T1WI and intermediate to high signal on T2WI. Lesions can have irregular margins with peripheral edematous changes. Lesions can show Gd-contrast enhancement.	Infection by the Gram-negative bacillus *Bartonella henselae* can result in self-limited regional adenitis. This infection usually occurs in patients < 30 years and is often related to contact with cats.
Parasitic infection	Parasitic infections can vary from cystic-appearing lesions to poorly marginated or circumscribed solid lesions depending on the infectious organism and stage of its life cycle.	Parasitic infections can occur in soft tissues in endemic regions or in immunocompromised patients.
Granuloma annulare	Poorly defined subcutaneous lesion with intermediate signal on T1WI, and heterogeneous low to slightly high signal on T2WI.	Benign inflammatory disorder that can involve the epidermis, dermis, and subcutaneous fat. Often occurs in children and young adults. Lesions can occur as localized, generalized, or subcutaneous forms. The localized type can appear as one or more lesions. The generalized type has a slightly wider distribution than the localized type. The subcutaneous type often affects children between 2 and 5 years.
Sarcoid (Fig. 18.44)	Sarcoid granulomas can also occur in subcutaneous fat and may be associated with superficial adenopathy. Lesions are often nodular with low to intermediate signal on T1WI, and intermediate to high signal on T2WI. Lesions usually show Gd-contrast enhancement. Sarcoid can also involve muscles as discrete lesions.	Chronic systemic granulomatous disease of unknown etiology in which noncaseating granulomas occur in various tissues and organs. Common sites of involvement include the lungs, lymph nodes, liver, spleen, skin, and eyes. **(See Atlas Chapter A 71)**
Giant cell reaction to foreign body	Lesions usually occur in soft tissue and often have low-intermediate signal on T1WI and low, intermediate, and/or high signal on T2WI. Lesions can show Gd-contrast enhancement. Sites of bone erosion and/or destruction may be seen, particularly with penetrating trauma. The MRI signal of the foreign body varies based on its composition.	Reactive granulomatous lesions can form adjacent to foreign bodies, and may simulate neoplasm.
Gout (Fig. 18.45)	Tophi have variable sizes and shapes, and have low-intermediate signal on T1WI, FS T2WI, and T2WI. Zones of high signal on T2WI can also be seen in tophi. Erosions of bone, synovial pannus, joint effusion, bone marrow, and soft tissue edema can be seen with MRI. Tophi may show heterogeneous, diffuse, or peripheral/marginal Gd-contrast enhancement patterns.	Gout is an inflammatory disease involving synovium resulting from deposition of monosodium urate crystals and occurs when the serum urate level exceeds its solubility in various tissues and body fluid. **(See Atlas Chapter A 32)**

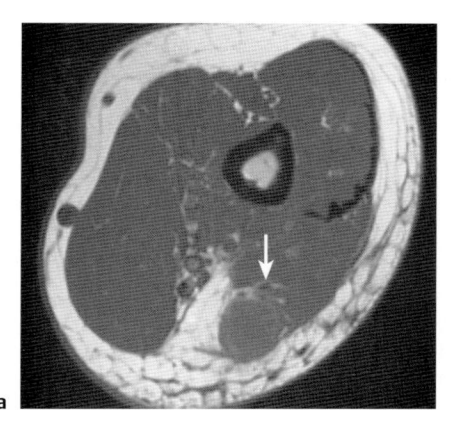

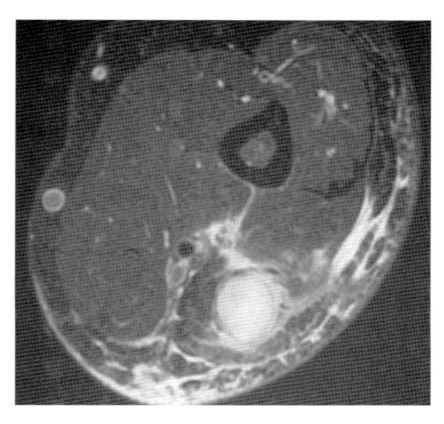

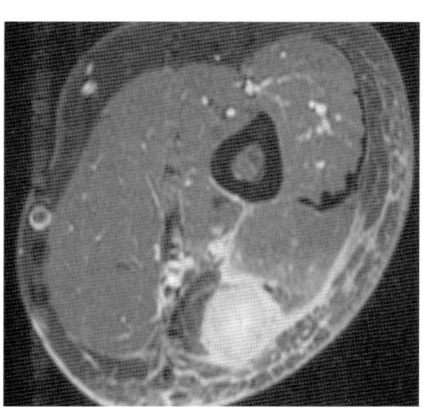

Figure 18.**43 a–c** A 45-year-old man with cat scratch disease with a granuloma involving a lymph node in the distal arm. The nodular lesion has intermediate signal on axial T1WI (**a**) and slightly high to high signal on axial FS T2WI (**b**). The lesion shows Gd-contrast enhancement on axial FS T1WI (**c**). Irregular zones of inflammatory reaction are seen in the soft tissues peripheral to the nodular lesion.

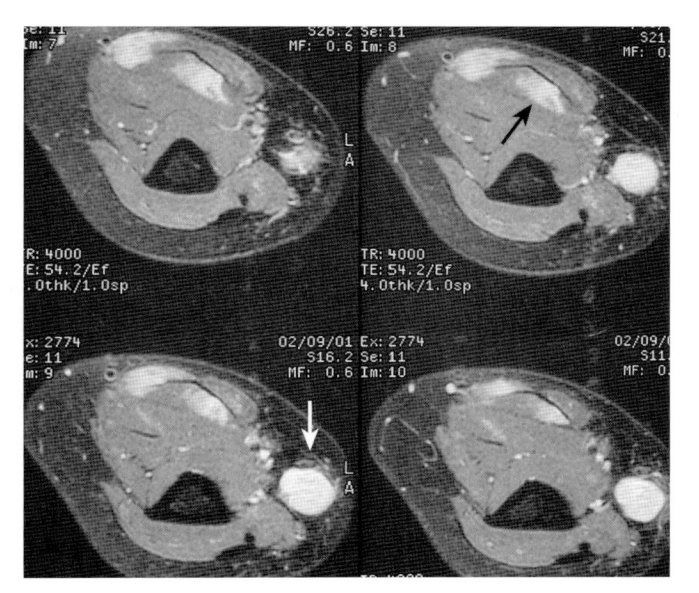

Figure 18.**44** A 49-year-old woman with sarcoid granulomas in the subcutaneous fat and within the biceps brachii muscle at the distal arm. The lesions have slightly irregular margins, and have high signal on axial FS T2WI.

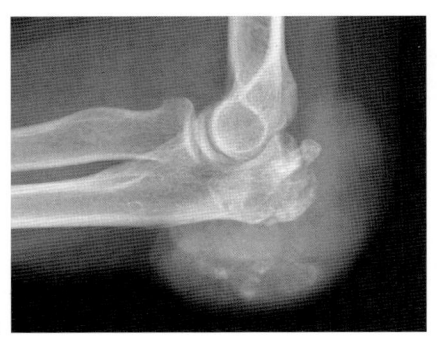

Figure 18.**45 a–c** A 57-year-old woman with gout and a large tophus containing several calcifications in the superficial soft tissues at the elbow associated with bone erosion as seen on a lateral radiograph (**a**). The tophus has intermediate signal on sagittal T1WI (**b**) and mixed high, slightly high, intermediate, and low signal on sagittal FS T2WI (**c**).

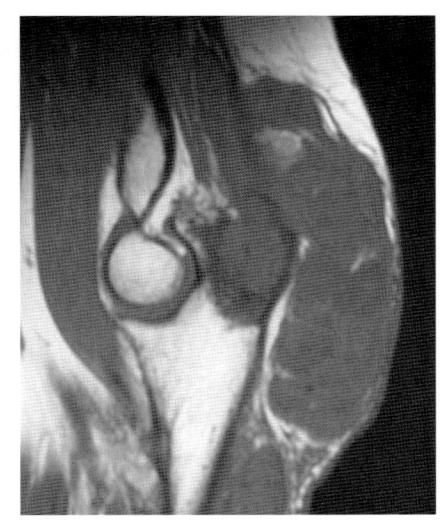

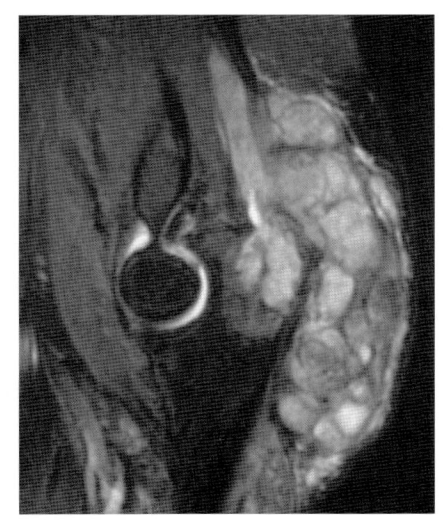

Table 18 (Continued)   Tumors and tumorlike lesions of the superficial soft tissues including subcutaneous fat

Lesion	MRI Findings	Comments
Rheumatoid arthritis (Fig. 18.46)	MRI can show diffuse and/or localized zones of synovial hypertrophy; soft tissue swelling; zones of erosion and/or destruction of hyaline cartilage, menisci, subchondral bone, tendons and/or ligaments; bursal fluid collections containing "rice bodies," other extra-articular cysts; intraosseous cystic-like areas, joint effusion, and rheumatoid nodules. With tendon and ligament involvement, abnormal increased signal is seen on PDWI and T2WI. Tendons and ligaments may be thickened from partial tearing or thinned. Tenosynovitis is usually seen with fluid and hypertrophied synovium within tendon sheaths.	Rheumatoid arthritis is a chronic multisystem disease of unknown etiology in which there is a persistent inflammatory synovitis that typically involves peripheral joints in a symmetric distribution. The inflammatory synovitis associated with rheumatoid arthritis typically results in progressive destruction of cartilage and bone, leading to joint dysfunction. **(See Atlas Chapter A 70)**
Kimura disease	Poorly marginated subcutaneous lesions with intermediate signal on T1WI and slightly high to high signal on T2WI. Lesions often show prominent Gd-contrast enhancement.	Inflammatory autoimmune disorder involving the superficial soft tissues composed of enlarged lymph nodes with eosinophilic infiltration, often occurs in Asian males between 10 and 30 years.

Other

Lesion	MRI Findings	Comments
Giant cell tumor of the tendon sheath (Fig. 18.47)	Lesions usually have well-defined margins and are often adjacent to a tendon/tendon sheath. Lesions have low-intermediate or intermediate signal on T1WI and PDWI and mixed low, intermediate and/or high signal on T2WI and FS T2WI. Zones of low signal on T2WI often correspond to sites of hemosiderin deposition. Lesions often show Gd-contrast enhancement in either homogeneous or heterogeneous pattern.	Giant cell tumors of the tendon sheath and pigmented villonodular synovitis (PVNS) represent benign proliferative lesions of synovium (tendon sheaths, joints, and bursae). Giant cell tumors of the tendon sheaths can occur as localized nodular lesions attached to tendon sheaths outside of joints (hands, feet) or within joints (infrapatellar portion of knee joint); or as a diffuse form near/outside of large joints such as the knee, ankles, etc. **(See Atlas Chapter A 30)**
Fibroma of the tendon sheath (Fig. 18.48)	Lesions are ovoid or fusiform and well-circumscribed, and are often located adjacent to tendons of the fingers, hands, wrists, and feet. Lesions usually have low-intermediate signal on T1WI. On T2WI, lesions can have a slightly heterogeneous low-intermediate signal in half, intermediate signal in a third, or mixed low and intermediate signal and/or high signal in the remainder. Lesions can show diffuse or peripheral Gd-contrast enhancement.	Fibromas of the tendon sheath are benign, small fibrous nodules involving tendons and tendon sheaths of the fingers, hands, wrists, or feet. **(See Atlas Chapter A 23)**
Xanthoma	Xanthomas in tendons often appear as zones of fusiform enlargement with diffuse heterogeneous signal **(Atlas Figs. 505, 506)** Xanthomas usually contain multiple longitudinally oriented linear zones or striations with intermediate signal on T1WI and PDWI, and intermediate to slightly high signal on T2WI and FS T2WI interspersed among bands of low signal within the enlarged tendons **(Atlas Fig. 506)** On axial images, xanthomas often have a stippled or reticulated pattern on T1WI and T2WI resulting from collagen bundles with low signal surrounded by higher signal from lipid deposits, foamy histiocytes, and inflammatory reaction. **(Atlas Fig. 506)**	Xanthomas represent localized accumulations of lipids within normal structures such as tendons, skin, and bone. Xanthomas are considered reactive lesions and are not true neoplasms. They often occur in the setting of types I, II, and III hyperlipoproteinemia. **(See Atlas Chapter A 77)**

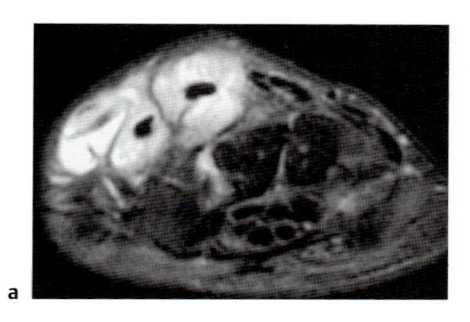

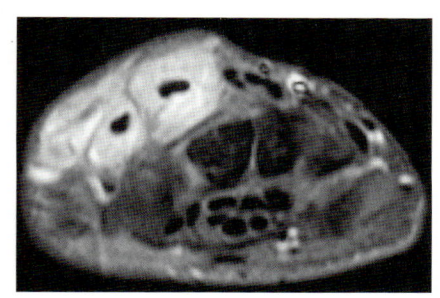

Figure 18.**46 a, b** A 48-year-old woman with rheumatoid arthritis. Pannus is seen in the tendon sheaths of 3 extensor tendons which has high signal on axial FS T2WI (**a**), and shows prominent Gd-contrast enhancement on axial FS T1WI (**b**).

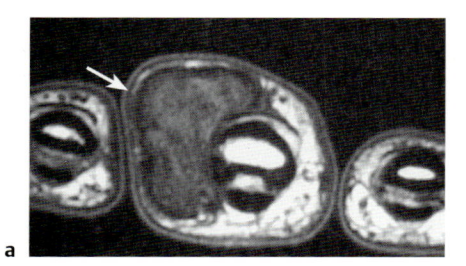

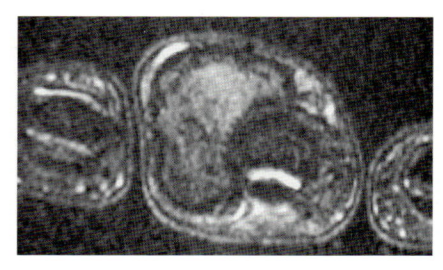

Figure 18.**47 a, b** A 28-year-old man with a giant cell tumor of the tendon sheath involving a finger. An ovoid lesion with well-defined margins is seen adjacent to a flexor tendon sheath and middle phalanx. The lesion has low-intermediate signal on axial (**a**) T1WI, and mixed high, intermediate, and low signal on axial FS T2WI (**b**).

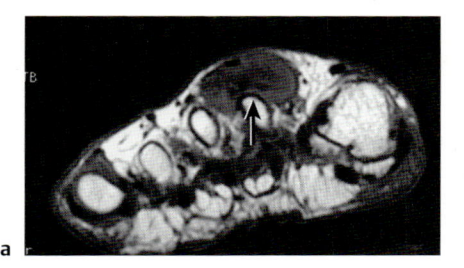

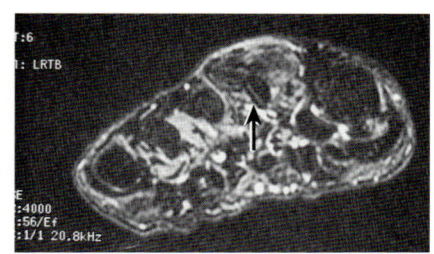

Figure 18.**48 a, b** A 63-year-old woman with a fibroma involving an extensor tendon sheath in the foot. The lesion has zones of low and intermediate signal on coronal (**a**) T1WI as well as on coronal FS T2WI (**b**).

References

Melanoma
Kalkman E, Baxter G. Melanoma. *Clin Radiol* 2004;59:313–326.

Squamous Cell Carcinoma
Bolzoni A, Cappiello J, Piazza C, et al. Diagnostic accuracy of magnetic resonance imaging in the assessment of mandibular involvement in oral-oropharyngeal squamous cell carcinoma. *Arch Otolaryngol Head Neck Surg* July 2004;130:837–843.

Goo HW, Kim EAR, Pi SY, Yoon CH. MR imaging of squamous cell carcinoma complicating chronic osteomyelitis of the femur. *AJR* February 2002;178:512–516.

Merkel Cell Carcinoma
Anderson SE, Beer KT, Banic A, et al. MRI of Merkel cell carcinoma: histologic correlation and review of the literature. *AJR* 2005;185: 1441–1448.

O'Rourke H, Meyers SP, Katzman PJ. Merkel cell carcinoma of the foot: case report and review of the literature. *J Foot Ankle Surg* May-June 2007;46(3):196–200.

Epithelioid Sarcoma
Dion E, Forest M, Brasseur JL, Amoura Z, Grenier P. Epithelioid sarcoma mimicking abscess: review of the MRI appearances. *Skeletal Radiol* 2001;30:173–177.

Herr MJ, Hamsen WS, Amadio PC, Scully SP. Epithelioid sarcoma of the hand. *Clin Orthop Relat R* 2005;431:193–200.

Kato H, Hatori M, Watanabe M, Kokubun S. Epithelioid sarcomas with elevated serum CA125: report of two cases. *Jpn J Clin Oncol* 2003;33: 141–144.

Myoepithelial Carcinoma
Darvishian F, Lin O. Myoepithelial cell-rich neoplasms. Cytologic features of benign and malignant lesions. *Cancer (Cancer Cytopathology)* December 25, 2004;102(6):355–361.

Hornick JL, Fletcher CDM. Myoepithelial tumors of soft tissue. A clinicopathologic and immunohistochemical study of 101 cases with evaluation of prognostic parameters. *Am J Surg Pathol* September 2003;27(9):1183–1196.

Hornick JL, Fletcher CDM. Cutaneous myoepithelioma: a clinicopathologic and immunohistochemical study of 14 cases. *Human Pathol* January 2004;35(1):14–24.

Venkatraman L, Sinnathuray AR, Raut V, Brooker DS, McCluggage WG. Soft tissue myoepithelioma: a case report. *Pathology* 2002;34: 451–454.

Granular Cell Tumor
Blacksin MF, White LM, Hameed M, Kandel R, Patterson FR, Benevenia J. Granular cell tumor of the extremity: magnetic resonance imaging characteristics with pathologic correlation. *Skeletal Radiol* 2005; 34:625–631.

Elkousy H, Harrelson J, Dodd L, Martinez S, Scully S. Granular cell tumors of the extremities. *Clin Orthop Relat R* 2000;380:191–198.

Pleomorphic Hyalinizing Angiectatic Tumor
Folpe AL, Weiss SW. Pleomorphic hyalinizing angiectatic tumor. Analysis of 41 cases supporting evolution from a distinctive precursor lesion. *Am J Surg Pathol* 2004;28:1417–1425.

Lee JC, Jiang WY, Karpinski RHS, Moore ED. Pleomorphic hyalinizing angiectatic tumor of soft parts. *Surgery* 2005;137:119–121.

Weiss SW. Pleomorphic hyalinizing angiectatic tumor of soft parts. In: Fletcher CDM, Unni KK, eds. *World Health Organization Classification of tumors. Pathology and Genetics of Tumors of Soft Tissue and Bone.* Lyon, France: IARC Press; 2002:191.

Hypothenar Hammer Injury of the Ulnar Artery

Blum AG, Zabel JP, Kohlmann R, et al. Pathologic conditions of the hypothenar eminence: evaluation with multidetector CT and MR imaging. *RadioGraphics* 2006:26:1021–1044.

Drape JL, Feydy A, Guerini H, et al. Vascular lesions of the hand. *Eur J Radiol* 2005;56:331–343.

Cat Scratch Disease

Dong PR, Seeger LL, Yao L, Panosian CB, Johnson BL, Eckhardt JJ. Uncomplicated cat-scratch disease: findings at CT, MR imaging and radiography. *Radiology* 1995;195:837–839.

Gielen J, Wang XL, Vanhoenacker F, et al. Lymphadenopathy at the medial epitrochlear region in cat-scratch disease. *Eur Radiol* 2003;13: 1363–1369.

Mele FM, Friedman M, Reznik AM. MR imaging of the knee: findings in cat scratch disease. *AJR* 1996;166:1232–1233.

Granuloma Annulare

Bancroft LW, Perniciaro C, Berquist TH. Granuloma annulare: radiographic demonstration of progressive mutilating arthropathy with vanishing bones. *Skeletal Radiol* 1998;27:211–214.

Chung S, Frush DP, Prose NS, Shea CR, Laor T, Bisset GS. Subcutaneous granuloma annulare: MR imaging features in six children and literature review. *Radiology* 1999;210:845–849.

Kransdorf MJ, Murphey MD, Temple HT. Subcutaneous granuloma annulare: radiologic appearance. *Skeletal Radiol* 1998;27:266–270.

Kimura Disease

Choi AH, Lee GK, Kong KY, et al. Imaging findings of Kimura's disease in the soft tissue of the upper extremity. *AJR* 2005;184:193–199.

Huang GS, Lee HS, Chiu YC, Yu CC, Chen CY. Kimura's disease of the elbows. *Skeletal Radiol* 2005;34:555–558.

Table 19 Lesions involving peripheral nervous tissue		
Lesion	**MRI Findings**	**Comments**
Benign lesions		
Schwannoma (Fig. 19.1)	Circumscribed or lobulated lesions, low-intermediate signal on T1WI, high signal on T2WI and FS T2WI, usually show prominent Gd-contrast enhancement. High signal on T2WI and Gd-contrast enhancement can be heterogeneous in large lesions due to cystic degeneration and/or hemorrhage.	Encapsulated neoplasms arising asymmetrically from nerve sheath, most common type of intradural extramedullary neoplasms involving the spine, usual presentation in adults with pain and radiculopathy, paresthesias, and lower extremity weakness. Multiple schwannomas seen with neurofibromatosis type 2 (NF2). **(See Atlas Chapter A 72)**
Neurofibroma (Figs. 19.2, 19.3)	Solitary neurofibromas are spheroid or lobulated lesions +/− irregular margins, low-intermediate signal on T1WI, high signal on T2WI and FS T2WI, usually show prominent Gd-contrast enhancement. High signal on T2WI and Gd-contrast enhancement can be heterogeneous in large lesions +/− erosion of adjacent bone. **Plexiform neurofibromas** usually appear as curvilinear and multinodular lesions involving multiple nerve branches, and have low to intermediate signal on T1WI and intermediate, slightly high to high signal on T2WI and FS T2WI +/− bands or strands of low signal. Lesions usually show Gd-contrast enhancement.	Unencapsulated neoplasms involving nerve and nerve sheath, usual presentation in adults with pain and radiculopathy, paresthesias, and lower extremity weakness. Multiple neurofibromas seen with neurofibromatosis type 1 (NF1). **(See Atlas Chapter A 56)**
Neurothekeoma (Fig. 19.4)	Neurothekeomas can occur as circumscribed lesions with low-intermediate signal on T1WI, high signal on T2WI, and heterogeneous Gd-contrast enhancement.	Neurothekeoma, also referred to as nerve sheath myxoma, is considered to be a neurofibroma with prominent myxoid matrix separated into lobules by fibrous connective tissue. **(See Atlas Chapter A 56)**
Granular cell tumor (Fig. 19.5)	Tumors can have circumscribed and/or irregular margins, and contain low-intermediate signal on T1WI and PDWI, and slightly high to high signal on T2WI and FS T2WI. Tumors can also have low-intermediate signal on T2WI. Tumors can show prominent Gd-contrast enhancement.	Rare benign schwannian neoplasms that contain cells with diffuse granular cytoplasm, and are immunoreactive to S-100, but not to HMB-45. Tumors are often located in the dermis/subcutis, and occasionally within muscle. Occur more commonly in females compared with males, adults over 30 years old.
Traumatic neuroma (Fig. 19.6)	Traumatic neuromas can appear as bulbous lesions at the end of a transected nerve (terminal neuroma) or as fusiform swelling of an intact nerve (spindle neuroma). Lesions often have low-intermediate signal on T1WI, intermediate signal on PDWI, and mildly heterogeneous intermediate to high signal on T2WI and FS T2WI	Non-neoplastic lesions that result from complete or partial transection of nerves. The proximal end of the damaged or transected nerve undergoes a benign proliferative process that can be painful. Terminal neuromas refer to traumatic neuromas that result from transection or avulsion of nerves and occur 1–12 months after injury. Spindle neuromas refer to focal swelling of intact nerves damaged by chronic friction or irritation. **(See Atlas Chapter A 57)**
Avulsed nerve root (Fig. 19.7)	Nerve root avulsions may be seen as discontinuous nerves with bulbous ends within dura or extradural fluid collections. Post-traumatic nerve root pouch cysts may also be seen.	Spinal injury can affect the integrity of bone, ligaments, disks, spinal cord, as well as the connection of the nerve roots to the spinal cord.
Morton neuroma (Fig. 19.8)	Lesions located in neurovascular bundle within the intermetatarsal space on the plantar side of the transverse metatarsal ligament. Lesions appear as nodular zones with low-intermediate signal on T1WI and PDWI that is isointense or slightly hyperintense relative to muscle. Lesions often have low to intermediate signal on T2WI that is hypointense or isointense relative to fat. Lesions can have intermediate, slightly high, or high signal on FS T2WI. Lesions can show Gd-contrast enhancement that is often more conspicuous with fat-suppression.	Non-neoplastic lesions that result from perineural fibrosis of a plantar digital nerve near the metatarsal head. **(See Atlas Chapter A 51)**

306 Table 19 Lesions involving peripheral nervous tissue

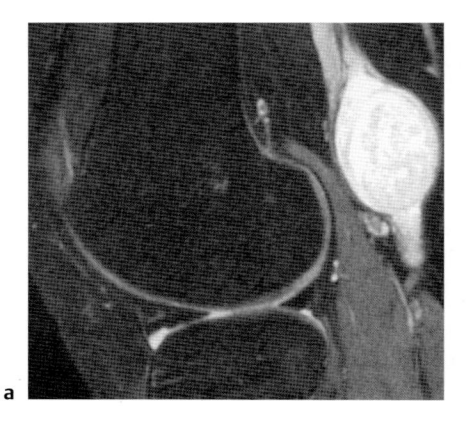

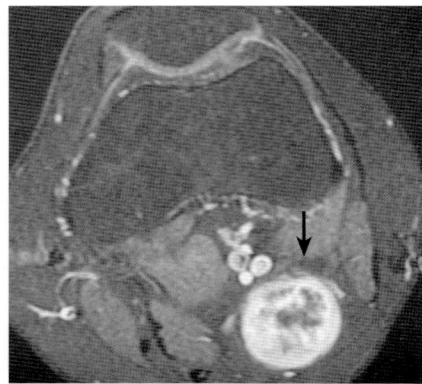

Figure 19.**1 a, b** A 17-year-old female with a schwannoma involving the tibial nerve at the dorsal knee. A well-circumscribed ovoid lesion is seen along the nerve that has high signal on sagittal FS T2WI (**a**) and shows prominent Gd-contrast enhancement on axial FS T1WI (**b**).

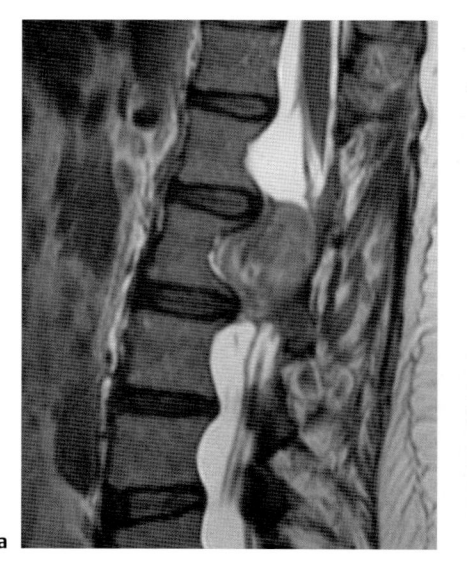

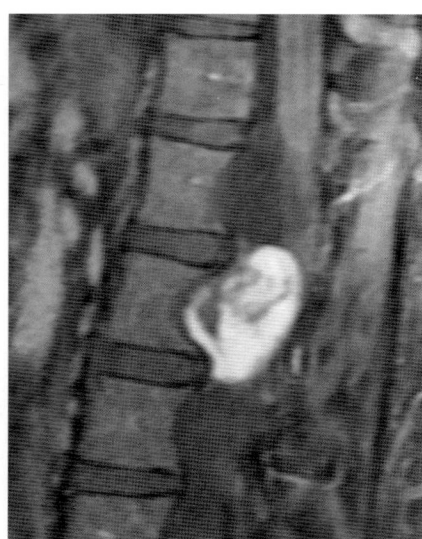

Figure 19.**2 a–d** A 52-year-old woman with NF1 and a large left paraspinal neurofibroma extending through a widened intervertebral foramen resulting in compression of the thecal sac. Note also the scalloping of the dorsal margins of the vertebral bodies from dural ectasia. The lesion has heterogeneous intermediate and slightly high signal on sagittal (**a**) and axial (**c**) T2WI, and shows heterogeneous Gd-contrast enhancement on sagittal (**b**) and axial (**d**) FS T1WI.

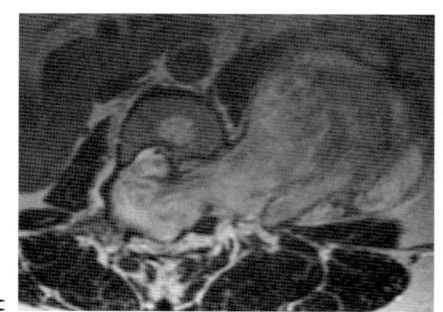

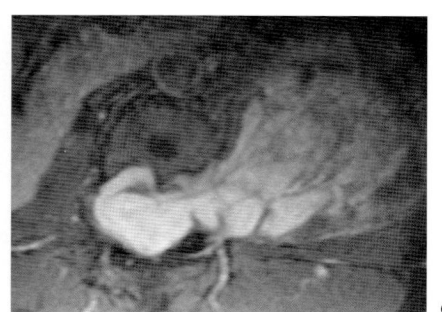

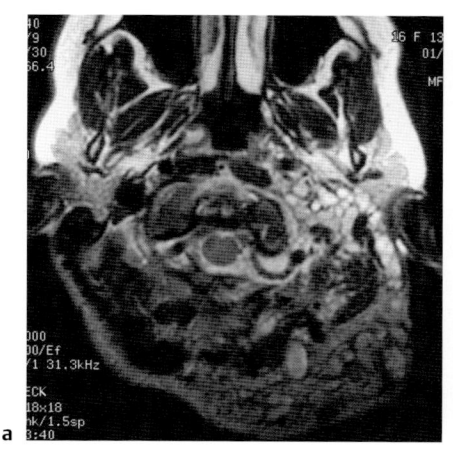

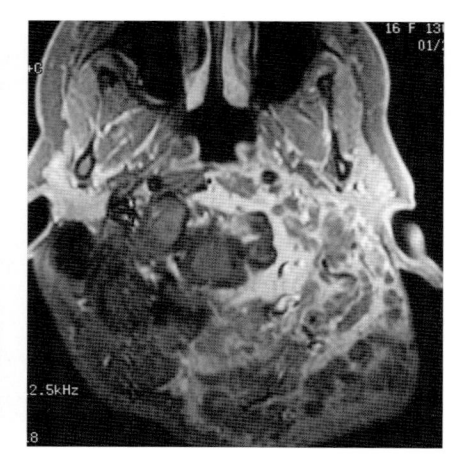

Figure 19.**3 a, b** A 16-year-old female with a plexiform neurofibroma involving the posterior scalp and skull. The tumor appears as curvilinear and multinodular zones with intermediate, slightly high to high signal separated by curvilinear zones of low signal on axial T2WI (**a**) and shows heterogeneous Gd-contrast enhancement on axial FS T1WI (**b**).

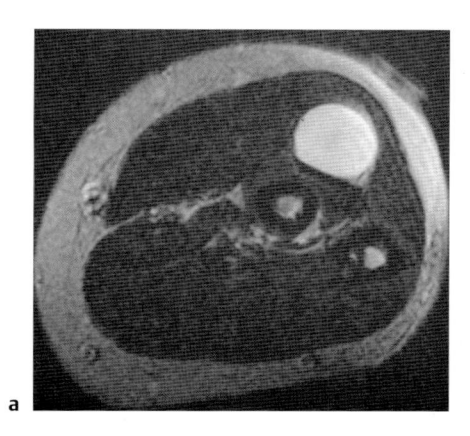

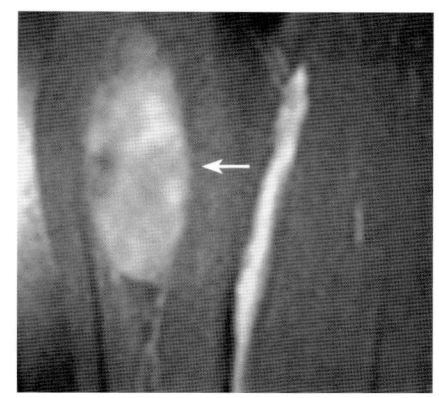

Figure 19.**4 a, b**   A 38-year-old man with a neurothekeoma involving the flexor digitorum superficialis muscle of the proximal forearm. The lesion has high signal on axial T2WI (**a**) and shows moderate heterogeneous Gd-contrast enhancement on sagittal FS T1WI (**b**).

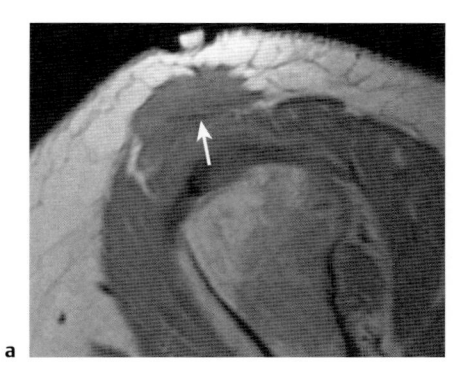

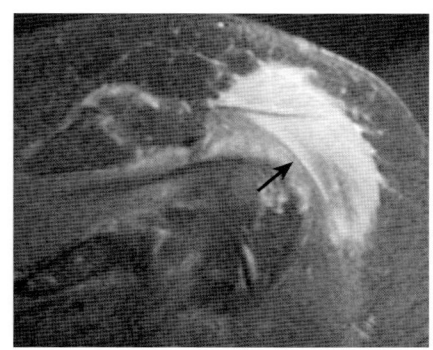

Figure 19.**5 a, b**   A 56-year-old woman with a granular cell tumor involving the subcutaneous fat and superficial portion of the deltoid muscle. The tumor has irregular margins and contains low-intermediate signal on sagittal PDWI (**a**) and shows prominent Gd-contrast enhancement on coronal FS T1WI (**b**).

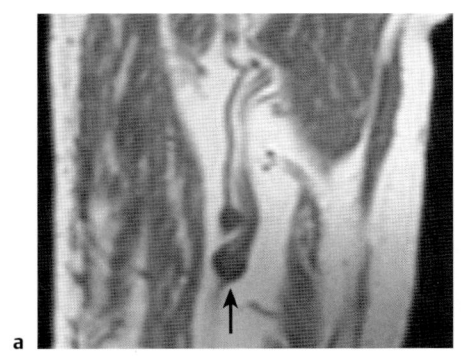

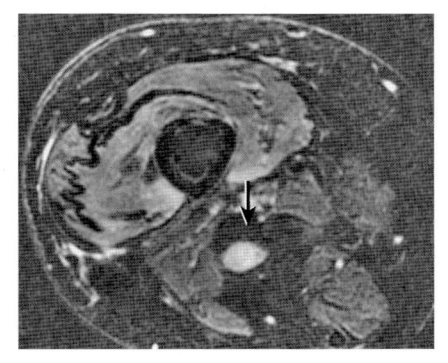

Figure 19.**6 a, b**   A 60-year-old man with a traumatic neuroma involving the sciatic nerve in the thigh after an amputation of the leg. Bulbous dilatation of the distal transected sciatic nerve is seen that has low-intermediate signal on sagittal T1WI (**a**) and high signal on axial FS T2WI (**b**).

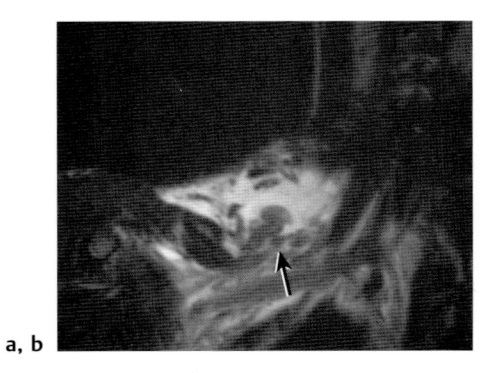

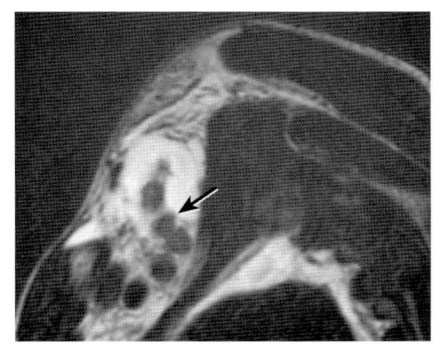

Figure 19.**7 a, b**   A 15-year-old male with traumatic avulsion of multiple nerves of the right brachial plexus. Multiple nodular low signal structures representing retracted torn nerve endings are seen within high signal fluid on coronal (**a**) and sagittal (**b**) FS T2WI.

Figure 19.**8**   Morton neuroma between the third and fourth digits. The nodular lesion has low–intermediate signal on coronal T1WI.

Table 19 (Continued) Lesions involving peripheral nervous tissue

Lesion	MRI Findings	Comments
Lipoma of nerve (fibrolipomatous hamartoma) (Fig. 19.9)	Well-circumscribed fusiform-shaped lesions involving nerves. On T1WI, PDWI, and T2WI a network of cylindrical longitudinally oriented thin curvilinear signal voids with 1–3 mm diameters is seen within a background of intermediate to high signal. This "coaxial cable-like" appearance is secondary to the combination of nerve fascicles with varying degrees of fatty infiltration, and epineural and perineural fibrosis. The degree of fatty proliferation varies among patients. Lesions may follow the branching patterns of nerves.	Rare benign lesions with varying degrees of fibrous and fatty (mature adipocytes) infiltration of the epineurium (nerve sheath) of peripheral nerves as well as within the interfascicular connective tissue (perineurium) of nerves. **(See Atlas Chapter A 22)**
Paraganglioma (Fig. 19.10)	Spheroid or lobulated lesion with intermediate signal on T1WI, intermediate-high signal on T2WI and FS T2WI, +/− tubular zones of flow voids, usually show prominent Gd-contrast enhancement, +/− foci of high signal on T1WI from mucin or hemorrhage, +/− peripheral rim of low signal (hemosiderin) on T2WI.	Neoplasms that arise from paraganglion cells of neural crest origin. Usually occur at carotid body, jugular foramen, middle ear, and along vagus nerve. Rarely occur in spine. **(See Atlas Chapter A 66)**
Ganglioneuroma (Fig. 19.11)	Tumors are well-circumscribed with low-intermediate signal on T1WI and slightly high to high signal on T2WI and FS T2WI. Small foci or strands of low signal on T2WI may be seen secondary to calcifications and fibrous tissue, respectively. Tumors show mild to marked heterogeneous Gd-contrast enhancement. MRI can show extension of these tumors into the spinal canal.	Rare benign lesions of the sympathetic nervous system composed of ganglion cells and schwannian stroma, and typically lack neuroblasts and mitotic figures. **(See Atlas Chapter A 55)**

Malignant lesions

Lesion	MRI Findings	Comments
Malignant peripheral nerve sheath tumor (MPNST) (Fig. 19.12)	These lesions usually have heterogeneous signal on T1WI and T2WI; as well as heterogeneous Gd-contrast enhancement because of necrosis and hemorrhage. Some malignant peripheral nerve sheath tumors (MPNSTs) are similar in appearance to benign nerve sheath tumors.	Malignant tumors of the peripheral nerve sheath that contain mixtures of packed hyperchromatic spindle cells with elongated nuclei and slightly eosinophilic cytoplasm, mitotic figures, and zones of necrosis. Approximately 50% of MPNSTs occur in patients with NF1, followed by de novo evolution from peripheral nerves. Malignant peripheral nerve sheath tumors infrequently arise from schwannomas, ganglioneuroblastomas/ganglioneuromas, and pheochromocytomas. **(See Atlas Chapter A 56)**
Primitive neuroectodermal tumor/extraskeletal Ewing sarcoma (Fig. 19.13)	Tumors usually have low-intermediate signal on T1WI and PDWI, heterogeneous slightly high to high signal on T2WI and FS T2WI. Margins of the lesions are often ill-defined. Lesions typically show prominent irregular Gd-contrast enhancement.	Extracranial primitive neuroectodermal tumors (extracranial PNETs) are malignant tumors of bone and soft tissue composed of undifferentiated small cells with round nuclei. These tumors are similar to Ewing sarcoma, except that extracranial PNETs usually show varying degrees of neural differentiation. **(See Atlas Chapter A 20)**

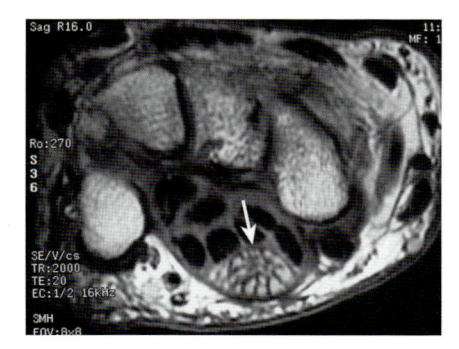

Figure 19.**9** A 9-year-old boy with a fibrolipomatous hamartoma (lipomatosis of the nerve) involving the median nerve at the wrist. Cylindrical, longitudinally oriented, thin, curvilinear zones of low signal are seen against a background of intermediate to high signal on axial PDWI.

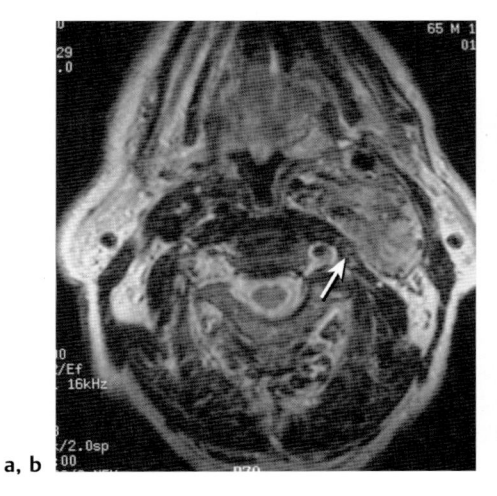

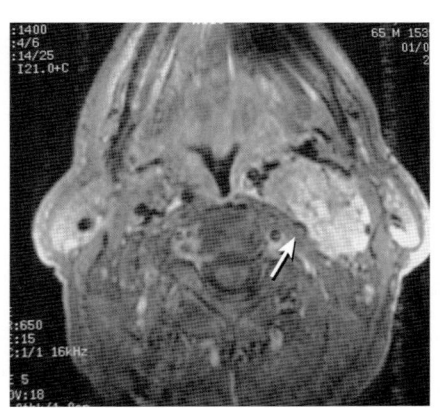

Figure 19.**10a, b** A 65-year-old man with a paraganglioma at the left common carotid artery bifurcation in the neck, also referred to as a carotid body tumor. The ovoid tumor splays the proximal external carotid artery from the internal carotid artery, and has heterogenous slightly high and intermediate signal on axial T2WI (**a**). The tumor shows prominent Gd-contrast enhancement on axial FS T1WI (**b**). Multiple tortuous and punctate zones of signal void are seen within the peripheral and central portions of the tumor.

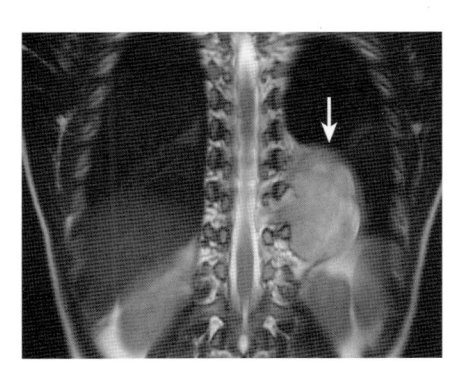

Figure 19.**11** A 10-year-old boy with a left paraspinal ganglioneuroma. The tumor has well-circumscribed margins and has heterogeneous intermediate, slightly high to high signal on coronal T2WI.

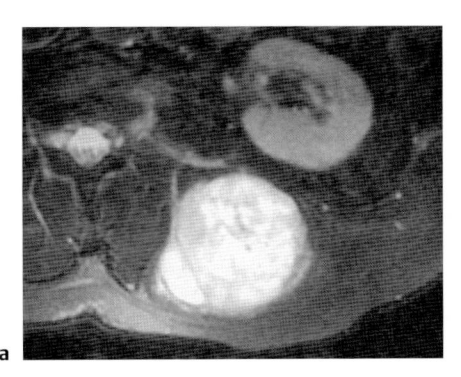

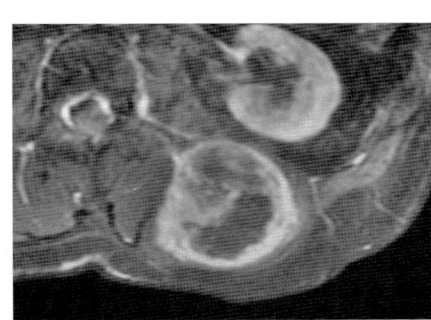

Figure 19.**12a, b** Malignant peripheral nerve sheath tumor in the left posterior paraspinal muscles of a 51-year-old man. The tumor has high signal on axial FS T2WI (**a**) and shows heterogeneous Gd-contrast enhancement on axial FS T1WI (**b**) as well as zones of central necrosis.

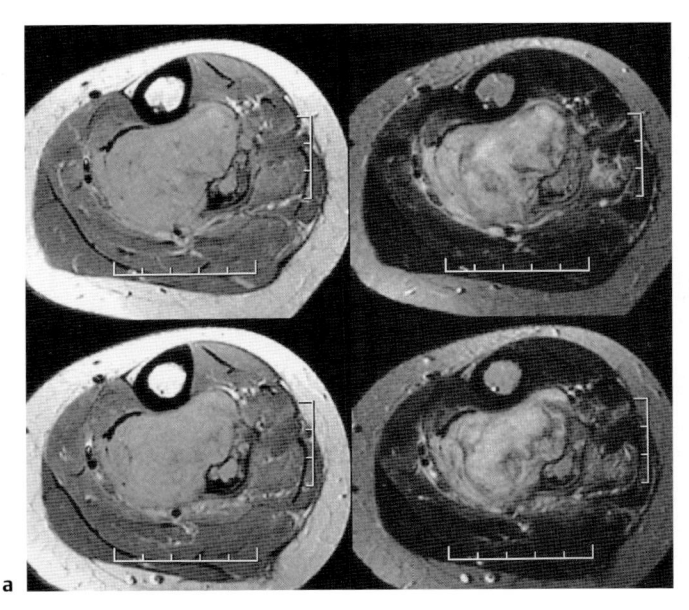

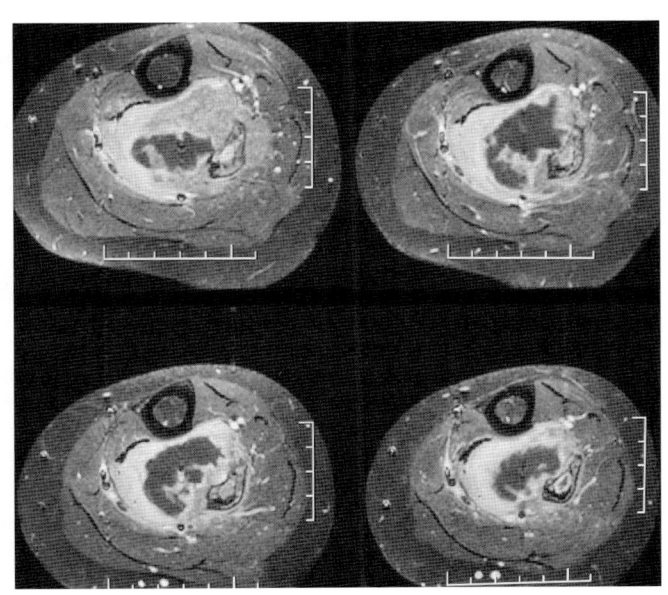

Figure 19.**13a, b** An 11-year-old boy with Ewing sarcoma/PNET involving the proximal fibula. The tumor has poorly defined margins and is associated with cortical destruction and prominent extraosseous tumor extension. The tumor contains zones with intermediate and slightly high signal on axial PDWI (**a**, *images on left*) and slightly high to high signal on axial T2WI (**a**, *images on right*). The tumor shows prominent irregular Gd-contrast enhancement on axial FS T1WI (**b**) as well as zones of central necrosis.

Table 19 (Continued) Lesions involving peripheral nervous tissue

Lesion	MRI Findings	Comments
Neuroblastoma/ganglioneuroblastoma (Fig. 19.14)	Tumors can have distinct or indistinct margins, and have low-intermediate signal on T1WI, homogeneous or heterogeneous intermediate, slightly high, and/or high signal on T2WI and FS T2WI. Zones of high signal on T2WI may occur from sites of hemorrhage or necrosis. Foci of low signal on T2WI may be seen secondary to calcifications and blood products. Tumors can show mild to marked heterogeneous Gd-contrast enhancement. MRI can show extension of these tumors into the spinal canal as well as into bone marrow.	Neuroblastomas and ganglioneuroblastomas are malignant tumors of the sympathetic nervous system that consist of neoplastic neuroectodermal cells derived from the neural crest. Neuroblastomas are highly malignant undifferentiated tumors whereas ganglioneuroblastomas are intermediate-grade malignant tumors. **(See Atlas Chapter A 55)**
Lymphoma of nerve (Fig. 19.15)	Lymphoma involving nerves can have intermediate signal on T1WI, high signal on FS T2WI, and show Gd-contrast enhancement.	Non-Hodgkin lymphoma (NHL) represents a group of lymphoid tumors whose neoplastic cells frequently originate at extranodal sites and spread in an unpredictable pattern. NHL can infiltrate soft tissues such as muscle, nerves, dermis, and epidermis. **(See Atlas Chapter A 47)**
Merkel cell tumor (Fig. 19.16)	Tumors can have circumscribed margins, and have low-intermediate signal on T1WI and PDWI and slightly high to high signal on T2WI. Zones of necrosis with high signal on T2WI may occur within the tumors. Tumors can show Gd-contrast enhancement.	Rare primary malignant neuroendocrine neoplasms that involve the skin and dermis usually in adults over 60 years. Tumor cells are small and contain neurosecretory cytoplasmic granules secondary to neural crest origin.

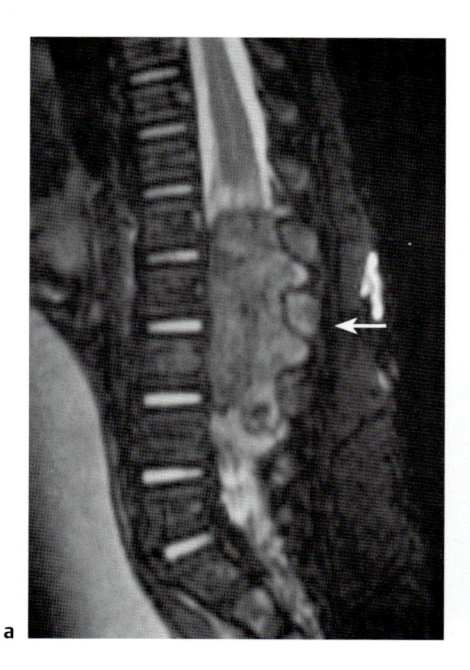

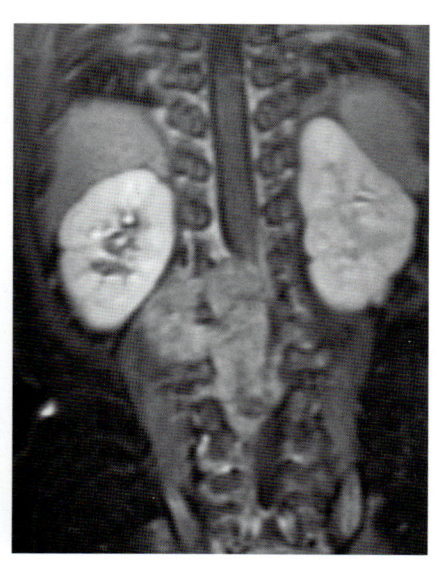

Figure 19.**14 a, b** A 10-month-old boy with a right paraspinal neuroblastoma that extends into the spinal canal resulting in spinal cord compression. The tumor has heterogeneous intermediate and slightly high signal on sagittal FS T2WI (**a**) and shows heterogeneous Gd-contrast enhancement on coronal FS T1WI (**b**).

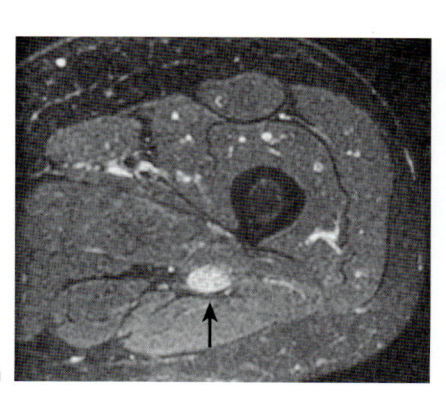

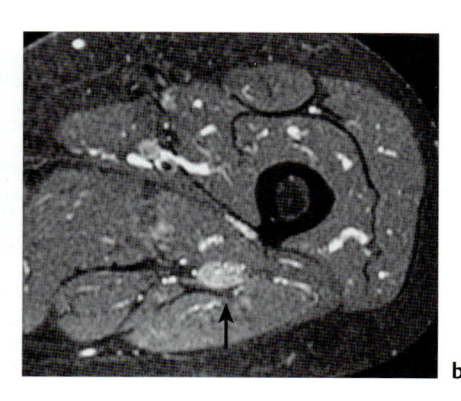

Figure 19.**15 a, b** A 70-year-old woman with B cell NHL involving the sciatic nerve. The lymphoma has high signal on axial FS T2WI (**a**) and shows Gd-contrast enhancement on axial FS T1WI (**b**).

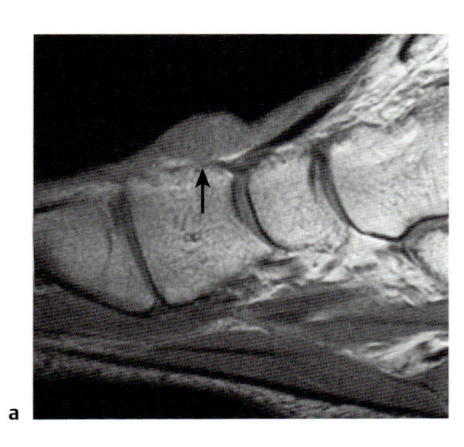

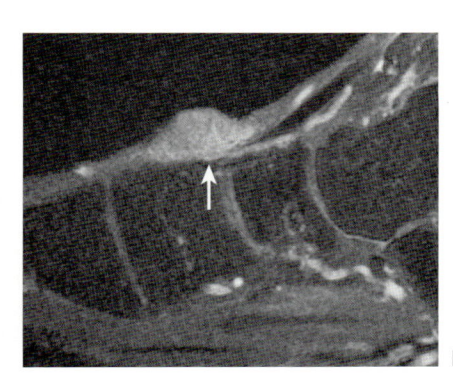

Figure 19.**16 a, b** A 72-year-old man with a Merkel cell tumor involving the dorsal superficial soft tissues of the foot. The tumor has low-intermediate signal on sagittal PDWI (**a**) and shows moderate Gd-contrast enhancement on sagittal FS T1WI (**b**).

References

Granular Cell Tumor
Blacksin MF, White LM, Hameed M, Kandel R, Patterson FR, Benevenia J. Granular cell tumor of the extremity: magnetic resonance imaging characteristics with pathologic correlation. *Skeletal Radiol* 2005;34: 625–631.

Elkousy H, Harrelson J, Dodd L, Martinez S, Scully S. Granular cell tumors of the extremities. *Clin Orthop Relat R* 2000;380:191–198.

Merkel Cell Carcinoma
Anderson SE, Beer KT, Banic A, et al. MRI of Merkel cell carcinoma: histologic correlation and review of the literature. *AJR* 2005;185: 1441–1448.

O'Rourke H, Meyers SP, Katzman PJ. Merkel cell carcinoma of the foot: case report and review of the literature. *J Foot Ankle Surg* May-June 2007;46(3):196–200.

Table 20 Lesions that contain fat

Lesion	MRI Findings	Comments
Congenital		
Lipomyelocele/lipomyelo-meningocele (Fig. 20.1)	Unfolded caudal neural tube (neural placode) covered by a lipoma. Usually contiguous with the dorsal subcutaneous fat through congenital defects (spina bifida) in the posterior elements of the involved vertebrae and/or sacrum. With lipomyelomeningocele, the dorsal lipoma that extends into the spinal canal is asymmetric resulting in rotation of the placode and meningocele.	Failure of closure of the caudal neural tube results in an unfolded neural tube covered by a lipoma which is typically contiguous with the dorsal subcutaneous fat. The subcutaneous fat is intact, although the lipoma often protrudes dorsally. Features associated with lipomyeloceles and lipomyelomeningoceles include: tethered spinal cord, dorsal bony dysraphism, and deficient dura posteriorly at the site of the neural placode. Not associated with Chiari II malformations. Diagnosis usually in childhood, occasionally as adults.
Intradural lipoma/spinal lipoma (Fig. 20.2)	Focal dorsal dysraphic spinal cord attached to a lipoma; has high signal on T1WI. Lipoma often extends from the central canal of the spinal cord to the pial surface, intact dorsal dural margins and posterior vertebral elements.	Intradural lipomas often occur in the cervical or thoracic regions. **(See Atlas Chapter A 43)**
Benign lesions		
Lipoma—intraosseous (Fig. 20.3)	Lesions are typically well-circumscribed intramedullary lesions that often have a peripheral thin border of low signal on T1WI, PDWI, and T2WI. Lesions often have high signal on T1WI and PDWI and intermediate-high signal on T2WI, which is isointense to subcutaneous fat. Suppression of fat signal typically occurs with short Tan inversion recovery (STIR) and frequency selective FS T1WI or FS T2WI. Cystic zones are seen in approximately two-thirds of intraosseous lipomas and range from 2 to 35 mm. Calcifications, when present, usually appear as zones of low signal or signal void.	Lipomas in bone are uncommon benign hamartomas composed of mature white adipose tissue without cellular atypia. **(See Atlas Chapter A 43)**
Lipoma—soft tissue (Fig. 20.4)	Superficial lipomas in subcutaneous fat often have circumscribed margins and have MRI signal comparable to subcutaneous fat on T1WI, PDWI, T2WI, and FS T2WI. Lipomas may also be localized within and/or between muscles. Nonfatty thin septa may be present within superficial or deep-seated lipomas. These thin septa may show slightly high to high signal on FS T2WI. Lipomas often show no Gd-contrast enhancement. Minimal to mild Gd-contrast enhancement may, however, be seen along the thin nonfatty septae.	Lipomas are common benign hamartomas in soft tissue that are composed of mature white adipose tissue without cellular atypia. **(See Atlas Chapter A 43)**
Lipomatosis (Fig. 17.21)	Infiltrating adipose tissue or multiple lobules of fat can be seen in muscles, fascial planes, and/or subcutaneous fat.	Diffuse proliferation of mature adipose tissue. Can occur as several types. The diffuse type typically affects the soft tissues of an extremity or trunk in children with or without associated osseous hypertrophy. Multiple symmetric lipomatosis (Madelung disease) usually occurs in the neck, trunk, and pelvis of adult men (peak incidence in the 5th decade. Shoulder girdle lipomatosis usually occurs in women and involves the muscles at one shoulder and adjacent chest wall. Adiposis dolorosa (Dercum syndrome) usually occurs in obese postmenopausal women who have multiple painful fatty lesions in the extremities or trunk.

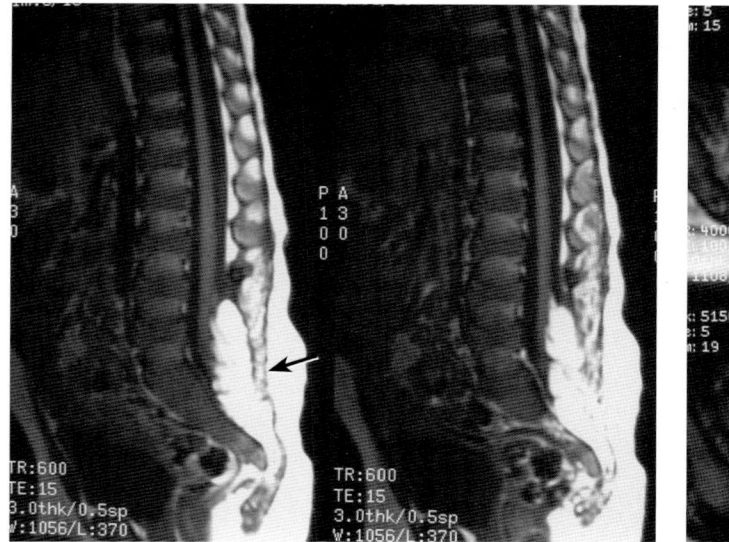

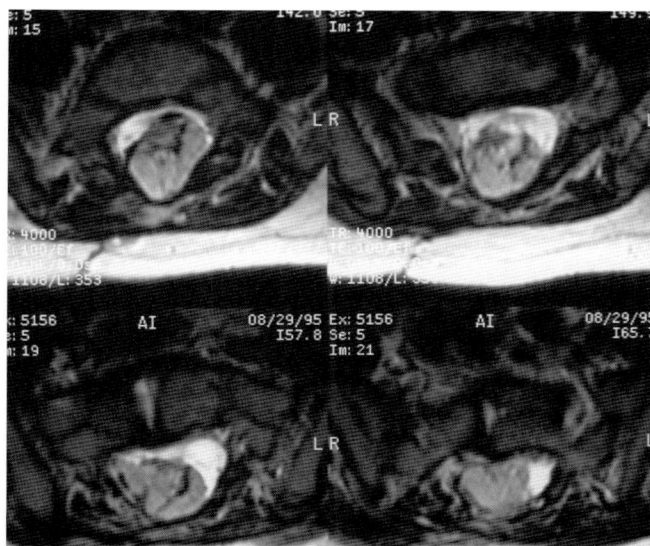

Figure 20.**1 a, b** A lipomyelocele, which represents an unfolded neural tube covered by a lipoma, is seen between congenital bony defects at the posterior elements on sagittal T1WI (**a**) and axial T2WI (**b**).

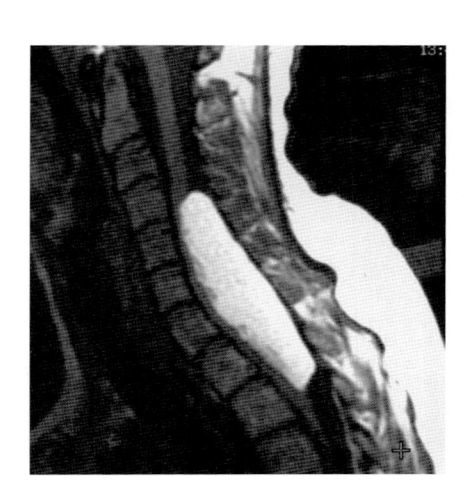

Figure 20.**2** Intradural lipoma involving the dorsal portion of the cervical and upper thoracic spinal cord. The lipoma has high signal on sagittal T1WI.

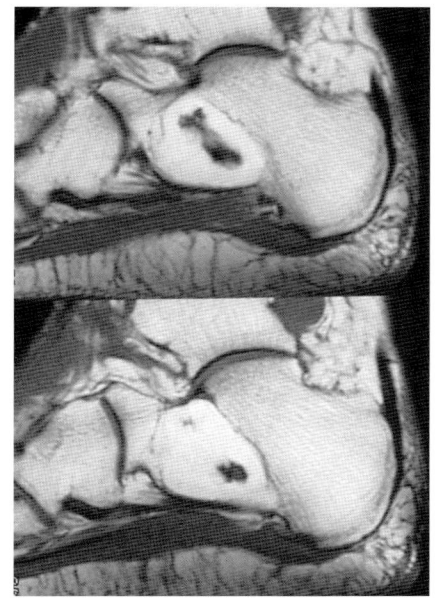

Figure 20.**3** A 47-year-old woman with an intraosseous lipoma of the calcaneus that has thin margins of low signal surrounding a central zone of mostly high fat signal as well as several zones of low signal on sagittal T1WI.

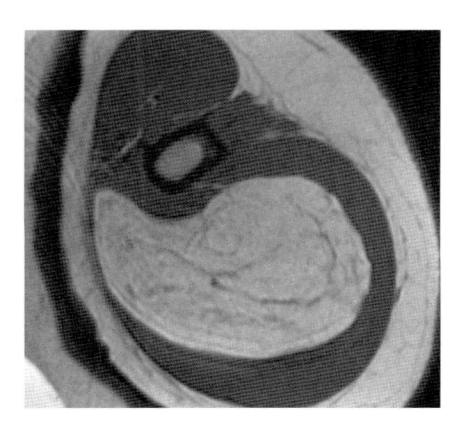

Figure 20.**4** A 43-year-old woman with an intramuscular lipoma in the triceps brachii muscle of the arm that has high signal on axial T1WI.

Table 20 (Continued) Lesions that contain fat

Lesion	MRI Findings	Comments
Lipoma—atypical lipoma (Fig. 20.5)	Atypical lipomas are less common than the classic benign lipoma. They often contain cystic/necrotic zones, calcifications, thick septa, and/or nodular zones that may or may not show Gd-contrast enhancement. Most atypical lipomas contain >75% fat, whereas liposarcomas often have <75% fat. Distinguishing between atypical lipomas and low-grade liposarcomas with MRI, however, can be difficult and challenging.	Osseous or chondroid metaplasia with myxoid changes can be associated with lipomas. These **atypical lipomas** have been labeled as **chondroid lipomas, osteolipomas,** or **benign mesenchymomas. Chondroid lipomas** nign adipose tumors that contain mature fat, lipoblasts, and chondroid matrix. **Spindle cell** and **pleomorphic lipomas** are lipoma variants that have overlapping histologic features of varying proportions of mature fat cells, spindle cells, hyperchromatic spheroid cells, collagen and multinucleated giant cells. Lipomas with high fibrous tissue content have been labeled as fibrolipomas. **(See Atlas Chapter A 43)**
Hibernoma (Fig. 20.6)	Well-defined soft tissue lesions that often have intermediate to high signal on T1WI (hypo- or isointense relative to fat), slightly high signal on T2WI, slightly hyperintense signal relative to fat on FS T2WI and STIR. Mild signal heterogeneity, internal septations, and/or branching-serpentine, slow-flow vascular channels may be seen on T1WI and T2WI. Lesions can show Gd-contrast enhancement within branching-serpentine vascular channels.	Rare benign lesions derived from brown adipose tissue intermixed with white adipose tissue. **(See Atlas Chapter A 43)**
Fibrolipomatous hamartoma of nerve (Fig. 20.7)	Fusiform-shaped lesions involving nerves containing a network of cylindrical, longitudinally oriented, thin, curvilinear signal voids with 1–3 mm diameters are seen against a background of intermediate to high signal on T1WI, PDWI, and T2WI. This "coaxial cable-like" lesion may follow the branching patterns of nerves.	Fibrolipomatous hamartomas are rare benign lesions with varying degrees of fibrous and fatty infiltration of the epineurium of peripheral nerves as well as within the interfascicular connective tissue of nerves. Frequently involve the median nerve followed by the ulnar nerve, radial nerve, brachial plexus, sciatic nerve, nerves of the lower extremity. **(See Atlas Chapter A 22)**
Lipoblastoma (Fig. 20.8)	Lesions are often circumscribed, although some have margins that infiltrate adjacent muscle or subcutaneous tissues. Lesions typically contain zones with MRI signal approximating that of fat on T1WI and T2WI. Fatty zones within the lesions may have signal slightly lower than normal fat on T1WI as well as higher signal on FS T2WI and STIR resulting from the differing fat contents and shapes of immature lipoblasts compared with mature adipocytes. Intralesional bands and/or nodular zones with low-intermediate to slightly high signal on T1WI and T2WI may be seen in large lesions. Variable degrees of Gd-contrast enhancement can be seen, particularly in the nonlipomatosis portions.	Rare benign mesenchymal tumors that contain embryonal white fat, and typically occur during infancy and early childhood. **(See Atlas Chapter A 42)**

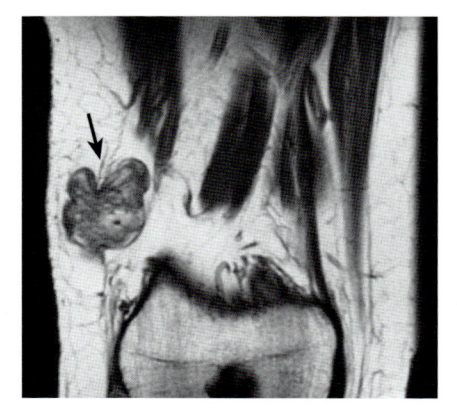

Figure 20.5 A 57-year-old woman with a chondroid/myxoid lipoma in the soft tissues of the distal lateral thigh. The lesion has lobulated well-defined margins and has heterogeneous low, intermediate, and high signal on coronal T1WI.

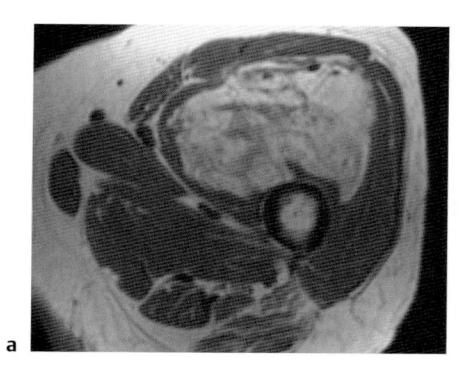

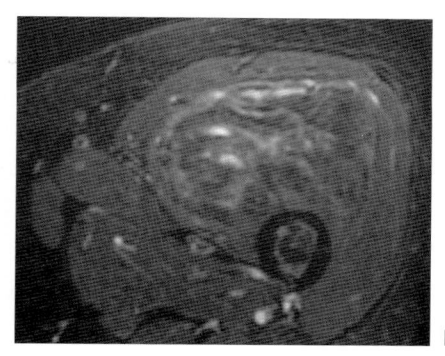

Figure 20.**6 a, b** A 71-year-old woman with a hibernoma involving the vastus muscles of the proximal thigh. The lesion has well-defined margins and contains mostly fat signal on axial T1WI (**a**) as well as curvilinear and small nodular zones of low signal. The signal of the fatty portions of the lesion is suppressed on axial FS T2WI (**b**).

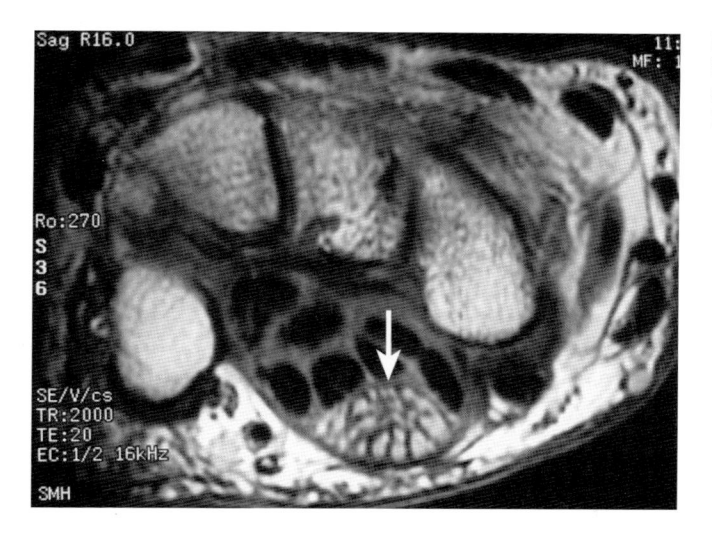

Figure 20.**7** A 59-year-old man with a fibrolipomatous hamartoma involving the median nerve at the wrist. Cylindrical, longitudinally oriented, thin, curvilinear zones of low signal are seen against a background of intermediate to high signal on axial PDWI.

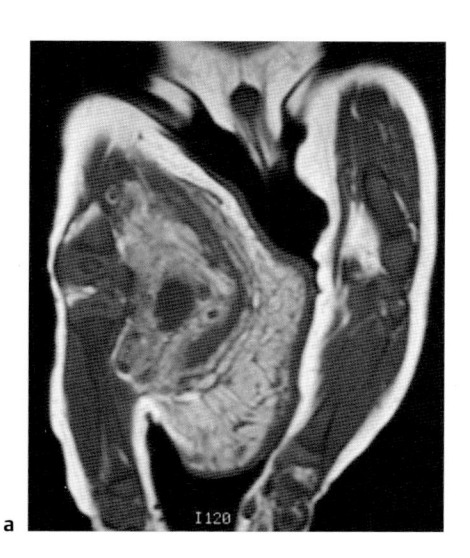

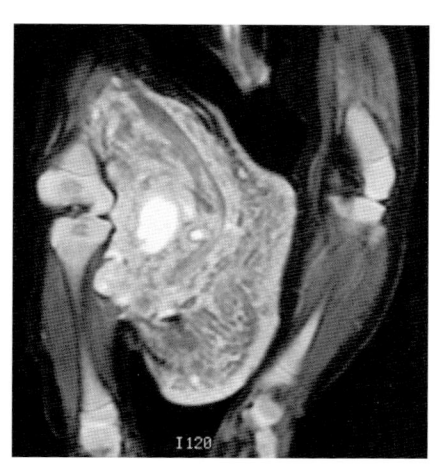

Figure 20.**8 a, b** A 3-month-old boy with a large lipoblastoma involving the thigh. The lesion infiltrates adjacent muscles and subcutaneous tissues, and contains zones with MRI signal approximating that of fat on coronal T1WI (**a**). Many of the fatty zones have signal slightly lower than subcutaneous fat on T1WI as well as higher signal on coronal STIR (**b**).

Table 20 (Continued) Lesions that contain fat

Lesion	MRI Findings	Comments
Epidural lipomatosis (Fig. 20.9)	Increased extradural fat is seen within the spinal canal with resultant narrowing of the thecal sac.	Epidural lipomatosis is a condition in which there is prominent deposition of unencapsulated mature adipose tissue in the epidural space. May be related to obesity, chronic use of steroid medication, or endogenous hypercortisolemia. Thoracic 60%, lumbar 40%. **(See Atlas Chapter A 43)**
Spinal angiolipoma	Lesions are typically epidural, and often have intermediate to high signal on T1WI and high signal on T2WI. Usually show prominent Gd-contrast enhancement.	Very rare benign lesions composed of mature adipocytes and various-sized blood vessels ranging from capillaries, small to large veins, and arteries.
Hemangioma (Figs. 20.10, 20.11)	**Hemangiomas in bone:** Lesions are often well-circumscribed and often have intermediate to high signal on T1WI, PDWI, T2WI, and FS T2WI. On T1WI, hemangiomas usually have signal equal to or greater than adjacent normal marrow secondary to fatty components. Hemangiomas usually show Gd-contrast enhancement (mild to prominent). Extraosseous extension of hemangiomas may lack adipose tissue, with resulting intermediate signal on T1WI. Pathologic fractures associated with intraosseous hemangiomas usually result in low-intermediate marrow signal on T1WI. **Hemangiomas in soft tissue:** Lesions can have either well-circumscribed margins or irregular margins. They usually have low-intermediate signal or heterogeneous low-intermediate and high signal on T1WI and PDWI. Hemangiomas often have defined margins with high signal on T2WI, and high signal on FS T2WI except for zones of fat within the lesions. Lesions usually show prominent Gd-contrast enhancement.	Benign hamartomatous lesions of bone and soft tissues composed of capillary, cavernous, and/or malformed venous vessels, with or without varying amounts of mature adipose tissue. **(See Atlas Chapter A 34)**
Dermoid (Fig. 20.12)	Circumscribed lesions that may have identifiable walls with low signal on T1WI and T2WI. The contents of dermoid cysts can have low, intermediate, and/or high signal on T1WI and T2WI. Fluid–fluid and fat–fluid levels may be seen within dermoids. Lesions may show enhancement at the wall margins, but not centrally. Dermoids may be associated with anomalies such as skeletal dysraphism and dorsal dermal sinus.	Ectoderm-lined inclusion cysts that contain hair, sebaceous and sweat glands, and squamous epithelium. These lesions slowly enlarge, but are not considered to be neoplasms. **(See Atlas Chapter A 15)**

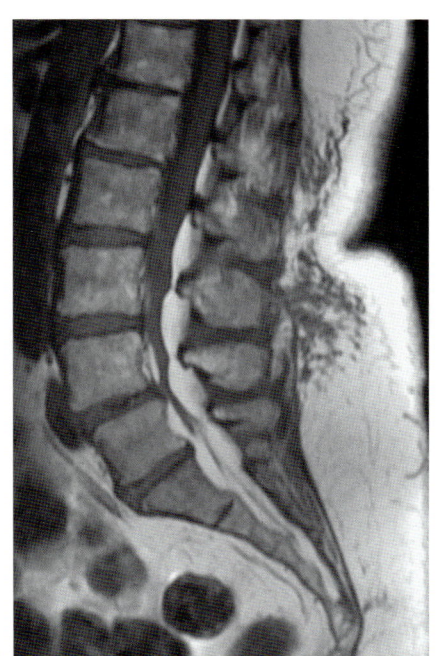

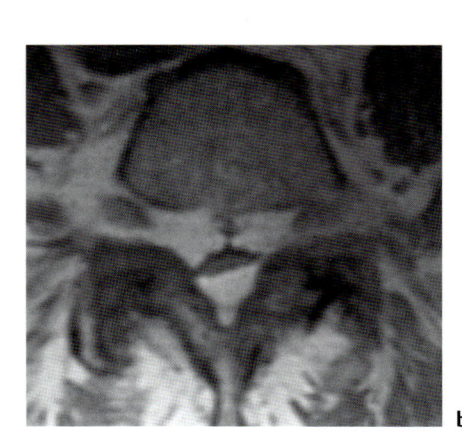

Figure 20.9 a, b Epidural lipomatosis in a 52-year-old man. Prominent epidural fat is seen in the lumbar spinal canal causing narrowing of the thecal sac on sagittal T1WI (**a**) and axial PDWI (**b**).

Dermoid **317**

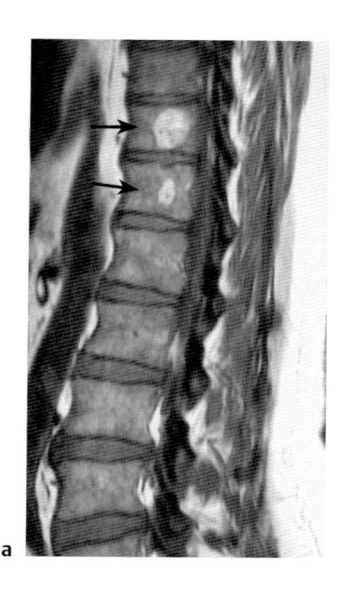

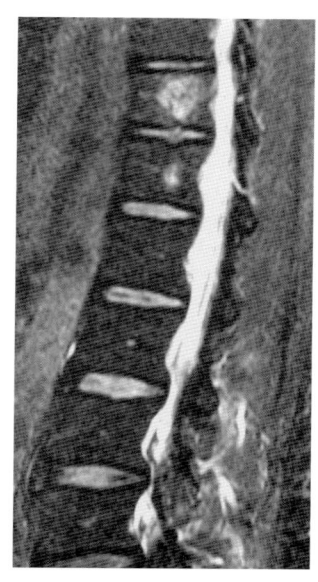

Figure 20.**10 a, b**   Hemangiomas in the T12 and L1 vertebral bodies. The hemangiomas have spheroid configurations and have mostly high signal on sagittal (**a**) and sagittal FS T2WI (**b**).

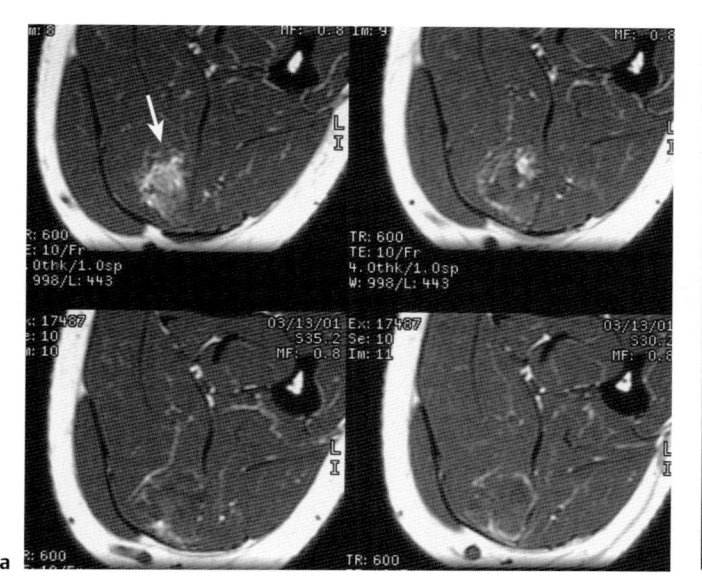

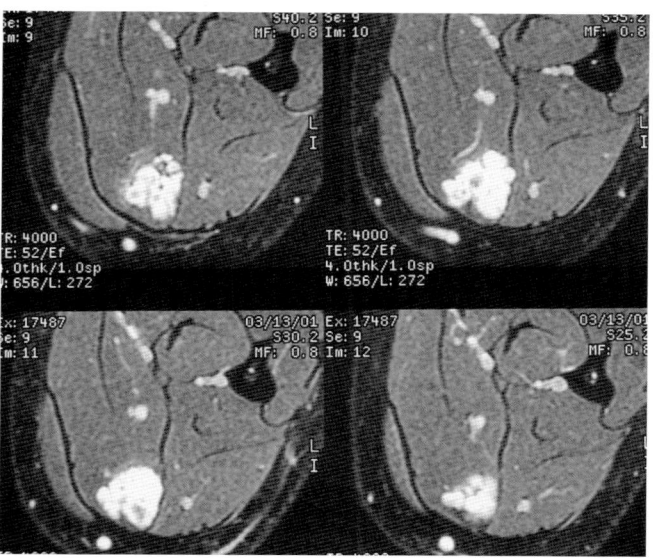

Figure 20.**11 a, b**   Intramuscular hemangioma in the soleus muscle of the leg. The lesion has slightly lobulated margins and contains zones of intermediate and high signal on axial T1WI (**a**) and high signal on axial FS T2WI (**b**).

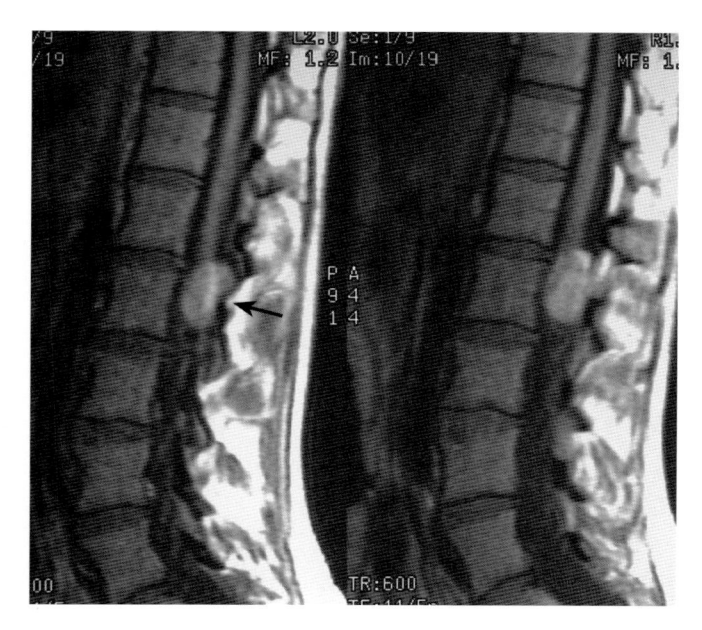

Figure 20.**12**   A 27-year-old woman with a dermoid in the posterior lumbar spinal canal. The lesion has high signal on sagittal T1WI.

Table 20 (Continued) Lesions that contain fat

Lesion	MRI Findings	Comments
Teratoma (Fig. 20.13)	Lesions usually have circumscribed margins and can contain various combinations and proportions of zones with low, intermediate, and/or high signal on T1WI, PDWI, T2WI, and FS T2WI. Lesions can contain teeth and zones of bone formation, as well as amorphous, clump-like, and/or curvilinear calcifications with low signal on T1WI, PDWI, T2WI, and FS T2WI. Fluid–fluid and fat–fluid levels may be seen within teratomas. Gd-contrast enhancement is usually seen in solid portions and septa. Invasion of adjacent tissue and bone destruction, as well as metastases are findings associated with malignant teratomas.	Teratomas are neoplasms that arise from displaced embryonic germ cells (multipotential germinal cells), and contain various combinations of cells and tissues derived from more than one germ layer (endoderm, mesoderm, ectoderm). **(See Atlas Chapter A 76)**
Muscle infarct (Fig. 20.14)	In the early phases of ischemia and infarction, poorly defined zones of increased signal on T2WI and FS T2WI can be seen in the involved muscles. Remote infarcts are seen as fatty replacement of muscle tissue.	Zones of ischemic injury and death involving muscle can result from trauma, corticosteroid treatment, chemotherapy, radiation treatment, diabetes, occlusive vascular disease, collagen vascular and other autoimmune diseases. **(See Atlas Chapter A 37)**
Denervation of muscle (Fig. 20.15)	In the early phases of denervation within 15 days, involved muscles can have low signal on T1WI, and slightly high to high signal on T2WI and FS T2WI without involvement of the adjacent fascia and subcutaneous fat. After one year, fatty replacement of the involved muscles with atrophy can be seen.	Early phases of denervation results in neurogenic edema. In chronic and complete muscle denervation after 1 year, atrophy and fatty replacement of muscle typically occurs. Parsonage–Turner syndrome is one type of denervation that results in an acute painful shoulder from injury of the brachial plexus and damage to the suprascapular nerve (C 5, C 6) with involvement of the supraspinatus and/or infraspinatus muscles. Quadrilateral space syndrome results from damage or injury to the axillary nerve (C 5, C 6) that can affect the teres minor and deltoid muscles.
Lipoma arborescens (Fig. 20.16)	Usually appears as multiple nodular or frond-like deposits with fat signal within hypertrophied synovium, often associated with a joint effusion.	Lipoma arborescens, also referred to as diffuse synovial lipoma, represents a disorder in which there are multiple villous or frond-like zones of fatty deposition in synovium within a joint, tendon sheath, and/or bursa. **(See Atlas Chapter A 43)**
Liposclerosing myxofibrous tumor (Fig. 20.17)	Lesions have well-defined margins with variable thickness of low signal on T1WI and T2WI. Lesions often have low to intermediate signal on T1WI and intermediate to high signal on T2WI and FS T2WI. Small zones with signal equal to fat can be seen at the periphery of these lesions.	Uncommon benign fibro-osseous lesions that contain varying proportions with histologic features of lipoma, fibroxanthoma, myxoma, fibrous dysplasia, bone cyst, myxofibroma, fat necrosis, and/or ischemic ossification. Most of the lesions occur in the intertrochanteric region of the femur. **(See Atlas Chapter A 45)**
Xanthoma (Fig. 20.18)	Often appear as zones of fusiform enlargement of tendons with diffuse heterogeneous signal **(Atlas Figs. 505, 506).** Usually contain multiple longitudinally oriented linear zones or striations with intermediate signal on T1WI and PDWI, and intermediate to slightly high signal on T2WI and FS T2WI interspersed among bands of low signal within the enlarged tendons **(Atlas Fig. 506)** On axial images, xanthomas often have a stippled or reticulated pattern on T1WI and T2WI resulting from collagen bundles with low signal surrounded by higher signal from lipid deposits, foamy histiocytes, and inflammatory reaction. **(Atlas Fig. 506)**	Xanthomas represent localized accumulations of lipids within normal structures such as tendons, skin, and bone. Xanthomas are considered reactive lesions and are not true neoplasms, and often occur in the setting of types I, II, and III hyperlipoproteinemia. **(See Atlas Chapter A 77).**

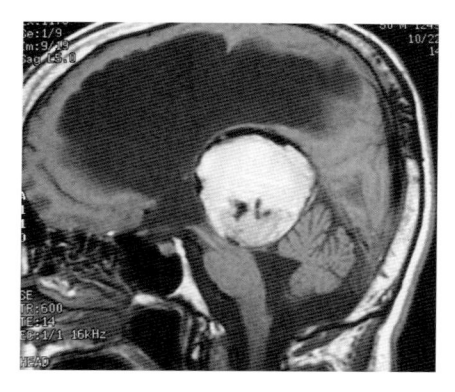

Figure 20.**13** A 50-year-old man with an intracranial teratoma in the pineal recess. The lesion has a peripheral rim of low signal surrounding internal contents with mostly high signal as well as small zones of low signal on T1WI.

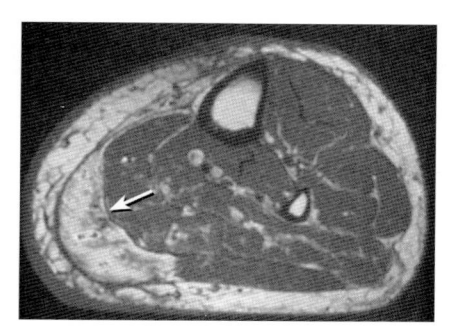

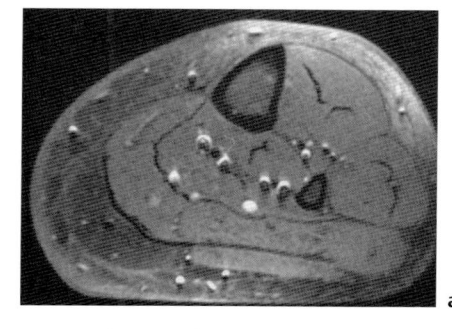

Figure 20.**14 a, b** A 60-year-old man with a remote infarct involving the medial gastrocnemius muscle. There is diffuse high signal on axial T1WI (**a**) in the muscle secondary to fatty atrophy resulting from the infarct which has corresponding low signal on axial FS T1WI (**b**).

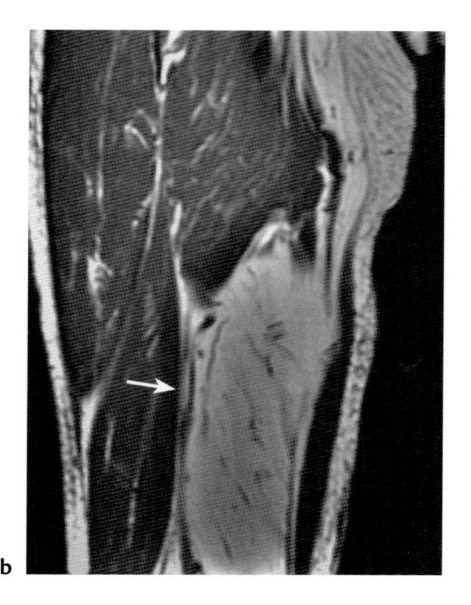

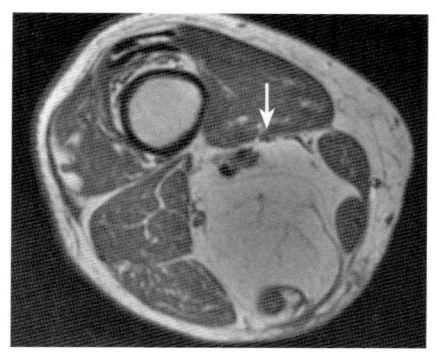

Figure 20.**15 a, b** Denervation in an 82-year-old man with a history of polio. Extensive fatty replacement is seen involving the semimembranosus muscle on coronal (**a**) and axial (**b**) T1WI.

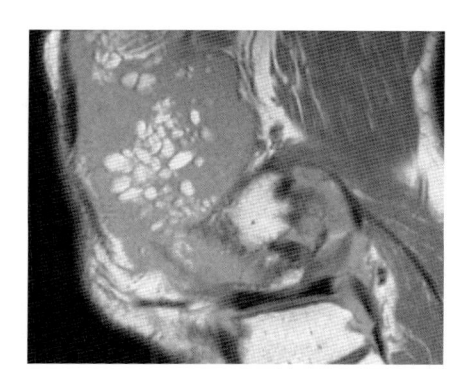

Figure 20.**16** A 37-year-old man with lipoma arborescens at the knee. Multiple nodular and frond like/villous deposits with fat signal are seen within hypertrophied synovium on sagittal PDWI.

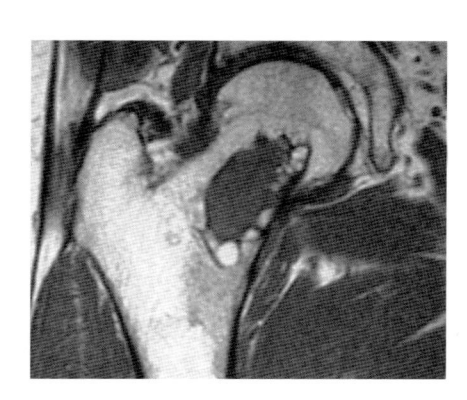

Figure 20.**17** A 61-year-old man with a liposclerosing myxofibrous tumor in the intertrochanteric portion of the femur. The lesion has well-defined margins with thin low signal margins on coronal T1WI. The internal portion of the lesion has mostly low-intermediate signal as well as small peripheral zones with high fat signal.

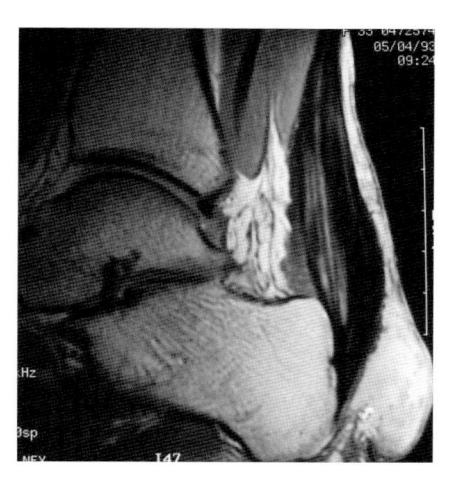

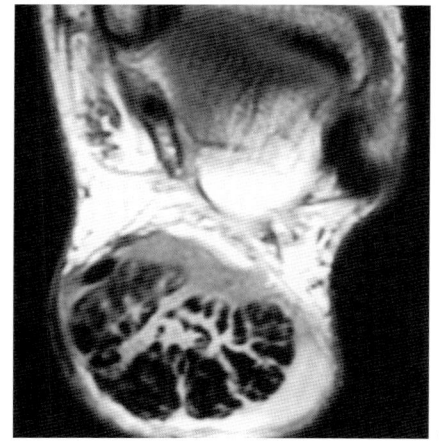

Figure 20.**18 a, b** Xanthoma involving the Achilles' tendon. Sagittal (**a**) and axial (**b**) T1WI shows striated zones with increased signal within an enlarged tendon.

Table 20 (Continued) **Lesions that contain fat**

| Lesion | MRI Findings | Comments |

Malignant

Liposarcoma (Figs. 20.19–20.21) | **Well-differentiated type:** tumors contain up to 75% overall fat signal, as well as thick nonadipose septae and/or nodular nonadipose zones. Nonadipose zones can have low-intermediate signal on T1WI and PDWI and low, intermediate, and/or high signal on T2WI. Tumor margins are usually smooth, well-defined, and/or lobulated. Nonadipose portions of these tumors can show varying degrees of Gd-contrast enhancement. MRI features that are more commonly associated with well-differentiated liposarcomas compared with lipomas include large tumor size and presence of Gd-contrast enhancing nonadipose thick septa or nodular/patchy zones. **Myxoid type:** These tumors usually have predominantly low signal on T1WI, and may contain smaller proportions of high fat signal in lacy, amorphous, and/or linear configurations. Most myxoid liposarcomas contain < 26% fat. Some myxoid liposarcomas do not contain fatty zones. Tumors can have heterogeneous or homogeneous high signal on PDWI, T2WI, and some have a multiloculated pattern. Low signal septa may be present on T2WI. Tumors usually show Gd-contrast enhancement in varying degrees and patterns, or rarely none at all. **Pleomorphic type:** Tumors often have relatively well-defined margins, and have heterogeneous/mixed low, intermediate, and/or high signal on T1WI, PDWI, and T2WI. Less than 26% of the tumor volumes have fat signal. Tumors usually show prominent Gd-contrast enhancement in a heterogeneous pattern. **Round cell liposarcomas:** Tumors can have relatively well-defined margins (72%) or poorly defined margins (28%), and have heterogeneous/mixed low, intermediate, and/or high signal on T1WI, PDWI, and T2WI. Most round cell liposarcomas contain < 26% fat. Tumors usually show prominent Gd-contrast enhancement (61%) in a heterogeneous pattern that may be globular or nodular. **Dedifferentiated liposarcomas:** Tumors have a component with features of a well-differentiated liposarcoma as well as a focal nonlipomatous mass. These tumors frequently occur in the retroperitoneum and are large (mean = 19.3 cm). Tumors can have well-defined, relatively well-defined, and/or irregular/poorly defined margins. Tumors often have heterogeneous/mixed low, intermediate, and/or high signal on T1WI, PDWI, and T2WI. Hemorrhage and necrosis can be seen in the nonlipomatous portions. Tumors often show prominent Gd-contrast enhancement in nonlipomatous portions in a heterogeneous or homogeneous pattern. | Malignant mesenchymal tumors containing portions showing differentiation into adipose tissue. Liposarcomas are classified into five sub-types (well-differentiated [40–54%], myxoid [23%], pleomorphic [5–7%], dedifferentiated [10%], and round cell [6%]). **(See Atlas Chapter A 44)**

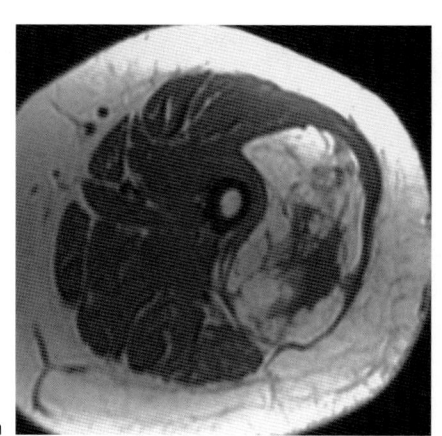

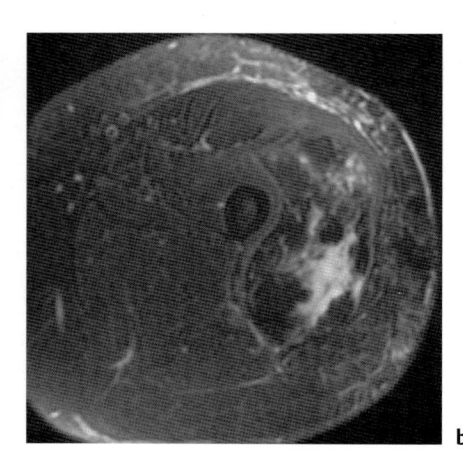

Figure 20.**19 a, b** A 57-year-old woman with a well-differentiated low-grade liposarcoma involving the vastus lateralis muscle of the thigh. The tumor has high fat signal on axial T1WI (**a**) as well as zones with low-intermediate signal. The nonfatty portions of the tumor have high signal on axial FS T2WI (**b**).

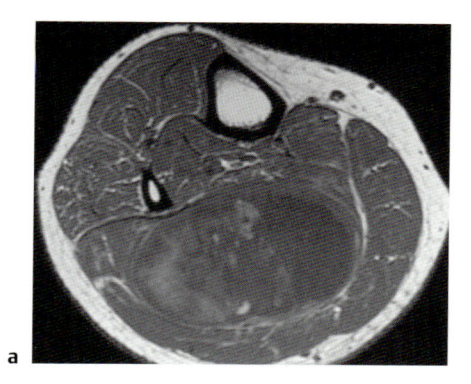

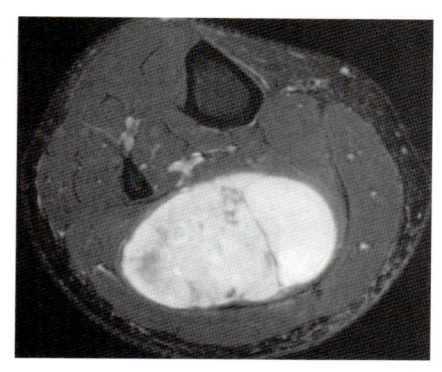

Figure 20.**20 a, b** A 34-year-old woman with a myxoid liposarcoma in the posterior calf. The tumor has circumscribed margins and contains mostly low-intermediate signal on axial T1WI (**a**) as well as small irregular zones of high fat signal. Most of the tumor has high signal on axial (**b**) FS T2WI secondary to the myxoid components. The signal from the zones of fat is suppressed on FS T2WI.

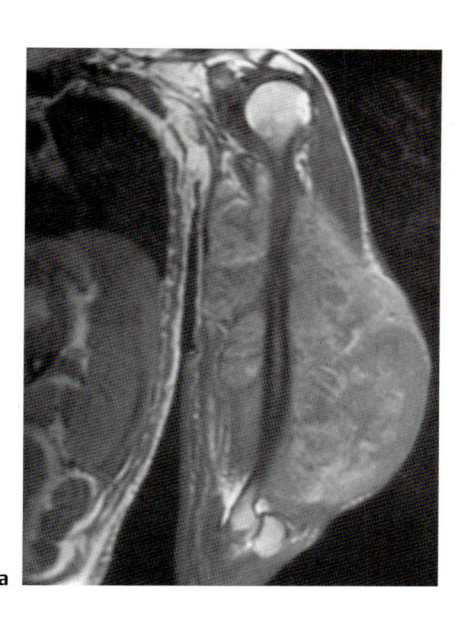

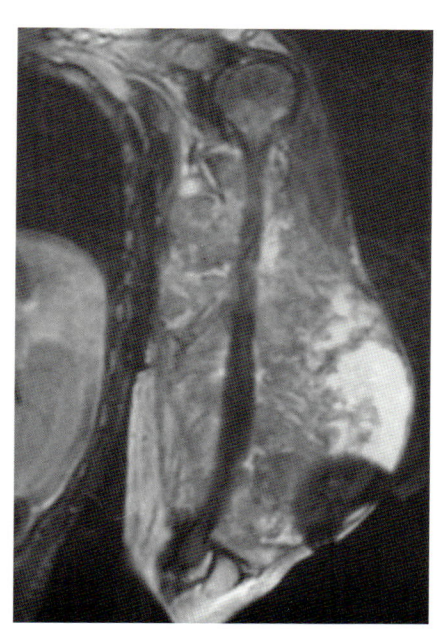

Figure 20.**21 a, b** A 43-year-old man with a high-grade pleomorphic liposarcoma involving the left arm. The tumor has heterogeneous intermediate and slightly high signal on coronal T1WI (**a**) and mixed low-intermediate, slightly high, and high signal on coronal FS T2WI (**b**).

References

Lipomatosis

Amine B, Leguilchard F, Benhamou CL. Dercum's disease (adiposis dolorosa): a new case - report. *Joint Bone Spine* 2004;71:147–149.

Drevelegas A, Pilavaki M, Chourmouzi D. Lipomatous tumors of soft tissue: MR appearance with histological correlation. *Eur J Radiol* 2004;50:257–267.

Haloi AK, Ditchfield M, Penington A, Phillips R. Facial infiltrative lipomatosis. *Pediatr Radiol* 2006;36:1159–1162.

Klein FA, Smith MJ, Kasenetz I. Pelvic lipomatosis: 35-year experience. *J Urol* May 1988;139(5):998–1001.

Murphy MD, Carroll JF, Flemming DJ, Pope TL, Gannon FH, Kransdorf MJ. Benign musculoskeletal lipomatous lesions. *RadioGraphics* September–October 2004;24(5):1433–1466.

Sener RN. Epidural, paraspinal, and subcutaneous lipomatosis. *Pediatr Radiol* 2003;33:655–657.

Torigian DA, Siegelman ES. CT findings of pelvic lipomatosis of nerve. *AJR* March 2005;184:94–96.

Spinal Angiolipoma

Leu NH, Chen CY, Shy CG, et al. MR imaging of an infiltrating spinal epidural angiolipoma. *AJNR* May 2003;24:1008–1011.

Gelabert-González M, Agulleiro-Díaz J, Reyes-Santías RM. Spinal extradural angiolipoma, with a literature review. *Childs Nerv Syst* 2002; 18:725–728.

Klisch J, Spreer J, Bloss HG, Baborie A, Hubbe U. Radiological and histological findings in spinal intramedullary angiolipoma. *Neuroradiology* 1999;41:584–587.

Denervation of Muscle

Bredella MA, Tirman PFJ, Fritz RC, Wischer TK, Stork A, Genant HK. Denervation syndromes of the shoulder girdle: MR imaging with electrophysiologic correlation. *Skeletal Radiol* 1999;28:567–572.

Cothan RL, Helms C. Quadrilateral space syndrome: incidence of imaging findings in a population referred for MRI of the shoulder. *AJR* 2005;184:989–992.

Atlas

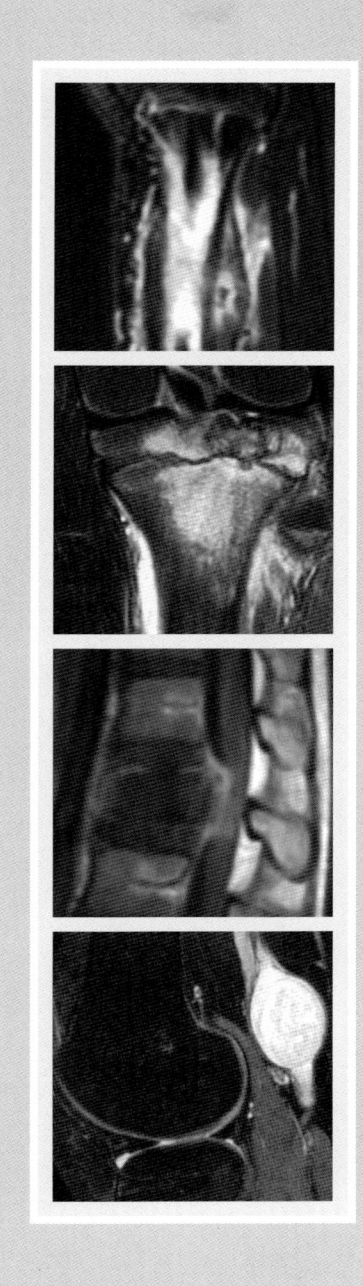

A 1 Adamantinoma (Also Referred to as Extragnathic Adamantinoma, Adamantinoma of Long Bones, Juvenile Intracortical Adamantinoma)[3]

ICD-O Code

9261/3

Definition

Adamantinomas are rare, low-grade malignant bone tumors consisting of epithelial cells surrounded by spindle cells and osteofibrous tissue that often involve the shaft of the tibia.[2–4,9,10,12,13]

Frequency of Occurrence

Adamantinomas of long bones account for < 1 % of primary bone tumors.[3,4,7,8,12,13]

Age at Presentation

From 3 to 86 years, median = 19–25 years, average = 35 years, most common in 3rd and 4th decades.[3,4,7,8,12,13]

Gender Ratio (M/F)

1/1 to 2/1[3,4,9,12]

Location

Lesions usually occur in the tibia (mid-diaphysis > distal metaphysis), but much more rarely in the fibula, ulna, femur, radius, humerus, metatarsals, capitate, ischium, and ribs.[2–4,9,12,13] Tumors in the tibia involve the anterior cortex in 86 % of cases.[13] Tumors occasionally involve only the posterior or posteromedial tibial cortex.[13]

Signs and Symptoms[2–4]

Tumors can present as localized swelling with or without pain. Pathologic fractures occur in up to 10 % of cases.[13] The duration of symptoms ranges from months to years.

Gross Pathologic Findings

These tumors are considered as low-grade, malignant neoplasms of epithelial origin. Tumors are well-circumscribed, fleshy, fibrous lesions, which are often more than 5 cm in length and may contain cystic zones with or without hemorrhage.[2–6,10,12,13] Tumors can involve bone cortex, with or without marrow involvement.[2–6,10,12,13]

Histopathologic Findings[2–6,10,12,13]

Tumors often have variable proportions of epithelial-like and mesenchymal-like components. Tumor cells can appear as large polygonal cells with euchromatin, fusiform cells, and/or small cells with poorly defined cytoplasm. Mitotic figures are usually uncommon. Collagenized zones may be present, and regions of giant cell reaction can be seen in hemorrhagic portions.[2,3] Two major histologic patterns have also been described which are at the opposite ends of a spectrum: the classic adamantinoma type and the osteofibrous dysplasia-like type.[13] The classic type contains aggregates of epithelial cells which proportionally dominate the osteofibrous background.[13] There are four differentiation patterns of the classic form: basiloid, squamoid, tubular, and spindle cell.[2,3] More than one of these patterns often occurs in a single lesion.[2,3] The basiloid pattern is made up of lobules of cuboid or columnar cells.[2,3] The squamoid type contains zones of squamous differentiation with keratinization.[2,3] The tubular pattern consists of loose fascicles of elongated cells adjacent to bone trabeculae lined by osteoblasts.[2,3] The spindle cell pattern includes cells in storiform, herringbone, or cartwheel arrangements, often with abundant collagen.[2,3] The osteofibrous dysplasia-type adamantinoma contains proportionally dominant osteofibrous tissue relative to minimal scattered keratin-positive epithelial tumor cells.[2,3,13] Lesions can be associated with fibrous dysplasia-like regions.[2,3,13] Tumors have been reported to show immunoreactivity to basal epithelial keratins 1, 5, 13, 14, and 19, vimentin in spindle cells, and carcinoembryonic antigen.[2,3]

Tumor Genetics

Tumors may show two balanced translocations, t(1;13;22)(q22;p13) and t(15;17)(q12;p13),[2,10] and another translocation has been reported, t(7;13)(q32 q14).[2] Gains of chromosomes 7, 8, 12, and 19 have also been reported.[3] Aneuploid zones and TP53 gene abnormalities have been observed in the epithelial portions of the tumors.[2,3]

Findings on Plain Films (Roentgenograms)[1–3,5,6,13,14]

Lesions appear as eccentric circumscribed zones of radiolucency involving the cortex, which occur as either a solitary focus or in a "saw-tooth" and/or multinodular pattern (Fig. **1**). The involved cortex is often thickened.[13] Tumors can extend into the marrow resulting in a honeycomb radiolucent appearance. Extra-osseous soft tissue lesions and periosteal bone formation may occasionally be seen with adamantinomas.

MRI Findings[1,5,13]

Adamantinomas can appear either as a solitary lobulated focus (73 %) or in a multinodular pattern of signal alteration in bone cortex (27 %), with or without marrow involvement (Fig. **1**). Tumors can extend longitudinally within bone from 2 to 21 cm, mean = 9 cm.[13] With MRI, 60 % of adamantinomas have been shown to involve bone cortex and marrow compared with 40 % that showed only cortical involvement.[13] Tumor foci in bone typically have low-intermediate signal on T1WI and PDWI, and slightly high to high signal on T2WI and FS T2WI. Tumor signal on T2WI and FS T2WI can be homogeneous (62 %) or heterogeneous (38 %).[13] After Gd-contrast administration, lesions usually show prominent enhancement.[13] Adamantinomas with a multinodular pattern have enhancing nodules which have high signal on T2WI and FS T2WI separated by zones of low signal from intervening cortical bone.[13] Tumor destruction of the outer cortical margins was observed in 32 % of cases.[13] Only 9 % of adamantinomas showed tumor extension into the adjacent soft tissues.[13]

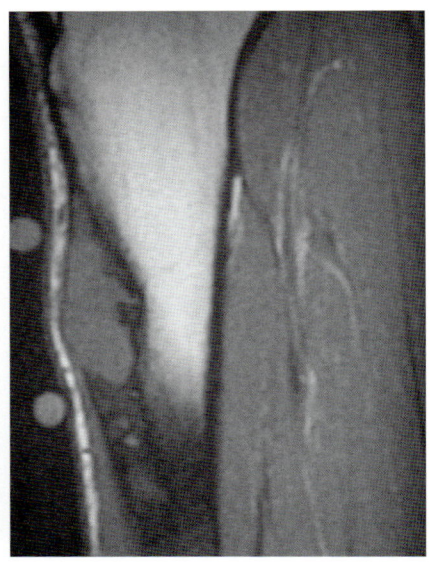

Figure **1 a–d** A 23-year-old woman with an adamantinoma of the tibial diaphysis. AP radiograph (**a**) shows a radiolucent lesion in the tibia. MRI shows the tumor to have low-intermediate signal on T1WI (**b**), high signal on T2WI (**c**), and Gd-contrast enhancement on FS T1WI (**d**). There is expansion of the cortical bone at the site of the tumor, as well as tumor extension toward the marrow.

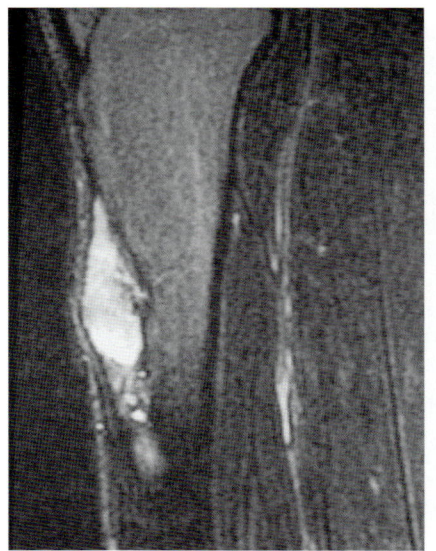

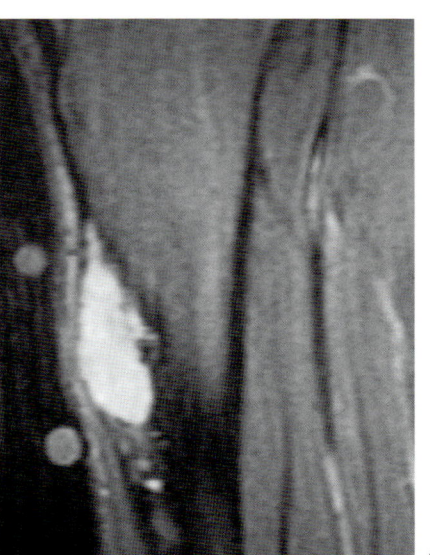

Differential Diagnosis

Osteofibrous dysplasia, fibrous dysplasia, metastatic disease, eosinophilic granuloma, aneurysmal bone cyst, chondromyxoid fibroma, non-ossifying fibroma, osteomyelitis.

Treatment and Prognosis[2–4,12,13]

Wide excision with bone grafting is the optimal treatment. Where resection is incomplete, local recurrence has been reported to occur in 32% of cases and lung metastases in 25%.[13] Metastatic disease and paraneoplastic syndromes have also been reported. Lesions are considered to be resistant to radiation treatment. The mortality rate is ~15% of patients suffering from adamantinomas.

References

1 Conway WF, Hayes CW. Miscellaneous lesion of bone. *Radiol Clin North Am* 1993;31(2):339–358.
2 Forest M. Adamantinoma. In: Forest M, Tomeno B, Vanel D, eds. *Orthopedic Surgical Pathology: Diagnosis of Tumors and Pseudotumoral Lesions of Bone and Joints* Edinburgh: Churchill Livingstone; 1998:385–393.
3 Hogendoorn PCW, Hashimoto H. Adamantinoma. In: Fletcher CDM, Unni KK, Mertens F, eds. *World Health Organization Classification of Tumours. Pathology and Genetics of Tumours of Soft Tissue and Bone* Geneva: IARC Press; 2002:333–334.
4 Huvos AG. Adamantinoma of extragnathic bones. In: Huvos, AG, ed. *Bone Tumors: Diagnosis, Treatment, and Prognosis* 2nd ed. Philadelphia, Pa: W.B. Saunders; 1991:677–693.
5 Judmaier W, Peer S, Krejzi T, Dessl A, Kuhberger R. MR findings in tibial adamantinoma—a case report. *Acta Radiol* 1998;39:276–278
6 Kumar D, Mulligan ME, Levine AM, Dorfman HD. Classic adamantinoma in a 3-year-old. *Skeletal Radiol* 1998;27:406–409.
7 Mulder JD, Schutte HE, Kroon HM, Taconis WK. Introduction. In: *Radiologic Atlas of Bone Tumors* Amsterdam: Elsevier; 1993:3–6.
8 Mulder JD, Schutte HE, Kroon HM, Taconis WK. The Diagnosis of Bone Tumors. In: *Radiologic Atlas of Bone Tumors* Amsterdam: Elsevier; 1993:9–46.
9 Mulder JD, Schutte HE, Kroon HM, Taconis WK. Adamantinoma. In: *Radiologic Atlas of Bone Tumors* Amsterdam: Elsevier; 1993: 255–262.

10 Salisbury JR. Bone neoplasms containing epithelial and epitheloid cells. In: Helliwell TR, ed. *Pathology of Bone and Joint Neoplasms* Philadelphia, Pa: W.B. Saunders; 1999:345–368.

11 Unni KK. Introduction and scope of study. In: *Dahlin's Bone Tumors: General Aspects and Data on 11 087 Cases* 5th ed. Philadelphia, Pa: Lippincott, Williams & Wilkins; 1996:1–9.

12 Unni KK. Adamantinoma of long bones. In: *Dahlin's Bone Tumors: General Aspects and Data on 11 087 Cases* 5th ed. Philadelphia, Pa: Lippincott, Williams & Wilkins; 1996:333–342.

13 Van der Woude HJ, Hazelbag HM, Bloem JL, Taminiau AHM, Hogendoorn PCW. MRI of adamantinoma of long bones in correlation with histopathology. *AJR Am J Roentgenol* 2004;183:1737–1744.

14 Young JWR, Aisner SC, Resnik CS, Levine AM, Dorfman HD, Whitley NO. Case Report 660. *Skeletal Radiol* 1991;20:152–156.

A 2　Aneurysmal Bone Cyst

Definition

Aneurysmal bone cysts (ABCs) are tumor-like expansile bone lesions containing cavernous spaces filled with blood.[1,10,13,21,27,30,32,40] Two-thirds of ABCs are primary bone lesions but may otherwise be secondary to other bone lesions/tumors such as giant cell tumors, chondroblastomas, osteoblastomas, osteosarcomas, chondromyxoid fibromas, nonossifying fibromas, fibrous dysplasia, fibrosarcomas, malignant fibrous histiocytomas, and metastatic disease.[10,13,32,40] Solid ABCs are also referred to as **giant cell reparative granulomas**[14,32]

Frequency of Occurrence

ABCs account for ~11% of primary tumor-like lesions of bone.[25–27,40]

Age at Presentation

From 1 to 25 years, median = 14 years.[13,25–27,32] As many as 75–85% occur in patients below 25 years.[13,25,26] Patients with aneurysmal bone cysts tend to be younger than patients with giant cell tumors.[40] ABCs occasionally occur in older adults up to 67 years of age.[25,26]

Gender Ratio (M / F)

1 / 1 to 1 / 1.3 [13,16,32]

Location[8,10,13,16,19,21,22,29,32–34,40]

ABCs occur in many different bones, often involving the metaphyseal regions of long bones, and posterior elements of vertebrae. Long bones represent ~50–60% of cases, vertebrae ~20–30%, and short tubular and flat bones ~20%. Distal femur or proximal tibia > cervical vertebrae > thoracic vertebrae > proximal femur > sacrum, proximal fibula, carpal bones > proximal humerus, distal tibia, distal fibula > scapula, iliac bones > craniofacial bones. Most lesions are eccentric within medullary bone, although cortically centered lesions occur in up to 18% of cases.[16,33] In the spine, the posterior elements are usually involved in nearly all cases (lamina in 80%, pedicles in 59%), and the vertebral bodies in 71%.[29] Lesions in the sacrum usually involve more than one segment.[29] Multiple sites of involvement occur in 8% of cases.[16] Solid ABCs (giant cell reparative granulomas) occur in the femur > ulna > tibia > humerus, radius, fibula > other bones; metaphyseal > diaphyseal > juxtaarticular > metadiaphyseal locations; most often they are eccentric within medullary bone.[14] Aneurysmal cysts rarely occur in soft tissues[19,34]

Signs and Symptoms[10,13,16,27,32,40]

Patients can present with local pain and swelling (weeks to months), or with pathologic fractures in up to 25% of cases. Spinal lesions can be associated with spinal cord compression[13,32]

Gross Pathologic Findings[6,8,10,13,14,21,27,30,32,40]

Lesions often appear as sponge-like tissue in bone with cavities ranging in size from millimeters to 2 cm, filled with unclotted blood. A thin layer of periosteal bone covers the lesion. Solid components of aneurysmal bone cysts have friable and/or fibrous tissue with zones of hemorrhage.

Histopathologic Findings[6,8,10,13,14,21,27,30,32,40]

Primary ABCs typically have cavernous spaces filled with blood. Fibrous septae lined by fibroblastic cells as well as strands of woven bone are present between dilated capillaries or sinusoids. Osteoclastic giant cells and hemosiderin-laden macrophages are also often present in the septae lining the blood channels. The outer expansile margins of the lesion are limited by periosteal connective tissue and/or periosteal bone. A solid variant of ABC (or giant cell reparative granuloma) contains spindle-cells and osteoclasts surrounding zones of hemorrhage and necrosis.[14,32] Zones of woven bone are also present.[14,32] Careful evaluation of all ABCs should be made for the presence of co-existent bone tumors to enable appropriate treatment planning.

Lesion Genetics

Chromosomal rearrangements involving the short arm of chromosome 17 with five different chromosomes have been reported.[32] Many ABCs probably result from acquired chromosomal rearrangements with clonal proliferations from activation of a 17 p oncogene.[32]

Findings on Plain Films (Roentgenograms) and Computed Tomography[1–5,7–13,15–18,21,22,27,28,31–33,35,36,40]

Lesions often appear as solitary, expansile radiolucent lesions that are often eccentric within medullary bone with narrow zones of transition, with or without sclerotic borders adjacent to normal bone (Figs. **2–7**). Outer expanded margins of lesions often have a thin shell of bone which may partially demineralize. Lesions may have associated extra-osseous soft tissue components. Invasion of the growth plate can occur in children. CT can show subtle subperiosteal calcification and internal features such as small trabeculae and fluid–fluid levels.

Findings on Radionuclide Bone Scans

ABCs are usually associated with increased radiopharmaceutical accumulation, often with a rim-like pattern.

MRI Findings[2–5,7–9,11,12,15,16,18,22,23,27,28,31–33,35–38,40]

ABCs often have a low signal rim on T1-, PD-, and T2-weighted images adjacent to normal medullary bone, and between extra-osseous soft tissues (Figs. **2–6**). Various combinations of low, intermediate, and/or high signal on these images are usually seen within ABCs as well as fluid–fluid levels. Variable Gd-contrast enhancement is seen at the margins of lesions as well as involving the internal septae. The solid types of ABCs (or giant cell reparative granuloma) can also have heterogene-

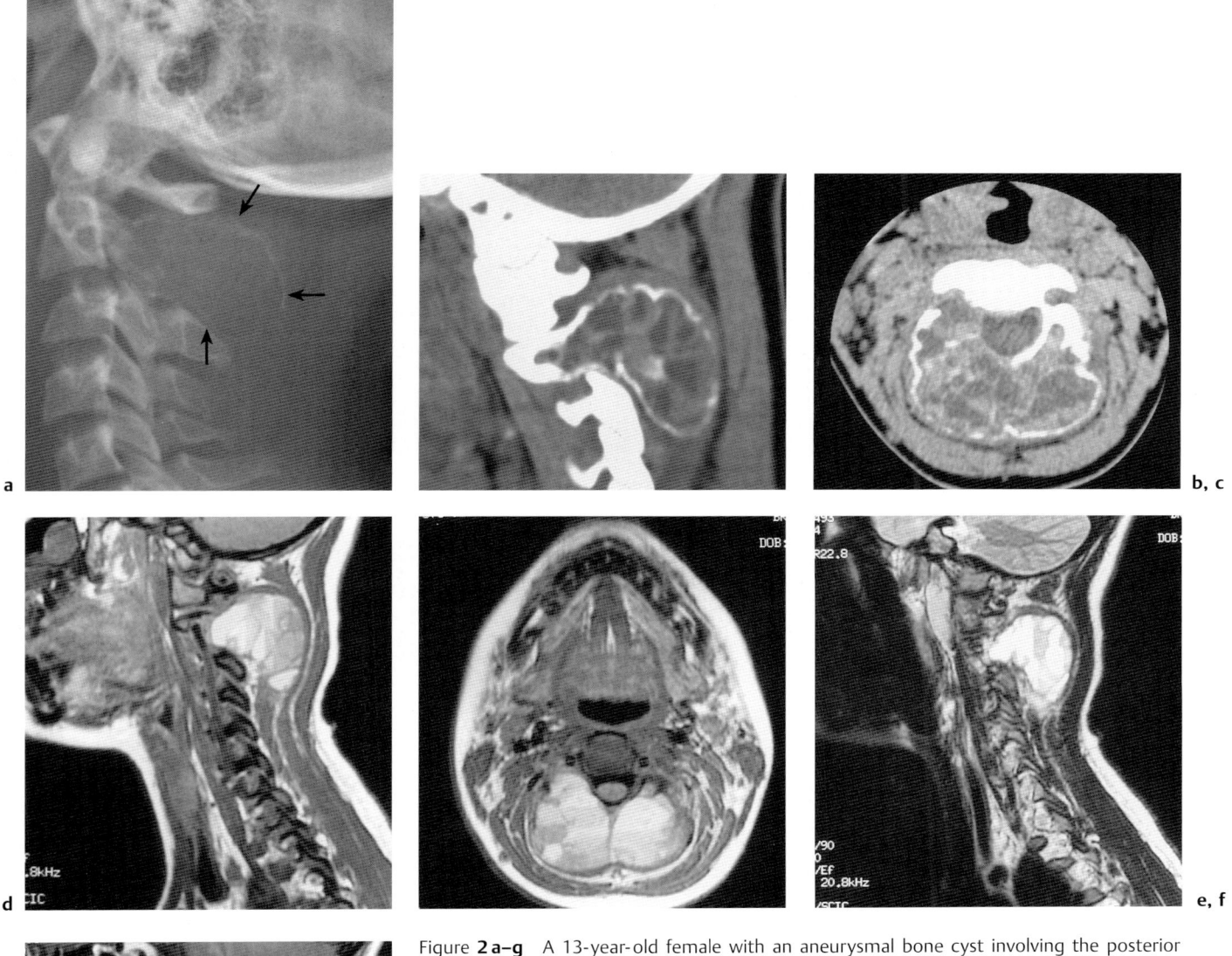

Figure 2a–g A 13-year-old female with an aneurysmal bone cyst involving the posterior elements of C2. Lateral radiograph (a), and sagittal (b) and axial (c) CT scans show an expansile radiolucent lesion involving the posterior elements of C2. Fluid–fluid levels in the lesion are seen on the CT images. MRI shows the expansile lesion to contain multiple fluid–fluid levels on sagittal (d) and axial (e) T1WI, and sagittal (f) T2WI. The lesion shows multiple lobules with peripheral rimlike Gd-contrast enhancement on sagittal (g) T1WI.

Figure **3 a–d** A 10-year-old female with an aneurysmal bone cyst in the right acetabulum. AP radiograph (**a**) shows a geographic radiolucent lesion. MRI shows the lesion to contain a fluid–fluid level on axial (**b**) T2WI. The lesion shows thin, peripheral rimlike Gd-contrast enhancement on coronal (**c**) and axial (**d**) FS T1WI.

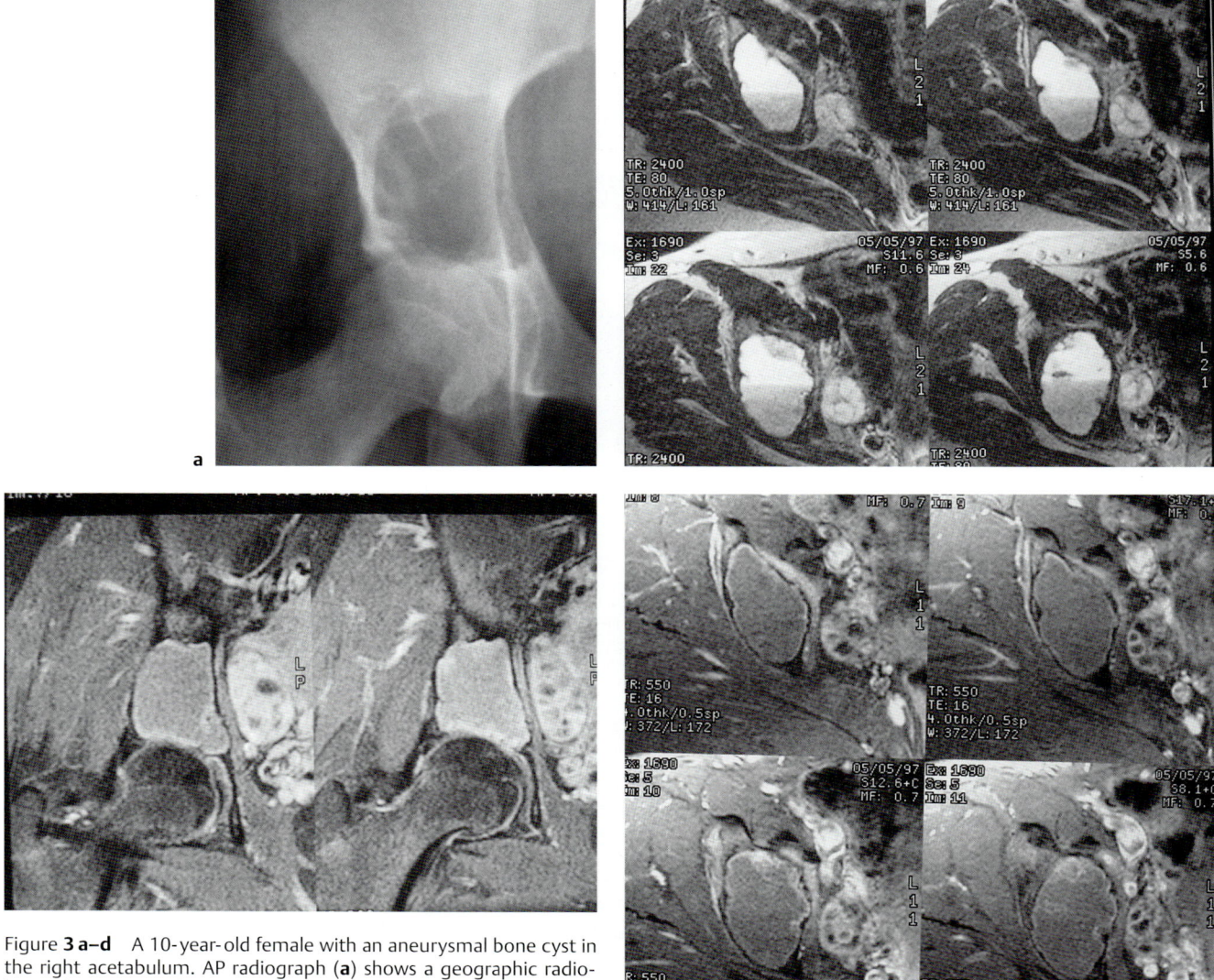

ous low, intermediate, and/or high signal on T1WI, PDWI, and T2WI, as well as peripheral rim-like and central Gd-contrast enhancement on FS T1WI (Fig. **7**).

Differential Diagnosis[9,10,16,20,21,24,37,38]

Giant cell tumor, unicameral bone cyst with hemorrhage, osteoblastoma, brown tumor-hyperparathyroidism, fibrous dysplasia, eosinophilic granuloma, enchondroma, chondroblastoma, metastasis, plasmacytoma, chondromyxoid fibroma, telangiectatic osteosarcoma, osteomyelitis, hemophilic pseudotumor, juxta-articular cysts in rheumatoid arthritis.

Treatment and Prognosis[5,7,8,10,13,16,28,29,40]

Resection or curettage are the most common methods of treatment. Local recurrence can occur in 10–44% of patients.[16] Up to 90% of recurrences occur in the first 2 years.[16] Embolization of ABCs has also been performed as a primary treatment or in preparation for surgical excision.

Treatment and Prognosis **331**

Figure **4a–e** An 11-year-old male with an aneurysmal bone cyst involving the medial proximal shaft of the femur. AP radiograph (**a**) shows a geographic radiolucent expansile lesion. Coronal (**b**) T1WI shows the lesion to have circumscribed margins, and contains mostly intermediate signal with several foci of high signal. Coronal (**c**) and sagittal (**d**) FS T2WI shows the lesion to be multiseptated with fluid–fluid levels containing high and low-intermediate signal. The lesion has expanded and thinned cortical margins as well as high signal in the adjacent soft tissues. The lesion shows peripheral rimlike and septal Gd-contrast enhancement on coronal (**e**) FS T1WI.

Figure **5a–e** A 14-year-old female with an aneurysmal bone cyst in the proximal lateral right tibia. AP radiograph (**a**) shows a geographic radiolucent lesion. MRI shows the lesion to have low to intermediate signal as well as a small focus of high signal on coronal (**b**) T1WI. The lesion contains multiple fluid–fluid levels on coronal (**c**) and axial (**d**) FS T2WI. The lesion shows multiple lobules with peripheral rimlike Gd-contrast enhancement on axial (**e**) FS T1WI.

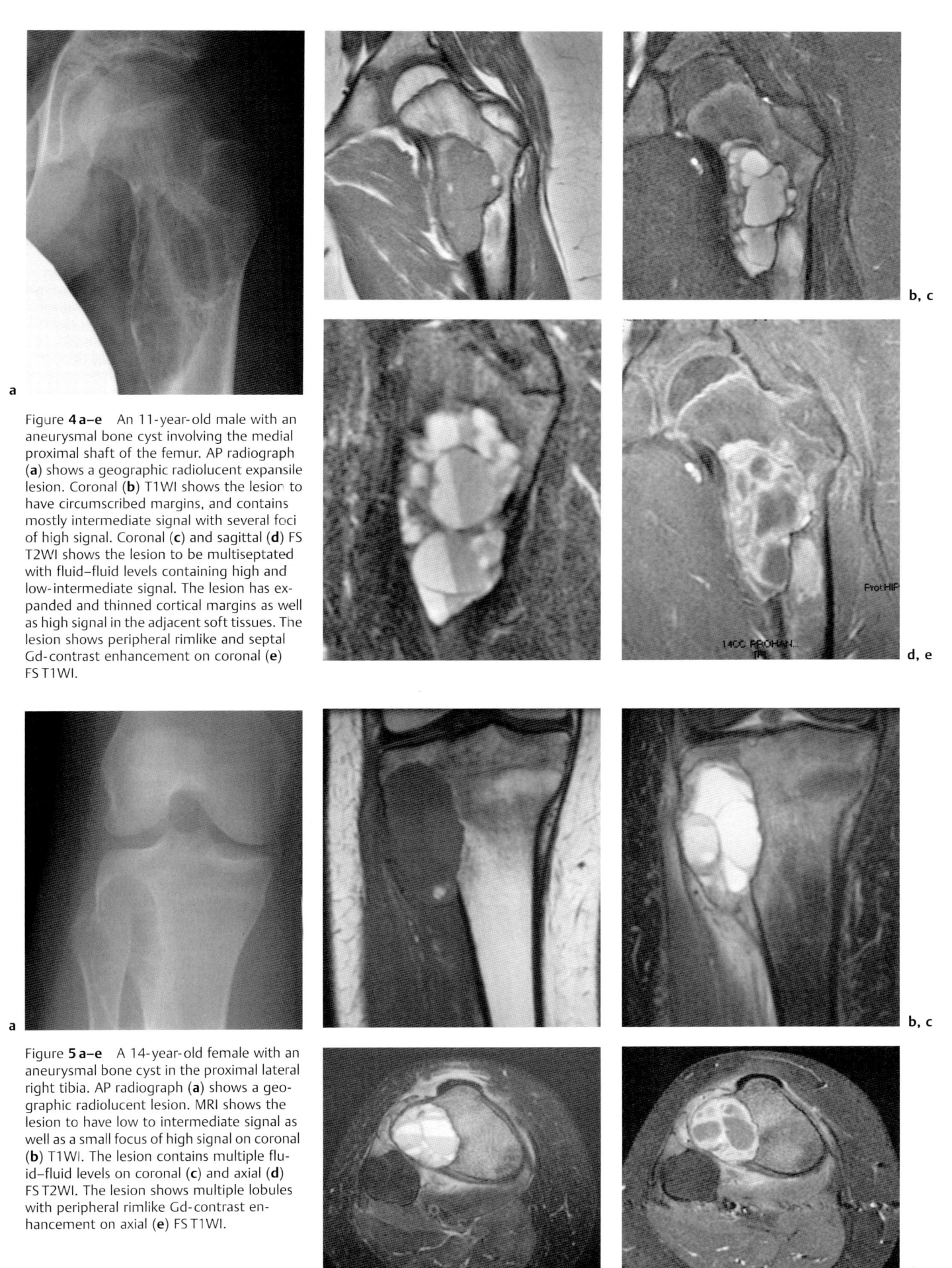

A 3   Bone Cyst (Also Referred to as Simple Bone Cyst, Unicameral Bone Cyst, Solitary Bone Cyst)

Definition

Bone cysts are intramedullary cavities filled with serous or serosanguinous fluid.[1,3,4]

Frequency of Occurrence

Simple or unicameral bone cysts (UBCs) represent ~9% of primary tumor-like lesions of bone.[7]

Age at Presentation

From 1 to 30 years, median = 11 years.[8] Approximately 85% of cases occur in the first two decades.[4] Lesions can also occur in older adults up to 62 years of age.[8,9]

Gender Ratio (M/F)

2/1 to 3/1.[3,4,9]

Location

Lesions are located in the proximal humerus > distal femur > proximal femur > iliac bone > tibia > fibula, calcaneus > radius, ulna > other sites.[3,9]

Signs and Symptoms

UBCs may be initially seen as incidental findings on radiographs or present from pathologic fractures in up to 70% of cases.[3,9] Locations within bone: metadiaphyseal > diaphyseal > metaphyseal.[9] Only 3% of UBCs involve the epiphysis.[9]

Gross Pathologic Findings

UBCs often show a slight bulge in the overlying thinned bone cortex with intact periosteum.[1,3,9] The underlying cyst may have a bluish appearance under the thinned cortex.[9] UBC content is usually clear, yellow-green, and serous, and when associated with pathologic fracture is sero-sanguineous.[1,3,9,11] The inner walls of the UBCs often have a thin glistening, whitish or reddish-brown appearance.[3,9] The inner surface frequently has ridges.[11] Partial or complete septa may be occasionally seen.[11] Usually, one cystic compartment is seen, except for lesions associated with prior fracture or recurrent lesions which may have several compartments.[1,3,9] When complete septa are present, these bone cysts have been referred to as multicameral.[11]

Histopathologic Findings

The cyst walls are composed of a thin continuous or wavy layer of fibrous tissue with fibroblasts, collagen fibers, multinucleated giant cells, with or without zones of hemorrhage or hemosiderin.[1,3,9,11] Immature bone or osteoid trabeculae surrounded by osteoblasts may be seen at the cyst walls.[1] Focal deposits of eosinophilic material in the inner cyst walls derived from fibrin may be seen with calcifications and occasional ossification resembling cementum.[1,9,11] Cyst fluid often contains prostaglandins, interleukin-1, proteolytic enzymes, and alkaline and acid phosphatases.[1] UBCs with pathologic fractures usually show callus and granulation tissue, as well as giant cells, cholesterol crystals, and hemosiderin.[1,9,11]

Lesion Genetics

Cells in these lesions are typically diploid.[1] A complex chromosomal rearrangement involving chromosomes 4, 6, 8, 12, 16, and 21 has been reported in a single case.[1,4]

Findings on Plain Films (Roentgenograms) and Computed Tomography

UBCs are geographic, medullary, radiolucent lesions with well-defined margins that are typically located in the metaphysis and/or diaphysis[1-4,6,9-11] (Figs. **8, 11–13**). UBCs rarely involve the epiphysis.[1,2,9] The margins may be smooth or slightly lobulated.[1,9] Lobulated or trabeculaed margins of UBCs result from ridges on the inner surface of the cortex.[1] In tubular bones, mild to moderate expansion of bone may occur with thinning of the overlying cortex.[1-4,6,9-11] The thinned cortex results in increased susceptibility to pathologic fracture[1-4,6,9-11] (Figs. **12–14**). Periosteal reaction and a "fallen-leaf" fracture fragment are often seen with UBCs complicated by pathologic fracture[1,2,6] (Figs. **12–14**). No matrix mineralization is present in UBCs. No extra-osseous soft tissue mass is associated with UBCs.[1-4,6,9-11]

CT scans may show fluid–fluid levels and fibrous septa.[1]

MRI Findings

UBCs often have a peripheral rims of low signal on T1-, PD-, and T2-weighted images adjacent to normal medullary bone, and between extra-osseous soft tissues[1,2,6,9,10] (Figs. **8–14**). UBCs usually contain fluid with low to low-intermediate signal on T1WI; low-intermediate, intermediate, or slightly high signal on PDWI, and high signal on T2WI.[1,2,6,9,10] Fluid–fluid levels may occur.[1] In tubular bones, mild to moderate expansion of bone may occur with variable thinning of the overlying cortex.[2] For UBCs without pathologic fracture, thin, peripheral Gd-contrast enhancement can be seen at the margins of lesions.[6]

UBCs with pathologic fracture can have heterogeneous or homogeneous low-intermediate to high signal on T1WI, and heterogeneous or homogeneous high signal on T2WI and FS T2WI[6] (Figs. **12–14**). MRI features associated with UBCs complicated by fracture include internal septations in 100%, and fluid–fluid levels or hemorrhage in 61%.[6] After Gd-contrast administration, UBCs with fracture can show irregular peripheral enhancement up to 1-cm thick, nodular enhancing zones, and enhancement at internal septations.[6] Juxtacortical soft tissue and periosteal enhancement also commonly occur with recent pathologic fractures of UBCs.[6]

Differential Diagnosis

Enchondroma, aneurysmal bone cyst, fibrous dysplasia, non-ossifying fibroma, Brodie abscess, chondromyxoid fibroma, giant cell tumor, chondrosarcoma.

Differential Diagnosis 335

Figure **8 a–e**   A 17-year-old male with a unicameral bone cyst involving the proximal di-metaphyseal portion of the humerus. AP radiograph (**a**) shows a geographic radiolucent slightly expansile lesion. Coronal (**b**) T1WI shows the lesion to have intermediate signal, and coronal (**c**) and axial (**d**) FS T2WI shows the lesion to have high signal with expanded and thinned cortical margins as well as thin, high periosteal signal. The intramedullary lesion shows peripheral rimlike Gd-contrast enhancement, as well as at the periosteum on axial (**b**) FS T1WI.

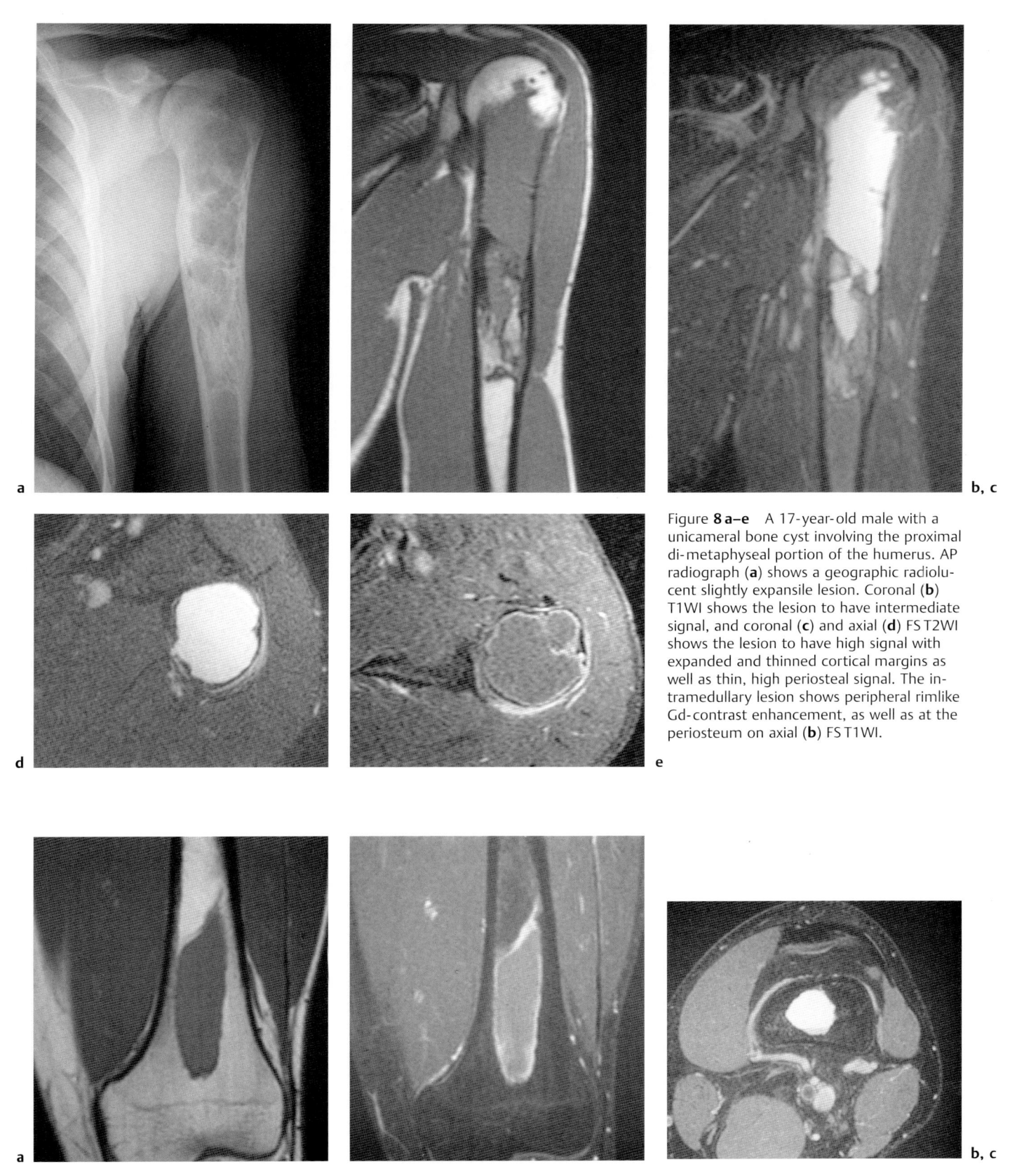

Figure **9 a–c**   A 16-year-old male with a unicameral bone cyst in the distal di-metaphyseal portion of the femur. Coronal PDWI (**a**) shows a well-circumscribed lesion with intermediate signal. The lesion shows peripheral rimlike Gd-contrast enhancement on coronal FS T1WI (**b**). The lesion has high signal on FS T2WI (**c**) and contains a fluid–fluid level.

336 A 3 – Bone Cyst

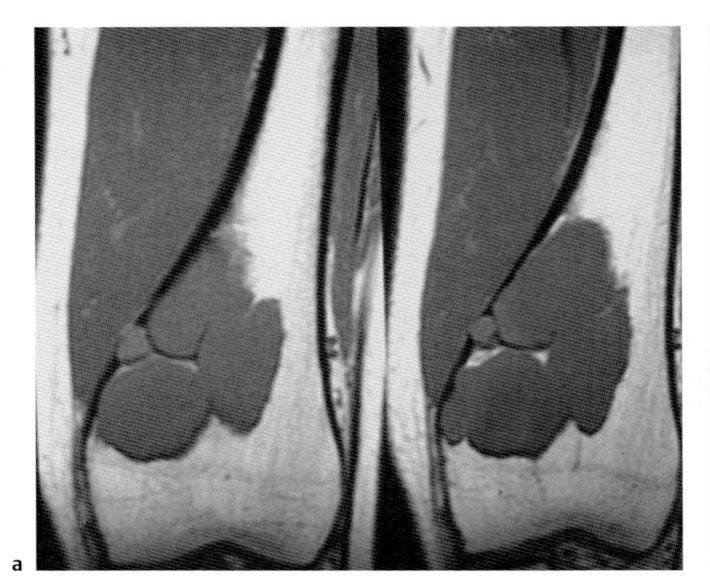

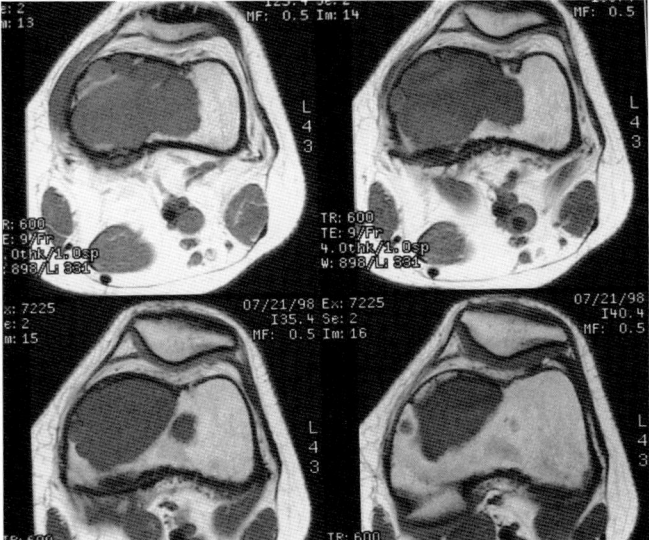

Figure **10 a–c** A 17-year-old female with a unicameral bone cyst in the distal di-metaphyseal portion of the femur. Coronal (**a**) and axial (**b**) T1WI shows a well-circumscribed lesion with low-intermediate signal, and high signal on axial (**c**) FS T2WI. Several thin septa are seen as well as several small fluid–fluid levels. Thinning of the cortex with slight expansion is also noted.

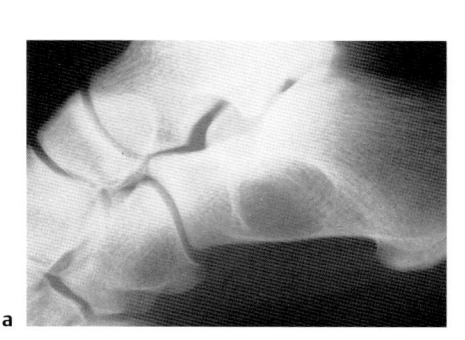

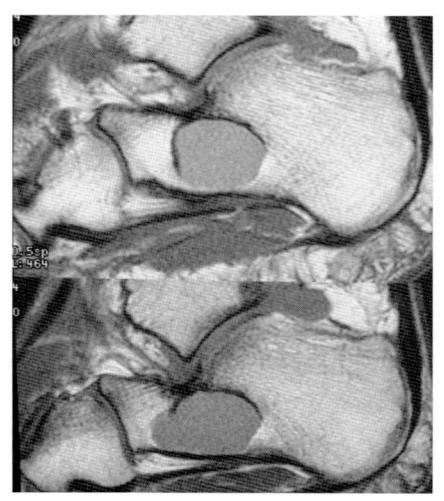

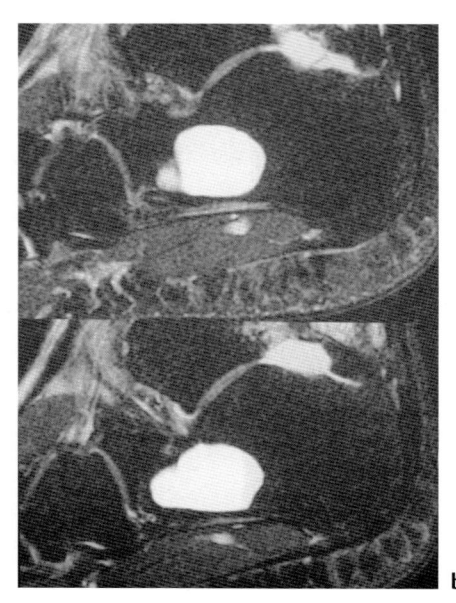

Figure **11 a, b** A 17-year-old male with a unicameral bone cyst in the calcaneus bone. Lateral radiograph shows a geographic radiolucent lesion. The lesion has intermediate signal on sagittal PDWI (**a**), and high signal on sagittal FS T2WI (**b**), as well as a small fluid–fluid level.

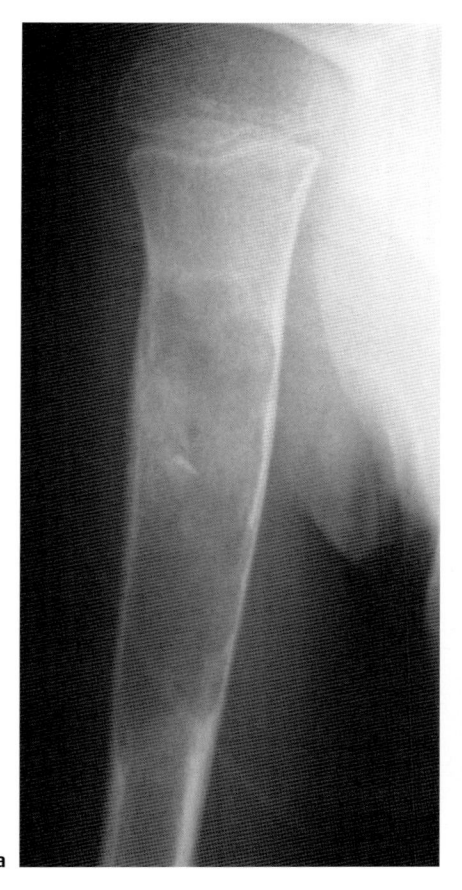

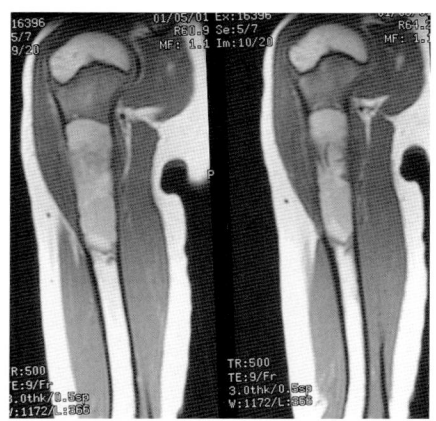

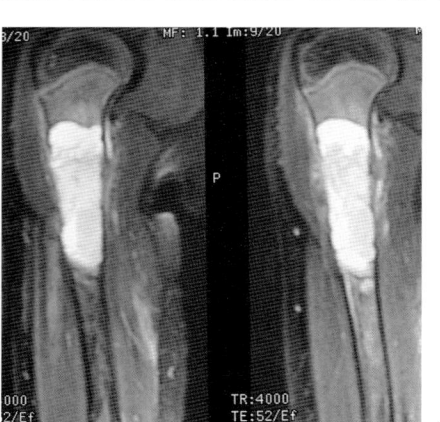

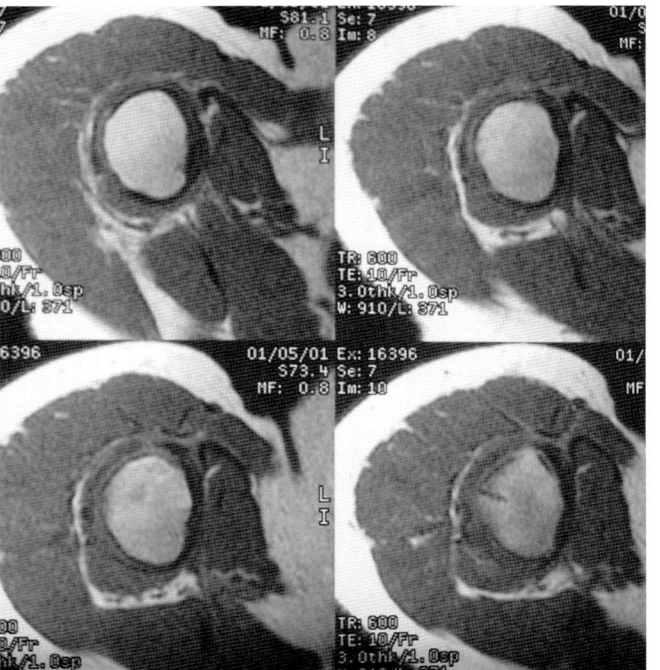

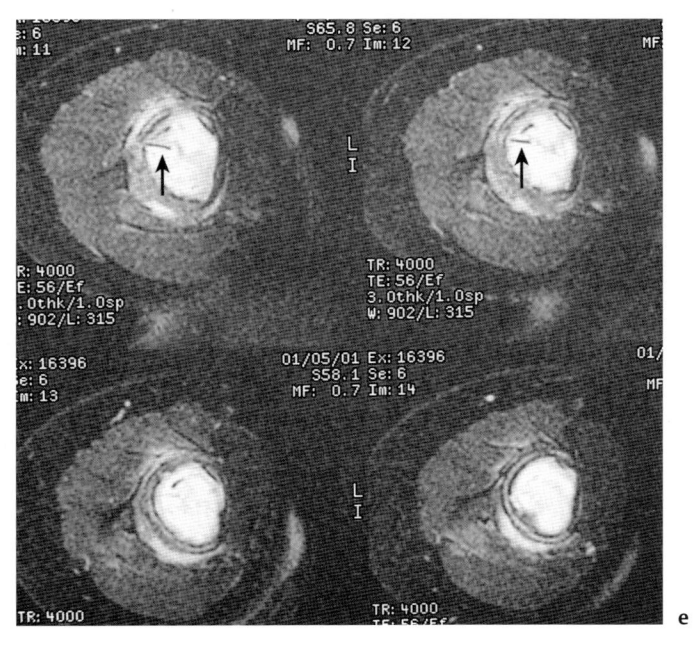

Figure 12 a–e A 9-year-old male with a pathologic fracture at a unicameral bone cyst involving the proximal di-metaphyseal portion of the humerus. AP radiograph (**a**) shows a radiolucent geographic lesion with a "fallen fragment." The lesion has heterogeneous intermediate and high signal on coronal (**b**) and axial (**d**) T1WI, and coronal (**c**) and axial (**e**) FS T2WI. The "fallen fragments" are also seen (**d**, **e**).

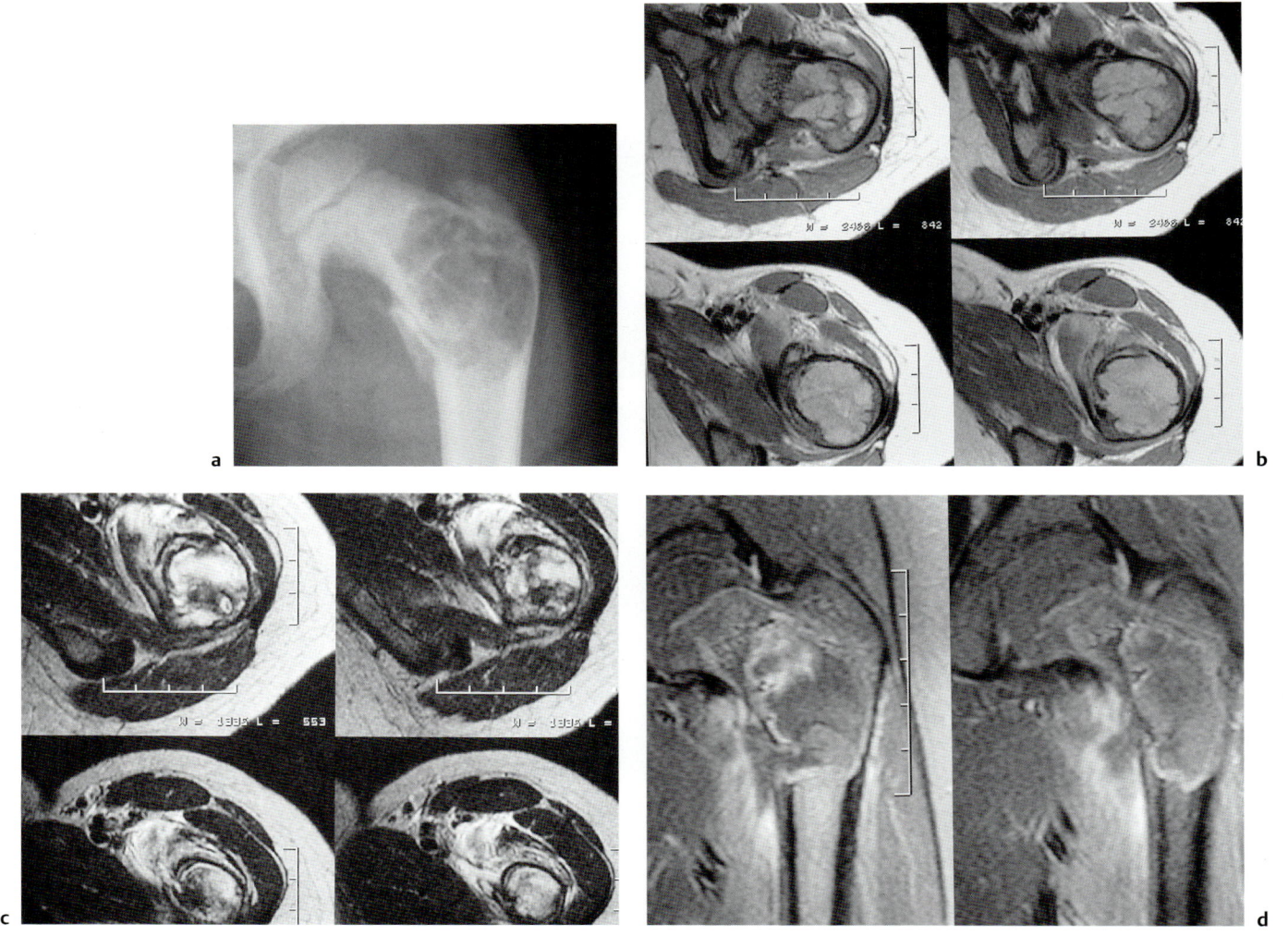

Figure 13 a–d A 4-year-old female with a pathologic fracture at a unicameral bone cyst involving the intertrochanteric region of the femur. AP radiograph (**a**) shows a radiolucent geographic lesion with cortical fracture. The lesion has heterogeneous intermediate and slightly high signal on axial PDWI (**b**) mixed low, intermediate, and high signal on axial T2WI (**c**). The lesion shows irregular peripheral Gd-contrast enhancement on coronal FS T1WI (**d**), as well as in the adjacent soft tissues.

Prognosis and Treatment

Up to 70% of UBCs are associated with pathologic fracture.[3,9] Surgical treatment consists of curettage and placement of bone graft material.[9,12] In patients with pathologic fractures secondary to UBCs, surgery is usually performed after ample callus has formed.[9] Local recurrence after surgery may occur in 15–40% of cases.[1] Injection of steroids, such as methylprednisolone into the lesion after drainage of cyst contents has given similar results.[1,9,11,12] Percutaneous grafting with allograft and/or bone substitutes has also been recently utilized in the treatment of bone cysts.[12]

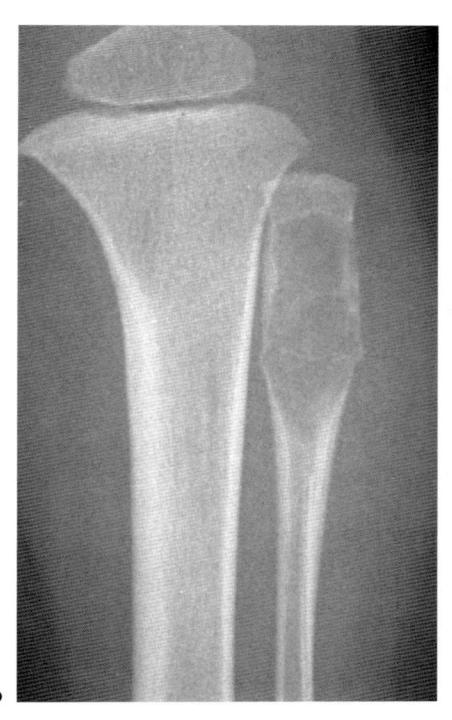

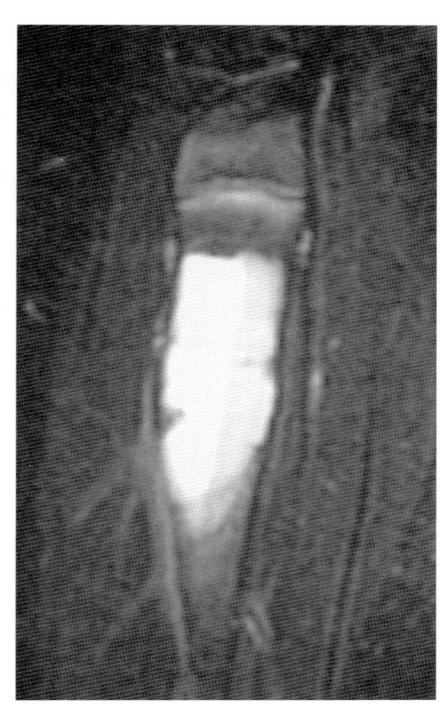

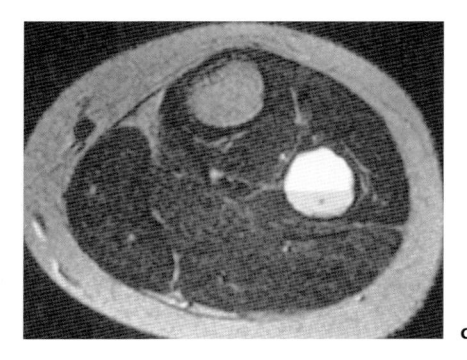

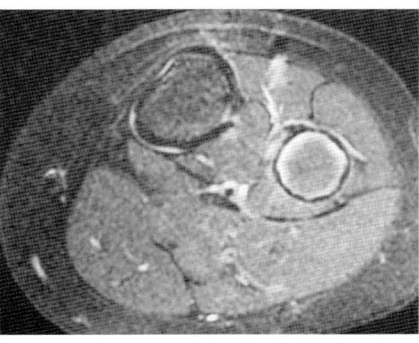

Figure 14 a–d   A 1-year-old female with a pathologic fracture at a unicameral bone cyst involving the proximal di-metaphyseal portion of the fibula. AP radiograph (**a**) shows a fracture at a geographic radiolucent slightly expansile lesion. The lesion has high signal on sagittal FS T2WI (**b**) and axial T2WI (**c**) with a fluid–fluid level. The lesion shows peripheral rimlike Gd-contrast enhancement on axial FS T1WI (**d**), as well as thin periosteal enhancement.

References

1. Forest M Simple bone cyst. In: Forest M, Tomeno B, Vanel D, eds. *Orthopedic Surgical Pathology: Diagnosis of Tumors and Pseudotumoral Lesions of Bone and Joints* Edinburgh: Churchill Livingstone; 1998:519–529.
2. Haims AH, Desai P, Present D, Beltran J. Epiphyseal extension of a unicameral bone cyst. *Skeletal Radiol* 1997;26:51–54.
3. Huvos AG. Simple bone cyst and aneurysmal bone cyst. In: Huvos AG, ed. *Bone Tumors: Diagnosis, Treatment, and Prognosis* 2nd ed. Philadelphia, Pa: W.B. Saunders; 1991:727–738.
4. Kalil RK, Araujo ES. Simple bone cyst. In: Fletcher CDM, Unni KK, Mertens F, eds. *World Health Organization Classification of Tumours. Pathology and Genetics of Tumours of Soft Tissue and Bone* Geneva: IARC Press; 2002:340.
5. Lee JH, Reinus WR, Wilson AJ. Quantitative analysis of the plain radiographic appearance of unicameral bone cysts. *Invest Radiol* 1999;34:28–37.
6. Margau R, Babyn P, Cole W, Smith C, Lee F. MR imaging of simple bone cysts in children: not so simple. *Pediatr Radiol* 2000; 30: 551–557.
7. Mulder JD, Schutte HE, Kroon HM, Taconis WK. Introduction. In: *Radiologic Atlas of Bone Tumors* Amsterdam: Elsevier; 1993:3–6.
8. Mulder JD, Schutte HE, Kroon HM, Taconis WK. The diagnosis of bone tumors. In: *Radiologic Atlas of Bone Tumors* Amsterdam: Elsevier; 1993:9–46.
9. Mulder JD, Schutte HE, Kroon HM, Taconis WK. Solitary bone cyst. In: *Radiologic Atlas of Bone Tumors* Amsterdam: Elsevier; 1993:579–590.
10. Sullivan RJ, Meyer JS, Dormans JP, Davidson RS. Diagnosing aneurysmal and unicameral bone cysts with magnetic resonance imaging. *Clin Orthop Relat Res* 1999;366:186–190.
11. Unni KK. Conditions that commonly simulate primary neoplasms of bone. In: *Dahlin's Bone Tumors: General Aspects and Data on 11 087 Cases* 5th ed. Philadelphia, Pa: Lippincott, Williams & Wilkins; 1996: 355–432.
12. Wilkins RM. Unicameral bone cysts. *J Am Acad Orthop Surg* 2000;8: 217–224.

A 4 Angiofibroma (Also Referred to as Juvenile Nasopharyngeal Angiofibroma)

Definition

Angiofibromas are benign fibrovascular tumors that are locally destructive and typically occur in male adolescents.[3,4]

Frequency of Occurrence

Occurrence is 1 in 5000, and accounts for 0.05 % of neoplasms of the head and neck.[4,6] Angiofibromas are the most common benign tumor of the nasopharynx.[6]

Age at Presentation

From 8 to 25 years, mean = 15.3–15.5 years.[4,11]

Gender Ratio (M / F)

Angiofibromas almost exclusively involve male adolescents.[3,4] Rare cases have been reported in females.[5]

Location

These lesions typically occur in the nasopharynx near and/or within the pterygopalatine fossa and pterygomaxillary fissure.[3] Lesions may show locally aggressive growth patterns with bone remodeling and extension into adjacent paranasal sinuses, infratemporal fossa, orbit via the inferior orbital fissure, and intracranially via the foramen rotundum, pterygoid canal, or superior orbital fissure.[3] Tumor extension into the pterygoid canal with invasion of the pterygoid process and greater wing of the sphenoid has been reported to occur in up to 60 % of cases.[8] Sphenoid sinus invasion has been reported to occur in up to two-thirds of cases.[6] Intracranial extension occurs in up to 36 % of cases and is typically extradural.[4] Extracranial extension usually occurs toward the nasal cavity and infratemporal fossa, and occasionally toward the nasopharyngeal mucosa, base of the pterygoids, and/or vascular spaces of the clivus.[4]

Signs and Symptoms

These lesions are frequently associated with epistaxis and/or nasal obstruction.[3]

Gross Pathologic Findings

Lesions are firm, pink-white lesions.[14] The cut surface is yellow-white with white trabeculations.[14]

Histopathologic Findings

Angiofibromas contain cells with round, ovoid, and/or short spindle-shaped nuclei[14] as well as stromal cells with stellate nuclei.[14] Lesions typically also contain fibrous tissue and prominent vascular channels.[14]

Findings on Plain Films (Roentgenograms) and Computed Tomography

Angiofibromas often have circumscribed margins, and usually have soft tissue attenuation.[3,6–8,10,13,14] These lesions usually show contrast enhancement.[1,3,4,6,7,13,14] Lesions are commonly associated with erosion and/or remodeling of adjacent bone, particularly the pterygopalatine fossa.[3,4,6–8,13,14]

MRI Findings

Angiofibromas are usually circumscribed lesions with sharp margins which may be lobulated.[1,4,5,7,8,10,13,14] Lesions typically have low-intermediate signal on T1WI, and heterogeneous slightly high to high signal on T2WI[1,4,5,7,8,10,13,14] (Figs. **15**, **16**). Flow voids on T2WI may be seen in the lesions representing blood vessels.[1,4,5,7,8,10,13,14] After Gd-contrast administration, lesions show prominent enhancement.[1,4,5,7,8,10,13,14]

Differential Diagnosis

Hypervascular nasal polyps, lymphoma, nasopharyngeal carcinoma, rhabdomyosarcoma, parotid neoplasm, hemangioma, metastatic disease.[14]

Prognosis and Treatment

Conventional arteriography is often used for diagnosis as well as for embolization with or without subsequent surgery.[3,5,11–13,15] Endoscopically assisted surgical techniques have been used.[4,9,10] Large, late-stage angiofibromas have been treated with preoperative embolization, surgical excision, and radiosurgery.[2] New craniofacial or subcranial techniques and infratemporal fossa approaches with osteotomies can allow greater surgical access to large angiofibromas, including those which involve the skull base and intracranial compartment.[15] Findings associated with recurrence of angiofibromas include high tumor growth rate at the time of surgery and incomplete surgical resection because of sphenoid invasion.[8] Residual lesions seen with MRI after treatment can undergo spontaneous resolution.[1,10] Advanced angiofibromas can be treated with radiotherapy, after which they tend to regress slowly over several months.[12] Angiofibromas that regress slowly have an increased recurrence risk.[12]

References

1. Chagnaud C, Petit P, Bartoli J, et al. Postoperative follow-up of juvenile nasopharyngeal angiofibromas: assessment by CT scan and MR imaging. *Eur Radiol* 1998;8(5):756–764.
2. Dare AO, Gibbons KJ, Proulx GM, Fenstermaker RA. Resection followed by radiosurgery for advanced juvenile nasopharyngeal angiofibroma: report of two cases. *Neurosurgery* 2003;52(5):1207–1211.
3. Eich GF, Hoeffel JC, Tschäppeler H, Gassner I, Willi UV. Fibrous tumours in children: imaging features of a heterogeneous group of disorders. *Pediatr Radiol* 1998;28:500–509.
4. El-Banhawy OA, El-Dien A, El-Hafiz S, Am T. Endoscopic-assisted midfacial degloving approach for type III juvenile angiofibroma. *Int J Pediatr Otorhinolaryngol* 2004;68:21–28.

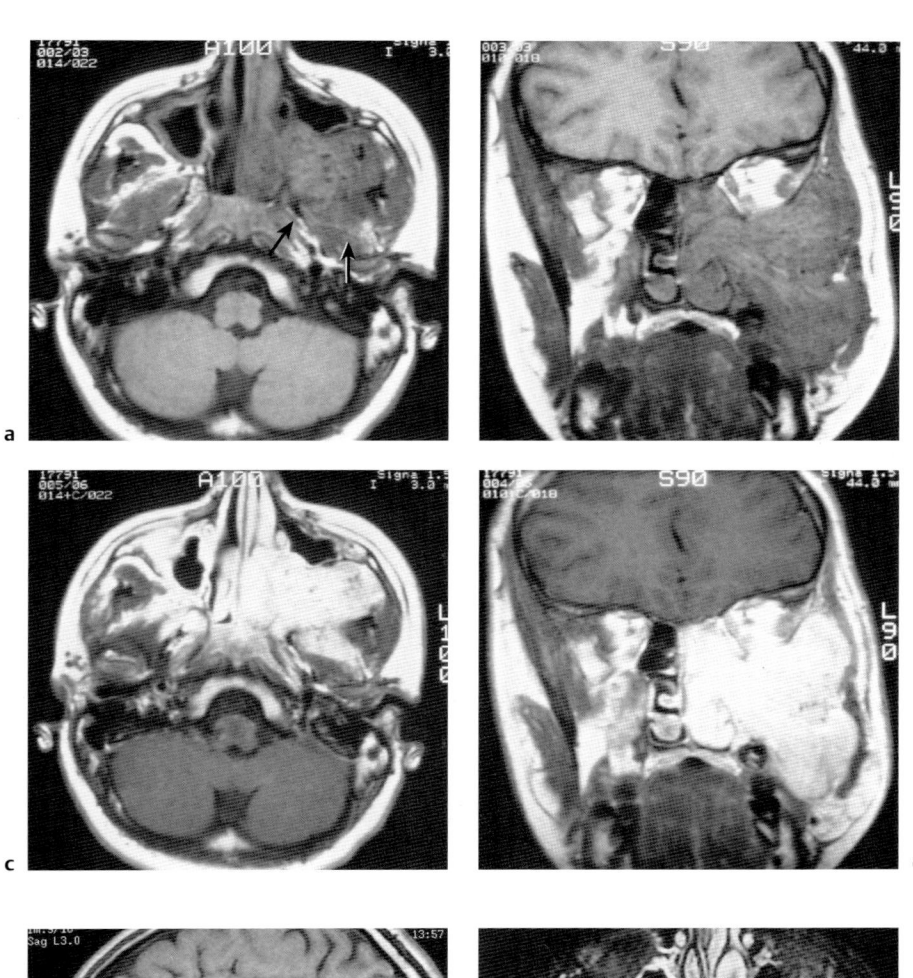

Figure 15 a–d A 15-year-old male with an angiofibroma involving the left nasal cavity, left sphenopalatine foramen, and left pterygomaxillary fissure associated with bone remodeling and erosion at the orbit and maxillary sinus. The lesion has intermediate signal on axial (**a**) and coronal (**b**) T1WI, and contains several flow voids. The lesion shows prominent Gd-contrast enhancement on axial (**c**) and coronal (**d**) T1WI.

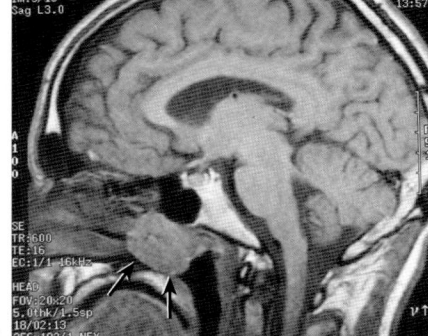

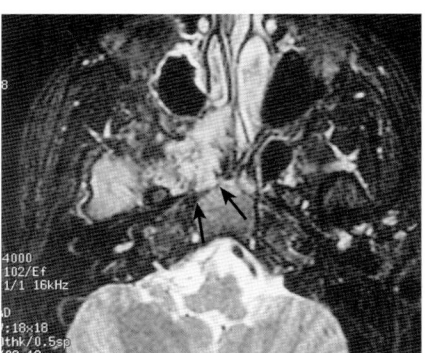

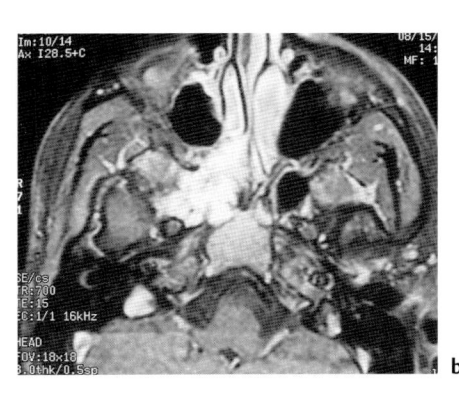

FigureFigure 16 a–c An 18-year-old man with angiofibroma involving the right nasal cavity, right sphenopalatine foramen, and right pterygomaxillary fissure with bone erosion and remodeling of the dorsal portion of the right maxillary sinus. The lesion has intermediate signal on sagittal FS T2WI (**a**), check edited text.and predominantly high signal with small foci of low signal on axial FS T2WI (**b**). The lesion shows prominent Gd-contrast enhancement on axial FS T1WI (**c**).

5 Jones BV, Koch BL. Magnetic resonance imaging of the pediatric head and neck. *Top Magn Reson Imaging* 1999;10(6):348–361.

6 Laine FJ, Nadel L, Braun IF. CT and MR imaging of the central skull base. Part 2. Pathologic spectrum. *Radiographics* 1990;10(5): 797–821.

7 Lloyd G, Howard D, Lund VJ, Savy L. Imaging for juvenile angiofibroma. *J Laryngol Otol* 2000;114(9):727–730.

8 Lloyd G, Howard D, Phelps P, Cheesman A. Juvenile angiofibroma: the lessons of 20 years of modern imaging. *J Laryngol Otol* 1999; 113(2): 127–134.

9 Nicolai P, Berlucchi M, Tomenzoli D, et al. Endoscopic surgery for juvenile angiofibroma: when and how. *Laryngoscope* 2003;113(5): 775–782.

10 Önerci TM, Yücel OT, Öðretmenoðlu O. Endoscopic surgery in treatment of juvenile nasopharyngeal angiofibroma. *Int J Pediatr Otorhinolaryngol* 2003;67:1219–1225.

11 Paris J, Guelfucci B, Moulin G, Zanaret M, Triglia JM. Diagnosis and treatment of juvenile nasopharyngeal angiofibroma. *Eur Arch Otorhinolaryngol* 2001;258(3):120–124.

12 Reddy KA, Mendenhall WM, Amdur RJ, Stringer SP, Cassisi NJ. Long-term results of radiation therapy for juvenile nasopharyngeal angiofibroma. *Am J Otolaryngol* 2001;22(3):172–175.

13 Schick B, Kahle G. Radiological findings in angiofibroma. *Acta Radiol* 2000;41(6):585–593.

14 Seo CS, Han MH, Chang KH, Yeon KM. Angiofibroma confined to the pterygoid muscle region: CT and MR demonstration. *AJNR Am J Neuroradiol* 1996;17:374–376.

15 Tewfik TL, Tan AK, al Noury K, et al. Juvenile nasopharyngeal angiofibroma. *J Otolaryngol* 1999;28(3):145–151.

A 5   Angiomatoid Fibrous Histiocytoma (Also Referred to as Angiomatoid Malignant Fibrous Histiocytoma)

ICD-O Code
8836/1

Definition
Angiomatoid fibrous histiocytoma (AFH) is considered to be a low-grade fibrohistiocytic neoplasm.[1–3,5]

Frequency of Occurrence
AFH accounts for 1.6% of primary, malignant soft tissue tumors.[7]

Age at Presentation
From 2 to 71 years, mean = 20 years.[2,3]

Gender Ratio (M/F)
1/1.3[3]

Location
Lesions occur in the upper extremity > lower extremity > trunk > hand and wrist > proximal limb girdle > hip and buttocks > head and neck.[3,6,7] Lesions are often located in the deep dermis and subcutis.[2,4,6]

Signs and Symptoms
AFH often presents as painless slow-growing masses in the superficial soft tissues.[2,6] Rarely, systemic signs of anemia, weight loss, and fever may occur from tumor production of cytokines.[2]

Gross Pathologic Findings
AFH ranges from less than 1 cm to 12 cm, median = 2 cm.[2,3] Lesions can be firm, tan-gray, and multinodular with circumscribed margins.[2] Blood-filled cystic spaces are often present within these neoplasms.[2]

Histopathologic Findings
AFH typically contains nodules of spindle-shaped or epithelioid cells with ovoid vesicular nuclei associated with increased mitotic activity, as well as blood-filled cystic spaces that are not lined by endothelial cells (pseudoangiomatoid spaces). Lesions may have a thick, fibrous pseudocapsule and a pericapsular lymphoplasmacytic response.[2,3]

Tumor Genetics
A deletion involving chromosome 11 (q24) and rearrangements involving chromosomes 2, 12, 16, and 17 have been reported in a single case.[2] A gene fusion product (FUS/ATF1 protein) has

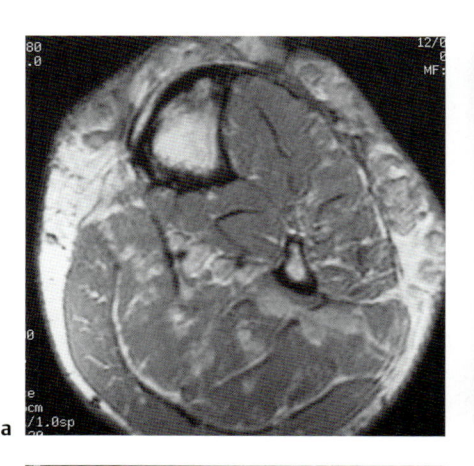

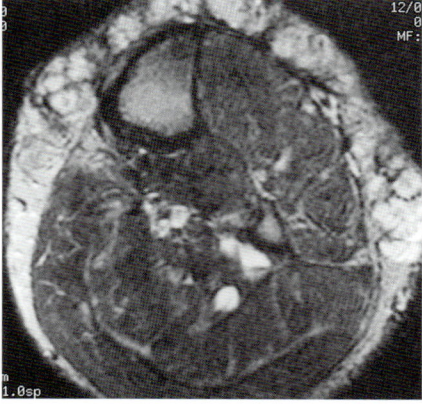

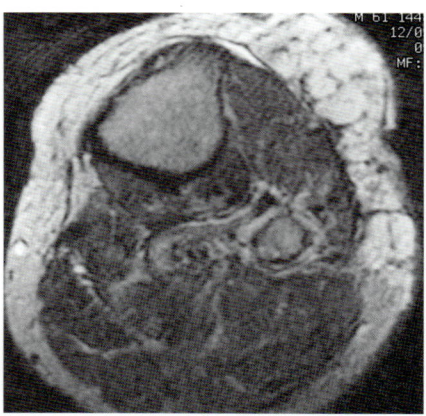

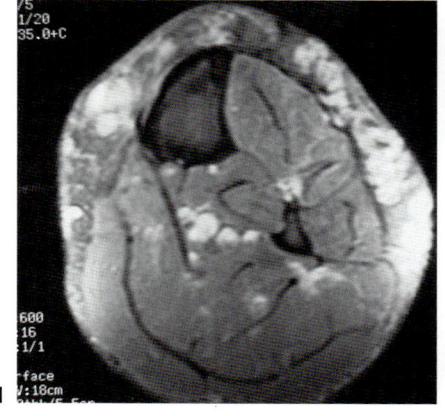

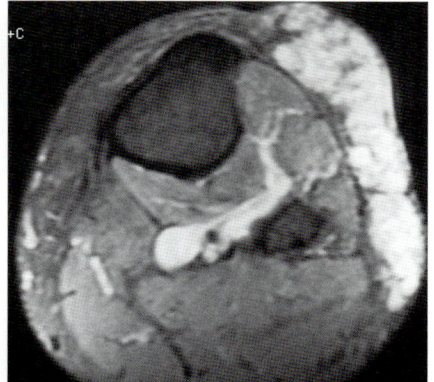

Figure 17 a–e   A 61-year-old man with an angiomatoid fibrous histiocytoma in the subcutaneous fat of the leg. Axial PDWI (**a**) and T2WI (**b, c**) show multinodular lesions in the subcutaneous fat which have intermediate signal on PDWI, and heterogeneous high signal on T2WI. The multinodular lesions show prominent Gd-contrast enhancement on FS T1WI (**d, e**).

been found resulting from translocation of the chromosome band 16p11 (FUS gene) to chromosome band 12q13 (ATF1 gene).[2]

MRI Findings

AFH can appear as multinodular lesions in the dermis or superficial soft tissues (Fig. 17). Lesions can have heterogeneous low-intermediate signal on T1WI and PDWI, and heterogeneous high signal on T2WI. Fluid–fluid levels may be seen secondary to hemorrhage. Thin septa with low signal on T2WI may be seen between the multiple nodular zones with high signal. After Gd-contrast administration, AFH can show prominent heterogeneous enhancement.

Differential Diagnosis

Malignant fibrous histiocytoma, myxoid liposarcoma, lymphangioma, hemangioma, hemangioendothelioma, angiosarcoma.

Prognosis and Treatment

Cases of AFH typically have a non-aggressive clinical course, unlike malignant fibrous histiocytomas.[2,3] AFH is treated by surgical excision with wide margins.[2] Local recurrence ranges from 2 to 11% of cases.[2] Metastatic disease is uncommon, occurring in less than 1%.[2]

References

[1] Daw NC, Billups CA, Pappo AS, et al. Malignant fibrous histiocytoma and other fibrohistiocytic tumors in pediatric patients: the St Jude Children's research hospital experience. *Cancer* 2003;97:2839–2847

[2] Fanburg-Smith JC, Cin PD. Angiomatoid fibrous histiocytoma. In: Fletcher CDM, Unni KK, Mertens F, eds. *World Health Organization Classification of Tumours. Pathology and Genetics of Tumours of Soft Tissue and Bone* Geneva: IARC Press; 2002:194–195.

[3] Fanburg-Smith JC, Miettinen M. Angiomatoid "malignant" fibrous histiocytoma: a clinicopathologic study of 158 cases and further exploration of the myoid type. *Hum Pathol* 1999;30:1336–1343.

[4] Hasegawa T, Seki K, Ono K, Hirohashi S. Angiomatoid (malignant) fibrous histiocytoma: a peculiar low-grade tumor showing immunophenotypic heterogeneity and ultrastructural variations. *Pathol Int* 2000;50:731–738.

[5] Lagace R, Aurias A. Does malignant fibrous histiocytoma exist? *Ann Pathol* 2002;22:29–34.

[6] Kransdorf MJ, Murphey MD. Malignant fibrous and fibrohistiocytic tumors. In: *Imaging of Soft Tissue Tumors* 2nd ed. Philadelphia, Pa: Lippincott, Williams & Wilkins; 2006:257–297.

[7] Kransdorf MJ. Malignant soft-tissue tumors in a large referral population: distribution of diagnoses by age, sex, and location. *AJR Am J Roentgenol* 1995;164:129–134.

A6 Angiosarcoma (Also Referred to as Malignant Hemangioendothelioma, High-Grade Hemangioendothelioma, Hemangiosarcoma, Angioendothelioma, Angiofibrosarcoma, and Hemangioendotheliosarcoma)

ICD-O Code

9120/3

Definition

Angiosarcomas are primary malignant tumors composed of neoplastic blood vessels in bone and/or soft tissues.[1,4–7,10,11,14,15,17,18] These tumors can be associated with Paget disease, radiation treatment, bone infarcts, knee and hip prostheses, synthetic vessel grafts, prior trauma or surgery, osteomyelitis, and hereditary disorders (neurofibromatosis type 1, Maffucci disease, achondroplasia).

Frequency of Occurrence

Angiosarcomas represent less than 1% of malignant bone tumors,[7,12,13,16,17] and account for 2% of malignant soft tissue tumors.[8,9]

Age at Presentation

Bone: from 10 to 82 years, median = 47 years.[12–14,16]

Soft tissue lesions: from 5 to 97 years, mean = 49 years.[8,9,11]

Gender Ratio (M/F)

Bone: 1.4/1 to 2/1.[3,7,14,17]

Soft tissue lesions: 1.1/1 to 1.7/1.[9,11]

Location

Bone. Common locations include: vertebrae, pelvic bones, tibia, humerus, femur, skull, and others.[14–16] Tumors are multifocal in 20–30% of cases.[15,16] In tubular bones, tumors are often diaphyseal or metadiaphyseal, and rarely are epiphyseal alone.[14]

Soft tissue. Angiosarcomas of soft tissue occur most commonly in the skin, subcutaneous tissues, breast, liver spleen, and bone.[10,11] Such angiosarcomas occur less frequently in skeletal muscle, retroperitoneum, mesentery, and mediastinum.[10,11] Locations of these angiosarcomas have been reported in order of decreasing frequency as follows: head and neck, trunk, lower extremity, hip and buttocks, upper extremity, hand and wrist, foot and ankle, retroperitoneum.[8,9]

Signs and Symptoms

Bone lesions. Tumors can be associated with localized tenderness and dull pain, from several weeks' to several years' duration.[3,7,14,15,17]

Soft tissue lesions. Tumors often present as enlarging painful mass-lesions of several weeks' duration, which may contain zones of hemorrhage, and may be associated with anemia or coagulopathy.[10,11,18]

Gross Pathologic Findings

Angiosarcomas are soft, bloody, fleshy and spongy tumors in bone cortex, medulla, and/or soft tissues.[6,7,11]

Histopathologic Findings[1–7,11,15,17,18]

Tumors contain neoplastic cells with varying atypia lining vascular spaces and channels. Endothelial cells are often pleomorphic with hyperchromatic nuclei and prominent nucleoli. Undifferentiated zones containing spindle and/or epithelioid cells may be present. Angiosarcomas are often immunoreactive to von Willebrand factor, CD 31, CD 34, vimentin, and Ulex Europaeus.[11,15,18]

Tumor Genetics

Angiosarcomas in soft tissues typically show various complex cytogenetic aberrations.[18] Of the various chromosomal rearrangements that have been reported, the most frequent involve gains of 5 pter-p11, 8 p12-qter, and 20 pter-q12; losses involving 4 p, 7 p15-pter, and Y, as well as 22 q abnormalities.[18] KRAS 2 and TP53 mutation have been reported for angiosarcomas that result from exposure to vinyl chloride and thorium dioxide.[18] Translocations involving chromosomes 1 and 3 have been reported for epithelioid hemangioendotheliomas of bone.[15]

Findings on Plain Films (Roentgenograms) and Computed Tomography

Bone.[1–3,6,14,15] Tumors are typically osteolytic lesions. Zones of sclerosis and reactive bone formation occur in 10%.[14] Broad, poorly-defined zones of transition and presence of an extraosseous soft tissue tumor are features commonly seen with higher grades of malignancy. Multifocal lesions in adjacent bones may occur. Angiosarcomas may be associated with bone infarcts.[1]

Soft tissue. Tumors can have low-intermediate attenuation on CT.[2]

MRI Findings

Bone. Tumors have low-intermediate signal on T1WI, and mixed low, intermediate, and/or high signal on T2WI.[2,15] Tumors can show prominent Gd-contrast enhancement.[2]

Soft tissue. Tumors have low-intermediate signal on T1WI, and mixed low, intermediate, and/or high signal on T2WI[10] (Fig. **18**). Tumors can show prominent Gd-contrast enhancement in a homogeneous or heterogeneous pattern.[10]

Differential Diagnosis

Bone. Metastases, myeloma/plasmacytoma, lymphoma, eosinophilic granuloma, osteomyelitis, Kaposi sarcoma, cystic angiomatosis, fibrosarcoma, aneurysmal bone cyst.

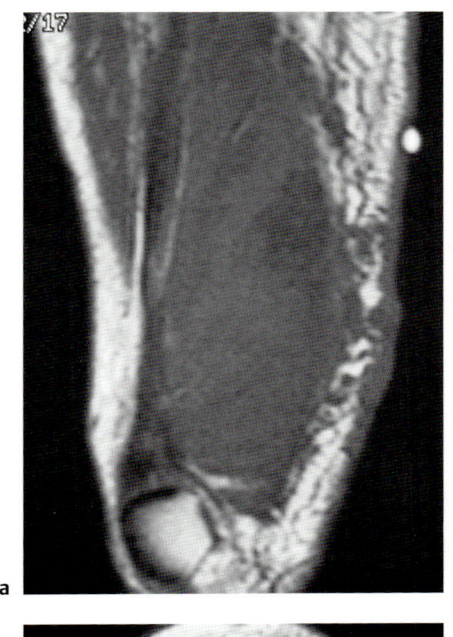

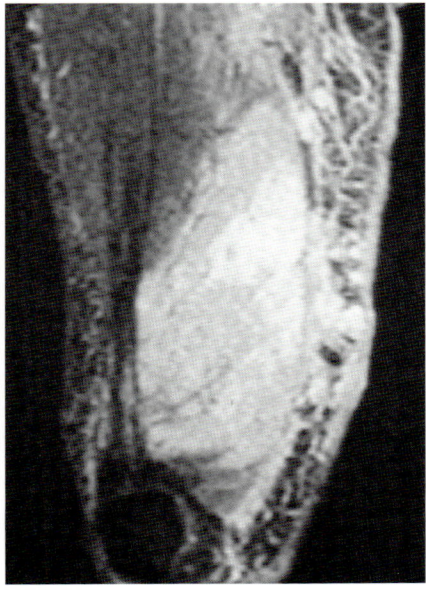

Figure **18 a–e** A 74-year-old man with an angiosarcoma in the medial anterior thigh involving the vastus medialis muscle. The tumor has low-intermediate signal on coronal (**a**) and axial (**c**) T1WI, heterogeneous high signal on coronal STIR (**b**), and mixed low, intermediate, and/or high signal on axial T2WI (**d**). The tumor shows prominent Gd-contrast enhancement on FS T1WI (**e**).

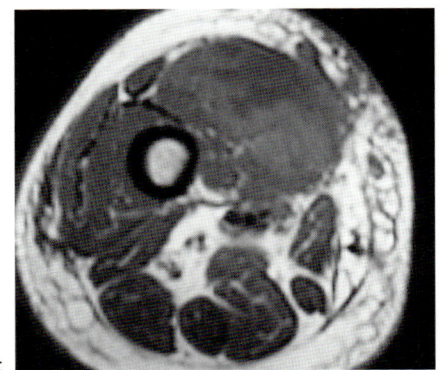

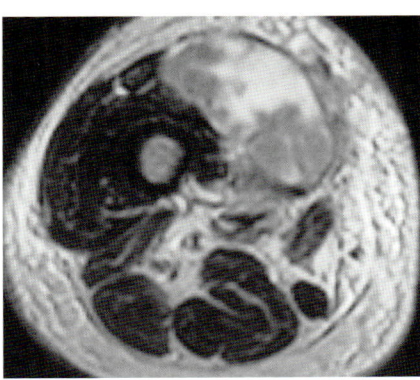

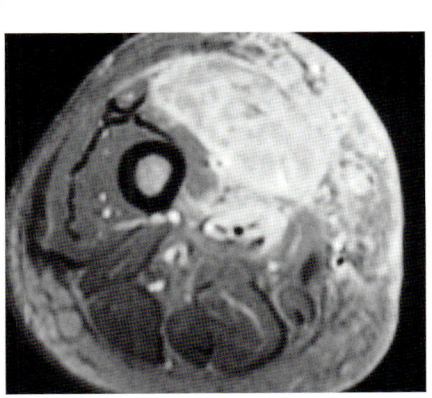

Soft tissue. Liposarcoma, dermatofibrosarcoma, malignant peripheral nerve sheath tumor, malignant fibrous histiocytoma, synovial sarcoma, melanoma, leiomyosarcoma, lymphoma, metastatic disease, sarcoid, granular cell tumor.

Prognosis and Treatment

Angiosarcomas in bone. Prognosis depends on histologic grade of angiosarcomas.[7,15] High-grade lesions typically have a poor prognosis.[7] Metastases occur in the skeleton, pleura, lung, and lymphatics.[6,7] Treatment is typically surgery with adjuvant chemotherapy.[6,7] Angiosarcomas are moderately responsive to radiation treatment.[6,7] The overall survival rate has been reported to be ~ 20 % for high-grade lesions.[6] Multifocal tumors can have a higher survival rate.[15]

Angiosarcomas in soft tissue. Angiosarcomas in soft tissue are very aggressive tumors that are locally invasive and can result in metastatic disease to the lungs, lymph nodes, bone, and soft tissues.[10,11,18] Poor prognosis is associated with older patient ages, larger tumor size, retroperitoneal tumor location, and/or high Ki67 values.[11,18] Tumors are treated with surgery, and up to 20 % have local recurrence.[10,18]

References

1 Abdelwahab IF, Klein MJ, Hermann G, Springfield D. Angiosarcomas associated with bone infarcts. *Skeletal Radiol* 1998;27:546–551.
2 Bourekas EC, Cohen ML, Kamen CS, Tarr RW, Lanzieri CF, Lewin JS. Malignant hemangioendothelioma (angiosarcoma) of the skull: plain film, CT, and MR appearance. *AJNR Am J Neuroradiol* 1996;17: 1946–1948.
3 Conway WF, Hayes CW. Miscellaneous lesion of bone. *Radiol Clin North Am* 1993;31(2):339–358.
4 Darby AJ. Vascular neoplasms of bone. In: Helliwell TR, ed. *Major Problems in Pathology: Pathology of Bone and Joint Neoplasms* 1st ed. Philadelphia, Pa: W.B. Saunders; 1999:37:337.
5 Das Gupta TK, Chaudhuri PK. Tumors of vascular and perivascular tissue. In: Das Gupta TK, Chaudhuri PK, eds. *Tumors of the Soft Tissues.* 2nd ed. Stamford, Conn.: Appleton & Lange; 1998:420–425.
6 Forest M. Vascular tumors. In: Forest M, Tomeno B, Vanel D, eds. *Orthopedic Surgical Pathology: Diagnosis of Tumors and Pseudotumoral Lesions of Bone and Joints.* Edinburgh: Churchill Livingstone; 1998:345–362.
7 Huvos AG. Angiosarcoma of Bone (Epithelioid Hemangioendothelioma; Malignant Hemangioendothelioma). In: Huvos AG, ed. *Bone Tumors: Diagnosis, Treatment, and Prognosis* 2nd ed. Philadelphia, Pa: WB Saunders; 1991:579–594.
8 Kransdorf MJ, Murphey MD. Soft tissue tumors in a large referral population: prevalence and distribution of diagnoses by age, sex, and location. In: *Imaging of Soft Tissue Tumors* 2nd ed. Philadelphia, Pa: WB Saunders; 2006:6–37.
9 Kransdorf MJ. Malignant soft-tissue tumors in a large referral population: distribution of diagnoses by age, sex, and location. *AJR Am J Roentgenol* 1995;164:129–134.

10. Kransdorf MJ, Murphey MD. Vascular and Lymphatic Tumors. In: *Imaging of Soft Tissue Tumors* 2nd ed. Philadelphia, Pa: Lippincott, Williams & Wilkins; 2006:150–188.
11. Meis-Kindblom JM, Kindblom LG. Angiosarcoma of soft tissue: a study of 80 cases. *Am J Surg Pathol* 1998;22(6):683–697.
12. Mulder JD, Schutte HE, Kroon HM, Taconis WK. Introduction. In: *Radiologic Atlas of Bone Tumors* Amsterdam: Elsevier; 1993:3–6.
13. Mulder JD, Schutte HE, Kroon HM, Taconis WK. The diagnosis of bone tumors. In: *Radiologic Atlas of Bone Tumors* Amsterdam: Elsevier; 1993:9–46.
14. Mulder JD, Schutte HE, Kroon HM, Taconis WK. Hemangio-endothelioma and Hemangio-endotheliosarcoma. In: *Radiologic Atlas of Bone Tumors* Amsterdam: Elsevier; 1993:241–248.
15. Roessner A, Boehling T. Angiosarcoma. In: Fletcher CDM, Unni KK, Mertens F, eds. *World Health Organization Classification of Tumours. Pathology and Genetics of Tumours of Soft Tissue and Bone* Geneva: IARC Press; 2002:322–323.
16. Unni KK. Introduction and scope of study. In: *Dahlin's Bone Tumors: General Aspects and Data on 11 087 Cases* 5th ed. Philadelphia, Pa: Lippincott, Williams & Wilkins; 1996:1–9.
17. Unni KK. Hemangioendothelioma (Hemangiosarcoma) and Hemangiopericytoma. In: *Dahlin's Bone Tumors: General Aspects and Data on 11 087 Cases* 5th ed. Philadelphia, Pa: Lippincott, Wiliams & Wilkins; 1996:317–331.
18. Weiss SW, Lasota J, Miettinen MM. Angiosarcoma of soft tissue. In: Fletcher CDM, Unni KK, Mertens F, eds. *World Health Organization Classification of Tumours. Pathology and genetics of tumours of soft tissue and bone* Geneva: IARC Press; 2002:175–177.

A 7 Chondroblastoma

ICD-O Code
9230/0

Definition
Chondroblastomas are benign cartilaginous tumors with chondroblast-like cells and areas of chondroid matrix formation usually involving the epiphysis.[2,4,5,9,12,16,19] Chondroblastomas usually present before cessation of endochondral bone growth.[2,4,5,9,12,16,19]

Frequency of Occurrence
From 5 to 9% of benign bone lesions, 1–3% of all bone lesions.[5,9,14–16,18,19]

Age at Presentation[4,5,9,14–16,18,19]
From 3 to 73 years, median = 17 years; mean = 16 years for lesions in long bones; mean = 28 years in other bones. Most cases are diagnosed between the ages of 5 and 25 years.[8,9] Chondroblastomas are rare in children below 10 years old and adults older than 60 years.[4]

Gender Ratio (M/F)
1.5 to 2/1.[5,14–16,19,21]

Location[5,6,16,19]
Lesions are located in the epiphyseal regions of long bones (40%), or involve both the epiphyseal and adjacent metaphyseal regions (60%). More than 70% occur in long bones but may also occur in apophyses (such as greater trochanter, etc.) Most lesions are mono-ostotic. Proximal humerus > proximal and distal femur > proximal tibia > talus > calcaneus > bony pelvis > ribs > vertebrae > skull. Chondroblastomas rarely occur in the spine and craniofacial bones.[16] Spinal tumors most often involve the thoracic vertebrae and usually involve both the body and pedicles.[6]

Signs and Symptoms[1,2,4–6,9–11,16,19,21]
Tumors can be associated with swelling and pain in the region of the lesion for several months to years in duration. Pathologic fractures are uncommon. Spinal tumors can be associated with spinal cord compression.[6]

Gross Pathologic Findings[2,4,5,9,11,16,19,21]
Chondroblastomas are relatively small, well-demarcated neoplasms ranging in size from 1 to 7 cm. Chondroblastomas are mottled gritty and/or soft lesions that range from gray-yellow to gray-brown. Lesion can contain calcifications, areas of hemorrhage and/or cystic changes. Chondroblastomas can be associated with aneurysmal bone cysts in 10–40% of cases.

Histopathologic Findings[2,4,5,7–11,16,19,21]
Chondroblastomas are composed of nearly uniform oval or polyhedral cells with oval grooved nuclei and small volumes of pink cytoplasm separated by scant interstitial matrix. Pericellular fine calcifications are often seen in a "chicken wire" or "lattice-like" pattern. In most cases, normal mitotic activity is observed. Most chondroblastomas show chondroid differentiation ranging from multiple small foci to extensively distributed. Areas of necrosis and hemorrhage may be present surrounded by multinucleated giant cells. Vascular invasion is rare. Cystic regions and secondary aneurysmal bone cysts may represent small or large proportions of the entire lesions. Lesions are often immunoreactively positive for S-100 protein (expressed by chondrocytes and chondroblasts), vimentin, and fibronectin; and occasionally positive for cytokeratin, actin, and epithelial membrane protein.

Tumor Genetics
Most chondroblastomas are diploid tumors with low proliferative fractions.[9] Structural anomalies involving chromosomes 5 and 8 have been reported.[2,9] Structural abnormalities involving 11 p15, similar to giant cell tumors, have also been reported.[2] Aggressive chondroblastomas are associated with unbalanced translocations involving chromosomes 2, 5, 8, and 21; and rearrangements involving chromosome band 8 q21.[2,9]

Findings on Plain Films (Roentgenograms) and Computed Tomography[1–11,13,16,17,19]
Chondroblastomas are geographic lytic lesions that often involve the epiphysis with or without metaphyseal involvement (Figs. **19–22, 24**). Tumors are often eccentric, ranging from 1 to 7 cm in diameter. Lesions may have thin sclerotic margins, cortical bone expansion, endosteal expansion, and/or periosteal reaction. Matrix mineralization (punctate, ring-like, or arc-like) may be seen in 25 to 33% of cases on plain films.[2,21] A higher percentage of mineralization can be seen with CT.[2] Chondroblastomas can also occur in apophyses.

Findings on Radionuclide Bone Scans[3]
Lesions usually are associated with increased radiopharmaceutical accumulation.

MRI Findings[1,6–8,10,13,16,17,20]
Chondroblastomas often have fine lobular margins, and typically have low-intermediate heterogeneous signal on T1WI, and mixed low, intermediate, and/or high signal on T2WI (Figs. **19–25**). Areas of low signal on T2WI are secondary to chondroid matrix mineralization, and/or hemosiderin (Figs. **22, 23, 25**). Lobular, marginal or septal Gd-contrast enhancement patterns can be seen. Tumors may have thin margins of low signal on T2WI representing sclerotic borders. Cortical destruction is uncommon. Perilesional zones with high signal on T2WI and Gd-contrast enhancement are commonly seen in bone marrow as well as periosteal locations, indicating reactive hyperemia and/or edema[21] (Figs. **20–25**). These perilesional MRI

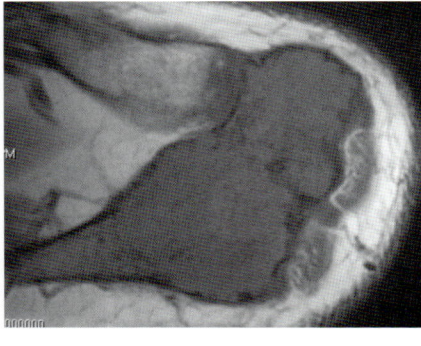

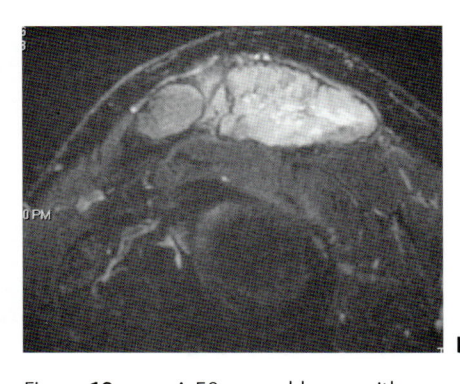

Figure 19 a–e A 50-year-old man with chondroblastoma in the acromion. Axial CT shows a radiolucent expansile lesion in the acromion (**a**). The lesion has fine lobular margins, and low-intermediate heterogeneous signal on axial T1WI (**b**), and mixed low, intermediate, and high signal on sagittal FS T2WI (**c**). The lesion shows prominent Gd-contrast enhancement on sagittal (**d**) and axial (**e**) FS T1WI.

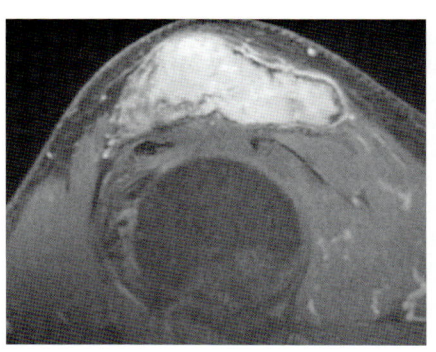

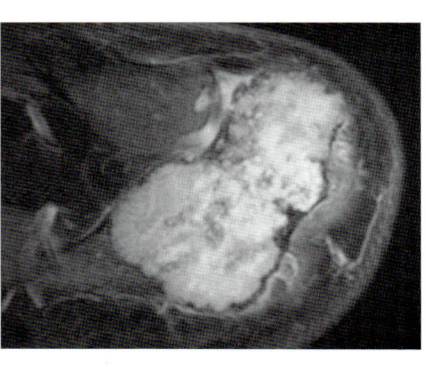

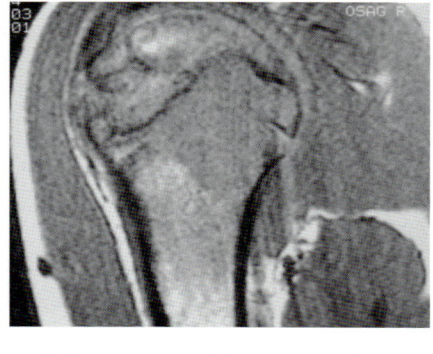

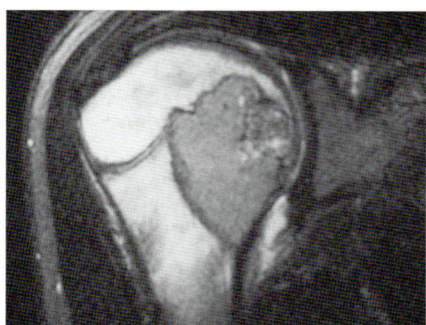

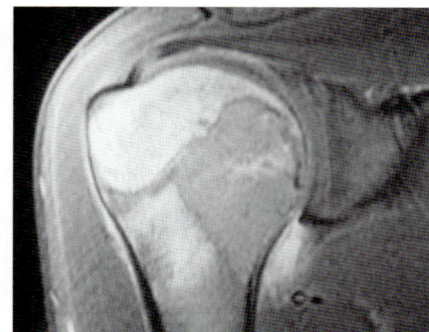

Figure 20 a–d A 15-year-old male with chondroblastoma involving the physeal plate, epiphysis, and metaphysis of the proximal humerus. Axial CT shows a radiolucent lesion in the humerus (**a**). The lesion has low-intermediate signal on coronal T1WI (**b**), and mixed intermediate and high signal on coronal T2WI (**c**), and is surrounded by high signal on T2WI in the adjacent marrow. The lesion shows moderate Gd-contrast enhancement on coronal FS T1WI (**d**), as well as prominent enhancement in the adjacent marrow.

findings have been shown to be correlated with inflammatory reaction associated with elevated tumor prostaglandin levels.[22] Aneurysmal bone cysts can be seen associated with chondroblastomas (Figs. **23**, **24**). In spinal tumors, bone expansion can result in spinal cord compression.[6]

Differential Diagnosis

Giant cell tumor, clear cell chondrosarcoma, enchondroma, aneurysmal bone cyst, chondromyxoid fibroma, enchondroma, eosinophilic granuloma, degenerative or post-traumatic cyst/intra-osseous ganglion, ischemic necrosis.

Treatment and Prognosis[2,4,5,9,11,16,19,21]

Standard treatment is curettage with or without bone grafts, which produces successful results in 80–90% of patients.[9,21] Local recurrence typically ranges from 5 to 38% of cases, and usually occurs within 2 years. Because of difficulty in complete surgical resection, chondroblastomas may recur in up to 50% of patients.[9] Recurrences can be treated with repeat curettage or resection. Although chondroblastomas are sensitive to radiation, this type of treatment is not used because of the risk of malignant transformation into sarcoma. Rare metastases have been reported to the lungs.[9]

Treatment and Prognosis 349

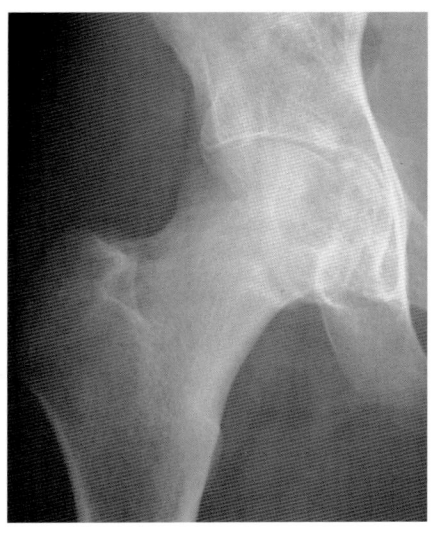

Figure **21 a–d** A 17-year-old male with chondroblastoma in the proximal femur. AP radiograph (**a**) shows a geographic radiolucent lesion in the epiphysis medially. With MRI, the lesion is located mostly in the epiphysis, but also involves the physeal plate and a small portion of the metaphysis. The lesion has expanded and thinned the medial margin of the femoral head. The lesion has slightly lobulated margins, and has low-intermediate signal on coronal T1WI (**b**), and slightly high signal on coronal FS T2WI (**c**), as well as in the adjacent marrow. The lesion shows moderate heterogeneous Gd-contrast enhancement on coronal FS T1WI (**d**), as well as prominent enhancement in the adjacent marrow.

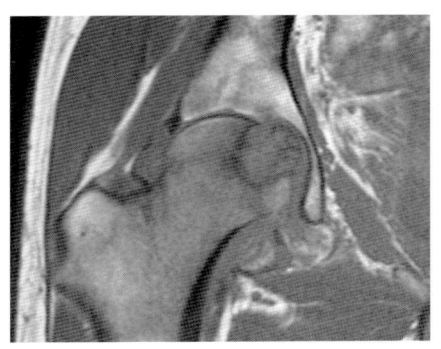

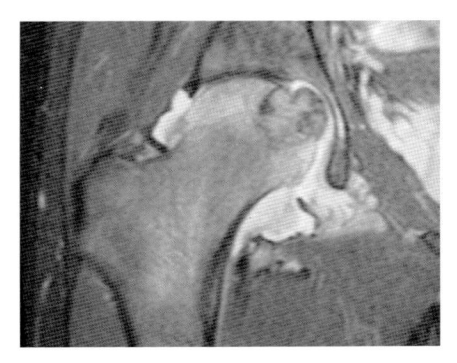

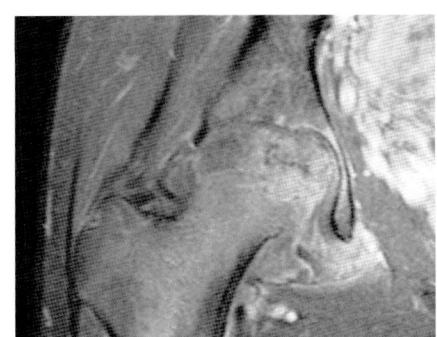

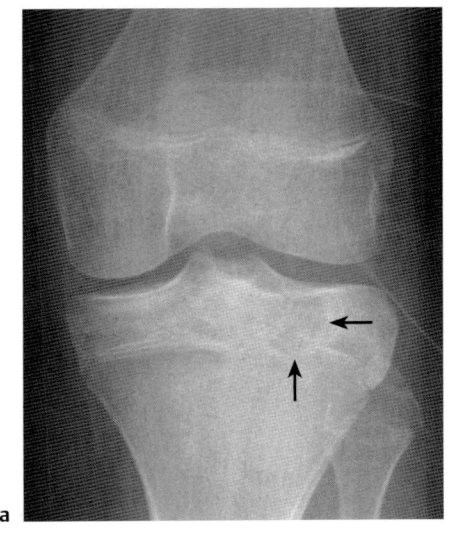

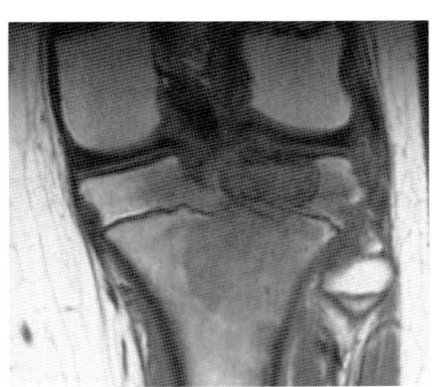

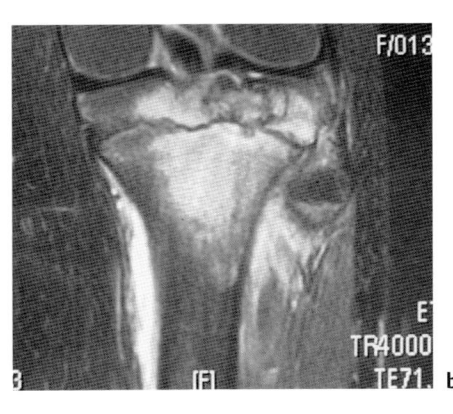

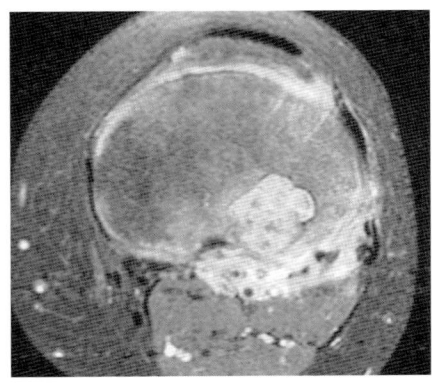

Figure **22 a–e** A 13-year-old female with chondroblastoma in the tibia. The lesion has slightly lobulated margins and is located at the physeal plate with extension into both the epiphysis and metaphysis. AP radiograph (**a**) shows a slightly radiolucent zone in the epiphysis with thin sclerotic margins. The lesion has low-intermediate signal on coronal (**b**) T1WI, and high and low signal on coronal (**c**) and axial (**d**) FS T2WI, as well as in the adjacent marrow. The lesion shows zones of prominent Gd-contrast enhancement on axial (**e**) FS T1WI, as well as mild enhancement in the adjacent marrow.

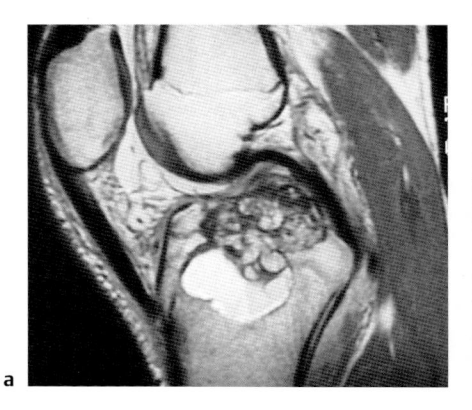

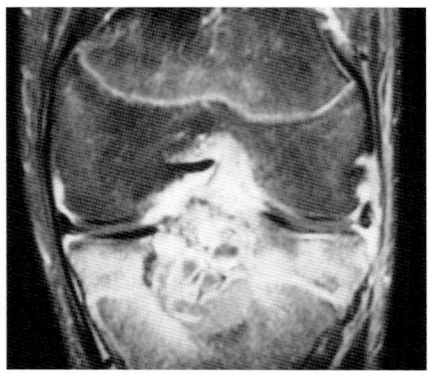

Figure 23 a, b A 17-year-old male with chondroblastoma in the tibia with a secondary aneurysmal bone cyst. The lesion has slightly lobulated margins and is located at the physeal plate with extension into both the epiphysis and metaphysis. The lesion has mixed low, intermediate, and high signal on sagittal T2WI (**a**). Multiple lobules with high signal on T2WI are seen in both the metaphyseal and epiphyseal regions of the lesion, representing a secondary aneurysmal bone cyst. The lesion shows lobular and septal zones of prominent Gd-contrast enhancement on coronal FS T1WI (**b**), as well as in the adjacent marrow.

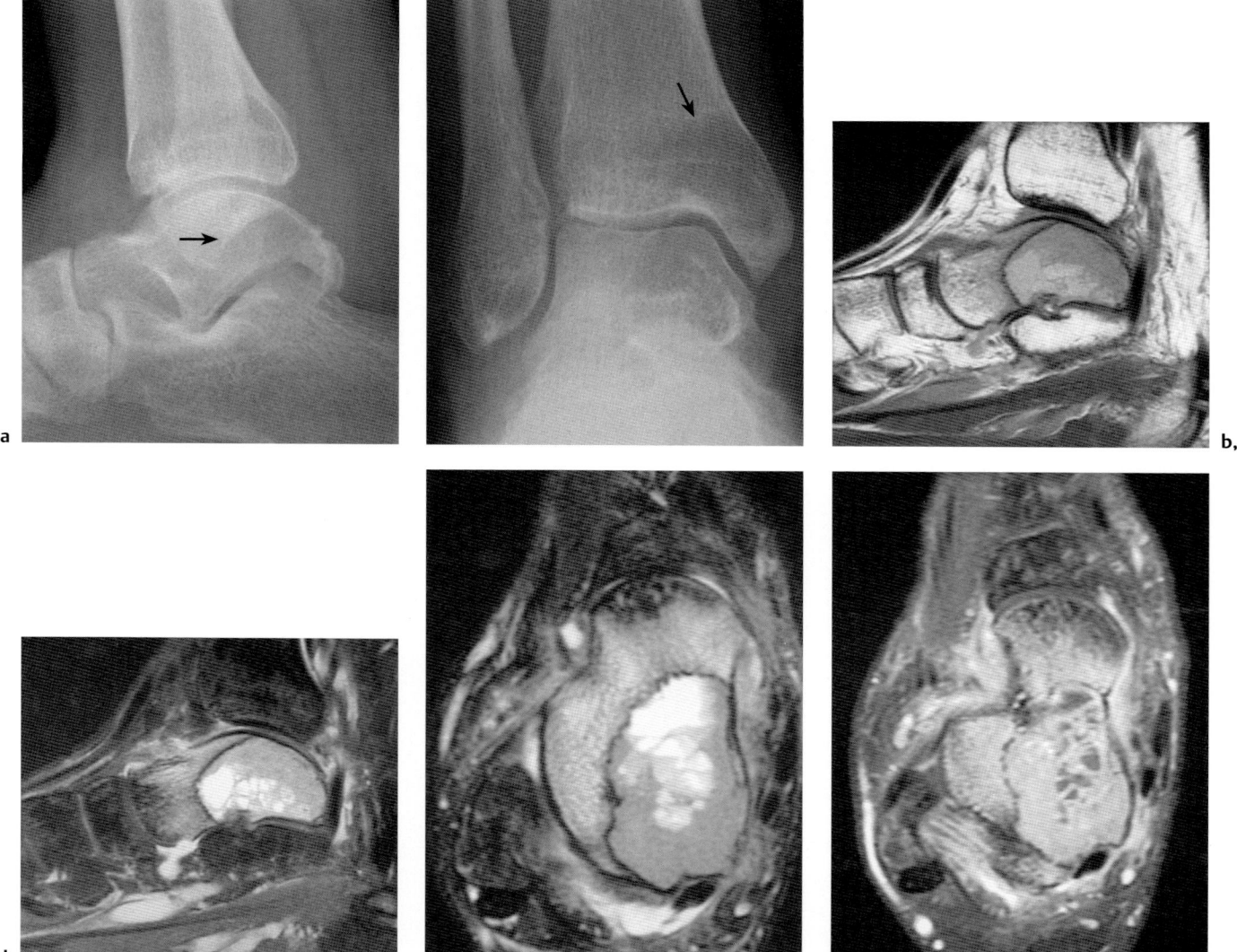

Figure 24 a–f A 20-year-old man with chondroblastoma in the talus with a secondary aneurysmal bone cyst. Lateral (**a**) and AP (**b**) radiographs shows a radiolucent zone in the thin sclerotic margins in the talus. The lesion has a thin peripheral zone of low signal on sagittal (**c**) PDWI, and sagittal (**d**) and axial (**e**) FS T2WI. The lesion has low-intermediate signal on PDWI (**c**), and zones of both intermediate and high signal on FS T2WI (**d**, **e**), as well as high signal in the adjacent marrow. Multiple locules of high signal on FS T2WI represent secondary aneurysmal bone cyst. The lesion shows zones of prominent Gd-contrast enhancement on axial FS T1WI (**f**), as well as in the adjacent marrow.

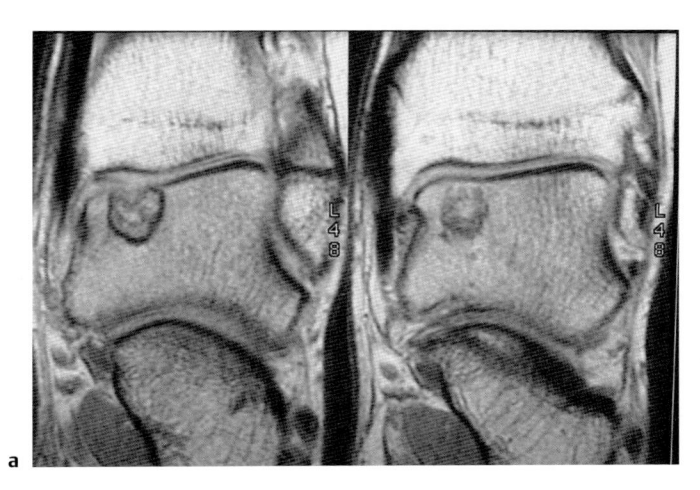

Figure **25 a–c** A 15-year-old male with chondroblastoma in the talus with associated fracture. Coronal PDWI (**a**) and T2WI (**b**) show a small circumscribed lesion in the upper talus with a fracture deformity at the upper margin. The lesion contains mixed low, intermediate, and high signal on PDWI and T2WI centrally, and is surrounded by a thin rim of low signal. The lesion shows prominent Gd-contrast enhancement on coronal FS T1WI (**c**), as well as in the adjacent marrow.

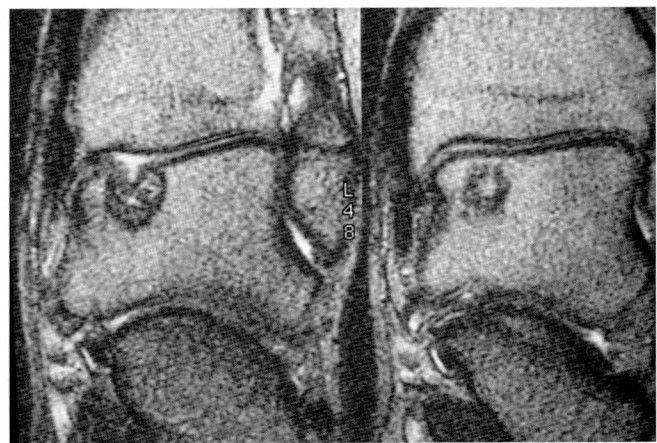

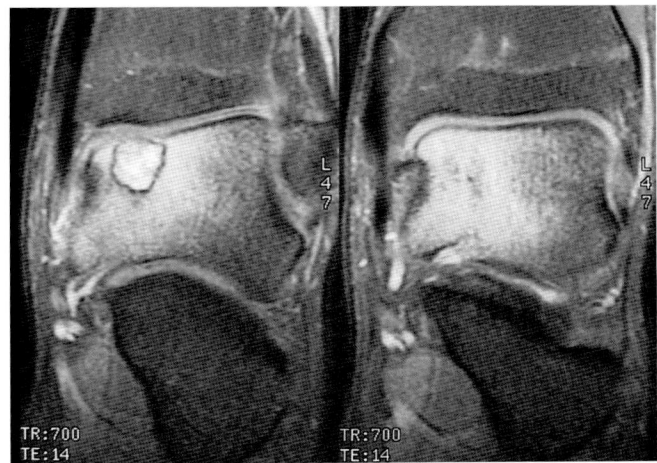

References

1. Flowers CH, Rodriguez J, Naseem M, Reyes MM, Verano AS. MR of benign chondroblastoma of the temporal bone. *AJNR Am J Neuroradiol* 1995;16:414–416.
2. Forest M. Chondroblastoma. In: Forest M, Tomeno B, Vanel D, eds. *Orthopedic Surgical Pathology: Diagnosis of Tumors and Pseudotumoral Lesions of Bone and Joints* Edinburgh: Churchill Livingstone; 1998:207–218.
3. Giudici MA, Moser RP, Kransdorf MJ. Cartilaginous bone tumors. *Radiol Clin North Am* 1993;31(2):237–259.
4. Helliwell TR. Central cartilaginous neoplasms of bone. In: Helliwell TR, ed. *Major Problems in Pathology: Pathology of Bone and Joint Neoplasms*. Vol 37. 1st ed. Philadelphia, Pa: W.B. Saunders; 1999: 209–210.
5. Huvos AG. Chondroblastoma and clear-cell chondrosarcoma. In: Huvos AG, ed. *Bone Tumors: Diagnosis, Treatment, and Prognosis* 2nd ed. Philadelphia, Pa. W.B. Saunders; 1991:295–315.
6. Ilaslan H, Sundaram M, Unni KK. Vertebral chondroblastoma. *Skeletal Radiol* 2003;32:66–71.
7. Jee WH, Park YK, McCauley TR, et al. Chondroblastoma: MR characteristics with pathologic correlation. *J Comput Assist Tomogr* 1999; 23(5):721–726.
8. Kaim AH, Hügli R, Bonél HM, Jundt G. Chondroblastoma and clear-cell chondrosarcoma: radiological and MRI characteristics with histopathological correlation. *Skeletal Radiol* 2002;31:88–95.
9. Kilpatrick SE, Parisien M, Bridge JA. Chondroblastoma. In: Fletcher CDM, Unni KK, Mertens F, eds. *World Health Organization Classification of Tumours. Pathology and Genetics of Tumours of Soft Tissue and Bone* Geneva: IARC Press; 2002:241–242.
10. Ly JQ, LaGatta LM, Beall DP. Calcaneal chondroblastoma with secondary aneurysmal bone cyst. *AJR Am J Roentgenol* 2004;182:130.
11. Mangham DC. Giant cell tumor of bone and giant cell-containing lesions of bone. In: Helliwell TR, ed. *Major Problems in Pathology: Pathology of Bone and Joint Neoplasms*. Vol 37. 1st ed. Philadelphia, Pa: W.B. Saunders; 1999:37:315–319.
12. Meyer JS, Dormans JP. Differential diagnosis of pediatric musculoskeletal masses. *Magn Reson Imaging Clin N Am* 1998;6(3):561–577
13. Miller SL, Hoffer FA. Malignant and benign bone tumors. *Radiol Clin North Am* 2001;39(4):673–699.
14. Mulder JD, Schutte HE, Kroon HM, Taconis WK. Introduction. In: *Radiologic Atlas of Bone Tumors* Amsterdam: Elsevier; 1993:3–6.
15. Mulder JD, Schutte HE, Kroon HM, Taconis WK. The diagnosis of bone tumors. In: *Radiologic Atlas of Bone Tumors* Amsterdam: Elsevier; 1993:9–46.
16. Mulder JD, Schutte HE, Kroon HM, Taconis WK. Chondroblastoma. In: *Radiologic Atlas of Bone Tumors* Amsterdam: Elsevier; 1993: 461–473.
17. Muntané A, Valls C, de Miquel MA, Pons LC. Chondroblastoma of the temporal bone: CT and MR appearance. *AJNR Am J Neuroradiol* 1993;14:70–71.
18. Unni KK. Introduction and scope of study. In: *Dahlin's Bone Tumors: General Aspects and Data on 11 087 Cases* 5th ed. Philadelphia, Pa: Lippincott, Williams & Wilkins; 1996:1–9.
19. Unni KK. Benign chondroblastoma. In: *Dahlin's Bone Tumors: General Aspects and Data in 11 087 Cases* 5th ed. Lippincott, Williams & Wilkins;1996:47–57.
20. Weatherall PT, Maale GE, Mendelsohn DB, Sherry CS, Erdman WE, Pascoe HR. Chondroblastoma: classic and confusing appearance at MR imaging. *Radiology* 1994;190(2):467–474.
21. Wold LE, Adler CP, Sim FH, Unni KK. Chondroblastoma. In: *Atlas of Orthopedic Pathology*. 2nd ed. Philadelphia, Pa: W.B. Saunders; 2003: 232–237.
22. Yamamura S, Sato K, Sugiura H, et al. Prostaglandin levels of primary bone tumor tissues correlate with peritumoral edema demonstrated by magnetic resonance imaging. *Cancer* 1997;79:255–261.

A 8 Chondroma, Intramedullary Type: Enchondroma (Also Referred to as Intra-osseous Chondroma or Central Chondroma)

ICD-O code

9220/0

Definitions

Solitary enchondromas are benign lesions composed of hyaline cartilage located in the medullary portion of bones.[2,5,6,8,12,13,15]

Multiple enchondromatosis / Ollier disease.[2,5,6,8,9,12,13,15] Multiple enchondromatosis is a genetic cartilage dysplasia involving endochondral formed bone resulting in multiple enchondromas. Ollier disease results from anomalies of endochondral bone formation with enchondromas located predominantly, or only, in limbs on one side. Short and long tubular bones of the limbs are primarily affected.

Metachondromatosis is a rare disorder that includes the combination of enchondromatosis and osteochondromatosis.[2,5,6,8,12,13,15]

Maffucci syndrome refers to a very rare disease with simultaneous occurrence of multiple enchondromas and cutaneous or visceral hemangiomas of soft tissue.[2,5-9,12,13,15]

Frequency of Occurrence

Chondromas represent 10–25% of benign bone tumors.[5,6,8,10-12,14,15] Enchondromas are intramedullary chondromas, and represent ~24 to 40% of all chondromas; they can be solitary (88%) or multiple (12%). Ollier disease is a dyschondroplasia involving endochondrally formed bone resulting in multiple enchondromas (enchondromatosis). Metachondromatosis is a combination of enchondromatosis and osteochondromatosis, and is rare. Maffucci disease refers to a syndrome with multiple enchondromas and soft tissue hemangiomas, and is very rare.

Age at Presentation

Enchondroma: from 3 to 83 years, median = 35 years, mean = 38–40 years, peaks in 3rd and 4th decades[8,10-12,14,15]

Ollier disease: from 1 to 63 years, median = 12 years.[2,9,12]

Maffucci syndrome: occurs in children and adults.[7,8]

Gender Ratio (M/F)

Enchondroma: 0.8 / 1 to 1.1 / 1.[5,6,8,10-12,14,15]

Ollier disease: 1 / 1.[2,9]

Maffucci syndrome: 1 / 1.[2,7,9]

Location

Solitary enchondroma.[6,10-12] Locations include: phalanx (hands) (~30%) > femur > metacarpals > humerus > tibia > ribs > metatarsals > phalanx (feet) > fibula > ulna > other sites. Intra-osseous locations: diaphyseal (58%) > meta-diaphyseal (39%) > epiphyseal-equivalent zones (3%). Central (80%) > eccentric location within bone.

Multiple enchondromatosis / Ollier disease, Maffucci syndrome. Lesions are most frequently located in the small bones of the hands and feet.[7,9,12] In Ollier disease, lesions are usually located predominantly or only in limbs on one side.[9,12] In Maffucci syndrome, hemangiomas in the soft tissues may be near or distant from the enchondromas.[7,12]

Signs and Symptoms[2,5,6,12,13,15]

Solitary enchondromas are usually asymptomatic unless bone cortex is fractured or eroded causing focal pain (40%). Lesions in hands or feet are often associated with deformities and/or pathologic fractures.

Gross Pathologic Findings[2,5-8,12,15]

Enchondromas are typically lobulated or nodular, bluish-white, firm lesions with varying degrees of matrix mineralization causing gritty texture.

Histopathologic Findings[2,5-8,12,15]

Lesions contain varying-sized lobules of hyaline cartilage separated by normal marrow (fat and trabeculae) and fibrous strands. Cartilage cells are relatively few among the abundant intercellular matrix, which is comprised of varying proportions of hyaline chondroid and mucinous/myxoid components. Chondrocytes are relatively uniform in size with small, rounded nuclei in vacuolated cytoplasm. Mitotic figures are rare or absent. Varying degrees of matrix mineralization are usually seen. Lesions are immunoreactive to S-100 protein, and types I, II, and VI collagen.[2]

Lesion Genetics

These lesions have been reported to have diploid or near-diploid cells with structural abnormalities involving chromosomes 6 and 12.[8] Patients with Ollier disease have been reported to have mutations involving the PTHR1 gene which encodes a receptor for parathyroid hormone.[9] Maffucci syndrome is a nonhereditary mesodermal dysplasia.[7]

Findings on Plain Films (Roentgenograms) and Computed Tomography[2,4,5,9,12,13,15]

Enchondromas are usually well-circumscribed radiolucent lesions, often containing chondroid matrix mineralization (Figs. **26, 27, 30, 31, 33–35**). In small bones, cortex can be eroded and thinned on the endosteal side, with or without associated bone expansion. In large bones, expansion is minimal or not seen. CT is more sensitive than plain films in detecting subtle matrix mineralization and erosion of cortex (Fig. **33**). In patients with Maffucci syndrome, hemangiomas in the soft tissues may contain phleboliths.[7,12]

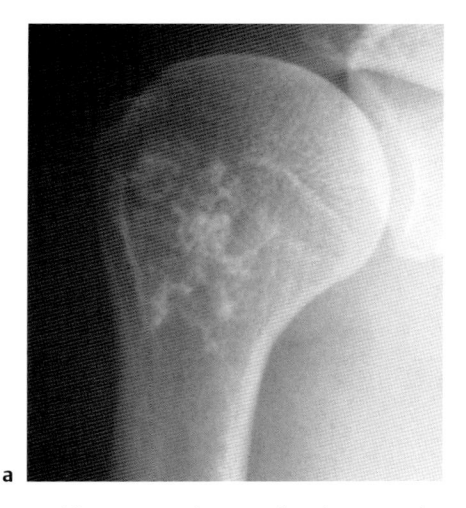

Figure **26 a–c** A 40-year-old woman with an enchondroma in the proximal humerus. AP radiograph (**a**) shows chondroid matrix mineralization in the lesion. The lesion has lobulated circumscribed margins and contains nodular zones with intermediate signal separated by thin curvilinear zones of low signal on sagittal PDWI (**b**). On sagittal FS T2WI (**c**), the lesion has predominantly high signal with foci and bands of low signal.

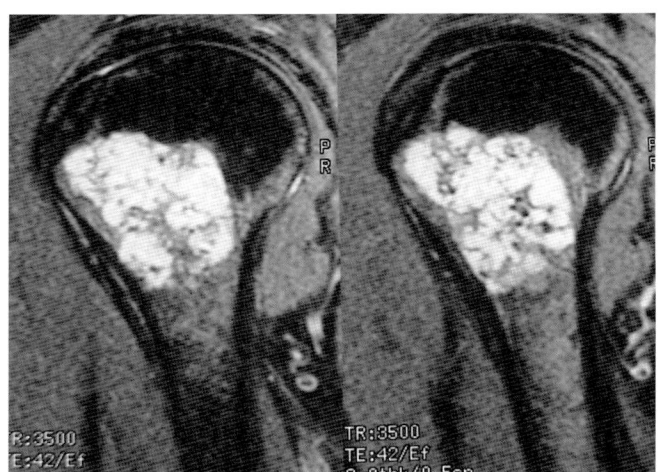

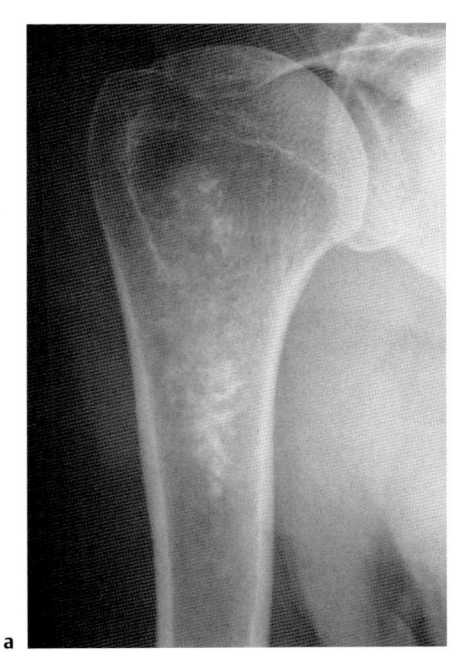

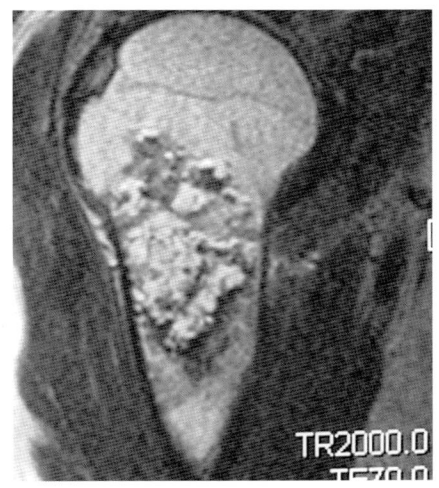

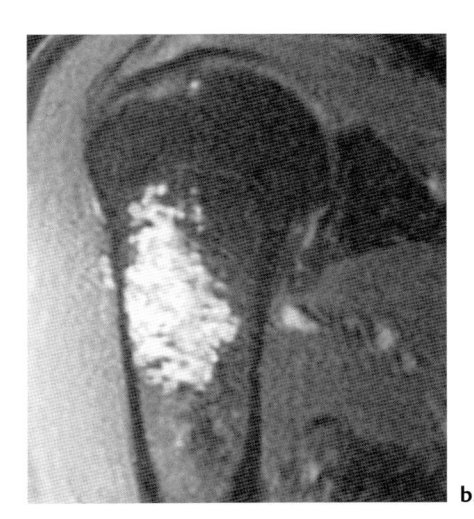

Figure **27 a–c** A 50-year-old man with an enchondroma in the proximal humerus. AP radiograph (**a**) shows chondroid matrix mineralization in the lesion. On coronal T2WI (**b**), the lesion has predominantly high signal with foci and bands of low signal. The lesion shows prominent Gd-contrast enhancement on FS T1WI (**c**).

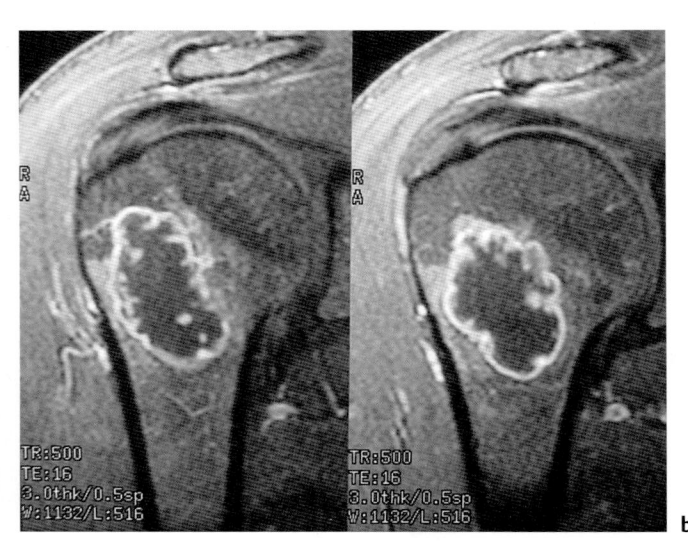

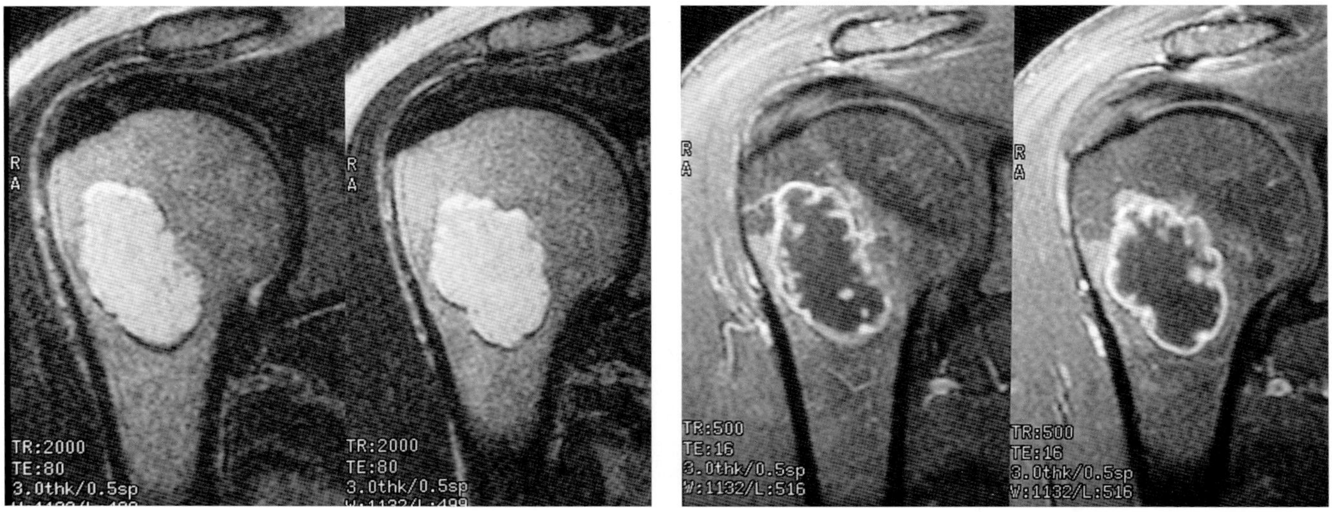

Figure **28 a, b** A 44-year-old woman with an enchondroma in the proximal humerus. The lesion has lobulated circumscribed margins and has high signal on coronal T2WI (**a**) surrounded by a thin rim of low signal. The lesion shows thin lobulated peripheral Gd-contrast enhancement on coronal FS T1WI (**b**).

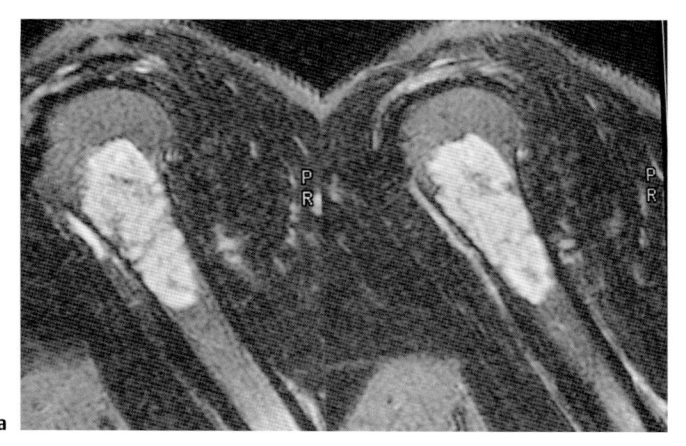

Figure **29 a, b** A 48-year-old man with an enchondroma in the proximal humerus. The lesion has lobulated circumscribed margins and contains predominantly high signal with curvilinear zones of low signal on sagittal T2WI (**a**). The lesion shows both heterogeneous central and peripheral curvilinear patterns of Gd-contrast enhancement on coronal FS T1WI (**b**).

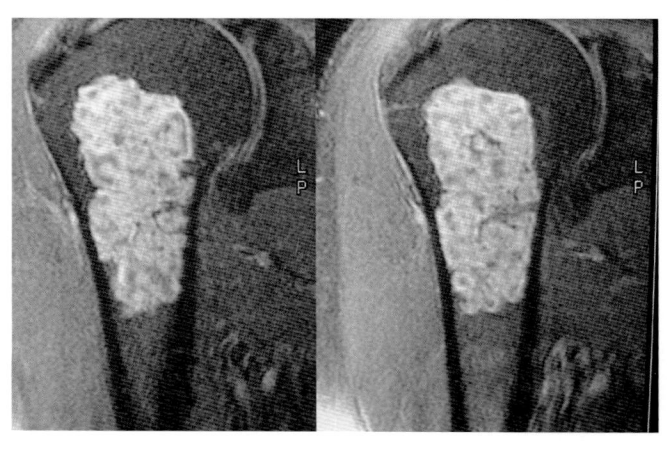

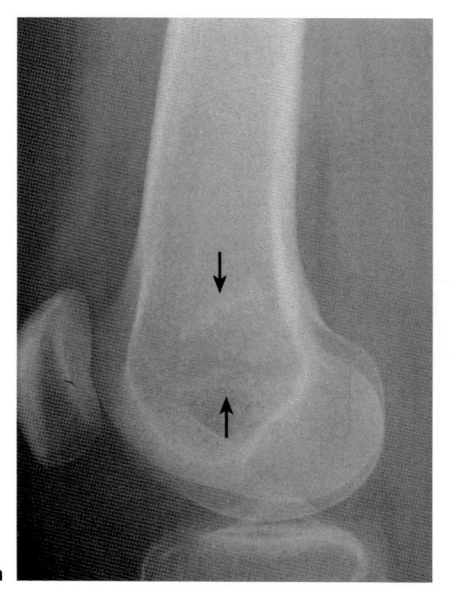

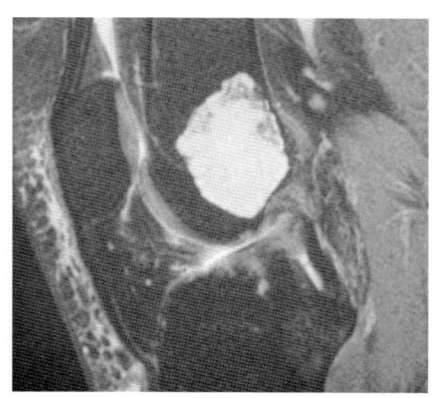

Figure **30 a, b** A 39-year-old woman with an enchondroma in the distal femur. Lateral radiograph (**a**) shows faint chondroid matrix mineralization in the lesion. The lesion has lobulated circumscribed margins and contains high signal on sagittal FS T2WI (**b**).

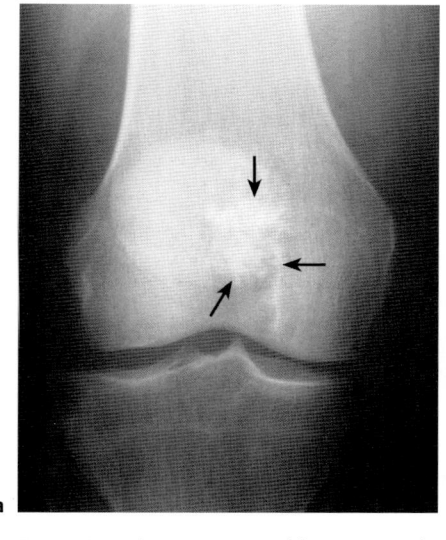

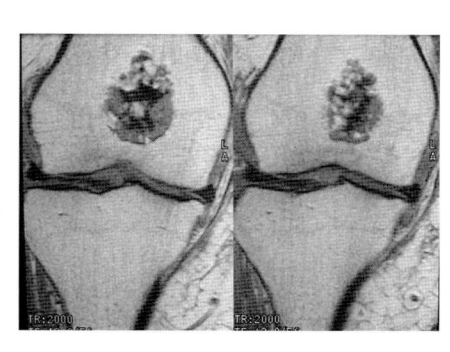

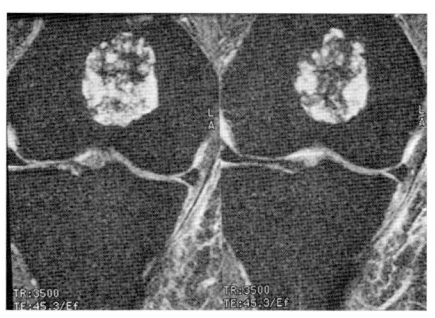

Figure **31 a, b** A 66-year-old woman with an enchondroma in the distal femur. AP radiograph (**a**) shows chondroid matrix mineralization in the lesion. The lesion has lobulated circumscribed margins and contains zones of low, intermediate, and slightly high signal on coronal (**b**) PDWI, and zones of high and low signal on coronal (**c**) FS T2WI.

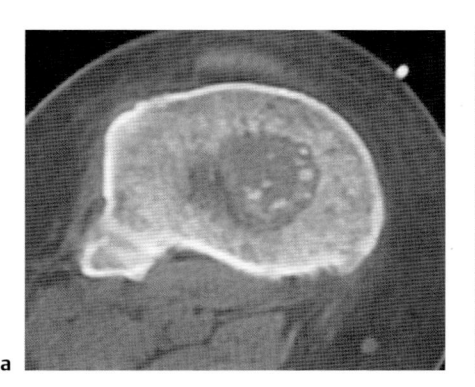

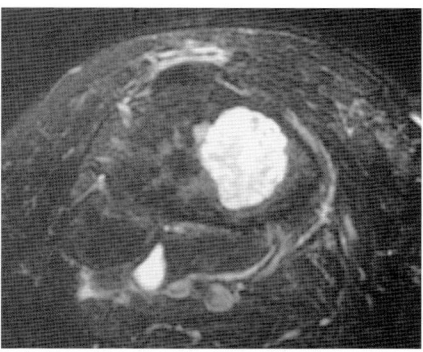

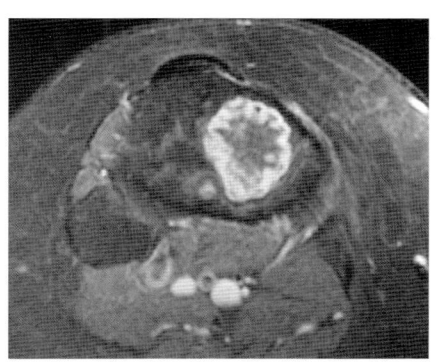

Figure **32 a–c** A 45-year-old woman with an enchondroma in the proximal tibia. Axial CT image (**a**) shows a circumscribed radiolucent lesion containing chondroid matrix. The lesion has lobulated circumscribed margins and contains high signal on axial (**b**) FS T2WI. The lesion shows lobulated peripheral Gd-contrast enhancement on axial (**c**) FS T1WI.

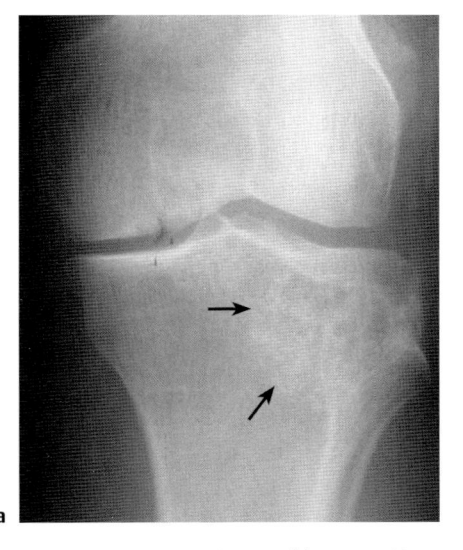

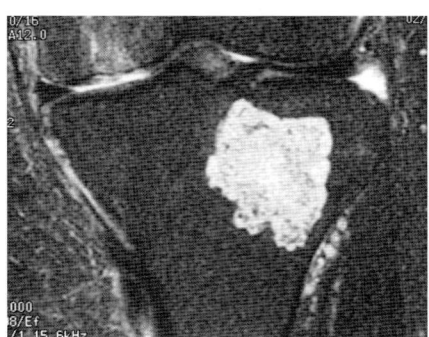

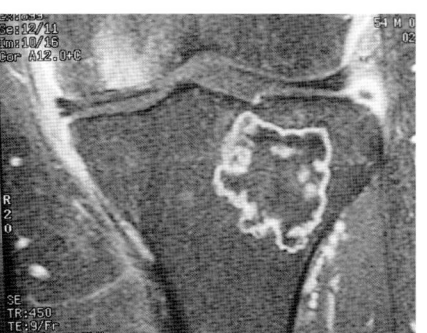

Figure **33 a–c** A 54-year-old man with an enchondroma in the proximal tibia. AP radiograph (**a**) shows a lesion containing chondroid matrix. The lesion has lobulated circumscribed margins and contains high signal on coronal (**b**) FS T2WI. The lesion shows lobulated peripheral Gd-contrast enhancement on coronal (**c**) FS T1WI.

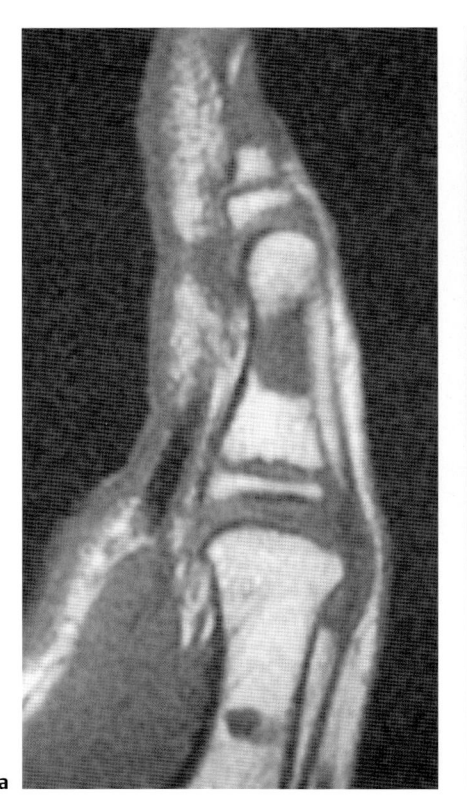

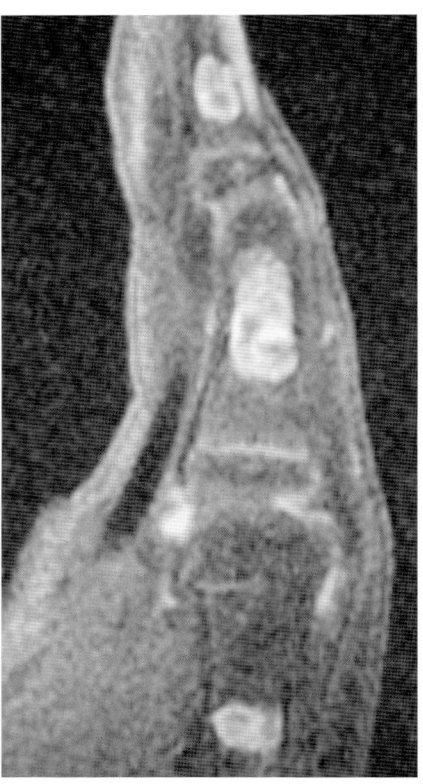

Figure **34 a, b** An 11-year-old female with an Ollier disease. Sagittal (**a**) T1WI shows single enchondromas in the metacarpal bone, proximal and middle phalanges, which have low-intermediate signal. The lesions show nodular and lobulated peripheral Gd-contrast enhancement on sagittal (**b**) FS T1WI.

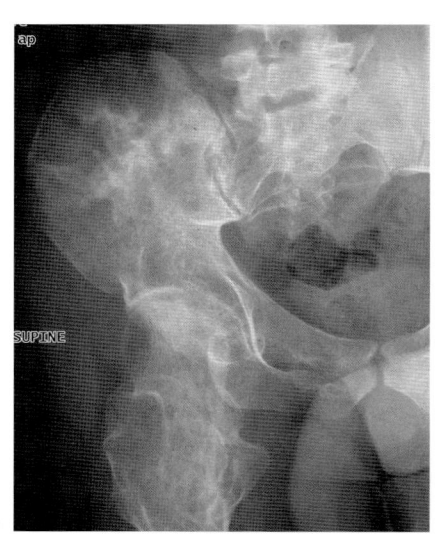

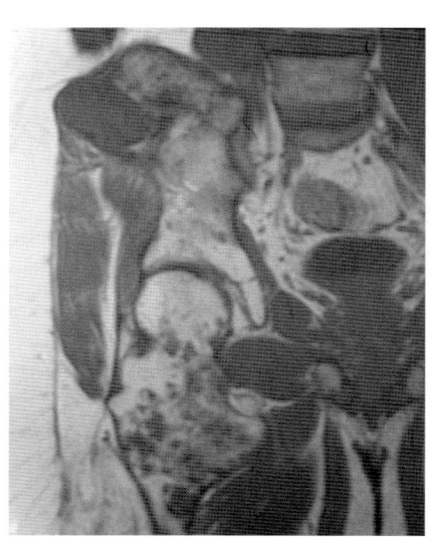

Figure **35 a–c** A 29-year-old man with Ollier disease. AP radiograph (**a**) shows multiple enchondromas involving the iliac bone, ischium, pubic bone, and femur. The lesions have low-intermediate signal on coronal (**b**) T1WI, and high signal on coronal (**c**) FS T2WI. The lesions show nodular and lobulated peripheral Gd-contrast enhancement on coronal (35 d) FS T1WI

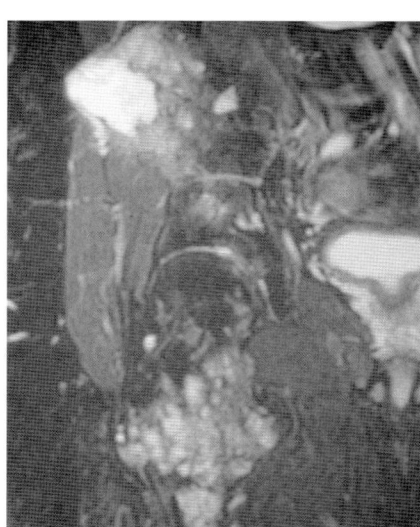

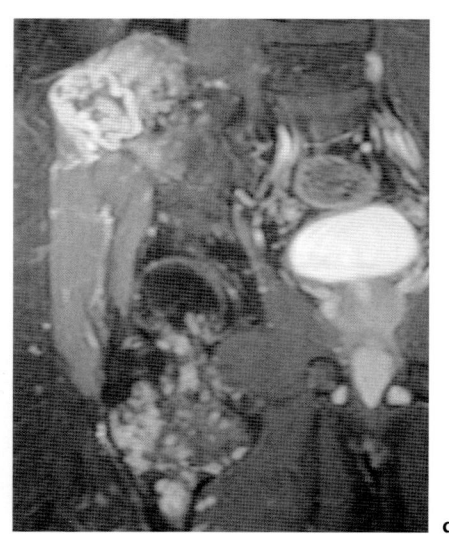

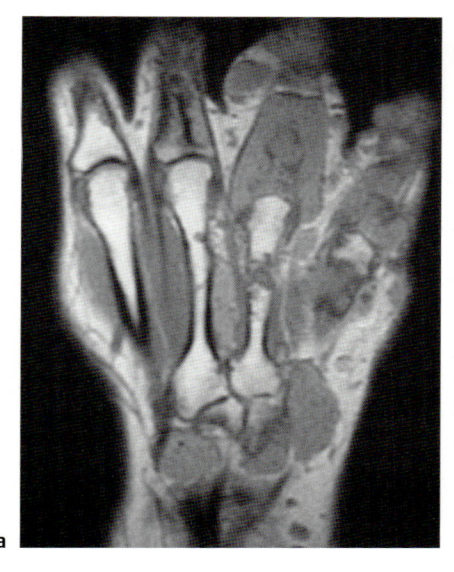

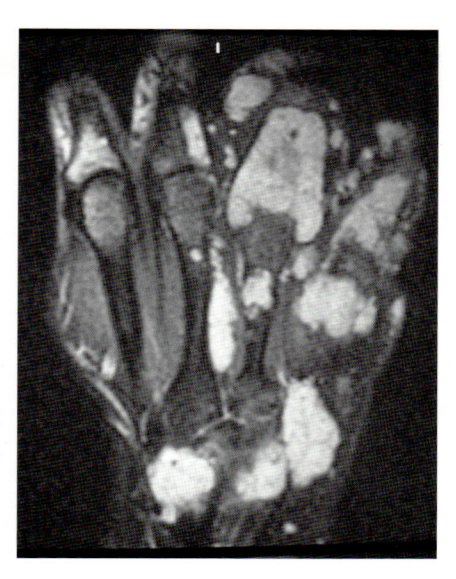

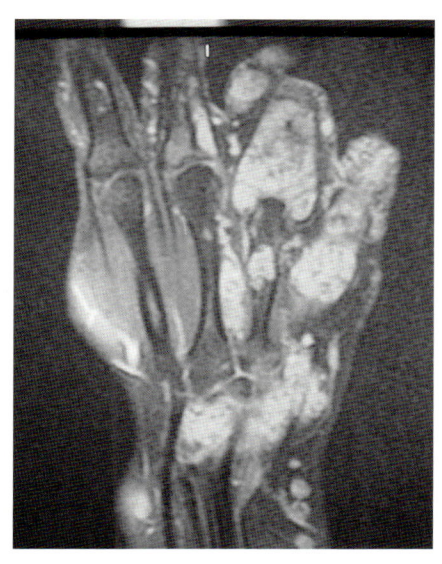

Figure 36 a–c A 20-year-old woman with Maffucci syndrome who has multiple intra-osseous enchondromas and soft tissue hemangiomas involving the wrist and hand. Multiple intra-osseous lesions and circumscribed extra-osseous soft tissue lesions are seen, which have mostly intermediate signal on coronal PDWI (**a**) and high signal on coronal FS T2 W (**b**). Some of the intra-osseous lesions are associated with cortical expansion. The lesions show prominent Gd-contrast enhancement on coronal FS T1WI (**c**).

MRI Findings[1,3,4,13]

Enchondromas often appear as lobulated, intramedullary lesions with well-defined borders ranging in size from 3 to 16 cm, mean = 5 cm (Figs. **26–36**). Mild endosteal scalloping can be seen. Lesions usually have low-intermediate signal on T1WI and intermediate signal on PDWI. On T2WI and fat-suppressed T2WI, lesions usually have predominantly high signal with foci and/or bands of low signal representing areas of matrix mineralization and fibrous strands. No zones of abnormal high signal on T2WI are typically seen in the marrow outside the borders of the lesions. Lesions typically show Gd-contrast enhancement in various patterns (peripheral curvilinear lobular, central nodular/septal and peripheral lobular, or heterogeneous diffuse). Patients with Maffucci syndrome usually have multiple enchondromas as well as multiple hemangiomas in the soft tissues, which typically have high signal on FS T2WI and prominent Gd-contrast enhancement (Fig. **36**).

Deep endosteal scalloping (greater than two-thirds cortical thickness), cortical destruction, extrao-sseous soft tissue mass, and periosteal reaction are features commonly associated with chondrosarcoma and not with enchondroma. Pathologic fractures are less common with enchondromas compared with chondrosarcomas. Using fast, contrast-enhanced MRI, enchondromas reportedly have delayed enhancement (after 10 s to 2 min from the start of arterial enhancement) compared with chondrosarcomas, which show enhancement in the first 10 seconds. Using early and exponential features of dynamic contrast enhancement may enable confirmation of the diagnosis of chondrosarcoma and exclusion of enchondroma.

Differential Diagnosis

Chondrosarcoma, bone infarct, unicameral bone cyst, aneurysmal bone cyst, fibrous dysplasia, giant cell tumor, chondroblastoma, chondromyxoid fibroma.

Treatment and Prognosis[2,5,6,8,9,12,15]

Solitary enchondromas are benign lesions that can increase in size during childhood and adolescence. After completion of endochondral bone growth, enchondromas typically do not enlarge. If growth of enhcondromas occurs in adults, low-grade chondrosarcoma should be excluded. Degeneration of enchondromas to chondrosarcoma may occur in 1 % of solitary enchondromas and up to 56 % in patients with multiple enchondromas (multiple enchondromatosis, Ollier disease, and Maffucci syndrome).[2,5–9,12,15] The risk of developing chondrosarcoma is greater for patients with Maffucci syndrome than for patients with Ollier disease.[8] Chondrosarcomas have been reported in 15–56 % of patients with Maffucci syndrome.[7] The hemangiomas in Maffuci syndrome can also degenerate into sarcomas in 3–5 % of cases.[7] Removal can be accomplished by en-bloc resection or curettage with or without bone grafts.

References

1 Aoki J, Sone S, Fujioka F, et al. MR of enchondroma and chondrosarcoma: rings and arcs of Gd-DTPA enhancement. *J Comput Assist Tomogr* 1991;15:1011–1016.
2 Forest M. Chondroma. In: Forest M, Tomeno B, Vanel D, eds. *Orthopedic Surgical Pathology: Diagnosis of Tumors and Pseudotumoral Lesions of Bone and Joints* Edinburgh: Churchill Livingstone; 1998: 191–205.
3 Geirnaerdt MJ, Hogendoorn Pancras CW, Bloem JL, Taminiau Antonie HM, van der Woude HJ. Cartilaginous tumors: fast contrast-enhanced MR imaging. *Radiology* 2000;214(2):539–546.
4 Giudici MA, Moser RP, Kransdorf MJ. Cartilaginous bone tumors. *Radiol Clin North Am* 1993;31(2):237–259.
5 Helliwell TE. Central cartilaginous neoplasms of bone. In: Helliwell TR, ed. *Major Problems in Pathology: Pathology of Bone and Joint Neoplasms* 1st ed. Philadelphia, Pa: W.B. Saunders; 1999;37: 193–214.
6 Huvos AG. Solitary and multiple osteochondromas and enchondromas; juxtacortical chondroma; Maffucci's disease. In: Huvos AG, ed. *Bone Tumors: Diagnosis, Treatment, and Prognosis* 2nd ed. Philadelphia, Pa: W.B. Saunders Co.; 1991:276–279.

7. Kransdorf MJ, Murphey MD. Vascular and lymphatic tumors. In: Kransdorf MJ, Murphey MD. *Imaging of Soft Tissue Tumors* 2nd ed. Philadelphia, Pa: W.B. Saunders 2006:150-188.
8. Lucas DR, Bridge JA. Chondromas, enchondroma, periosteal chondroma, and enchondromatosis. In: Fletcher CDM, Unni KK, Mertens F, eds. *World Health Organization Classification of Tumours. Pathology and Genetics of Tumours of Soft Tissue and Bone* Geneva: IARC Press; 2002:237-240.
9. Mertens F, Unni KK. Enchondromatosis: Ollier's disease and Maffucci syndrome. In: Fletcher CDM, Unni KK, Mertens F, eds. *World Health Organization Classification of Tumours. Pathology and Genetics of Tumours of Soft Tissue and Bone* Geneva: IARC Press; 2002:356-357.
10. Mulder JD, Schutte HE, Kroon HM, Taconis WK. Introduction. In: *Radiologic Atlas of Bone Tumors* Amsterdam: Elsevier; 1993:3-6.
11. Mulder JD, Schutte HE, Kroon HM, Taconis WK. The diagnosis of bone tumors. In: *Radiologic Atlas of Bone Tumors.* Amsterdam: Elsevier; 1993:9-46.
12. Mulder JD, Schutte HE, Kroon HM, Taconis WK. Intraosseous chondroma. In: *Radiologic Atlas of Bone Tumors* Amsterdam: Elsevier; 1993:421-434.
13. Murphey MD, Flemming DJ, Boyea SR, Bojescul JA, Sweet DE, Temple HT. From the archives of the AFIP. Enchondroma versus chondrosarcoma of the appendicular skeleton: differentiating features. *Radiographics* 1998;18:1213-1237.
14. Unni KK. Introduction and scope of study. In: *Dahlin's Bone Tumors: General Aspects and Data on 11 087 Cases* 5th ed. Philadelphia, Pa: Lippincott, Williams & Wilkins; 1996:1-9.
15. Unni KK. Chondroma. In: *Dahlin's Bone Tumors: General Aspects and Data on 11 087 Cases* 5th ed. Philadelphia, Pa: Lippincott, Williams & Wilkins;1996:25-45.

A 9 Chondroma, Periosteal or Juxtacortical Type
(Also Referred to as Periosteal or Juxtacortical Chondroma, Surface Chondroma, and Juxtacortical/Parosteal Chondroma)

ICD-O Code
9221/0

Definition
Juxtacortical chondromas are benign protuberant hyaline cartilaginous tumors that arise from the periosteum and are superficial to bone cortex.[1–4,7–9,12]

Frequency of Occurrence[5–7,11,12]
Juxtacortical chondromas account for <1% of bone lesions. Juxtacortical chondromas represent ~5–12% of chondromas, which also include enchondroma, osteochondroma (exostosis), and capsular, synovial, and tendon-sheath types.

Age at Presentation
From 4 to 77 years, median = 26 years.[7]

Gender Ratio (M/F)
1.3/1 to 2/1[2,7]

Location
Lesions occur in the hand and foot bones > femur > tibia > humerus > others.[1,3,4,7] Juxtacortical chondromas occur most frequently at the surface of the diaphyseal portions of bone, followed by the metadiaphyseal and metaphyseal regions.[7] Lesions rarely occur in the epiphyseal region alone.[7]

Signs and Symptoms
Juxtacortical chondromas can be present as slow-growing, painless or dull-aching, bony protrusions.[2–4,7–10,12,13]

Gross Pathologic Findings[1–4,7,8,12,13]
Juxtacortical chondromas contain lobules of bluish-white hyaline cartilage adjacent to the cortex with variable calcification. Lesions range in size from 1 to 14 cm, although most are less than 5 cm. The mean size of juxtacortical chondromas is 2.6–4 cm, median size = 2.5 cm.

Histopathologic Findings[1–4,7,8,12,13]
Juxtacortical chondromas contain lobulated hyaline cartilage that lacks nuclear atypia. Lesions often contain foci of calcification (50%), ossification, and myxoid material. Peripheral areas of cellular pleomorphism may be seen occasionally.[3]

Tumor Genetics
Lesions typically show a diploid pattern with low proliferative activity.[4] Structural alterations involving chromosomes 6 and 12 have been reported.[4]

Findings on Plain Films (Roentgenograms) and Computed Tomography[1–3,7–10,12,13]
Juxtacortical chondromas often appear as soft tissue lesions with or without calcifications (Figs. **37**, **39**). Lesions are associated with erosion and radiolucent scalloping of the underlying cortex. Periosteal thickening is seen at the base and at the periphery of the lesion adjacent to normal cortex and trabeculae (saucer-configuration). Rarely, a thin shell of periosteal bone can be seen along the outer margin of the lesion. Lesions typically do not prominently extend into the medullary space.

MRI Findings[1,9,10,13]
Lesions are located at the bone surface and are usually lobulated with low-intermediate signal on T1WI, which is hypo- or isointense relative to muscle (Figs. **37–41**). Lesions usually have heterogeneous predominantly high signal on T2WI. Lesions are surrounded by low signal borders on T2WI representing thin sclerotic reaction. Areas of low signal on T2WI are secondary to matrix mineralization. Edema is not typically seen in nearby medullary bone.[13] Lesions often show a peripheral pattern of Gd-contrast enhancement which correlates to fibrovascular bundles surrounding the cartilage lobules.[13] Chondromas can also occur in a subperiosteal location (Fig. **41**).

Differential Diagnosis
Fibrous cortical defect, periosteal chondrosarcoma, periosteal osteosarcoma, parosteal osteosarcoma, periosteal/cortical desmoid, synovial chondroma, aneurysmal bone cyst.

Treatment and Prognosis
Standard treatment is en-bloc resection or local excision that includes the periosteum, lesion, and fibrous capsule.[1,2,8] Recurrence is treated by en-bloc excision with bone grafting if necessary.

Figure 37 a–f A 14-year-old male with a sessile type of juxtacortical/periosteal chondroma involving the humerus. AP radiograph (**a**) and axial CT image (**b**) show a lesion with chondroid matrix at the medial outer cortical surface of the proximal humeral diaphysis. Irregular cortical thickening is seen at the base of the lesion. The lesion has intermediate signal on axial (**c**) PDWI, and heterogeneous predominantly high signal as well zones of intermediate and low signal on axial (**d**) T2WI, and sagittal (**e**) FS T2WI. Periosteal thickening at the base of the lesion is seen as irregular zones of low signal at the outer cortical margin. The lesion shows irregular zones of Gd-contrast enhancement on axial (**f**) FS T1WI.

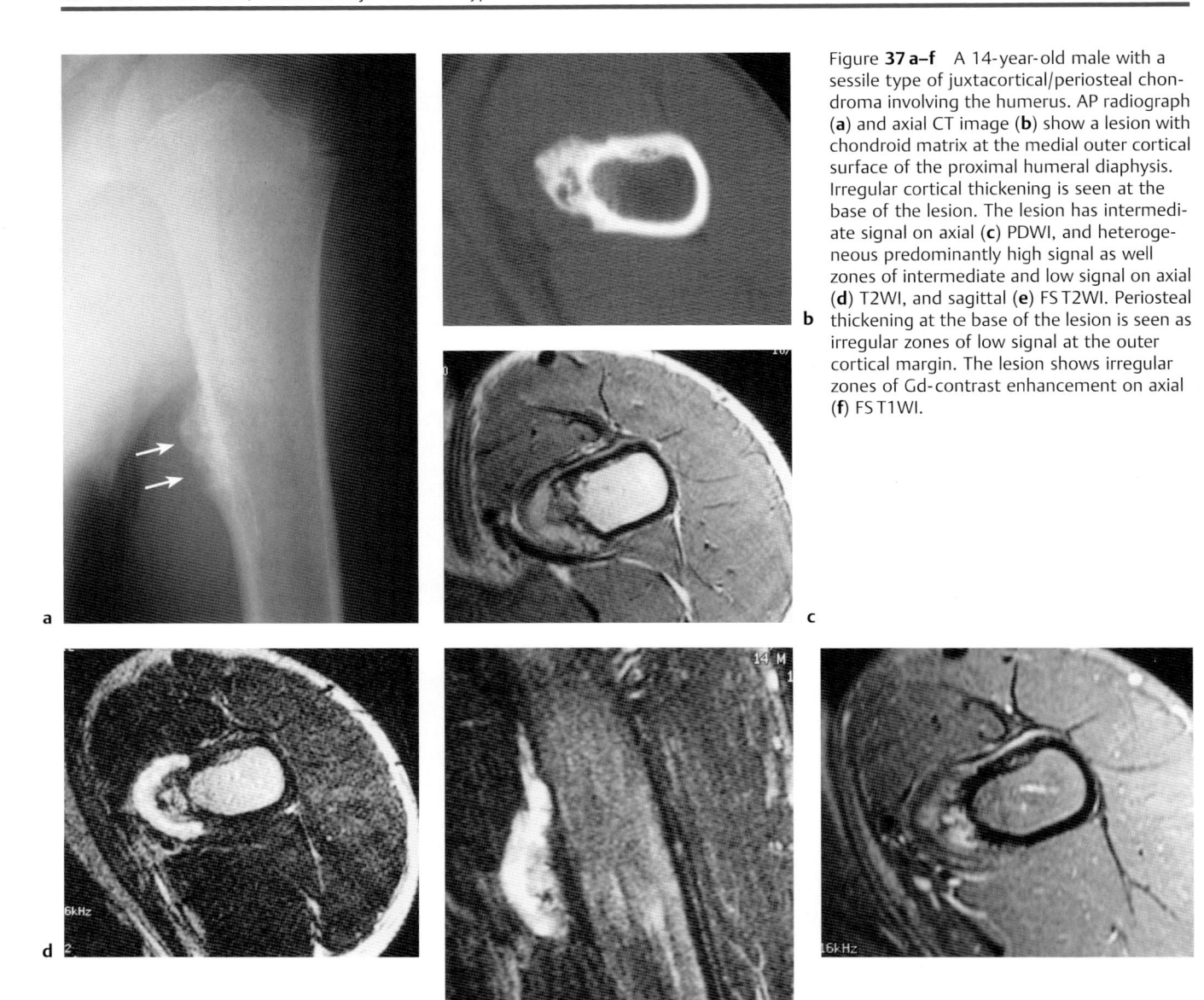

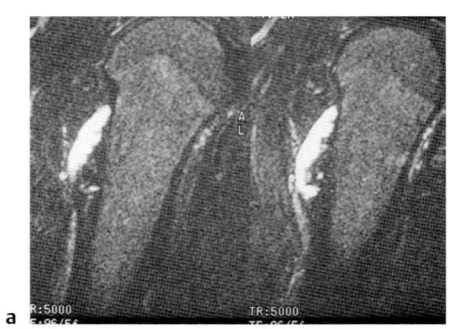

Figure 38 a–e A 28-year-old man with a sessile-type juxtacortical/periosteal chondroma involving the metadiaphyseal region of the humerus. The lesion has heterogeneous predominantly high signal as well zones of intermediate and low signal on sagittal (**a, c**) FS T2WI and axial (**b**) T2WI. The lesion has intermediate signal on axial (**b**) PDWI. Periosteal thickening at the base of the lesion is seen as irregular zones of low signal at the outer cortical margin. The lesion shows irregular zones of Gd-contrast enhancement on sagittal (**d**) T1WI and sagittal (**e**) FS T1WI.

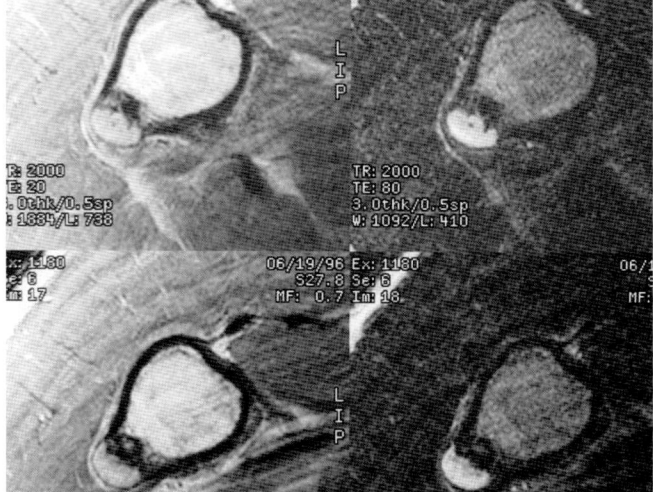

Figure 38 c–e ▷

Treatment and Prognosis **361**

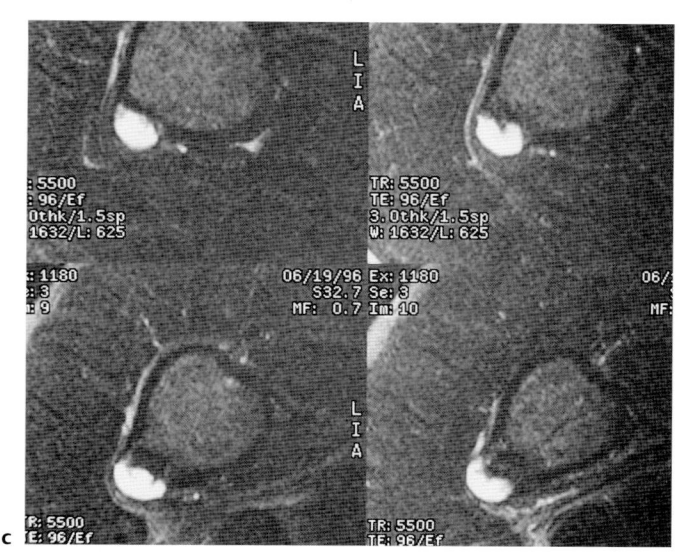

Figure **38 c–e**

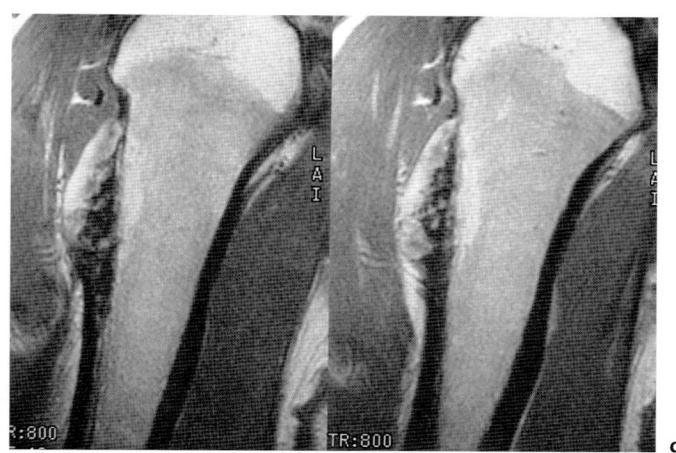

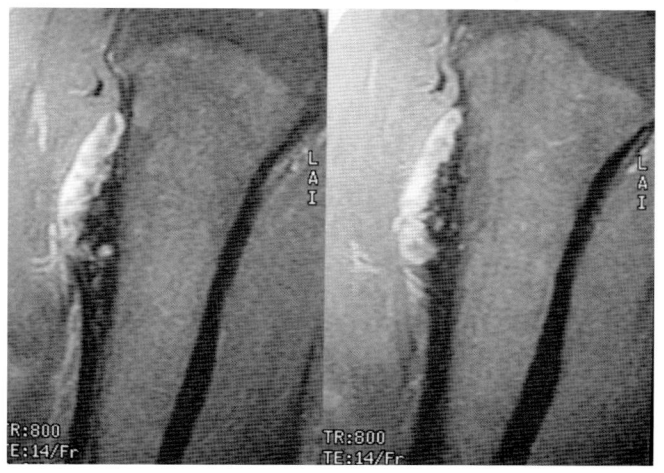

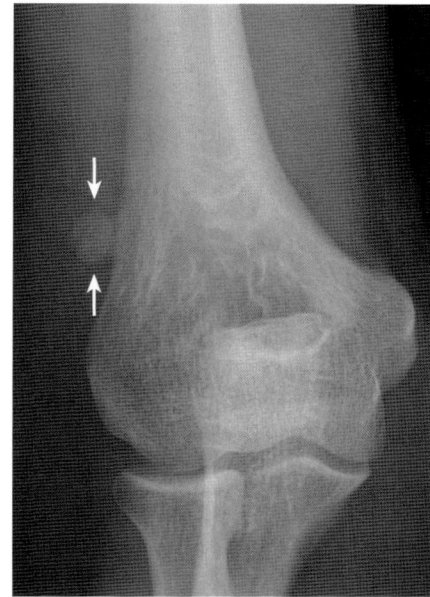

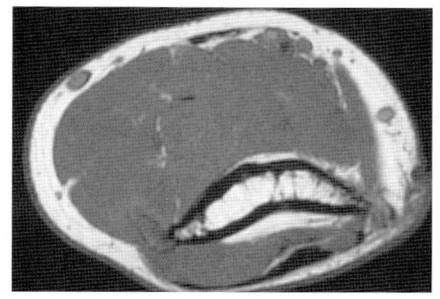

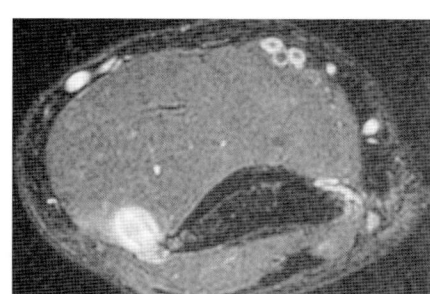

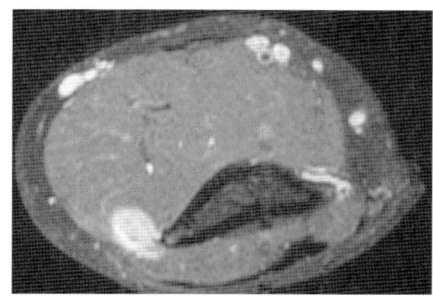

Figure **39 a–d** A 40-year-old man with a juxtacortical/periosteal chondroma involving the distal humerus. AP radiograph (**a**) shows a pedunculated mineralized lesion arising from an intact outer cortical surface. The lesion has low-intermediate signal on axial (**b**) T1WI, and high signal on axial (**c**) FS T2WI. Slight periosteal thickening is seen at the base of the lesion. The lesion shows prominent Gd-contrast enhancement on axial (**d**) FS T1WI.

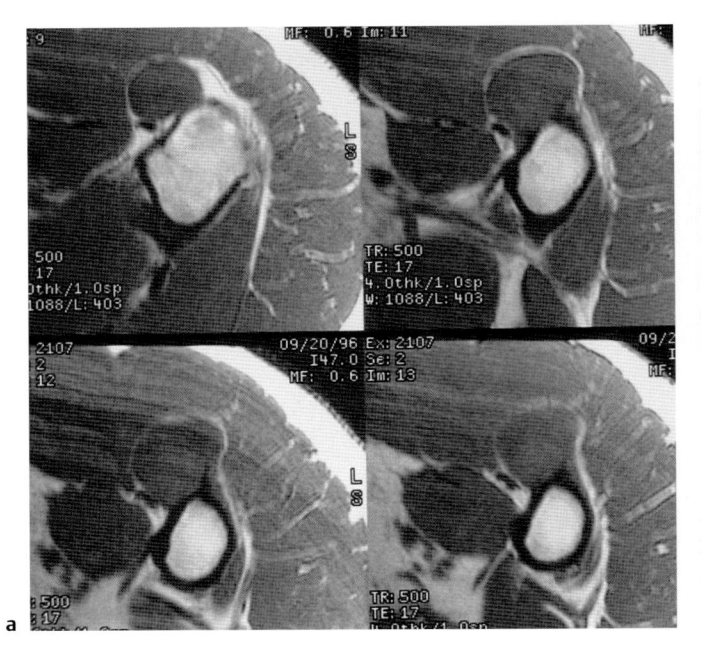

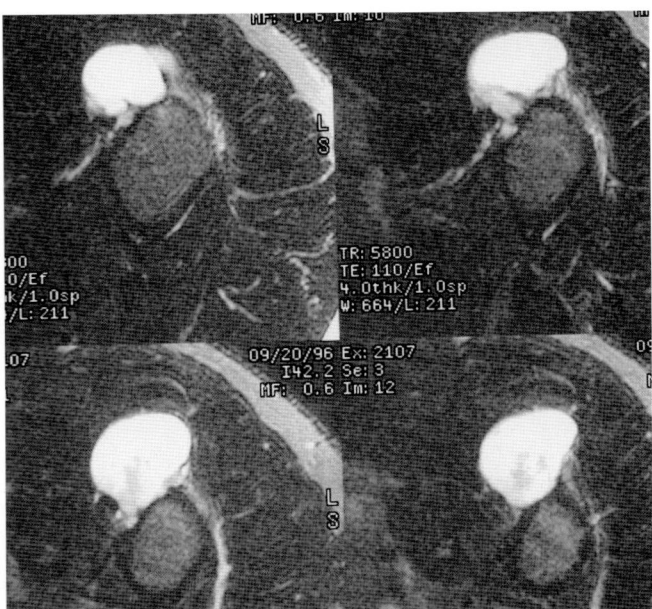

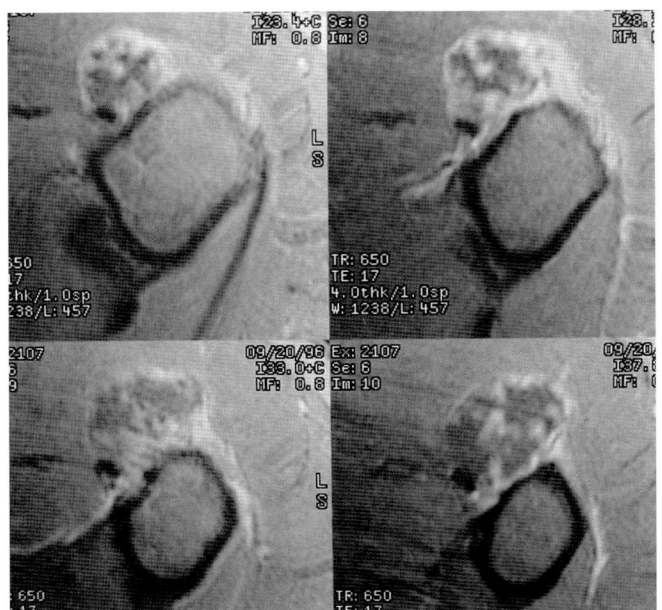

Figure **40 a–c** A 28-year-old man with a juxtacortical/periosteal chondroma involving the proximal humerus. The lesion has low-intermediate signal on axial (**a**) T1WI, and high signal on axial (**b**) FS T2WI. The lesion shows nodular and lobulated peripheral Gd-contrast enhancement on axial (**c**) FS T1WI.

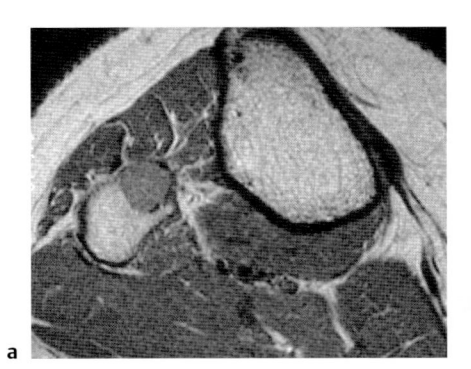

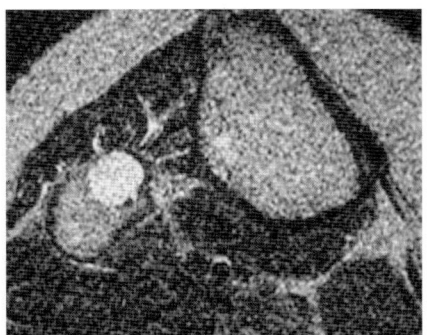

Figure **41 a–e** A 29-year-old woman with a subperiosteal chondroma involving the proximal fibula. The lesion has intermediate signal on axial (**a**) PDWI, and high signal on axial (**b**) T2WI and axial (**c**) FS T2WI. The lesion shows lobulated peripheral Gd-contrast enhancement on axial (**d**) and sagittal (**e**) FS T1WI.

Figure **38 c–e** ▷

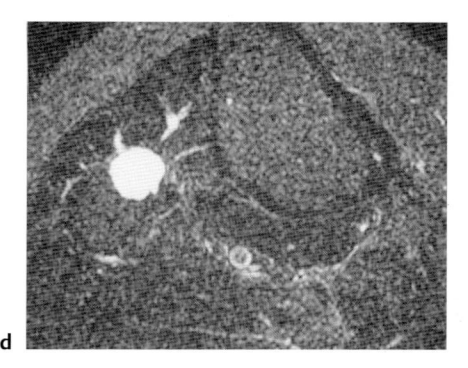

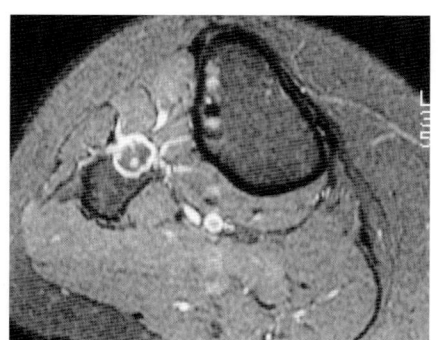

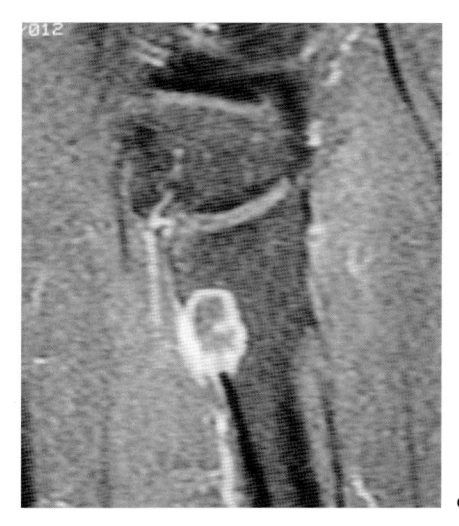

Figure 41 c–e

References

1. Brien EW, Mirra JM, Luck JV Jr. Benign and malignant cartilage tumors of bone and joint: their anatomic and theoretical basis with an emphasis on radiology, pathology and clinical biology. II. Juxtacortical cartilage tumors. *Skeletal Radiol* 1999;28:1–20.
2. Forest M. Chondroma. In: Forest M, Tomeno B, Vanel D, eds. *Orthopedic Surgical Pathology: Diagnosis of Tumors and Pseudotumoral Lesions of Bone and Joints.* Edinburgh: Churchill Livingstone; 1998: 200–201.
3. Huvos AG. Solitary and multiple osteochondromas and enchondromas; juxtacortical chondroma; Maffucci's disease. In: Huvos AG, ed. *Bone Tumors: Diagnosis, Treatment, and Prognosis* 2nd ed. Philadelphia, Pa: W.B. Saunders; 1991:276–279.
4. Lucas DR, Bridge JA. Chondromas: enchondroma, periosteal chondroma, and enchondromatosis. In: Fletcher CDM, Unni KK, Mertens F, eds. *World Health Organization Classification of Tumours. Pathology and Genetics of Tumours of Soft Tissue and Bone* Geneva: IARC Press; 2002:237–240.
5. Mulder JD, Schutte HE, Kroon HM, Taconis WK. Introduction. In: *Radiologic Atlas of Bone Tumors* Amsterdam: Elsevier; 1993:3–6.
6. Mulder JD, Schutte HE, Kroon HM, Taconis WK. The diagnosis of bone tumors. In: *Radiologic Atlas of Bone Tumors* Amsterdam: Elsevier; 1993:9–46.
7. Mulder JD, Schutte HE, Kroon HM, Taconis WK. Surface chondroma. In: *Radiologic Atlas of Bone Tumors* Amsterdam: Elsevier; 1993: 435–437.
8. Reid RP. Bone neoplasms and tumor-like lesions on the bone surface. In: Helliwell TR, ed. *Major Problems in Pathology: Pathology of Bone and Joint Neoplasms* Vol 37. 1st ed. Philadelphia, Pa: W.B. Saunders; 1999:230–231.
9. Robinson P, White LM, Sundaram M, et al. Periosteal chondroid tumors: radiologic evaluation with pathologic correlation. *AJR Am J Roentgenol* 2001;177:1183–1188.
10. Tillich M, Lindbichler F, Reittner P, Weybora W, Linhart W, Fotter R. Childhood periosteal chondroma: femoral neck thickening and remote hyperostosis as clues to plain film diagnosis. *Pediatr Radiol* 1998;28:899.
11. Unni KK. Introduction and scope of study. In: *Dahlin's Bone Tumors: General Aspects and Data in 11 087 Cases* 5th ed. Philadelphia, Pa: Lippincott, Williams & Wilkins; 1996:1–9.
12. Unni KK. Chondroma. In: *Dahlin's Bone Tumors: General Aspects and Data on 11 087 Cases* 5th ed. Philadelphia, Pa: Lippincott, Williams & Wilkins; 1996:25–45.
13. Woertler K, Blasius S, Brinkschmidt C, Hillmann A, Link TM, Heindel W. Periosteal chondroma: MR characteristics. *J Comput Assist Tomogr* 2001;25(3):425–430.

A 10 Chondromyxoid Fibroma

ICD-O Code
9241/0

Definition
Chondromyxoid fibromas are rare, benign, slow-growing bone lesions that contain chondroid, myxoid, and fibrous components.[4–6,11,18,20,26,27]

Frequency of Occurrence
Chondromyxoid fibromas represent 2 to 4% of primary benign bone lesions, and < 1% of primary bone lesions[16–18,25,26,27]

Age at Presentation
Most chondromyxoid fibromas occur between the ages of 1 and 40 years, median = 17 years, and peak incidence in the 2nd to 3rd decades.[16–18,25–27] Eighty percent of these tumors occur in patients less than 30 years old.[18] Tumors occasionally occur in older patients up to 79 years.[18]

Gender Ratio (M/F)
1/1 to 1.6/1 [16,17,25–27]

Location[4–6,11,17,18,20,26,27]
Chondromyxoid fibromas occur in the tibia > femur > pelvic bones > ankle and foot > fibula > ulna > ribs > humerus > skull > other bones, including vertebrae. In tubular bones, tumors occur most frequently in the metadiaphyseal and metaphyseal regions.[18]

Signs and Symptoms
Gradual onset of localized swelling and pain with or without restriction of movement; duration can be from 2 weeks to 10 years.[4–6,11,18,20,26,27]

Gross Pathologic Findings[4,6,11,18,20,26,27]
Lesions range in size from 1 to 13 cm, with an average of 3 cm. Chondromyxoid fibromas appear as lobulated, white to gray-white, firm and semitranslucent lesions with smooth surfaces and circumscribed borders. Erosion of the overlying bone is commonly seen.

Histopathologic Findings[4,6–8,10–15,18–22,26,27]
Chondromyxoid fibromas appear as a mixture of various proportions of myxoid, chondroid, and fibrous components with lobular patterns of growth. Scattered giant cells can be seen at the periphery of the lobules. Mitotic figures are uncommon. Small foci of calcification can be seen in a minority of lesions. Abrupt demarcation of the lesion with adjacent noninvolved bone is commonly seen.

Lesion Genetics
Abnormalities involving bands q13 and q25 of chromosome 6 have been reported.[20] Rearrangements involving chromosomes 2 and 5 have also been reported.[4] Chondromyxoid fibromas are associated with a unique genetic expression pattern composed of extensive diffuse hydrated proteoglycans, and focal regions of collagen types II, I, III, and VI.[20]

Findings on Plain Films (Roentgenograms) and Computed Tomography[1–4,6,9,11–15,18,19,21,22,24,26,27]
Chondromyoid fibromas are radiolucent, well-circumscribed lesions containing apparent "ridges" and "septa" with abrupt zones of transition (Figs. 42, 43). The apparent ridges and septa represent erosions and indentations on normal bone from the adjacent lesions. Tumors may have thin sclerotic margins, with or without peripheral thick reactive sclerotic margins. Expansion and thinning of overlying cortex is commonly seen, with or without periosteal reaction. Lesions are usually eccentric in long bones. In small bones, lesions often involve the full bone diameter. Matrix mineralization is uncommon (seen in 13% of lesions, best seen with CT).

Findings on Radionuclide Bone Scans
Lesions usually are associated with increased radiopharmaceutical accumulation.

MRI Findings[1–3,8–10,12–15,18,19,21–24,27]
Lesions are often slightly lobulated with low-intermediate signal on T1WI, intermediate signal on PDWI, and heterogeneous predominantly high signal on T2WI secondary to myxoid and hyaline chondroid components with high water content (Figs. 42, 43). MR signal heterogeneity on T2WI is related to the proportions of myxoid, chondroid, and fibrous components within the lesions. Thin, low signal septa within lesions on T2WI are secondary to fibrous strands. Lesions are surrounded by low signal borders representing thin sclerotic reaction. Edema is not typically seen in adjacent medullary bone. Lesions show prominent diffuse Gd-contrast enhancement.

Differential Diagnosis
Giant cell tumor, aneurysmal bone cyst, unicameral bone cyst, nonossifying fibroma / fibrous cortical defect, fibrous dysplasia, enchondroma, eosinophilic granuloma, chondroblastoma, desmoplastic fibroma.

Treatment and Prognosis
Standard treatment is block resection or curettage and bone grafting.[4,5,9,11,18,20,26] Recurrence is seen in 10–25% of cases.[6,20,26]

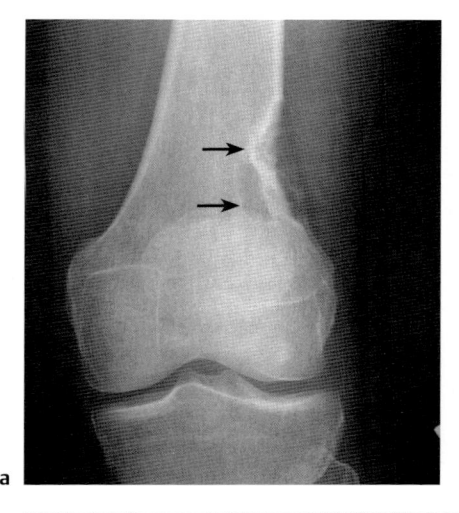

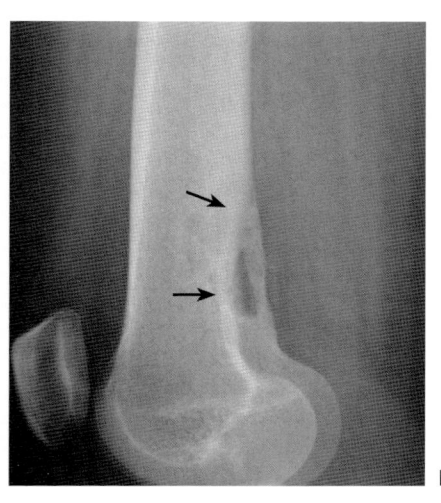

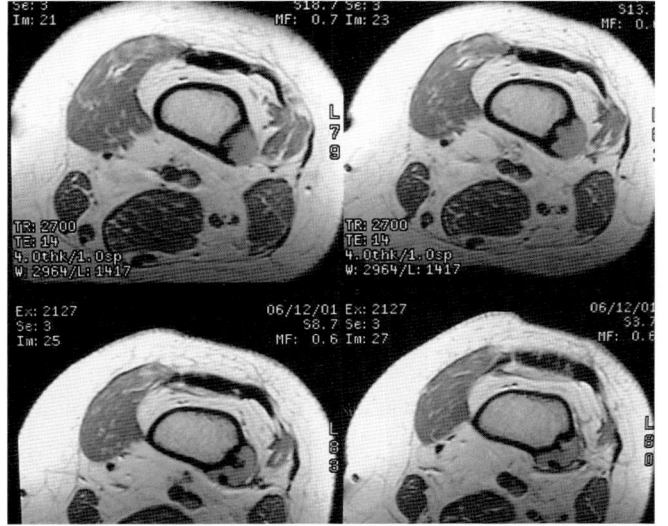

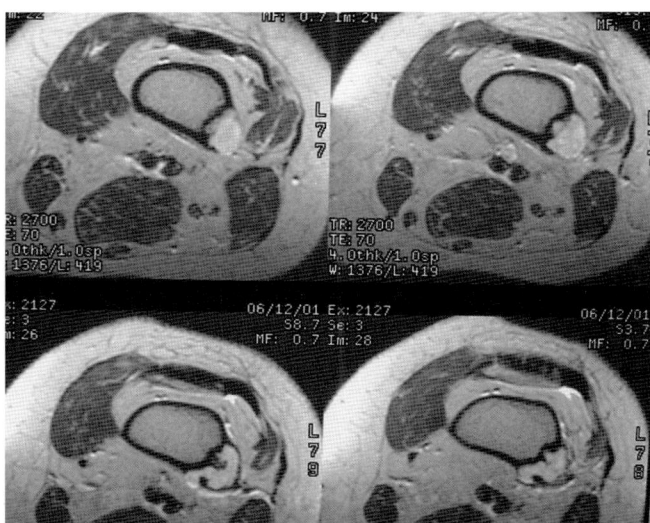

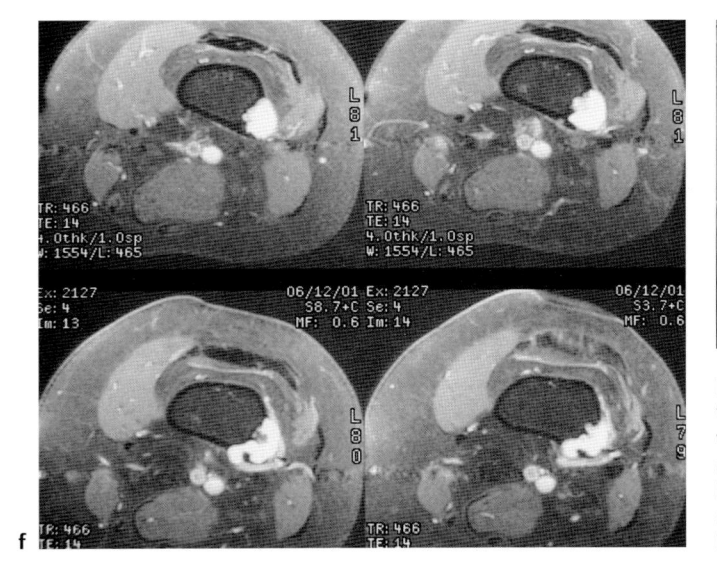

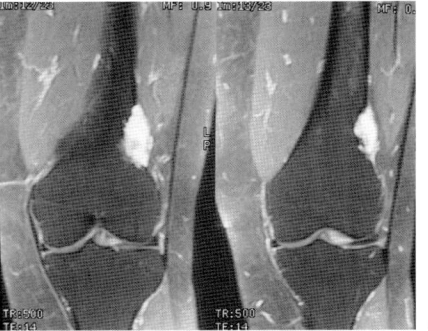

Figure **42 a–f** A 39-year-old woman with chondromyxoid fibroma in the distal femur. AP (**a**) and lateral (**b**) radiographs show a radiolucent, well-circumscribed, eccentric lesion in the femur with ridges associated with slight expansion and thinning of the overlying cortex. The lesion has intermediate signal on axial (**c**) PDWI, and high signal on axial (**d**) T2WI. The lesion shows prominent diffuse Gd-contrast enhancement on coronal (**e**) and axial (**f**) FS T1WI.

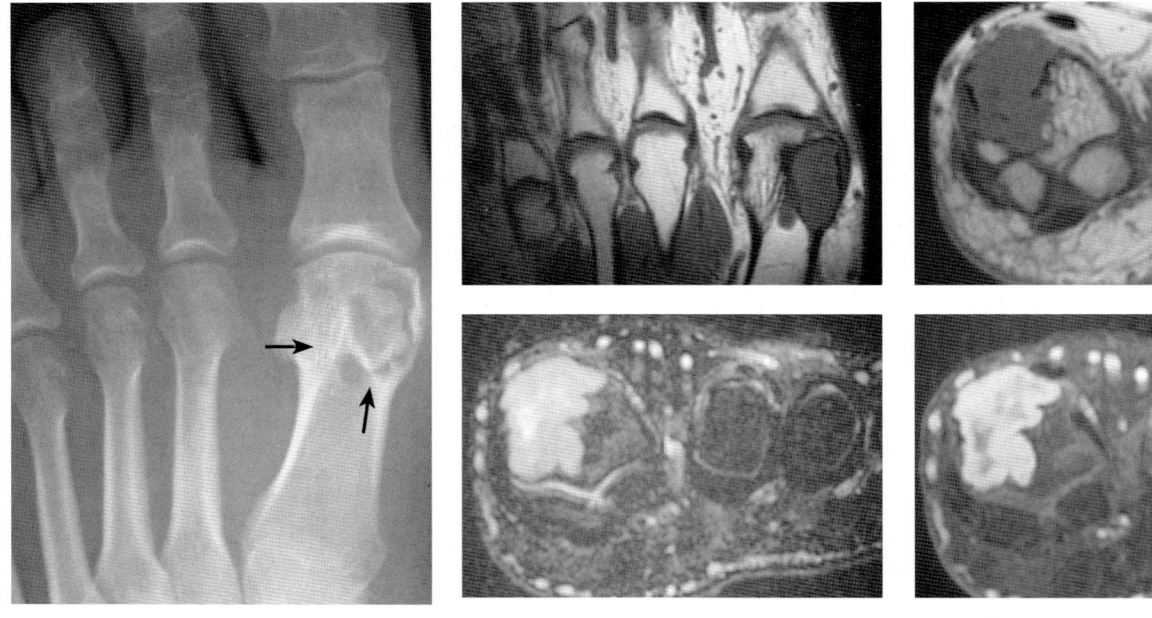

Figure **43 a–f** A 34-year-old man with chondromyxoid fibroma in the distal 1st metatarsal bone. AP radiograph (**a**) shows a radiolucent, well-circumscribed lesion in the metatarsal head with thin sclerotic margins associated with slight expansion and thinning of the overlying cortex. The lesion has low-intermediate signal on coronal (**b**) and axial (**c**) T1WI, and heterogeneous high signal on axial (**d**) FS T2WI. The lesion shows prominent diffuse Gd-contrast enhancement on axial (**e**) and coronal (**f**) FS T1WI.

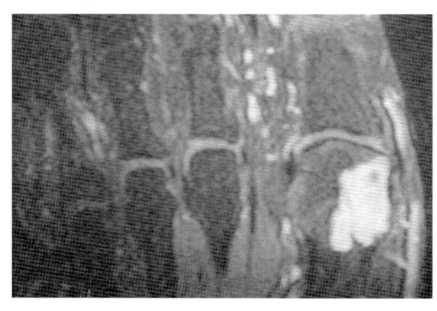

References

1. Adams MJ, Spencer GM, Totterman S, Hicks DG. Quiz: Case Report 776. *Skeletal Radiol* 1993;22:358–361.
2. Brat HG, Renton P, Sandison A, Cannon S. Chondromyxoid fibroma of the sacrum. *Eur Radiol* 1999;9:1800–1803.
3. Bruder E, Zanetti M, Boos N, von Hochstetter AR. Chondromyxoid fibroma of two thoracic vertebrae. *Skeletal Radiol* 1999;28:286–289.
4. Forest M. Chondromyxoid fibroma. In: Forest M, Tomeno B, Vanel D, eds. *Orthopedic Surgical Pathology: Diagnosis of Tumors and Pseudotumoral Lesions of Bone and Joints.* Edinburgh: Churchill Livingstone; 1998:223–231.
5. Helliwell TR. Central cartilaginous neoplasms of bone. In: Helliwell TR, ed. *Major Problems in Pathology: Pathology of Bone and Joint Neoplasms* Vol 37. 1st ed. Philadelphia, Pa: W.B. Saunders; 1999: 193–214.
6. Huvos AG. Chondromyxoid fibroma; myxoma of the facial skeleton; myxoma and fibromyxoma of extragnathic bones. In: Huvos AG, ed. *Bone Tumors Diagnosis, Treatment, and Prognosis* 2nd ed. 1991: 319–330.
7. Keel SB, Bhan AK, Liebsch NJ, Rosenberg AE. Chondromyxoid fibroma of the skull base: a tumor which may be confused with chordoma and chondrosarcoma: a report of three cases and review of the literature. *Am J Surg Pathol* 1997;21(5):577–582.
8. LeMay DR, Sun JK, Mendel E, Hinton DR, Giannotta SL. Chondromyxoid fibroma of the temporal bone. *Surg Neurol* 1997;48:148–152.
9. Lopez-Ben R, Siegal GP, Hadley MN. Chondromyxoid fibroma of the cervical spine: case report. *Neurosurgery* 2002;50(2):409–411.
10. Macdonald D, Fornasier V, Holtby R. Chondromyxoid fibroma of the acromium with soft tissue extension. *Skeletal Radiol* 2000;29: 168–170.
11. Mangham DC. Giant cell tumor of bone and giant cell-containing lesions of bone. In: Helliwell TR, ed. *Major Problems in Pathology: Pathology of Bone and Joint Neoplasms* Vol 37. 1st ed. Philadelphia, Pa: W.B. Saunders; 1999:304–329.
12. Marin C, Gallego C, Manjón P, Martinez-Tello FJ. Juxtacortical chondromyxoid fibroma: imaging findings in three cases and a review of the literature. *Skeletal Radiol* 1997;26:642–649.
13. Mehta S, Szklaruk J, Faria SC, Raymond AK, Whitman GJ. Chondromyxoid fibroma of the sacrum and iliac bone. *AJR Am J Roentgenol* 2006;186:467–469.
14. Mitchell M, Sartoris DJ, Resnick D. Case report 713. *Skeletal Radiol* 1992;21:252–255.
15. Mizuno K, Sasaki T, Prado G, et al. Chondromyxoid fibroma of the scapula associated with aneurysmal bone cyst. *Radiat Med* 1999; 17(5):383–387.
16. Mulder JD, Schutte HE, Kroon HM, Taconis WK. Introduction. In: *Radiologic Atlas of Bone Tumors* Amsterdam: Elsevier; 1993:3–6.
17. Mulder JD, Schutte HE, Kroon HM, Taconis WK. The diagnosis of bone tumors. In: *Radiologic Atlas of Bone Tumors.* Amsterdam: Elsevier; 1993:9–46.
18. Mulder JD, Schutte HE, Kroon HM, Taconis WK. Chondromyxoid fibroma. In: *Radiologic Atlas of Bone Tumors* Amsterdam: Elsevier; 1993:475–482.
19. O'Connor PJ, Gibbon WW, Hardy G, Butt WP. Chondromyxoid fibroma of the foot. *Skeletal Radiol* 1996;25:143–148.
20. Ostrowski ML, Spjut HJ, Bridge JA. Chondromyxoid fibroma. In: Fletcher CDM, Unni KK, Mertens F, eds. *World Health Organization Classification of Tumours. Pathology and Genetics of Tumours of Soft Ttissue and Bone* Geneva: IARC Press; 2002:243–245.
21. Park SH, Kong KY, Chung HW, Kim CJ, Lee SH, Kang HS. Juxtacortical chondromyxoid fibroma arising in an apophysis. *Skeletal Radiol* 2000;29:466–469.
22. Patino-Cordoba JI, Turner J, McCarthy SW, Fagan P. Chondromyxoid fibroma of the skull base. *Otolaryngol Head Neck Surg* 1998;118(3): 415–418.

23 Soler R, Rodríguez E, Suárez I, Gayol A. Magnetic resonance imaging of chondromyxoid fibroma of the fibula. *Eur J Radiol* 1994;18:210–211.
24 Tarhan NC, Yologlu Z, Tutar NU, Coskun M, Agildere AM, Arikan U. Chondromyxoid fibroma of the temporal bone: CT and MRI findings. *Eur Radiol* 2000;10:1678–1680.
25 Unni KK. Introduction and scope of study. In: *Dahlin's Bone Tumor: General Aspects and Data on 11 087 Cases* 5th ed. Philadelphia, Pa: Lippincott, Williams & Wilkins; 1996:1–9.
26 Unni KK. Chondromyxoid Fibroma. In: *Dahlin's Bone Tumors: General Aspects and Data on 11 087 Cases* 5th ed. Philadelphia, Pa: Lippincott, Williams & Wilkins; 1996:59–69.
27 Wu CT, Inwards CY, O'Laughlin S, Rock MG, Beabout JW, Unni KK. Chondromyxoid fibroma of bone: a clinicopathologic review of 278 cases. *Hum Pathol* 1998;29(5):438–446.

A 11 Chondrosarcoma

ICD-O Codes

Central, primary, and secondary: 9220/3

Peripheral: 9221/3

Dedifferentiated: 9243/3

Mesenchymal: 9240/3

Clear cell: 9242/3

Definition

Chondrosarcomas are malignant tumors containing cartilage formed within sarcomatous stroma. Chondrosarcomas can contain areas of calcification/mineralization, myxoid material, and/or ossification. Primary chondrosarcomas (62–86%) represent lesions occurring without pre-existent lesions, whereas secondary chondrosarcomas arise from formerly benign cartilaginous lesions (enchondroma, enchondromatosis / Ollier disease, Maffucci syndrome / multiple enchondromas [soft tissue hemangiomas], osteochondroma, multiple osteochondromas / exostoses, synovial chondromatosis), or other lesions (Paget disease, fibrous dysplasia, prior irradiation, repetitive trauma).[15,39] Periosteal chondrosarcomas are rare malignant cartilage tumors that occur on the surface of bone.[2,9,15] Chondrosarcomas rarely arise within synovium.[37]

Chondrosarcomas are also classified according to their (1) site of origin (osseous vs. extra-osseous); (2) locations in bone (central or intramedullary [75%] or peripheral or surface/cortical based [25%]); and (3) histology. There are five major histologic variants of chondrosarcomas: conventional, clear cell, dedifferentiated, mesenchymal, and myxoid.[1,2,8,9,15,23,25,27,29–31,33–35,39]

Frequency of Occurrence

Bone: Chondrosarcomas represent from 12 to 21% of malignant bone lesions, 21–26% of primary sarcomas of bone, 9–14% of all bone tumors, 6% of skull base tumors, and 0.15% of all intracranial tumors.[1,8,29,30,33,39] Chondrosarcomas are predominantly osseous lesions (96%), and rarely occur as primary extra-osseous tumors (4%)[15] or arise within synovium.[37]

Soft tissue: Chondrosarcomas represent 2.1% of malignant soft tissues, and < 1% of all soft tissue tumors.[19,20]

Age at Presentation

Bone: from 5 to 91 years, mean = 40 years, median = 26–59 years.[1,15,28–30,33,38]

Soft tissue: from 22 to 71 years, mean = 49 years.[20]

Gender Ratio (M/F)

Bone: 1.3 / 1 to 2 / 1.[8,15,29,30,33,38,39]

Soft tissue: 1.4 / 1.[20]

Location

Bone:
- For **conventional intra-osseous chondrosarcomas,** tumors occur in the femur > pelvic bones > humerus > ribs > tibia > craniofacial bones > sternum > scapula > vertebrae > feet > hands.[8,15,29,30,33,39] In long bones, chondrosarcomas involve the metaphysis (49%), diaphysis (36%), or epiphysis (15%).[31]
- **Peripheral chondrosarcoma** refers to a chondrosarcoma that arises from a cartilaginous exostosis or osteochondroma.[31] Common locations include the scapula, iliac bone, tibia, femur, pubic bone, and rib.[31]
- **Periosteal chondrosarcomas (juxtacortical chondrosarcomas)** have histologic features of a low-grade conventional chondrosarcoma, and occur on the surface of bones (distal femoral metadiaphysis > proximal humeral metadiaphysis > proximal femoral meta-diaphysis > iliac wing).[31,33,39,40]
- For **dedifferentiated chondrosarcomas**, common sites include pelvic bones, femur, and humerus.[28,39]
- The rare, **clear cell chondrosarcoma** usually involves the epiphyseal region of long bones, (proximal femur > proximal humerus > distal femur > proximal tibia > other sites.[4,9,33,39]
- For **mesenchymal chondrosarcomas**, common sites of involvement include: craniofacial bones, iliac bone, ribs, and vertebrae.[9,33,34]

Soft tissue: Tumors occur in the lower extremity > trunk > hip and buttocks > foot and ankle > upper extremity > proximal limb girdle > head and neck > hand and wrist > retroperitoneum.[20,23,26] Myxoid chondrosarcomas often occur in the deep subcutis or deeper soft tissues (80% are located in proximal extremities or limb girdles, and 20% involve the trunk).[26] Up to one-third of mesenchymal chondrosarcomas occur as primary tumors in the soft tissues.[9,33,34] Chondrosarcomas rarely arise within synovium.[37]

Signs and Symptoms

Bone: Chondrosarcomas can be painless or result in local pain, swelling, and tenderness; with or without pathologic fracture.[2,8,13,15,25,28,31,33,34,39]

Soft tissue: Extraskeletal chondrosarcomas often present as enlarging soft tissue masses which may be associated with pain and tenderness, as well as restricted range of motion for tumors near joints.[19,23]

Gross Pathologic
Findings[2,3,5, 6, 8,9,13,15,19,21,25,26,28,31,33–35,39]

Chondrosarcomas often appear as lobulated, pearly, bluish-white, translucent tumors, associated with areas of calcification/ossification and slimy mucoid material. Destructive changes are often seen in the involved bone. Clear cell chondrosarcomas are usually gray-red and soft, with or without cystic spaces, and can involve the epiphysis. Periosteal chondrosarcomas are typically large (> 5 cm) tumors covered by a fibrous layer, which is located on the surfaces of bones and usually appears as lobulated gray-white tissue with or without yellowish calcifications or ossifications.[2,9,15] For extraskeletal myxoid chondrosarcomas, tumors range in size from 1 to 25 cm, with a median size of 7 cm.[26]

Histopathologic Findings[3,5–9,13–15,19,25,26,28,31,33–35]

Histologic findings of chondrosarcoma need to be correlated with radiographic findings for appropriate diagnosis and treatment because of the discordance between biologic behavior and histologic features.

Conventional chondrosarcoma (70–75%).[1–3,8,15,33] Tumors contain multiple atypical chondrocytes which vary in size and often contain large hyperchromatic nuclei, as well as large cartilage cells with large single nuclei or multiple nuclei. Nuclear atypia is often mild to moderate. Tumor cells permeate and surround bony trabeculae in the marrow compartment. Hyaline cartilage is present in lesions as well as extracellular matrix, usually containing mucinous material and/or myxoid changes. Necrosis may be present in high-grade tumors. Mitotic figures are uncommon. Grade 1 lesions (27–61%) have moderate cytologic atypia and are hypercellular compared with enchondromas. Grade 2 chondrosarcomas (33–60%) are hypercellular relative to grade 1 lesions. Nuclei in grade 2 lesions are hyperchromatic and enlarged. Grade 3 (3–31%) chondrosarcomas are less common and have marked hypercellularity with bizarrely shaped nuclei. Conventional chondrosarcomas are typically intra-osseous tumors. Peripheral chondrosarcomas refer to chondrosarcomas that arise from osteochondromas, and usually have histologic features similar to a conventional intra-osseous chondrosarcoma.[31]

Clear cell chondrosarcoma (1–2%).[3,4,9,15,18,25,33,39] These tumors typically occur in patients older than 18 years after cessation of endochondral bone growth, age range 14–84 years, mean = 37 years, peaking in the 4th and 5th decades.[3,9,15,18,25,33,39] These tumors occur two to three times more frequently in males than females.[9,25] Tumor cells vary in appearance from immature chondroblasts to mature chondrocytes. Neoplastic cells have clear cytoplasm and centrally positioned nuclei with few mitotic figures. Multinucleated osteoclast-like giant cells may also be seen. Tumor matrix and/or zones having histology similar to conventional chondrosarcoma are often present. The cartilage may be calcified or ossified. Woven bone may form in the stroma. Clear cell chondrosarcomas are sometimes referred to as "malignant chondroblastoma." Clear cell chondrosarcomas are slow-growing neoplasms.

Dedifferentiated chondrosarcoma (6–11%).[1,3,9,28,33] This tumor type occurs as either primary and secondary chondrosarcomas, usually in patients ranging in age from 29 to 85 years, with the average between 50 and 60 years.[1,9,15,28] Male to female ratios of 1.5/1 to 2/1 have been reported.[9] Lesions have mixtures of high-grade spindle cells and low-grade or high-grade malignant cartilage cells.

Mesenchymal chondrosarcoma (2–10%).[1,3,5,6,33,34] Patients with these tumors range in age from 5 to 74 years, with peak occurrences in the 2nd and 3rd decades. Both genders are equally affected.[33,34] Tumors contain sheets of undifferentiated small cells with oval nuclei associated with an extracellular reticulin network. Small to large foci of cartilage are seen in the lesions, with or without reactive osteoid and bone formation. This type can also occur as extra-osseous tumors in soft tissues.

Myxoid chondrosarcoma (12%).[5–7,26,33] Patients with these tumors range in age from 6 to 89 years, median = 52 years, and mean = 49 years.[7,26,33] A male to female ratio of 2/1 has been reported[26,33] Lesions are considered low-grade tumors, and are also known as chordoid sarcoma. Tumors can contain abundant myxoid/mucoid stroma with strands and/or foci of cells with small hyperchromatic nuclei and moderate cytoplasm containing glycogen granules. In addition, relatively well-differentiated cartilage cells are usually seen. Areas of hemorrhage and cysts are often seen in extra-osseous tumors. Matrix mineralization/calcification is rarely seen. Typically, minimal or no mitotic activity is seen in tissue samples. These tumors often occur as extra-osseous tumors in the soft tissues of the extremities (thigh most common), and rarely in bone.[26] Extraskeletal myxoid chondrosarcomas are associated with a chromosomal translocation: t(9;22) (q22–31;q11–12).[14,33]

Periosteal chondrosarcoma (1–2%). These tumors are also referred to as juxtacortical chondrosarcomas. They are located on the surfaces of bones, are typically large (> 5 cm), and have histologic features similar to conventional chondrosarcomas[2,9,15,21,33,40]

Tumor Genetics

Chondrosarcomas have been reported to be associated with loss of chromosomes or chromosome segments including: 1 p36, 1 p13–22, 4, 5 q13–31, 6 q22-qter, 9 p22-pter, 10 p, 10 q24-qter, 11 p13-pter, 18 p, 18 q22-qter, and 22 q13.[2] Chromosomal gains have also been reported at 7 p13-pter, 12 q15-qter, 19, 20 pter-q11, and 21 q.[2] Deletions from chromosome 13 q have been shown to be associated with increased risk of metastatic disease.[2] Trisomy 22 has been detected in primary conventional chondrosarcomas.[2]

Findings on Plain Films (Roentgenograms) and Computed Tomography[2–4,8–13,15,17,18,25,28,31–34,36,39,40]

Central conventional chondrosarcoma. Tumors usually appear as areas of radiolucency involving medullary bone secondary to destruction, and endosteal scalloping. Areas of cortical bone destruction occur late and periosteal reaction is usually minimal. Cartilaginous matrix mineralization, variously described as "arcs," "rings," "punctate," "popcorn," "flocculent," "fluffy," and/or "cotton wool" configurations, is common. Margins of the tumor tend to become less well-defined with increasing grade of tumor. Tumors may be associated with expansion of bone (Figs. **44**, **46**, **47**, **49**, **52–54**).

Peripheral chondrosarcoma. These tumors are associated cartilaginous cap thicknesses of osteochondromas exceeding 2 cm, as well as erosive and/or destructive bony changes, soft tissue mass, chondroid mineralization, and/or thickening of cortex at sites of attachment to bone (Fig. **57**).

Periosteal chondrosarcoma.[21,33,40] These tumors vary in size from 5 to 11 cm. The bone cortex is either thinned or thickened but not destroyed. Lesions occasionally involve medullary bone. Juxtacortical soft tissue components of the lesion can have chondroid calcifications, with or without radial periosteal bone formation, and/or a thin peripheral rim of periosteal bone.

Figure **44 a–d** A 42-year-old woman with a chondrosarcoma involving the clivus. Axial CT image (**a**) shows the lesion to have prominent chondroid matrix mineralization. The lesion erodes the clivus and extends dorsally compressing the pons. The tumor has low-intermediate signal on axial (**b**) T1WI, and mostly high signal with foci of low signal on axial (**c**) T2WI. The tumor shows prominent heterogeneous Gd-contrast enhancement on axial (**c**) T1WI.

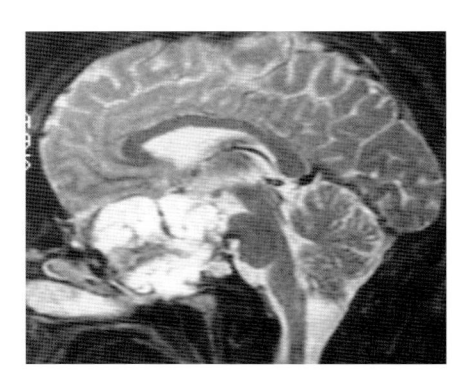

Figure **45** Chondrosarcoma involving the ethmoid and sphenoid paranasal sinuses with extension into the nasal cavity. The lesion has mostly high signal with bands of low signal on sagittal FS T2WI.

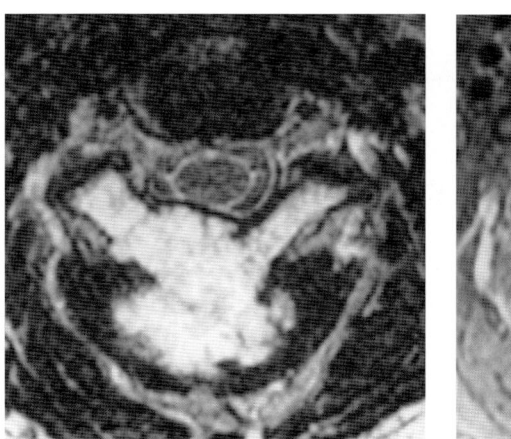

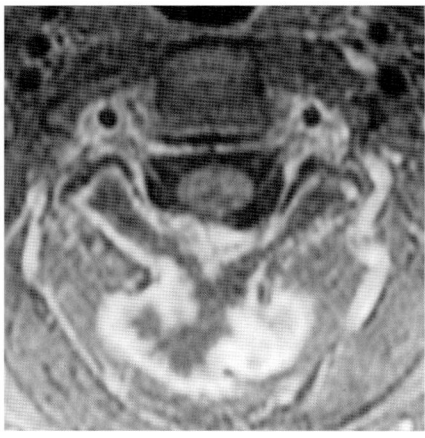

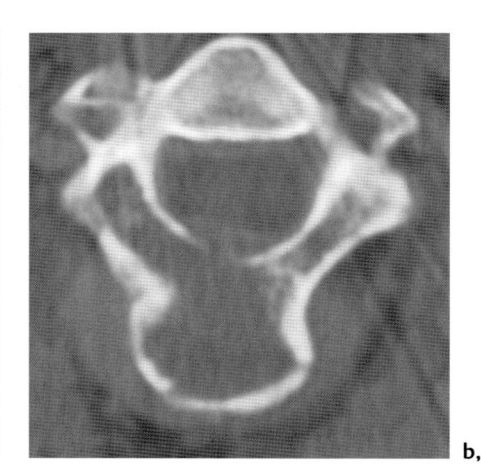

Figure **46 a–c** A 50-year-old man with chondrosarcoma involving the posterior elements of C 3. The tumor has high signal with thin bands of low signal on axial T2WI (**a**). The lesion shows irregular nodular and curvilinear patterns of Gd-contrast enhancement on axial FS T1WI (**b**). Axial CT image (**c**) shows a radiolucent expansile lesion involving the posterior elements.

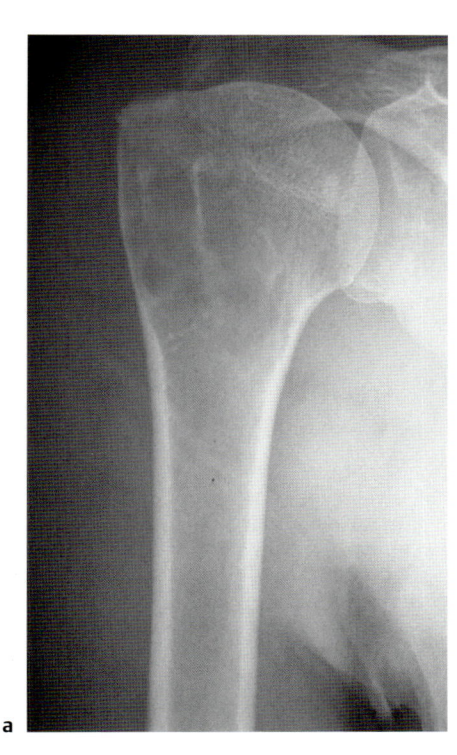

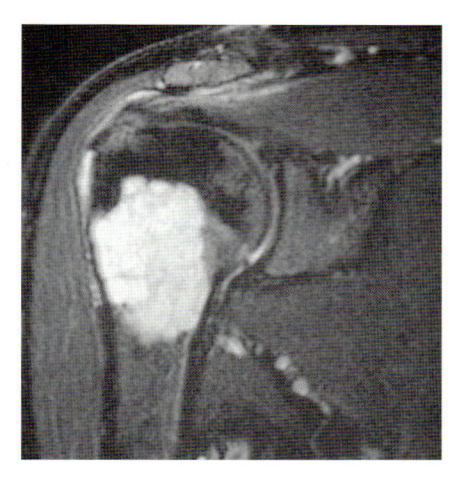

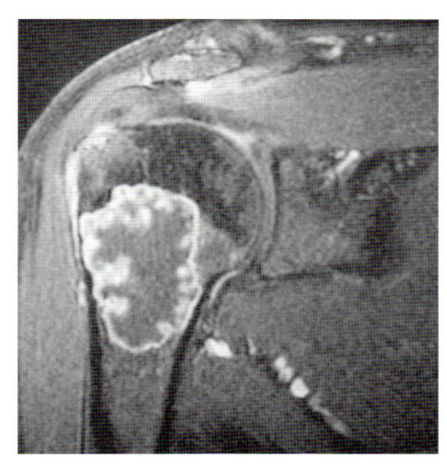

Figure **47 a–c**   A 45-year-old woman with a low-grade chondrosarcoma involving the proximal humerus. AP radiograph (**a**) shows a radiolucent lesion with chondroid matrix mineralization. The lesion has lobulated, circumscribed margins and contains high signal on coronal (**b**) FS T2WI. The lesion shows lobulated peripheral Gd-contrast enhancement on coronal (**c**) FS T1WI.

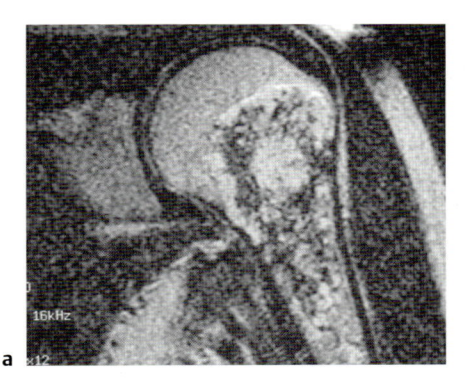

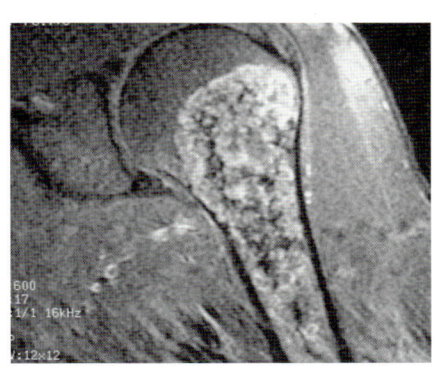

Figure **48 a, b**   A 55-year-old woman with a low-grade chondrosarcoma involving the proximal humerus. The lesion has lobulated, circumscribed and irregular margins, and contains low, intermediate, and high signal on coronal T2WI (**a**). The lesion shows heterogeneous diffuse Gd-contrast enhancement on coronal (**b**) FS T1WI.

Clear cell chondrosarcoma. Tumors appear as lytic lesions involving the epiphyseal regions/ends of long bone, and usually range from 3 to 7.5 cm, mean 5 cm. Lesions can also occur in or extend into metaphyseal or diaphyseal regions. Matrix mineralization is seen in 30% of cases. Lesions may have a sclerotic rim. Large lesions (>3 cm) often are associated with cortical destruction. Lesions are most commonly located in the proximal humerus or proximal femur. Lesions occur in patients who are typically older than those with chondroblastoma.

Dedifferentiated chondrosarcoma. These tumors usually appear as multifocal radiolucent zones in medullary bone with endosteal scalloping. Cartilaginous matrix mineralization is common. Areas of cortical bone destruction are commonly seen with extension into adjacent soft tissues (Fig. **54**).

Mesenchymal chondrosarcoma. These tumors are often large, predominantly lytic lesions with irregular borders. Minimal matrix mineralization is seen in 75%. These neoplasms can also occur as extra-osseous tumors.

Extra-osseous myxoid chondrosarcoma. These tumors appear as soft tissue masses, usually without matrix mineralization (Fig. **59**).

Findings on Radionuclide Bone Scans

Lesions are typically associated with increased radiopharmaceutical accumulation.

MRI Findings[2–4,10,11,13,16–19,21,26–28,31–34,36–40]

Conventional chondrosarcomas. Lesions range from 3 to 28 cm in size, mean = 8 cm. Lesions usually have low-intermediate signal on T1WI, intermediate signal on PDWI, and heterogeneous predominantly high signal on T2WI (Figs. **44–53**, **58**). Zones of low signal on T2WI are related to the presence and degree of matrix mineralization and/or fibrous tissue. Lesions often have lobulated margins, with or without internal septations. Peritumoral high signal on T2WI in marrow and periosteal soft tissues may be seen associated with chondrosarcomas, and typically not with enchondromas.[16] Chondrosarcomas usually show contrast-enhancement in patterns ranging from lobulated peripheral and/or septal, or homogeneous versus het-

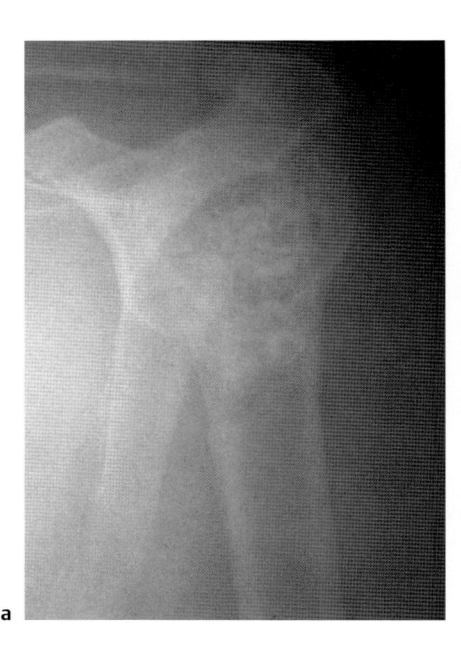

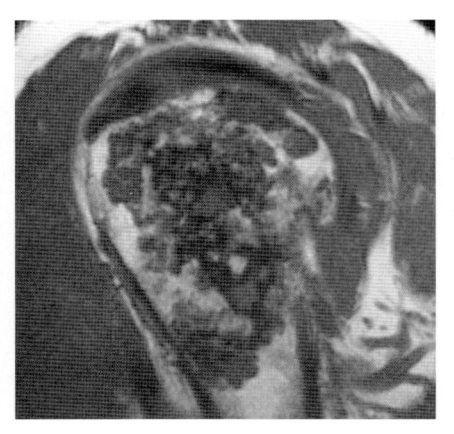

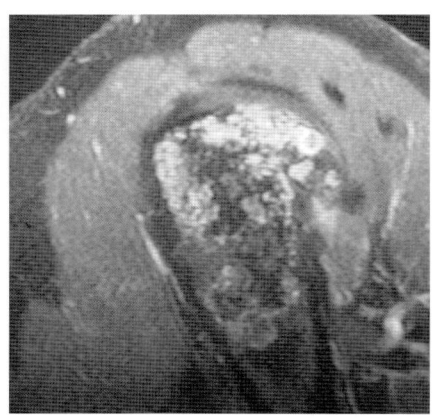

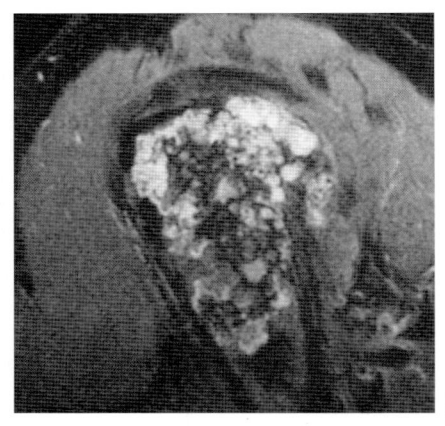

Figure **49 a–d** A 70-year-old man with a chondrosarcoma involving the proximal humerus. Oblique lateral radiograph (**a**) shows a lesion containing prominent chondroid matrix mineralization. The lesion has lobulated, circumscribed and irregular margins, and contains low-intermediate signal on sagittal (**b**) T1WI, and heterogeneous low, intermediate, and high signal on sagittal (**c**) FS-T2WI. The lesion shows heterogeneous diffuse Gd-contrast enhancement on sagittal (**d**) FS T1WI.

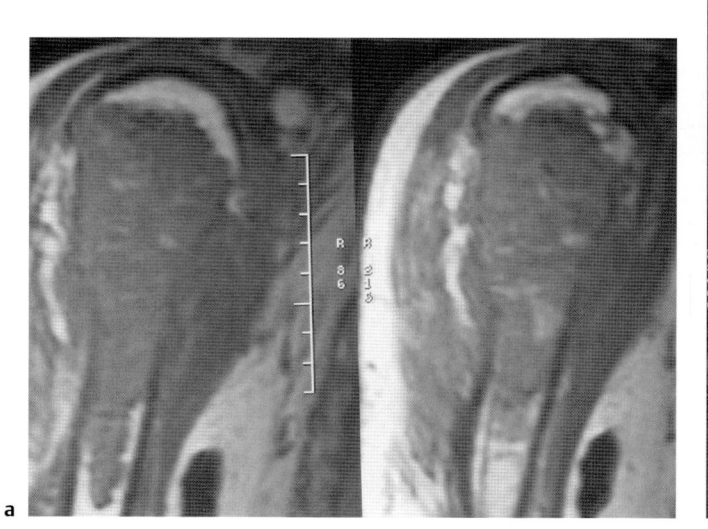

Figure **50 a, b** An 88-year-old man with a dedifferentiated chondrosarcoma involving the proximal humerus. The lesion has both lobulated circumscribed and irregular margins, and contains low-intermediate signal on sagittal (**a**) T1WI. The lesion shows prominent heterogeneous Gd-contrast enhancement on axial (**b**) FS T1WI which through the cortex. Sense unclear, something missing?

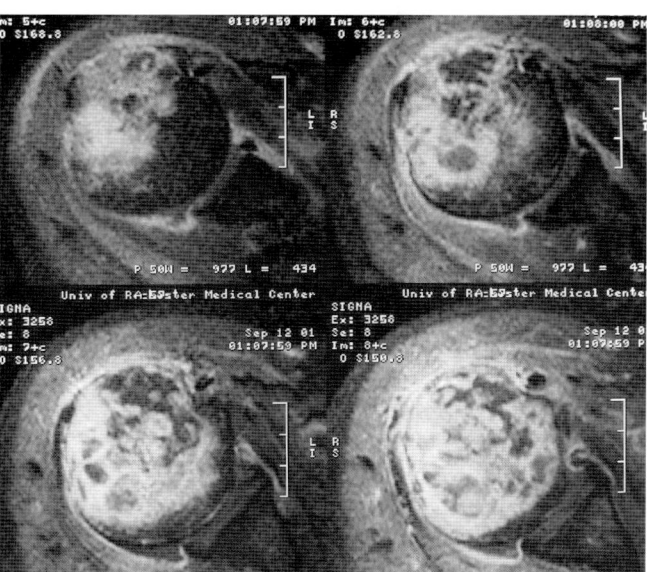

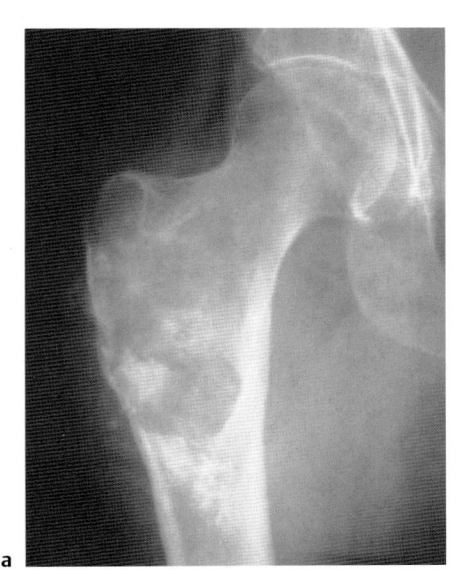

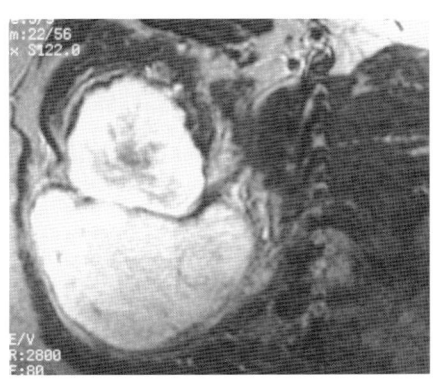

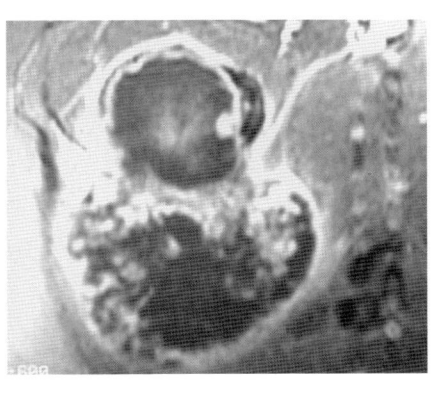

Figure **51 a–c** A 34-year-old man with a high-grade, myxoid chondrosarcoma involving the proximal femur, with cortical destruction and extra-osseous extension of tumor dorsally. AP radiograph (a) shows a radiolucent lesion containing mineralized chondroid matrix. The lesion has irregular circumscribed margins and contains high signal on axial (**b**) FS T2WI. The lesion shows lobulated irregular peripheral Gd-contrast enhancement on axial (**c**) FS T1WI.

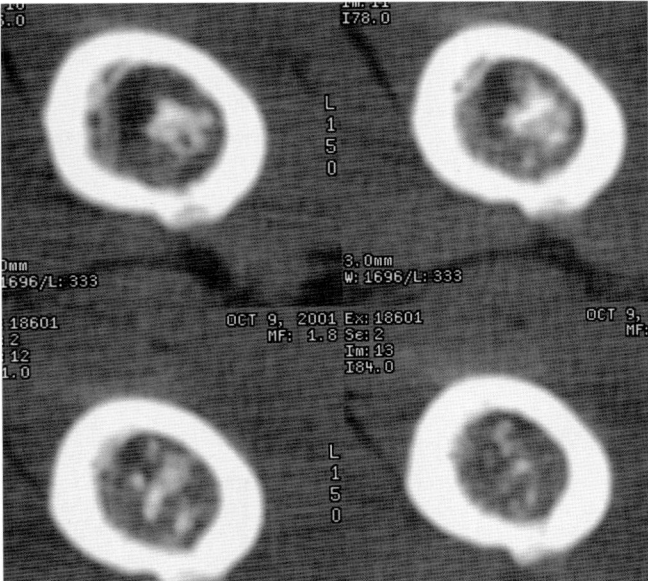

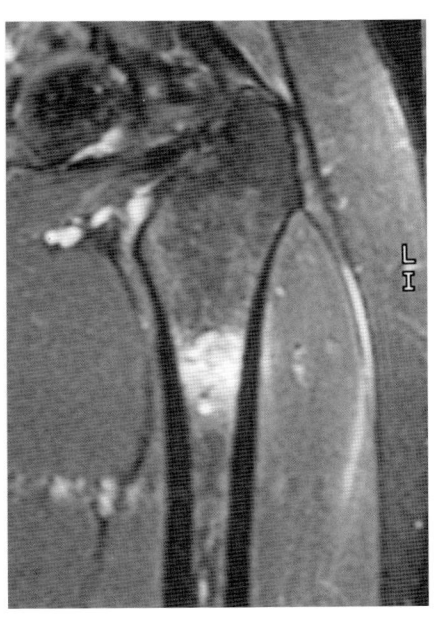

Figure **52 a, b** A 41-year-old man with a low-grade chondrosarcoma involving the proximal diaphysis of the femur. Axial CT images (a) show intramedullary chondroid matrix mineralization. The lesion has lobulated circumscribed margins and contains high signal on coronal (**b**) FS T2WI.

erogeneous depending on the degree of matrix mineralization and/or necrosis.[10,11,27] MRI can readily show sites of cortical destruction and extension of tumor into the adjacent soft tissues.

Peripheral chondrosarcomas. MRI can easily demonstrate the thickness of cartilaginous caps of osteochondromas, as well as erosive and/or destructive changes involving osteochondromas. Cartilage cap thickness exceeding 2 cm is commonly associated with malignant degeneration or dedifferentiation of osteochondromas into secondary chondrosarcomas. Lesions have low-intermediate signal on T1WI, intermediate signal on PDWI, and heterogeneous intermediate-high signal on T2WI (Figs. **56, 57**). Lesions show heterogeneous contrast enhancement, with or without Gd-contrast enhancement of adjacent soft tissues, suggesting tumor invasion.

Periosteal chondrosarcomas.[21,33,40] These tumors vary in size from 4 to 11 cm. The bone cortex is either thinned or thickened but not destroyed. Lesions occasionally involve medullary bone. Juxtacortical soft tissue components of the lesion can have chondroid calcifications, with or without radial periosteal bone formation, and/or a thin peripheral rim of periosteal bone. Lesions have low-intermediate signal on T1WI, intermediate signal on PDWI, and heterogeneous intermediate-high signal on T2WI (Fig. **55**). Lesions show heterogeneous contrast enhancement. Gd-contrast enhancement of adjacent soft tissues may be seen from tumor invasion.

Clear cell chondrosarcomas.[4,18,33] Lesions usually are seen near the ends of long bones, with or without extension into metaphyseal and diaphyseal regions. Smaller lesions may be well circumscribed; larger lesions may have associated cortical disruption and extension into adjacent soft tissues. Lesions typically have low-intermediate signal on T1WI and heterogeneous intermediate-high signal on T2WI. Lesions usually show prominent Gd-contrast enhancement.

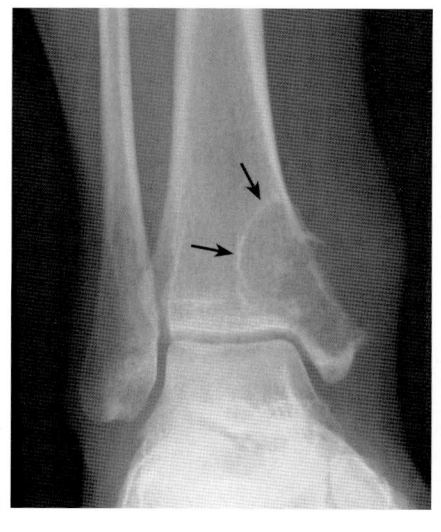

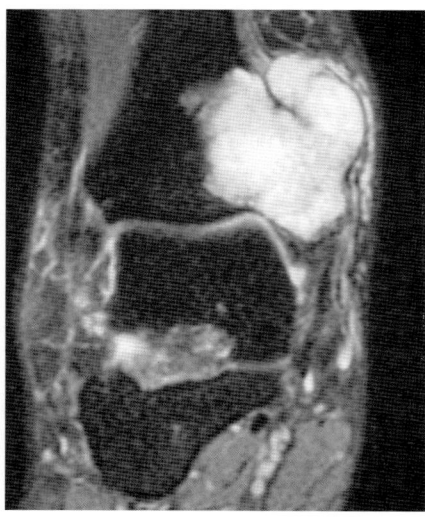

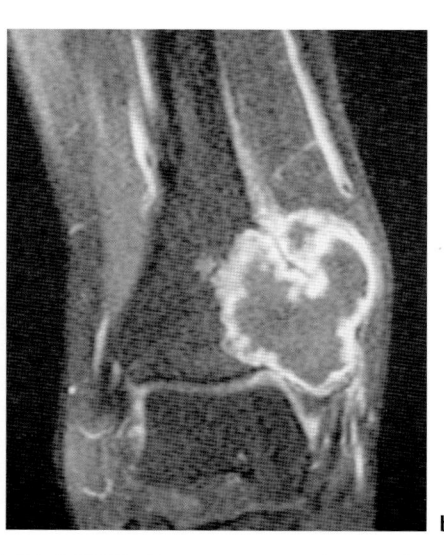

Figure **53 a–c** A 44-year-old woman with a grade 2 chondrosarcoma involving the distal tibia. AP radiograph (**a**) shows a radiolucent intramedullary lesion with erosion and destruction of cortical bone. The tumor has lobulated, circumscribed margins and contains mostly high signal on coronal (**b**) FS T2WI. The tumor extends into the adjacent soft tissues through a zone of cortical destruction. The tumor shows irregular peripheral lobular Gd-contrast enhancement on coronal (**c**) FS T1WI.

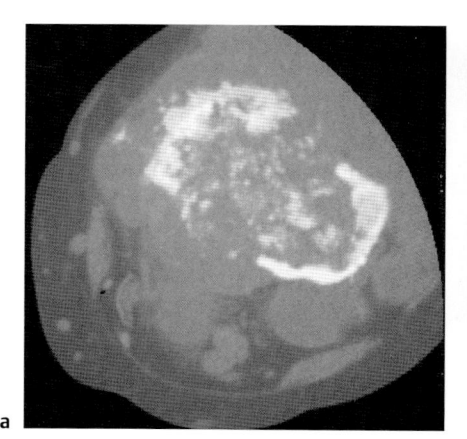

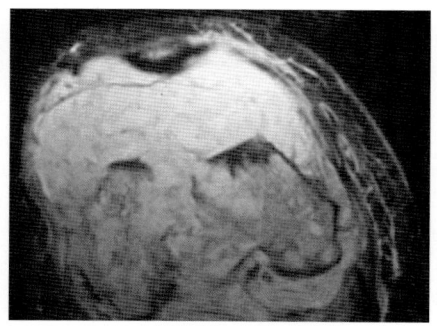

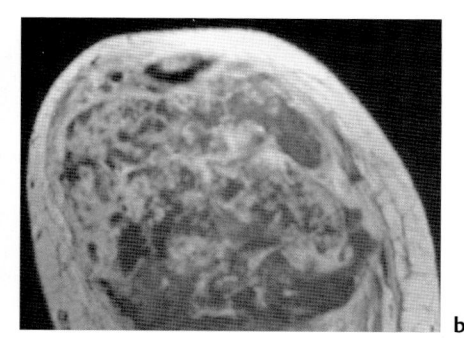

Figure **54 a–c** A 60-year-old woman with a dedifferentiated chondrosarcoma involving the distal femur. Axial CT image (**a**) shows a radiolucent lesion with chondroid matrix mineralization and associated zones of cortical destruction. The tumor has heterogeneous high signal on axial (**b**) FS T2WI. Extensive cortical destruction is seen with tumor extension from the marrow into the knee joint and adjacent soft tissues. The lesion shows irregular heterogeneous Gd-contrast enhancement on axial (**c**) T1WI.

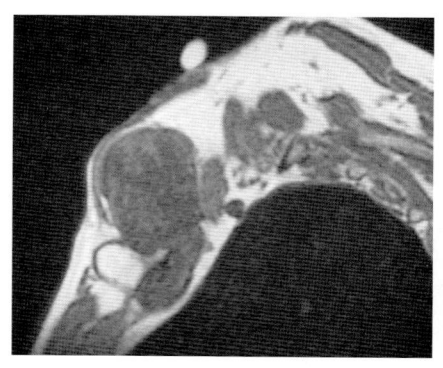

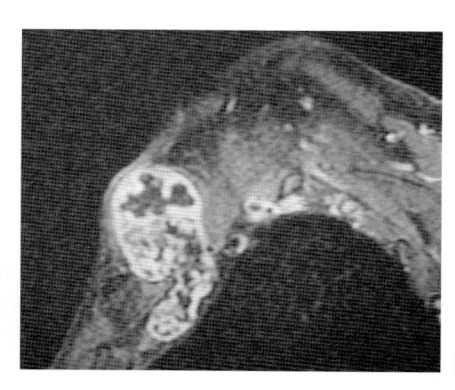

Figure **55** A 40-year-old man with a low-grade, perisoteal chondrosarcoma along the cortical surface of the clavicle. The lesion has circumscribed margins and contains intermediate signal on sagittal (**a**) T1WI, and shows irregular peripheral and central lobular Gd-contrast enhancement on axial sagittal (**b**) FS T1WI.

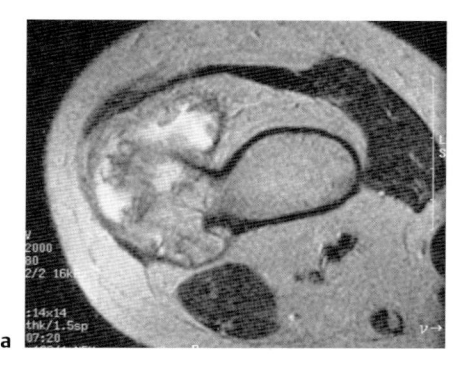

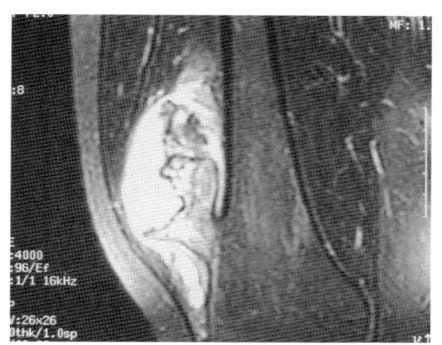

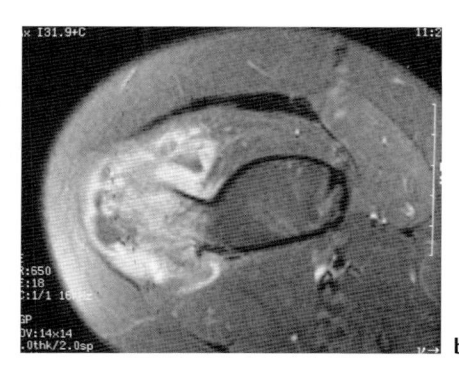

Figure **56 a–c**   An 18-year-old woman with a secondary low-grade chondrosarcoma arising from an osteochondroma at the distal femur. The thickened cartilaginous cap of the tumor has irregular circumscribed margins and contains heterogeneous slightly high and high signal with small foci of low signal on axial (**a**) T2WI, and high signal on coronal (**b**) FS T2W1. Zones of cortical destruction are seen at the osteochondroma adjacent to the malignant cartilaginous cap. The lesion shows irregular heterogeneous Gd-contrast enhancement on axial (**c**) FS T1WI.

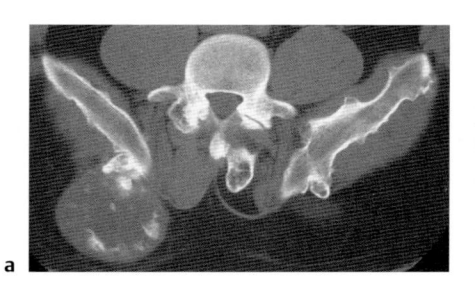

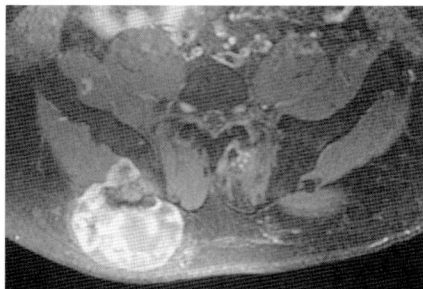

Figure **57 a, b**   A 30-year-old man who has multiple hereditary exostoses (osteochondromas) and a secondary low-grade chondrosarcoma arising from an osteochondroma at the posterior right iliac bone. Axial CT image (**a**) shows the tumor to have soft tissue attenuation as well as foci of chondroid mineralization. The thickened cartilaginous cap of the tumor has circumscribed margins and shows irregular heterogeneous Gd-contrast enhancement on axial (**b**) FS T1WI.

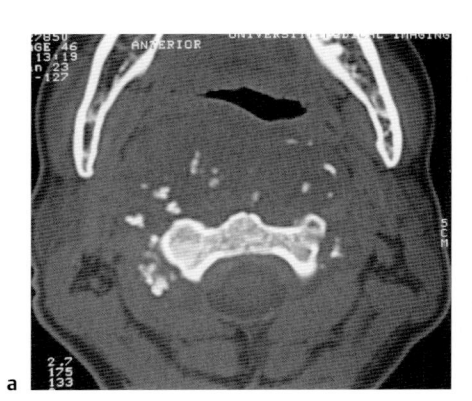

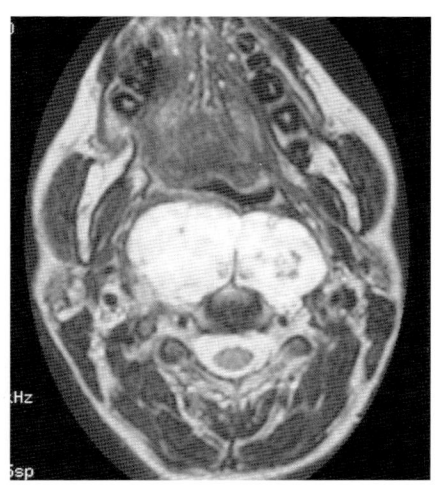

Figure **58**   A 44-year-old woman with a well-differentiated extra-osseous chondrosarcoma located ventral to the cervical spine. Axial CT image (**a**) shows the tumor to have soft tissue attenuation as well as foci of chondroid mineralization. The tumor has circumscribed margins and contains mostly high signal on axial T2WI (**b**) as well as small zones of low signal.

Dedifferentiated chondrosarcomas.[28,33] Lesions usually have low-intermediate signal on T1WI and PDWI, and heterogeneous predominantly high signal on T2WI (Figs. **50, 54**). Zones of low signal on T2WI are related to the presence and degree of matrix mineralization and/or fibrous tissue. Lesions often have irregular poorly-defined margins and associated cortical destruction. Lesions usually show heterogeneous contrast enhancement. MRI can readily show sites of extension of the lesion into the adjacent soft tissues.

Mesenchymal chondrosarcomas.[17,28,33,36] Tumors are usually destructive lesions commonly associated with extra-osseous soft tissue masses. Lesions have low-intermediate signal on T1WI, intermediate signal on PDWI, and heterogeneous intermediate-high or slightly high signal on T2WI. Foci of low signal on T1WI and T2WI can be seen secondary to chondroid matrix mineralization. Lesions typically show heterogeneous Gd-contrast enhancement.[36] Mesenchymal chondrosarcomas can arise in soft tissues (Fig. **60**) or bone.[36]

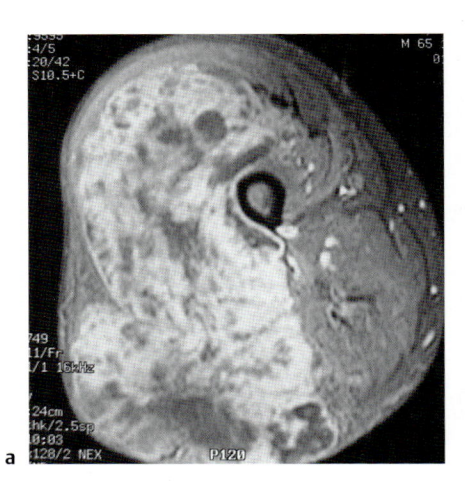

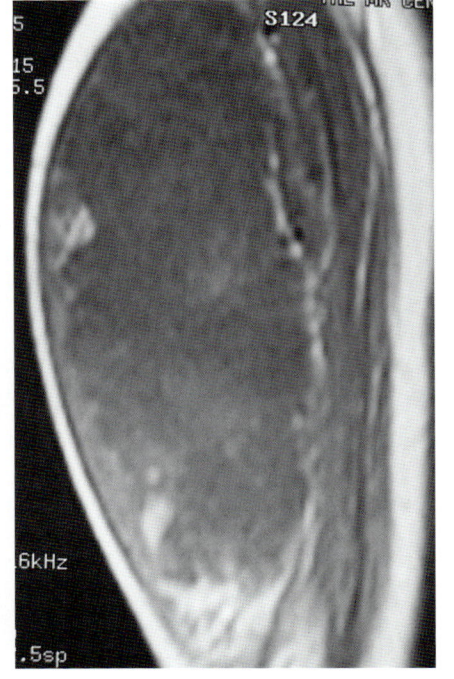

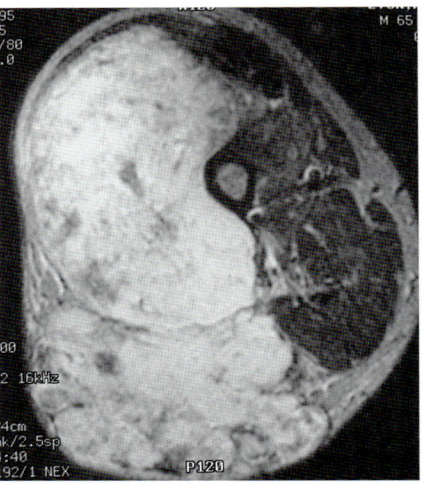

Figure **59 a, b** A 65-year-old man with an extra-osseous myxoid chondrosarcoma in the distal thigh. The lesion has circumscribed margins and contains heterogeneous mostly high signal with small foci of low signal on axial (**a**) T2WI. The lesion shows prominent irregular heterogeneous Gd-contrast enhancement on axial (**b**) FS T1WI.

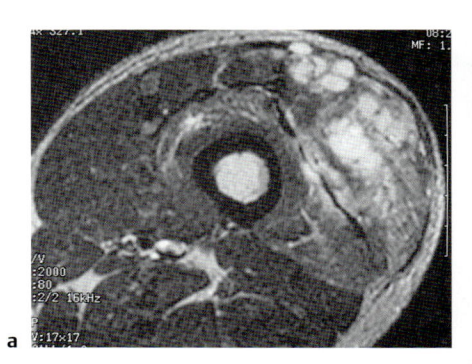

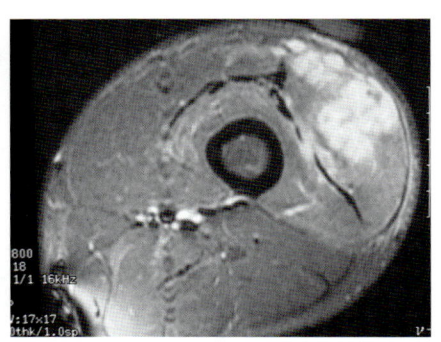

Figure **60 a, b** An 18-year-old man with an extra-osseous mesenchymal chondrosarcoma involving the vastus lateralis and adjacent soft tissues in the distal thigh. The tumor has poorly defined margins and has heterogeneous mostly high signal on axial T2WI (**a**). The lesion shows prominent irregular Gd-contrast enhancement on axial FS T1WI (**b**).

Myxoid chondrosarcomas.[19,33] These tumors can occur in bone (Fig. **51**) or arise in soft tissues (Fig. **59**). In soft tissues, tumors often have lobulated margins and range in size from 4 to 7 cm. Lesions usually have low-intermediate signal on T1WI and PDWI, and predominantly high signal on T2WI. Hemorrhagic foci in myxoid chondrosarcomas can show intermediate to high signal on T1WI and T2WI. Myxoid chondrosarcomas show heterogeneous contrast enhancement.

Differential Diagnosis

Enchondroma, fracture callus, fibrous dysplasia, chondroblastoma, chondromyxoid fibroma, chondroblastic osteosarcoma, osteoblastoma, bone infarct, chordoma. The distinction between an enlarging symptomatic enchondroma and a low-grade chondrosarcoma can be difficult based on imaging features.

Treatment and Prognosis

Conventional chondrosarcomas.[1,3,8,13,33] Treatment often consists of en-bloc surgical resection, with or without limb salvage procedures in long bones.[1,3,8,38] These tumors are usually resistant to radiation.[8] Fractionated proton beam radiation has also been used.[1] The prognosis for grade 1 and 2 lesions is related to the extent of resection. The 5-year survival rates for grade 1 tumors range from 71 to 94%, 40 to 75% for grade 2 tumors, and 15 to 44% for grade 3 tumors.[1,2,8,33] Local recurrence usually occurs within 3 years after surgery.[1] Metastatic risk is high for grade 3 lesions with rates of 75–85% at 5 years.[8]

Peripheral chondrosarcomas. These tumors are treated with en bloc resection.[31] The 5-year survival rate ranges from 80 to 90%.[31]

Periosteal chondrosarcomas. Treatment typically consists of wide resection.[9,31,33] These tumors are usually well-differentiated chondrosarcomas and often have a favorable prognosis.[9,31]

Clear cell chondrosarcomas. These tumors are considered a low-grade malignancy.[4,9,13,31,33] Treatment is en bloc or wide resection, which is associated with a 16% recurrence rate and 8% mortality.[4,9,31,33] A 5-year survival rate of 92% has been reported.[9] Local recurrence may occur up to 15 years after initial surgery.[38] Metastases occur in 15–25% of patients and are commonly located in the lungs, brain, and bone.[9,13,33]

Dedifferentiated chondrosarcomas. These are aggressive malignant neoplasms with 5-year survival of 8 to 13%, median survival of 6 months.[1,2,9,13,38] Metastases are common and are often located in the lungs, bones, and visceral organs.[9,13] Standard treatment is radical resection, followed by radiation and chemotherapy.[9,13]

Mesenchymal chondrosarcomas. These tumors are aggressive sarcomas with 5-year survival rates between 40 and 60% and 10-year survival rates of 25–30%.[1,9,19,33] A mean survival rate of 38 months has been reported.[15,17] Metastases occur in 60% of cases, and occur most frequently in lung, lymph nodes, and bone.[1] Treatment usually consists of wide surgical excision.[6,9,17,33]

Myxoid chondrosarcomas. The 5-year survival rate is 90%, and the 10-year survival rate ranges from 45 to 78%.[19,26,33] Metastases occur in 46% of patients.[26] Histologic grading is not reliable for prognosis.[26] Treatment usually consists of wide surgical excision.[6,33] Radiation and chemotherapy have not been effective to date.[6]

References

1. Barnes L. Pathobiology of selected tumors of the base of the skull. *Skull Base Surg* 1991;1:207–216.
2. Bertoni F, Bacchini P, Hogendoorn PCW. Chondrosarcoma. In: Fletcher CDM, Unni KK, Mertens F, eds. *World Health Organization Classification of Tumours. Pathology and Genetics of Tumours of Soft Tissue and Bone* Geneva: IARC Press; 2002:247–251.
3. Brien EW, Mirra JM, Kerr R. Benign and malignant cartilage tumors of bone and joint: their anatomic and theoretical basis with an emphasis on radiology, pathology and clinical biology. *Skeletal Radiol* 1997;26:325–353.
4. Cannon CP, Nelson SD, Seeger SD, Eckardt JJ. Clear cell chondrosarcoma mimicking chondroblastoma in a skeletally immature patient. *Skeletal Radiol* 2002;31:369–372.
5. Das Gupta TK, Chaudhuri PK. Pathology of soft tissue sarcoma. In: Das Gupta TK, Chaudhuri PK, eds. *Tumors of the Soft Tissues* 2nd ed. New York, NY: Appleton and Lange; 1998:63–200.
6. Das Gupta TK, Chaudhuri PK. Heterotopic bone and cartilage. In: Das Gupta TK, Chaudhuri PK, eds. *Tumors of the Soft Tissues* 2nd ed. New York, NY: Appleton and Lange; 1998:465–469.
7. Dei Tos AP, Wadden C, Fletcher Christopher DM. Extraskeletal myxoid chondrosarcoma: an immunohistochemical reappraisal of 39 cases. *Appl Immunohistochem Mol Morphol* 1997;5(2):73–77.
8. Forest M. Chondrosarcoma. In: Forest M, Tomeno B, Vanel D, eds. *Orthopedic Surgical Pathology: Diagnosis of Tumors and Pseudotumoral Lesions of Bone and Joints* Edinburgh: Churchill Livingstone; 1998:233–256.
9. Forest M. Chondrosarcoma: variants. In: Forest M, Tomeno B, Vanel D, eds. *Orthopedic Surgical Pathology: Diagnosis of Tumors and Pseudotumoral Lesions of Bone and Joints.* Edinburgh: Churchill Livingstone; 1998:261–288.
10. Geirnaerdt MJ, Hogendoorn PC, Bloem JL, Taminiau AH, van der Woude HJ. Cartilaginous tumors: fast contrast-enhanced MR imaging. *Radiology* 2000;214(2):539–546.
11. Hanna SL, Magill HL, Parham DM, Bowman LC, Fletcher BD. Childhood chondrosarcoma: MR imaging with gadolinium-DTPA. *Magn Reson Imaging* 1990;8(5):669–672.
12. Hassounah M, Al-Mefty O, Akhtar M, Jinkins JR, Fox JL. Primary cranial and intracranial chondrosarcoma—a survey. *Acta Neurochir (Wien)* 1985;78:123–132
13. Helliwell TR. Central cartilaginous neoplasms of bone. In: Helliwell TR, ed. *Major Problems in Pathology: Pathology of Bone and Joint Neoplasms.* Vol 37. 1st ed. Philadelphia, Pa: W.B. Saunders 1999: 193–214.
14. Hieken TJ, Levine EA. Molecular biology of soft tissue tumors. In: Das Gupta TK, Chaudhuri PK, eds. *Tumors of the Soft Tissues.* 2nd ed. New York, NY: Appleton and Lange; 1998:201–225.
15. Huvos AG. Chondrosarcoma including spindle-cell (dedifferentiated) and myxoid chondrosarcoma; mesenchymal chondrosarcoma. In: Huvos AG, ed. *Bone Tumors: Diagnosis, Treatment, and Prognosis* 2nd ed. Philadelphia, Pa: W.B. Saunders; 1991:343–362.
16. Janzen L, Logan PM, O'Connell JX, Connell DG, Munk PL. Intramedullary chondroid tumors of bone: correlation of abnormal peritumoral marrow and soft-tissue MRI signal with tumor type. *Skeletal Radiol* 1997;26:100–106.
17. Johnson DBS, Breidahl W, Newman JS, Devaney K, Yahanda A. Extraskeletal mesenchymal chondrosarcoma of the rectus sheath. *Skeletal Radiol* 1997;26:501–504.
18. Kaim AH, Hugli R, Borel HM, Jundt G. Chondroblastoma and clear cell chondrosarcoma: radiological and MRI characteristics with histopathologic correlation. *Skeletal Radiol* 2002;31:88–95.
19. Kransdorf MJ, Murphey MD. Extraskeletal osseous and cartilaginous tumors. In: *Imaging of Soft Tissue Tumors* 2nd ed. Philadelphia, Pa: W. B. Saunders; 2006:437–480.
20. Kransdorf MJ. Malignant soft-tissue tumors in a large referral population: distribution of diagnoses by age, sex, and location. *AJR Am J Roentgenol* 1995;164:129–134.
21. Kumta SM, Griffith JF, Chow Louis TC, Leung PC. Primary juxtacortical chondrosarcoma dedifferentiating after 20 years. *Skeletal Radiol* 1998;27:569–573.
22. Lee YY, Van Tassel P. Craniofacial chondrosarcomas: imaging findings in 15 untreated cases. *AJNR Am J Neuroradiol* 1989;10:165–170.
23. Lucas DR, Heim S. Extraskeletal myxoid chondrosarcoma. In: Fletcher CDM, Unni KK, Mertens F, eds. *World Health Organization Classification of Tumours. Pathology and Genetics of Tumours of Soft Tissue and Bone* Geneva: IARC Press; 2002:213–215.
24. Mack MG, Vogl TJ. MR-guided ablation of head and neck tumors. *Magn Reson Imaging Clin N Am* 2002;10(4):707–713.
25. McCarthy EF, Freemont A, Hogendoorn PCW. Clear cell chondrosarcoma. In: Fletcher CDM, Unni KK, Mertens F, eds. *World Health Organization Classification of Ttumours. Pathology and Genetics of Tumours of Soft Tissue and Bone* Geneva: IARC Press; 2002:257–258.
26. Meis-Kindblom JM, Bergh P, Gunterberg B, Kindblom LG. Extraskeletal myxoid chondrosarcoma: a reappraisal of its morphologic spectrum and prognostic factors based on 117 cases. *Am J Surg Pathol* 1999;23(6):636–650.
27. Meyers SP, Hirsch WL Jr, Curtin HD, Barnes L, Sekhar LN, Sen C. Chondrosarcomas of the skull base: MR imaging features. *Radiology* 1992;184(1):103–108.
28. Milchgrub S, Hogendoorn PCW. Dedifferentiated chondrosarcoma. In: Fletcher CDM, Unni KK, Mertens F, eds. *World Health Organization Classification of Tumours. Pathology and Genetics of Tumours of Soft Tissue and Bone* Geneva: IARC Press; 2002:252–254.
29. Mulder JD, Schutte HE, Kroon HM, Taconis WK. Introduction. In: *Radiologic Atlas of Bone Tumors* Amsterdam: Elsevier; 1993:3–6.
30. Mulder JD, Schutte HE, Kroon HM, Taconis WK. The diagnosis of bone tumors. In: *Radiologic Atlas of Bone Tumors* Amsterdam: Elsevier; 1993:9–46.
31. Mulder JD, Schutte HE, Kroon HM, Taconis WK. Chondrosarcoma. In: *Radiologic Atlas of Bone Tumors* Amsterdam: Elsevier; 1993:139–191.
32. Murphey MD, Flemming DJ, Boyea SR, Bojescul JA, Sweet DE, Temple HT. From the archives of the AFIP. Enchondroma versus chondrosarcoma of the appendicular skeleton: differentiating features. *Radiographics* 1998;18:1213–1237.
33. Murphey MD, Walker EA, Wilson AJ, Kransdorf MJ, Temple HT, Gannon FH. From the archives of the AFIP. Imaging of primary chondrosarcoma: radiologic-pathologic correlation. *Radiographics* 2003;23:1245–1278.

34 Nakashima Y, Park YK, Sugano O. Mesenchymal chondrosarcoma. In: Fletcher CDM, Unni KK, Mertens F, eds. *World Health Organization Classification of Tumours. Pathology and Genetics of Tumours of Soft Tissue and Bone* Geneva: IARC Press; 2002:255–256.

35 Salisbury JR. Bone neoplasms containing epithelial and epithelioid cells. In: Helliwell TR, ed. *Major Problems in Pathology: Pathology of Bone and Joint Neoplasms* Vol 37. 1st ed. Philadelphia, Pa: W.B. Saunders; 1999:359–360.

36 Shinaver CN, Mafee MF, Choi KH. MRI of mesenchymal chondrosarcoma of the orbit: case report and review of the literature. *Neuroradiology* 1997;39:296–301.

37 Taconis WK, van der Heul RO, Taminiau AMM. Synovial chondrosarcoma: report of a case and review of the literature. *Skeletal Radiol* 1997;26:682–685.

38 Unni KK. Introduction and scope of study. In: *Dahlin's Bone Tumors: General Aspects and Data in 11 087 Cases* 5th ed. Philadelphia, Pa: Lippincott, Williams & Wilkins; 1996:1–9.

39 Unni KK. Chondrosarcoma (primary, secondary, dedifferentiated, and clear cell). In: *Dahlin's Bone Tumors: General Aspects and Data in 11 087 Cases* 5th ed. Philadelphia, Pa: Lippincott, Williams & Wilkins; 1996:71–106.

40 Vanel D, De Paolis M, Monti C, Mercuri M, Picci P. Radiological features of 24 periosteal chondrosarcomas. *Skeletal Radiol* 2001; 30:208–212.

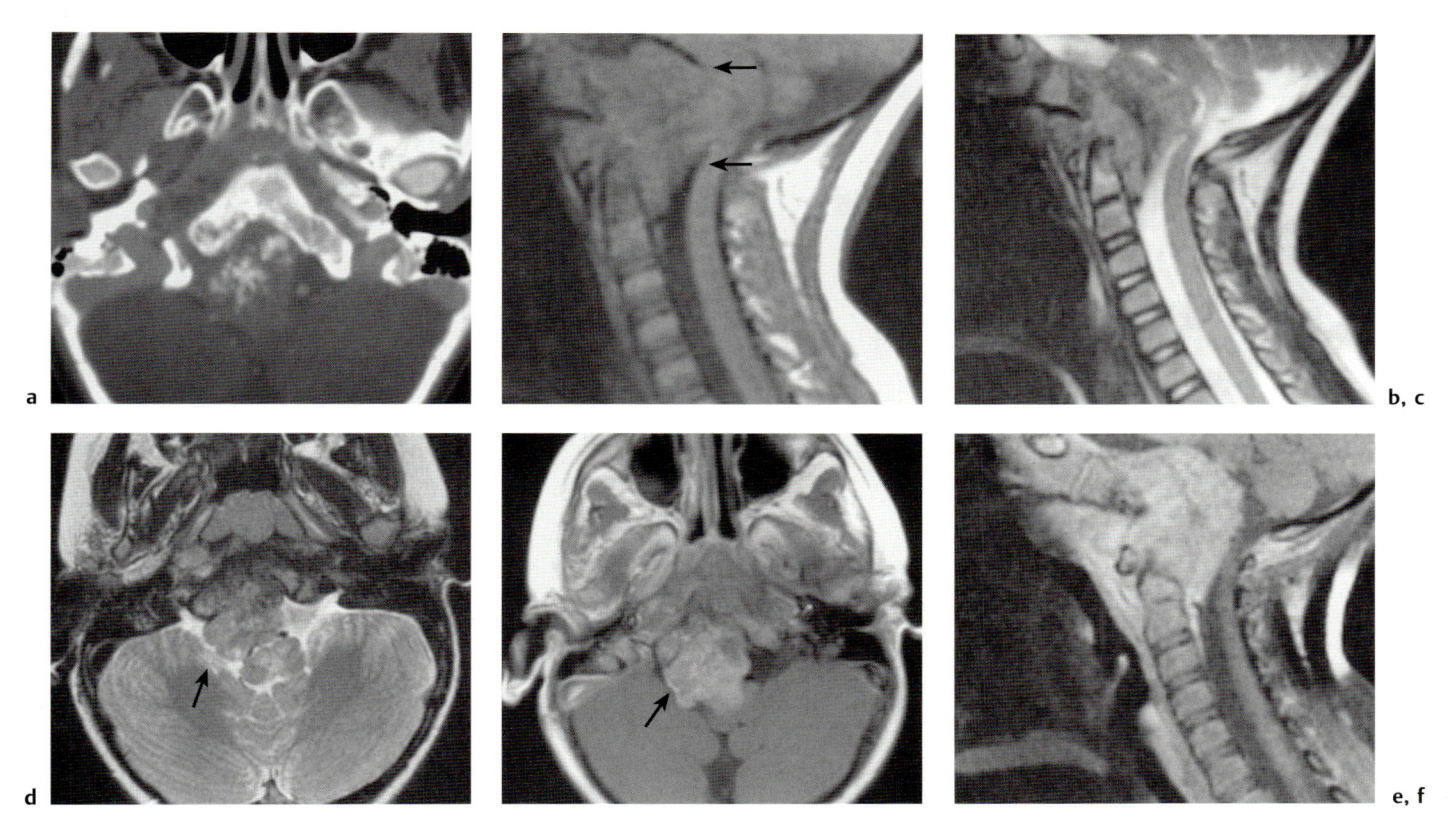

Figure **63 a–f** A 4-year-old female with a sarcomatoid chordoma involving the lower clivus and upper dens as well as the adjacent soft tissues at the craniovertebral junction, with extension dorsally causing compression of the medulla and upper spinal cord. Axial CT image (**a**) shows mineralization within the tumor and erosive changes at the dorsal margin of the clivus. The tumor has intermediate and low signal on sagittal (**b**) T1WI and sagittal (**c**) and axial (**d**) T2WI. The tumor shows heterogeneous moderate Gd-contrast enhancement on axial (**e**) T1WI and sagittal (**f**) FS T1WI.

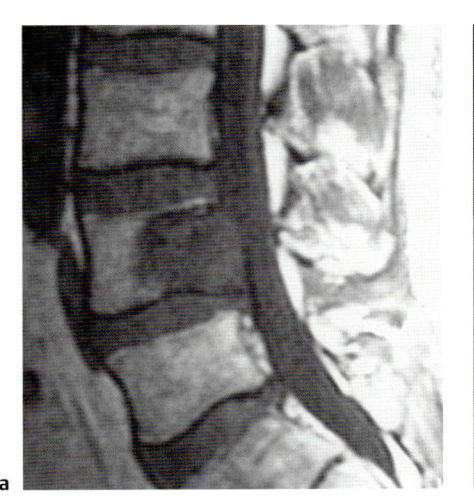

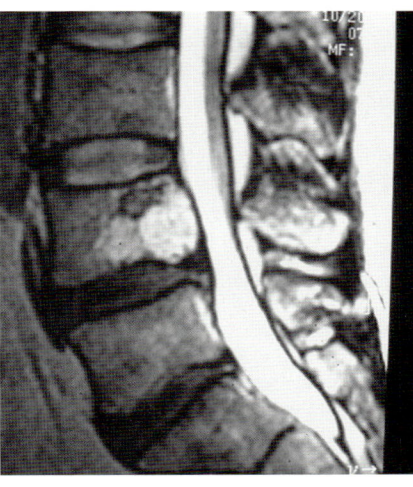

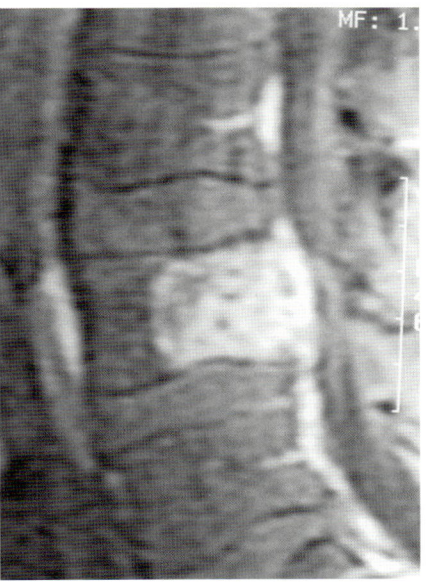

Figure **64 a–c** A 48-year-old man with a chordoma involving the dorsal portion of the L 4 vertebral body. The tumor has low-intermediate signal on sagittal T1WI (**a**), and heterogeneous mostly high signal with small zones of low signal on sagittal T2WI (**b**). The tumor shows prominent heterogeneous Gd-contrast enhancement on FS T1WI (**c**).

Treatment and Prognosis[1,10,13,14,17,21–23,25,27,28]

Average survival for chondroid chordomas (16 years) is greater than for conventional chordomas (4 years). Morbidity and mortality are usually secondary to local recurrence and extension. Distant metastasis is uncommon. Systemic metastases occur in 7–14% of cases and are frequently located in lung, bone, lymph nodes, liver, and skin.[2,6] New aggressive surgical approaches have shown improved outcome.[6,13,21–23] Combined treatment of surgery and radiation is routinely used.[2,6] Proton beam radiation and stereotactic radiosurgery have also been used to treat chordomas of the skull base.[1,10]

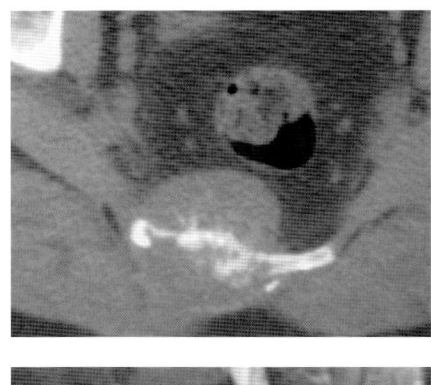

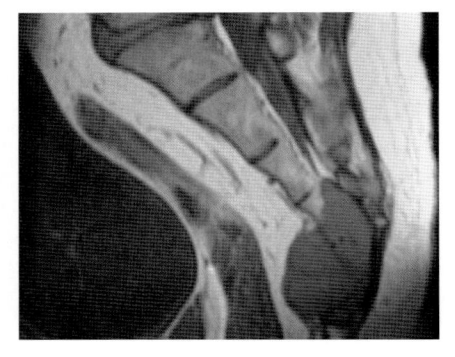

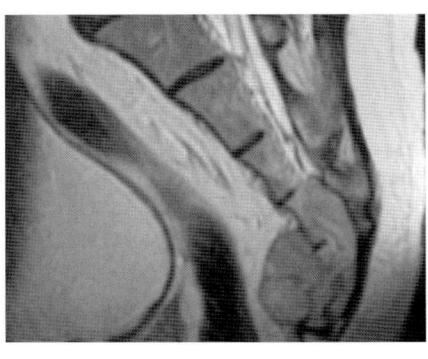

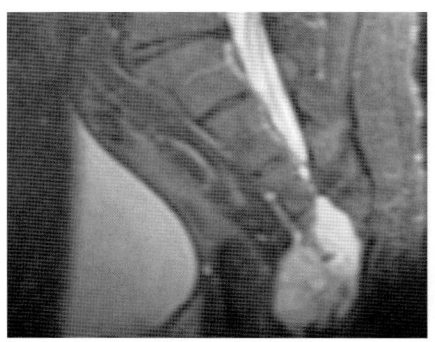

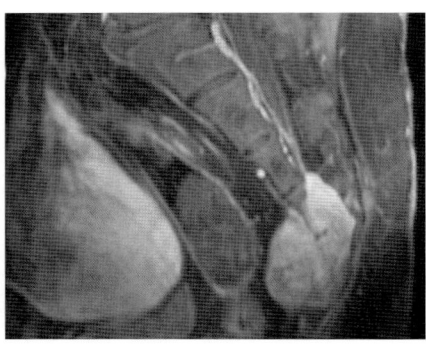

Figure **65 a–e** A 40-year-old man with chordoma involving the sacrum. The tumor has intermediate attenuation and is associated with bone destruction on axial CT (**a**). The tumor has mostly intermediate signal on sagittal T1WI (**b**), intermediate to slightly high signal on sagittal T2WI (**c**), and mostly high signal on sagittal FS T2WI (**d**). The tumor shows prominent Gd-contrast enhancement on sagittal FS T1WI (**e**).

References

1. Austin-Seymour M, Munzenrider J, Goitein M, et al. Fractionated proton radiation therapy of chordoma and low-grade chondrosarcoma of the base of the skull. *J Neurosurg* 1989;70:13–17.
2. Barnes L. Pathobiology of selected tumors of the base of the skull. *Skull Base Surg* 1991;1(4):207–216.
3. Delank KS, Kriegsmann J, Drees P, Eckardt A, Eysel P. Metastasizing chordoma of the lumbar spine. *Eur Spine J* 2002;11:167–171.
4. Diel J, Ortiz O, Losada RA, Price DB, Hayt MW, Katz DS. The sacrum: pathologic spectrum, multi-modality imaging, and subspecialty approach. *Radiographics* 2001;21:83–104.
5. Doucet V, Peretti-Viton P, Figarella-Branger D, Manera L, Salamon G. MRI of intracranial chordomas. Extent of tumour and contrast enhancement: criteria for differential diagnosis. *Neuroradiology* 1997;39:571–576.
6. Erdem E, Angtuaco EC, Van Hemert R, Park JS, Al-Mefty O. Comprehensive review of intra-cranial chordoma. *Radiographics* 2003;23:995–1009.
7. Forest M. Chordoma. In: Forest M, Tomeno B, Vanel D, eds. *Orthopedic Surgical Pathology: Diagnosis of Tumors and Pseudotumoral Lesions of Bone and Joints* Edinburgh: Livingstone Churchill; 1998:397–410.
8. Heffelfinger MJ, Dahlin DC, MacCarty CS, Beabout JW. Chordomas and cartilaginous tumors at the skull base. *Cancer* 1973;32:410–420.
9. Huvos AG Chordoma. In: Huvos AG, ed. *Bone Tumors: Diagnosis, Treatment, and Prognosis* 2nd ed. Philadelphia, Pa: W.B. Saunders; 1991:599–617.
10. Kondziolka D, Lunsford LD, Flickinger JC. The role of radiosurgery in the management of chordoma and chondrosarcoma of the cranial base. *Neurosurgery* 1991;29(1):38–46.
11. Laine FJ, Nadel L, Braun IF. CT and MR imaging of the central skull base. Part 2. Pathologic spectrum. *Radiographics* 1990;10(5):797–821.
12. Larson TC III, Houser OW, Laws ER Jr. Imaging of Cranial Chordomas. *Mayo Clin Proc* 1987;62:886–893.
13. Meyers SP, Hirsch WL Jr, Curtin HD, Barnes L, Sekhar LN, Sen C. Chordomas of the skull base: MR features. *AJNR Am J Neuroradiol* 1992;13:1627–1636.
14. Mirra JM, Nelson SD, Rocca CD, Mertens F. Chordoma. In: Fletcher CDM, Unni KK, Mertens F, eds. *World Health Organization Classification of Tumours. Pathology and Genetics of Tumours of Soft Tissue and Bone* Geneva: IARC Press; 2002:316–317.
15. Mulder JD, Schutte HE, Kroon HM, Taconis WK. Introduction. In: *Radiologic Atlas of Bone Tumors* Amsterdam: Elsevier; 1993:3–6.
16. Mulder JD, Schutte HE, Kroon HM, Taconis WK. The diagnosis of bone tumors. In: *Radiologic Atlas of Bone Tumors* Amsterdam: Elsevier; 1993:9–46.
17. Mulder JD, Schutte HE, Kroon HM, Taconis WK. Chordoma. In: *Radiologic Atlas of Bone Tumors* Amsterdam: Elsevier; 1993: 267–274.
18. Oot RF, Melville GE, New Paul FJ, et al. The role of MR and CT in evaluating clival chordomas and chondrosarcomas. *AJR Am J Roentgenol* 1988;151:567–575.
19. Rich TA, Schiller A, Suit HD, Mankin HJ. Clinical and pathologic review of 48 cases of chordoma. *Cancer* 1985;56:182–187.
20. Salisbury JR. Bone neoplasms containing epithelial and epithelioid cells. In: Helliwell TR, ed. *Major Problems in Pathology: Pathology of Bone and Joint Neoplasms* Vol 37. 1st ed. Philadelphia, Pa: W.B. Saunders 1999:352–360.
21. Sekhar LN, Schramm VL, Jones NF. Subtemporal-preauricular infratemporal fossa approach to large lateral and posterior cranial base neoplasms. *J Neurosurg* 1987;67:488–499.
22. Sekhar LN, Janecka IP, Jones NF. Subtemporal–infratemporal and basal subfrontal approach to extensive cranial base tumours. *Acta Neurochir (Wien)* 1988;92:83–92.
23. Sen CN, Sekhar LN, Schramm VL, Janecka IP. Chordoma and Chondrosarcoma of the cranial base: an 8-year experience. *Neurosurgery* 1989;25(6):931–941.
24. Smith J, Ludwig RL, Marcove RC. Sacrococcygeal chordoma: a clinicoradiological study of 60 patients. *Skeletal Radiol* 1987;16:37–44.
25. Smolders D, Wang X, Drevelengas A, Vanhoenacker F, DeSchepper AM. Value of MRI in the diagnosis of non-clival, non-sacral chordoma. *Skeletal Radiol* 2003;32:343–350.
26. Sze G, Uichanco LS III, Brant-Zawadzki MN, et al. Chordomas: MR imaging. *Radiology* 1988;166(1):187–191.
27. Unni KK. Introduction and scope of study. In: *Dahlin's Bone Tumors: General Aspects and Data on 11 087 Cases* 5th ed. Philadelphia, Pa: Lippincott, Williams & Wilkins; 1996:1–9.
28. Unni KK. Chordoma. In: *Dahlin's Bone Tumors: General Aspects and Data on 11 087 Cases* 5th ed. Philadelphia, Pa: Lippincott, Williams & Wilkins; 1996:291–303.

5 Kransdorf MJ, Murphey MD. Malignant fibrous and fibrohistiocytic tumors. In: *Imaging of Soft Tissue Tumors* 2nd ed. Philadelphia, Pa: W. B. Saunders; 2006:257–297.
6 Linn SC, West RB, Pollack JR, et al. Gene expression patterns and gene copy number changes in dermatofibrosarcoma protuberans. *Am J Pathol* 2003;163(6):2383–2395.
7 Ono I, Kaneko F. Magnetic resonance imaging for diagnosing skin tumors. *Clin Dermatol* 1995;13:393–399.
8 Sun LM, Wang CJ, Huang CC, et al. Dermatofibrosarcoma protuberans: treatment results of 35 cases. *Radiother Oncol* 2000;57:175–181.
9 Torreggiani WC, Al-Ismail K, Munk PL, Nicolaou S, O'Connell JX, Knowling MA. Dermatofibrosarcoma protuberans: MR imaging features. *AJR Am J Roentgenol* 2002;178:989–993.
10 Weiss SW, Goldblum JR. Fibrohistiocytic Tumors of Intermediate Malignancy. In: Weiss SW, Goldblum JR, eds. *Enzinger and Weiss' Soft Tissue Tumors* 4th ed. St. Louis, Mo: Mosby; 2001:491–534.

A 14 Dermatomyositis

Definition

Dermatomyositis is a nonsupperative, autoimmune inflammatory disease of unknown etiology, involving muscle fibers, skin, and blood vessels. This disorder is considered a systemic vasculopathy. Dermatomyositis can be associated with other connective tissue diseases such as scleroderma and mixed connective tissue disease.

Frequency of Occurrence

Incidence 2–8 per million, prevalence 4–60 per million.[9]

Age at Presentation

Juvenile dermatomyositis: children between 2 and 15 years.[5,13]

Adult dermatomyositis: peak incidence in 5th decade.[10]

Gender Ratio

Dermatomyositis occurs more often in females than males.

Location

Muscles of shoulder and pelvis are the most common locations, often symmetric.[5]

Signs and Symptoms

Patients may have these signs and symptoms: proximal lower extremity muscle weakness followed by proximal upper extremity weakness; myalgia and muscle tenderness; heliotropic rash (upper eyelids) with periorbital edema; scaling erythematous eruptions or red patches (Gottron papules on knuckles, elbows, and knees); and elevated levels of serum creatine phosphokinase.[2,4,9,13] Skin rashes can also be observed on the elbows, neck, upper chest, and shoulders.[9]

Gross Pathologic Findings

Swelling, edema, and/or ischemia are seen in affected muscles in the early stages of the disease.[4] Muscle atrophy and fatty infiltration are seen in the late or chronic phases.

Histopathologic Findings

In the active phase of this disease, a humoral immune response occurs against vascular endothelium with deposition of the C5b-9 membrane component of complement. Associated with these findings are resultant abnormalities of the endomysial capillary bed and ischemic muscle injury.[1,4,9] Inflammatory infiltrates with collections of B cells can be observed at vessels in skeletal muscle.[4,8] Positive reactions with antibodies to the Mi-2 antigen are relatively specific for dermatomyositis.[9] In later phases of the disease, fatty infiltration occurs in the ischemic muscles as well as muscle atrophy.[2,6,9,10]

Findings on Plain Films (Roentgenograms) and Computed Tomography

In the acute stages, soft tissue swelling and subcutaneous edema may be observed as indistinctness of fat and soft tissue planes (Fig. 71). In the chronic phases, irregular or amorphous deposits of calcium/minerals are seen in the subcutaneous soft tissues in up to 50% of cases, which is associated with muscle atrophy(Figs. 69, 70, 72).[5] The subcutaneous calcifications are sometimes referred to as milk of calcium (Fig. 72).[13] Radiographic findings of arthritis are usually absent.

MRI Findings

In the acute and subacute phases of the disease, poorly defined zones of high signal on T2WI and FS T2WI are seen in muscles, subcutaneous fat, and fascia resulting from ischemic or infarcted muscle secondary to vasculitis (Figs. 70, 71).[2,5,7] Enlargement of the involved muscles often occurs. Zones of low signal on T2WI in subcutaneous fat can be seen corresponding to areas of calcifications seen on radiographs and CT scans (Figs. 69, 70, 72). Milk of calcium collections have variable signal on T1WI and T2WI, depending on the relative proportions of fluid and fluid–calcium levels (Fig. 72).[13]

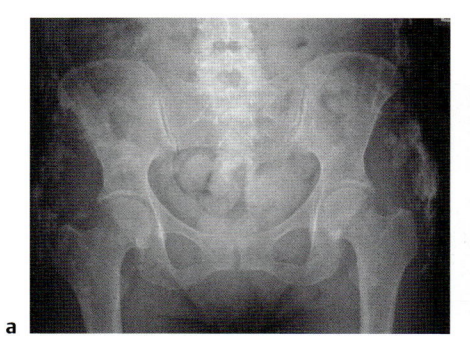

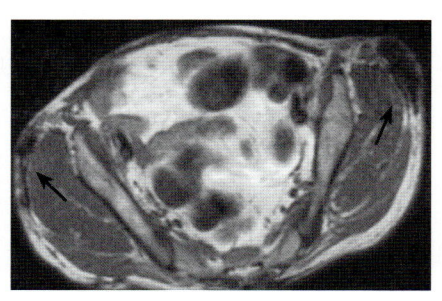

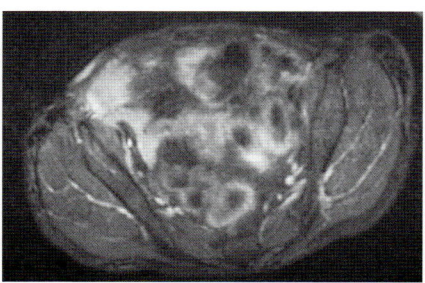

Figure **69 a–c** A 42-year-old man with dermatomyositis involving the pelvic and thigh regions. AP radiograph (**a**) shows irregular amorphous deposits of calcium/minerals in the subcutaneous soft tissues. Zones of low signal on axial T1WI (**b**) and axial FS T2WI (**c**) are seen in the subcutaneous fat corresponding to areas of calcification seen on the radiograph.

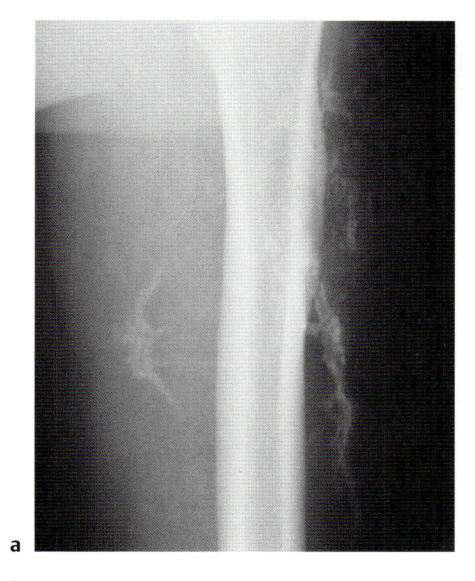

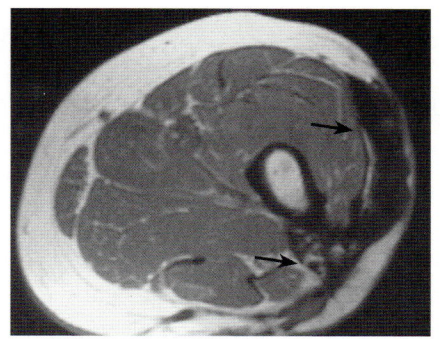

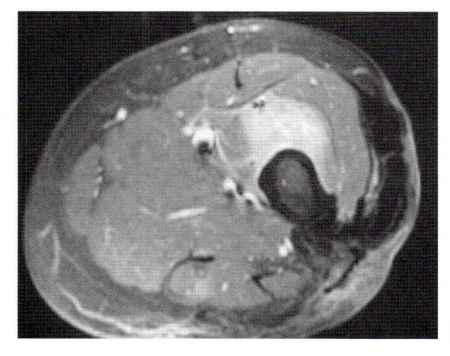

Figure **70 a–c** A 60-year-old man with dermatomyositis involving the thigh. AP radiograph (**a**) shows irregular amorphous deposits of calcium/minerals in the subcutaneous soft tissues. Zones of low signal on axial T1WI (**b**) are seen in the subcutaneous fat corresponding to areas of calcification seen on the radiograph. After Gd-contrast administration, a poorly defined zone of enhancement is also seen in the vastus intermedius muscle on axial FS T1WI (**c**) secondary to active inflammation.

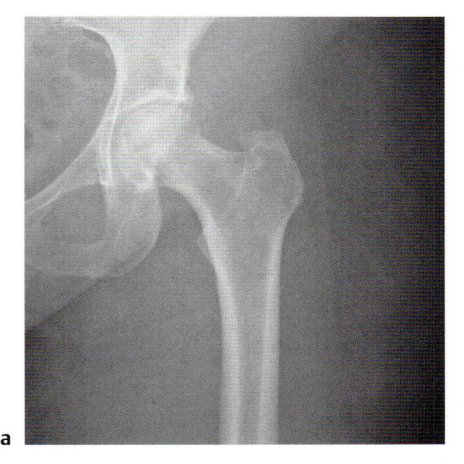

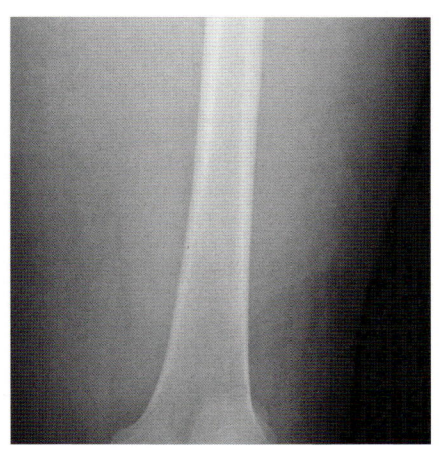

Figure **71 a–e** A 78-year-old woman with dermatomyositis involving the thigh. AP radiographs (**a**, **b**) show edematous changes in the soft tissues without calcification. Zones of abnormal low signal on axial T1WI (**c**) are seen in the subcutaneous fat, which have corresponding high signal on axial FS T2WI (**d**). Poorly defined zones of abnormal high signal on FS T2WI (**d**) and abnormal Gd-contrast enhancement on FS T1WI (**e**) are seen in the thigh muscles secondary to active inflammation.

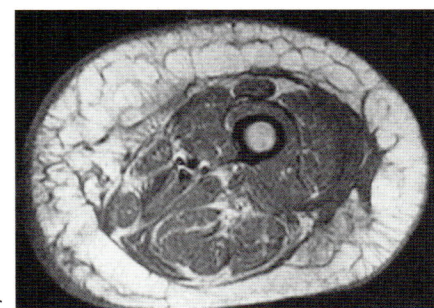

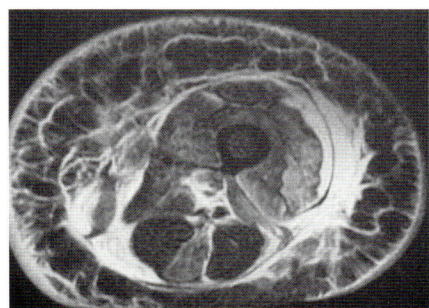

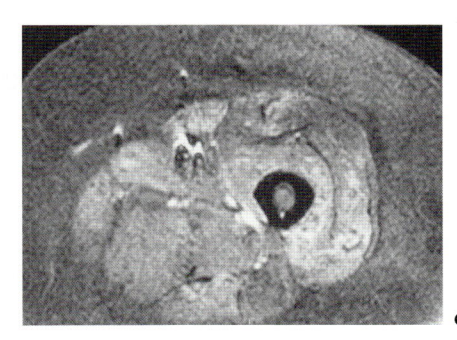

Poorly defined zones of low signal can occur in the subcutaneous fat on T1WI (Figs. **69–72**). After Gd-contrast administration, poorly defined zones of enhancement can be seen in muscles, fascia, and/or subcutaneous fat if there is active inflammation and/or ischemia–infarction (Figs. **70, 71**). Subcutaneous and intermuscular calcium-containing collections often have mild peripheral enhancement.[2,13] Muscle atrophy with fatty infiltration can be seen in the chronic phases. Patients with inactive disease may have no signal abnormalities evident with MRI.[6]

Hydrogen MR spectroscopy can show decreased choline-to-lipid and creatine-to-lipid ratios in chronic phases.[3] P-31 MR spectroscopy shows inefficient energy metabolism or impaired oxidative metabolism indices in muscles of patients with myopathic dermatomyositis, and during exercise in muscles of patients with amyopathic variant of dermatomyositis.[1,11]

Differential Diagnosis

Healed necrotizing fasciitis, radiation injury, post-traumatic injury, cellulitis, pyomyositis, polymyositis, graft versus host disease, deep venous thrombosis, rhabdomyolysis, acute deinnervation, sickle cell crisis, Duchenne muscular dystrophy (chronic dermatomyositis), Becker muscular dystrophy (chronic dermatomyositis), congenital muscular dystrophy (chronic dermatomyositis), spinal muscular atrophy (chronic dermatomyositis).

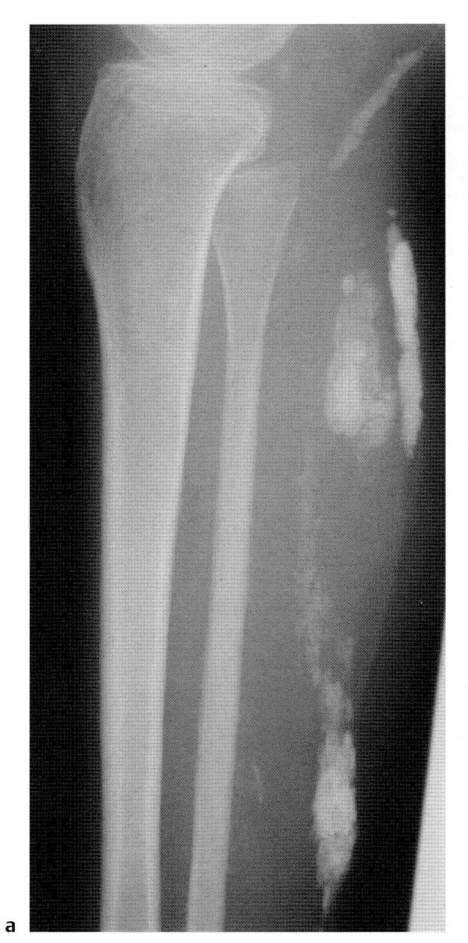

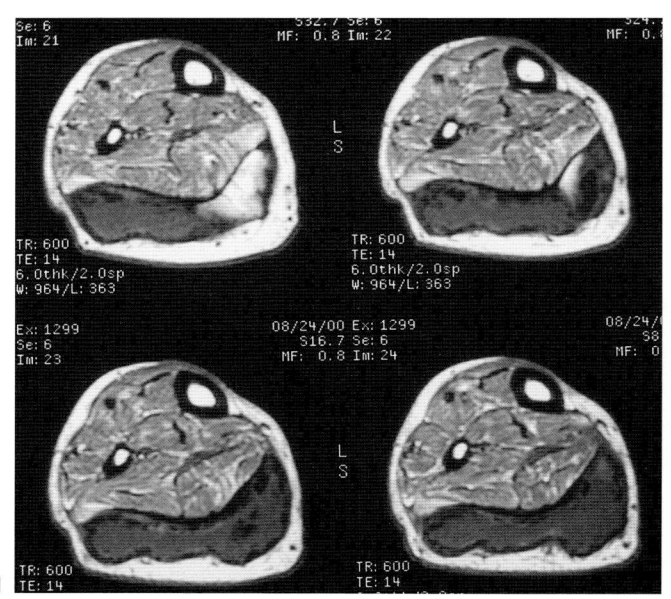

Figure 72 a–e A 49-year-old woman with dermatomyositis involving the leg. Lateral radiograph (**a**) shows irregular amorphous deposits of calcium/minerals in the dorsal subcutaneous soft tissues. A zone of abnormal intermediate and low signal surrounded by a shaggy rim of low signal is seen on sagittal (**b**) and axial (**d**) T1WI. This zone has mostly high signal with irregular zones of low signal centrally surrounded by a thick irregular rim of low signal on sagittal (**c**) and axial (**e**) FS T2WI.

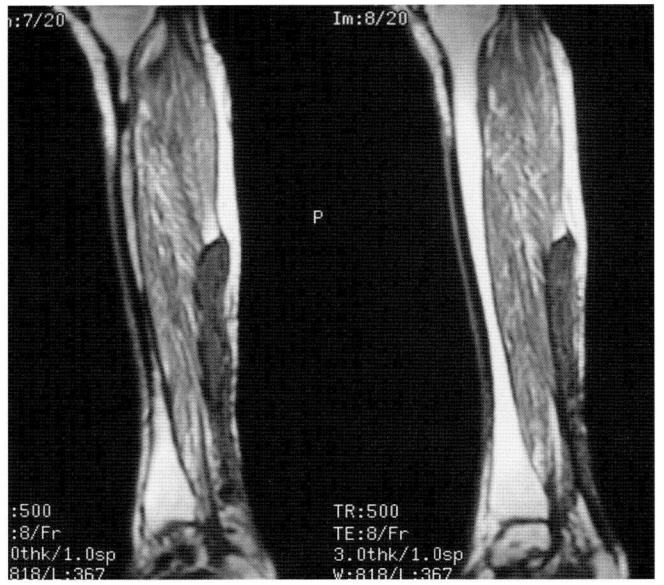

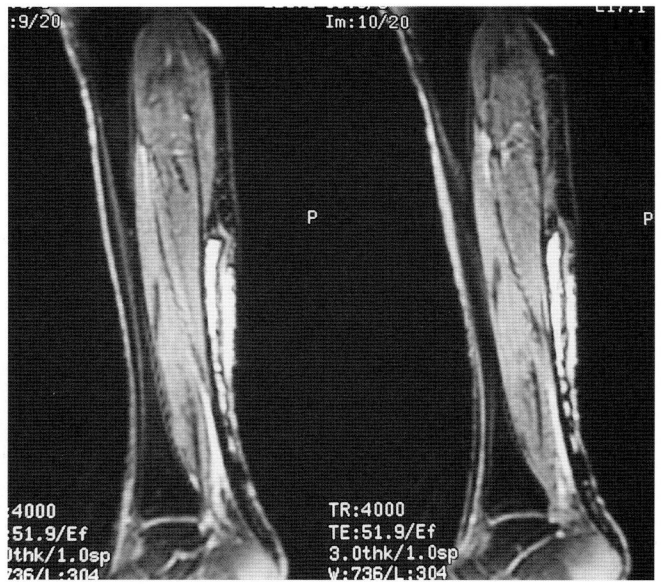

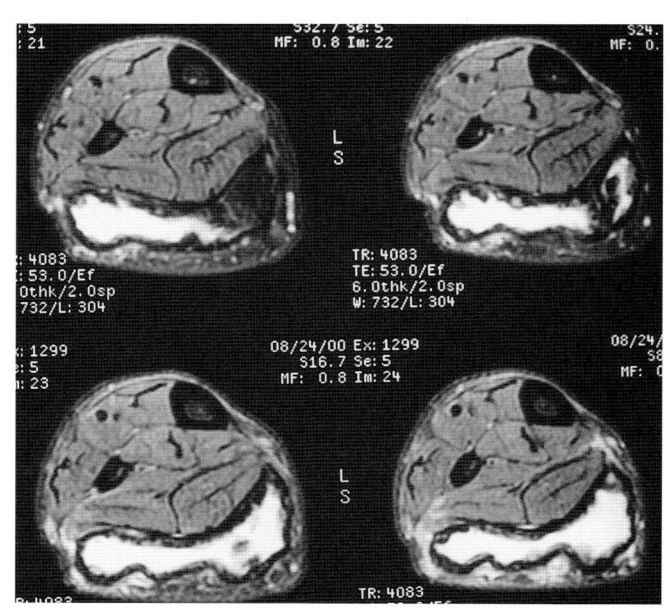

Prognosis and Treatment

MRI is useful in determining the extent and degree of active and chronic disease, as well as response to therapy.[5,6,12] Treatment often consists of corticosteroids and other immunosuppressive drugs.[9] Monoclonal antibodies directed toward the B-cells involved in the aberrant immune response are under investigation.[9] Patients with dermatomyositis have an increased risk of developing cancer relative to the general population.[4,14]

References

1. Cea G, Bendahan D, Manners D, et al. Reduced oxidative phosphorylation and proton efflux suggest reduced capillary blood supply in skeletal muscle of patients with dermatomyositis and polymyositis: a quantitative 31P-magnetic resonance spectroscopy and MRI study. *Brain* 2002;125(7):1635-1645.
2. Chan WP, Liu GC. Pictorial Essay: MR imaging of primary skeletal muscle diseases in children. *AJR Am J Roentgenol* 2002;179(4):989-997.
3. Chung YL, Smith EC, Williams SC, et al. In vivo proton magnetic resonance spectroscopy in polymyositis and dermatomyositis: a preliminary study. *Eur J Med Res* 1997;2(11):483-487.
4. Cotran RS, Kumar V, Collins T, Aster J, Kumar V. Diseases of immunity. In: Cotran RS, Kumar V, Collins T, eds. *Pathologic Basis of Disease* 6th ed. Philadelphia, Pa: W.B. Saunders; 1999:188-259.
5. Hanlon R, King S. Overview of the radiology of connective tissue disorders in children. *Eur J Radiol* 2000;33(2):74-84.
6. Hernandez RJ, Sullivan DB, Chenevert TL, Keim DR. MR imaging in children with dermatomyositis: musculoskeletal findings and correlation with clinical and laboratory findings. *AJR Am J Roentgenol* 1993;161(2):359-366.
7. Kimball AB, Summers RM, Turner M, et al. Magnetic resonance imaging detection of occult skin and subcutaneous abnormalities in juvenile dermatomyositis. Implications for diagnosis and therapy. *Arthritis Rheum* 2000;43(8):1866-1873.
8. Lofberg M, Liewendahl K, Lamminen A, Korhola O, Somer H. Antimyosin scintigraphy compared with magnetic resonance imaging in inflammatory myopathies. *Arch Neurol* 1998;55(7):987-993.
9. Mastaglia FL, Garlepp MJ, Phillips BA, Zilko PJ. Inflammatory myopathies: clinical, diagnostic and therapeutic aspects. *Muscle Nerve* 2003;27(4):407-425.
10. May DA, Disler DG, Jones EA, Balkissoon AA, Manaster BJ. Abnormal signal intensity in skeletal muscle at MR imaging: patterns, pearls, and pitfalls. *Radiographics* 2000;20:S 295-S 315.
11. Park JH, Vital TL, Ryder NM, et al. Magnetic resonance imaging and P-31 magnetic resonance spectroscopy provide unique quantitative data useful in the longitudinal management of patients with dermatomyositis. *Arthritis Rheum* 1994;37(5):736-746.
12. Revelon G, Rahmouni A, Jazaerli N, et al. Acute swelling of the limbs: magnetic resonance pictorial review of fascial and muscle signal changes. *Eur J Radiol* 1999;30:11-21.
13. Samson C, Soulen RL, Gursel E. Milk of calcium fluid collections in juvenile dermatomyositis: MR characterisitics. *Pediatr Radiol* 2000;30:28-29.
14. Weiss SW, Goldblum JR. Osseous soft tissue tumors. In: Weiss SW, Goldblum JR, eds. *Enzinger and Weiss Soft Tissue Tumors* 4th ed. St. Louis, Mo: Mosby; 2001:1389-1417.

A 15 Dermoid and Epidermoid

Definition

Dermoids are ectoderm-lined inclusion cysts that contain hair, sebaceous and sweat glands, and squamous epithelium.[9] Dermoids slowly enlarge, although are not considered to be neoplasms.[9] Dermoids can be congenital lesions that arise between 3 and 5 weeks of gestation when surface ectoderm fails to separate completely from the adjacent neural tube.[3,9] Dermoids can also form as a result of invagination or sequestration of surface ectoderm at sites of dermal fusion (face, eyes, ears) during gestation.[3,9] In older patients, dermoids may occur from displacement of skin into deeper structures from trauma, surgery, or lumbar puncture.[3,9]

Epidermoids are ectoderm-lined inclusion cysts that contain only squamous epithelium.[9] Epidermoids slowly enlarge, although are not considered to be neoplasms.[9] Congenital epidermoid cysts arise later in gestation than dermoids, and tend to be more superficial and lateral relative to dermoids.[9] In older patients, epidermoids may occur from displacement of skin into deeper structures from trauma, surgery, or lumbar puncture.[9]

Frequency of Occurrence

Dermoids and epidermoids account for up to 5% of intracranial masses and up to 2% of intraspinal tumors.[3,9] Dermoid cysts are the most common orbital lesions in children.[9] Dermoids also commonly occur as ovarian lesions.

Age at Presentation

Dermoids and epidermoids can be congenital lesions, or can occur in children or adults as acquired lesions resulting from displacement of skin elements into deeper tissues from trauma, surgery, or other medical procedures such as lumbar puncture.[9] Dermoid cysts are often diagnosed in the 2nd to 3rd decades, whereas epidermoids often present in the 3rd to 4th decades.[3,9]

Gender Ratio

Males are slightly more affected than females.[9]

Location

Dermoids: orbits (zygomaticofrontal and frontoethmoidal sutures, supraorbital ridge, lateral eyebrow), posterior cranial fossa (cisterna magna, 4th ventricle, prepontine cistern), suprasellar cistern, spine, ovary, and other soft tissues.[3,9] Spinal dermoids can be extradural, intradural-extramedullary, or intramedullary.[3] Spinal dermoids are located in the lumbosacral region (60%), followed by the thoracic and cervical regions.[3] Some spinal dermoids are associated with a dorsal dermal sinus.[9] Dermoid cysts rarely occur within the cerebral ventricles, brain parenchyma, and brainstem.[4]

Epidermoids: intradiploic space (often involving the temporal or parietal bones), intradural extra-axial intracranial lesions (cerebellopontine angle cistern / congenital cholesteatoma, middle cranial fossa), extramedullary spinal lesions, soft tissues of the extremities.[9] Acquired cholesteatomas are secondary epidermoids that occur in the middle ear from retraction pockets or displaced epithelium from outside to inside the pars flaccida of the tympanic membrane.[9] Epidermoid cysts rarely occur within the cerebral ventricles, brain parenchyma, and brainstem.[4]

Signs and Symptoms

Dermoids are slow-growing lesions that are often asymptomatic.[3,9] Dermoids may be associated with chronic erosive changes involving adjacent bones. Rupture of dermoids within the central nervous system can result in seizures and other significant neurologic events because of severe chemical meningitis.[9] Large dermoids in the posterior cranial fossa may cause hydrocephalus.[9] Dermoids in the spinal canal can be associated with progressive lower extremity neurologic deficits and bladder sphincter dysfunction.[7] Approximately 20% of dermoids involving the spine are associated with a dorsal dermal sinus.[7] Other clinical features associated with spinal dermoids include sacral dimple, tufts of hair, and spina bifida.[7]

Epidermoids are slow-growing lesions that are often asymptomatic.[9] Epidermoids may be associated with chronic erosive changes involving adjacent bones. Rupture of epidermoids within the central nervous system can result in seizures and other significant neurologic events because of severe chemical meningitis.[9] Epidermoids typically do not cause hydrocephalus. Acquired cholesteatomas in the middle ear are often associated with conductive hearing loss that results from erosions of the ossicular chain.

Gross Pathologic Findings

Dermoids. Lesions typically appear as unilocular cysts containing viscous yellow, green, and/or brown fluid containing keratin, hair, and various fat metabolites and cholesterol crystals.[3]

Epidermoids. Lesions are nodular or multilobulated, with a capsule containing a thin lining of stratified squamous epthilelium.[4,9] The cyst's contents often appear waxy, shiny, and smooth due to keratin.[9]

Histopathologic Findings

Dermoids. Lesions usually have a capsule containing connective tissue lined by stratified squamous epithelium with dermal appendages such as hair follicles, hair, sebaceous glands, and sweat glands.[3] Calcifications may occur in the cyst walls.[3] Cyst contents often include keratin, hair, and various fat metabolites and cholesterol crystals.[3] Occasionally bone and/or cartilage may be present inside these lesions.[3]

Epidermoids. Lesions have thin walls with flat squamous cells.[9] The contents of an epidermoid arise from debris from the desquamated squamous epithelial cells and include keratin, cholesterol, and other lipids.[9]

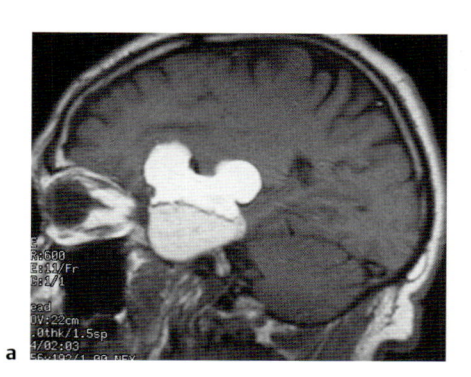

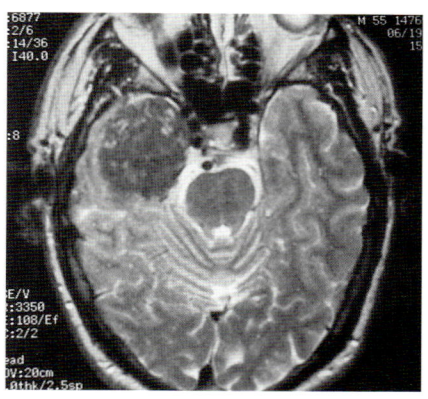

Figure **73 a, b** A 55-year-old man with a dermoid in the right middle cranial fossa. Sagittal (**a**) T1WI show a circumscribed extra-axial lesion, which has heterogeneous mostly high signal with a thin low signal septum. The lesion has mixed low and high signal on axial (**b**) T2WI.

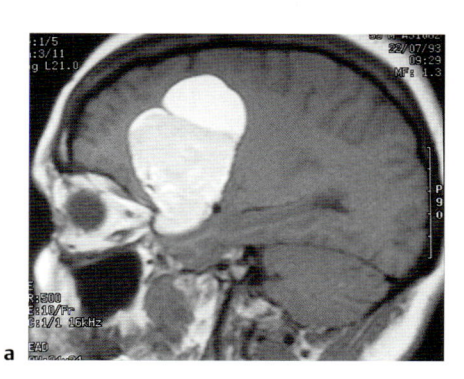

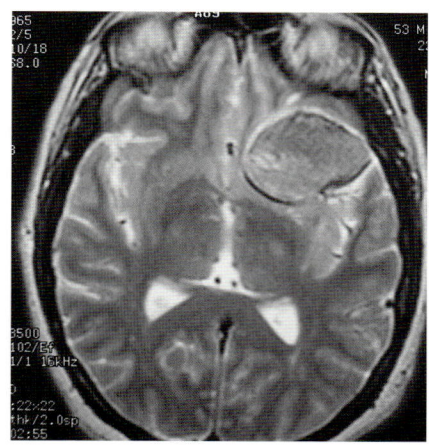

Figure **74 a, b** A 53-year-old man with a dermoid in the left middle and anterior cranial fossae, as well as the suprasellar cistern. Sagittal (**a**) T1WI shows a circumscribed, lobulated, extra-axial lesion which has heterogeneous high, intermediate, and low signal surrounded by a thin rim of low signal. The lesion has mixed low and high signal on axial T2WI and is surrounded by a thin rim of low signal (**b**).

Findings on Plain Films (Roentgenograms) and Computed Tomography

Dermoids.[2–4,9,11] Dermoid cysts can produce erosions of adjacent bone.[9] Dermoids within bone can cause erosion and/or expansion of the involved bone, with or without sclerotic margins.[9] On CT, dermoids are often circumscribed unilocular lesions which usually have thick walls that may or may not contain calcifications[9] (Fig. **76**). The contents of dermoids can have low attenuation (−60 HU to −90 HU) similar to fat, resulting from sebaceous and other lipid material.[2,9] Fat–fluid levels can occur within dermoids.[9] Dermoids may rupture, and zones of low attenuation similar to fat can be seen near or distant to the primary lesion.[3] Less frequently, some dermoids may have low attenuation similar to water, or high attenuation similar to hemorrhage.[4,9,11]

Epidermoids.[9,13] Epidermoid cysts can produce erosions of adjacent bone.[9] Epidermoids within bone can cause erosion and/or expansion of the involved bone, with or without sclerotic margins[9] (Fig. **78**). On CT, epidermoids are circumscribed and/or lobulated lesions that have thin imperceptible walls.[9] Epidermoids typically have low attenuation similar to water.[9] Infrequently, some epidermoids have high attenuation similar to hemorrhage from high protein content and high viscosity.[13]

MRI Findings

Dermoids.[3,4,7,9,11] Dermoid cysts are circumscribed lesions which may have identifiable walls with low signal on T1WI and T2WI.[9] The contents of dermoid cysts can have low, intermediate and/or high signal on T1WI and T2WI[3,4,7,9,11] (Figs. **73–76**). After Gd-contrast administration, dermoids may show enhancement at the wall margins, but not centrally.[9] Dermoids may be associated with anomalies such as skeletal dysraphism and dorsal dermal sinus.[9] Dermoids may rupture into the subarachnoid space, and zones of high signal on T1WI similar to fat can be seen near or distant to the primary lesion[3] (Fig. **75**). Ruptured dermoids may incite an inflammatory meningitis and may be associated with adhesive arachnoiditis involving the cauda equina.[3,9]

Epidermoids.[1,2,4–6,8,12–14] Epidermoid cysts are circumscribed lesions which may have slightly lobulated margins. Epidermoids usually have low signal or low-intermediate signal on T1WI, and high signal on T2WI and FS T2WI that may approximate cerebrospinal fluid (CSF)[1,2,4–6,8,12,14] (Figs. **77–81**). Lesions occasionally contain foci of high signal on T1WI (Fig. **81**). With FLAIR, epidermoids typically show higher signal than CSF.[5] Epidermoids typically show very high signal on diffusion-weighted images,[1,5,12] which may result from T2 shine-through effect or diffusion restriction.[5] Apparent diffusion coefficient mapping can allow distinction between these possibilities (Fig. **77**). Infrequently, epidermoids have been shown to have high signal on T1WI, and/or low signal on T2WI secondary to cyst contents with high protein content and high viscosity.[13] Epidermoids may show minimal peripheral Gd-contrast enhancement, but no enhancement is typically seen centrally.[6,9] Intracranial epidermoids are soft lesions which may be associated with displacement of adjacent brain tissue and other neurologic structures, but hydrocephalus does not typically occur.[6] Ruptured epidermoids may incite an inflammatory meningitis and may be associated with adhesive arachnoiditis involving the cauda equina.[9]

392 A 15 – Dermoid and Epidermoid

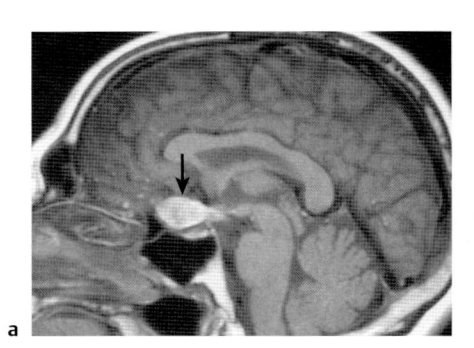

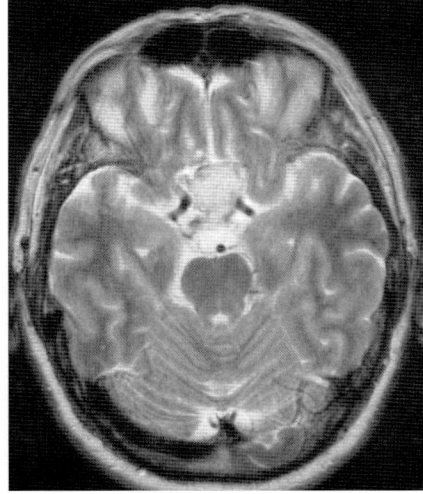

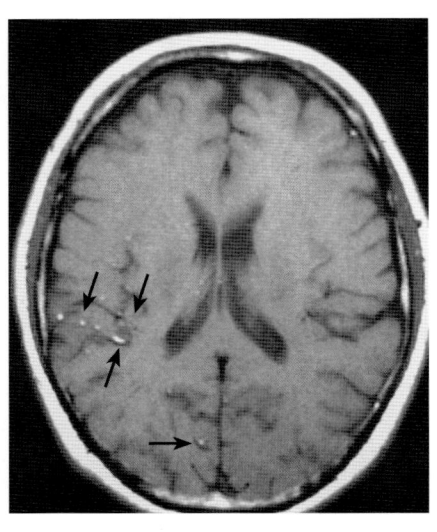

Figure **75 a–c** A 53-year-old man with a leaking dermoid in the suprasellar cistern. Sagittal (**a**) and axial (**c**) T1WI show an extra-axial lesion, which has heterogeneous slightly high signal. Check as edited. The lesion has heterogeneous slightly high signal on axial T2WI (**b**). Multiple small foci with high signal on T1WI are seen in the subarachnoid space representing droplets from the leaking dermoid.

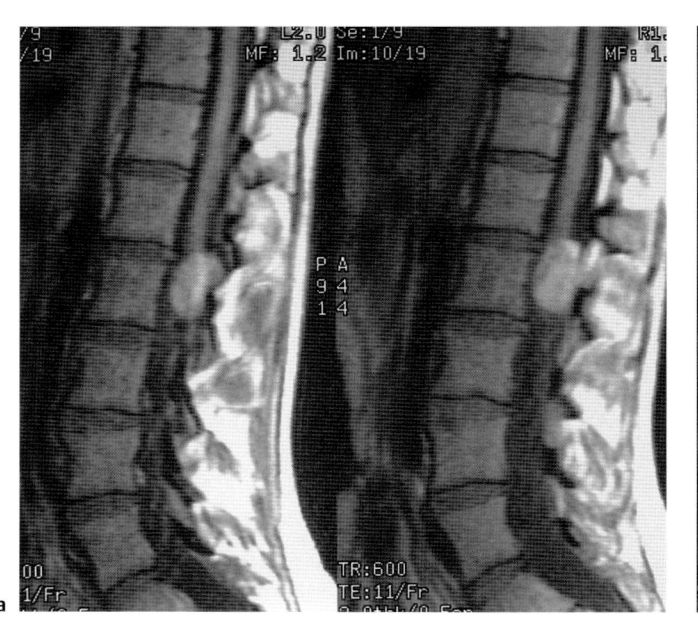

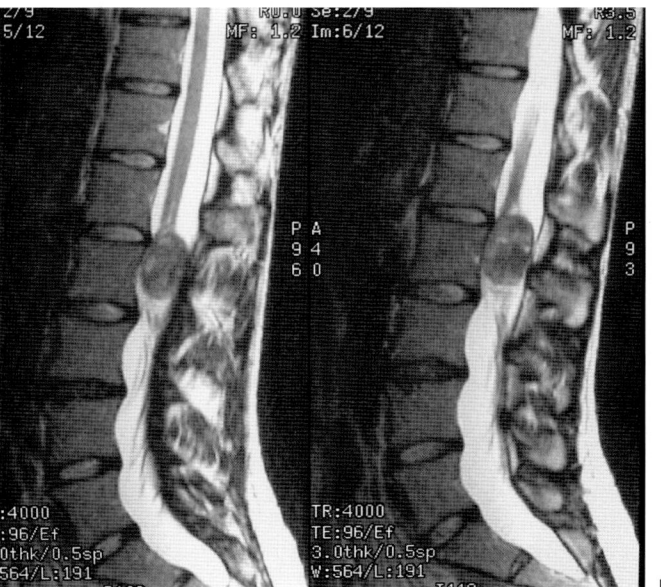

Figure **76 a–c** A 27-year-old woman with a dermoid in the posterior lumbar spinal canal. The lesion has high signal on sagittal T1WI (**a**), and low-intermediate signal on sagittal (**b**) T2WI. Axial CT image (**c**) shows the lesion to contain multiple calcifications.

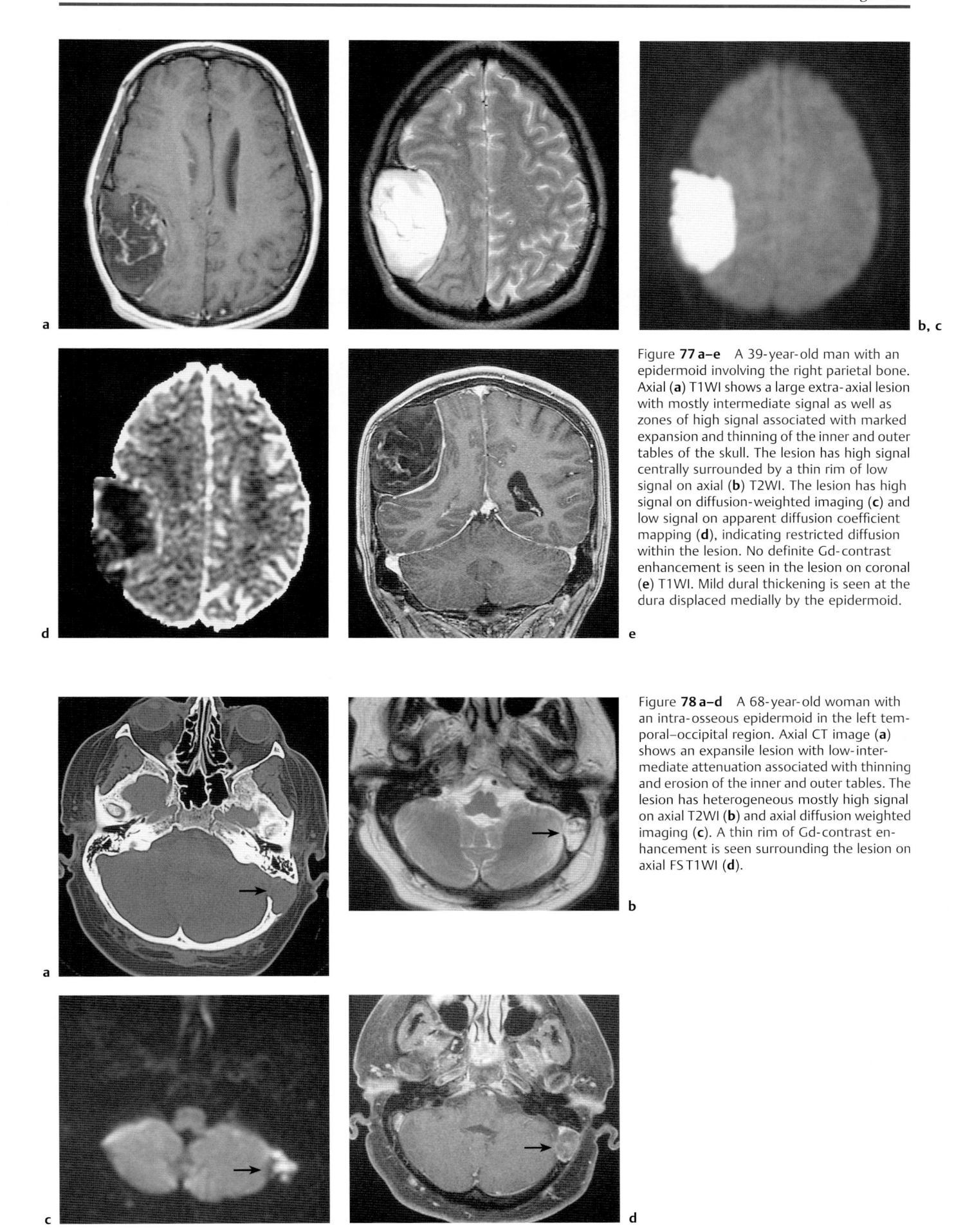

Figure 77 a–e A 39-year-old man with an epidermoid involving the right parietal bone. Axial (**a**) T1WI shows a large extra-axial lesion with mostly intermediate signal as well as zones of high signal associated with marked expansion and thinning of the inner and outer tables of the skull. The lesion has high signal centrally surrounded by a thin rim of low signal on axial (**b**) T2WI. The lesion has high signal on diffusion-weighted imaging (**c**) and low signal on apparent diffusion coefficient mapping (**d**), indicating restricted diffusion within the lesion. No definite Gd-contrast enhancement is seen in the lesion on coronal (**e**) T1WI. Mild dural thickening is seen at the dura displaced medially by the epidermoid.

Figure 78 a–d A 68-year-old woman with an intra-osseous epidermoid in the left temporal–occipital region. Axial CT image (**a**) shows an expansile lesion with low-intermediate attenuation associated with thinning and erosion of the inner and outer tables. The lesion has heterogeneous mostly high signal on axial T2WI (**b**) and axial diffusion weighted imaging (**c**). A thin rim of Gd-contrast enhancement is seen surrounding the lesion on axial FS T1WI (**d**).

Figure 79 a–c A 38-year-old man with an epidermoid along the endocranial surface of the clivus. The lesion has slightly lobulated margins and has low-intermediate signal on sagittal T1WI (**a**) and high signal on axial T2WI (**b**). The lesion has mixed, mostly intermediate signal on axial FLAIR images (**c**).

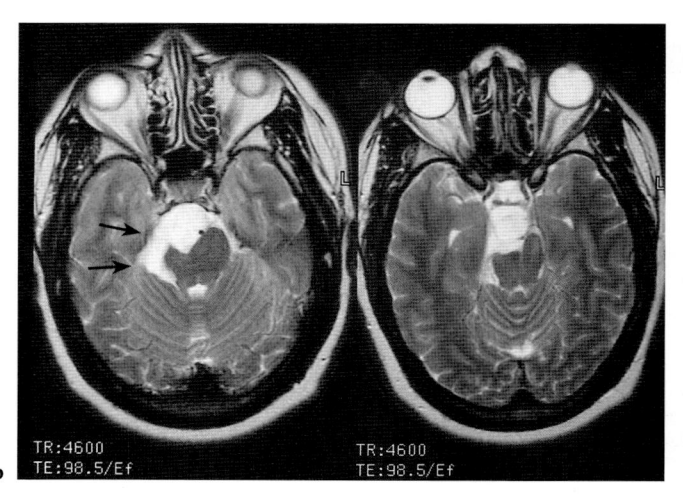

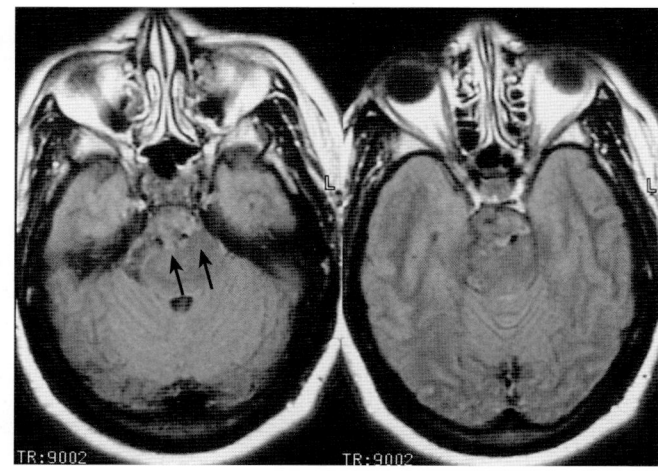

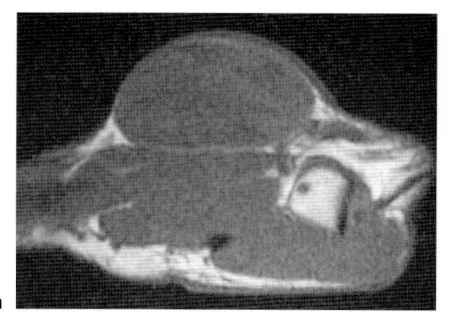

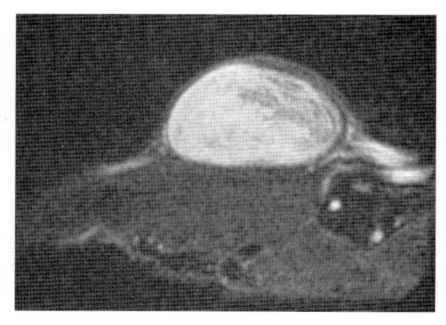

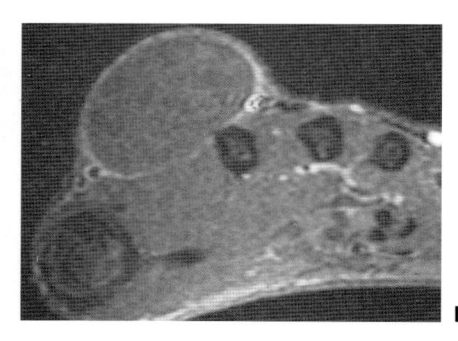

Figure 80 a–c A 35-year-old man with an epidermoid involving the dorsal soft tissues of the hand. The lesion has intermediate signal on sagittal (**a**) T1WI, and heterogeneous mostly high signal on sagittal (**b**) FS T2WI. The lesion shows no Gd-contrast enhancement on axial (**c**) T1WI.

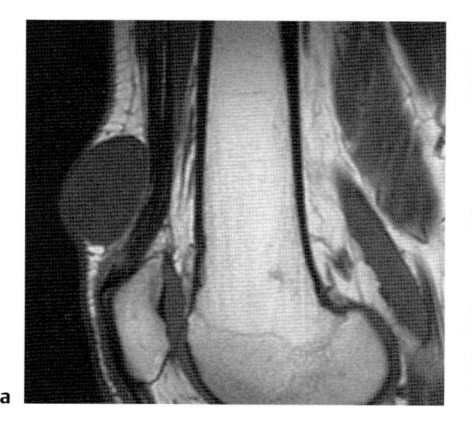

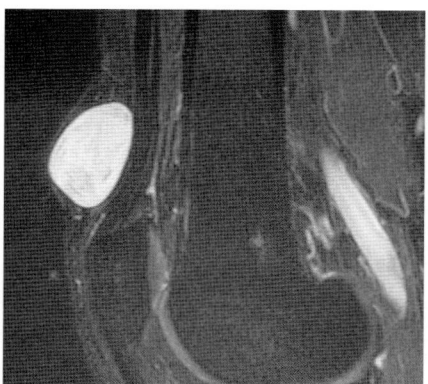

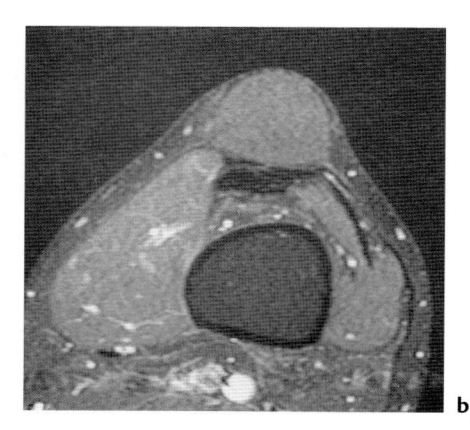

Figure 81 a–c A 25-year-old man with an epidermoid involving the anterior soft tissues at the knee. The lesion has low-intermediate signal on sagittal (**a**) Saggital what? and high signal on sagittal (**b**) FS T2WI. The lesion shows no Gd-contrast enhancement on axial (**c**) T1WI.

Differential Diagnosis

Teratomas, lipomas, liposarcomas, granulomas, fat necrosis, sebaceous cyst.[3]

Prognosis and Treatment

Both dermoids and epidermoids are usually treated with gross total resection.[4,7,8,12,13] Postoperative steroids may be beneficial to minimize the potential of meningitis when these lesions involve the central nervous system.[8]

References

1. Bergui M, Zhong J, Bradac GB, Sales S. Diffusion-weighted images of intracranial cyst-like lesions. *Neuroradiology* 2001;43:824–829.
2. Bonneville F, Sarrazin JL, Marsot-Dupuch K, et al. Unusual lesions of the cerebellopontine angle: a segmental approach. *Radiographics* 2001;21(2):419–438.
3. Calabrò F, Capellini C, Jinkins JR. Rupture of spinal dermoid tumors with spread of fatty droplets in the cerebrospinal fluid pathways. *Neuroradiology* 2000;42:572–579.
4. Caldarelli M, Colosimo C, Di Rocco C. Intra-axial dermoid/epidermoid tumors of the brainstem in children. *Surg Neurol* 2001;56(2):97–105.
5. Chen S, Ikawa F, Kurisu K, Arita K, Takaba J, Kanou Y. Quantitative MR evaluation of intracranial epidermoid tumors by fast fluid-attenuated inversion recovery imaging and echo-planar diffusion-weighted imaging. *AJNR Am J Neuroradiol* 2001;22(6):1089–1096.
6. Kallmes DF, Provenzale JM, Cloft HJ, McClendon RE. Typical and atypical MR imaging features of intracranial epidermoid tumors. *AJR Am J Roentgenol* 1997;169(3):883–887.
7. Mhatre P, Hudgins PA, Hunter S. Dermoid cyst in the lumbosacral region. Radiographic findings. *AJR Am J Roentgenol* 2000;174(3):874–875.
8. Scarrow AM, Levy EI, Gerszten PC, Kulich SM, Chu CT, Welch WC. Epidermoid cyst of the thoracic spine: case history. *Clin Neurol Neurosurg* 2001;103(4):220–222.
9. Smirniotopoulos JG, Chiechi MV. Teratomas, dermoids, and epidermoids of the head and neck. *Radiographics* 1995;15:1437–1455.
10. Szklaruk J, Tamm EP, Choi H, Varavithya V. MR imaging of common and uncommon large pelvic masses. *Radiographics* 2003;23(2):403–424.
11. Tateshima S, Numoto RT, Abe S, Yasue M, Abe T. Rapidly enlarging dermoid cyst over the anterior fontanel: a case report and review of the literature. *Childs Nerv Syst* 2000;16:875–878.
12. Teksam M, Casey SO, Michel E, Benson M, Truwit CL. Intraspinal epidermoid cyst: diffusion-weighted MRI. *Neuroradiology* 2001;43:572–574.
13. Timmer FA, Sluzewski M, Treskes M, van Rooij WJJ, Teepen JLJM, Wijnalda D. Chemical analysis of an epidermoid cyst with unusual CT and MR characteristics. *AJNR Am J Neuroradiol* 1998;19:1111–1112.
14. Zamani AA. Cerebellopontine angle tumors: role of magnetic resonance imaging. *Top Magn Reson Imaging* 2000;11(2):98–107.

A 16 Desmoid Tumor (Also Referred to as Fibromatosis, Superficial and Deep Types Involving Soft Tissues; Desmoplastic Fibroma; Desmoid Tumor within Bone)

Desmoid is derived from the Greek word "desmos" meaning band or tendon.[3]

ICD-O Code

Palmar/plantar fibromatosis: 8821/1

Aggressive fibromatosis: 8821/1

Abdominal (mesenteric) fibromatosis: 8822/1

Desmoplastic fibroma of bone: 8823/0

Definition

Desmoid tumors or fibromatoses represent a group of soft tissue lesions comprised of benign fibrous tissue with elongated or spindle-shaped cells adjacent to collagen.[2,3,5,7,8,10–14, 17,27,31,32,39,41] Lesions are categorized by location as superficial (palmar—Dupuytren contracture, plantar—Ledderhose disease, penile—Peyronie disease) or deep (extra-abdominal, abdominal, or intra-abdominal).[1,3,5,10,11,14,15,17,20,22,31–33,35,37,39,43,44] Aggressive fibromatosis is a type that usually occurs in the deep soft tissues and consists of proliferation of fibrous tissue that infiltrates adjacent tissues.[11,20,31] Aggressive fibromatosis has a greater tendency to recur locally after surgery compared with circumscribed desmoid tumors.[11,20,31] Desmoids rarely occur in bone and are referred to as desmoplastic fibroma.[2,4, 6–9,12,13,16,26,28,30,36,41,42] Desmoid tumors can occur in association with Gardner syndrome and Turcot syndrome.[3,17,28,30,34] Fibromatosis coli is a benign form of infantile fibromatosis involving the distal sternocleidomastoid muscle, which can occur after abnormal intrauterine positioning or difficult deliveries.[17,29]

Frequency of Occurrence

Bone: Desmoplastic fibromas account for <1% of bone lesions[9,23,24,40,41]

Soft tissue:
- **Superficial fibromatosis.** These lesions account for 1.5% of benign soft tissue tumors.[19]
- **Dupuyten contracture (palmar fibromatosis).** These lesions affect 1–2% of the population, up to 20% of patients older than 60 years of age.[17]
- **Plantar fibromatosis.** These lesions account for ~1% of benign soft tissue tumors.[18,19]
- **Deep fibromatosis (adults).** These lesions account for 5% of benign soft tissue tumors.[18,19] The incidence is 2–4 per million per year[11,20]
- **Deep fibromatosis (children).** These lesions are rare.[39]
- **Fibromatosis coli.** These lesions are rare and occur in 0.4% of live births.[17,29]

Age at Presentation

Superficial fibromatosis: from 17 to 65 years, mean = 41 years.[18,19]

Dupuyten contracture (palmar fibromatosis): usually affects adults > 60 years.[10,17]

Plantar fibromatosis: from 20 to 60 years.[10,17]

Deep fibromatosis (adults): from 13 to 60 years, mean = 34 years[18,19,31]; peak age between 25 and 35 years.[20]

Deep fibromatosis (children): from 6 months to 8 years, mostly in first 2 years.[14,39]

Fibromatosis coli: most cases are diagnosed in infants below 6 months.[29]

Desmoplastic fibroma: from 1 to 71 years, mean = 20 years, median = 34 years, peaks in 2nd decade.[9,12,13,25,26,41]

Gender Ratio (M/F)

Superficial fibromatosis: 2/1.[19]

Dupuytren contracture: 3–4/1.[10,17]

Plantar fibromatosis: 1/1.[10, 17]

Deep fibromatosis (adults): 1/1.4 to 1/2.[19,31]

Deep fibromatosis (children): predominantly occurs in males.[14]

Fibromatosis coli: 1/1.[29]

Desmoplastic fibroma: 1/1 to 2/1.[9,13,41]

Location

Bone:
- **Desmoplastic fibroma** is a rare bone tumor that represents the intra-osseous version of desmoid tumor (fibromatosis). These lesions are usually present in the dimetaphyseal region, although can be seen in the diaphyseal or epiphyseal regions.[9,13] Mandible > iliac bone > humerus > tibia > vertebrae > ulna > scapula > femur.[13,16] Lesions in the skull have also been reported.[4,30]

Soft tissue:
- **Superficial fibromatosis.** Lesions occur in the foot and ankle > hand and wrist > trunk.[19] Duputyren contracture involves the palmar aponeurosis, often at the distal palmar crease (fourth > fifth > third > second rays, bilateral in 50%); plantar fibromatosis involves the plantar aponeurosis (usually medial, bilateral in 35%), and Peyronie / fibromatosis involves the penis.[10,17]
- **Deep fibromatosis (adults) / abdominal desmoids.** These lesions occur in the mesentery, retroperitoneum.[3,20] Desmoid tumors also occur in the abdominal wall at musculoaponeurotic structures.[3,20] Common sites include the rectus, oblique, and tranversalis muscles, and/or fascia.[3]
- **Deep fibromatosis / extra-abdominal desmoids (adults).** These lesions occur in the chest wall, paraspinal tissues, pelvic wall, mediastinum, extremities (lower extremity > foot and ankle > hand and wrist > upper extremity), head and neck, and mediastinum.[3,11] Locations for deep fibromatosis have been reported in order of decreasing frequency as:

trunk > lower extremity > foot and ankle > retroperitoneum > head and neck, hip and buttocks, hand and wrist, upper extremity.[19] For aggressive fibromatosis, involvement occurs in the upper extremity in 25 to 40% of cases, lower extremity in 20–30%, head and neck in 20–30%, and trunk in 10–15%.[27]

- **Deep fibromatosis (children).** Common sites include: head and neck (tongue, mandible, maxilla, mastoid), trunk, and proximal extremities.[14] Intra-abdominal desmoids in children are uncommon.[14]
- **Fibromatosis coli.** Lesions are characteristically located at the distal lower portion of the sternocleidomastoid muscle.[17,29]

Signs and Symptoms

Dupuytren contracture. These lesions occur as subcutaneous soft tissue nodules in the palmar aspect of hand, usually at the distal skin crease.[17] These lesions can restrict movement.[17]

Plantar Fibromatosis. These lesions occur as subcutaneous firm soft-tissue nodule or nodules (~33%) in the plantar aspect of the foot.[17]

Deep fibromatosis (adults and children). Patients can have solitary firm lesions noticed in skeletal muscle and/or adjacent fascia or aponeurosis.[3,11,17] Lesions are usually not painful.[3,11,17,31,32] Lesions can also be seen in the trunk, tongue, head, and neck.[3,17,31]

Fibromatosis coli. Infants often present with a firm mass in the lower third of the sternocleidomatoid muscle 2–4 weeks after birth.[17,29] The affected muscle is thickened and shortened in length, resulting in cervicofacial asymmetry.[29] Torticollis is seen in up to 20% of infants with fibromatosis coli.[17] Fibromatosis coli can be seen in association with other developmental abnormalities such as forefoot anomalies (metatarsus adductus, talipes equinovarus) and hip dysplasia with congenital hip dislocation.[17,29]

Desmoplastic fibromas. These lesions are usually asymptomatic until they become large, or because of pathologic fracture.[12,41] Pathologic fractures occur in 12% of desmoplastic fibromas.[2]

Gross Pathologic Findings

Dupuytren contracture. Lesions can appear as nodules or poorly defined nodular aggregates of gray-white or yellow firm tissue.[10,17]

Plantar fibromatosis. Lesions can appear as nodules or poorly defined nodular aggregates of gray-white or yellow firm tissue.[10,17]

Deep fibromatosis. These lesions are usually firm and gritty, and on cut surface are glistening white to light gray.[11,17] Lesions lack a true capsule. Lesions range from 2 to 20 cm in size.[11]

Fibromatosis coli. Lesions typically appear as fusiform, tan gritty masses involving the lower sternocleidomastoid muscle, and usually measure <5 cm in length and <2 cm in width.[29]

Desmoplastic fibroma. Lesions are usually firm, rubbery, and gray-white with a variegated whorled pattern.[8,13]

Histopathologic Findings

Dupuytren contracture. Lesions typically consist of benign fibrous tissue with elongated or plump spindle-shaped cells with little variability in appearance containing normochromatic nuclei with small nucleoli.[10] Mitotic figures are infrequent.[10] The spindle-shaped cells are usually associated with moderate or large amounts of collagen.[10,17]

Plantar fibromatosis. Lesions typically consist of benign fibrous tissue with elongated or plump spindle-shaped cells of little variability in appearance, which contain normochromatic nuclei with small nucleoli.[10] Mitotic figures are infrequent.[10] The spindle-shaped cells are often associated with moderate to large amounts of collagen.[10,17] Occasional multinucleated giant cells may be seen.[10]

Deep fibromatosis (adults and children). These lesions are often poorly marginated with infiltrative margins, and contain varying proportions of elongated spindle-shaped or fibroblast-like cells surrounded by dense bands of collagen.[3,11,14,31] Nuclei are usually small and pale, and contain between one and three nucleoli.[11,31] Mitoses are infrequent[3,11,14] Lesions can infiltrate adjacent tissue including muscle, which may result in reactive multinucleated giant cells.[11,31] Lesions tend to be more invasive/aggressive in children than in adults.[17] These lesions may be associated with Gardner syndrome and Turcot syndrome.[3,17,28,31] These tumors are immunoreactive to vimentin, muscle specific and smooth muscle actin as well as beta-catenin.[11]

Fibromatosis coli. Lesions contain groups of plump, spindle-shaped cells within myxoid and/or collagenous ground substance.[29] The relative proportions of spindle cells, myxoid material, and collagen can vary depending on the time of evaluation.[29] Long standing lesions often have less spindle cells and relatively larger amounts of collagen compared with earlier stage lesions.[29] Multinucleated skeletal myocytes, plump fibroblastic and myofibroblastic cells may also be seen in fine needle aspirates or surgical specimens.[29]

Desmoplastic fibroma. These lesions contain varying proportions of wavy bands of collagen and elongated spindle-shaped cells containing spindly-appearing nuclei. Mitotic figures are typically absent or rare.[8,13]

Lesion Genetics

Superficial fibromatoses often have near-diploid kartyotypes, as well as gains of chromosomes 7 or 8.[10] Desmoid-type fibromatoses and desmoplastic fibromas of bone can have cells with trisomies for chromosomes 8 and/or 20 in ~30% of lesions.[8,11] Inactivation of the APC tumor suppressor gene on chromosome 5q has been reported in patients with familial polyposis, and occasionally in patients with sporadic desmoid tumors.[11] Patients with sporadic desmoid tumors have been reported to have mutations affecting beta-catenin, altering the normal inhibiting influence of the APC gene product effect.[11]

Findings on Plain Films (Roentgenograms) and Computed Tomography

Superficial fibromatosis. On plain films a small soft tissue lesion may be seen, whereas on CT a focal lesion with soft tissue attenuation may be observed.

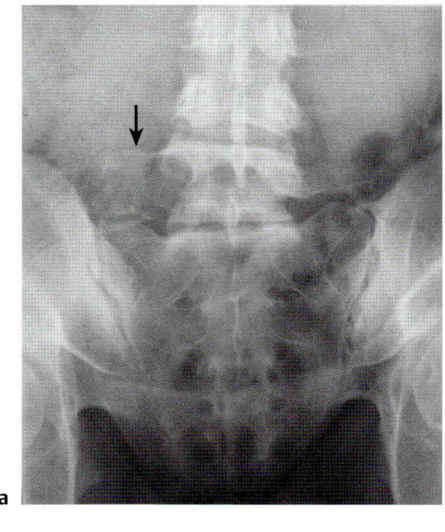

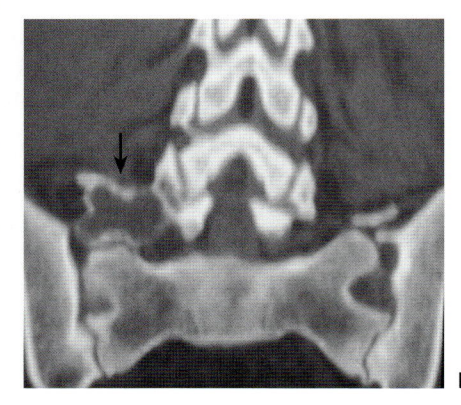

Figure **82 a–e** Desmoplastic fibroma involving the L5 vertebral body, right pedicle and transverse process. AP radiograph (**a**), and coronal (**b**) and axial (**c**) CT images show an expansile, radiolucent lesion with a thin peripheral shell of bone. The lesion has mostly intermediate signal on axial PDWI (**d**) and mixed signal with zones of intermediate, slightly high, high, and low signal on axial T2WI (**e**).

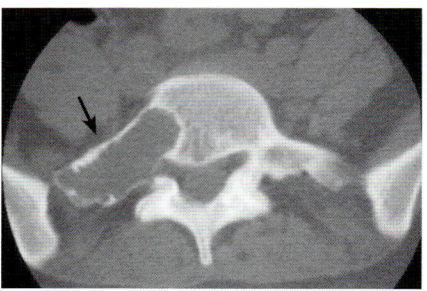

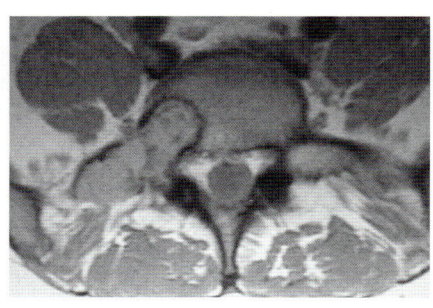

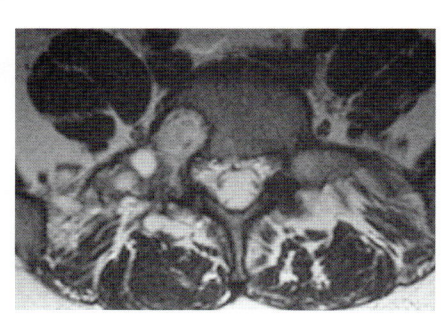

Deep fibromatosis (adults and children). Desmoids may appear on plain films as poorly-defined soft tissue lesions, which may cause bone erosion, periosteal reaction, and/or bone deformation.[17,27] In children, bowing of bone can occur.[17,27] Calcifications are uncommon.[20] On CT, desmoids can appear as soft tissue lesions with attenuation usually similar to or slightly increased relative to muscle.[3,5,14,27] Occasionally, attenuation of the lesions may be lower than muscle. Margins of lesions can be distinct and/or poorly defined.[3,5,14,27] Lesions show variable enhancement.[27] CT readily shows sites of bone erosion.[27,31]

Fibromatosis coli. On CT, fusiform swelling of the lower sternocleidomastoid muscle is usually seen.[17]

Desmoplastic fibroma.[6–9,12,13,23,41] Desmoplastic fibromas are typically radiolucent, lobulated, centrally located lesions with abrupt zones of transition, with or without: trabeculated appearance at borders, bone expansion with thinning of cortex, reactive sclerosis, and/or periosteal reaction (Fig. **82**). The lesions typically do not have matrix mineralization. CT is more accurate than plain films in defining the extent of bone destruction.[23]

MRI Findings

Dupuytren contracture. Lesions (10–55 mm) are seen along the flexor tendons. Lesions have low-intermediate signal on T1WI and T2WI.

Plantar fibromatosis. Lesions are usually present along the medial portion of the plantar aponeurosis. Lesions often have well-defined borders to superficial fat and somewhat ill-defined margins with adjacent deep muscles. Invasion of muscles is seen in 15 % of cases. Lesions have heterogeneous low-intermediate signal on T1WI, PDWI, and T2WI, slightly high to high signal on fat suppressed T2WI or STIR (Fig. **83**). Lesions show various degrees of heterogeneous Gd-contrast enhancement.

Deep fibromatosis (adults and children).[1,3,14,15,17,20,21,27,31,33,34,39,43,44] Lesions can have distinct and/or poorly defined margins and can cross fascial compartments.[20] Lesions usually have homogeneous or heterogeneous low-intermediate signal on T1WI, intermediate signal on PDWI, and variable intermediate-high signal on T2WI (with or without zones of low signal) and slightly high to high signal on FS T2WI (Figs. **84–86**). Myxoid zones in the lesions can have high signal on T1WI and T2WI. Tumors with high cellularity tend to show higher signal on T2WI than lesions with larger proportions of collagen. Lesions show variable degrees and patterns (heterogeneous vs. homogenous) of Gd-contrast enhancement. Pattern or degree of Gd-contrast enhancement by desmoids does not enable prediction of rate of tumor recurrence.

Fibromatosis coli.[17] Lesions usually appear as fusiform enlargement of the lower sternocleidomastoid muscle.[17] No discrete focal lesions are usually seen in the enlarged lower sternocleidomastoid muscle.[17] The involved muscle can have low-intermediate signal on T1WI, PDWI, and T2WI; and low, intermediate and/or slightly high signal on FS T2WI[17] (Fig. **87**).

Desmoplastic fibroma.[2,4,9,16,23,41,42] Desmoplastic fibromas are lobulated lesions with abrupt zones of transition. Lesions usually have low-intermediate signal on T1WI, intermediate signal on PDWI, and heterogeneous intermediate to high signal on T2WI (Fig. **82**). Lesions may have internal or peripheral zones of low signal on T1WI and T2WI secondary to dense collagenous parts of the lesions and/or foci with high signal on T2WI from cystic zones. Thin curvilinear zones of low signal on T2WI can be seen

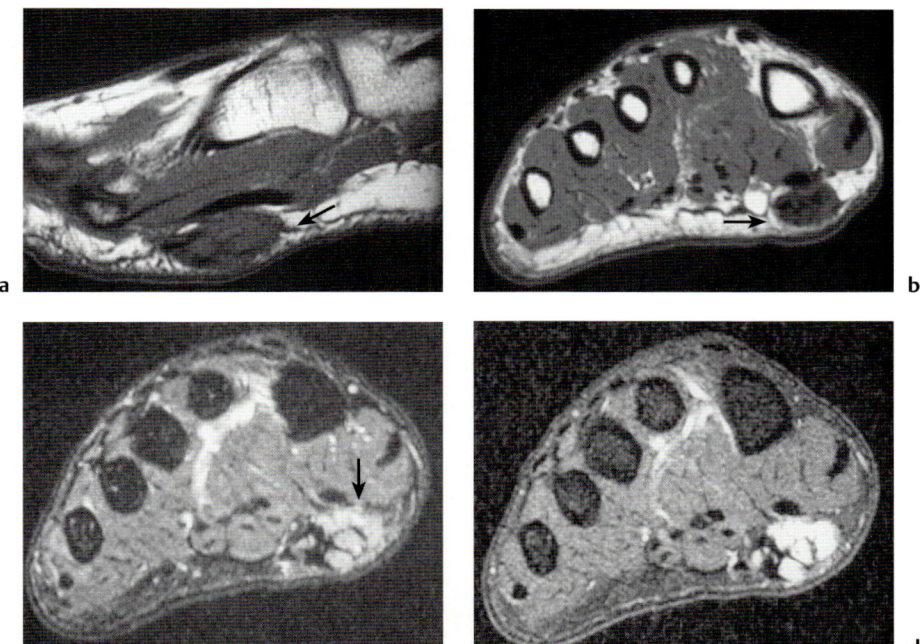

Figure **83 a–d** Desmoid tumor (plantar fibromatosis) involving the superficial soft tissues at the plantar aspect of the foot. The lesion has intermediate and low signal on sagittal (**a**) and axial (**b**) T1WI, and heterogeneous mostly high signal on axial FS T2WI (**c**). The lesion shows prominent Gd-contrast enhancement on axial FS T1WI (**d**).

at the margins of the lesions. Lesions show variable degrees and patterns of Gd-contrast enhancement.[5,23] Gd-contrast enhancement typically occurs in the more cellular portions of the lesions compared with the hypocellular and collagenous parts. Cortical disruption and soft tissue extension are commonly seen.

Differential Diagnosis

Superficial fibromatosis. Post-traumatic scar involving tendon or aponeurosis, giant cell tumor of tendon sheath, fibroma of tendon sheath, granuloma, gout.

Deep fibromatosis. Malignant fibrous histiocytoma, liposarcoma, leiomyosarcoma, malignant Schwannoma, synovial sarcoma, fibrosarcoma, rhabdomyosarcoma, epitheloid sarcoma, Kaposi sarcoma, clear cell sarcoma, malignant granular cell tumor, nodular fasciitis, neurofibroma, Schwannoma, giant cell tumor of tendon sheath, granular cell tumor, leiomyoma, fibroma of tendon sheath, proliferative fasciitis, dermatomyositis, hematoma, proliferative myositis, heterotopic bone formation.

Desmoplastic fibroma. Nonossifying fibroma, fibrous dysplasia, low-grade fibrosarcoma, unicameral or aneurysmal bone cyst, chondromyxoid fibroma, giant cell tumor, lymphoma, myeloma, metastatic lesion.

Treatment and Prognosis

Dupuytren contracture. These lesions are slow-growing.[10] Surgical excision is the standard treatment.[10] The risk of local recurrence is related to the extent of surgical resection.[10] Dermatofasciectomy with subsequent skin grafting usually produces the lowest recurrence rate.[10]

Plantar fibromatosis. These lesions are slow-growing.[10] Surgical excision is the standard treatment.[10] The risk of local recurrence is related to the extent of surgical resection, presence of multiple nodules, and presence of bilateral lesions.[10] Dermatofasciectomy with subsequent skin grafting usually produces the lowest recurrence rate.[10]

Deep fibromatosis. These lesions are more aggressive and infiltrative than superficial fibromatosis with regard to growth rate, size, and invasion of adjacent tissues.[11,14,27,31] Deep fibromatosis in children tends to be more aggressive and invasive than in adults.[14,17] Surgical excision with wide margins of normal-appearing tissue is the optimal treatment to include areas of tumor invasion not palpable at surgery or defined with imaging.[11,14,17] Local recurrence ranges from 25 to 77% of patients.[17,32] Radiation has been used as adjuvant therapy.[14,31,32] Chemotherapy has also been used as adjuvant treatment in children.[14,31,38,39] Lesions typically do not metastasize.[11,17,20,32,39] Lesions can invade neurovascular bundles and joints causing contractures. Severe morbidity from prolonged recurrences may require limb amputation.[32,39]

Fibromatosis coli. Lesions can initially grow rapidly, followed by progressively slower growth rates.[17] Lesions can then regress from 5 months to 2 years after diagnosis.[17] Most lesions are successfully treated with passive stretching and physiotherapy.[29] However, persistent masses are found in 10–15% of patients with associated abnormal cervicocranial posture despite passive stretching; and surgical tenotomy may be needed.[29] Up to 90% of patients have normal function after treatment with either passive stretching, physiotherapy, and/or tenotomy.[29] Patients older than 1 year with fibromatosis coli are typically less responsive to treatment than younger infants.[29]

Desmoplastic fibroma. These tumors are slowly progressive and locally aggressive.[2,7,8,26,30] The lesions can be treated with en bloc resection and/or definitive curettage with or without bone grafts.[7,8,26,30] Local recurrence has been reported to be 17% for en bloc resection,[2] and up to 47–72% for currettage.[2,7,8] Local recurrence can occur up to 8 years after treatment.[8] Radiation is not recommended because of the potential for dedifferentiation and/or malignant degeneration.[13]

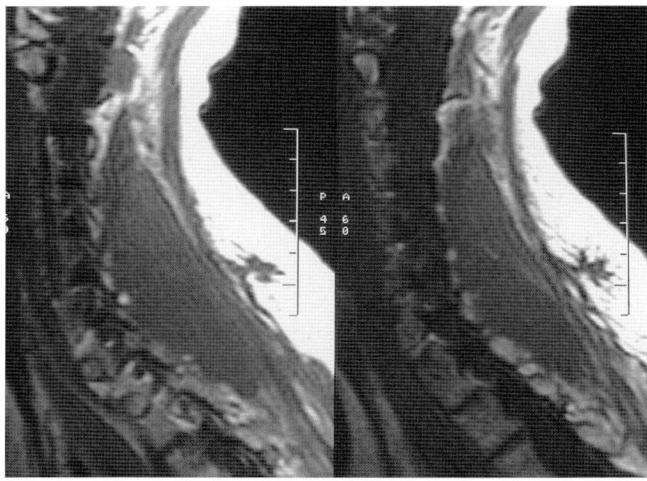

Figure **84 a–f** A 20-year-old woman with Turcot syndrome and multiple desmoid tumors involving the posterior paraspinal muscles of the cervical and upper thoracic spine (**a**, **b**, **c**) and lumbar spine (**d**, **e**, **f**). Sagittal (**a**, **d**) T1WI shows fusiform lesions with low-intermediate signal which have high signal on sagittal (**b**, **e**) T2WI. The lesions show prominent Gd-contrast enhancement on sagittal (**c**, **f**) FS T1WI.

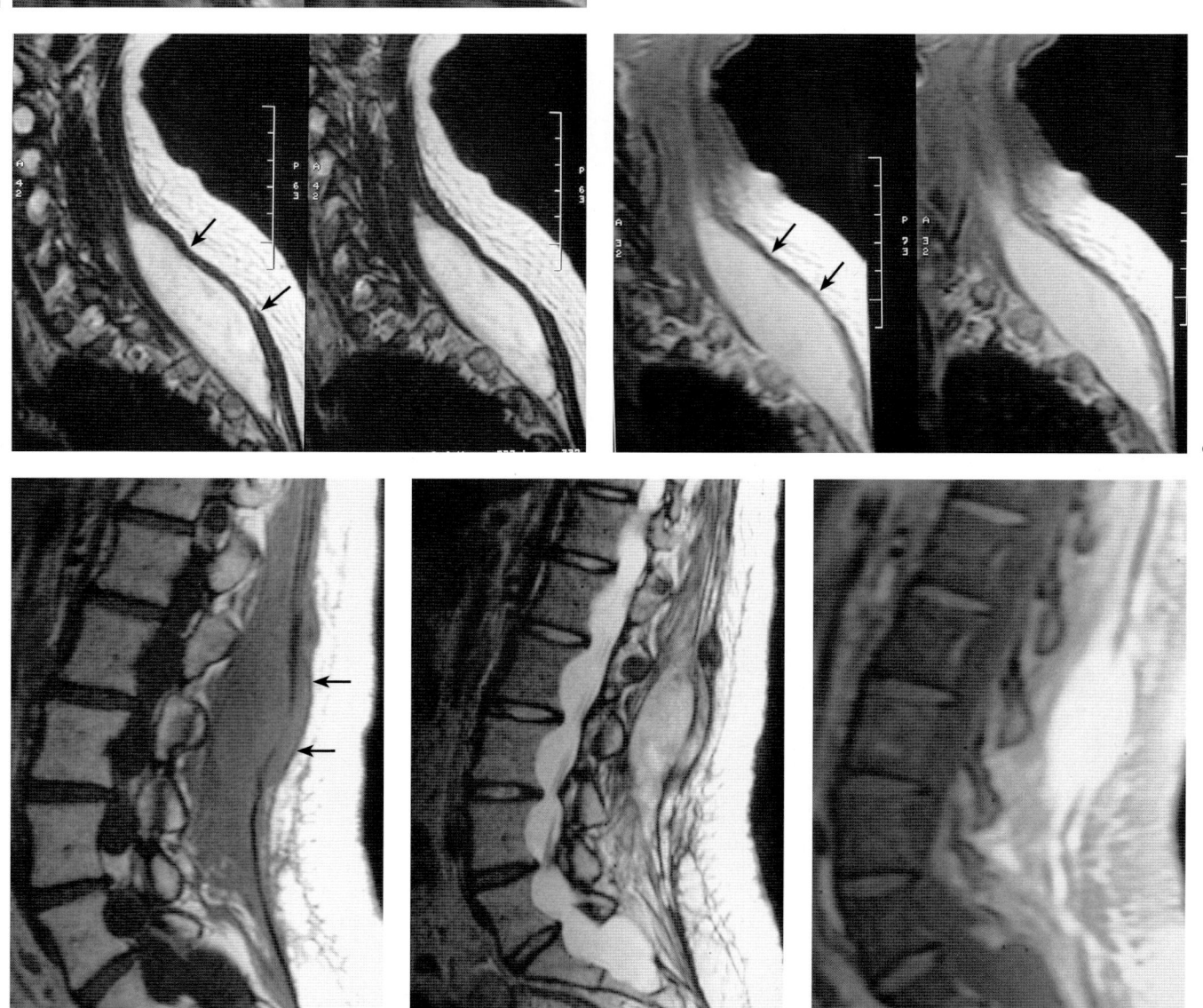

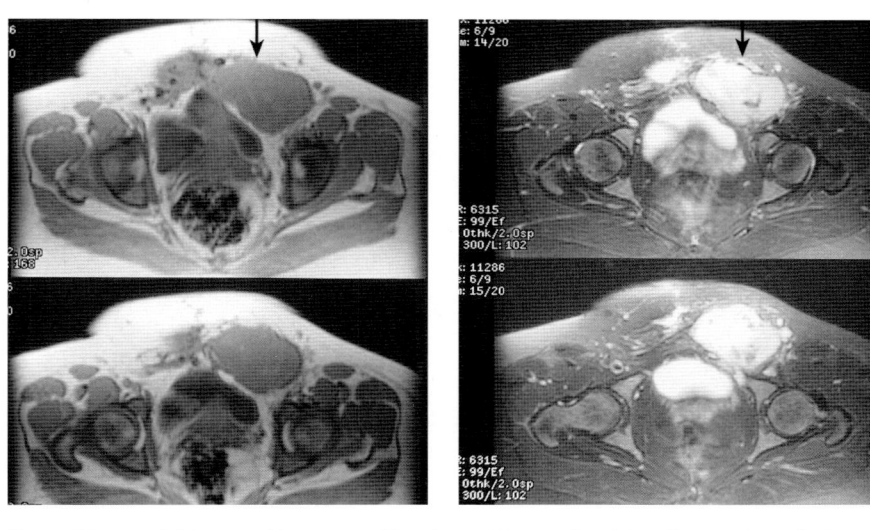

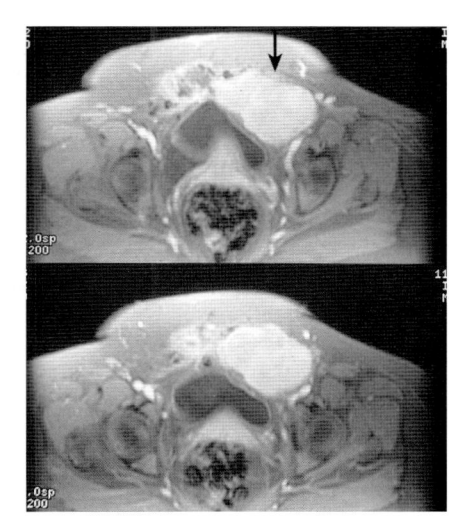

Figure **85 a–c** A 31-year-old woman with a desmoid tumor involving the anterior soft tissues at the pelvis. The lesion has intermediate signal on axial PDWI (**a**), and high signal on axial FS T2WI (**b**). The lesion shows prominent Gd-contrast enhancement on axial FS T1WI (**c**).

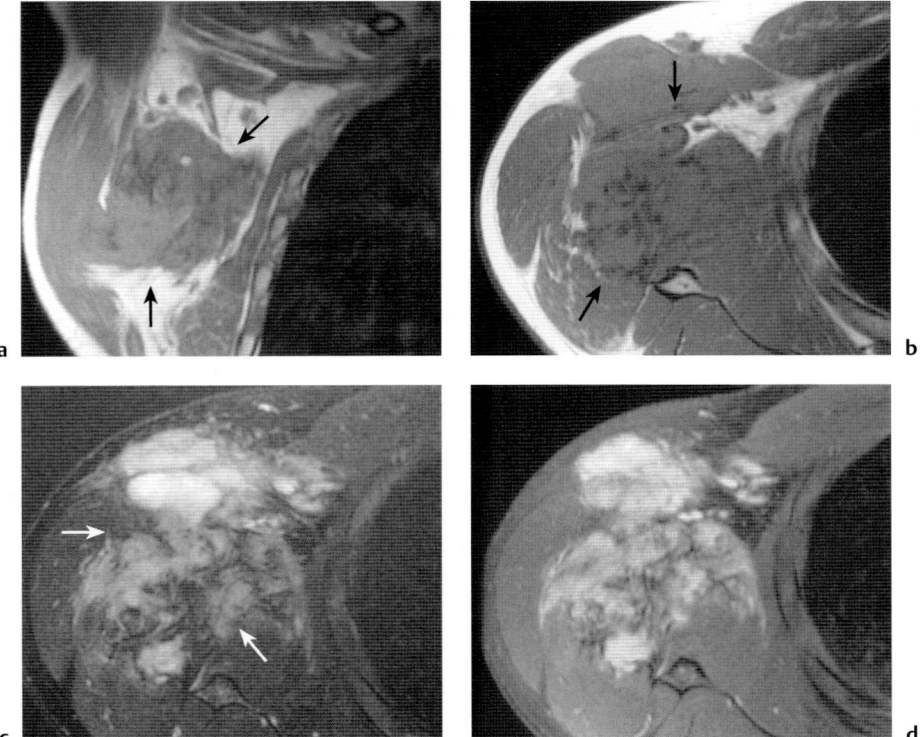

Figure **86 a–d** A 32-year-old man with aggressive fibromatosis involving the soft tissues in the right axilla. MRI shows a lobulated lesion with indistinct margins which has intermediate signal on coronal (**a**) and axial (**b**) T1WI, and slightly high and high signal on axial (**c**) FS T2WI. Foci and thin curvilinear zones of low signal are also seen on T1WI and FS T2WI. The lesion shows prominent heterogeneous Gd-contrast enhancement on axial (**d**) FS T1WI.

References

1. Bissett GS III. MR imaging of soft-tissue masses in children. *Magn Reson Imaging Clin N Am* 1996;4(4):697–719.
2. Bohm P, Krober S, Greschniok A, Laniado M, Kaiserling E. Desmoplastic fibroma of the bone. A report of two patients, review of the literature, and therapeutic implications. *Cancer* 1996;78:1011–1023.
3. Casillas J, Sais GJ, Greve JL, Iparraguirre MC, Morillo G. Imaging of intra- and extraabdominal desmoid tumors. *Radiographics* 1991;11(6):959–968.
4. Celli P, Cervoni L, Trillo G. Desmoplastic fibroma of the skull. Case report and review of the literature. *Neurochirurgie* 1997;43:260–264.
5. Chaudhuri B, Das Gupta TK. Pathology of soft tissue sarcoma. In: Das Gupta TK, Chaudhuri PK, eds. *Tumors of the Soft Tissues* 2nd ed. New York, NY: Appleton and Lange; 1998:88–95.
6. Crim JR, Gold RH, Mirra JM, Eckardt JJ, Bassett LW. Desmoplastic fibroma of bone: radiographic analysis. *Radiology* 1989;172:827–832.
7. Forest M. Desmoplastic fibroma of bone. In: Forest M, Tomeno B, Vanel D, eds. *Orthopedic Surgical Pathology: Diagnosis of Tumors and Pseudotumoral Lesions of Bone and Joints* Edinburgh: Churchill Livingstone; 1998:303–316.
8. Fornasier V, Pritzker KPH, Bridge JA. Desmoplastic fibroma of bone. In: Fletcher CDM, Unni KK, Mertens F, eds. *World Health Organization Classification of Tumours. Pathology and Genetics of Tumours of Soft Tissue and Bone* Geneva: IARC Press; 2002:288.
9. Frick MA, Sundaram M, Unni KK, et al. Imaging findings in desmoplastic fibroma of bone: distinctive T2 characteristics. *AJR Am J Roentgenol* 2005;184:1762–1767.

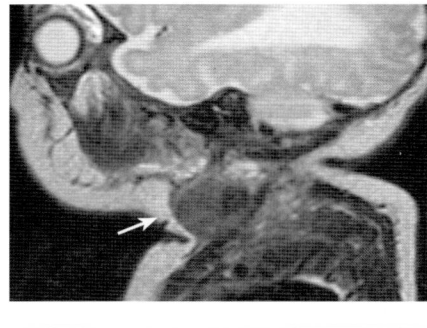

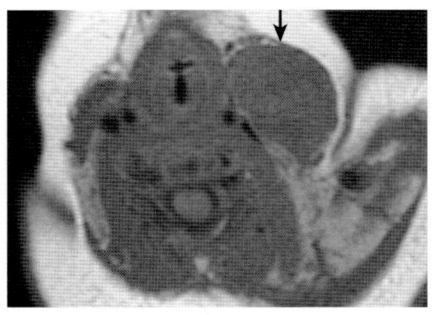

Figure **87 a–d** A 5-week-old male infant with fibromatosis coli involving the left sternoclavicular muscle. There is fusiform thickening of the left sternoclavicular muscle which has low-intermediate signal on sagittal T2WI (**a**), intermediate signal on axial T1WI (**b**), and mixed low, intermediate, and slightly high signal on axial FS T2WI (**c**). Minimal Gd-contrast enhancement is seen on coronal FS T1WI (**d**).

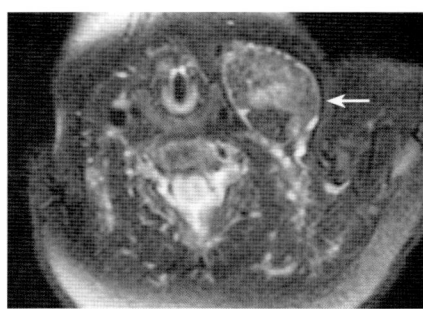

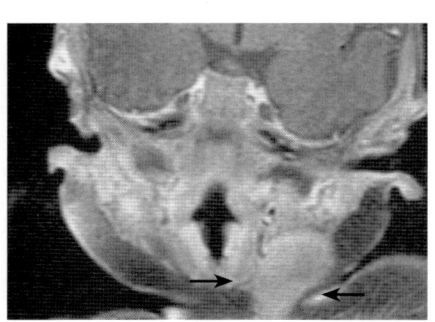

10 Goldblum J, Fletcher JA. Superficial fibromatoses. In: Fletcher CDM, Unni KK, Mertens F, eds. *World Health Organization Classification of Tumours. Pathology and Genetics of Tumours of Soft Tissue and Bone* Geneva: IARC Press; 2002:81–82.

11 Goldblum J, Fletcher JA. Desmoid-type fibromatoses. In: Fletcher CDM, Unni KK, Mertens F, eds. *World Health Organization Classification of Tumours. Pathology and Genetics of Tumours of Soft Tissue and Bone* Geneva: IARC Press; 2002:83–84.

12 Huvos AG. Desmoplastic fibroma and periosteal "desmoid". In: Huvos AG, ed. *Bone Tumors: Diagnosis, Treatment, and Prognosis*, 2nd ed. Philadelphia, Pa: W.B. Saunders; 1991:404–405.

13 Kilpatrick SE, Unni KK. Spindle cell lesions of bone. In: Helliwell TR, ed. *Major Problems in Pathology: Pathology of Bone and Joint Neoplasms*. Vol 37. 1st ed. Philadelphia, Pa: W.B. Saunders, 1999: 239–240.

14 Kingston CA, Owens CM, Jeanes A, Malone M. Pictorial essay—Imaging of desmoid fibromatosis in pediatric patients. *AJR Am J Roentgenol* 2002;178:191–199.

15 Kobayashi H, Kotoura Y, Hosono M, et al. MRI and scintigraphic features of extraabdominal desmoid tumors. *Clin Imaging* 1997; 21(1):35–39.

16 Kong KY, Kang HS, Jung HW, Kim JJ, Lee CK. MR findings of desmoplastic fibroma of the spine. A case report. *Acta Radiol* 2000;41: 89–91.

17 Kransdorf MJ, Murphey MD. Benign fibrous and fibrohisiocytic tumors. In: *Imaging of Soft Tissue Tumors* 2nd ed. Philadelphia, Pa: W.B. Saunders; 2006:189–256.

18 Kransdorf MJ, Murphy MD. Soft tissue tumors in a large referral population: prevalence and distribution of diagnoses by age, sex, and location. In: *Imaging of Soft Tissue Tumors* 2nd ed. Philadelphia, Pa: W.B. Saunders; 2006:6–37.

19 Kransdorf MJ. Benign soft-tissue tumors in a large referral population: distribution of specific diagnoses by age, sex, and location. *AJR Am J Roentgenol* 1995;164:395–402.

20 Lee JC, Thomas JM, Phillips S, Fisher C, Moskovic E. Aggressive fibromatosis: MRI features with pathologic correlation. *AJR Am J Roentgenol* 2006;186:247–254.

21 Lee JK, Glazer HS. Controversy in the MR imaging appearance of fibrosis. *Radiology* 1990;177:21–22.

22 Lewis JJ, Boland PJ, Leung DH, Woodruff JM, Brennan MF. The enigma of desmoid tumors. *Ann Surg* 1999;229:866–873.

23 Mahnken AH, Nolte-Ernsting CC, Wildberger JE, Wirtz DC, Gunther RW. Cross-sectional imaging patterns of desmoplastic fibroma. *Eur Radiol* 2001;11:1105–1110.

24 Mulder JD, Schutte HE, Kroon HM, Taconis WK. Introduction. In: *Radiologic Atlas of Bone Tumors* Amsterdam: Elsevier; 1993:3–6.

25 Mulder JD, Schutte HE, Kroon HM, Taconis WK. The diagnosis of bone tumors. In: *Radiologic Atlas of Bone Tumors* Amsterdam: Elsevier ; 1993:9–46.

26 Mulder JD, Schutte HE, Kroon HM, Taconis WK. Desmoplastic fibroma. In: *Radiologic Atlas of Bone Tumors* Amsterdam: Elsevier; 1993:541–547.

27 Mulder JD, Schutte HE, Kroon HM, Taconis WK. Fibromatosis. In: *Radiologic Atlas of Bone Tumors* Amsterdam: Elsevier; 1993:639–646.

28 Mullins KJ, Rubio A, Meyers SP, Korones DN, Pilcher WH. Malignant ependymomas in a patient with Turcot's syndrome: case report and management guidelines. *Surg Neurol* 1998;49:290–294.

29 O'Connell. Fibromatosis coli. In: Fletcher CDM, Unni KK, Mertens F, eds. *World Health Organization Classification of Tumours. Pathology and Genetics of Tumours of Soft Tissue and Bone* Geneva: IARC Press; 2002:61–62.

30 Pensak ML, Nestok BR, VanLoveren H, Shumrick KA. Desmoplastic fibroma of the temporal bone. *Am J Otol* 1997;18:627–631.

31 Perez-Cruet MJ, Burke JM, Weber R, DeMonte F. Aggressive fibromatosis involving the cranial base in children. *Neurosurgery* 1998; 43(5):1096–1102.

32 Pignatti G, Barbanti-Brodano G, Ferrari D, et al. Extraabdominal desmoid tumor: a study of 83 cases. *Clin Orthop Relat Res* 2000; 375:207–213.

33 Quinn SF, Erickson SJ, Dee PM, et al. Walling MR imaging in fibromatosis: results in 26 patients with pathologic correlation. *AJR Am J Roentgenol* 1991;156:539–542.

34 Rai AT, Nguyen TP, Hogg JP, Gabriele FJ. Aggressive fibromatosis of the neck in a patient with Gardner's syndrome. *Neuroradiology* 2001;43:650–652.

35 Romero JA, Kim EE, Kim CG, Chung WK, Isiklar I. Different biologic features of desmoid tumors in adults and juvenile patients: MR demonstration. *JComput Assist Tomogr* 1995;19:782–787.

36 Shuto R, Kiyosue H, Hori Y, Miyake H, Kawano K, Mori H. CT and MR imaging of desmoplastic fibroma *Eur Radiol* 2002;12:2474–2476.

37 Siegel MJ. Magnetic resonance imaging of musculoskeletal soft tissue masses. *Radiol Clin North Am* 2001;39(4):714–715.

38 Skapek SX, Hawk BJ, Hoffer F, et al. Combination chemotherapy using vinblastine and methotrexate for the treatment of progressive desmoid tumor in children. *J Clin Oncol* 1998;16:3021–3027.

39 Spiegel DA, Dormans JP, Meyer JS, et al. Aggressive fibromatosis from infancy to adolescence. *J Pediatr Orthop* 1999;19(6):776–784.

40 Unni KK. Introduction and scope of study. In: *Dahlin's Bone Tumors: General Aspects and Data on 11087 Cases* 5th ed. Philadelphia, Pa: Lippincott, Williams & Wilkins; 1996:1–9.

41 Unni KK. Fibrosacroma and desmoplastic fibroma. In: *Dahlin's Bone Tumors: General Aspects and Data on 11087 Cases* 5th ed. Philadelphia, Pa: Lippincott, Williams & Wilkins; 1996:197–210.

42 Vanhoenacker FM, Hauben E, De Beuckeleer LH, Willemen D, Van Marck E, De Schepper AM. Desmoplastic fibroma of bone: MRI features. *Skeletal Radiol* 2000;29:171–175.

43 Van Slyke MA, Moser RP Jr, Madewell JE. MR imaging of periarticular soft-tissue lesions. *Magn Reson Imaging Clin N Am* 1995;3(4):662–664.

44 Weatherall PT. Benign and malignant masses. *Magn Reson Imaging Clin N Am* 1995;3(4):669–694.

A 17 Elastofibroma

ICD-O Code

8820/0

Definition

Elastofibromas are benign, slow-growing fibroblastic tumorlike lesions that contain large amounts of enlarged coarse elastic fibers.[1-6,9-13] These lesions typically occur in patients over 50 years old, and most are located between the lower scapula and chest wall.[1-6,9-13] The etiology of these lesions is uncertain.[2] It has been suggested that these lesions are not true neoplasms but are fibroblastic pseudotumors that result from repetitive trauma or friction between the lower scapula and adjacent chest wall, or result from focal abnormal elastogenesis.[2,6] A genetic predisposition to these lesions has been shown in some cases.[2,6,9]

Frequency of Occurrence

Elastofibromas are rare and account for 0.3% of benign soft tissue tumors.[5-8] These lesions are typically asymptomatic and have been suggested to be more common than previously reported.[11] Lesions smaller than 3 cm have been found at autopsy in 24% of women and 11% of men older than 55 years.[11]

Age at Presentation

From 48 to 74 years, mean = 61 years,[8] median = 70 years.[3] Peak occurrence is in the 7th and 8th decades.[2]

Gender Ratio (M/F)

1/1 to 1/2 [6,8]

Location

The most common sites are the trunk between lower scapula and chest wall (96%) > lower extremity (2%), hip and buttock (2%).[8] Bilateral parascapular lesions are not uncommon.[4,6,9] Other reported sites include the deltoid muscle, thoracic wall, axilla, infra-olecranon fossa, thigh, hand, foot, spinal canal, joints, greater trochanter region, viscera, gastrointestinal tract, and sclera.[1,2,9,10]

Signs and Symptoms

Elastofibromas are slow-growing lesions that rarely cause pain and tenderness.[2,6] Parascapular lesions may be associated with limitation in range of motion of the shoulder.[1]

Gross Pathologic Findings[1,2,4-6]

Elastofibromas are usually gray-white or gray-tan rubbery lesions with internal zones of yellow fat, and often range from 2 to 15 cm in size.[1,2,4-6] Lesions typically have ill-defined margins.[1,2,4,5]

Histopathologic Findings[1,2,4-6,9-11]

Elastofibromas contain mixtures of hyalinized collagenous tissue with scattered fibroblasts, large numbers of elastic fibers, entrapped mature fat cells, and small amounts of mucoid stroma.[1,2,4,5,9-11] The elastic fibers are typically hypereosinophilic.[2,6] Elastic fibers can be branched or unbranched, large and coarse, and/or organized into linear arrangements of small globules or serrated disks which may have a "pipe-cleaner" or "beads on a string" appearance.[2,6]

Lesion Genetics

These lesions have been found to commonly have abnormalities involving the short arm of chromosome 1.[2]

Findings on Plain Films (Roentgenograms) and Computed Tomography[1,4,5,9,10]

These lesions frequently have a lenticular shape with or without well-defined margins. They often have mostly soft tissue attenuation similar to skeletal muscle, as well as variable amounts of low attenuation from intralesional fatty deposits. Chronic erosions may be seen in adjacent bones.[1]

MRI Findings[1,3-5,9-13]

Lesions often range from 5 to 10 cm, and frequently have a lenticular shape with or without well-defined margins. On T1WI and T2WI, lesions often have mostly intermediate signal that is isointense to muscle, as well as variable amounts of high signal from intralesional fatty deposits (Fig. **88**). After Gd-contrast administration, lesions usually show variable degrees of enhancement, often in a heterogeneous pattern.

Differential Diagnosis

Atypical lipoma, liposarcoma, hemangioma, hematoma, desmoid, neurofibroma, lymphangioma, hamartoma, cicatricial fibroma, malignant fibrous histiocytoma.[9,11]

Treatment and Prognosis

Elastofibromas are slow-growing benign lesions that are cured by complete excision.[2] Local recurrence is rare.[2,9] These lesions have been reported to have no malignant potential[9] Core or fine-needle biopsies can be useful in excluding the diagnosis of sarcoma and avoiding surgery.[3,4,13]

References

1 Bae SJ, Shin MJ, Kim SM, Cho KJ. Intra-articular elastofibroma of the shoulder joint. *Skeletal Radiol* 2002;31:171–174.
2 Hashimoto H, Bridge JA. Elastofibroma. In: Fletcher CDM, Unni KK, Mertens F, eds. *World Health Organization Classification of Tumours. Pathology and Genetics of Tumours of Soft Tissue and Bone* Geneva: IARC Press; 2002:56–57.
3 Hayes AJ, Alexander N, Clark MA, Thomas JM. Elastofibroma: a rare soft tissue tumour with a pathognomonic anatomical location and clinical symptom. *Eur J Surg Oncol* 2004;30:450–453.

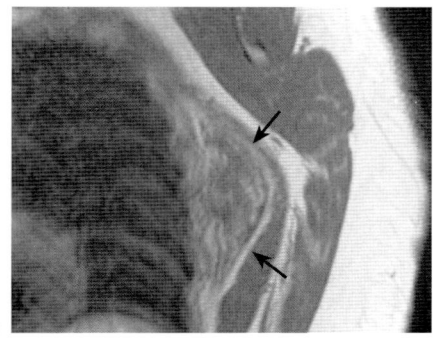

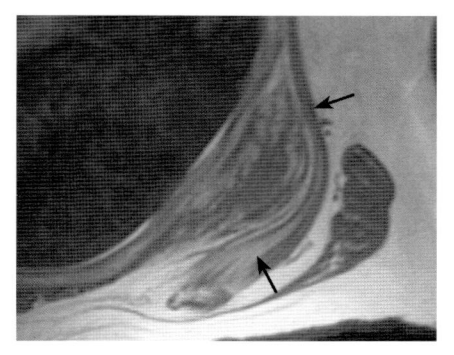

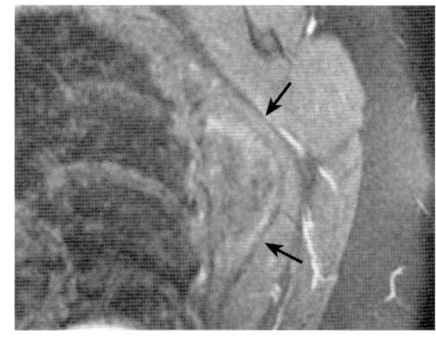

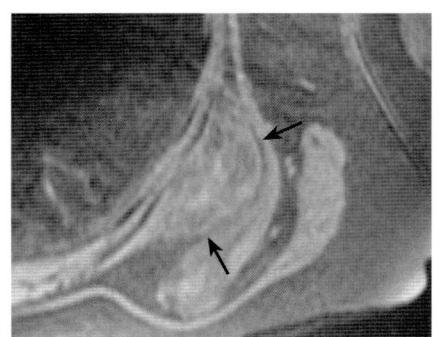

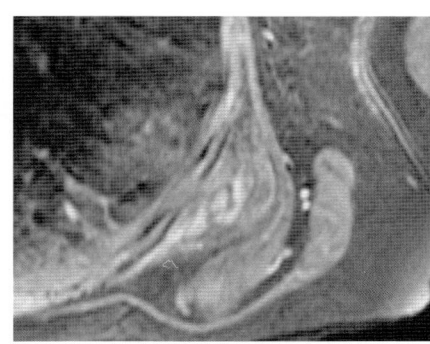

Figure **88 a–d** Elastofibroma located between the lower scapula and chest wall in a 68-year-old woman. Coronal (**a**) and axial (**b**) T1WI show a lens-shaped lesion, which has mixed intermediate and high signal. The high signal zones represent intralesional fat as seen on coronal (**c**) FS T1WI and axial (**d**) FS T1WI. The lesion shows a heterogeneous pattern of Gd-contrast enhancement on FS T1WI (**e**).

4 Hsieh SC, Shih Tiffany TF, Li YW. Bilateral elastofibroma dorsi two case reports. *Clin Imaging* 1999;23(1):47–50.

5 Kransdorf MJ, Meis JM, Montgomery E. Elastofibroma: MR and CT appearance with radiologic–pathologic correlation. *AJR Am J Roentgenol* 1992;159:575–579.

6 Kransdorf MJ, Murphey MD. Benign fibrous and fibrohistiocytic tumors. In: Kransdorf MJ, Murphey MD, eds. *Imaging of Soft Tissue Tumors* 2nd ed. Philadelphia, Pa: W.B. Saunders; 2006:189–256.

7 Kransdorf MJ, Murphy MD. Soft tissue tumors in a large referral population: prevalence and distribution of diagnoses by age, sex, and location. In: Kransdorf MJ, Murphey MD, eds. *Imaging of Soft Tissue Tumors* 2nd ed. Philadelphia, Pa: W.B. Saunders; 2006:6–37.

8 Kransdorf MJ. Benign soft-tissue tumors in a large referral population: distribution of specific diagnoses by age, sex, and location. *AJR Am J Roentgenol* 1995;164:395–402.

9 Naylor MF, Nascimento AG, Sherrick AD, McLeod RA. Elastofibroma dorsi: radiologic findings in 12 patients. *AJR Am J Roentgenol* 1996;167:683–687.

10 Nishida A, Uetani M, Okimoto T, Hayashi K, Hirano T. Bilateral elastofibroma of the thighs with concomitant subscapular lesions. *Skeletal Radiol* 2003;32:116–118.

11 Schick S, Zembsch A, Gahleitner A, et al. Atypical appearance of elastofibroma dorsi on MRI: case report and review of the literature. *J Comput Assist Tomogr* 2000;24(2):288–292.

12 Yu JS, Weis LD, Vaughan LM, Resnick D. MRI of elastofibroma dorsi. *J Comput Assist Tomogr* 1995;19(4):601–603.

13 Zembsch A, Schick S, Trattnig S, Walter J, Amann G, Ritschl P. Elastofibroma dorsi. Study of two cases and magnetic resonance imaging findings. *Clin Orthop Relat Res* 1999; (364):213–219.

A 18 Eosinophilic Granuloma (Also Referred to as Langerhans Cell Histiocytosis, Formerly Histiocytosis X)

ICD-O Code

Langerhans cell histiocytosis: 9751/1

Langerhans cell histiocytosis (unifocal): 9752/1

Langerhans cell histiocytosis (multifocal): 9753/1

Langerhans cell histiocytosis (disseminated): 9754/3

Definition[8,9,13,21,23,25]

Single or multiple eosinophilic granulomas are benign, tumor-like lesions consisting of Langerhans cells (histiocytes) and variable amounts of lymphocytes, polymorphonuclear cells, and eosinophils. Langerhans cells are mononuclear cells involved in both immune and nonimmune inflammatory responses. Langerhans cells are derived from bone marrow stem cells (CD 34+) and perform important roles in immune regulation. There are three types of Langerhans cell histiocytosis: a localized type involving bone or lung, **eosinophilic granuloma**; and two systemic types, the acute–subacute fulminant **Letterer–Siwe disease**, and a chronic disseminated form, **Hand–Schüller–Christian disease**

Frequency of Occurrence

Eosinophilic granulomas[8,9,13,19,23–25] account for 70% of Langerhans cell histiocytosis, 1% of primary bone lesions, and 8% of tumor-like lesions; 5–20 per million children per year in the United States, 1–2 per million in the Netherlands, 1 per 200 000 children per year younger than 15 years.

Letterer–Siwe disease accounts for 10% of Langerhans cell histiocytosis.[23]

Hand–Schüller–Christian disease accounts for 20% of Langerhans cell histiocytosis.[23]

Age at Presentation

Eosinophilic granuloma. From 1 to 60 years, median = 10 years, average = 13.5 years, peak incidence is between 5 and 10 years; 80–85% occur in patients less than 30 years, and 60% occur in children less than 10 years.[8,9,13,17–19,23–25] Lesions involving the mandible tend to occur in older patients, average age = 26 years.[13]

Letterer–Siwe disease. This usually occurs in children younger than 3 years.[19,23]

Hand–Schüller–Christian disease. This occurs in children from 1 to 5 years.[23]

Gender Ratio (M / F)

Eosinophilic granuloma: 1.1 / 1 to 2 / 1.[13,19,23]

Letterer–Siwe disease: 1 / 1.[23]

Hand–Schüller–Christian disease: 1.3 / 1.[23]

Location

Eosinophilic granuloma.[1,3,8,9,12,13,19,23] Lesions occur in the skull / craniofacial bones > femur > iliac bone > rib > vertebrae > humerus > tibia > other bones. Intra-osseous locations are diaphyseal (two-thirds) > metadiaphyseal > metaphyseal > epi-metaphyseal.[19] In vertebrae, the vertebral body is the most common location for eosinophilic granulomas.[13,19,20,22] Involvement of the posterior elements is rare.[1,3,19,20,22]

Letterer–Siwe disease. This disease often involves multiple organs such as the liver, spleen, lymph nodes, lungs, and bone.[23]

Hand–Schüller–Christian disease. Lesions are located in the liver, spleen, lymph nodes, skin, and bones.[23]

Signs and Symptoms

Eosinophilic granuloma.[1–4,8–13,15,19–23,25] The clinical manifestations depend on the sites of bony involvement. Signs and symptoms include localized pain and swelling, exophthalmos (orbital lesion), otitis media (temporal bone), diabetes insipidus (sella turcica), and spinal or neural compression (vertebral lesions). Pathologic fractures of long bones are uncommon.

Letterer–Siwe disease. This disease is associated with hepatosplenomegaly, lymphadenopathy, anemia, petechiae, osseous lesions, and/or skin rashes.[23]

Hand–Schüller–Christian disease. This disease is associated with otitis media, exophthalmos (25%), polyuria / diabetes insipidus (< 50%) from lesions at the skull base or direct involvement of the pituitary gland or stalk, palpable skull lesions, bleeding and loosening of teeth from mandibular or maxillary lesions, hepatosplenomegaly, lymphadenopathy, eczema, xanthomatosis, anemia, low-grade fevers, and elevated erythrocyte sedimentation rates.[23,25] The clinical triad of this disease includes exophthalmos, diabetes insipidus, and radiolucent bone lesions.[25]

Gross Pathologic Findings

Eosinophilic granulomas are often soft yellow-brown lesions, with or without areas of hemorrhage or cysts associated with zones of bone destruction.[8,9,13,19,21,23,25]

Letterer–Siwe disease occurs as osseous / soft tissue lesions plus hepatosplenomegaly and lymphadenopathy.[23,25]

Hand–Schüller–Christian disease occurs as osseous / soft tissue lesions plus hepatosplenomegaly and lymphadenopathy.[23,25]

Histopathologic Findings

Lesions of Langerhans cell histiocytosis have variable cellular compositions of Langerhans cells, macrophages, osteoclast-like giant cells, polymorphonuclear cells, and eosinophilic leukocytes.[8,9,13,14,16,19,21,23,25] Langerhans cells have folded or indented nuclei with homogeneous pink granular cytoplasm. Eosinophilic leukocytes have irregular bilobed or indented nuclei and are a prominent feature of the lesions. Langerhans cell histiocytes are typically immunoreactive to S-100, CD 1 a, and CD 68.[8,13,14] CD 1 a is a membrane glycoprotein that is a marker for Langerhans cells.[8,14] CD 68 is a glycoprotein in lysosomes of histiocytes and monocytes/macrophages, and positive immunoreactivity can be seen with Langerhans cell histiocytosis as well as non-Langerhans histiocyte subpopulations, such as with Erdheim–Chester disease.[8,14] With electron microscopy, 20% of Langerhans cell histiocytes have cytoplasm that contains X bodies, also referred to as Birbeck granules.[8,13,14,25]

Findings on Plain Films (Roentgenograms) and Computed Tomography

Langerhans cell histiocytosis involving bone.[4,6,8,9,12,13,19,20,22,23,25]: Lesions are typically radiolucent with either well-circumscribed or poorly-defined margins, with or without sclerotic margins, and with or without associated soft tissue mass (Figs. **89, 92, 94–97**). In the healing phases, lesions may have sclerotic margins.

- **Long Bones.** Lesions usually are radiolucent zones in diaphyseal or metadiaphyseal regions, endosteal scalloping and cortical lucent are common. Periosteal reaction is common, with or without extension into adjacent soft tissues. Lesions may be associated with pathologic fractures.[4,6,8,9,12,13,15,19,21–23,25]
- **Flat bones.** Eosinophilic granulomas in flat bones often appear as poorly-defined radiolucent lesions.[23]
- **Skull.** Lesions can have unequal erosion of the inner and outer tables giving a "beveled edge" appearance, with or without a central small sclerotic zone referred to as a "button sequestrum."[12,20,22,23]
- **Mandible.** Zones of lucency with "floating teeth" may be seen.[6,23]
- **Spine.** Lesions are typically located in the vertebral bodies and occasionally in the posterior elements.[3,12,22,23] Occasional collapse of the vertebral body may result.[22,23] Lesions rarely cause significant spinal canal compression. Disk spaces are usually preserved.

Findings on Radionuclide Bone Scans

Lesions show variable radiopharmaceutical accumulation (55% show increased uptake, 35% show normal uptake, and 10% show decreased uptake).

MRI Findings[1–3,5–7,11,12,16,19,20,22,23,26]

Langerhans cell histiocytosis usually appears as focal intramedullary lesion(s) associated with trabecular and cortical bone destruction. Lesions typically have low-intermediate signal on T1WI and PDWI; and heterogeneous slightly-high to high signal on T2WI[1–3,5–7,11,12,16,19,20,22,23,26] (Figs. **89–97**). Poorly defined zones of high signal on T2WI are usually seen in the marrow peripheral to the portions of the lesions associated with radiographic evidence of bone destruction, indicating reactive inflammatory and edematous changes.[2,5,26]

Extension of lesions from the marrow into adjacent soft tissues through areas of cortical disruption are commonly seen as well as linear periosteal zones of high signal on T2WI.[1–3,5,7,11,12,16,19,20,22,23]

Lesions typically show prominent Gd-contrast enhancement in marrow and in extra-osseous soft tissue portions of the lesions.[6,11,12,20,23] Poorly defined zones of Gd-contrast enhancement are also seen in the marrow peripheral to the portions of the lesions associated with radiographic evidence of bone destruction, indicating reactive inflammatory and edematous changes.[2,5,11,12,16,22,23] These perilesional MRI findings have been shown to be correlated with inflammatory reaction associated with elevated tumor prostaglandin levels.[26]

Lesions involving the skull often are associated with scalp and dural enhancement representing reactive inflammation[12,20] (Figs. **89, 90**).

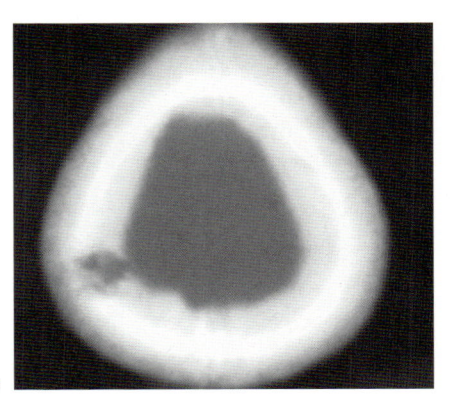

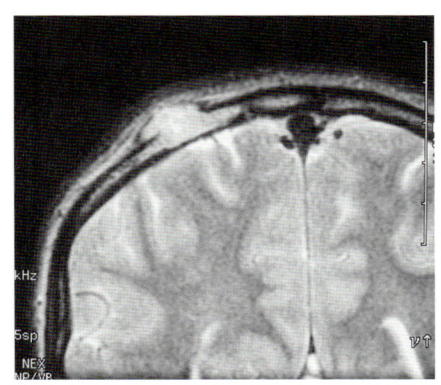

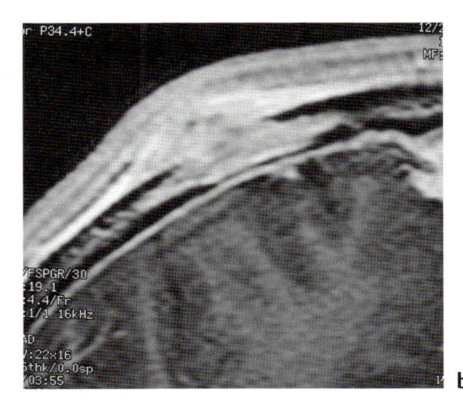

Figure **89 a–c** A 14-year-old female with an eosinohilic granuloma involving the skull. Axial CT image (**a**) shows a radiolucent lesion with slightly irregular margins. The lesion has high signal on coronal T2WI (**b**), and extends from the marrow into the scalp through a zone of cortical destruction. Poorly defined zones of high signal on T2WI are seen in the marrow peripheral to the portions of the lesions associated with radiographic evidence of bone destruction. The lesion shows prominent Gd-contrast enhancement in marrow and in the extra-osseous soft tissue portion of the lesion on coronal T1WI (**c**). Poorly defined zones of Gd-contrast enhancement are also seen in the marrow peripheral to the portions of the lesion that are associated with radiographic evidence of bone destruction.

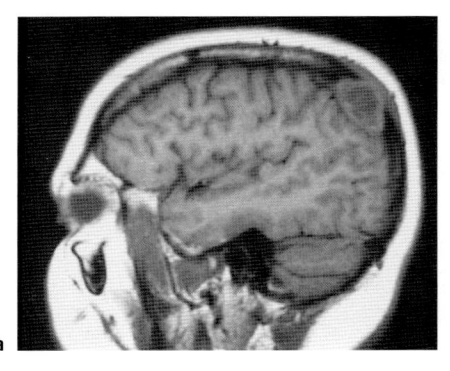

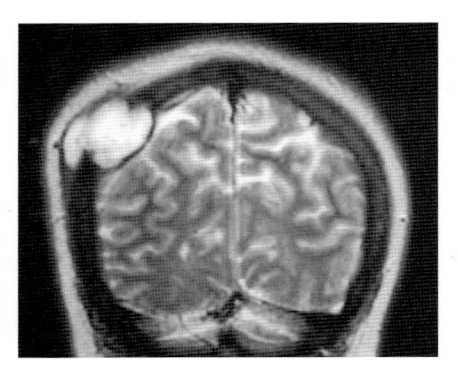

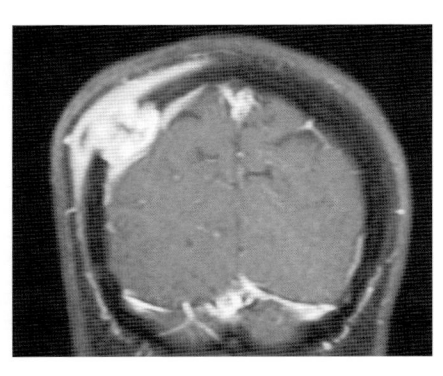

Figure **90 a–c** 20-year-old woman with an eosinophilic granuloma involving the right parietal bone. The lesion has low-intermediate signal on sagittal (**a**) T1WI, and high signal on coronal (**b**) T2WI. Intracranial and extracranial extension of the lesion is seen through areas of cortical disruption. The lesion shows prominent Gd-contrast enhancement in the marrow, intracranial and extracranial portions of the lesion as well as the dura on coronal (**c**) FS T1WI.

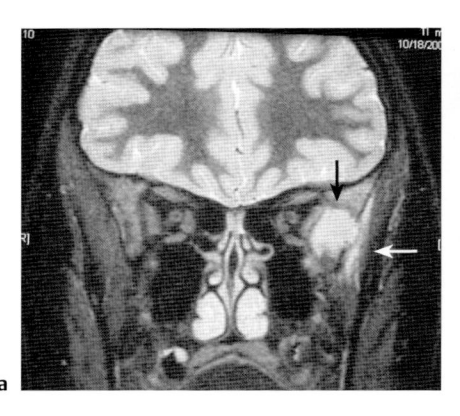

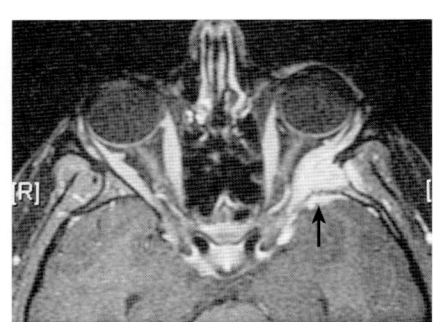

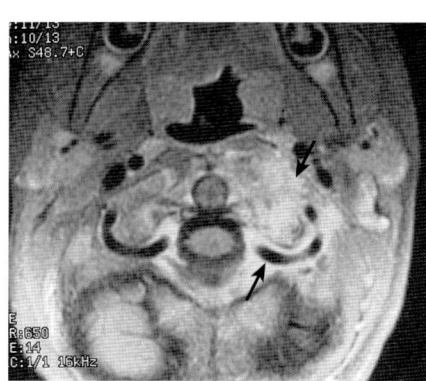

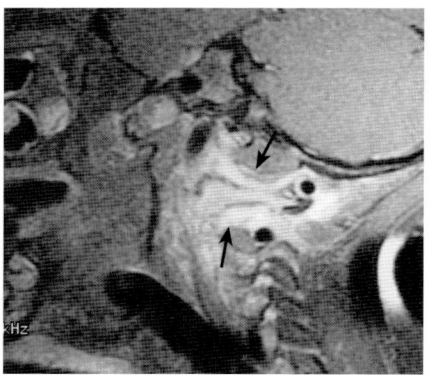

Figure **91 a, b** A 13-year-old female with an eosinophilic granuloma involving the left zygoma, with associated bone destruction and extra-osseous extension into the orbit and lateral soft tissues. The lesion has high signal on coronal STIR (**a**), and shows prominent Gd-contrast enhancement on axial FS T1WI (**b**).

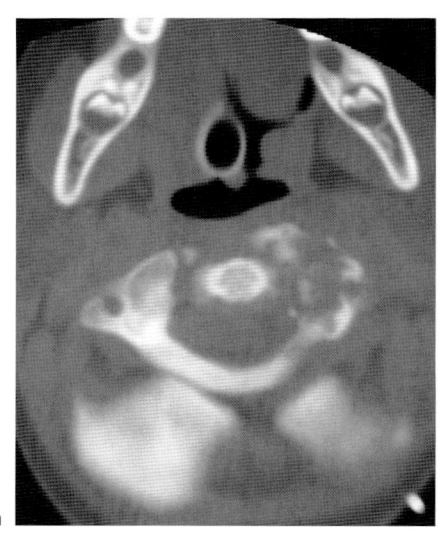

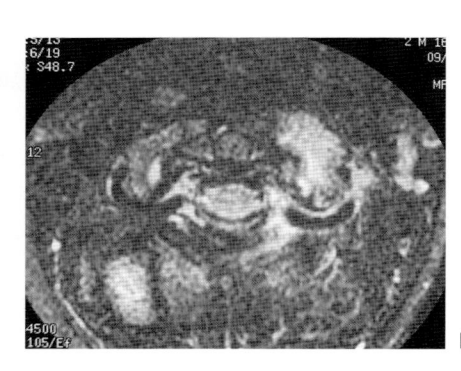

Figure **92 a–d** A 2-year-old male with an eosinophilic granuloma involving the articular mass and pedicle of C 1. The lesion is radiolucent with poorly defined margins on axial CT (**a**). The lesion has high signal on axial FS T2WI (**b**). The lesion shows prominent Gd-contrast enhancement in marrow and in the extra-osseous soft tissue portions on axial (**c**) and sagittal (**d**) FS T1WI.

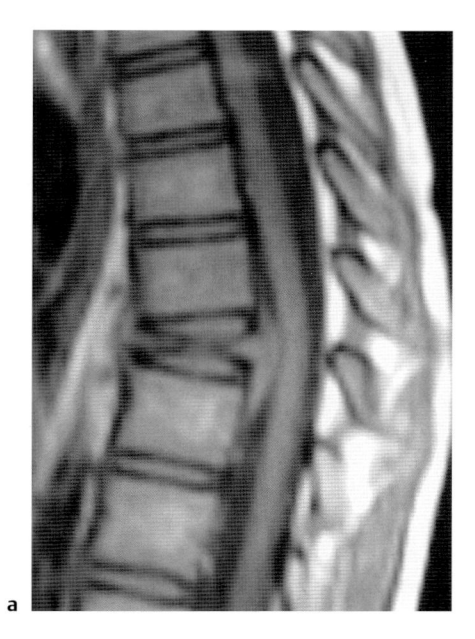

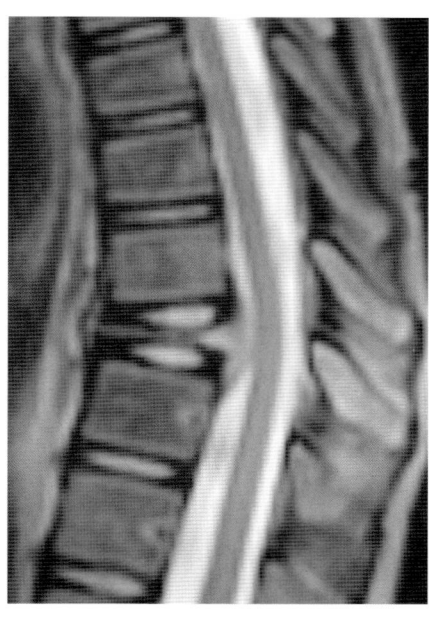

Figure **93 a, b** An 11-year-old female with an eosinophilic granuloma involving the T9 vertebral body with collapse. The lesion has low-intermediate signal on sagittal T1WI (**a**), and heterogeneous slightly high to high signal on sagittal T2WI (**b**).

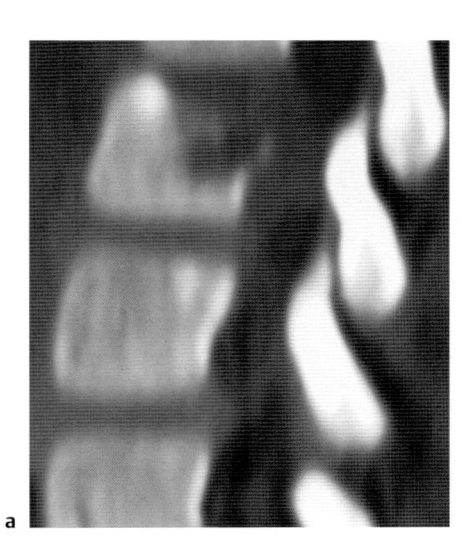

Figure **94 a–d** A 6-year-old male with an eosinophilic granuloma involving the L3 vertebral body. Sagittal CT image (**a**) shows a radiolucent lesion with poorly defined margins and cortical destruction. The lesion has low-intermediate signal on sagittal T1WI (**b**), and heterogeneous slightly high to high signal on sagittal FS T2WI (**c**).

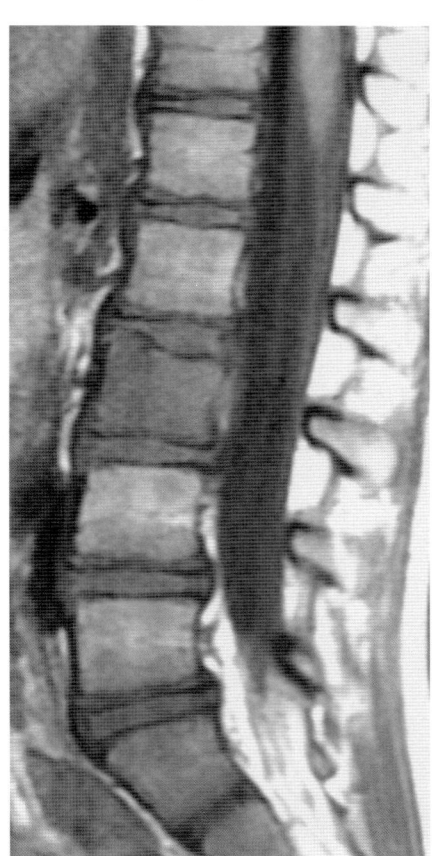

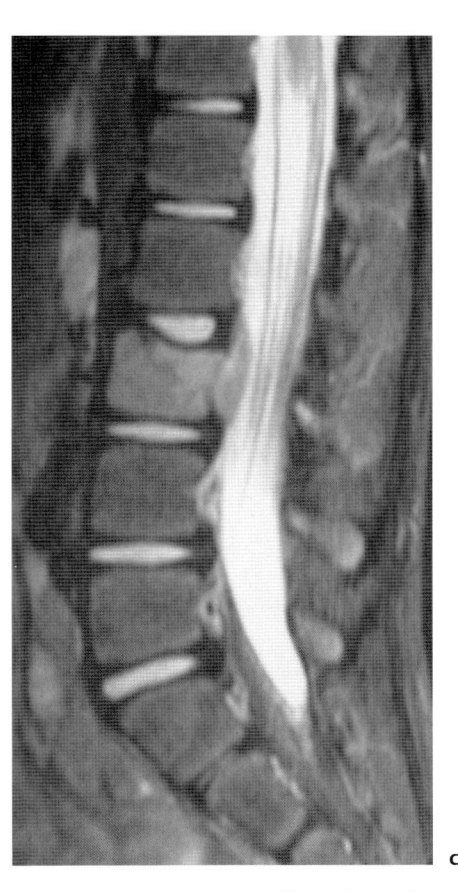

Figure **94 d** ▷

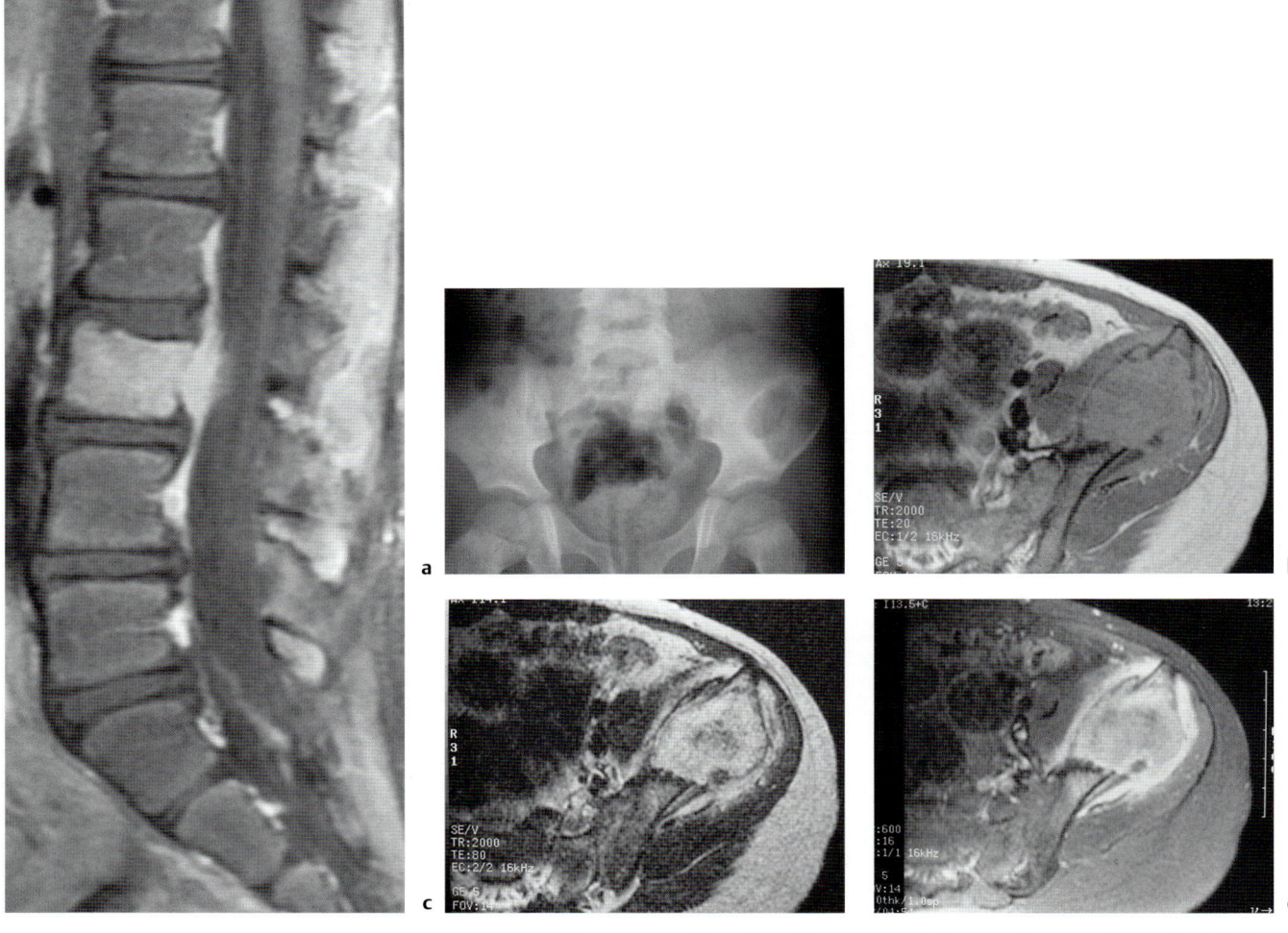

Figure **94 d** The lesion shows prominent Gd-contrast enhancement in the marrow as well as an extra-osseous portion, which extends into the anterior epidural soft tissues on sagittal FS T1WI (**d**).

Figure **95 a–d** A 4-year-old male with an eosinophilic granuloma involving the left iliac bone. AP radiograph (**a**) shows a radiolucent lesion with thin sclerotic margins. The lesion has intermediate signal on axial PDWI (**b**), and heterogeneous slightly high to high signal on axial T2WI (**c**). The lesion expands the bone and is associated with cortical disruption and extra-osseous extension. The lesion shows prominent Gd-contrast enhancement in marrow and in extra-osseous soft tissue portions on axial FS T1WI (**d**).

Differential Diagnosis

For Langerhans cell histiocytosis: osteomyelitis, Ewing sarcoma, lymphoma, telangiectatic osteosarcoma, giant cell tumor, desmoplastic fibroma, chondromyxoid fibroma, plasmacytoma/myeloma, metastatic lesion. In healing phases: fibrous cortical defect, nonossifying fibroma.

Treatment and Prognosis

Eosinophilic granuloma.[1,3,8–10,13,19,21–23,25] Lesions with low morbidity can be followed conservatively by observation. Spontaneous regression and reactivation can occur.[13] Prognosis for lesions involving the skull base is worse than for other craniofacial locations.[13] Treatment of more clinically symptomatic lesions may include excision, curettage, steroid injection, and radiation.[1,3,8–10,13,19,21–23,25] For cervical lesions, immobilization can often result in successful outcomes.[3,22] Progression of eosinophilic granuloma involving the spine may require radiation.[3] In the spinal cases with instability or neurologic deficits, surgery is often required.[3,22] Chemotherapy has also been used.[22]

Letterer–Siwe disease. This disease can have a rapidly progressive clinical course with high morbidity and mortality from involvement of multiple organ systems.[23] Patients usually receive chemotherapy.[23] Death is often secondary to sepsis within 1 to 2 years.[23]

Hand–Schüller–Christian disease. Prognosis depends on extent and distribution of organ systems involved.[23] In severe cases, mortality can be 15%, often resulting from anemia, thrombocytopenia/hemorrhage, pneumonia, and pulmonary fibrosis.[24] Disease may be chronic and may extend over 25 years.[23]

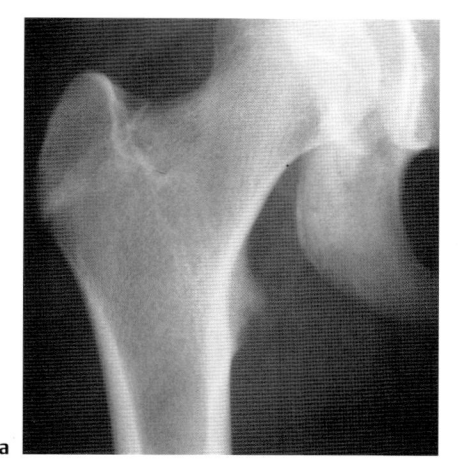

Figure **96 a–c** A 13-year-old female with an eosinophilic granuloma involving the lesser trochanter. A radiolucent focus is seen at the lesser trochanter on an AP radiograph (**a**). A poorly defined zone of signal alteration is seen in the marrow associated with cortical disruption and extra-osseous extension. The lesion has heterogeneous slightly high to high signal on axial FS T2WI (**b**). The lesion shows prominent Gd-contrast enhancement on coronal FS T1WI (**c**).

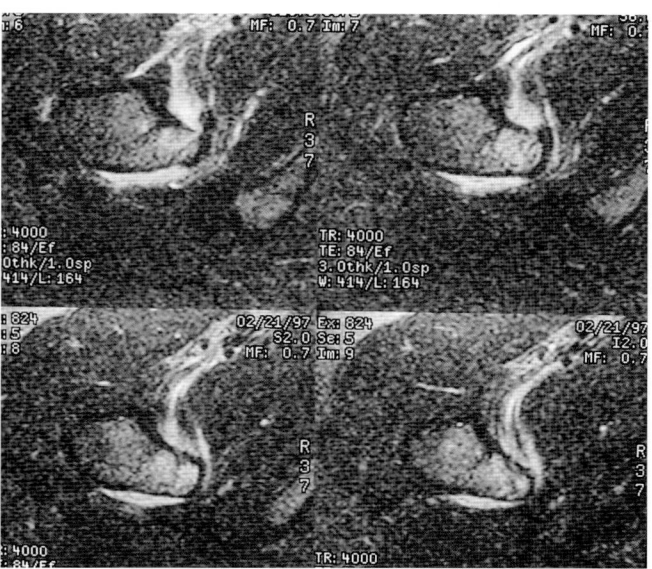

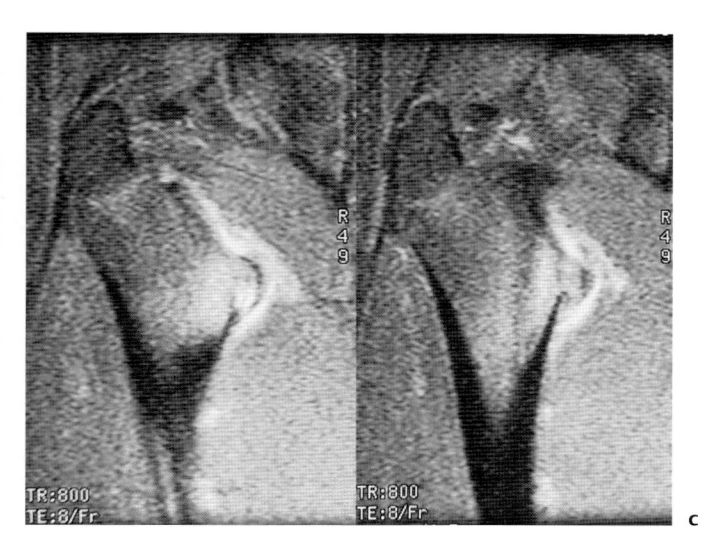

References

1 Acciarri N, Paganini M, Fonda C, Gaist G, Padovani R. Langerhans' cell histiocytosis of the spine causing cord compression: case report. *Neurosurgery* 1992;31:965–968.

2 Beltran J, Aparisi F, Bonmati LM, Rosenberg ZS, Present D, Steiner GC. Eosinophilic granuloma: MRI manifestations. *Skeletal Radiol* 1993; 22:157–161.

3 Bertram C, Madert J, Eggers C. Eosinophilic granuloma of the cervical spine. *Spine* 2002;27:1408–1413.

4 Conway WF, Hayes CW. Miscellaneous lesions of bone. *Radiol Clin North Am* 1993;31:339–358.

5 Davies AM, Pikoulas C, Griffith J. MRI of eosinophilic granuloma. *Eur J Radiol* 1994;18:205–209.

6 David R, Oria RA, Kumar R, et al. Radiologic features of eosinophilic granuloma of bone. *AJR Am J Roentgenol* 1989;153:1021–1026.

7 De Schepper AM, Ramon F, Van Marck E. MR imaging of eosinophilic granuloma: report of 11 cases. *Skeletal Radiol* 1993;22:163–166.

8 DeYoung BR, Unni KK. Langerhans' cell histiocytosis. In: Fletcher CDM, Unni KK, Mertens F, eds. *World Health Organization Classification of Tumours. Pathology and Genetics of Tumours of Soft Tissue and Bone* Geneva: IARC Press; 2002:345–346.

9 Forest M. Eosinophilic granuloma. In: Forest M, Tomeno B, Vanel D. eds. *Orthopedic Surgical Pathology: Diagnosis of Tumors and Pseudotumoral Lesions of Bone and Joints* Edinburgh: Churchill Livingstone; 1998:555–566.

10 Ghanem I, Tolo VT, D'Ambra P, Malogalowkin MH. Langerhans' cell histiocytosis of bone in children and adolescents. *J Pediatr Orthop* 2003;23:124–130.

11 Hayes CW, Conway WF, Sundaram M. Misleading aggressive MR imaging appearance of some benign musculoskeletal lesions. *Radiographics* 1992;12:1119–1134.

12 Hindman BW, Thomas RD, Yound LW, Yu L. Langerhans' cell histiocytosis: unusual skeletal manifestations observed in thirty-four cases. *Skeletal Radiol* 1998;27:177–181.

13 Huvos AG. Langerhans' cell granulomatosis; Langerhans' cell histiocytosis; solitary and multifocal eosinophilic granuloma of bone. In: Huvos AG, ed. *Bone Tumors: Diagnosis, Treatment, and Prognosis* 2nd ed. Philadelphia, Pa: W.B. Saunders; 1991:695–706.

14 Kenn W, Eck M, Allolio B, et al. Erdheim–Chester disease: evidence for a disease entity different from Langerhans' cell histiocytosis? Three cases with detailed radiological and immunohistochemical analysis. *Hum Pathol* 2000;31(6):734–739.

15 Miller SL, Hoffer FA. Malignant and benign bone tumors. *Radiol Clin North Am* 2001;39(4):693–694.

16 Monroc M Ducou le Pointe H, Haddad S, Josset P, Montagne JP. Soft tissue signal abnormality associated associated with eosinophilic granuloma. Correlation of MR imaging with pathologic findings. *Pediatr Radiol* 1994;24:328–332.

17 Mulder JD, Schutte HE, Kroon HM, Taconis WK. Introduction. In: *Radiologic Atlas of Bone Tumors* Amsterdam: Elsevier; 1993:3–6.

18 Mulder JD, Schutte HE, Kroon HM, Taconis WK. The diagnosis of bone tumors. In: *Radiologic Atlas of Bone Tumors* Amsterdam: Elsevier; 1993:9–46.

19 Mulder JD, Schutte HE, Kroon HM, Taconis WK. Langerhans' histiocytosis (histiocytosis X). In: *Radiologic Atlas of Bone Tumors* Amsterdam: Elsevier; 1993:653–670.

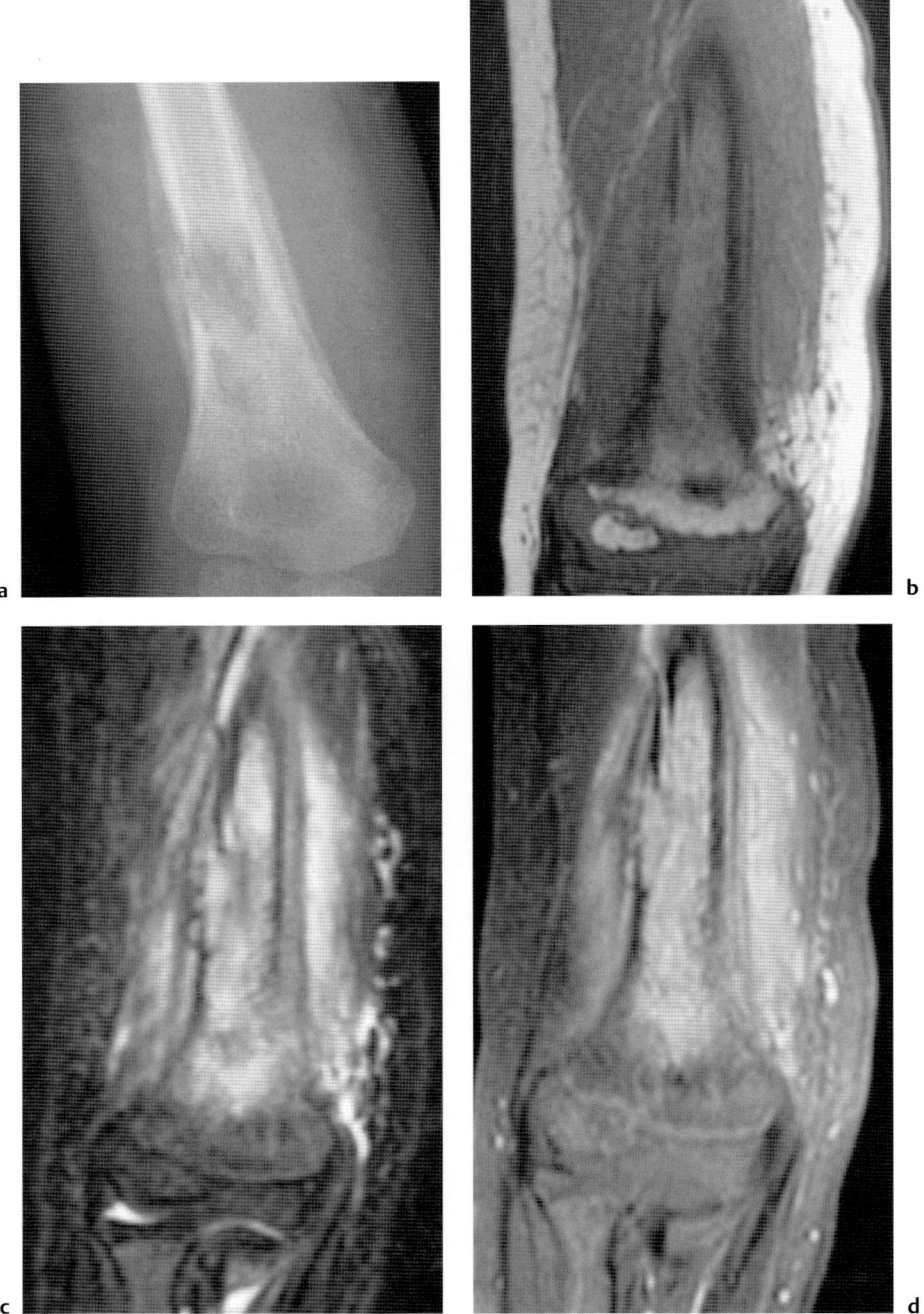

Figure **97 a–d** A 5-year-old male with an eosinophilic granuloma involving the distal humeral diaphysis. AP radiograph (**a**) shows a radiolucent, intramedullary lesion with irregular margins and prominent periosteal reaction. The periosteal reaction medially contains several zones of lucency. The lesion has low-intermediate signal on coronal T1WI (**b**) and heterogeneous high signal on coronal FS T2WI (**c**). A zone of cortical destruction is seen, as well as poorly defined extra-osseous zones with high signal on FS T2WI. Prominent abnormal Gd-contrast enhancement is seen in the marrow, periosteal reaction, and extra-osseous soft tissues on coronal FS T1WI (**d**).

20 Okamoto K, Ito J, Furusawa T, Sakai K, Tokiguchi S. Imaging of calvarial eosinophilic granuloma. *Neuroradiology* 1999;41:723–728.

21 Perlman EJ. Ewing's sarcoma, lymphoma, and Langerhans' cell proliferations. In: Helliwell TR, ed. *Major Problems in Pathology: Pathology of Bone and Joint Neoplasms.* Vol 37. 1st ed. Philadelphia, Pa: W.B. Saunders;1999:279–303.

22 Scarpinati M, Artico M, Artizzu S. Spinal cord compression by eosinophilic granuloma of the cervical spine. Case report and review of the literature. *Neurosurg Rev* 1995;18:209–212.

23 Stull MA, Kransdorf MJ, Devaney KO. From the archives of the AFIP – Langerhans' cell histiocytosis of bone. *Radiographics* 1992;12(4):801–823.

24 Unni KK. Introduction and scope of study. In: Unni KK, ed. *Dahlin's Bone Tumors: General Aspects and Data on 11 087 Cases* 5th ed. Philadelphia, Pa: Lippincott, Williams & Wilkins; 1996:1–9.

25 Unni KK. Conditions that commonly simulate primary neoplasms of bone. In: Unni KK, ed. *Dahlin's Bone Tumors: General Aspects and Data on 11 087 Cases* 5th ed. Philadelphia, Pa: Lippincott, Williams & Wilkins; 1996:355–432.

26 Yamamura S, Sato K, Sugiura H, et al. Prostaglandin levels of primary bone tumor tissues correlate with peritumoral edema demonstrated by magnetic resonance imaging. *Cancer* 1997;79:255–261.

A 19 Erdheim–Chester Disease (Also Referred to as Chester–Erdheim Disease, Lipoid Granulomatosis, and Lipogranulomatosis)

Definition

Erdheim–Chester disease is a rare, multisystem, non-Langerhans cell histiocytic disorder of unknown etiology that usually affects adults.[1-13] In this disease, collections of foamy macrophages can be seen within various tissues and organs of the musculoskeletal, pulmonary, cardiac, gastrointestinal, and central nervous systems.[1-13] Lesions have also been reported in lymph nodes, retroperitoneum, kidneys, breast, aorta, and orbits.[2,3,5]

Frequency of Occurrence

Erdheim–Chester disease is rare.[1,2,13]

Age at Presentation

From 7 to 84 years,[1,7,13] average = 53 years.[4,7,13] Most common in 4th to 7th decades.[3,6]

Gender Ratio (M/F)

1/1 to 1.3/1.[2,13]

Location

Common sites in bone include the femur, tibia, radius, humerus, elbow, ulna, carpus.[1,2,4,13] Lesions infrequently involve flat bones and the axial skeleton.[13] Skeletal abnormalities are often bilateral, and usually involve the diaphyseal and metaphyseal regions.[2] Epiphyseal abnormalities are uncommon.[3] Lesions are less frequently seen in the axial skeleton.[7] Lesions in the central nervous system can occur in the cerebrum, hypothalamus, cerebellum, and choroid plexus; they rarely involve the spinal or cranial dura.[1,2,4,5,13] Orbital lesions can be intraconal or extraconal, or involve eyelids the periorbital soft tissues.[3,6,13]

Signs and Symptoms

Lesions can present as a localized asymptomatic mass.[1] Intraosseous lesions can be associated with bone pain, which occurs in up to 50% of patients and usually in the lower extremities.[2,13] Patients may also have joint pain and keloid formation.[3,4] Extensive infiltration of tissues or organs with foamy macrophages can result in organ failure or multisystem dysfunction.[1-4] Patients may have fever, weight loss, and/or malaise.[7,13] Lesions in the brain can produce symptoms (limb weakness, paraplegia, ataxia, numbness, nystagmus, etc.) mimicking multiple sclerosis.[4,5] Involvement of the hypothalamus and pituitary stalk can result in diabetes insipidus.[2,4,5,7] Involvement of the heart and/or pericardium can produce cardiac failure.[2] Lesions in the orbit can cause exophthalmos.[2,7,13] Orbital involvement is often bilateral and painless.[13] Xanthoma-like lesions involving the eyelids can occur and are referred to as xanthelasmas.[13] Shortness of breath secondary to pulmonary fibrosis from lung involvement can progress to cardiorespiratory failure.[2,7]

Gross Pathologic Findings

In bone, there is usually replacement of fatty marrow with varying degrees of fibrous tissue and collections of lipid-laden macrophages.[2,6] Infiltration of bone with foamy lipid-laden histiocytes of Erdheim–Chester disease often results in intramedullary zones of osteosclerosis.[2]

Histopathologic Findings

Specimens show xanthomatous or xanthogranulomatous lesions containing foamy lipid-laden histiocytes with small bland nuclei; also Touton-like giant cells, multinucleated giant cells, fibrosis/dense collagen, chronic inflammatory cells lymphocytes and histiocytes), and occasional scattered eosinophils.[1,4-6,13] Zones of osteonecrosis may be present.[9] Foamy histiocytes are usually immunoreactive to the histiocytic antigen CD 68, and show variable or no reactivity to S 100.[2,5,7-9,12,13] Unlike Langerhans cell histiocytosis, Erdheim–Chester lesions lack immunoreactivity to CD 1 a and OKT6, and also lack intracytoplasmic Birbeck bodies on electron microscopy.[1,2]

Findings on Plain Films (Roentgenograms) and Computed Tomography

Bone. Abnormalities often consist of diffuse and/or poorly-defined zones of coarsened trabecular thickening, increased medullary density, and cortical thickening, primarily involving the diaphyses and metaphyses[2-5,7,10-13] (Fig. **98**). The epiphyseal regions are less commonly affected.[3,5,13] Up to one-third of patients have a mixed osteosclerotic and osteolytic pattern.[3,10,13] Zones of cortical destruction may be seen occasionally with lesions in long bones.[10] Lesions are often osteolytic in flat bones such as the skull, ribs, and mandible.[7]

Orbits. On CT, intraobital lesions may be intraconal or extraconal and usually have low and/or intermediate attenuation.[3,5] Lesions may have circumscribed margins or occur as diffuse infiltrative abnormalities within orbital fat.[3] Lesions may also cause eyelid xanthelasmas.[3]

MRI Findings

Bone. Lesions can appear as irregular zones with low and/or intermediate signal on T1WI and PDWI, and mixed low, intermediate and/or high signal on T2WI and FS T2WI within marrow[3,6,7] (Fig. **98**). Zones of cortical destruction with or without extra-osseous lesion extension may be seen occasionally with lesions in long bones.[10] After Gd-contrast administration, heterogeneous enhancement may be seen in the involved marrow and zones of extra-osseous extension if present.[10]

Orbits. Abnormalities can appear as intraconal or extraconal lesions with low to intermediate signal on T1WI and PDWI, and variable low, intermediate and/or high signal on T2WI and FS T2WI[6,7] (Fig. **99**). After Gd-contrast administration, enhancement is often seen in the involved marrow or soft tissue lesion zones.

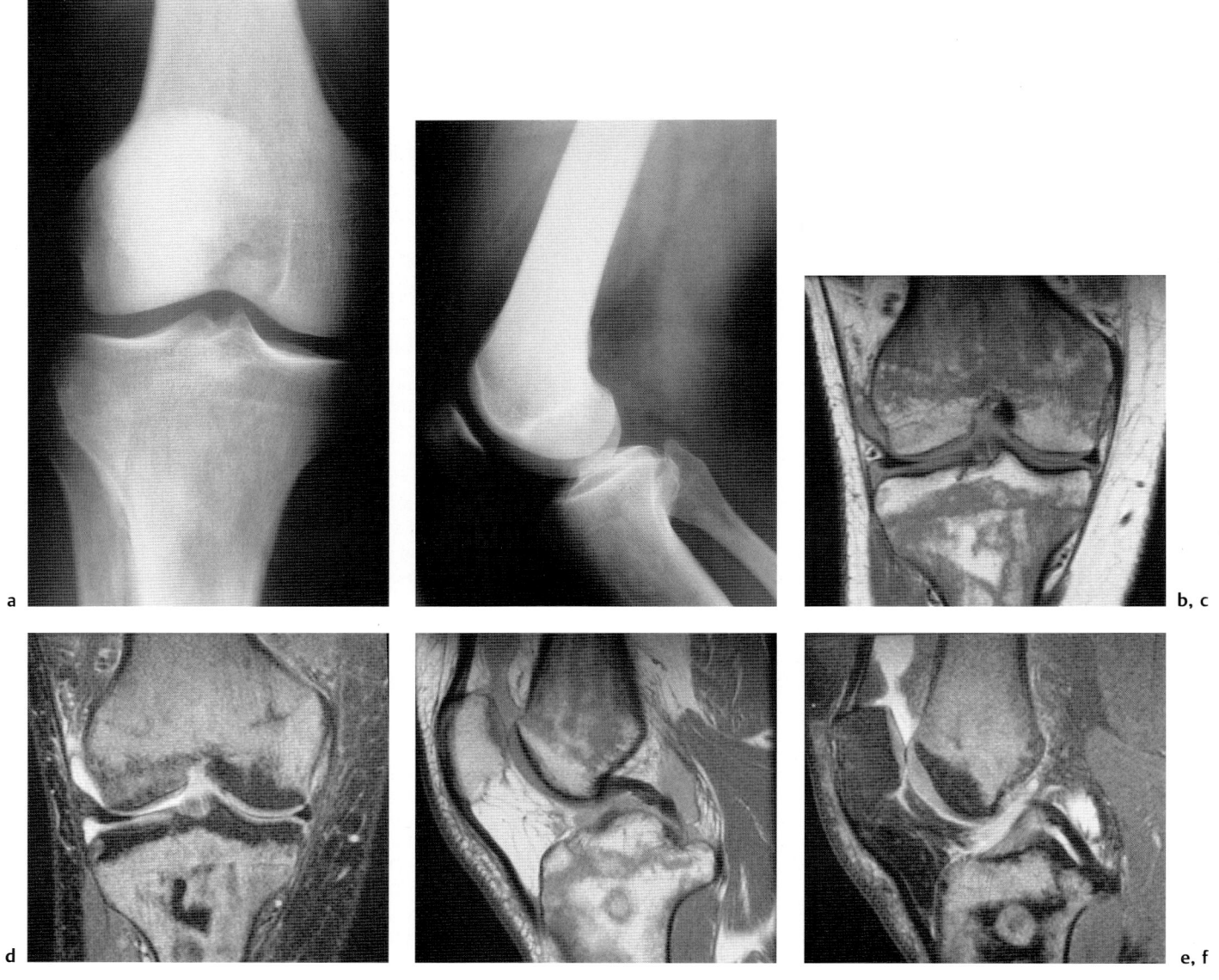

Figure **98 a–f** A 39-year-old man with Erdheim–Chester disease with bone marrow involvement. AP (a) and lateral (b) radiographs show increased medullary density, coarsened trabecular thickening, and cortical thickening. Irregular zones with intermediate signal on coronal (c) and sagittal (e) PDWI, and slightly high signal on coronal (d) and sagittal (f) FS T2WI are seen within the marrow in the epiphyseal, metaphyseal, and metadiaphyseal regions.

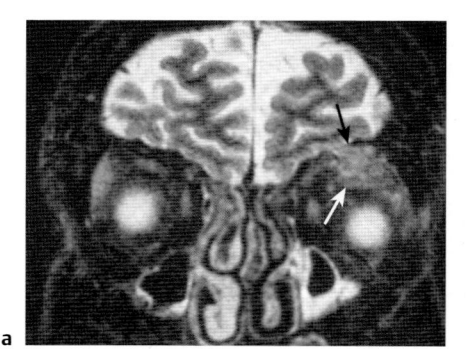

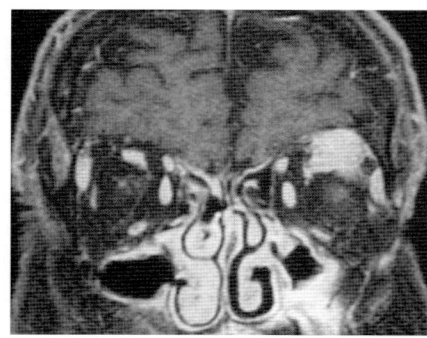

Figure **99 a, b** Erdheim–Chester disease in the upper left orbit involving the superior rectus muscle and intraconal fat. The lesion has slightly high signal on coronal STIR (a), and shows prominent Gd-contrast enhancement on coronal FS T1WI (b).

Dura. Abnormalities can appear as circumscribed epidural, intradural, and/or subdural lesions with low to intermediate signal on T1WI, and variable low, intermediate and/or high signal on T2WI and FS T2WI.[1] After Gd-contrast administration, cranial and spinal dural lesions may or may not show contrast enhancement.[1,5]

Differential Diagnosis

Langerhans cell histiocytosis, Hand–Schüller–Christian disease, lymphoma, Castelman disease, sarcoidosis, Wegener granulomatosis, tuberculosis, chronic osteomyelitis, fibrous dysplasia, bone infarct, Gaucher disease, mucopolysaccharidoses, Paget disease.[1,3,10,12]

Prognosis and Treatment

The prognosis of Erdheim–Chester disease depends on the extent and location of disease.[2] Erdheim–Chester disease has been treated with surgical debulking, prednisone, cyclosporine, vincristine, vinblastine, cyclophosphamide, and/or doxorubicin.[2,6,7,12,13] Radiation treatment may be useful for lesions in the brain parenchyma and other locations.[4,6,12,13] Immunotherapy with agents such as interferon-[alpha]2a has also been used.[6,7,12,13] Multisystem disease can progress to result in death from respiratory distress, pulmonary fibrosis, renal and/or heart failure.[3,4,6,7,12] Thirty-seven percent of patients died after a mean follow-up interval of 32 months.[13]

References

1 Albayram S, Kizilkilic O, Zulfikar Z, Islak C, Kocer N. Spinal dural involvement in Erdheim–Chester disease: MRI findings. *Neuroradiology* 2002;44:1004–1007.
2 Al-Quran S, Reith J, Bradley J, Rimsza L. Erdheim–Chester disease: case report, PCR-based analysis of clonality, and review of literature. *Mod Pathol* 2002;15(6):666–672.
3 Bancroft LW, Berquist TH. Erdheim–Chester disease: radiographic findings in five patients. *Skeletal Radiol* 1998;27:127–132.
4 Bohlega S, Alwatban J, Tulbah A, Bakheet SM, Powe J. Cerebral manifestation of Erdheim–Chester disease: clinical and radiologic findings. *Neurology* 1997;49(6):1702–1705.
5 Caparros-Lefebvre D, Pruvo JP, Remy M, Wallaert B, Petit H. Neuroradiologic asoects of Erdheim–Chester disease. *AJNR Am J Neuroradiol* 1995;16:735–740.
6 De Abreu MR, Chung CB, Biswal S, Haghighi P, Hesselink J, Resnick D. Erdheim–Chester disease: MR imaging, anatomic, and histopathologic correlation of orbital involvement. *AJNR Am J Neuroradiol* 2004;25:627–630.
7 Gottlieb R, Chen A. MR findings of Erdheim Chester disease. *J Comput Assist Tomogr* 2002;26(2):257–261.
8 Kenn W, Eck M, Allolio B, et al. Erdheim–Chester disease: evidence for a disease entity different from Langerhans' cell histiocytosis? Three cases with detailed radiological and immunohistochemical analysis. *Hum Pathol* 2000;31(6):734–739.
9 Kim NR, Ko YH, Choe YH, Lee HG, Huh B, Ahn GH. Erdheim–Chester disease with extensive marrow necrosis: a case report and literature review. *Int J Surg Pathol* 2001;9(1):73–79.
10 Kushihashi T, Munechika H, Sekimizu M, Fujimaki E. Erdheim–Chester disease involving bilateral lower extremities. MR features. *AJR Am J Roentgenol* 2000;174(3):875–876.
11 Murray D, Marshall M, England E, Mander J, Chakera TMH. Erdheim–Chester disease. *Clin Radiol* 2001;56:481–484.
12 Shamburek RD, Brewer HB, Gochuico BR. Erdheim–Chester disease: a rare multisystem histiocytic disorder associated with interstitial lung disease. *Am J Med Sci* 2001;321(1):66–75.
13 Veyssier-Belot C, Cacoub P, Caparros-Lefebvre D, et al. Erdheim–Chester disease: clinical and radiology characteristics of 59 cases. *Medicine* 1996;75(3):157–169.

A 20 Ewing Sarcoma

ICD-O Code

9260/3

Definition

Ewing sarcoma is a malignant primitive tumor of bone comprised of undifferentiated small cells with round nuclei.[3,7,8,20,21,25,26] **Extracranial primitive neuroectodermal tumors (extracranial PNETs)** of bone and soft tissue are mostly similar to Ewing sarcoma, except that extracranial PNETs usually show varying degrees of neural differentiation.[3,7,8,20,21,25,26]

Frequency of Occurrence

Ewing sarcoma accounts for 6–11% of primary malignant bone tumors, and 5–7% of primary bone tumors.[18-20,24-26] Ewing sarcoma usually occurs in Caucasians and Hispanics, and rarely occurs in Blacks and Asians.[7,8,26] The annual incidence in the United States is 2.1 per million.[7] Ewing sarcoma rarely occurs in the soft tissues, representing 1% of malignant soft tissues and <1% of all soft tissue tumors.[7,11]

Age at Presentation

Ewing sarcoma in bone: usually occurs in patients ranging from 1 to 30 years, median = 14 years; 75% in first 2 decades, > 90% in patients < 25 years; peaks in 2nd decade.[7,8,18-20,24-26]

Extraskeletal Ewing sarcoma: from 11 to 42 years, mean = 25 years.[11]

Gender Ratio (M/F)

3/2[8,11,25,26]

Location

Bone. Tumors are located in the femur > iliac bone > rib > tibia > humerus > fibula > vertebra, sacrum > scapula > radius, ulna > craniofacial bones.[4,7,8,18-20,24-26] Ewing sarcoma rarely involves the phalanges, bones of the feet, or calcaneous.[8] Ewing sarcoma occurs most frequently within the central medullary portions of bone (84%), versus eccentric locations within bone (11%), intracortical locations (5%) or subperiosteal locations (<1%).[20] In long bones, tumors are located in the diaphyseal region (57%), metadiaphyseal region (33%), metaphyseal region (6%), epi-metadiaphyseal zone (3%), or epi-metaphyseal region (1%).[20] In vertebrae, tumors involve the body (54%), arch (23%), body and arch (23%).[20]

Soft tissues. Tumors occur in the trunk > lower extremity > retroperitoneum > hip, buttocks > proximal limb girdle > upper extremity, head and neck.[11]

Signs and Symptoms

Pain and swelling for several months are common clinical symptoms[7,8,21,25,26] Fever may result from tumor necrosis.[7,21,26] Patients may also have anemia, leukocytosis, and elevated erythrocyte sedimentation rates.[7,21,25,26] Pathologic fracture is uncommon.[25,26] Up to 35% of patients have metastases at presentation.[7]

Gross Pathologic Findings

Ewing sarcoma occurs typically as soft gray-white moist tumors, often with areas of hemorrhage and/or necrosis associated with bone destruction and extra-osseous soft tissue mass.[2,3,7,8,26] Periosteal reactive ossification, "Codman Triangles," are commonly seen in Ewing tumors in long bones.[3,7,8,25,26]

Histopathologic Findings[2,3,7-9,20,21,25,26]

Ewing sarcoma consists of sheets of at least two cell populations. Cells can have spherical to ellipsoid shapes with round to oval nuclei and finely granular, ill-defined or well-defined cytoplasm. In addition, smaller cells with hyperchromatic nuclei and eosinophilic cytoplasm are also commonly seen. The mitotic rate tends to be low. Little intercellular stroma is common, except for widely separated strands of fibrous tissue. Lesions show little to no reticulin fibers within the cellular portions of the lesions. Zones of acute and/or chronic inflammation, necrosis, reactive fibrous and osseous tissue in Ewing tumors may complicate histopathologic interpretation.

Extracranial PNET shows histology similar to Ewing sarcoma except for evidence of neural differentiation (Homer Wright pseudorosettes), as well as by immunohistochemistry (higher rate of reactivity to neuron-specific enolase, synaptophysin, chromogranin, and S-100 compared with undifferentiated Ewing sarcoma) and electron microscopy (occasional cytoplasmic processes containing neurosecretory granules.)[3,7,8,21,26]

Other Ewing tumors have histopathologic and immunohistochemical features that are intermediate between the most undifferentiated forms of Ewing sarcoma and extracranial PNET.[3,7,8,21,26]

Ewing tumors/extracranial PNET show positive immunohistochemical reaction to the MIC 2 (CD 99) gene product in up to 95% of cases.[3,7,21,26] The MIC 2 gene product is a membrane-bound glycoprotein that is probably involved in cell adhesion processes.[21] The MIC 2 gene is located on the sex chromosomes and is not related to the t(11;22) translocation.[3,21]

Tumor Genetics

Ewing tumors and extracranial PNET commonly show translocations involving chromosomes 11 and 22 at. t(11;22) (q24;q12).[3,7,21,26] Using reverse transcriptase with the polymerase chain reaction, the genes and gene products at the translocation break points on chromosomes 11 and 22 have been identified.[3,21] The t(11;22) translocation results in the fusion of the FLI-1 gene at 11q24 to the EWS gene at 22q12.[3,21,26] The hybrid protein that results from translation of the gene fusion has been detected in almost all Ewing sarcomas and extracranial PNETs.[3,21,26] This translocation is also seen in peripheral neuroepithelioma, Askin tumor (extracranial PNET involving the thoracic wall) and extra-osseous Ewing sarcoma.

Findings on Plain Films (Roentgenograms) and Computed Tomography[1,3,5,6,8,16,20–22,25,26,29]

Ewing sarcoma often appears as a central radiolucent lesion with poorly defined margins (permeative > "moth-eaten" appearance), irregular zones of cortical destruction, and interrupted lamellated ("onion skin") or perpendicular ("hair on end") periosteal reaction (Figs. **100, 102–106**). Codman triangles can be seen at the borders of tumor periosteal reaction with zones of cortical destruction and extra-osseous tumor extension (Figs. **105, 106**). Lesions occur in diaphysis > metadiaphysis. Sclerosis can be seen in combination with lytic regions in a minority of cases. CT can show a thin striated periosteal reaction perpendicular to the long axis of bones, also referred to as the "hair on end" appearance (Figs. **100, 104**).

Extra-osseous soft tissue masses and extent of lesions are better seen with CT than with plain films. Extra-osseous soft tissue masses typically do not show ossification or calcification (Figs. **107, 108**).

Findings on Radionuclide Bone Scans

Ewing sarcoma typically shows increased radiopharmaceutical accumulation of both technetium-99 m methylene diphosphonate and gallium-67-citrate. Soft tissue components of the lesions may show mild uptake.

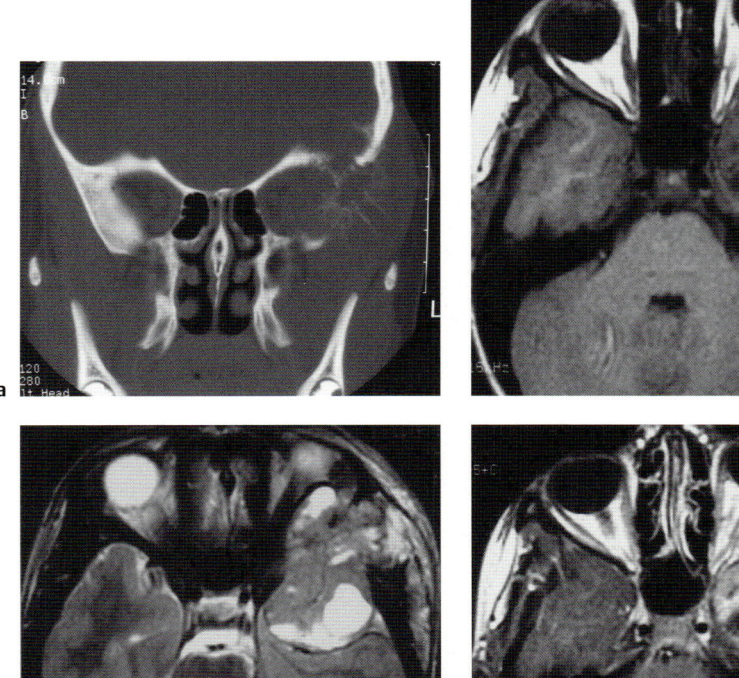

Figure **100 a–d** An 11-year-old female with Ewing sarcoma involving the left frontal and zygomatic bones with tumor extension intracranially as well as into the left orbit. Coronal (**a**) CT image shows a soft tissue tumor, containing perpendicular striated periosteal reaction associated with bone destruction. The tumor has zones of low and intermediate signal on axial (**b**) T1WI, heterogeneous intermediate and high signal on axial (**c**) T2WI with small foci of low signal. The tumor shows prominent irregular Gd-contrast enhancement on axial T1WI (**d**).

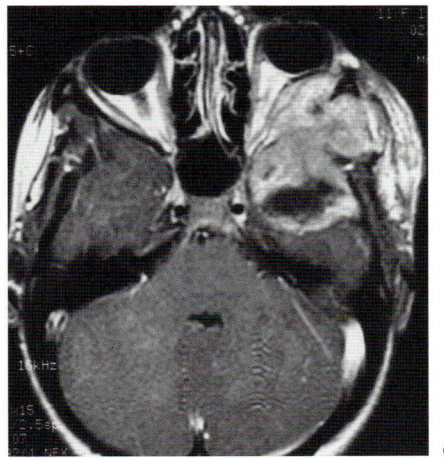

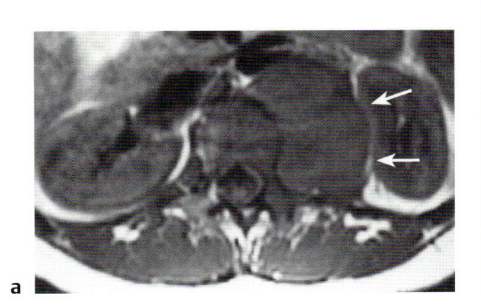

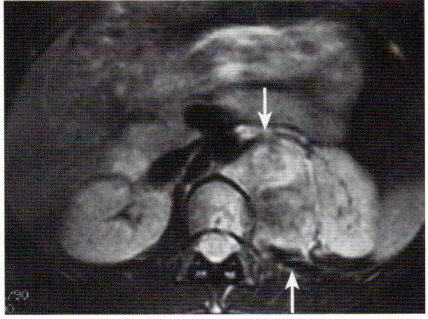

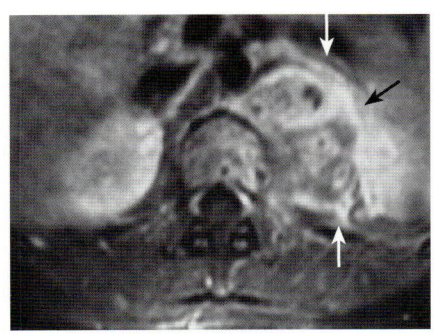

Figure **101 a–c** A 16-year-old female with Ewing sarcoma involving a vertebral body with extension laterally into the adjacent soft tissues on the left. Axial (**a**) T1WI shows the tumor to have low-intermediate signal. The tumor has heterogeneous mostly slightly high and high signal on axial (**b**) FS T2WI, and shows heterogeneous Gd-contrast enhancement on axial (**c**) FS T1WI.

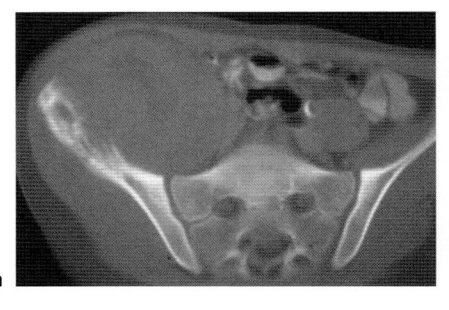

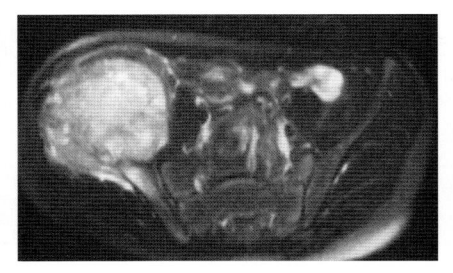

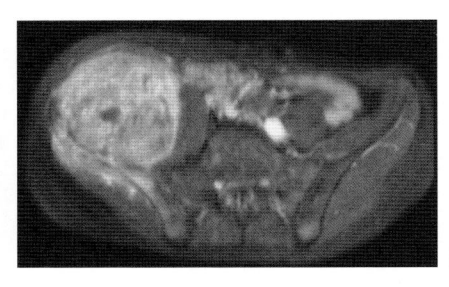

Figure 102 a–c A 10-year-old male with Ewing sarcoma involving the right iliac bone associated with bone destruction and extra-osseous tumor extension. Axial CT image (**a**) shows a permeative, radiolucent lesion involving the iliac bone associated with a large extra-osseous mass. The tumor has heterogeneous mostly slightly high and high signal on axial FS T2WI (**b**). The tumor shows heterogeneous Gd-contrast enhancement on axial FS T1WI (**c**).

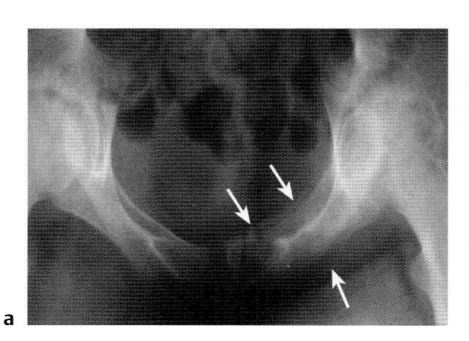

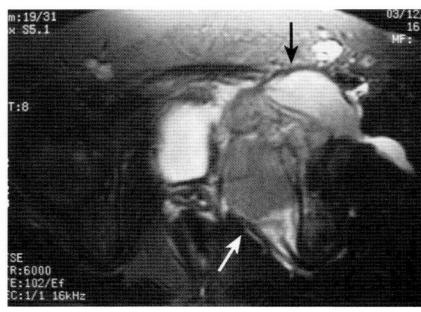

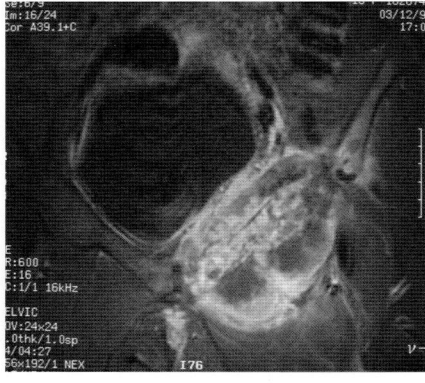

Figure 103 a–c A 13-year-old female with Ewing sarcoma involving the left pubic bone. AP radiograph (**a**) shows a permeative, radiolucent lesion with periosteal reaction. The tumor is associated with cortical destruction and extra-osseous tumor extension (**b**, **c**). The tumor has heterogeneous slightly high to high signal on axial FS T2WI (**b**). The tumor shows prominent irregular Gd-contrast enhancement on coronal FS T1WI (**c**).

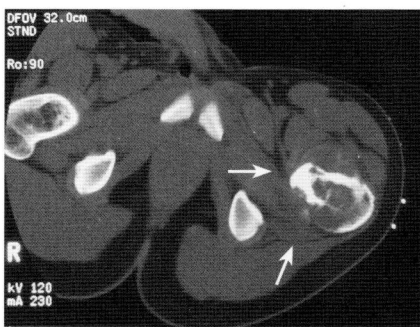

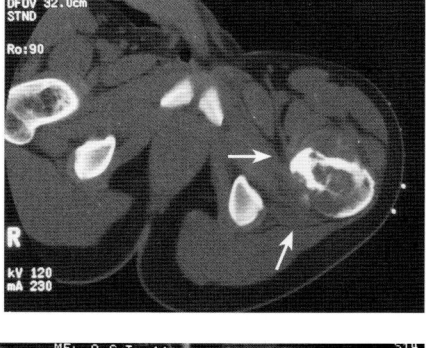

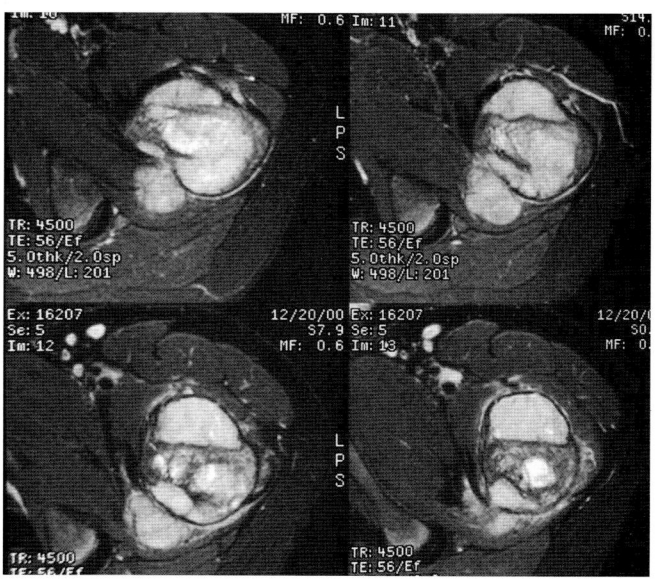

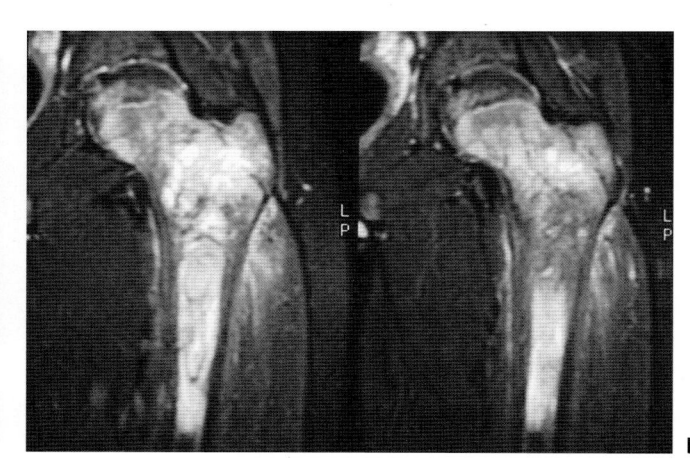

Figure 104 a–c A 15-year-old male with Ewing sarcoma involving the proximal left femur. Axial CT image (**a**) shows a permeative, radiolucent tumor in the femur associated cortical destruction and extra-osseous tumor extension, which contains minimal striated periosteal reaction. The tumor has poorly defined margins, and has mostly high signal on coronal (**b**) and axial (**c**) FS T2WI. Zones of cortical destruction and extra-osseous tumor extension are also seen with MRI.

Figure 105 a–e A 9-year-old male with Ewing sarcoma involving the proximal tibia. AP (**a**) and lateral (**b**) radiographs show a permeative, radiolucent lesion in the proximal diaphyseal and metadiaphyseal portions of the tibia associated with irregular zones of cortical destruction and lamellated "onion skin" periosteal reaction. Codman triangles are seen at the proximal and distal borders of tumor periosteal reaction (**a**, **b**). The tumor has poorly defined margins and has heterogeneous slightly high to high signal on axial T2WI (**c**). Curvilinear thin zones of low signal on axial T2WI (**c**) represent elevated periosteum. The tumor shows prominent irregular Gd-contrast enhancement on axial (**d**) and coronal (**e**) FS T1WI. Zones of cortical destruction and extra-osseous tumor extension are also seen with MRI.

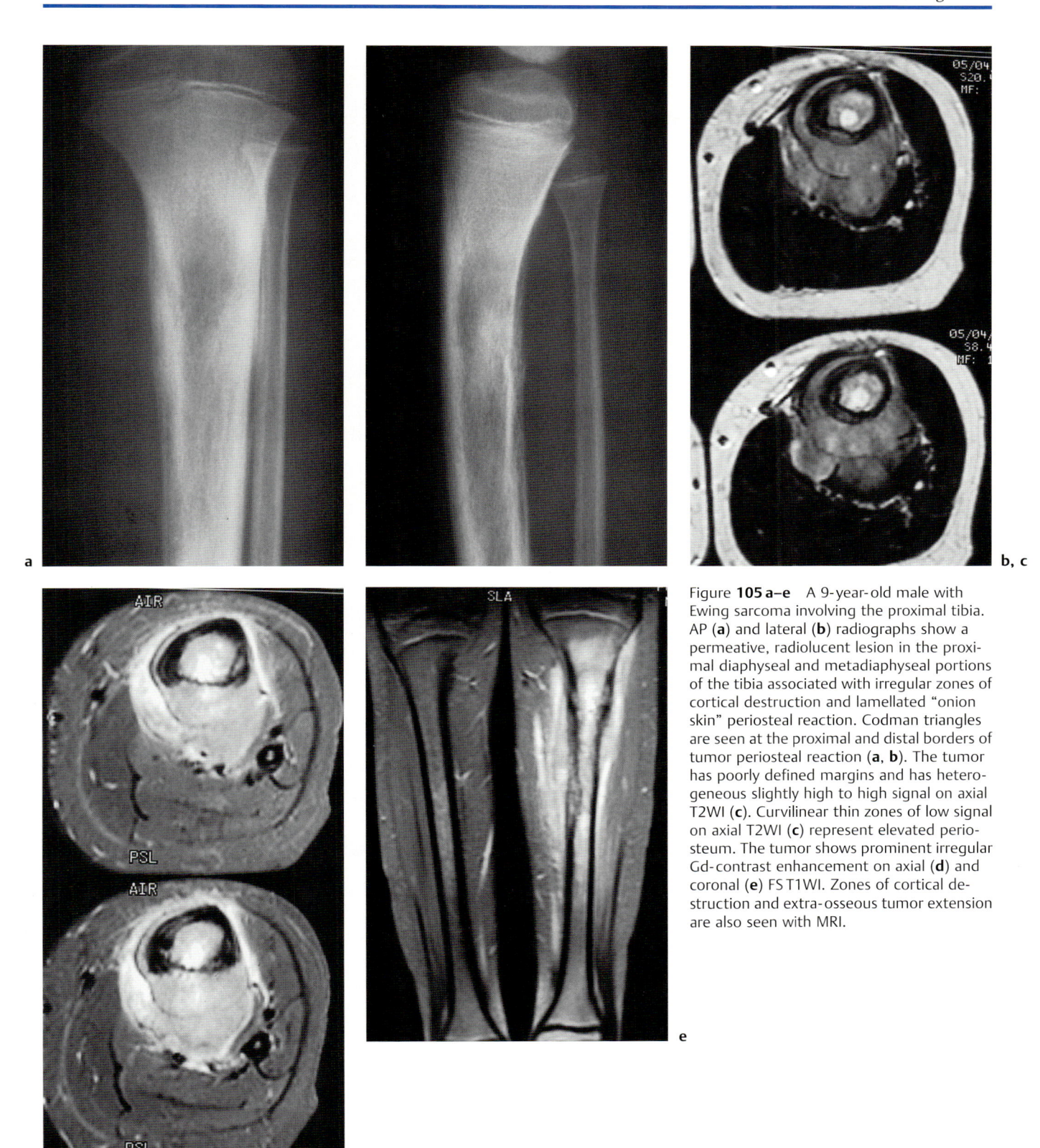

MRI Findings[1,3,4,6,10,12–17,20,22,23,25–29]

Lesions usually have low-intermediate signal on T1WI and PDWI, heterogeneous slightly high to high signal on T2WI and FS T2WI (Figs. **100–108**). Margins of the lesions are often ill defined. Lesions typically show prominent irregular Gd-contrast enhancement. MRI shows areas of cortical destruction; as well as the size, extent, and configuration of extra-osseous soft tissue masses (Figs. **100–103, 105–107**). Dynamic Gd-contrast enhancement can allow differentiation between rapidly-enhancing tumors with higher mean initial slope values compared with reactive intramedullary and non-neoplastic soft tissue edema. On T2WI, thin striated zones of low signal can be sometimes be seen oriented perpendicular to the long axis of the involved bone, representing the "hair on end" appearance of periosteal or reactive bone formation within extra-

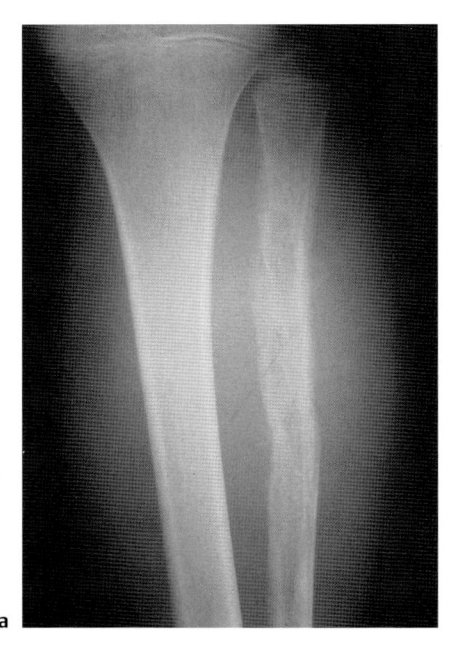

Figure **106 a–c** An 11-year-old male with Ewing sarcoma / PNET involving the proximal fibula. AP radiograph (**a**) shows a permeative, radiolucent lesion in the proximal diaphyseal and metadiaphyseal portions of the fibula associated with irregular zones cortical destruction and lamellated "onion skin" periosteal reaction. Codman triangles are seen at the proximal and distal borders of tumor periosteal reaction (**a**). The tumor has poorly defined margins and is associated with cortical destruction and prominent extra-osseous tumor extension. The tumor contains zones with intermediate and slightly high signal on axial PDWI (**b**, images on left), and slightly high to high signal on axial T2WI (**b**, images on right). Curvilinear thin zones of low signal represent elevated periosteum and tumor periosteal reaction (**b**). The tumor shows prominent irregular Gd-contrast enhancement on axial FS T1WI (**c**), as well as zones of central necrosis.

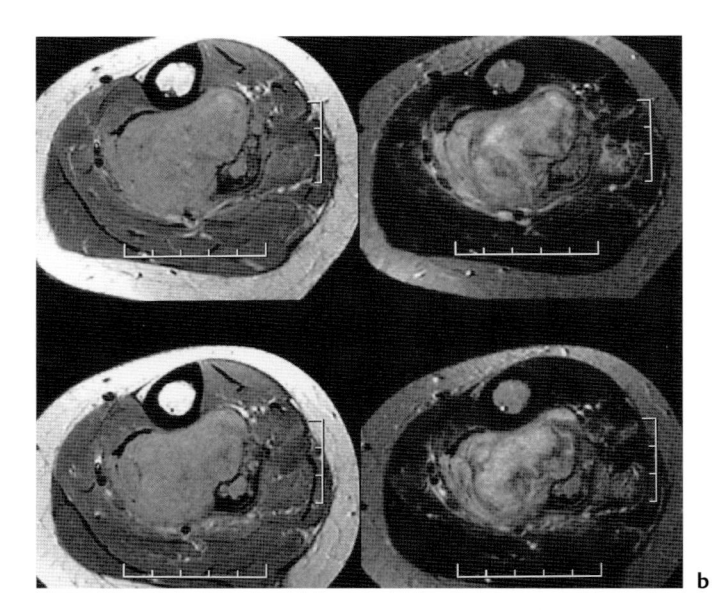

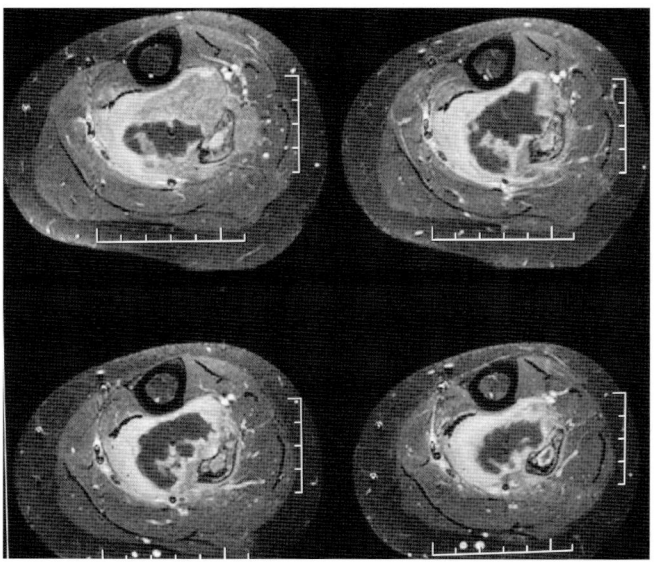

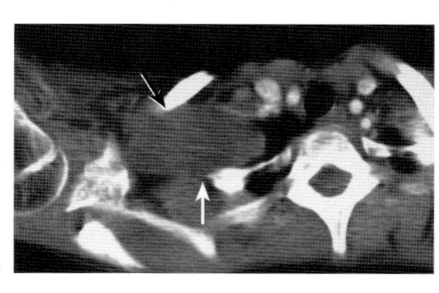

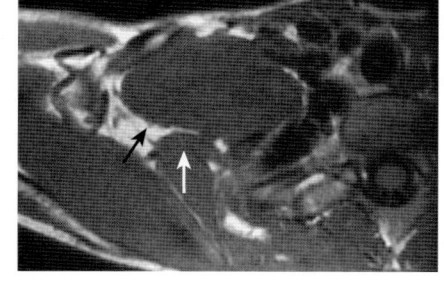

Figure **107 a–d** An 11-year-old female with an extra-osseous Ewing sarcoma in the soft tissues adjacent to the right clavicle. Axial CT image (**a**) shows a circumscribed lesion with intermediate attenuation. The tumor has intermediate signal on axial T1WI (**b**), and high signal on axial FS T2WI (**c**). The tumor shows moderate Gd-contrast enhancement on axial FS T1WI (**d**).

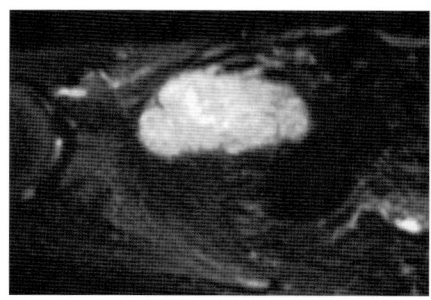

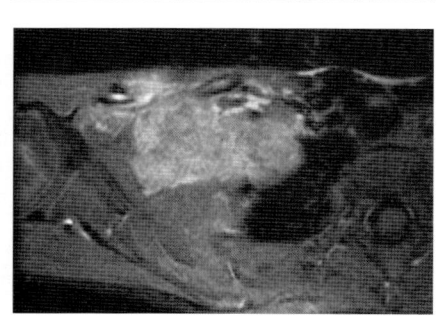

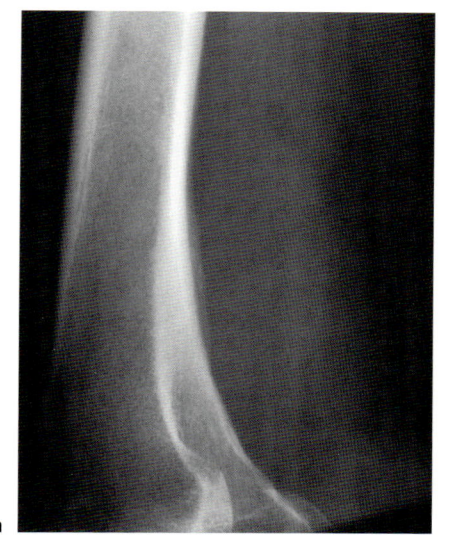

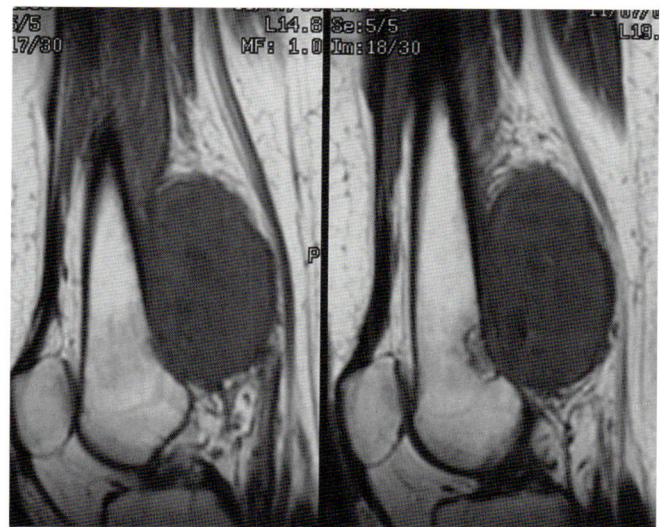

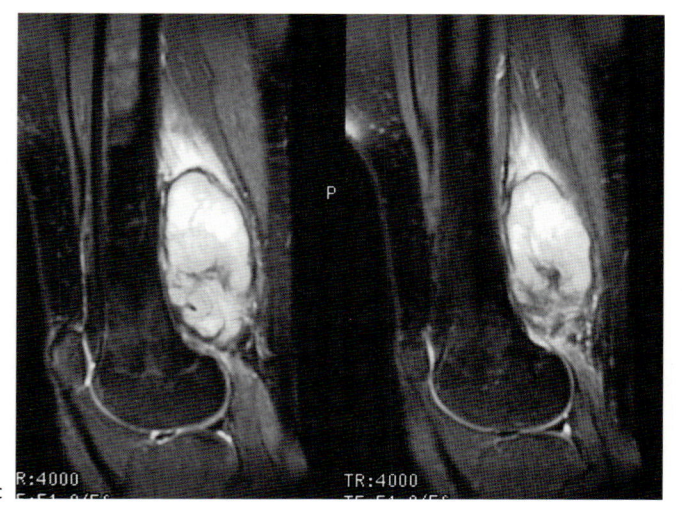

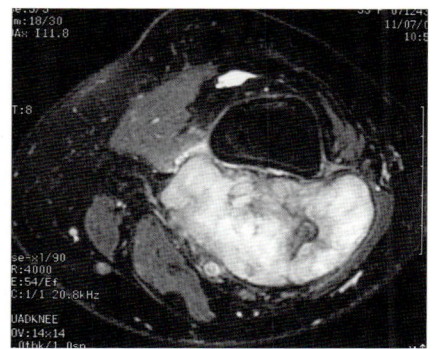

Figure **108 a–d** 54-year-old woman with an extra-osseous Ewing sarcoma in the distal posterior thigh. Lateral radiograph (**a**) shows a mass with soft tissue opacity dorsal to the distal femur. The tumor has mostly intermediate signal with several small foci of low signal on sagittal (**b**) T1WI. The tumor has mostly high signal on sagittal (**c**) and axial (**d**) FS T2WI, and also contains curvilinear zones of low signal. Poorly defined zones of high signal on FS T2WI are seen in the soft tissues peripheral to the tumor. The tumor extends up to the femoral cortex and is associated with minimal periosteal reaction but no cortical destruction or intramedullary invasion.

osseous tumor extension, which may or may not be under an elevated layer of periosteum[29] These findings correspond to those seen with CT.[29] The soft tissue components of Ewing sarcoma in flat bones tend to be larger than in long bones.

After chemotherapy and/or radiation treatment, dynamic Gd-contrast enhanced MRI can be used to evaluate treatment response by defining remaining viable tumor from zones of necrosis by initial enhancement slope analysis and/or shapes of the time-intensity enhancement curves in regions of interest.[4,15,27,28] Viable tumor typically has rapid, early Gd-DTPA enhancement compared with areas of necrosis.

Differential Diagnosis

Osteomyelitis, myeloma, metastatic disease, osteosarcoma, non-Hodgkin lymphoma, giant cell tumor, eosinophilic granuloma, giant cell tumor, chondrosarcoma, fibrosarcoma, malignant fibrous histiocytoma.[20]

Treatment and Prognosis

Ewing sarcoma is a highly malignant tumor.[3,7,8,20,21,26] Important prognostic features include the tumor size, stage, and anatomic location.[26] Up to 35% of patients have metastases at presentation.[3,7] Metastatic disease is common to the lungs, bone, and lymph nodes.[3,7,8,26] The presence of metastases at diagnosis is associated with poor survival (5-year survival of ~25% compared with 65% for localized disease at diagnosis).[3] Large tumors and those that arise in the pelvis also have poor outcomes.[26] Treatment is based on primary (neoadjuvant) chemotherapy, radiation, resection of the primary tumor, as well as postsurgical adjuvant chemotherapy and/or radiation.[3,7,8,20,21,26] Histologic response to neoadjuvant chemotherapy has been shown to be useful for estimating prognosis[3,21] After neoadjuvant chemotherapy, tumors that show 100% necrosis show 3-year survival rates up to 100%.[21] Tumors that show more than 70% necrosis after chemotherapy have 87% survival with median follow-up of 3.5 years.[21] Tumors that show less than 70% necrosis after chemotherapy have 35% survival.[21] Patients with Ewing sarcoma have an 8.5-fold increased risk for developing other types of cancer, and a 100-fold increase for developing a bone or soft tissue sarcoma within the radiated field.[3]

References

1. Carlotti CG Jr, Drake J, Hladky JP, Teshima I, Becker LE, Rutka JT. Primary Ewing's sarcoma of the skull in children. *Pediatr Neurosurg* 1999;31:307–315.
2. Chaudhuri B, Das Gupta TK. Pathology of soft tissue sarcoma. In: Das Gupta TK, Chaudhuri PK, eds. *Tumors of the Soft Tissues* 2nd ed. New York, NY: Appleton and Lange 1998:155.
3. Coindre JM. Ewing sarcoma. In: Forest M, Tomeno B, Vanel D, eds. *Orthopedic Surgical Pathology: Diagnosis of Tumors and Pseudotumoral Lesions of Bone and Joints* Edinburgh: Churchill Livingstone; 1998:441–457.
4. Dyke JP, Panicek DM, Healey JH, et al. Osteogenic and Ewing's sarcomas: estimation of necrotic fraction during induction chemotherapy with dynamic contrast-enhanced MR imaging. *Radiology* 2003;228: 271–278.
5. Eggli KD, Quiogue T, Moser RP. Ewing's sarcoma. *Radiol Clin North Am* 1993;31:325–337.
6. Fletcher BD. Imaging pediatric bone sarcomas: diagnosis and treatment-related issues. *Radiol Clin North Am* 1997;35(6):1477–1486.
7. Grier HE. The Ewing family of tumors—Ewing's sarcoma and primitive neuroectodermal tumors. *Pediatr Clin North Am* 1997;44(4): 991–1004.
8. Huvos AG. Ewing's Sarcoma. In: Huvos AG, ed. *Bone Tumors: Diagnosis, Treatment, and Prognosis* 2nd ed. Philadelphia, Pa: W.B. Saunders; 1991:523–542.
9. Jaffe N. Soft tissue sarcomas in children. In: Das Gupta TK, Chaudhuri PK, eds. *Tumors of the Soft Tissues* 2nd ed. New York, NY: Appleton and Lange; 1998:589–591.
10. Kransdorf MJ, Murphey MD. Neurogenic tumors. In: *Imaging of Soft Tissue Tumors* 2nd ed. Philadelphia, Pa: W.B. Saunders; 2006: 328–380.
11. Kransdorf MJ. Malignant soft-tissue tumors in a large referral population: distribution of specific diagnoses by age, sex, and location. *AJR Am J Roentgenol* 1995;164:129–134.
12. Lang P, Honda G, Roberts T, et al. Musculoskeletal neoplasm: perineoplastic edema versus tumor on dynamic postcontrast MR images with spatial mapping of instantaneous enhancement rates. *Radiology* 1995;197:831–839.
13. MacVicar AD, Olliff JF, Pringle J, Pinkerton CR, Husband Janet ES. Ewing's sarcoma: MR imaging of chemotherapy-induced changes with histologic correlation. *Radiology* 1992;184(3):859–864.
14. Meyer JS, Dormans JP. Differential diagnosis of pediatric musculoskeletal masses. *Magn Reson Imaging Clin N Am* 1998;6(3):570–571.
15. Miller SL, Hoffer FA, Reddick WE, et al. Tumor volume or dynamic contrast-enhanced MRI for prediction of clinical outcome of Ewing's sarcoma family of tumors. *Pediatr Radiol* 2001;31:518–523.
16. Miller SL, Hoffer FA. Malignant and benign bone tumors. *Radiol Clin North Am* 2001;39(4):682–684.
17. Mukhopadhyay P, Gairola M, Sharma MC, Thulkar S, Julka PK, Rath GK. Primary spinal epidural extraosseous Ewing's sarcoma: report of five cases and literature review. *Australas Radiol* 2001;45:372–379.
18. Mulder JD, Schutte HE, Kroon HM, Taconis WK. Introduction. In: *Radiologic Atlas of Bone Tumors.* Amsterdam: Elsevier; 1993:3–6.
19. Mulder JD, Schutte HE, Kroon HM, Taconis WK. The diagnosis of bone tumors. In: *Radiologic Atlas of Bone Tumors* Amsterdam: Elsevier; 1993:9–46.
20. Mulder JD, Schutte HE, Kroon HM, Taconis WK. Ewing's Sarcoma. In: *Radiologic Atlas of Bone Tumors* Amsterdam: Elsevier; 1993:193–214.
21. Perlman EJ. Ewing's sarcoma, lymphoma, and Langerhans' cell proliferations. In: Helliwell TR, ed. *Major Problems in Pathology: Pathology of Bone and Joint Neoplasms* Vol 37. 1st ed. Philadelphia, Pa: W.B. Saunders;1999:279–299.
22. Saifuddin A, Whelan J, Pringle Jean AS, Cannon SR. Malignant round cell tumours of bone: atypical clinical and imaging features. *Skeletal Radiol* 2000;29:646–651.
23. Shin JH, Lee HK, Rhim SC, Cho KJ, Choi CG, Suh DC. Spinal epidural extraskeletal Ewing sarcoma: MR findings in two cases. *AJNR Am J Neuroradiol* 2001;22:795–798.
24. Unni KK. Introduction and scope of study. In:*Dahlin's Bone Tumors: General Aspects and Data on 11 087 Cases* 5th ed. Philadelphia, Pa: Lippincott, Williams & Wilkins; 1996:1–9.
25. Unni KK. Ewing's Tumor. In: *Dahlin's Bone Tumors: General Aspects and Data on 11 087 Cases* 5th ed. Philadelphia, Pa: Lippincott, Williams & Wilkins; 1996:249–260.
26. Ushigome S, Machinami R, Sorensen PH. Ewing's sarcoma/primitive neuroectodermal tumour (PNET). In: Fletcher CDM, Unni KK, Mertens F, eds. *World Health Organization Classification of Tumours. Pathology and Genetics of Tumours of Soft Tissue and Bone* IARC Press; 2002:298–300.
27. Van der Woude HJ, Bloem JL, Verstraete KL, Taminiau AH, Nooy MA, Hogendoorn PC. Osteosarcoma and Ewing's sarcoma after neoadjuvant chemotherapy: value of dynamic MR imaging in detecting viable tumor before surgery. *AJR Am J Roentgenol* 1995;165: 593–598.
28. Van der Woude HJ, Bloem JL, Hogendoorn PC, Pancras CW. Preoperative evaluation and monitoring chemotherapy in patients with high-grade osteogenic and Ewing's sarcoma: review of current imaging modalities. *Skeletal Radiol* 1998;27:57–71.
29. Wenaden AET, Szyszko TA, Saifuddin A. Imaging of periosteal reactions associated with focal lesions of bone. *Clin Radiol* 2005;60: 439–456.

A 21 Nodular Fasciitis (Also Referred to as Pseudosarcomatous Fasciitis, Proliferative Fasciitis, Infiltrative Fasciitis, and Pseudosarcomatous Fibromatosis)

Definition

Nodular fasciitis is a benign, reactive soft tissue lesion comprised of proliferating fibroblasts.[2-4,6] These lesions usually occur in the subcutaneous tissue or muscle.[4,6] Less common forms of nodular fasciitis are lesions that extend into vessel lumens (intravascular fasciitis) or skull and adjacent soft tissues (cranial fasciitis).[4,6]

Frequency of Occurrence

Nodular fasciitis is a common lesion that accounts for 11% of benign soft tissue tumors and 7% of all soft tissue tumors.[6-8]

Age at Presentation

From 11 to 51 years, mean = 31 years.[6-3] Nodular fasciitis typically occurs in young adults aged less than 30 years, but can occur in children and older adults.[4,5,8] Cranial fasciitis often occurs in infants less than 2 years old.[4]

Gender Ratio (M/F)

1/1[1,4] to 1.2/1[8]

Location

Subcutaneous (80–90%) location predominates over intramuscular or fascial subtypes.[5-9] Nodular fasciitis occurs most frequently in the upper extremity, followed by the head and neck, trunk, lower extremity, hand and wrist, proximal limb, and hip/buttock.[8] Lesions that involve adjacent periosteum have been referred to as parosteal fasciitis. Nodular fasciitis that contains metaplastic bone has been referred to as ossifying fasciitis.[6] Cranial fasciitis is a version of nodular fasciitis that involves the scalp and usually presents in infancy.[4,6,9] Intravascular fasciitis is a rare form that involves medium-sized to small-sized arteries or veins.[4,6]

Signs and Symptoms

Nodular fasciitis often occurs as an enlarging palpable soft tissue lesion.[4,6] Lesions may show rapid growth over several weeks followed by slower rates of enlargement.[4,6] Lesions may or may not be associated with pain (50%).

Gross Pathologic Findings

Lesions usually range from 2 to 5 cm and often contain firm fibrous regions, myxoid zones, and occasional cystic zones.[2-4,6,9] Intravascular fasciitis may be nodular or plexiform.[4] Cranial fasciitis lesions can be circumscribed and firm, with or without myxoid of cystic zones.[4]

Histopathologic Findings

Lesions contain bland, plump, spindle-like cells (fibroblastic and myofibroblastic), often in a myxoid matrix. The spindle-like cells usually lack pleomorphism and nuclear hyperchromasia.[2-4,6,9] The mitotic rate can be moderate to high, simulating a sarcoma, although atypical mitoses are not usually seen.[2-4,6,9] Portions of the lesion may be highly cellular or less cellular in loose organization with myxoid material.[4,6] Multiple capillaries and inflammatory cells can be seen at the periphery of the lesions.[4,6] The histologic features of nodular fasciitis can mimic sarcoma.[2-4,6,9]

Nodular fasciitis can have positive immunohistochemical reactions to smooth muscle actin, muscle-specific actin, actin, and vimentin.[2,4] Nodular fasciitis rarely shows immunoreactivity to desmin, and typically does not show positive immunohistochemical reactions to S-100 or keratin.[2,4]

Lesion Genetics

Cells are typically diploid.[4] Rearrangements of 3 q21, losses of chromosomes 2 and 13, and a 2;15 translocation have been reported for these lesions.[4]

Findings on Plain Films (Roentgenograms) and Computed Tomography[1,4,6]

Nodular fasciitis can be seen as soft tissue lesions. Intramuscular lesions can have attenuation slightly less than muscle, as well as areas of low attenuation on CT secondary to myxoid zones when present (Fig. **109**). Cranial fasciitis may be associated with erosions of the outer and inner tables of the skull, with or without thin sclerotic margins.[4,6]

MRI Findings[1,5,6,10]

Nodular fasciitis often appears as well-circumscribed lesions in subcutaneous fat, muscles, or fascia (Figs. **109**, **110**). Lesions are often 4 cm or less in size. Lesions in subcutaneous fat or fascia may have mildly irregular or even stellate borders.

Lesions usually have intermediate signal on T1WI (slightly hyperintense relative to muscle) and PDWI; and homogeneous or mildly heterogeneous high signal on T2WI and FS T2WI (Figs. **109**, **110**). Surrounding edema is occasionally seen. Older lesions with high fibrous content may have intermediate signal on T2WI.

After Gd-contrast, lesions can show homogeneous or peripheral rim-like patterns of enhancement.

Differential Diagnosis

Sarcoma, hematoma, benign or malignant fibrous histiocytoma, Schwannoma, dermatofibroma (skin lesions).

Treatment and Prognosis

Nodular fasciitis lesions are usually self-limited.[4,6] Intravascular fasciitis and cranial fasciitis have similar indolent courses as nodular fasciitis.[4] Surgical excision is often utilized.[4,6] Recurrence after excision is rare (<2%).[4]

424 A 21 – Nodular Fasciitis

Figure **109 a–e** A 43-year-old man with intramuscular nodular fasciitis involving the deltoid muscle at the left shoulder. Axial CT image (**a**) shows the lesion to have attenuation that is slightly less than muscle, as well as areas of low attenuation. The lesion has intermediate signal on coronal (**b**) PDWI. The lesion has high signal on coronal (**c**) and sagittal (**d**) FS T2WI, which is surrounded by a thin rim of low signal and poorly defined zones of high signal in the adjacent soft tissues. The lesion shows prominent Gd-contrast enhancement on sagittal (**e**) FS T1WI.

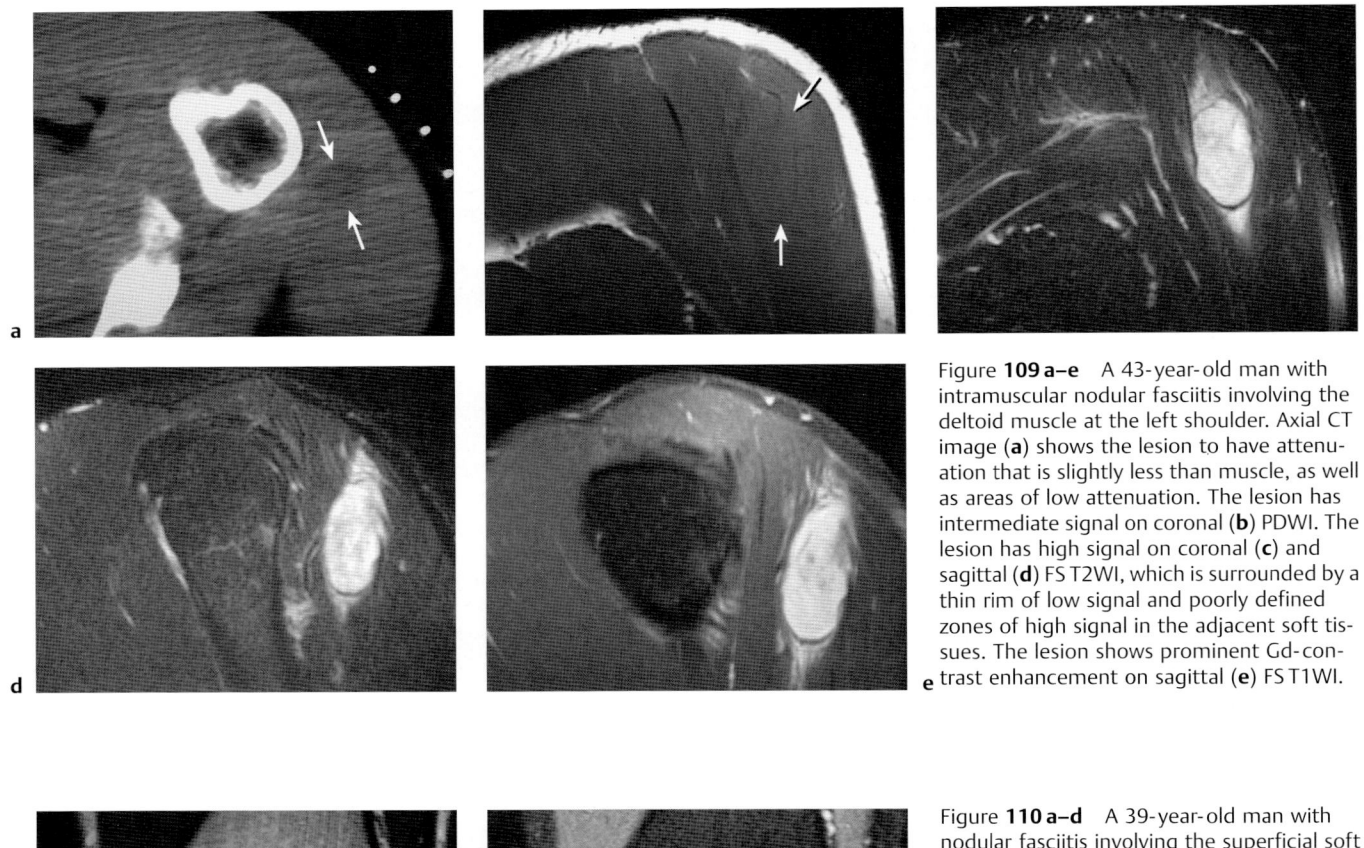

Figure **110 a–d** A 39-year-old man with nodular fasciitis involving the superficial soft tissues of the distal medial thigh. The lesion has circumscribed margins, and has intermediate signal on coronal (**a**) T1WI, and mildly heterogeneous high signal on coronal (**b**) and axial (**c**) FS T2WI. The lesion shows prominent Gd-contrast enhancement on axial (**d**) FS T1WI.

References

1 Bancroft LW, Peterson JJ, Kransdorf MJ, Nomikos GC, Murphey MD. Soft tissue tumors of the lower extremities. *Radiol Clin North Am* 2002;40:991–1011.
2 Das Gupta TK, Chaudhuri PK. Nodular fasciitis (pseudosarcomatous fasciitis). In: Das Gupta TK, Chaudhuri PK, eds. *Tumors of the Soft Tissues.* 2nd ed. New York, NY: Appleton and Lange; 1998:87–88.
3 Das Gupta TK, Chaudhuri PK. Tumors of the fibrous tissue. In: Das Gupta TK, Chaudhuri PK, eds. *Tumors of the Soft Tissues* 2nd ed. Appleton and Lange Pubs.; 1998:265–308.
4 Evans H, Bridge JA. Nodular fasciitis. In: Fletcher CDM, Unni KK, Mertens F, eds. *World Health Organization Classification of Tumours. Pathology and Genetics of Tumours of Soft Tissue and Bone* Geneva: IARC Press; 2002:48–49.
5 Jelinek J, Kransdorf MJ. MR imaging of soft-tissue masses: mass-like lesions that simulate neoplasms. *Magn Reson Imaging Clin N Am* 1995;3(4):727–741.
6 Kransdorf MJ, Murphey MD. Benign fibrous and fibrohistiocytic tumors. In: *Imaging of Soft Tissue Tumors* 2nd ed. Philadelphia, Pa: W.B. Saunders; 2006:189–256.
7 Kransdorf MJ, Murphey MD. Soft tissue tumors in a large referral population: prevalence and distribution of diagnoses by age, sex, and location. In: *Imaging of Soft Tissue Tumors* 2nd ed. Philadelphia, Pa: W.B. Saunders; 2006:6–37.
8 Kransdorf MJ. Benign soft-tissue tumors in a large referral population: distribution of specific diagnoses by age, sex, and location. *AJR Am J Roentgenol* 1995;164:395–402.
9 Reid RP. Bone neoplasms and tumor-like lesions on the bone surface. In: Helliwell TR, ed. *Major Problems in Pathology: Pathology of Bone and Joint Neoplasms.* Vol 37. 1st ed. Philadelphia, Pa: W.B. Saunders; 1999:215–235.
10 Sundaram M, Sharafuddin Melhem JA. MR imaging of benign soft-tissue masses. *Magn Reson Imaging Clin N Am* 1995;3(4):609–627.

A 22 Fibrolipomatous Hamartoma (Also Referred to as Nerve Lipoma, Neural Fibrolipoma, Lipofibromatous Hamartoma, Perineural Lipoma, Intraneural Lipoma, Lipofibroma, and Lipomatous Hamartoma)

ICD-O Code

8850/0

Definition

Fibrolipomatous hamartomas are rare, benign lesions with varying degrees of fibrous and fatty (mature adipocytes) infiltration of the epineurium (nerve sheath) of peripheral nerves as well as within the interfascicular connective tissue (perineurium) of nerves.[1–3,5–10]

Frequency of Occurrence

These lesions are rare and account for less than 1% of benign soft tissue tumors, and less than 1% of lipomas and lipoma variants.[3,4,9]

Age at Presentation

From 4 to 75 years,[5] mean = 24 to 40 years.[2,4,5] These lesions can also be congenital or occur in early childhood.[1,6]

Gender Ratio (M/F)

1.3/1[4] to 1/1.1[9]

Location

Lesions most frequently involve the median nerve and its digital branches (80%) followed by the ulnar nerve, radial nerve, brachial plexus, sciatic nerve, nerves of the lower extremity, ankle (superficial peroneal nerve), and feet (medial plantar nerve).[1,3–10] Lesions involving the median and ulnar nerves are usually solitary in 80% of cases.[9] Lesions involving the brachial plexus may be multifocal.[9]

Signs and Symptoms

Fibrolipomatosis hamartomas are soft, slowly enlarging lesions that often occur along the volar aspects of the wrist, hand, distal forearm, and foot.[1–3,5–10] Associated ipsilateral macrodactyly (macrodystrophia lipomatosa) may occur in up to two-thirds of patients (females > males) near the sites of fibrolipomatosis hamartomas.[1,2,6,10] The macrodactyly often involves the second or third digits of the hands or feet which are inervated by the involved nerves.[3,6,10] Initially, these lesions are usually painless without neurologic signs.[1,3,6,10] Eventually, these lesions can be associated with nerve compression resulting in pain, parathesia, and motor deficit.[1,3,6,10] Lesions in the wrist can cause carpal tunnel syndrome.[1,3,6,9]

Gross Pathologic Findings

Lesions are often yellow-tan, rubbery fusiform masses within the involved nerve sheaths.[1–3,6,7,9,10] Lesions may range from 5 to 30 cm in length, and up to 2.5 cm in diameter.[2,9]

Histopathologic Findings[6,7,10]

Infiltration of fat cells within the interfascicular connective tissue (perineurium) of enlarged nerves is typically seen, often in association with perineural and epineural fibrosis.[6,7,10] The perineural fibrous tissue is usually concentric around the nerve bundles.[6] Atrophy of nerve fibers can occur after many years. Fibrolipomatous hamartoma differs from neural sheath lipoma in that the latter does not have fatty cells intervening between the nerve fascicles. Rarely, metaplastic bone formation may occur in these lesions.[5,6]

Findings on Plain Films (Roentgenograms) and Computed Tomography

Lesions can appear as a subcutaneous fusiform mass with fatty tissue attenuation containing serpentine structures with soft tissue attenuation representing thickened nerve bundles.[2,10] Bone hypertrophy (macrodactyly) may be seen adjacent to the lesion.[10] Rarely, metaplastic bone formation may occur in these lesions and appear as calcifications on radiographs or CT examinations.[5]

MRI Findings

Lesions are well-circumscribed and fusiform-shaped, involving nerves.[1–3,5,7,10] On T1WI, PDWI, and T2WI a network of cylindrical, longitudinally-oriented, thin curvilinear zones of low signal of 1 to 3 mm in diameter is seen within a background of intermediate to high signal[1–3,5,7,10] (Figs. **111, 112**). This typical appearance, likened to a coaxial cable, is secondary to the combination of nerve fascicles with varying degrees of fatty infiltration, and epineural and perineural fibrosis.[1–3,5,7,10] The enlarged median nerves often contain 15 to 16 of these "coaxial cables," representing bundles of axons encased in epineural fibrous tissue.[9] Fibrolipomatous hamartomas of the ulnar nerve are usually smaller and contain fewer neural bundles (usually three or four) than lesions involving median nerves.[9] The degree of fatty proliferation varies among patients.[2,10] Lesions may follow the branching patterns of nerves.[2]

Lesions can show moderate to prominent Gd-contrast enhancement in fibrous tissue components of the lesions adjacent to spiculated low signal foci representing nerve fibers.[10]

Differential Diagnosis

Neural sheath lipoma, traumatic neuroma, plexiform neurofibroma, ganglion cyst, vascular malformation, atypical Schwannoma, hereditary hypertrophic interstitial neuritis of Dejerine–Sottas disease.[1,2,5,10]

Treatment and Prognosis

Surgical exploration with diagnostic biopsy is frequently performed for symptomatic lesions.[1–3,5,6,10] For patients with carpal tunnel syndrome, carpal release is commonly performed.[1,3,5,6,10] Complete resection can result in significant motor and sensory deficits.[1,3,6,7,10] Using MRI, preoperative diagnosis can usually be made, obviating the need for biopsy.[5,7]

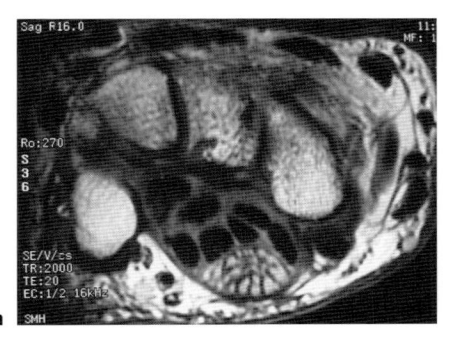

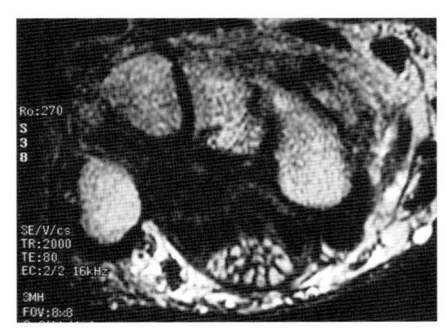

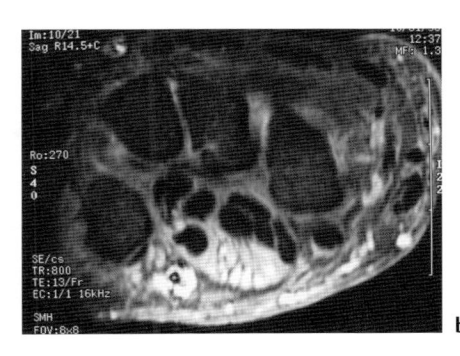

Figure 111 a–c A 59-year-old man with a fibrolipomatous hamartoma involving the median nerve at the wrist. Cylindrical, longitudinally oriented, thin curvilinear zones of low signal are seen within a background of intermediate to high signal on axial PDWI (**a**), and slightly high signal on axial T2WI (**b**). The lesion shows Gd-contrast enhancement on axial FS T1WI (**c**).

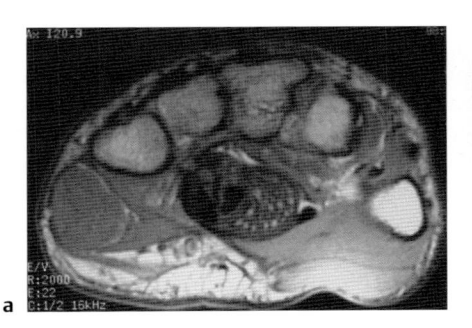

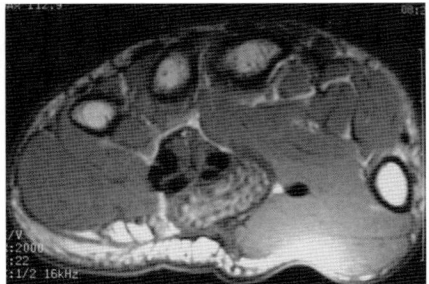

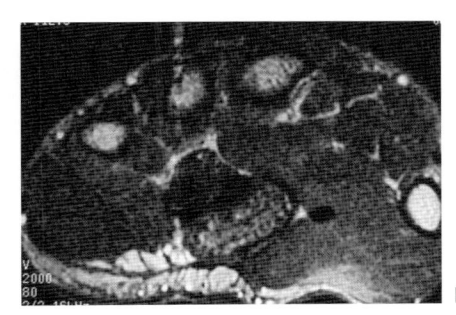

Figure 112 a–c A 16-year-old male with a fibrolipomatous hamartoma involving the median nerve at the wrist. Cylindrical, longitudinally oriented, thin curvilinear zones of low signal are seen within a background of intermediate to high signal on axial PDWI (**a**, **b**), and slightly high signal on axial T2WI (**c**).

References

1. Cavallaro MC, Taylor JA, Gorman JD, Haghighi P, Resnick D. Imaging findings in a patient with fibrolipomatous hamartoma of the median nerve. *AJR Am J Roentgenol* 1993;161:837–838.
2. De Maeseneer M, Jaovisidha S, Lenchik L, et al. Fibrolipomatous hamartoma: MR imaging findings. *Skeletal Radiol* 1997;26:155–160.
3. Kransdorf MJ, Murphey MD. Lipomatous tumors. In: *Imaging of Soft Tissue Tumors*. 2nd ed. Philadelphia, Pa: W.B. Saunders; 2006: 80–149.
4. Kransdorf MJ. Benign soft-tissue tumors in a large referral population: distribution of specific diagnoses by age, sex, and location. *AJR Am J Roentgenol* 1995;164:395–402.
5. Marom EM, Helms CA. Fibrolipomatous hamartoma: pathognomonic on MR imaging. *Skeletal Radiol* 1999;28:260–264.
6. Nielsen GP. Lipomatosis of nerve. In: Fletcher CDM, Unni KK, Mertens F, eds. *World Health Organization Classification of Tumours. Pathology and Genetics of Tumours of Soft Tissue and Bone* Geneva: IARC Press; 2002:24–25.
7. Ogose A, Hotta T, Higuchi T, Katsumi N, Koda H, Umezu H. Fibrolipomatous hamartoma in the foot: magnetic resonance imaging and surgical treatment. A report of two cases. *J Bone Joint Surg Am* 2002; 84-A(3):432–436.
8. Silverman TA, Enzinger FM. Fibrolipomatous hamartoma of nerve. A clinicopathologic analysis of 26 cases. *Am J Surg Pathol* 1985;9:7–14.
9. Toms AP, Anastakis D, Bleakney RR, Marshall TJ. Lipofibromatous hamartoma of the upper extremity: a review of the radiologic findings for 15 patients. *AJR Am J Roentgenol* 2006;186:805–811.
10. Van Breuseghem I, Scviot R, Pans S, Geusens E, Brys P, De Wever I. Fibrolipomatous hamartoma in the foot: atypical MR imaging findings. *Skeletal Radiol* 2003;32:651–655.

Fibroma of the Tendon Sheath

ICD-O Code

8810/0

Definition

Fibromas of the tendon sheath are benign, small, fibrous nodules involving tendons and tendon sheaths of the fingers, hands, wrists, or feet.[3,4]

Frequency of Occurrence

Fibromas of the tendon sheath represent ~1% of benign soft tissue tumors.[5,6]

Age at Presentation

From 15 to 81 years, mean = 35 years.[5,6]

Gender Ratio (M/F)

1.5/1 to 3/1.[3,5–7]

Location

As much as 98% of these lesions occur in the extremities, and 82% occur in the upper extremities.[2,3] Lesions are usually found along tendons of fingers (thumb, index, middle finger (49%), hands (21%), or wrist (12%).[3–6] Many of the remaining lesions involve the tendons at the plantar aspects of the feet, and anterior knee.[3–6] Rare sites of involvement include the arms, elbows, toes, temporomandibular joint, neck, and trunk.[3,9]

Signs and Symptoms[1–4,7–10]

Fibromas of the tendon sheath are typically slow-growing, with durations of months to years.[1–4,7–10] The lesions are often painless, although are occasionally associated with mild tenderness or pain.[3,7] Lesions are sometimes associated with trauma or limitation of tendon motion;[7] those involving the wrist may cause carpal tunnel syndrome.[3]

Gross Pathologic Findings

Lesions often range in size from 1 to 5 cm, mean = 2 cm.[7] Most lesions are less than 3 cm in diameter[3] and may have a multilobulated configuration.[3] Lesions are firm, circumscribed, gray-white nodular masses adjacent to tendon sheaths.[3,4,7] Erosion of adjacent bone may rarely occur.[3,7,10]

Histopathologic Findings

Lesions are composed of dense nodules of hypocellular fibrous connective tissue containing spindle-shaped fibroblasts in collagenous stroma separated by clefts.[3,4,7] Slitlike vascular channels may also be seen in these lesions.[3,4,7] Hypercellular regions may be seen in addition to the typical hypocellular areas, but these hypercellular zones lack nuclear hyperchromasia or coagulative necrosis.[3] Less frequently, other features such as myxoid change, cyst formation, stellate cells, dense hyalinization, chondroid and/or osseous metaplasia may be observed.[3]

Lesion Genetics

One of these lesions has been reported to have a translocation: t(2;11)(q31–32;q12).[3]

Findings on Plain Films (Roentgenograms) and Computed Tomography

Lesions may appear as ovoid or fusiform, superficial soft tissue masses which are infrequently associated with mild scalloping or remodeling of adjacent bone.[1,4,7,10] Lesions are usually seen at flexor tendons.[3,4]

MRI Findings[1,4,7,8]

Lesions are typically ovoid or fusiform, well circumscribed and located adjacent to tendons of the fingers, hands, wrists, feet, and other locations (Figs. 113, 114). Lesions are more common at the flexor tendons than at the extensor tendons.[3,4]

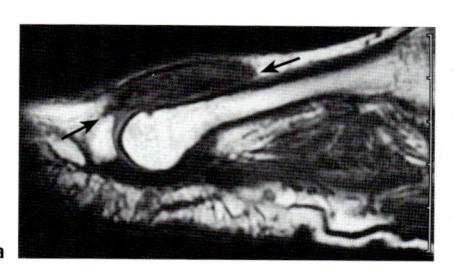

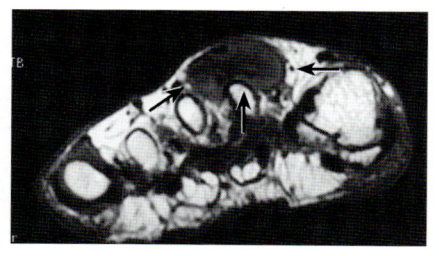

Figure 113 a–d A 63-year-old woman with a fibroma involving an extensor tendon sheath in the foot. The lesion has a fusiform shape with well-circumscribed margins, and has zones of low and intermediate signal on sagittal (a) and axial (b) T1WI, as well as on axial FS T2WI (c). The lesion shows heterogeneous Gd-contrast enhancement on axial FS T1WI (d).

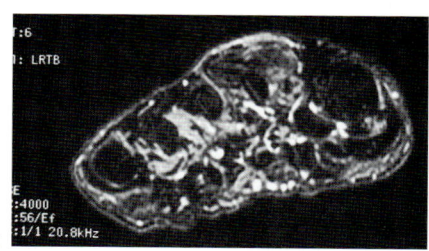

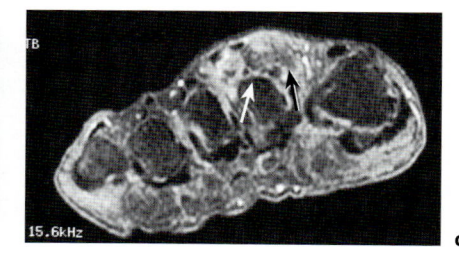

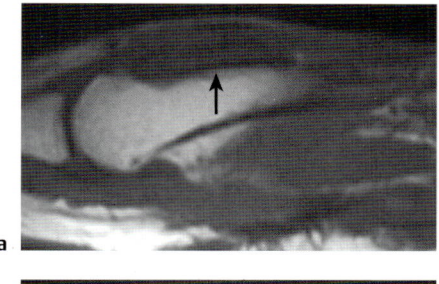

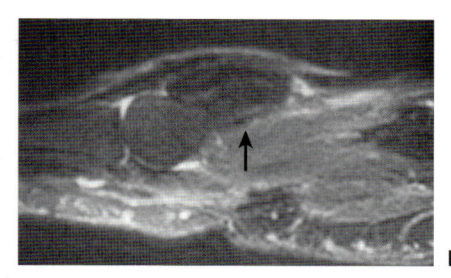

Figure **114 a–d** An 89-year-old woman with a fibroma involving an extensor tendon sheath in the hand. The lesion has well-circumscribed margins; and contains zones of low and intermediate signal on sagittal (**a**) and axial (**c**) T1WI, and mostly low signal on sagittal (**b**) and axial (**d**) FS T2WI.

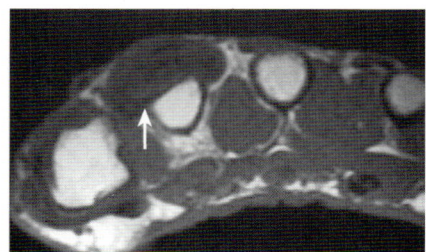

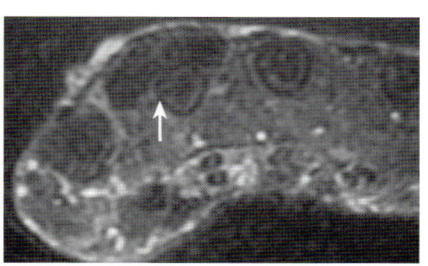

Lesions usually have low-intermediate signal on T1WI (equal to or less than skeletal muscle, 83%).[4] On T2WI, lesions have slightly heterogeneous low-intermediate signal in 50% of cases (equal to or less than skeletal muscle), intermediate signal that is hyperintense relative to muscle (33%), or mixed low and intermediate (17%).[4] Lesions can also have areas of high signal on FS T2WI. Lesions may be associated with remodeling or erosions of adjacent bone cortex (Fig. **114**). After Gd-contrast administration, lesions can show diffuse or peripheral enhancement patterns, or no discernable enhancement[4] (Fig. **113**, **114**).

Differential Diagnosis

Giant cell tumor of the tendon sheath (which is 2.7 times more common than fibroma of the tendon sheath),[4] hematoma, xanthoma, gout.

Treatment and Prognosis

Surgical resection is a common treatment for fibromas of the tendon sheath, usually for cosmetic reasons, pain, and/or limitation of motion.[3] Local recurrence can occur in up to 24% of patients from months to years after surgery.[3,7]

References

1 Bertolotto M, Rosenberg I, Parodi RC, et al. Case report: fibroma of the tendon sheath in the distal forearm with associated median nerve neuropathy—US, CT, and MR appearances. *Clin Radiol* 1996;51:370–372.
2 Chung EB, Enzinger FM. Fibroma of the tendon sheath. *Cancer* 1979;44:1945–1954.
3 Farshid G, Bridge JA. Fibroma of the tendon sheath. In: Fletcher CDM, Unni KK, Mertens F, eds. *World Health Organization Classification of Tumours. Pathology and Genetics of Tumours of Soft Tissue and Bone* Geneva: IARC Press; 2002:66.
4 Fox MG, Kransdorf MJ, Bancroft LW, Peterson JJ, Flemming DJ. MR imaging of fibroma of the tendon sheath. *AJR Am J Roentgenol* 2003; 180:1449–1453.
5 Kransdorf MJ. Benign soft-tissue tumors in a large referral population: distribution of specific diagnoses by age, sex, and location. *AJR Am J Roentgenol* 1995;164:395–402.
6 Kransdorf MJ, Murphey MD. Soft tissue tumors in a large referral population: prevalence and distribution of diagnoses by age, sex, and location. In: *Imaging of Soft Tissue Tumors* 2nd ed. Philadelphia, Pa: W.B. Saunders; 2006:6–37.
7 Kransdorf MJ, Murphy MD. Benign fibrous and fibrohistiocytic tumors. In: *Imaging of Soft Tissue Tumors* 2nd ed. Philadelphia: Pa: W.B. Saunders; 2006:189–256.
8 McGrory JE, Rock MG. Fibroma of the tendon sheath involving the patellar tendon. *Am J Orthop* 2000;29:465–467.
9 Misawa A, Okada K, Hirano Y, et al. Fibroma of the tendon sheath arising from the radio-ulnar joint. *Pathol Int* 1999;49:1089–1092.
10 Southwick GJ, Karamoskos P. Fibroma of the tendon sheath with bone involvement. *J Hand Surg* 1990;15(3):373–375.

A 24 Solitary Fibrous Tumor

ICD-O Code

8815/1

Definition

Solitary fibrous tumors (SFTs) are rare benign spindle-cell mesenchymal neoplasms that occur in a wide range of anatomic sites.[1-3] These fibroblastic tumors typically show a hemangiopericytoma-like branching vascular pattern.[1-3] Extrapleural SFTs morphologically resemble pleural SFTs, and have been termed hemangiopericytomas in the past.[1,3]

Frequency of Occurrence

These tumors are rare and have been reported to account for less than 2% of soft tissue tumors.[2,3]

Age at Presentation

From 20 to 77 years, median = 50 to 60 years.[2,3]

Gender Ratio (M/F)

1/1.[2,3]

Location

These lesions occur in the thoracic cavity (pleura > lung > mediastinum > diaphragm) > peritoneal/visceral/retroperitoneal > pelvis > head and neck > extremity > trunk.[2] Extrapleural SFTs occur in the subcutaneous tissue > deep soft tissues.[3]

Signs and Symptoms

Most SFTs are slow-growing, painless lesions.[3] Large SFTs may cause compression of adjacent anatomic structures, producing signs and symptoms based on location.[3,4] Extrathoracic SFTs are more likely to be symptomatic than thoracic lesions.[2] Osteoarthropathy (clubbing of fingers and arthritis) occurs in 10%, and symptomatic hypoglycemia occurs in 5% from tumoral secretion of insulin-like growth factors.[5]

Gross Pathologic Findings

SFTs are usually well-circumscribed, partially encapsulated lesions, which frequently have a whitish, firm, multinodular appearance.[1,3] Zones of hemorrhage and myxoid changes may be present.[2] Indistinct tumor margins and areas of tumor necrosis are associated with the infrequent, locally aggressive or malignant SFTs.[3]

Histopathologic Findings

SFTs contain short, round to spindle-shaped cells containing single vesicular nuclei with dispersed chromatin within scant cytoplasm.[1-3] Mitotic activity is typically low and rarely exceeds 3 per 10 high-power fields.[3,5] The spindle cells are separated by bands of hyalinized dense collagen intermixed with branching small- and medium-sized hemangiopericytoma-like vessels.[1-3,5]

SFTs typically have a patternless architecture with various combinations of hypercellular (tumor-cell rich) areas and hypocellular (collagen rich) zones.[1-3,5]

Malignant SFTs are hypercellular lesions with moderate or marked cellular atypia, increased mitotic activity (> 4 mitoses per 10 high-power fields), necrosis, and/or infiltrative tumor margins.[1,3,5]

Tumor cells are often immunoreactive to CD 34 (up to 95%) and CD 99 (70%).[3] Tumor cells can be immunoreactive to epithelial membrane antigen (35%), occasionally to Bcl-2 and smooth muscle actin, and rarely to desmin.[3,5] Lesions are usually negative for S 100 and cytokeratins.[1,5]

Lesion Genetics

These lesions are cytogenetically heterogeneous.[3] SFT has been associated with trisomy 21 and gains and losses in chromosomes[5]

Findings on Plain Films (Roentgenograms) and Computed Tomography

SFTs often have circumscribed margins on CT.[3] When present in the chest, SFTs can appear as a localized opacity on roentgenograms.[3] SFTs can have soft tissue attenuation that is slightly heterogeneous on CT.[3] SFTs can show contrast enhancement (Fig. **115**).

MRI Findings

SFTs usually have circumscribed margins. SFTs can have low to intermediate signal on T1WI and PDWI; low, intermediate, and/or slightly high signal on T2WI;[3] and heterogeneous slightly high to high signal on FS T2WI (Figs. **115, 116**). After Gd-contrast administration, SFTs can show prominent, slightly heterogeneous enhancement.

Differential Diagnosis

Hemangiopericytoma, synovial cell sarcoma, neurofibroma, Schwannoma, malignant or benign fibrous histiocytoma, fibrosarcoma, leiomyoma, angiosarcoma, rhabdomyosarcoma, epitheloid sarcoma, Kaposi sarcoma, hemangioendothelioma, clear cell sarcoma, nodular fasciitis.

Prognosis and Treatment

Thoracic and extrathoracic SFTs have similar clinical and pathologic features.[1] Treatment usually consists of surgical excision.[1,2] Most SFTs are benign, although up to 15% have aggressive behavior,[1,2,5] and typically have low rates of recurrence and metastasis after surgery.[1] SFTs in the extremities tend to have less aggressive behavior than SFTs elsewhere.[2] Surveillance is typically more intense for SFTs that are larger than 10 cm and those which contain histologically malignant portions (increased cellularity and mitotic activity).[1] Metastatic disease most frequently occurs in the lungs, bone, and liver.[2]

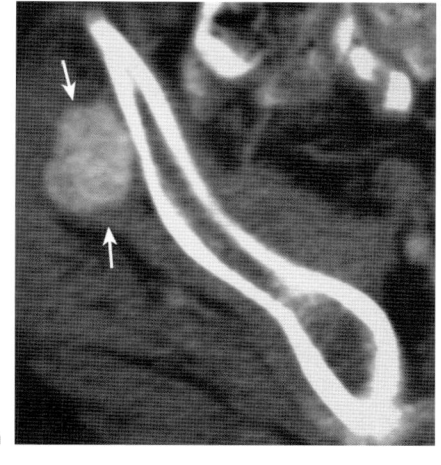

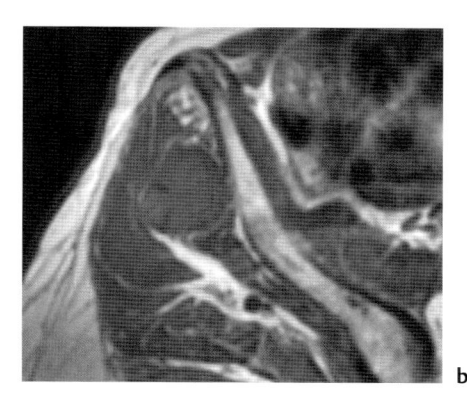

Figure **115 a–d** An 81-year-old man with a solitary fibrous tumor involving the gluteus mnimus muscle. The lesion has circumscribed margins, and shows contrast enhancement on axial CT (**a**). The lesion has intermediate signal on axial T1WI (**b**), high signal on axial FS T2WI (**c**), and shows prominent Gd-contrast enhancement on axial FS T1WI (**d**).

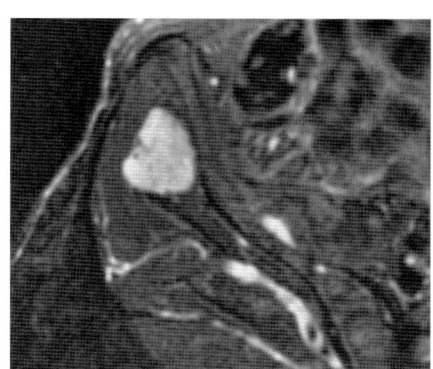

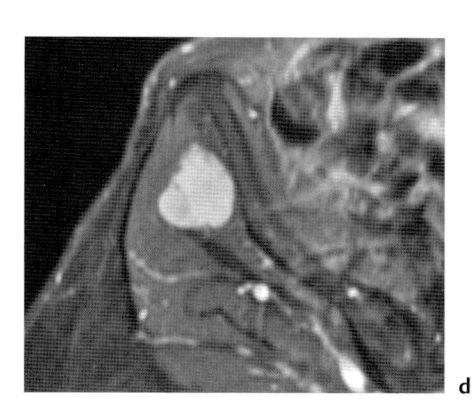

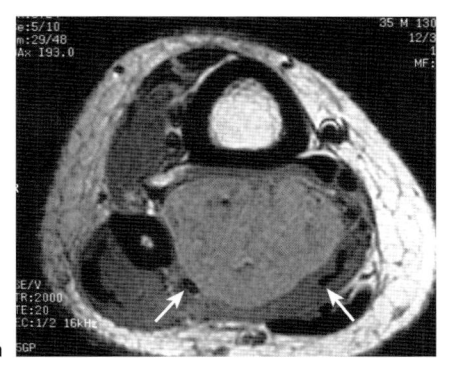

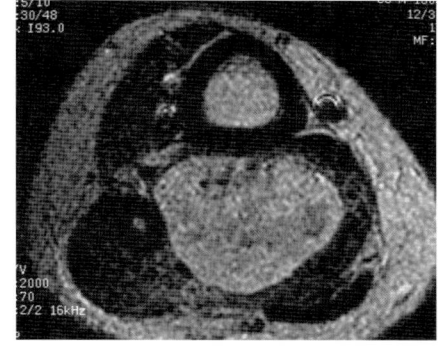

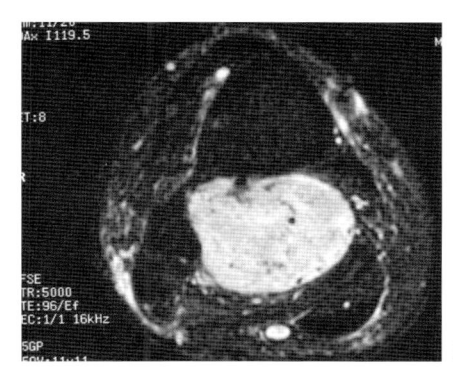

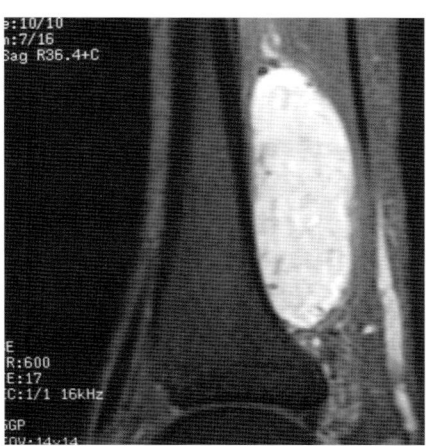

Figure **116 a–e** A 35-year-old man with a solitary fibrous tumor involving the soft tissues dorsal to the distal tibia. The lesion has circumscribed margins, and has intermediate signal on axial PDWI (**a**), slightly high signal on axial T2WI (**b**), and heterogeneous high signal on axial FS T2WI (**c**). The lesion shows prominent Gd-contrast enhancement on axial (**d**) and sagittal (**e**) FS T1WI.

also be associated with these tumors.[7,9-11,19,21] Low-grade lesions tend to be more circumscribed than higher-grade lesions.[7,9-11,19,21]

Fibrosarcomas of soft tissues. In adults, fibrosarcomas are firm masses, often gray-white and/or tan with relatively defined margins.[2,5,6,13,15,16] Zones of necrosis and/or hemorrhage can be seen in high-grade fibrosarcomas in adults.[5,6,13,15,16] Fibrosarcomas in young children are usually lobulated, firm and rubbery tumors, often with poorly defined margins, with or without areas of necrosis, hemorrhage, cystic degeneration, mucinous and/or myxoid changes.[2]

Histopathologic Findings

Fibrosarcomas of bone. Lesions are composed of intertwined bundles of fibroblast-like spindle cells often arranged in a "herringbone pattern."[7,9-11,19,21] The intercellular substance contains varying amounts of collagen fibers. Lesions are graded on the basis of the cytologic features of the tumor cells and cellularity of the tumors.[7,9-11,19,21]

- **Grade 1 tumors** (5%) are well-differentiated neoplasms composed of elongated fibroblastic spindle cells with ovoid or elongated nuclei with only very few mitoses. Abundant collagen fibers are present in the intercellular substance.
- **Grade 2 tumors** (65%) are moderately differentiated neoplasms with greater cellularity than grade 1 lesions. The nuclei of the spindle cells are more atypical in appearance with more mitoses than grade 1 lesions. Less collagen is seen than in grade 1 tumors.
- **Grade 3 and 4 tumors** (30%) have greater cellularity than the lower-grade fibrosarcomas. The spindle cells are greater in number with higher mitotic activity compared with lower-grade fibrosarcomas. Small tumor cells may also be seen in some of the high-grade lesions. Tumor cells have pleomorphic and hyperchromatic nuclei. Areas of necrosis are often seen in the lesions. Intercellular collagen is usually minimal for grade 3 lesions or not visualized in grade 4 lesions.

Fibrosarcomas of soft tissues.[2,4,6,13,15,16] Lesions have anaplastic fibroblastic spindle cells with varying degrees of nuclear pleomorphism, and mitotic activity. Amounts of intercellular collagen and reticulin are also variable. Congenital and infantile fibrosarcomas have similar histologic features compared with the adult types, except that the lesions tend to have a more fasciculated pattern. Immunohistochemical reactivity to vimentin is usually observed for both infantile and adult types, whereas immunoreactivity to smooth muscle actin is less frequent.[2,5]

- **Differentiated soft tissue fibrosarcomas (grades 1 and 2).** The spindle-shaped tumor cells are present in an interwoven intercellular substance of abundant collagen. Mitotic figures are rare.
- **Undifferentiated soft tissue fibrosarcomas (grades 3 and 4).** The tumor cells have atypical features / anaplasia and multiple mitotic figures. The amounts of intercellular collagen and reticulin are markedly diminished compared with the more well-differentiated fibrosarcomas. Giant cells with single or multiple nuclei are also seen in grade 3 and 4 tumors. Unlike malignant fibrous histiocytomas, the giant cells in fibrosarcomas do not have growth patterns such as matted, storiform, or pinwheel configurations.
- **Myxofibrosarcoma.** These tumors have a myxoid component containing hyaluronic acid, which occupies more than 50% of the lesion volume; as well as spindle cells, bizarre giant cells, and spheroid histiocytic cells with foamy cytoplasm.[16] Low-grade tumors have infrequent mitotic figures.[16]

These tumors often have curvilinear, thin-walled blood vessels with adjacent aggregates of tumor cells, lymphocytes, and plasma cells.[16] High-grade tumors contain fascicles and/or sheets of malignant pleomorphic and spindle cells with frequent atypical mitoses, zones of necrosis, and hemorrhage.[16]

- **Low-grade fibromyxoid sarcoma.**[6] These tumors contain whorled patterns of bland spindle cells, dense collagenous zones, and myxoid nodules.[6] Mitoses are uncommon.[6] Arcades of small blood vessels are often observed as well as small arteriole-sized vessels with adjacent sclerosis.[6] In ~40% of cases, dense zones of hyaline collagen are surrounded by cuffs of spindle cells, referred to as giant collagen rosettes.[6]
- **Sclerosing epithelioid fibrosarcoma.**[1,15] These tumors contain small epithelioid cells with spheroid, ovoid, or angulated nuclei within clear to eosinophilic cytoplasm.[15] Few mitoses are typically observed.[15] The tumor cells are often arranged in nests, cords, strands, or acini within abundant acidophilic collagen matrix.[15] The collagen matrix can occur as thick bands, in lace-like configurations, and/or hyalinized fibrous zones.[15]
- **Postradiation fibrosarcomas.** Lesions are often seen 4–15 years after radiation treatment of greater than 4000 cGy.[3] Histologic features are similar to other fibrosarcomas of soft tissue and bone.[3] Additional postradiation findings are often seen in the adjacent tissue, such as bone infarcts, fat and muscle necrosis/atrophy, and intimal vascular proliferation.

Tumor Genetics

Infantile fibrosarcoma of soft tissue is often associated with a chromosomal translocation, t(12;15) (p13;q26), which results in oncogenic activation of the NTRK3 gene.[2] Adult fibrosarcomas often have various different types of chromosomal rearrangements.[5] Myxofibrosarcomas and low-grade fibromyxoid sarcomas often have supernumerary ring chromosomes.[6,16]

Findings on Plain Films (Roentgenograms) and Computed Tomography

Fibrosarcomas of bone.[7-11,19,21] Tumors are usually radiolucent with permeative or "moth-eaten" appearance, sometimes in combination with a more geographic pattern. Tumor margins are usually irregular and indistinct, although some of the borders may be more sharply defined. Typically no sclerotic margins are seen. Areas of cortical destruction are usually present, with or without associated extra-osseous soft tissue masses.

Fibrosarcomas of soft tissues (adults). Tumors appear as soft tissue lesions without matrix mineralization; with or without associated bone erosion, destruction or deformity[13]

Fibrosarcomas of soft tissues (infants and young children). Tumors appear as soft tissue lesions without matrix mineralization, rarely associated bone destruction.[4,13]

MRI Findings

Fibrosarcomas of bone.[21] Fibrosarcomas are often intramedullary lesions with irregular margins, with or without associated cortical destruction and/or extra-osseous soft tissue masses. Lesions usually have low-intermediate signal on T1WI and PDWI, and heterogeneous intermediate, slightly high, and/or high signal on T2WI (Fig. **117**). After Gd-contrast administration, lesions usually show heterogeneous prominent enhancement.